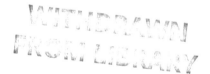

# Basics of
# ANESTHESIA

## SEVENTH EDITION

# Basics of
# ANESTHESIA

**SEVENTH EDITION**

## Manuel C. Pardo, Jr., MD

*Professor of Anesthesia and Perioperative Care, Residency Program Director,
University of California, San Francisco, School of Medicine, San Francisco,
California*

## Ronald D. Miller, MD, MS

*Professor Emeritus of Anesthesia, Department of Anesthesia and Perioperative
Care, University of California, San Francisco, School of Medicine, San Francisco,
California*

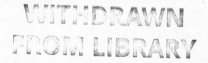
ELSEVIER

# ELSEVIER

1600 John F. Kennedy Blvd.
Ste 1800
Philadelphia, PA 19103-2899

BASICS OF ANESTHESIA, SEVENTH EDITION

ISBN: 978-0-323-40115-9

---

### Notices

---

Previous editions copyrighted in 2011, 2007, 2000, 1994, 1989, 1984.

**Library of Congress Cataloging-in-Publication Data**
Names: Pardo, Manuel, Jr., 1965- editor. | Miller, Ronald D., 1939- editor.
  | Preceded by (work): Miller, Ronald D., 1939- Basics of anesthesia.
Title: Basics of anesthesia / [edited by] Manuel C. Pardo, Jr., Ronald D.
  Miller.
Description: Seventh edition. | Philadelphia, PA : Elsevier, [2018] |
  Preceded by Basics of anesthesia / Ronald D. Miller, Manuel C. Pardo Jr.
  6th ed. c2011. | Includes bibliographical references and index.
Identifiers: LCCN 2017001280 | ISBN 9780323401159 (hardcover : alk. paper)
Subjects: | MESH: Anesthesia
Classification: LCC RD81 | NLM WO 200 | DDC 617.9/6--dc23 LC record
available at https://lccn.loc.gov/2017001280

*Executive Content Strategist:* Dolores Meloni
*Senior Content Development Specialist:* Ann R. Anderson
*Publishing Services Manager:* Patricia Tannian
*Senior Project Manager:* Sharon Corell
*Book Designer:* Ryan Cook

Printed in Canada.

Last digit is the print number:   9  8  7  6  5  4  3  2  1

Working together
to grow libraries in
developing countries

www.elsevier.com • www.bookaid.org

# CONTRIBUTORS

**Amr E. Abouleish, MD, MBA**
Professor
Department of Anesthesiology
The University of Texas Medical Branch
Galveston, Texas

**Meredith C.B. Adams, MD, MS**
Assistant Professor
Department of Anesthesiology
Director
Pain Medicine Fellowship
Medical College of Wisconsin
Milwaukee, Wisconsin

**Dean B. Andropoulos, MD, MHCM**
Professor
Department of Anesthesiology and Pediatrics
Vice Chair
Department of Anesthesiology
Baylor College of Medicine
Houston, Texas

**Jeffrey L. Apfelbaum, MD**
Professor and Chair
Department of Anesthesia and Critical Care
University of Chicago Medicine
Chicago, Illinois

**Sheila R. Barnett, MD**
Associate Professor of Anaesthesia
Harvard Medical School
Vice Chair
Perioperative Medicine
Department of Anesthesiology, Critical Care, and Pain Medicine
Beth Israel Deaconess Medical Center
Boston, Massachusetts

**Charles B. Berde, MD, PhD**
Professor of Anaesthesia (Pediatrics)
Harvard Medical School
Chief
Division of Pain Medicine
Department of Anesthesiology, Perioperative and Pain Medicine
Boston Children's Hospital
Boston, Massachusetts

**Michael P. Bokoch, MD, PhD**
Clinical Insructor and Liver Transplant Anesthesia Fellow
Department of Anesthesia and Perioperative Care
University of California, San Francisco, School of Medicine
San Francisco, California

**Kristine E. W. Breyer, MD**
Assistant Professor
Department of Anesthesia and Perioperative Care
University of California, San Francisco, School of Medicine
San Francisco, California

**Richard Brull, MD, FRCPC**
Professor
Department of Anesthesia
University of Toronto
Toronto, Ontario, Canada

**Vincent W.S. Chan, MD, FRCPC, FRCA**
Professor
Department of Anesthesia
University of Toronto
Toronto, Ontario, Canada

**Tony Chang, MD**
*Staff Anesthesiologist*
*Swedish Medical Center*
*Seattle, Washington*

**Frances Chung, MBBS, FRCPC**
*Professor*
*Department of Anesthesiology*
*University Health Network*
*Toronto Western Hospital*
*Toronto, Ontario, Canada*

**Neal H. Cohen, MD, MPH, MS**
*Vice Dean*
*School of Medicine*
*Professor*
*Department of Anesthesia and Perioperative Care*
*University of California, San Francisco, School of Medicine*
*San Francisco, California*

**Daniel J. Cole, MD**
*Professor of Clinical Anesthesiology*
*Department of Anesthesiology*
*Ronald Reagan UCLA Medical Center*
*Los Angeles, California*

**Wilson Cui, MD, PhD**
*Assistant Professor*
*Department of Anesthesia and Perioperative Care*
*University of California, San Francisco, School of Medicine*
*San Francisco, California*

**Andrew J. Deacon, B Biomed Sci (Hons), MBBS, FANZCA**
*Staff Specialist*
*Department of Anaesthesia and Pain Medicine*
*The Canberra Hospital*
*Garran, ACT, Australia*

**David M. Dickerson, MD**
*Assistant Professor*
*Department of Anesthesia and Critical Care*
*University of Chicago Medicine*
*Chicago, Illinois*

**Karen B. Domino, MD, MPH**
*Professor and Vice Chair for Clinical Research*
*Department of Anesthesiology and Pain Medicine*
*University of Washington*
*Seattle, Washington*

**Kenneth Drasner, MD**
*Professor Emeritus*
*Department of Anesthesia and Perioperative Care*
*University of California, San Francisco, School of Medicine*
*San Francisco, California*

**Talmage D. Egan, MD**
*Professor and Chair*
*Department of Anesthesiology*
*University of Utah School of Medicine*
*Salt Lake City, Utah*

**Helge Eilers, MD**
*Professor*
*Department of Anesthesia and Perioperative Care*
*University of California, San Francisco, School of Medicine*
*San Francisco, California*

**John Feiner, MD**
*Professor*
*Department of Anesthesia and Perioperative Care*
*University of California, San Francisco, School of Medicine*
*San Francisco, California*

**Alana Flexman, MD**
*Clinical Assistant Professor*
*Anesthesia, Pharmacology, and Therapeutics*
*The University of British Columbia*
*Vancouver, British Columbia, Canada*

**Elizabeth A.M. Frost, MD**
*Professor*
*Department of Anesthesiology, Perioperative and Pain Medicine*
*Icahn School of Medicine at Mount Sinai*
*New York, New York*

**William R. Furman, MD, MMHC**
*Professor and Acting Chair*
*Department of Anesthesiology*
*Dartmouth College*
*Geisel School of Medicine*
*Vice President*
*Regional Perioperative Service Line*
*Dartmouth Hitchcock Medical Center*
*Lebanon, New Hampshire*

**Steven Gayer, MD, MBA**
*Professor of Anesthesiology and Ophthalmology*
*Department of Anesthesiology*
*University of Miami Miller School of Medicine*
*Miami, Florida*

**Sarah Gebauer, MD, BA**
*Assistant Professor*
*Department of Anesthesiology and Critical Care Medicine and*
*Department of Internal Medicine*
*Division of Palliative Care*
*University of New Mexico*
*Albuquerque, New Mexico*

**Rebecca M. Gerlach, MD FRCPC**
*Assistant Professor*
*Department of Anesthesia and Critical Care*
*Interim Director for Anesthesia Perioperative Medicine Clinic*
*University of Chicago Medicine*
*Chicago, Illinois*

**David B. Glick, MD, MBA**
*Professor*
*Department of Anesthesia and Critical Care*
*Medical Director*
*Post-Anesthesia Care Unit*
*University of Chicago Medicine*
*Chicago, Illinois*

**Erin A. Gottlieb, MD**
*Assistant Professor*
*Department of Anesthesiology*
*Baylor College of Medicine*
*Director of Clinical Operations*
*Division of Pediatric Cardiovascular Anesthesiology*
*Texas Children's Hospital*
*Houston, Texas*

**Andrew T. Gray, MD, PhD**
*Professor*
*Department of Anesthesia and Perioperative Care*
*University of California, San Francisco, School of Medicine*
*San Francisco, California*

**Melissa Haehn, MD**
*Assistant Professor*
*Department of Anesthesia and Perioperative Care*
*University of California, San Francisco, School of Medicine*
*San Francisco, California*

**Jin J. Huang, MD**
*Assistant Professor*
*Department of Anesthesia and Perioperative Care*
*University of California, San Francisco, School of Medicine*
*San Francisco, California*

**Lindsey L. Huddleston, MD**
*Assistant Professor*
*Department of Anesthesia and Perioperative Care*
*University of California, San Francisco, School of Medicine*
*San Francisco, California*

**Robert W. Hurley, MD, PhD**
*Professor and Vice Chairman*
*Department of Anesthesiology*
*Director*
*F&MCW Comprehensive Pain Program*
*Medical College of Wisconsin*
*Milwaukee, Wisconsin*

**Omar Hyder, MD, MS**
*Staff Anesthesiologist*
*Department of Anesthesia, Critical Care, and Pain Medicine*
*Massachusetts General Hospital*
*Boston, Massachusetts*

**Andrew Infosino, MD**
*Professor*
*Department of Anesthesia and Perioperative Care*
*University of California, San Francisco, School of Medicine*
*San Francisco, California*

**Ken B. Johnson, MD**
*Professor*
*Department of Anesthesiology*
*University of Utah School of Medicine*
*Salt Lake City, Utah*

**Tae Kyun Kim, MD, PhD**
*Associate Professor*
*Department of Anesthesia and Pain Medicine*
*Pusan National University*
*School of Medicine*
*Busan, Korea*

**Kerry Klinger, MD**
*Assistant Professor*
*Department of Anesthesia and Perioperative Care*
*University of California, San Francisco, School of Medicine*
*San Francisco, California*

**Anjali Koka, MD**
*Instructor in Anaesthesia*
*Harvard Medical School*
*Department of Anesthesiology, Perioperative and Pain Medicine*
*Boston Children's Hospital*
*Boston, Massachusetts*

**Catherine Kuza, MD**
*Assistant Professor*
*Department of Anesthesiology and Critical Care Medicine*
*Keck School of Medicine of the University of Southern California*
*Los Angeles, California*

**Benn Lancman, MBBS, MHumFac, FANZCA**
*Visiting Clinical Instructor*
*Department of Anesthesia and Perioperative Care*
*University of California, San Francisco, School of Medicine*
*San Francisco, California*
*Associate Clinical Instructor*
*School of Medicine*
*University of Sydney*
*Sydney, NSW, Australia*

**Chanhung Z. Lee, MD, PhD**
*Professor*
*Department of Anesthesia and Perioperative Care*
*University of California, San Francisco, School of Medicine*
*San Francisco, California*

**Linda L. Liu, MD**
*Professor*
*Department of Anesthesia and Perioperative Care*
*University of California, San Francisco, School of Medicine*
*San Francisco, California*

**Jennifer M. Lucero, MD**
*Assistant Professor*
*Department of Anesthesia and Perioperative Care*
*University of California, San Francisco, School of Medicine*
*San Francisco, California*

**Alan J.R. Macfarlane, BSc (Hons), MBChB (Hons), MRCP, FRCA**
*Consultant Anaesthetist*
*Department of Anaesthesia*
*Glasgow Royal Infirmary and Stobhill Ambulatory Hospital*
*Honorary Senior Clinical Lecturer*
*Department of Anaesthesia, Critical Care, and Pain Medicine*
*University of Glasgow, Great Britain*

**Vinod Malhotra, MD**
*Professor and Vice-Chair for Clinical Affairs*
*Department of Anesthesiology*
*Professor of Anesthesiology in Clinical Urology*
*Weill Cornell Medical College*
*Clinical Director of the Operating Rooms*
*New York-Presbyterian Hospital*
*Weill-Cornell Medical Center*
*New York, New York*

**Mitchell H. Marshall, MD**
*Clinical Professor and Chief of Anesthesiology Service*
*New York University Langone Hospital for Joint Diseases*
*Department of Anesthesiology, Perioperative Care, and Pain Medicine*
*New York University School of Medicine*
*New York, New York*

**Mary Ellen McCann, MD, MPH**
*Senior Associate in Perioperative Anesthesia*
*Associate Professor of Anaesthesia*
*Harvard Medical School*
*Department of Anesthesiology Perioperative and Pain Medicine*
*Boston Children's Hospital*
*Boston, Massachusetts*

**Joseph H. McIsaac, III, MD, MS**
*Associate Clinical Professor*
*Department of Anesthesiology*
*University of Connecticut School of Medicine*
*Farmington, Connecticut*
*Chief of Trauma Anesthesia*
*Department of Anesthesiology*
*Hartford Hospital*
*Hartford, Connecticut*

**Rachel Eshima McKay, MD**
*Professor*
*Department of Anesthesia and Perioperative Care*
*University of California, San Francisco, School of Medicine*
*San Francisco, California*

**Lingzhong Meng, MD**
*Professor of Anesthesiology and Neurosurgery*
*Chief*
*Division of Neuro Anesthesia*
*Department of Anesthesiology*
*Yale University School of Medicine*
*New Haven, Connecticut*

**Ronald D. Miller, MD, MS**
*Professor Emeritus of Anesthesia*
*Department of Anesthesia and Perioperative Care*
*University of California, San Francisco, School of Medicine*
*San Francisco, California*

**Cynthia Newberry, MD**
*Assistant Professor*
*Department of Anesthesiology*
*University of Utah School of Medicine*
*Salt Lake City, Utah*

**Dorre Nicholau, MD, PhD**
*Professor*
*Department of Anesthesia and Perioperative Care*
*University of California, San Francisco, School of Medicine*
*San Francisco, California*

**Shinju Obara, MD**
*Associate Professor*
*Surgical Operation Department*
*Anesthesiology and Pain Medicine*
*Fukushima Medical University Hospital*
*Fukushima, Japan*

**Howard D. Palte, MBChB, FCA(SA)**
*Assistant Professor*
*Department of Anesthesiology*
*University of Miami*
*Miami, Florida*

**Anup Pamnani, MD**
Assistant Professor of Anesthesiology
Department of Anesthesiology
Weill Cornell Medical College
New York, New York

**Manuel C. Pardo, Jr., MD**
Professor and Vice Chair
Residency Program Director
Department of Anesthesia and Perioperative Care
University of California, San Francisco, School of Medicine
San Francisco, California

**Krishna Parekh, MD**
Assistant Professor
Department of Anesthesia and Perioperative Care
University of California, San Francisco, School of Medicine
San Francisco, California

**James P. Rathmell, MD**
Professor of Anaesthesia
Harvard Medical School
Chair
Department of Anesthesiology, Perioperative and Pain
Medicine
Brigham and Women's Health Care
Boston, Massachusetts

**Amy C. Robertson, MD, MMHC**
Assistant Professor
Department of Anesthesiology
Vanderbilt University Medical Center
Nashville, Tennessee

**David Robinowitz, MD, MHS, MS**
Associate Professor
Department of Anesthesia and Perioperative Care
University of California, San Francisco, School of Medicine
San Francisco, California

**Mark D. Rollins, MD, PhD**
Professor
Department of Anesthesia and Perioperative Care
Director
Obstetric and Fetal Anesthesia
University of California, San Francisco, School of Medicine
San Francisco, California

**Andrew D. Rosenberg, MD**
Professor and Chair and Dorothy Reaves Spatz, MD, Chair
Department of Anesthesiology, Perioperative Care, and Pain
Medicine
New York University School of Medicine
New York, New York

**Patricia Roth, MD**
Professor
Department of Anesthesia and Perioperative Care
University of California, San Francisco, School of Medicine
San Francisco, California

**Scott R. Schulman, MD, MHS**
Professor of Anesthesia, Surgery, and Pediatrics
Department of Anesthesia and Perioperative Care
University of California, San Francisco, School of Medicine
San Francisco, California

**David Shimabukuro, MDCM**
Professor
Department of Anesthesia and Perioperative Care
University of California, San Francisco, School of Medicine
San Francisco, California

**Mandeep Singh, MBBS, MD, MSc, FRCPC**
Assistant Professor
Department of Anesthesiology
Toronto Western Hospital
University Health Network
Toronto, Ontario, Canada

**Peter D. Slinger, MD, FRCPC**
*Professor and Staff Anesthesiologist*
*Department of Anesthesia*
*University of Toronto*
*Toronto General Hospital*
*Toronto, Ontario, Canada*

**Sulpicio G. Soriano, II, MD**
*Professor*
*Department of Anesthesia, Critical Care, and Pain Medicine*
*Harvard Medical School*
*Endowed Chair in Pediatric Neuroanesthesia*
*Boston Children's Hospital*
*Boston, Massachusetts*

**Scott Springman, MD**
*Professor*
*Department of Anesthesiology*
*Medical Director*
*Outpatient Surgical Services*
*University of Wisconsin School of Medicine and Public Health*
*Madison, Wisconsin*

**Randolph H. Steadman, MD, MS**
*Professor and Vice Chair of Education*
*Director*
*Liver Transplant Anesthesiology*
*Department of Anesthesiology and Perioperative Medicine*
*University of California, Los Angeles*
*David Geffen School of Medicine*
*Los Angeles, California*

**Erica J. Stein, MD**
*Associate Professor*
*Department of Anesthesiology*
*Wexner Medical Center at The Ohio State University*
*Columbus, Ohio*

**Marc Steurer, MD, DESA**
*Associate Professor*
*Department of Anesthesia and Perioperative Care*
*University of California, San Francisco, School of Medicine*
*Vice Chief*
*Department of Anesthesia and Perioperative Care*
*Zuckerberg San Francisco General Hospital and Trauma Care*
*San Francisco, California*

**Bobbie Jean Sweitzer, MD, FACP**
*Professor of Anesthesiology*
*Director*
*Perioperative Medicine*
*Northwestern University Feinberg School of Medicine*
*Chicago, Illinois*

**James Szocik, MD**
*Clinical Associate Professor*
*Department of Anesthesiology*
*University of Michigan*
*Ann Arbor, Michigan*

**Magnus Teig, MB, ChB, MRCP, FRCA**
*Clinical Associate Professor*
*Department of Anesthesiology*
*University of Michigan*
*Ann Arbor, Michigan*

**Kevin K. Tremper, PhD, MD**
*Professor and Chair*
*Department of Anesthesiology*
*University of Michigan*
*Ann Arbor, Michigan*

**Avery Tung, MD, FCCM**
*Professor and Quality Chief for Anesthesia*
*Department of Anesthesia and Critical Care*
*University of Chicago*
*Chicago, Illinois*

**John H. Turnbull, MD**
*Assistant Professor*
*Department of Anesthesia and Perioperative Care*
*University of California, San Francisco, School of Medicine*
*San Francisco, California*

**Arthur Wallace, MD, PhD**
*Professor*
*Department of Anesthesia and Perioperative Care*
*Chief*
*Anesthesiology Service*
*San Francisco Veterans Affairs Medical Center*
*University of California, San Francisco*
*San Francisco, California*

**Stephen D. Weston, MD**
*Assistant Professor*
*Department of Anesthesia and Perioperative Care*
*University of California, San Francisco, School of Medicine*
*San Francisco, California*

**Elizabeth L. Whitlock, MD, MSc**
*Clinical Instructor and Postdoctoral Research Fellow*
*Department of Anesthesia and Perioperative Care*
*University of California, San Francisco, School of Medicine*
*San Francisco, California*

**Victor W. Xia, MD**
*Clinical Professor*
*Department of Anesthesiology and Perioperative Medicine*
*University of California, Los Angeles*
*David Geffen School of Medicine*
*Los Angeles, California*

**Edward N. Yap, MD**
*Assistant Professor*
*Department of Anesthesia and Perioperative Care*
*University of California, San Francisco, School of Medicine*
*San Francisco, California*

# FOREWORD

The first edition of *Basics of Anesthesia*, edited by Robert K. Stoelting and Ronald D. Miller, was my first textbook of anesthesia. As an anesthesia resident at the University of California, San Francisco (UCSF), I relied on *Basics of Anesthesia* to provide concise coverage of fundamental principles and developments in our field. Drs. Stoelting's and Miller's co-editorship of the book continued through the fifth edition. The sixth edition, published in 2011 by Dr. Miller and new co-editor, Manuel C. Pardo, Jr., featured a companion website, Expert Consult, that presented the complete text and illustrations in an online format. This seventh edition of *Basics of Anesthesia* represents the culmination of Dr. Miller's 33-year stewardship of the book. We should admire his determined leadership to publish a textbook that offers the anesthesia community an invaluable educational resource reflecting the ever-evolving practice of anesthesia. This book is symbolic of Dr. Miller's uncompromising desire for all anesthesia learners and providers to walk in his path, in "the Pursuit of Excellence," which was the title of his Rovenstine Lecture at the Annual Meeting of the American Society of Anesthesiology in 2008.

Michael A. Gropper, MD, PhD
Professor and Chair
UCSF Department of Anesthesia and
Perioperative Care

# PREFACE TO THE SEVENTH EDITION

The *Basics of Anesthesia* continues its tradition of providing updated and concise information for the entire community of anesthesia learners. In this seventh edition, editors Ronald D. Miller and Manuel C. Pardo, Jr., have added four new chapters and rigorously updated all content to reflect evolving developments in the specialty. The editors are pleased to welcome the contribution of more than 30 new authors, mostly from the United States, but also from Japan, Australia, Canada, South Korea, and the United Kingdom.

This edition marks the transition to a new lead editor, Manuel C. Pardo, Jr., Professor of Anesthesia and Perioperative Care and Director of the Anesthesia Residency Program at the University of California, San Francisco. Dr. Pardo has worked alongside retiring lead editor, Dr. Miller, to identify emerging trends and chronicle advances in anesthesia care. In this edition the editors have eliminated the History chapter and added four new chapters: Chapter 12, "Anesthetic Neurotoxicity"; Chapter 49, "Palliative Care"; Chapter 50, "Sleep Medicine and Anesthesia"; and Chapter 51, "New Models of Anesthesia Care: Perioperative Medicine, the Perioperative Surgical Home, and Population Health." The editors elected to provide more in-depth coverage to the prior edition's chapter on "Trauma, Bioterrorism, and Natural Disasters," which has been split into two chapters: Chapter 42, "Anesthesia for Trauma," and Chapter 43, "Human-Induced and Natural Disasters." Multiple chapters have been restructured to promote clarity and organization of the material. In addition, we have continued to make extensive use of color figures, illustrations, and tables to present concepts in a focused manner. Each chapter has "Questions of the Day," which are designed to promote reflection on the chapter content. Many questions focus on understanding relevant basic concepts as well as analyzing challenging clinical situations.

We are extremely thankful to the authors of the current and previous editions of *Basics of Anesthesia* for their commitment to the excellence of the book. The editors also gratefully acknowledge the expertise of editorial analyst Tula Gourdin, who managed the communication with the authors, editors, and publisher and ensured that no detail was overlooked throughout the entire publication process. We also wish to acknowledge our publisher, Elsevier, and the dedication of their staff, including executive content strategists William R. Schmitt and Dolores Meloni, senior content development specialist Ann Ruzycka Anderson, and senior project manager Sharon Corell.

Ronald D. Miller
Manuel C. Pardo, Jr.

# CONTENTS

# Contents

# Basics of
# ANESTHESIA

## SEVENTH EDITION

# INTRODUCTION

# 1 SCOPE OF ANESTHESIA PRACTICE

## Ronald D. Miller and Manuel C. Pardo, Jr.

The specialty of anesthesiology has evolved dramatically since the first public demonstration of ether use in the 19th century. Originally, the emphasis was completely on providing surgical anesthesia. As surgical procedures became more diverse and complex, other associated skills were developed. For example, airway management, including endotracheal intubation, was required to provide controlled ventilation to patients who had respiratory depression and paralysis from neuromuscular blocking drugs. These practices required the development of a "recovery room," which was later termed a *postoperative* or *postanesthesia care unit* (PACU) (Chapter 39). The skills that anesthesiologists used in the recovery room evolved and progressed into intensive care units (ICUs) and the specialty of critical care medicine (Chapter 41). The development of regional anesthesia created opportunities for treatment of some chronic pain syndromes (Chapters 40 and 44). Anesthesiology also evolved into a recognized medical specialty (as affirmed by the American Medical Association and the American Board of Medical Specialties), providing continuous improvement in patient care based on the introduction of new drugs and techniques made possible in large part by research in the basic and clinical sciences.

## DEFINITION OF ANESTHESIOLOGY AS A SPECIALTY

A more formal definition of the specialty of anesthesiology is provided by The American Board of Anesthesiology (ABA).[1] The ABA defines anesthesiology as a discipline within the practice of medicine dealing with but not limited to:

1. Assessment of, consultation for, and preparation of patients for anesthesia.
2. Relief and prevention of pain during and following surgical, obstetric, therapeutic, and diagnostic procedures.
3. Monitoring and maintenance of normal physiology during the perioperative period.
4. Management of critically ill patients including those receiving their care in an intensive care unit.
5. Diagnosis and treatment of acute, chronic, and cancer-related pain.
6. Management of hospice and palliative care.
7. Clinical management and teaching of cardiac, pulmonary, and neurologic resuscitation.
8. Evaluation of respiratory function and application of respiratory therapy.
9. Conduct of clinical, translational, and basic science research.
10. Supervision, instruction, and evaluation of performance of both medical and allied health personnel involved in perioperative or periprocedural care, hospice and palliative care, critical care, and pain management.
11. Administrative involvement in health care facilities and organizations, and medical schools as appropriate to the ABA's mission.

As with other medical specialties, anesthesiology is represented by professional societies (American Society of Anesthesiologists, International Anesthesia Research Society), scientific journals (Anesthesiology, Anesthesia & Analgesia), a residency review committee with delegated authority from the Accreditation Council for Graduate Medical Education (ACGME) to establish and ensure compliance of anesthesia residency training programs with published standards, and a medical specialty board, the ABA, that establishes criteria for becoming a certified specialist in anesthesiology. The ABA, in conjunction with other specialty boards, has also developed criteria for maintenance of certification, which includes a program of continual self-assessment and lifelong learning, along with periodic assessment of professional standing, cognitive expertise in practice performance, and improvement.[1] This describes the American system. Other countries and societies have their systems to certify specialists in anesthesiology. Some countries work in a collective manner to educate and certify specialists in anesthesiology (e.g., European Society of Anesthesia).

## EVOLUTION OF ANESTHESIA AS A MULTIDISCIPLINARY MEDICAL SPECIALTY

In the last 50 years, the medical specialty of anesthesiology has progressively extended its influence outside the operating rooms. Initially, the most important non–operating room patient care skills developed by anesthesia providers have been in pain management (Chapters 40 and 44) and adult critical care medicine (Chapter 41). Beginning in the 1980s, anesthesia residency training required rotation experiences in these areas. In 1985, the ABA began issuing subspecialty certificates in critical care medicine to candidates who had completed at least a year of specialty training, thus becoming the first recognized subspecialty of anesthesiology. Pain medicine became the second subspecialty to be formally recognized when the ABA began issuing certificates in 1991. By this time, residency programs required rotations in multiple specialty areas, and fellowship programs in many areas were being developed. This reflected the progressive complexity of health care as well as extensive specialization in all fields of medicine.

## Pain Management

Pain management is required in the perioperative setting (Chapter 40) as well as for chronic pain conditions (Chapter 44). The management of perioperative pain has become more complex as the relationship between postoperative pain control and functional outcomes (e.g., mobility after joint replacement surgery) has become more tightly linked. In addition, the increasing use of neuraxial and regional anesthesia techniques (Chapters 17 and 18) for postoperative pain management has led to increasingly specialized acute pain management services usually managed by anesthesiology.

An outpatient-based pain management center typically takes care of patients with chronic pain on an outpatient basis with occasional consultations in the hospital itself (e.g., for patients with chronic pain who require surgery that leads to acute and chronic pain). Many specialties are involved in chronic pain management, including neurology, neurosurgery, medicine, psychiatry, physical medicine, and physical therapy.

## Critical Care Medicine

Critical care medicine has significantly increased in complexity over the 30 years it has been recognized as a distinct subspecialty of anesthesiology (see Chapter 41). Increasingly, data from large randomized clinical trials are used to develop patient care protocols.[2] The categorization of ICU patients is most often arranged by one or more specialties (e.g., medical, surgical, neurosurgical, cardiac). Because so many specialties can or need to be involved, the critical care medicine specialist may have his or her initial residency training in several different specialties, including anesthesiology, medicine, surgery, neurology, pulmonary medicine, nephrology, or emergency medicine. In many institutions, anesthesiologists are in local leadership roles in critical care medicine.

## Pediatric Anesthesia

Since the 1980s, anesthesia residency training has included rotations in pediatric anesthesia (see Chapter 34), and separate pediatric anesthesia fellowships have been offered for many years. However, subspecialty certification by the ABA has only been issued since 2013. In 2009, the ABA and the American Board of Pediatrics launched a combined integrated training program in both pediatrics and anesthesiology that would take 5 years instead of the traditional 6 years. In pediatric hospitals, the role of pediatric anesthesiologists is very clear. However, the practice (and staffing challenges) becomes more complex when pediatric and adult surgeries are performed in the same hospital. Typical questions include how young must a patient be when only pediatric anesthesiologists deliver anesthesia (i.e., instead of anesthesiologists whose practice is mostly adult patients)? How should anesthesia be covered when there are no pediatric anesthesiologists? In a few hospitals, pediatric anesthesiologists also manage patients in the pediatric ICUs.

## Cardiac Anesthesia

Cardiac anesthesia rotations have been required in residency for many years, and elective cardiac anesthesia fellowships have been available for at least as long (see Chapters 25 and 26). In 2006, the ACGME began to accredit adult cardiothoracic anesthesia fellowships, which led to increasing structure and standardization of the fellowships, including the requirement for echocardiography training. Anesthesiologists can obtain certification from the National Board of Echocardiography for perioperative transesophageal echocardiography as well as adult echocardiography. This certification is commonly achieved by cardiac anesthesiologists.

## Obstetric Anesthesia

Because of the unique physiology and patient care issues, and the painful nature of childbirth, obstetric anesthesia experiences have always been an essential component of anesthesia training programs (see Chapter 33). Similarly, anesthesia fellowship training in obstetric anesthesia has been offered for decades. In 2012, the ACGME began to accredit obstetric anesthesiology fellowships. Similar to the evolution of other ACGME anesthesia fellowships (i.e., critical care, pain medicine, pediatric anesthesia, and adult cardiothoracic anesthesia), this has resulted in standardized and structured training to develop future leaders in obstetric anesthesia. Currently, the ABA does not offer subspecialty certification in this area.

## Other Surgical Areas of Anesthesia

Anesthesia for the remaining surgical specialties is not associated with another certification process, although non-ACGME fellowship training may be available. These subspecialties include cardiothoracic (Chapter 27), colon and rectal (Chapters 28 and 29), general surgery, neurological (Chapter 30), ophthalmic (Chapter 31), oral and maxillofacial, urology, vascular, as well as hospice and palliative (Chapter 35). Anesthesia for the remaining surgical subspecialties is frequently delivered by anesthesiologists without additional special training other than that provided by a standard anesthesiology residency. Often, institutional patient volume dictates whether specialized anesthesia teams can deliver anesthesia. For example, institutions with large outpatient or neurosurgical surgery may have separate specialized teams.

## PERIOPERATIVE PATIENT CARE

### Preoperative Evaluation

Perioperative care includes preoperative evaluation, preparation in the immediate preoperative period, intraoperative care, PACU, acute postoperative pain management (Chapter 40), and possibly ICU care. Beginning in the late 1990s to early 2000s, most surgical patients were required to arrive the morning of surgery rather than the night before. This change frequently dictated that the anesthesia preoperative evaluation be performed during the morning of surgery. However, with complex patient medical risks and surgical procedures, many institutions created a preoperative clinic that allowed patients to be evaluated one or more days before the day of surgery. These clinics have become quite sophisticated (see Chapter 13) and are often managed by anesthesiologists. Patients may be evaluated directly by anesthesiologists, or the anesthesiologist may oversee care provided by nurses or nurse practitioners. Periodically, a patient will need additional evaluation by the primary care physician or other specialists for specific patient care issues.

### Operating Room Theaters

Operating room theaters are increasingly becoming management challenges (see Chapter 46). Matching operating room available time with predicted surgical complexity and length is an intellectual challenge in its own right.[1-4] "Throughput" is the term used to describe the efficiency of each patient's experience. For decades, surgical teams have been allowed to operate in two to three operating rooms at the same time. For the first time in decades, the risks of concurrent surgeries are being questioned.[5] Sometimes the throughput is delayed not because of the operating room availability but because of insufficient beds in the PACU. There are numerous steps in the perioperative pathway (e.g., preoperative evaluation, the accuracy of predicting length and complexity of surgical care, and patient flow in and out of PACUs) that can delay a patient's progress as scheduled. For example, patients may need to wait in the operating room when surgery is complete awaiting a bed in the PACU. Institutions are increasingly appointing perioperative or operating room directors who either manage the operating rooms or coordinate the entire perioperative process starting from the preoperative clinic until exit from the PACU. These positions can be administratively challenging and require considerable skill and clinical savvy. Such jobs are frequently held by an anesthesiologist, although sometimes the director might be a surgeon, nurse, or hospital administrator.

## Postanesthesia Care Unit

In a tertiary care hospital, the role of the PACU is pivotal (see Chapter 39). Not only are patients recovering from anesthesia and surgery, they also are receiving direction for appropriate care after their PACU time that spans from ICU to discharge. Even now, insufficient PACU beds are often a cause of delayed throughput in operating room theaters.[1-4] There are many scenarios that illustrate this basic problem. If the routine hospital beds are completely occupied, there is no place to transfer fully recovered patients in the PACU. If those patients stay in the PACU, there will then be no beds for patients who need recovery from operating room–based surgery and anesthesia. When this problem is anticipated, then surgery start times are delayed. In the future, as anesthesiologists take care of patients with more complex medical risks, more PACU beds will be required in hospitals. In addition to the quality of care, patient logistical management is key to the quality and efficiency of care in the perioperative period.

## TRAINING AND CERTIFICATION IN ANESTHESIOLOGY

### Postgraduate (Residency) Training in Anesthesiology

Postgraduate training in anesthesiology in the United States consists of 4 years of supervised experience in an approved program after the degree of doctor of medicine or doctor of osteopathy has been obtained. The first year of postgraduate training in anesthesiology consists of education in the fundamental clinical skills of medicine. The second, third, and fourth postgraduate years (clinical anesthesia years 1 to 3) are spent learning all aspects of clinical anesthesia, including subspecialty experience in obstetric anesthesia, pediatric anesthesia, cardiothoracic anesthesia, neuroanesthesia, anesthesia for outpatient surgery, recovery room care, regional anesthesia, and pain management. In addition to these subspecialty experiences, 4 months of training in critical care medicine is required. The duration and structure of anesthesiology education differ in countries around the world. Nevertheless, there is generalized international agreement on what constitutes adequate training in anesthesiology and its perioperative responsibilities.

The content of the educational experience during the clinical anesthesia years reflects the wide-ranging scope of anesthesiology as a medical specialty. Indeed, the anesthesiologist should function as the clinical pharmacologist and internist or pediatrician in the operating room. Furthermore, the scope of anesthesiology extends beyond the operating room to include acute and chronic pain management (see Chapters 40 and 44), critical care medicine (see Chapter 41), cardiopulmonary resuscitation (see Chapter 45), and research. More recently, anesthesia training programs have been given increasingly more flexibility. Programs can offer integrated residency and fellowship training, including options for significant research time. These more specialized training programs have the opportunity to produce leaders in subspecialty clinical areas and research. In addition, the ABA has supported the development of combined residency programs in anesthesia and internal medicine, anesthesia and pediatrics, and, most recently, anesthesia and emergency medicine. Clearly, anesthesia training programs are being encouraged to train anesthesiologists who can meet the challenges of the future.

Approximately 131 postgraduate training programs in anesthesiology are approved by the ACGME in the United States. Approved programs are reviewed annually by the Residency Review Committee (RRC) for Anesthesiology to ensure continued compliance with the published program requirements. The RRC for Anesthesiology consists of members appointed by the American Medical Association, the American Society of Anesthesiologists, and the ABA.

### American Board of Anesthesiology

The ABA was incorporated as an affiliate of the American Board of Surgery in 1938. After the first voluntary examination, 87 physicians were certified as diplomates of the ABA. The ABA was recognized as an independent board by the American Board of Medical Specialties in 1941. To date, more than 30,000 anesthesiologists have been certified as diplomates of the ABA based on completing an accredited postgraduate training program, passing a written and oral examination, and meeting licensure and credentialing requirements. These diplomates are referred to as "board-certified anesthesiologists," and the certificate granted by the ABA is characterized as the primary certificate. Starting on January 1, 2000, the ABA, like most other specialty boards, began to issue time-limited certificates (10-year limit). To recertify, all diplomates must participate in a program designated Maintenance of Certification in Anesthesiology (MOCA). In 2016, this program was newly redesigned as MOCA 2.0. Diplomates whose certificates are not time limited (any certificate issued before January 1, 2000) may participate voluntarily in MOCA. The MOCA program emphasizes continuous self-improvement (cornerstone of professional excellence) and evaluation of clinical skills and practice performance to ensure quality, as well as public accountability. The components include (1) professionalism and professional standing (unrestricted state license), (2) lifelong learning and self-assessment (formal and informal continuing medical education [CME], including patient safety), (3) assessment of knowledge, judgment, and skills (completing 30 MOCA minute pilot questions per calendar quarter), and (4) improvement in medical practice. This final component may include a variety of self-directed activities including simulation, quality improvement projects, or clinical pathway development.[6] Along with several other specialties, the ABA also issues certificates in pain medicine, critical care medicine, hospice and palliative medicine, sleep medicine, and pediatric anesthesiology to diplomates who complete 1 year of additional postgraduate training in the respective subspecialty, meet licensure and credentialing requirements, and pass a written examination. These certificates also have a 10-year time limit. Recertification requirements are continuing to evolve as part of the ABA transition to Maintenance of Certification in Anesthesiology for Subspecialties Program (MOCA-SUBS).

## Credentialing and Privileging

After completing residency and joining the medical staff of a hospital, the anesthesiologist must undergo the credentialing and privileging process, which allows appropriate institutions to collect, verify, and evaluate all data regarding a clinician's professional performance. Recently, three new concepts were developed on a joint basis by the ACGME and the American Board of Medical Specialties. General competencies (i.e., patient care, medical/clinical knowledge, practiced-based learning and improvement, interpersonal and communication skills, professionalism, and systems-based practice) are used by the medical staff to evaluate clinicians. Also, focused professional practice evaluation can be used to provide more thorough information about an individual clinician. The last new concept is ongoing professional practice evaluation. In essence, processes need to be developed to identify a problem as soon as possible.

## OTHER ANESTHETIC PROVIDERS

### Certified Registered Nurse Anesthetists

Certified registered nurse anesthetists (CRNAs) probably participate in more than 50% of the anesthetics administered in the United States, most often under the supervision of a physician. To become a CRNA, the candidate must earn a registered nurse degree, spend 1 year as a critical care nurse, and then complete 2 to 3 years of didactic and clinical training in the techniques of administration of anesthetics in an approved nurse anesthesia training program. The American Association of Nurse Anesthetists is responsible for the curriculum of nurse anesthesia training programs, as well as the establishment of criteria for certification as a CRNA. The activities of CRNAs frequently concern the intraoperative care of patients during anesthesia while working under the supervision (medical direction) of an anesthesiologist. This physician-nurse anesthetist team approach (anesthesia care team) is consistent with the concept that administration of anesthesia is the practice of medicine. In some situations CRNAs administer anesthesia without the supervision or medical direction of an anesthesiologist.

### Anesthesiologist Assistants

Anesthesiologist assistants complete a graduate-level program (about 27 months) and receive a master of medical science in anesthesia from an accredited training program (currently Case Western Reserve University, Emory University School of Medicine, Nova Southeastern University, South University, and University of Missouri).[3,7] Anesthesiologist assistants work cooperatively under the direction of the anesthesiologist as members of the anesthesia care team to implement the anesthesia care plan.

## QUALITY OF CARE AND SAFETY IN ANESTHESIA

### Continuous Quality Improvement

Quality is a difficult concept to define in the practice of medicine. It is generally agreed, however, that attention to quality improves patient safety and satisfaction with anesthetic care. Although the specialty of anesthesiology has had such emphasis for a long time, the National Academies of Sciences, Engineering, and Medicine (formerly the Institute of Medicine) drew attention to these issues in medicine overall in 2000 with their report "To Err Is Human."[4,8] New frequently used words became a routine part of our vocabulary (e.g., metrics of competency, ongoing measurement, standardization, checklists, timeouts, system approaches, and practice parameters).[5,6,9,10] Quality improvement programs in anesthesia are often guided by requirements of The Joint Commission (formerly the Joint Commission on Accreditation of Healthcare Organizations [JCAHO]). Quality of care is evaluated by attention to (1) structure (personnel and facilities used to provide care), (2) process (sequence and coordination of patient care activities such as performance and documentation of a preanesthetic evaluation, and continuous attendance to and monitoring of the patient during anesthesia), and (3) outcome. A quality improvement program focuses on measuring and improving these three basic components of care. In contrast to quality assurance programs designed to identify "outliers," continuous quality improvement (CQI) programs take a "systems" approach in recognition of the fact that random errors are inherently difficult to prevent. System errors, however, should be controllable and strategies to minimize them should be attainable. A CQI program may focus on undesirable outcomes as a way to identify opportunities for improvement in the structure and process of care.

Improvement in quality of care is often measured by a decrease in the rate of adverse outcomes (see Chapter 48). However, the relative rarity of adverse outcomes in anesthesia makes measurement of improvement difficult. To complement outcome measurement, CQI programs may focus on critical incidents and sentinel events. Critical incidents (e.g., ventilator disconnection) are events that cause or have the potential to cause injury if not noticed and corrected in a timely manner. Measurement of the occurrence rate of important critical incidents may serve as a substitute for rare outcomes in anesthesia and lead to improvement in patient safety. Sentinel events are isolated events that may indicate a systematic problem (syringe swap because of poor labeling, drug administration error related to keeping unneeded medications on the anesthetic cart).

The key factors in the prevention of patient injury related to anesthesia are vigilance, up-to-date knowledge, and adequate monitoring. Obviously, it is important to follow the standards endorsed by the American Society of Anesthesiologists. In this regard, American anesthesiology has been a leader within organized medicine in the development and implementation of formal, published standards of practice. These standards have significantly influenced how anesthesia is practiced in the United States (e.g., practice parameters).[6,10]

The publicity and emphasis on quality and safety have been intense for several years, but sometimes the standards are not implemented as rapidly and completely as desired. Recently suggestions have been made to attach credentialing requirements and penalties for failure to adhere to the required practices.[7,11] (See also Chapter 48.)

## ORGANIZATIONS WITH EMPHASIS ON ANESTHESIA QUALITY AND SAFETY

### Anesthesia Patient Safety Foundation

The Anesthesia Patient Safety Foundation (APSF) was established under the administration of Ellison C. Pierce, Jr., MD, during his year as president of the American Society of Anesthesiologists.[8,12] Initial financial support for formation of the APSF was provided by the American Society of Anesthesiologists, and this financial support continues to the present. In addition, APSF receives financial support from corporations, specialty societies, and individual donors. The purpose of APSF is to "assure that no patient shall be harmed by anesthesia." To fulfill this mission, the APSF provides research grants to support investigations designed to provide a better understanding of preventable anesthetic injuries and promotes national and international communication of information and ideas about the causes and prevention of harm from anesthesia. A quarterly APSF newsletter is the most widely distributed anesthesia publication in the world and is dedicated to discussion of anesthesia patient safety issues. Anesthesiology is the only specialty in medicine with a foundation dedicated solely to issues of patient safety. The National Patient Safety Foundation, formed in 1997 by the American Medical Association, is modeled after the APSF.

### Anesthesia Quality Institute

The Anesthesia Quality Institute (AQI) was formed in 2008 for the purpose of being a primary source of information for quality improvement in the practice of anesthesiology. It maintains data that can be used to "assess and improve patient care." Eventually, the AQI will be able to provide quality and safety data that could be used to meet regulatory requirements. The AQI is already being used as a source of data for clinical care, research, and societies that have improving quality of care as a goal. The AQI website describes the structure of the National Anesthesia Clinical Outcomes Registry (NACOR) and how data flow into and out of the AQI.[13]

### American Society of Anesthesiologists Closed Claims Project and Its Registries

The ASA Closed Claims Project and its Registries are a database of retrospective analyses of legal cases with adverse outcomes. This ongoing investigation has helped identify patient and practice risk areas that tend to have difficulties and require added attention from the specialty with regard to quality and safety.[5,9]

### Foundation for Anesthesia Education and Research

Although not directly involved with quality and safety, the Foundation for Anesthesia Education and Research (FAER) is an exceptionally important vehicle for support of research in the specialty of anesthesiology. FAER was established in 1986 with financial support from the American Society of Anesthesiologists. In addition, FAER receives financial support from corporations, specialty societies, and individual donors. The purpose of FAER is to encourage research, education, and scientific innovation in anesthesiology, perioperative medicine, and pain management. Over the years, FAER has funded numerous research grants and provided support for the development of academic anesthesiologists.

## PROFESSIONAL LIABILITY

Because of intense dedication to quality and safety, malpractice claims have been reduced both in frequency and magnitude. As a result, malpractice premiums have dramatically decreased over the last 20 years. Nevertheless the fundamental principles need to be understood. First, litigation still occurs. For example, 93 claims were filed in the United Kingdom over the years 1995 to 2007.[9,14] Sixty-two claims involved alleged drug administration errors in which muscle relaxants were the most common issue. Also, 19 claims involved patients being awake and paralyzed (see Chapter 47). With proper labeling and double-checking, such errors can be decreased. The anesthesiologist is clearly responsible for management and recovery from anesthesia. Physicians administering anesthetics are not expected to guarantee a favorable outcome to the patient but are required to exercise ordinary and reasonable care or skill in comparison to other anesthesiologists. That the anticipated result does not follow or that complications occur does not imply negligence (practice below the standard of care). Furthermore, an anesthesiologist is not responsible for an error in judgment unless it is viewed as inconsistent with the skill expected of every physician. As a specialist, however, an anesthesiologist is responsible for making medical judgments that are consistent with national, not local, standards. Anesthesiologists maintain professional liability (malpractice) insurance that provides financial protection in the event of a court judgment against them. Also, CRNAs can be held legally responsible for the technical aspects of the administration of anesthesia. It is likely, however, that legal responsibility for the actions of the CRNA will be shared by the physician responsible for supervising the administration of anesthesia.

The best protection for the anesthesiologist against medicolegal action lies in the thorough and up-to-date practice of anesthesia, coupled with interest in the patient by virtue of preoperative and postoperative visits plus detailed records of the course of anesthesia (automated information systems provide the resource to collect and record real-time actual data). Also, all anesthesia providers should be prepared to transition to anesthesia record keeping via automated information systems. Specifically, use of automated anesthetic records should be fully integrated into one's medical center information technology system. Unfortunately, implementation of electronic health records (EHRs) is difficult, costly, time-consuming, and fraught with many unintended consequences, including not meeting safety standards. However, a review of 2008-2014 national data reveals large gains in using EHRs with 75% of hospitals having at least a basic EHR system, up from 59% in 2013.[15] In the United States, at the forefront of implementation and use of health information technology is the Office of the National Coordinator (ONC) for Health Information Technology.

## Adverse Events

In the event of an accident or complication related to the administration of anesthesia, the anesthesiologist should promptly document the facts on the patient's medical record (see the APSF Adverse Event Protocol[16]) and immediately notify the appropriate agencies, beginning at the department level and continuing with one's own medical center quality improvement administration and risk management office. Patient treatment should be noted and consultation with other physicians sought when appropriate. The anesthesiologist should provide the hospital and the company that writes the physician's professional liability insurance with a complete account of the incident. The investigation and discussion of adverse events and complications may involve a root cause analysis (RCA) in collaboration with the physicians, nurses, and other staff involved with the patient's care.

## RISKS OF ANESTHESIA

Although patients may express a fear of dying during anesthesia, the fact is that anesthesia-related deaths have decreased dramatically in the last 2 decades.[11,17] Because fewer adverse events are being attributed to anesthesia, the professional liability insurance premiums paid by anesthesiologists have decreased.[12,18] The increased safety of anesthesia (especially for patients without significant coexisting diseases and undergoing elective surgery) is presumed to reflect the introduction of improved anesthesia drugs and monitoring (pulse oximetry, capnography), as well as the training of increased numbers of anesthesiologists. Despite the perceived safety of anesthesia, adverse events still occur, and not all agree that the mortality rate from anesthesia has improved as greatly as suggested. Improvement is based on a series of 244,000 surviving patients who underwent anesthesia and surgery. This series is the basis for estimating a mortality rate from anesthesia of 1 in 250,000.[14,19] It is likely that the safety of anesthesia and surgery can be improved by persuading patients to stop smoking, lose weight, avoid excess intake of alcohol, and achieve optimal medical control of essential hypertension, diabetes mellitus, and asthma before undergoing elective operations.

When perioperative adverse events occur, it is often difficult to establish a cause-and-effect mechanism. In many instances it is impossible to separate an adverse event caused by an inappropriate action of the anesthesiologist ("lapse of vigilance," breach in the standard of care) from an unavoidable mishap (maloccurrence, coincidental event) that occurred despite optimal care.[15,20] Examples of adverse outcomes other than death include peripheral nerve damage, brain damage, airway trauma (most often caused by difficult tracheal intubation), intraoperative awareness, eye injury, fetal/newborn injury, and aspiration. Difficult airway management has traditionally been perceived by anesthesiologists as the greatest anesthesia patient safety issue.[17,21] A survey of

> **Box 1.1** Patient Safety Concerns of Anesthesiologists in Large Group Practices
>
> 1. Distractions in the operating room
> 2. Production pressures
> 3. Communication (handoffs)
> 4. Medication safety
> 5. Postoperative respiratory monitoring, neuromuscular blocker monitoring

From Stoelting RK. Large anesthesia/practice management groups: how can APSF help everyone be safer? *APSF Newsletter.* 2016;30(3):45, 55-56. http://www.apsf.org.

large anesthesia groups has highlighted other concerns to patient safety (Box 1.1).

Improved monitoring of anesthetized patients hopefully will serve to further enhance the vigilance of the anesthesiologist and decrease the role of human error in anesthetic morbidity and mortality rates. Indeed, human error, in part resulting from lapses in attention (vigilance), accounts for a large proportion of adverse anesthesia events. A number of factors at work in the operating room environment serve to diminish the ability of the anesthesiologist to perform the task of vigilance. Prominent among these factors are sleep loss and fatigue with known detrimental effects on work efficiency and cognitive tasks (monitoring, clinical decision making). The RRC for Anesthesiology mandates that anesthesia residents not be assigned clinical responsibilities the day after 24-hour in-hospital call. The Health and Medicine Division (HMD) of the National Academies has made very specific recommendations regarding resident work hours and will no doubt make recommendations for physicians overall that could eventually be mandated. The emphasis on efficiency in the operating room ("production pressures") designed to improve productivity may supersede safety and provoke the commission of errors that jeopardize patient safety. At the same time, not all adverse events during anesthesia are a result of human error and therefore preventable.

## HAZARDS OF WORKING IN THE OPERATING ROOM

Anesthesiologists spend long hours in an environment (operating room) associated with exposure to vapors from chemicals (volatile anesthetics), ionizing radiation, and infectious agents (hepatitis viruses, human immunodeficiency virus). There is psychological stress from demands of the constant vigilance required for the care of patients during anesthesia. Furthermore, interactions with members of the operating team (surgeons, nurses) may introduce varying levels of interpersonal stress. Removal of waste anesthetic gases (scavenging)

has decreased exposure to trace concentrations of these gases, although evidence that this practice has improved the health of anesthesia personnel is lacking. Universal precautions are recommended in the care of every patient in an attempt to prevent the transmission of blood-borne infections, particularly by accidental needlestick injuries. Substance abuse, mental illness (depression), and suicide seem to occur with increased frequency among anesthesiologists, perhaps reflecting the impact of occupational stress.

Lastly, infection control for both patients and clinical personnel in the operating rooms require increasingly strict rules regarding specific procedures in the operating room such as washing hands.

## SUMMARY AND FUTURE OUTLOOK

This chapter reflects the constantly evolving and changing practice of anesthesia. Our responsibilities have grown in magnitude, scope, and depth. Although anesthesia practice is partly based on outpatient activities (see Chapters 37 and 44), it has also become a leading specialty with regard to inpatient medicine, especially the perioperative period including critical care medicine (see Chapter 41). Definitely more sophisticated technological tools and systems will be integrated in the practice of anesthesiology. In more recent years, the use of robots in the operating theater has become standard for specific surgeries.[18,22] The specialty will become even more valuable to medicine overall by attempting to anticipate future societal needs[15,20] and continuing to dedicate ourselves to the pursuit of excellence.[10] Lastly, this chapter has described the American organization and delivery of anesthesia. Every country in the world has or should subject their anesthesia practice to an intense and possibly similar type of analysis.

## QUESTIONS OF THE DAY

1. In the United States, which anesthesiology fellowships are accredited by the Accreditation Council for Graduate Medical Education? What is the impact of Accreditation Council for Graduate Medical Education accreditation on the structure of a fellowship program?
2. What are the sources of data in the National Anesthesia Clinical Outcomes Registry?
3. How has the Foundation for Anesthesia Education and Research helped to advance the specialty of anesthesiology?
4. What are the reasons for a decrease in anesthesia malpractice premiums over the past few decades? What steps can the anesthesia provider take to reduce the chance for a lawsuit after an adverse event?
5. What are the potential hazards of working in the operating room as an anesthesia provider?

## REFERENCES

1. American Board of Anesthesiology. http://www.theaba.org/PDFs/BOI/MOCA-BOI. Accessed April 28, 2016.
2. Matthay MA, Liu KD. New strategies for effective therapeutics in critically ill patients. *JAMA.* 2016;315(8):747–748.
3. Dexter F. A brief history of evidence-based operating room management: then and now. *Anesth Analg.* 2012;115:10–11.
4. Dexter F. High-quality operating room management research. *J Clin Anesth.* 2014;26:341–342.
5. Mello MM, Livingston EH. Managing the risks of concurrent surgeries. *JAMA.* 2016;315:1563–1564.
6. American Board of Anesthesiology. http://www.theaba.org/MOCA/MOCA-2-0-Part-4. Accessed April 28, 2016.
7. American Academy of Anesthesiologist Assistants. http://www.anesthetist.org.
8. Committee on Quality of Health Care in America, Institute of Medicine. *To Err Is Human.* Washington, DC: National Academy Press; 2000.
9. Spiess BD, Wahr JA, Nussmeier NA. Bring your life into FOCUS. *Anesth Analg.* 2010;110:283–287.
10. Miller RD. The pursuit of excellence. The 47th Annual Rovenstine Lecture. *Anesthesiology.* 2008;110:714–720.
11. Apfelbaum JL, Aveyard C, Cooper L, et al. Outsourcing anesthesia preparation. *Anesthesiol News.* 2009:1–6.
12. Pierce EC. The 34th Rovenstine Lecture: 40 years behind the mask: safety revisited. *Anesthesiology.* 1996;84:965–997.
13. Anesthesia Quality Institute. National Anesthesia Clinical Outcomes Registry. https://www.aqihq.org/introduction-to-nacor.aspx.
14. Cranshaw J, Gupta KJ, Cook TM. Litigation related to drug errors in anaesthesia: an analysis of claims against the NHS in England 1995-2007. *Anaesthesia.* 2009;64:1317–1323.
15. Adler-Milstein J, DesRoches C, Kralovec P, et al. Electronic health record adoption in US hospitals: progress continues, but challenges persist. *Health Aff (Milwood).* 2015;34(12):2174–2180.
16. Anesthesia Patient Safety Foundation (APSF). Clinical Safety. Adverse Event Protocol. http://www.apsf.org/resources_safety_protocol.php.
17. Cooper JB, Gaba DG. No myth: anesthesia is a model for addressing patient safety. *Anesthesiology.* 2002;97:1335–1337.
18. Hallinan JT. Once seen as risky, one group of doctors changes its ways. *The Wall Street Journal.* June 21, 2005.
19. Lagasse RS. Anesthesia safety: model or myth? A review of the published literature and analysis of current original data. *Anesthesiology.* 2002;97:1609–1617.
20. Miller RD. Report from the Task Force on Future Paradigms of Anesthesia Practice. *ASA Newsletter.* 2005;69:2–6.
21. Stoelting RK. APSF survey results identify safety issues priorities. *Spring APSF Newsletter.* 1999:6–7. http://www.apsf.org.
22. Berlinger NT. Robotic surgery: squeezing into tight places. *N Engl J Med.* 2006;354:2099–2101.

# 2

# LEARNING ANESTHESIA

Manuel C. Pardo, Jr.

The challenges of learning perioperative anesthesia care have grown considerably as the specialty, and medicine in general, have evolved. The beginning anesthesia trainee is faced with an ever-increasing quantity of knowledge, the need for adequate patient care experiences, and increased attention to patient safety as well as cost containment.[1] Most training programs begin with close clinical supervision by an attending anesthesiologist. More experienced trainees may offer their perspectives and practical advice. Some programs use a mannequin-based patient simulator or other forms of simulation to facilitate the learning process.[2] The practice of anesthesia involves the development of flexible patient care routines, factual and theoretical knowledge, manual and procedural skills, and the mental abilities to adapt to changing situations.[3]

## COMPETENCIES AND MILESTONES

The anesthesia provider must be skilled in many areas. The Accreditation Council for Graduate Medical Education (ACGME) developed its Outcome Project, which includes a focus on six core competencies: patient care, medical knowledge, professionalism, interpersonal and communication skills, systems-based practice, and practice-based learning and improvement (Table 2.1).[4] More recently, the ACGME has advanced the core competencies approach by adopting the Dreyfus model of skill acquisition to create a framework of "milestones" in the development of anesthesia residents during 4 years of training.[5,6] Table 2.2 shows an example of a milestone in the patient care competency. The milestones incorporate several aspects of residency training, including a description of expected behavior, the complexity of the patient and the surgical procedure, and the level of supervision needed by the resident.

**Table 2.1**   Competencies in Anesthesia Care

| Procedure Event/ Problem | Competency |
|---|---|
| Perform preoperative history and physical | Patient care, communication |
| Determine dose of neuromuscular blocking drug to facilitate tracheal intubation | Medical knowledge |
| Perform laryngoscopy and tracheal intubation | Patient care |
| Interact with surgeons and nurses in operating room | Professionalism, communication |
| Manage maintenance and emergence from anesthesia | Patient care |
| Patient with dental injury: refer to quality assurance committee | Systems-based practice |
| Patient with postoperative nausea: compare prophylaxis strategy with published literature | Practice-based learning and improvement |

## STRUCTURED APPROACH TO ANESTHESIA CARE

Anesthesia providers care for the surgical patient in the preoperative, intraoperative, and postoperative periods (Box 2.1). Important patient care decisions reflect on assessing the preoperative evaluation, creating the anesthesia plan, preparing the operating room, and managing the intraoperative anesthetic, postoperative care, and outcome. An understanding of this framework will facilitate the learning process.

### Preoperative Evaluation

The goals of preoperative evaluation include assessing the risk of coexisting diseases, modifying risks, addressing patients' concerns, and discussing options for anesthesia care (see Chapters 13 and 14). The beginning trainee should learn the types of questions that are the most important to understanding the patient and the proposed surgery. Some specific questions and their potential importance follow.

What is the indication for the proposed surgery? Is it elective or an emergency? The indication for surgery may have particular anesthetic implications. For example,

**Table 2.2**   Example of Anesthesia Resident Milestones: Patient Care Competency, Anesthetic Plan, and Conduct

| Level 1 | Level 2 | Level 3 | Level 4 | Level 5 |
|---|---|---|---|---|
| Formulates patient care plans that include consideration of underlying clinical conditions, past medical history, and patient, medical, or surgical risk factors Adapts to new settings for delivery of patient care | Formulates anesthetic plans for *patients undergoing routine procedures* that include consideration of underlying clinical conditions, past medical history, patient, anesthetic and surgical risk factors, and patient choice Conducts *routine* anesthetics, including management of commonly encountered physiologic alterations associated with anesthetic care, with *indirect supervision* | Formulates anesthetic plans for *patients undergoing common subspecialty procedures* that include consideration of medical, anesthetic, and surgical risk factors and that take into consideration a patient's anesthetic preference Conducts *subspecialty* anesthetics with *indirect supervision* but may require *direct supervision for more complex* procedures and patients | Formulates and tailors anesthetic plans that include consideration of medical, anesthetic, and surgical risk factors and patient preference for *patients with complex medical issues undergoing complex procedures with conditional independence* Conducts *complex* anesthetics with *conditional independence; may supervise others* in the management of complex clinical problems | *Independently* formulates anesthetic plans that include consideration of medical, anesthetic, and surgical risk factors as well as patient preference for *complex patients and procedures* Conducts *complex* anesthetic management *independently* |

Levels correspond to the following time points during residency:
Level 1: Resident has completed one postgraduate year of education.
Level 2: Resident is without significant experience in subspecialties of anesthesiology.
Level 3: Resident has experience in subspecialties of anesthesiology.
Level 4: Resident substantially fulfills milestones expected of an anesthesiology residency; designated as graduation target.
Level 5: Resident has advanced beyond performance targets defined for residency and is demonstrating "aspirational" goals.
From Anesthesiology Residency Review Committee. The Anesthesiology Milestone Project. https://www.acgme.org/Portals/0/PDFs/Milestones/AnesthesiologyMilestones.pdf. July 2015. Accessed May 2, 2016.

---

**Box 2.1** Phases of Anesthesia Care

**Preoperative Phase**
Preoperative evaluation
Choice of anesthesia
Premedication

**Intraoperative Phase**
Physiologic monitoring and vascular access
General anesthesia (i.e., plan for induction, maintenance, and emergence)
Regional anesthesia (i.e., plan for type of block, needle, local anesthetic)

**Postoperative Phase**
Postoperative pain control method
Special monitoring or treatment based on surgery or anesthetic course
Disposition (e.g., home, postanesthesia care unit, ward, monitored ward, step-down unit, intensive care unit)
Follow-up (anesthesia complications, patient outcome)

---

a patient requiring esophageal fundoplication will likely have severe gastroesophageal reflux disease, which may require modification of the anesthesia plan (e.g., preoperative nonparticulate antacid, intraoperative rapid-sequence induction of anesthesia).

A given procedure may also have implications for anesthetic choice. Anesthesia for hand surgery, for example, can be accomplished with local anesthesia, peripheral nerve blockade, general anesthesia, or sometimes a combination of techniques. The urgency of a given procedure (e.g., acute appendicitis) may preclude lengthy delay of the surgery for additional testing, without increasing the risk of complications (e.g., appendiceal rupture, peritonitis).

What are the inherent risks of this surgery? Surgical procedures have different inherent risks. For example, a patient undergoing coronary artery bypass graft has a significant risk of problems such as death, stroke, or myocardial infarction. A patient undergoing cataract extraction has an infrequent risk of major organ damage.

Does the patient have coexisting medical problems? Does the surgery or anesthesia care plan need to be modified because of them? To anticipate the effects of a given medical problem, the anesthesia provider must understand the physiologic effects of the surgery and anesthetic and the potential interaction with the medical problem. For example, a patient with poorly controlled systemic hypertension is more likely to have an exaggerated hypertensive response to direct laryngoscopy to facilitate tracheal intubation. The anesthesia provider may change the anesthetic plan to increase the induction dose of intravenously administered anesthetic (e.g., propofol) and administer a short-acting β-adrenergic blocker (e.g., esmolol) before instrumentation of the airway. Depending on the medical problem, the anesthesia plan may require modification during any phase of the procedure.

Has the patient had anesthesia before? Were there complications such as difficult airway management? Does the patient have risk factors for difficult airway management? Anesthesia records from previous surgery can yield much useful information. The most important fact is the ease of airway management techniques such as direct laryngoscopy. If physical examination reveals some risk factors for difficult tracheal intubation, but the patient had a clearly documented uncomplicated direct laryngoscopy for recent surgery, the anesthesia provider may choose to proceed with routine laryngoscopy. Other useful historical information includes intraoperative hemodynamic and respiratory instability and occurrence of postoperative nausea.

### Creating the Anesthesia Plan

After the preoperative evaluation, the anesthesia plan can be completed. The plan should list drug choices and doses in detail, as well as anticipated problems (Boxes 2.2 and 2.3). Many variations on a given plan may be acceptable, but the trainee and the supervising anesthesia provider should agree in advance on the details.

### Preparing the Operating Room

After determining the anesthesia plan, the trainee must prepare the operating room (Table 2.3). Routine operating room preparation includes tasks such as checking the anesthesia machine (see Chapter 15). The specific anesthesia plan may have implications for preparing additional equipment. For example, fiberoptic tracheal intubation requires special equipment that may be kept in a cart dedicated to difficult airway management.

### Managing the Intraoperative Anesthetic

Intraoperative anesthesia management generally follows the anesthesia plan but should be adjusted based on the patient's responses to anesthesia and surgery. The anesthesia provider must evaluate a number of different information pathways from which a decision on whether to change the patient's management can be made. The trainee must learn to process these different information sources and attend to multiple tasks simultaneously. The general cycle of mental activity involves observation, decision making, action, and repeat evaluation. Vigilance—being watchful and alert—is necessary for safe patient care, but vigilance alone is not enough. The anesthesia provider must weigh the significance of each observation and can become overwhelmed by the amount of information or by rapidly changing information. Intraoperative clinical events can stimulate thinking and promote an interactive discussion between the trainee and supervisor (Table 2.4).

---

**Box 2.2** Sample General Anesthesia Plan

**Case**
A 47-year-old woman with biliary colic and well-controlled asthma requires anesthesia for laparoscopic cholecystectomy.

**Preoperative Phase**
Premedication:
    Midazolam, 1-2 mg intravenous (IV), to reduce anxiety
    Albuterol, two puffs, to prevent bronchospasm

**Intraoperative Phase**
*Vascular Access and Monitoring*
Vascular access: one peripheral IV catheter
Monitors: pulse oximetry, capnography, electrocardiogram, noninvasive blood pressure with standard adult cuff size, temperature

*Induction*
Propofol, 2 mg/kg IV (may precede with lidocaine, 1 mg/kg IV)
Neuromuscular blocking drug to facilitate tracheal intubation (succinylcholine, 1-2 mg/kg IV) or nondepolarizing neuromuscular blocking drugs (rocuronium, 0.6 mg/kg)
Airway management
Face mask: adult medium size
Direct laryngoscopy: Macintosh 3 blade, 7.0-mm internal diameter (ID) endotracheal tube

**Maintenance**
Inhaled anesthetic: sevoflurane or desflurane
Opioid: fentanyl, anticipate 2-4 µg/kg IV total during procedure
Neuromuscular blocking drug titrated to train-of-four monitor (peripheral nerve stimulator) at the ulnar nerve[a]

*Emergence*
Antagonize effects of nondepolarizing neuromuscular blocking drug: neostigmine, 70 µg/kg, and glycopyrrolate, 14 µg/kg IV, titrated to train-of-four monitor
Antiemetic: dexamethasone, 4 mg IV, at start of procedure; ondansetron, 4 mg IV, at end of procedure
Tracheal extubation: when patient is awake, breathing, and following commands
Possible intraoperative problem and approach:
    Bronchospasm: increase inspired oxygen and inhaled anesthetic concentrations, decrease surgical stimulation if possible, administer albuterol through endotracheal tube (5-10 puffs), adjust ventilator to maximize expiratory flow

**Postoperative Phase**
Postoperative pain control: patient-controlled analgesia—hydromorphone, 0.2 mg IV; 6-min lockout interval, do not use basal rate
Disposition: postanesthesia care unit, then hospital ward

[a]Nondepolarizing neuromuscular blocking drug choices include rocuronium, vecuronium, pancuronium, atracurium, and cisatracurium.

---

**Box 2.3** Sample Regional Anesthesia Plan

**Case**
A 27-year-old man requires diagnostic right shoulder arthroscopy for chronic pain. He has no known medical problems.

**Preoperative Phase**
Premedication: midazolam, 1-2 mg intravenous (IV), to reduce anxiety

**Intraoperative Phase**
Type of block: interscalene
Needle: 22-gauge short-bevel, 5 cm long
Local anesthetic: 1.5% mepivacaine, 25 mL
Ancillary equipment: ultrasound machine with linear transducer, sterile sheath, ultrasound gel
Technique: chlorhexidine skin preparation, localize nerve in posterior triangle of neck, use ultrasound to guide in-plane needle insertion, inject local anesthetic
Intraoperative sedation and analgesia:
    Midazolam, 0.5-1 mg IV, given every 5-10 minutes as indicated
    Fentanyl, 25-50 µg IV, given every 5-10 minutes as indicated

**Postoperative Phase**
Postoperative pain control: when block resolves, may treat with fentanyl, 25-50 µg IV, as needed
Disposition: postanesthesia care unit, then home

## Patient Follow-up

The patient should be reassessed after recovery from anesthesia. This follow-up includes assessing general satisfaction with the anesthetic, as well as a review for complications such as dental injury, nausea, nerve injury, and intraoperative recall. There is increasing attention on the long-term impact of anesthesia, including the impact of "deep" levels of anesthesia, hypotension, and inhaled anesthetic dose on postoperative mortality rate.[7]

## LEARNING STRATEGIES

Learning during supervised direct patient care is the foundation of clinical training. Because the scope of anesthesia practice is so broad (see Chapter 1) and the competencies trainees are required to master are diverse, direct patient care cannot be the only component of the teaching program. Other modalities include lectures, group discussions, simulations, and independent reading. Lectures can be efficient methods for transmitting large amounts of information. However, the lecture format is not conducive to large amounts of audience interaction. Group discussions are most effective when they are small (fewer than 12 participants) and interactive. Journal clubs, quality assurance conferences, and problem-based case discussions lend themselves to this format. A teaching method termed *the flipped classroom* can combine aspects of lectures and group discussions.[8] One popular approach to the flipped classroom involves use of an online video lecture that must be viewed prior to the class session. Class time involves discussions or other active learning modalities that are only effective if the trainee has viewed the material beforehand. Simulations can

**Table 2.3** Operating Room Preparation

| Components | Preparation Tasks/Supplies and Equipment |
|---|---|
| **Basic Room Setup** | |
| Suction (S) | Check that suction is connected, working, and near the head of the bed. |
| Oxygen (O) | Check oxygen supply pressures (pipeline of approximately 50 psi and E-cylinder of at least 2000 psi). Check anesthesia machine (do positive-pressure circuit test). |
| Airway (A) | Two laryngoscope blades and handles |
| | Two endotracheal tubes of different sizes (one with and one without a stylet) |
| | Two laryngeal mask airways (LMA 3 and LMA 4) |
| | Two oral airways |
| | Two nasal airways |
| | Lidocaine or K-Y jelly |
| | Bite block and tongue depressor |
| | Tape |
| Intravenous access (I) | Two catheter sizes |
| | 1-mL syringe with 1% lidocaine |
| | Tourniquet, alcohol pads, gauze, plastic dressing, tape |
| Monitors (M) | Electrocardiographic pads |
| | Blood pressure cuff (correct size for patient) |
| | Pulse oximeter probe |
| | Capnography monitor (breathe into circuit to confirm function) |
| | Temperature probe |
| **Daily Drugs to Prepare** | |
| Premedicants | Midazolam, 2 mL at 1 mg/mL |
| Opioids | Fentanyl, 5 mL at 50 µg/mL |
| Induction drugs | Propofol, 20 mL at 10 mg/mL |
| | *or* |
| | Thiopental, 20 mL at 25 mg/mL |
| | Etomidate, 20 mL at 2 mg/mL |
| Neuromuscular blocking drugs | Succinylcholine, 10 mL at 20 mg/mL |
| | Rocuronium, 5 mL at 10 mg/mL |
| Vasopressors | Ephedrine, 10 mL at 5 mg/mL (dilute 50 mg/mL in 9 mL of saline) |
| | Phenylephrine, 10 mL at 100 µg/mL (dilute 10 mg in 100 mL of saline) |
| **Avoiding Drug Errors** | |
| Tips for prevention | Look twice at the source vial being used to prepare your drug. |
| | Some vials look alike, and some drug names sound the same. Always label your drugs as soon as they are prepared. Write the following on the label: drug name and concentration, date, time, your initials. |
| | Discard unlabeled syringes. |
| Conversion of % to mg/mL | Move decimal point one place to the right (1.0% = 10 mg/mL). |
| | By definition, 1% = 1 g/100 mL. |
| | 1% lidocaine is 1000 mg/100 mL, or 10 mg/mL. |
| Conversion of 1:200,000 | Memorize: 1:200,000 is 5 µg/mL (1:1000 is 1000 µg/mL or 1 mg/mL). |

**Table 2.4**   Examples of Intraoperative Events to Discuss

| Event | Questions to Consider | Possible Discussion Topics |
|---|---|---|
| Tachycardia after increase in surgical stimulation | Is the depth of anesthesia adequate? Could there be another cause for the tachycardia? Is the patient in sinus rhythm or could this be a primary arrhythmia? | Assessment of anesthetic depth Approaches to increasing depth of anesthesia Diagnosis of tachycardia |
| End-tidal $CO_2$ increases after laparoscopic insufflation | Is the patient having a potentially life-threatening complication of laparoscopy such as $CO_2$ embolism? What is the expected rise in end-tidal $CO_2$ with laparoscopic procedures? How should the mechanical ventilator settings be adjusted? | Complications of laparoscopy Mechanical ventilation modes Causes of intraoperative hypercarbia |
| Peripheral nerve stimulator indicates train-of-four 0/4 15 minutes prior to end of surgery | Is the nerve stimulator functioning properly? Is there a reason for prolonged neuromuscular blockade? Can the blockade be reversed safely? | Neuromuscular stimulation patterns Clinical implications of residual neuromuscular blockade Pharmacology of neuromuscular blockade reversal |

take several forms: task-based simulators to practice discrete procedures such as laryngoscopy or intravenous catheter placement, mannequin-based simulators to recreate an intraoperative crisis such as malignant hyperthermia or cardiac arrest, and computer-based simulators designed to repetitively manage advanced cardiac life support algorithms. Independent reading should include basic textbooks and selected portions of comprehensive textbooks as well as anesthesia specialty journals and general medical journals.

The beginning trainee is typically focused on learning to care for one patient at a time, that is, case-based learning. When developing an individual anesthesia plan, the trainee should also set learning goals for a case. For example, the patient in Box 2.2 has a history of asthma and requires laparoscopic surgery. Several questions could become topics for directed reading before the case or discussion during the case. *What complications of laparoscopic surgery can present intraoperatively? What are the manifestations? How should they be treated? How will the severity of the patient's asthma be assessed? What if the patient had wheezing and dyspnea in the preoperative area?* Trainees should regularly reflect on their practice and on how they can improve their individual patient care and their institution's systems of patient care.

## Learning Orientation Versus Performance Orientation

The trainee's approach to a learning challenge can be described as a "performance orientation" or a "learning orientation."[9] Trainees with a performance orientation have a goal of validating their abilities, while trainees with a learning orientation have the goal of increasing their mastery of the situation. Feedback is more likely to be viewed as beneficial for trainees with a learning orientation, while a trainee with a performance orientation is likely to view feedback as merely a mechanism to highlight an area of weakness. If the training setting is challenging and demanding, an individual with a strong learning orientation is more likely to thrive.

## TEACHING ANESTHESIA

The role of residents as teachers is increasingly recognized as crucially important to the training of medical students.[10] Residents will spend a significant amount of their time in teaching activities, even early in their own training. Many specialties have developed curricula to address this teaching role, which has a positive impact on both resident and student. One published approach consists of a series of workshops focused on six teaching skills: giving feedback, teaching around the case, orienting a learner, teaching a skill, teaching at the bedside, and delivering a minilecture.[11]

A clinical teaching approach that has been well described in several specialties is called the *One-Minute Preceptor* model.[12] It describes five sequential steps that can be used to structure brief clinical encounters. Table 2.5 lists the steps and an example relevant to an anesthesia student clerkship.

**Table 2.5** Example of One-Minute Preceptor Teaching Model in Anesthesia

You are working with a medical student on an anesthesia rotation. An otherwise healthy patient is receiving general anesthesia for laparoscopic cholecystectomy. After $CO_2$ insufflation and placement of the patient in Trendelenburg (head-down) position, the oxygen saturation decreases from 100% to 93%.

| Steps in Teaching | Dialogue With Student |
| --- | --- |
| Step 1. Get a commitment | Why do you think the oxygen saturation is decreasing? |
| Step 2. Probe for supporting evidence | What findings suggest that the endotracheal tube position changed? |
| Step 3. Teach general rules | Discuss how to approach acute hypoxemia during general anesthesia. |
| Step 4. Reinforce what was done well | You astutely observed other signs of endobronchial intubation such as elevated peak airway pressure. |
| Step 5. Correct mistakes | In the future, you would not give empiric bronchodilator therapy unless there are more definitive signs of bronchospasm. |

## QUESTIONS OF THE DAY

1. What is a "milestone" in the context of anesthesia residency training?
2. How would you adapt the sample general anesthesia plan in Box 2.2 if the patient had poorly controlled asthma and required emergency laparoscopic appendectomy?
3. What are the components of the One-Minute Preceptor teaching model?
4. You are working with a new anesthesia learner. How could you use the structure of Table 2.4 to develop questions and discussion topics for the following event: a healthy patient develops hypotension after induction of anesthesia and tracheal intubation?

## REFERENCES

1. Bould MD, Naik VN, Hamstra SJ. Review article: new directions in medical education related to anesthesiology and perioperative medicine. *Can J Anaesth.* 2012;59(2):136–150.
2. Murray DJ, Boulet JR. Simulation-based curriculum: the breadth of applications in graduate medical education. *J Grad Med Educ.* 2012;4(4):549–550.
3. Smith A, Goodwin D, Mort M, et al. Expertise in practice: an ethnographic study exploring acquisition and use of knowledge in anaesthesia. *Br J Anaesth.* 2003;91:319–328.
4. Leach DC. Competencies: from deconstruction to reconstruction and back again, lessons learned. *Am J Public Health.* 2008;98(9):1562–1564.
5. Khan K, Ramachandran S. Conceptual framework for performance assessment: competency, competence and performance in the context of assessments in healthcare–deciphering the terminology. *Med Teach.* 2012;34(11):920–928.
6. Anesthesiology Residency Review Committee. The Anesthesiology Milestone Project. July 2015. https://www.acgme.org/Portals/0/PDFs/Milestones/AnesthesiologyMilestones.pdf. Accessed May 2, 2016.
7. Willingham MD, Karren E, Shanks AM, et al. Concurrence of intraoperative hypotension, low minimum alveolar concentration, and low bispectral index is associated with postoperative death. *Anesthesiology.* 2015;123(4):775–785.
8. McLaughlin JE, Roth MT, Glatt DM, et al. The flipped classroom: a course redesign to foster learning and engagement in a health professions school. *Acad Med.* 2014;89(2):236–243.
9. Weidman J, Baker K. The cognitive science of learning: concepts and strategies for the educator and learner. *Anesth Analg.* 2015;121(6):1586–1599.
10. Post RE, Quattlebaum RG, Benich 3rd JJ. Residents-as-teachers curricula: a critical review. *Acad Med.* 2009;84(3):374–380.
11. Berger JS, Daneshpayeh N, Sherman M, et al. Anesthesiology residents-as-teachers program: a pilot study. *J Grad Med Educ.* 2012;4(4):525–528.
12. Furney SL, Orsini AN, Orsetti KE, et al. Teaching the one-minute preceptor. A randomized controlled trial. *J Gen Intern Med.* 2001;16(9):620–624.

# 3 ANESTHESIA AND HEALTH INFORMATION TECHNOLOGY

## David Robinowitz and Scott Springman

Anesthesia providers produce and record extraordinary amounts of physiologic, pharmacologic, and care management information. Since the previous edition of this text was published in 2011, there has been exponential growth in the use of computerized anesthesia information management systems (AIMS) both as a stand-alone system and as part of an overall patient care electronic health record (EHR). In the late 1990s, only a handful of academic anesthesia practices had an AIMS installation, with even fewer in private practice settings. However, by 2007 approximately 44% of academic medical centers had completed or were in the process of implementing AIMS. A 2014 follow-up survey estimated that 84% of U.S. academic medical centers would have an AIMS installed by the end of that year. The prediction was that within a few years, few anesthesia trainees would graduate from residency having used a paper anesthetic record.[1] EHRs will likely incorporate the growing number of adjunct electronic devices and other software, combining all into the global term *health information technology*, or *health IT*. Given the enormous impact of health IT on patient care, anesthesia providers must have an understanding of these technologies including their potential benefits and hazards. The scientific discipline that serves as the foundation of health IT is *medical informatics* (the branch of information science that relates to health care and biomedicine), which encompasses health informatics, medical computer science, and computers in medicine.

Given their special skills and knowledge, anesthesia providers should be key players in the development, assessment, selection, and deployment of perioperative health IT. Anesthesia teams now need a working knowledge of the applicable theory and practice of medical informatics. In this chapter, several key health IT topics

The editors and publisher would like to thank Dr. James Caldwell for contributing to this chapter in the previous edition of this work. It has served as the foundation for the current chapter.

for the anesthesia provider will be reviewed, with a focus on AIMS, including some considerations for managing the procurement and operation of information technology in an anesthetic practice.

## HISTORY OF ANESTHESIA DOCUMENTATION AND AIMS

The origins of the modern AIMS date back to the creation of the paper record in 1895 by neurosurgeon and physiologist Harvey Cushing and his medical school classmate E.A. Codman.[2] As pioneers of anesthesia quality improvement, Codman and Cushing had challenged each other to improve their anesthesia practice. In support of this goal, they were the first to collect and review physiologic data using written anesthesia records just 50 years after the discovery of anesthesia. About the same time, Cushing and others began to employ newly invented automated hemodynamic monitors with paper-based recordings, including noninvasive arterial blood pressure measurements. Over the subsequent 50 years, the anesthetic record maintained the same basic format for representation of hemodynamics, albeit with a slow and steady increase in the amount and types of data recorded. These two innovations—documentation of significant events during actual anesthesia and surgery coupled with automated real-time recordings of hemodynamic vital signs—formed the foundation of the modern AIMS.

The late 1970s and early 1980s saw the rollout and initial evaluation of the computerized anesthesia automated record keeper (AARK), but commercialization and widespread adoption were slowed by the limited availability of cheap and reliable computer hardware and software.[3] Yet, many benefits of AARKs became apparent, even within the limitations of this nascent technology. AARKs corrected limitations of paper records such as recall bias, illegible records, missing data or whole records (with regulatory and billing implications), and the lack of an audit trail for medical/legal purposes. Clinical studies of AARKs also revealed that they produced a more accurate record of hemodynamic variables than handwritten charts.[4] For instance, handwritten anesthetic records had increased "data smoothing" (i.e., recorded data were often approximated, leading to less variation between individually recorded data points) as compared to AARKs.

The 1990s and early 2000s heralded a proliferation of advanced computer hardware and software, such as local area networks, the Internet, digital hemodynamic monitors, medical communication protocols such as Health Level Seven International (HL7), and a significant reduction in the cost of computer processing power. Coupled with the voracious demand for more data that paper records could not satisfy, the relatively simple AARKs evolved into full-fledged AIMS, with numerous additional capabilities.

## THE DEMAND FOR DATA

In 2001, the Anesthesia Patient Safety Foundation (APSF) endorsed and advocated "the use of automated record keeping in the perioperative period and the subsequent retrieval and analysis of the data to improve patient safety."[5] There were also demands for anesthesia and perioperative data for such purposes as compliance documentation, research, quality assurance, and the streamlining of billing and administrative functions. However, U.S. federal government action may have most catalyzed the rapid pace of EHR adoption in this country in the 21st century. The Health Information Technology for Economic and Clinical Health (HITECH) Act, enacted as part of the American Recovery and Reinvestment Act of 2009, encouraged the adoption and appropriate use of health IT, including provisions for monetary incentives and penalties.

In 2011, the U.S. Department of Health and Human Services (HHS) Centers for Medicare & Medicaid Services (CMS) initiated the Medicare and Medicaid EHR Incentive Programs. Their Meaningful Use (MU) criteria encourage U.S. health care providers and organizations to adopt health IT through a staged process, via variable payments or penalties. For ongoing MU compliance, organizations must—by 2017—satisfy Stage 3 rules, which consolidate and update many of the Stage 1 and 2 requirements, as well as add requirements for privacy and security practices and the electronic submission of clinical quality measure (CQM) data for all providers (Box 3.1). Reporting compliance within the MU system is complex. For instance, there are specific reporting, incentive, and hardship exemption rules that may apply to anesthesia providers. Advice from the American Society of Anesthesiologists, HHS, Office of the National Coordinator for Health Information Technology (ONC), and health IT professionals may help navigate these requirements.[6,7] The requirements are dynamic, and in early 2016, in response to stakeholder feedback, the federal government was developing the Advancing Care Information program. This new program's intent is to simplify or replace the MU program, focusing on improving interoperability (see later) and creating user-friendly technology designed to support physician workflows. Up-to-date information about federal guidelines and requirements for health IT is available online.[8]

---

**Box 3.1** Objectives and Measures for Meaningful Use in 2017 and Beyond

- Protect patient health information
- Electronic prescribing (eRx)
- Clinical decision support (CDS)
- Computerized provider order entry (CPOE)
- Patient electronic access to health information
- Coordination of care through patient engagement
- Health information exchange (HIE)
- Public health and clinical data registry reporting

---

Discrete data collection and reporting within a health care organization is often cited as a key reason to implement health IT. Reporting supports analysis of workflows; guides efforts at utilization, scheduling, and resource management improvements; permits the measurement of costs, quality, and clinical outcomes; satisfies compliance regulations; serves research studies; and may be required by external public and private agencies. Important data will often reside across multiple systems, leading to the rise of the Data Warehouse, a central repository of integrated data, pooled from one or more separate sources.

Although local reporting has great potential, these local data are leading to the creation of national and international large databases, termed *data registries*.[9] Several observational data registries are focused on the fields of anesthesia and perioperative care: the Anesthesia Quality Institute (AQI), National Anesthesia Clinical Outcomes Registry (NACOR), the data registry of the Multicenter Perioperative Outcomes Group (MPOG), the Society for Ambulatory Anesthesia (SAMBA) database (SAMBA Outcomes Registry, SCOR), the Pediatric Regional Anesthesia Network, and the Society for Cardiovascular Anesthesiologists Adult Cardiac Anesthesia Module. These data registries can receive data directly from health IT, but several issues make sharing data from local health IT difficult. First, a significant investment of time and other resources is required to map local clinical concepts to the registry data schema. Another barrier to full harvesting of the information contained within these datasets is the inconsistency among the varieties of clinical taxonomies—a universally agreed-upon anesthesia "data dictionary" has yet to appear. A third issue is the missing or inaccurate data in health IT anesthesia documentation. This problem may be intractable without significant expense of resources or technological advances, because clinicians cannot be expected to be high-quality data-entry personnel while simultaneously administering anesthesia and caring for patients. Finally, much of health IT data is not discrete, structured, or categorized and rather is represented in plain text; that is, natural/human language. Until natural language processing (NLP, a field of artificial intelligence in which computer software understands human languages) matures, much of this information cannot be used to great extent.

Despite such challenges, there is significant potential for local and national registries with respect to quality improvement and health care research. These data can help describe the current state of clinical care and allow for benchmarking of process and outcome measures across multiple organizations, as well as sharing of lessons learned. Pooled data can also be analyzed to explore the relationships between specific patient care factors and clinical outcomes, especially when these outcomes are rare, although there are concerns that such observational, large cohort studies have significant shortcomings compared to traditional prospective randomized controlled trials.[10] But large datasets—often called *big data*—have helped big business in other fields visualize novel customer-product interrelationships and devise new strategies. Perhaps, big data techniques will be a cost- and time-effective way to augment prospective interventional studies and basic science research in anesthesia. Some anticipated uses of big data include modeling the risk of complications for perioperative patients and sending such information back to the EHR systems to inform clinical decision support (CDS) rules, possibly predicting problems before they actually occur. New computer techniques, such as machine learning or cognitive inference computing, may be able to use big data to draw conclusions from data in ways humans cannot.

## PROFESSIONAL PERFORMANCE DATA REPORTING WITH HEALTH IT

Electronic reporting of professional quality is a specific use of health IT data that is responsible for many reporting initiatives. The Physician Quality Reporting System (PQRS) receives quality information from individual eligible professionals and group practices for CMS. PQRS quality measures are designed to help eligible professionals and group practices assess their performance across a range of quality domains. In 2019, CMS plans to merge several current quality and value-based assessment systems (including MU and PQRS) into either Merit-based Incentive Payment Systems (MIPS) or advanced Alternative Payment Models (APMs) stemming from the recent Medicare Access and CHIP Reauthorization Act of 2015 (MACRA).[11]

Quality measure reporting is recognized as a critical feature of an EHR. Some systems give the option of recording quality documentation within the EHR itself. Conversely, perhaps this reporting should be conducted outside the EHR to reduce the risk of unwanted legal discovery. An alternative to direct documentation is membership in a CMS-approved *qualified clinical data registry* that has an option for collection and submission of PQRS quality measures data on behalf of individual providers. The AQI is currently designated as both a Patient Safety Organization, which meets criteria established in the Patient Safety Rule of the HHS and a qualified clinical data registry. Qualified clinical data registries and patient safety organizations have a high level of medicolegal discovery protection to encourage accurate reporting.[12] Because MPOG is also a 2015 qualified clinical data registry via its Anesthesiology Performance Improvement and Reporting Exchange registry (ASPIRE), NACOR and MPOG participants can leverage their participation in these data registries to also satisfy federal reporting requirements.

## FEATURES OF THE ELECTRONIC HEALTH RECORD IN ANESTHESIA AND PERIOPERATIVE CARE

The EHR is a longitudinal electronic record of patient health information generated by one or more encounters in any care delivery setting. Although there are significant realized and potential advantages of using EHRs for patients, providers, and the health care organization (Box 3.2), there are also many potential pitfalls. Careful design may make the difference between an effective EHR and a failed project. Because the fundamental purpose of the EHR is to support required clinical and administrative activities, the EHR should be intuitive and guide users as well as provide access to the right information at the right time to meet the needs of modern health care.

System feature requirements specific to AIMS include the AARK core functions (permanent recording of device data/device integration from hemodynamic monitors, anesthesia machines, and other clinical devices), capture of meta-data such as case events (e.g., in-the-room time; cardiopulmonary bypass time), documentation of preoperative evaluation (including the use of structured data to support reporting and CDS), management of perioperative orders, and integration with the patient's EHR and other records in various health IT systems. Key targets for integration include the following:

1. Medication data (requiring integration with pharmacy systems, which encompasses patient allergies, medication orders, administrations, interactions, formulary, and costs)
2. Laboratory and radiology systems (study orders and results, ability to record point-of-care test results)
3. Provider orders, notes, and consults
4. Nursing assessments including "ins and outs"
5. Billing functions (create charges to patient and their insurance plan)
6. Patient tracking (integration with admission/discharge/transfer application)
7. Perioperative management systems (e.g., case ordering, scheduling, utilization management)

For modular AIMS (components of a larger EHR), this integration may be operationalized via shared databases and routines (e.g., the AIMS module records medication orders and administrations in the enterprise database shared with the pharmacy and other clinical applications). For standalone AIMS, multiple interfaces (hardware and software) may be required to communicate data back and forth between the AIMS and the other health IT systems (described earlier) to avoid a perioperative information "black hole."

Perhaps the most important EHR feature is reliability. The EHR must be *fault tolerant*, meaning resistant to diverse challenges such as software "bugs," hacking,

---

**Box 3.2** Potential Benefits of Health Information Technology (Health IT)

- It provides legible documentation.
- Information is accessible anywhere inside or outside facility; accessible via mobile technology; accessible by patients and providers.
- Data entry is traceable (an audit trail).
- It offers better completeness and accuracy of information.
- Information is current, and data repository has the same information no matter how it is accessed.
- It decreases paperwork.
- It may improve care quality, reduce errors, improve coordination of care.
- It increases clinical efficiency, if constructed properly.
- It may eventually reduce overall health care costs.
- It facilitates research.
- It can facilitate teaching and learning.
- Automates many processes. Can apply rules and logic to 100% of documentation sessions. It never sleeps.
- It offers administrative efficiencies—including improving charge capture.
- Can provide real-time alerts, prompts, notifications, reminders.
- Patients can access their own health information.
- Health IT vendor is certified by CHPL and supports provider and organization attestation for Meaningful Use.

*CHPL*, Certified health IT product list.

---

hardware failures, network errors, and even natural disasters. Preparing for *business continuity* after a failure includes a fail-safe workflow (e.g., paper records with scanning) and redundant data storage. Two common models for protecting data are (1) *data mirroring*, in which an application on a local workstation works with locally stored data that are automatically copied to remote storage (or a *cloud*), and (2) the *client-server* model in which the local workstation (the *client*) works with data stored on a remote computer (the *server*). An advantage of data mirroring is that it may be resistant to brief network interruptions. Client-server architectures can simplify system management by centralizing software and data to ease maintenance and backup activities. Box 3.3 shows features that should be available in the EHR.

## HEALTH CARE INFORMATION PRIVACY AND SECURITY

Health care providers are morally and legally obligated to protect the privacy of their patients as well as the security of the EHR. The Health Insurance Portability and Accountability Act (HIPAA) Privacy, Security, and Breach Notification Rules are U.S. regulations that codify this obligation into law.[13] The Privacy Rule sets standards for when and how protected health information (PHI), may be used and disclosed in any medium, including

**Box 3.3** Some Desired Features and Capabilities in Health Information Technology

- Electronic document management
- Scanned document management
- Orders capability (computerized physician order entry, CPOE)
- Physiologic device data importation into EHR
- Exchanging information with other hospital processes and services: admission-discharge-transfer, scheduling, radiology, pharmacy, respiratory therapy, laboratory, blood bank, picture archiving and communication systems (PACS), emergency services
- Integration or communication with rehabilitation and long-term care facilities
- Staffing, concurrency checks
- Procedural documentation
- Templates that channel documentation, ensuring compliance with local organizational, national professional, and government guidelines, practice parameters, standards or requirements.
- Clinical decision-support checklists, alerts, reminders, emergency checklists and protocols
- "Scripting" or "macro" documentation allowing set-up and multi-item documentation for repetitive situations
- Structured handoffs
- Medication management
- Administrative reporting
- Mobile integration
- Charge capture
- Telemedicine
- Facility and professional charge capture and compliance checks and reports
- Patient communication and engagement (patient portals, care instructions, pathway guides, others)
- Structured discrete data (flowsheets, lists, checkboxes, buttons, etc.)
  - Categorized data, rather than free text
  - Facilitates reporting and data analysis
- Quality and outcomes analysis
  - Predictive modeling/analytics
  - Ability to export for data registries, population health projects
  - Data warehouse
  - Patient satisfaction surveys: HCAHAPS, Press-Ganey, others
  - Practice management reports

*HCAHAPS*, Hospital Consumer Assessment of Healthcare Providers and Systems survey; *CDS*, clinical decision support.

**Box 3.4** Protected Health Information

- Names
- Geographic subdivisions smaller than a state
- All elements of dates and the age of patients older than 89 years old
- Telephone and facsimile numbers, email or IP addresses, URLs
- Social security numbers, medical record numbers, health plan numbers, account numbers
- Device identifiers and serial numbers
- Biometric identifiers (e.g., fingerprints, voiceprints)
- Photographs of the face or other identifying objects, tattoos
- Any other unique identifying number, characteristic, or code

*IP*, Internet protocol; *URLs*, uniform resource locators.

The HHS Office for Civil Rights is responsible for administering and enforcing the HIPAA Security Rule. The details are complex and are described in detail on the HHS website.[14] In addition to HIPAA, other applicable federal, state, and local laws, as well as health care organizations' policies, may govern the protection of ePHI. Some key HIPAA provisions include the provision of an official notice of privacy rights to all patients, generally at "check-in" or on admission. Therefore, routine use of clinical data for anesthesia care generally does not require additional consent. However, patient authorization may be required for disclosure of PHI to other entities. Patients have a right to their own medical record as well as to limit access to their PHI. There are also laws that restrict changing information in the electronic record for fraudulent purposes. Modern EHRs should have extensive audit trails and integrity checks to detect alterations.

Data security is an evolving field, and as new system capabilities offer increased features, new vulnerabilities also emerge. HHS has raised the alarm about a recent increase in ePHI privacy breaches, detailed in a document on privacy and the security of ePHI produced by ONC.[15] Institutions and individual providers share responsibility in breach prevention. The security of health IT is a significant concern; for example, unknown hospital system hackers have held EHR data for ransom. Recommended ePHI privacy and security practices for individuals are summarized in Box 3.5.

At the health care organizational level, the security officer must perform a risk analysis, develop a risk mitigation plan, and approve electronic systems, such as an EHR. Purchasers of health IT must conduct security risk analyses upon installation or upgrade. The health care organization may also benefit from the work of the Health Information Trust Alliance (HITRUST), a U.S. organization that, in collaboration with health care, technology, and information security leaders, has established a Common Security Framework. This includes a prescriptive set

electronic, written, and oral. PHI includes any data that could be used to identify a patient, and when stored in digital form is termed electronic PHI (ePHI) (Box 3.4). The Security Rule requires certain precautions so that access to health IT systems is limited to those with legitimate purposes and proper authorization. The Breach Notification Rule requires health care providers and organizations to report any breach (a loss of patient privacy or failure of health IT security) to HHS, patients, and, in some cases, the media.

of controls that seek to harmonize the requirements of multiple regulations and standards and can be employed by organizations that create, access, store, or exchange sensitive and regulated data. MU Stage 3 includes provisions that the Food and Drug Administration will deliver new tools to help mobile health product developers manage health care data security. See Table 3.1 for the three main U.S. agencies involved in health IT oversight.

## SELECTED KEY TOPICS FOR HEALTH IT

### Interoperability

Health care data collection and management systems often consist of a core *application* (computer program) and separate modular applications or data sources (within the organization and outside the organization) that extend functionality. Some organizations take a predominantly *modular* approach and have many separate applications from multiple vendors in order to meet their complete health IT needs (e.g., the laboratory system, the orders system). When functions are largely centralized within the same general application, an organization may be said to have an *enterprise* system. The ability to communicate among the various modules and with outside applications and data sources is referred to as *interoperability*. With

high-level *interoperability*, organizations can share data even when using different types or versions of health IT.[16,17] Interoperability can be operationalized at different levels: software applications (1) may share information with built-in functionality, (2) may share data from application to application using standardized formats (e.g., HL7) or *application programming interfaces* (APIs), or (3) may interface remotely via *health information exchanges* (HIEs), which are large data stores that aggregate data from various health care organizations. Interoperability replaces inefficient paper workflows and reduces duplicative testing and medication mistakes. Interoperability also fosters better preventive care and chronic disease management, as well as improving provider communication.

In order to meet MU rules, modular software applications must be able to exchange and use electronic health information without special effort on the part of the user. The ONC has devised an "interoperability road map" to guide current and future development of a learning health system.[18] Interoperability also includes multiple device integration in which data from physiologic monitors, anesthesia machines, ventilators, intravenous pumps, medication dispensers, and other electronic devices are automatically captured by the EHR. The Internet of Things (IOT) is the broader trend in interoperability, in which many electronic devices (from home appliances, to vehicles, to personal health devices) are becoming interconnected, with resultant rapid growth in functionality (as well as increased security risks). Although interoperability is a challenging and resource-intensive process, it is a key promising feature of future health IT.

### System Design, User Interface, and Usability

The innumerable pieces of medical data in an EHR include laboratory test and imaging results, demographic information, billing and compliance data, scheduling, materials management, pharmacy data, physiologic data, and provider clinical documentation. Clinical assessment of patients might require users to find information on multiple screens, at different levels within the same application, or among several applications. A "hunt and peck"

---

**Box 3.5** Recommended Privacy and Security Practices for EHR Users

- Do not share passwords under any circumstances.
- Use a "strong" password (minimum of six characters, mix in uppercase, numbers, and symbols) on all computing devices including smartphones.
- Log out of computer systems when not in use.
- Destroy all papers containing PHI in a shredder or locked disposal bin.
- Do not leave PHI in any form lying around (better yet, avoid printing PHI).
- Do not send PHI over an unsecured email system, in social media, or leave messages with PHI on voicemail.

*EHR,* Electronic health record; *PHI,* protected health information.

---

**Table 3.1** Overview of Health Human Service Entities Applicable to EHR Oversight

| Federal Office/Agency | Website | Health IT-Related Responsibilities |
|---|---|---|
| Centers for Medicare and Medicaid Services (CMS) | www.cms.gov | Oversees Meaningful Use Program |
| Office for Civil Rights (OCR) | www.hhs.gov/ocr | Responsible for and enforces HIPAA Privacy, Security, and Breach Notification Rules |
| Office of the National Coordinator for Health Information Technology | www.HealthIT.gov www.healthit.gov/playbook | Support for the adoption and promotion of EHRs and Health Information Exchange (HIE) |

*EHRs,* Electronic health records; *HHS,* U.S. Department of Health and Human Services; *HIPAA,* Health Insurance Portability & Accountability Act of 1996.

approach, or presentation of data on screens in a way that impedes global comprehension, produces an enormous memory and cognitive burden on users and does not take into account *human factors.* In addition to reducing efficiency, poor *user interface and data visualization design* may impede efficient pattern recognition, clinical assessment, and accurate documentation. More broadly, poor user interface and system design can prevent clinicians from not only understanding what is happening to a patient but also being able to integrate information and predict and prepare for future events, a phenomenon termed *situational awareness.* Situational awareness was initially described in the field of aviation but has been applied to anesthesia. It is defined as the collective functioning of teams and applies to complex systems involving groups of clinicians and computer systems in perioperative care.[19]

In computer science and informatics, the user interface denotes all features of an information device with which a user may interact, including when and how the system invites interaction and how it responds to it. A good health IT user interface allows clinicians to quickly comprehend and process large amounts of information safely and efficiently. The user interface may be constrained by the overall design of the health IT system. Therefore, overall system design must be informed by the principles of *computer-human interaction. Human factors engineering* is the practice of considering the real-world needs and abilities of the technology user—expecting humans to act as humans—that is, to make mistakes as part of their normal interaction with the technology, and to have resource-constrained cognitive abilities and memory. One technique for improving human-computer system performance is *user-centered design*—an iterative technology development workflow—in which cycles of design and prototype development are informed by early user-based evaluation, such as simulation and evaluation of user interfaces during development. Although such iterative engineering practices may have larger up-front costs, there may be significant savings as technologies that are more acceptable to users are rolled out and expensive "re-dos" are avoided.

Design principles from industries other than computer science and aviation can also be successfully adapted to health IT. The industrial safety concept of a *hierarchy of controls* has been applied to health care and anesthesia IT, in which levels of intervention to defeat a hazard are described in order of most to least effective.[20] The most effective controls are those that simply *eliminate* a risk, that is, make it impossible for the bad outcome to occur. An example is a *hard stop* rule that does not permit ordering a medication with a lethal dose. The next level of intervention is *substitution,* in which a less hazardous process is substituted for the hazardous one, such as replacing anesthesia-drawn up medications with prefilled syringes with standardized concentrations, or in health

IT, replacing free text with specific check boxes or buttons. *Engineering the controls* refers to making it easier to avoid a hazard through system design. For example, the risk of a *COWPIE* (charting on wrong patient in EHR) can be reduced by including patient identification photographs in the EHR on various crucial screens or by requiring bar code scanning of identification bracelets for critical activites like blood product transfusion. The next level of danger avoidance is built on adminstrative or organizational practices and education, such as checklists prior to procedures (which can be built into AIMS workflows). The least effective level of control is at the individual level, such as training workers to always click on a link to check allergies prior to starting a case. Whenever possible, AIMS engineers and governance members should try to prevent hazards (e.g., patient safety, compliance issues, billing problems) at higher levels of control, and work with clinical and institutional leadership to eliminate, replace, or engineer them away.[21]

*Usability* is the extent to which a technology helps users achieve their goals in a satisfying, effective, and efficient manner within the constraints and complexities of their work environment. The American Medical Informatics Association (AMIA) has recommended usability principles in building EHRs. Several of these principles are particularly applicable to technology rolled out in the perioperative environment: *minimalism* (the ability to access core function quickly), *reversibility* (functionality to *undo* simple user errors), and *memory* (memory load reduction, to reduce the cognitive burden of operating the system, preserving memory capacity for core tasks).

The AMIA recommendation of *flexibility* highlights the usefulness of system customization. It is clear that usability may be increased by customizing the interface according to user preferences and roles. However, there are also benefits to standardizing user interfaces and system behaviors according to local and national norms, such that health IT developers must carefully balance the benefits of customization versus those of standardization. Although there is no single accepted evaluation tool for assessing usability of health IT, standardized questionnaires, simulation, and screen and video recording have been employed to evaluate user satisfaction, charting accuracy, situational awareness (effectiveness), and the number of "clicks" to complete a task (efficiency) in an old versus a new AIMS. Such testing should be performed both prior to implementation, and periodically after rollout with the goals of assessing and directing improvements in human interaction with the hardware, software, and human workflows that compose the total system.

An important corollary to usability concerns the *resiliency* of the users. When faced with low-usability, but mandated-to-be-used health IT systems, health care professionals will generally find a way to accomplish their goals, in spite of the system limitations. In such cases, although the health IT system may appear to be working successfully, the demands on the user's memory and attention (such as relying on system "*work-arounds*" or having their "face buried in the computer screen") may result in not only operating less efficiently but also in decreased situational awareness, clinical performance, and user satisfaction.[22]

## Clinical Decision Support

CDS is an important feature of effective modern health IT and one of the most touted reasons for organizations to purchase health IT:

> Clinical decision support provides clinicians, staff, patients, or other individuals with knowledge and person-specific information, intelligently filtered or presented at appropriate times, to enhance health and health care. CDS encompasses a variety of tools to enhance decision-making in the clinical workflow. These tools include computerized alerts and reminders to healthcare providers and patients; clinical guidelines; condition-specific order sets; focused patient data reports and summaries; documentation templates; diagnostic support; and contextually relevant reference information, among other tools.[8]

CDS may be *passive,* in which the system, by presenting the clinician with the right information at the right time, assists with decision making. Passive CDS includes the display of relevant laboratory results or vital signs, or providing quick access to appropriate checklists, protocols, standards, or policies and is tightly linked with user interface design. Passive CDS supports the basic levels of situational awareness: knowing what is happening now to one's patient. *Active* CDS uses logic (i.e., rules) to detect particular clinical scenarios and then execute actions, such as generating a warning, alert, or automated action. For example, an EHR can automatically monitor a patient's vital signs and laboratory results, and, when a significant anomaly is detected, such as signs of systemic inflammatory response syndrome, it generates a pop-up alert, sends a pager/smartphone alert, lights up a monitoring "dashboard," or suggests laboratory or medication orders. Active CDS can address failures of higher levels of situational awareness; that is, failure to integrate and analyze data from various sources to interpret a clinical situation. CDS may be implemented at the user level or may operate at a multipatient level, in real time, or over a longer period of time (e.g., an operating room efficiency dashboard).

CDS has many potential and realized benefits in managerial workflows, in process of care, and ultimately in care outcomes. In anesthesia, CDS has improved cardiac workup protocol adherence, warned of anticoagulation status before a regional block, sent near real-time reminders and notifications for intraoperative and critical care, and reduced some adverse outcomes, such as postoperative nausea and vomiting.[23,24] One significant limitation of CDS is that it cannot utilize information that is not accessible, such as medical history information from another, nonintegrated health system, nor data that have yet to be recorded in the EHR. What good is a drug-drug interaction alert that fails to appear because it does not *know* the patient's home medications or signals after the concerning medication has already been given? *Automation-induced complacency* describes the situation in which clinicians become overly dependent on alerts or other CDS and then fail to recognize and act on that same situation when CDS fails to warn them. Ensuring adequate EHR data and structure so that CDS is not a black box—that is, so that the provider understands how the CDS works and on what data it depends—may reduce these errors.

A 2016 National Patient Safety Goal to reduce unhelpful alerts and alarms addresses the inverse situation, in which too many or nonhelpful CDS warnings cause confusion and degradation of clinician performance through the phenomenon of *alert fatigue.* Given the consequences of alerts that fail to signal or warn inappropriately, CDS, especially active CDS, should be evaluated similarly to hemodynamic alarms or laboratory tests. They have measurable sensitivity and specificity, and in practice, coupled with the incidence of the issue to be detected, also have positive and negative predictive values; that is, what is the probability that the presence (or absence) of a CDS alert reflects the presence (or absence) of a true significant situation. To determine the impact of an active CDS intervention, health IT management should test it "in the background" and determine the warning characteristics, and once it has been rolled out, should measure the effect that the CDS tool has on health care provider behavior, such as ordering a new test or medication. One common sense recommendation is to avoid *hard stops* as much as possible, which can have the unintended consequence of completely stopping the ability of a user to perform productive work, a situation made exponentially worse when flawed design makes it impossible to satisfy the rule that led to the hard stop (a significant drawback for user satisfaction and effectiveness). If hard stops must be used for critical patient safety reasons, then it may be best to first test the rule as a caution or *soft stop,* observe for appropriate behavior, and, only when validated, turn on hard stop functionality.

## Transitioning to Health IT: From Paper Records to an AIMS, and Beyond

When transitioning from a traditional paper workflow, or when migrating to a new health IT system, decisions should be guided by such principles as usability, adding value to clinical work, supporting features such as CDS and reporting, and mitigating risks. These risks should not be underestimated, and an assessment of any IT system should include careful analysis and ongoing monitoring of untoward side effects (Box 3.6).

**Box 3.6** Possible Risks or Hazards of Health Information Technology

- Technology may paradoxically reduce direct communication between providers.
- IT can create more or new documentation work for clinicians.
- Information overload for clinicians may lead to cognitive errors.
- Traditional workflow may be significantly changed and fragmented by health IT.
- Documentation on wrong patient may be easier.
- E-work may cause provider distraction away from clinical work or from patient interaction.
- Copy-paste overuse may cause out-of-date information and bloated notes.
- Negative attitudes may be generated toward health IT.
- Loss or corruption of patient data can occur.
- Generation of new types of errors may be due to unanticipated system function and any disruption in traditional workflow or information transfer.
- Excessive costs include initial cost of system, ongoing costs for hardware and software licenses, network costs support, licenses and updates, facility IT support, and further development.
- A "hold harmless" clause in health IT vendor contracts may leave organizations liable for health IT-related clinical problems.
- There may be a persistence of paper workarounds.
- Overdependence on health IT can lead to *automation complacency.*
- Hidden dependencies cause unwanted, unanticipated changes in status of orders, patient electronic location.
- Alert fatigue, poor clinical correlation or specificity for medication or other alerts are potential problems.
- Poor user interface and usability can lead to errors and low user satisfaction.

*Health IT,* Health information technology.

**Box 3.7** Key Health Information Technology (IT) Issues to Investigate Prior to Selection or Implementation of an AIMS or Other Large Scale Health IT

- Will your health IT vendor(s) relationship be collaborative?
- What are reasonable estimates of cost over time? Closely examine financial agreements with software vendor, for acquisition, maintenance, and upgrades.
- Investigate requirements for and involvement with departmental level IT personnel, as well as need for clinician IT position supported by department and hospital. Very significant clinician time is required for planning and ongoing maintenance of all health IT software.
- Consider data, network and application dependability: minimizing software or hardware downtime, strategy for local and remote data back-ups, power reliability and back-up supply, data storage structure and physical location.
- Review remote access via network: Access via Internet? Access via mobile devices? Are users allowed to bring their own devices?
- Investigate access to applications: facility workstation numbers and locations, and ergonomics.
- Establish IT support: staffing, 24/7/365 support, on-site vs. remote support? Identify problem resolution response time for critical care areas such as operating room and critical care.
- Determine user sign-on and access (AKA: logon or authentication) system: Is access security defined at the user, role, department, or service level? If there are several standalone applications, is there a single sign-on (SSO) process? Is there an audit trail?
- How well do different components of local health IT integrate (interoperate) together? What are the inevitable limitations?
- Consider reporting capabilities, including provider generated, departmental management reports, health care system reports, and local, regional, professional, and national reporting requirements (including Meaningful Use).
- Determine how prior workflows must change. Can the software be modified to support existing workflows? Should some workflows change, or should such customization be avoided to support standardization?
- HIM (health information management) involvement for documentation policies

*AIMS,* Anesthesia information management systems.

Anesthesia and perioperative leaders have a central role to play in acquiring new AIMS or perioperative information management systems. They should be leaders in the consideration of new anesthesia and perioperative health IT and should work directly with potential vendors and application developers. Even if their health care organization is purchasing an enterprise-wide EHR, they still have the important role of sharing their evaluation of the AIMS and perioperative modules, and evaluating which components are acceptable (or not). Box 3.7 shows some issues to investigate during the selection and implementation of health IT, such as an AIMS. A basic checklist for large-scale health IT projects is shown in Box 3.8. Selected desirable features of perioperative health care technology are summarized in Box 3.9. Note the role of *change management,* the intersection of the new technology with the organization's culture, project communication, and implementation plan. Crucial "people factors" needed for a successful rollout include strongly committed leadership, a project champion with strong political and social skills, and early and frequent inclusion of end users in the project, from the initial design process to final evaluation. Users may be more drawn to a new system by their perception of the utility of the system—*what can it do?*—rather than by their perception of ease of use. But both are important, so project education not only should include how to use the system, but should demonstrate how the new tool can improve clinical care or the user's effectiveness and efficiency.[25]

When initiating a new AIMS or related health IT, remember that the primary goal of these systems is to improve the quality of the health of individual patients. Fundamental to

---

**Box 3.8** Basic Checklist for Health Information Technology Projects

**Implementation Project Planning**
- Allocation of resources
  - Equipment
  - Time
  - Money
  - Personnel
- Leadership
  - IT-Clinician partnership
  - Roles and accountability
- Goals
- Feature and gap analysis
- Timelines
- Milestones
- Change request management
- In-scope vs. out-of-scope decisions
- Vendor support
- Approach to workflow assessment and change
- Interprovider communication assessment
  - Organizational culture
- Pilot rollout vs. test and general rollout
- For enterprise systems: staged application rollout vs. "big-bang" implementation

**Prerollout training and testing**
- Shadow charting
- Usability assessment
- Use of simulation
- Mandatory training
- Initial and continuing education for providers
- "Super-users" and provider project "champions"
- Failure mode and effects analysis (FMEA)

---

**Box 3.9** Selected Desired Features in Perioperative Health Information Technology

- Support for preoperative clinic and perioperative surgical home
- Includes ambulatory and inpatient OR cases, OB, NORA (non-OR anesthesia), acute and chronic pain care, critical care
- Robust perioperative managerial, clinical workflow, and financial reports
- Perioperative management:
  - Status boards ("flight board") tracking of planned and in-progress patient flow for perioperative areas
  - Scheduling of patients, cases, and locations
  - Personnel assignments
  - Equipment and supply management

*NORA*, Non-operating room anesthesia; *OB*, obstetrics; *OR*, operating room.

---

this is that it support the quality, managerial, and financial "health" of the organization. However, when, in the interest of supporting these secondary goals, the burden of data entry becomes excessive, system usability and provider satisfaction will likely suffer. A recent American College of Physicians position paper highlights these tensions: "As value-based care and accountable care models grow, the primary purpose of the EHR should remain the facilitation of seamless patient care to improve outcomes while contributing to data collection that supports necessary analyses."[26] Although numerous stakeholders may wish to have additional data recorded in the medical record, it is the role of health IT governance and clinical leaders to prioritize these tasks according to institutional priorities. They must also advocate for overall usability, such that the act of using the new technology itself improves and does not degrade patient care.

## Legal Issues and Responsibilities of the AIMS User

Several cases in the literature have described the risks, such as legal liabilities, of using AIMS with design flaws or inadequate training or user practices. One of the most common apprehensions about AIMS concerns device integration, when transitioning from paper records to an AIMS. Providers have been concerned that the now-visible greater variation in autodocumented vital signs, and the inevitable data artifacts, will somehow present medicolegal risks. Although inaccurate autodocumentation, artifacts, and unnoticed data dropouts do present some risks, there is no historical evidence of significant medicolegal negative consequences to providers in general from the proper use of an AIMS.[27,28] In fact, the automatic recording of physiologic data may be welcomed by the specialty of anesthesia, because it removes the known problems of human filtering of data and improves the credibility of the record. Nonetheless, EHR users must understand the basic workflow of device data acquisition and be able to detect and correct failure of data capture. EHRs should also permit easy notation of artifact or data collection errors.

A case report of a patient undergoing a craniotomy illustrates these concerns.[29] According to legal records, upon returning from a break, the responsible anesthesia provider found that the device data/vital sign data stream had failed, without being noticed by the interim anesthesia provider who had covered the patient during the break. As a result, 93 minutes of data were not entered in the chart. The patient had postoperative quadriplegia, and the missing anesthetic documentation may have contributed to settling the case. The anesthesiologist did not recognize the interpretation of data transmission because the "active" window obscured the graphic display of data. This case emphasizes that monitoring devices occasionally fail and the need for the anesthesia provider to be vigilant.

Although improvements in AIMS design since this case include using CDS to display an alert when data flow is interrupted, ultimately, it is the responsibility of the health IT user to follow institutional, local, and national standards to create a complete and accurate anesthetic and medical record. Users may even need to periodically manually enter missing data or flag data gaps and artifacts according to the institutional policy. Such workflows also apply in cases of system or network downtime. When there are data issues, it is best to document fully and transparently what transpired, and to correct the record as soon as possible. Audit trails are discoverable and record the source of data and the time they were modified. Obviously, very late changes to an anesthetic record could have the appearance of impropriety.

its use as it applies to perioperative and critical care. The use of health IT is essential to the concept of a perioperative surgical home (PSH) (Box 3.9, and Chapter 51).

Acquisition and use of data will drive future changes in every organization. It is said that you can't manage what you can't measure. Once a large number of organizations contribute data about their patients into aggregated data pools, health IT may transform and improve patient care in ways far beyond current achievements.

## CONCLUSION AND THE FUTURE

Health IT is ubiquitous and inevitable, and evidence indicates that health IT does have real benefits,[30] but the design and details are crucial. Health IT should support both the clinical needs of providers and patients, as well as the financial and management needs of the organization. All anesthesia providers must understand how health IT impacts patient care. Anesthesia providers must be involved in IT decision making and development to ensure that current and future systems support the specific needs of perioperative care. Indeed, anesthesia trainees also have a role in advancing health IT, recognizing that IT systems can be useful for education and learning.[31,32] Health IT is still evolving rapidly and it is critical to monitor and study

## QUESTIONS OF THE DAY

1. What are the potential advantages of the electronic health record (EHR)?
2. What type of information is considered protected health information (PHI)?
3. What are the recommended information privacy and security practices for the anesthesia provider using an EHR?
4. Describe some examples of passive and active clinical decision support (CDS) in health care. What are the potential benefits and hazards of CDS?
5. What factors promote success in the transition from paper records to an electronic anesthesia information management system (AIMS)?

## REFERENCES

1. Stol IS, Ehrenfeld JM, Epstein RH. Technology diffusion of anesthesia information management systems into academic anesthesia departments in the United States. *Anesth Analg.* 2014;118(3): 644–650.
2. Molnar C, Nemes C, Szabo S, Fulesdi B. Harvey Cushing, a pioneer of neuroanesthesia. *J Anesth.* 2008;22(4):483–486.
3. Shah NJ, Tremper KK, Kheterpal S. Anatomy of an anesthesia information management system. *Anesthesiol Clin.* 2011;29(3):355–365.
4. Stabile M, Cooper L. Review article: the evolving role of information technology in perioperative patient safety. *Can J Anaesth.* 2013;60(2):119–126.
5. Directors ABO. APSF endorses use of automated record keepers. *Anesth Pat Safety Found Newsletter.* 2001;16(4).
6. Galvez JA, Rothman BS, Doyle CA, et al. A narrative review of meaningful use and anesthesia information management systems. *Anesth Analg.* 2015;121(3):693–706.
7. Centers for Medicare and Medicaid Services. EHR Incentive Programs. https://www.cms.gov/Regulations-and-Guidance/Legislation/EHRIncentivePrograms/index.html; 2016 Accessed 5/1/2016.

8. Office of the National Coordinator for Health Information Technology. Health IT.gov. Office of the National Coordinator for Health Information Technology. http://www.healthit.gov/; 2015 Accessed 5/1/2016.
9. Kheterpal S. In the land of the blind, the one-eyed man is king. *Anesthesiology.* 2014;120(3):523–525.
10. Vetter TR, Redden DT. The power and perils of big data: it all depends on how you slice, dice, and digest it. *Anesth Analg.* 2015;121(3):582–585.
11. Centers for Medicare & Medicaid Services (CMS). PQRS Measures. https://www.cms.gov/medicare/quality-initiatives-patient-assessment-instruments/pqrs/measurescodes.html; 2016 Accessed 8/24/2016.
12. Dutton RP. Making a difference: the Anesthesia Quality Institute. *Anesth Analg.* 2015;120(3):507–509.
13. Centers for Medicare & Medicaid Services (CMS). HIPAA Basics for providers: privacy, security, and breach notification rules. http://www.hhs.gov/hipaa/for-professionals/index.html; 2016 Accessed 5/1/2016.
14. U.S. Department of Health & Human Services (HHS). Health Information Privacy. www.hhs.gov/hipaa/for-professionals/security/laws-regulations/; 2016 Accessed 5/1/2016.

15. ONC. *Guide to Privacy and Security of Electronic Health Information V2.0. Office of the National Coordinator for Health Information Technology*; 2015.
16. HIMSS. What Is Interoperability?. http://www.himss.org/library/interoperability-standards/what-is-interoperability; www.healthit.gov/isa/; 2016 Accessed 5/1/2016.
17. Sittig DF, Wright A. What makes an EHR "open" or interoperable? *J Am Med Inform Assoc.* 2015;22(5):1099–1101.
18. Office of the National Coordinator for Health Information Technology (ONC). *Connecting Health and Care for the Nation. A Shared Nationwide Interoperability Roadmap*; 2015. www.healthit.gov/sites/default/files/hie-interoperability/nationwide-interoperability-roadmap-final-version-1.0.pdf.
19. Schulz CM, Endsley MR, Kochs EF, et al. Situation awareness in anesthesia: concept and research. *Anesthesiology.* 2013;118(3):729–742.
20. Nolan T. System changes to improve patient safety. *BMJ.* 2000;320:771–773.
21. Braun BRA, Donofrio K, Hafiz H, Loeb J. *The Joint Commission—Improving Patient and Worker Safety: opportunities for Synergy, Collaboration and Innovation*; 11/19/2012. http://www.jointcommission.org/improving_patient_worker_safety/. Accessed 5/1/2016.

22. Karsh BT, Weinger MB, Abbott PA, Wears RL. Health information technology: fallacies and sober realities. *J Am Med Inform Assoc.* 2010;17(6):617–623.

23. Epstein RH, Dexter F, Patel N. Influencing anesthesia provider behavior using anesthesia information management system data for near real-time alerts and post hoc reports. *Anesth Analg.* 2015;12(3):678–692.

24. Nair BG, Horibe M, Newman SF, et al. Anesthesia information management system-based near real-time decision support to manage intraoperative hypotension and hypertension. *Anesth Analg.* 2014;118(1):206–214.

25. Vigoda MM, Rothman B, Green JA. Shortcomings and challenges of information system adoption. *Anesthesiol Clin.* 2011;29(3):397–412.

26. Kuhn T, Basch P, Barr M, Yackel T. Clinical documentation in the 21st century: executive summary of a policy position paper from the American College of Physicians. *Ann Intern Med.* 2015;162(4):301–303.

27. Vigoda MM, Rembold SD. Implications of electronic discovery. *ASA Monitor.* 2011;75:20-21.

28. Mangalmurti SS, Murtagh L, Mello MM. Medical malpractice liability in the age of electronic health records. *N Engl J Med.* 2010;363(21):2060–2067.

29. Vigoda MM, Lubarsky DA. Failure to recognize loss of incoming data in an anesthesia record-keeping system may have increased medical liability. *Anesth Analg.* 2006;102(6):1798–1802.

30. Furukawa MF, Eldridge N, Wang Y, et al. Electronic health record adoption and rates of in-hospital adverse events. *J Patient Saf. Epub.* 2016 Feb 6.

31. Xie J. Up to speed: a role for trainees in advancing health information technology. *Pediatrics.* 2015;136(3):412–414.

32. Ehrenfeld JM, McEvoy MD, Furman WR, et al. Automated near-real-time clinical performance feedback for anesthesiology residents: one piece of the milestones puzzle. *Anesthesiology.* 2014;120(1):172–184.

# PHARMACOLOGY AND PHYSIOLOGY

# 4

# BASIC PHARMACOLOGIC PRINCIPLES

## Tae Kyun Kim, Shinju Obara, and Ken B. Johnson

The basic principles of pharmacology are a fundamental element of an anesthesia provider's knowledge base. This chapter provides an overview of key principles in clinical pharmacology used to describe anesthetic drug behavior. Box 4.1 lists definitions of some basic pharmacologic terms. Pharmacokinetic concepts include volumes of distribution, drug clearance, transfer of drugs between plasma and tissues, and binding of drugs to circulating plasma proteins. The section on pharmacokinetics introduces both the physiologic processes that determine pharmacokinetics and the mathematical models used to relate dose to concentration. Anesthesia providers rarely administer just one drug. Most anesthetics are a combination of several drugs with specific goals in analgesia, sedation, and muscle relaxation. Thus, pharmacodynamic interactions can profoundly influence anesthetic effect. Formulating the *right dose* of an anesthetic requires consideration of many patient factors: age; body habitus; sex; chronic exposure to opioids, benzodiazepines, or alcohol; presence of heart, lung, kidney, or liver disease; and the extent of blood loss or dehydration, among others. Two of these factors, body habitus and age, will be discussed as examples of patient factors influencing anesthetic drug pharmacology.

## PHARMACOKINETIC PRINCIPLES

Pharmacokinetics describes the relationship between drug dose and drug concentration in plasma or at the site of drug effect over time. The processes of absorption, distribution, and elimination (metabolism and excretion) govern this relationship. Absorption is not relevant to intravenously administered drugs but is relevant to all other routes of drug delivery. The time course of

The editors and publisher would like to thank Dr. Steven L. Shafer for contributing to this chapter in the previous edition of this work. It has served as the foundation for the current chapter.

**Box 4.1** Definitions of Basic Pharmacologic Terms

**Pharmacokinetics:** the relationship between drug dose and drug concentration at the site of drug action

 **Biophase:** the time delay between changes in plasma concentration and drug effect

 **Effect-site concentration:** a mathematically derived virtual location where an anesthetic drug exerts its effect

 **Front-end kinetics:** a description of intravenous drug behavior immediately following administration

 **Back-end kinetics:** a description of intravenous drug behavior when administered as continuous infusion, including the time period after termination of infusion

 **Context-sensitive half-time:** a description of the time required for drug concentration to decrease by 50% after termination of drug infusion, based on duration of infusion (context)

**Pharmacodynamics:** a description of what the drug does to the body including the relationship between drug concentration and pharmacologic effect

 **Dynamic range:** the drug concentration range in which changes in drug effect occur. Drug levels below the dynamic range are ineffective; levels above the dynamic range do not provide additional effect.

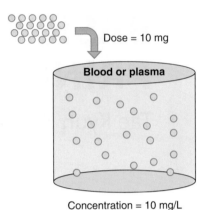

Concentration = 10 mg/L

Volume of distribution = 10 mg/(10 mg/L) = 1 L

**Fig. 4.1** Schematic of a single-tank model of distribution volume. The group of red dots at the top left represent a bolus dose that, when administered to the tank of water, evenly distribute within the tank. (Modified from Miller RD, Cohen NH, Eriksson LI, et al, eds. *Miller's Anesthesia.* 8th ed. Philadelphia: Saunders Elsevier; 2014:Fig. 24.1.)

intravenously administered drugs is a function of distribution volume and clearance. Estimates of distribution volumes and clearances are described by pharmacokinetic parameters. Pharmacokinetic parameters are derived from mathematical formulas fit to measured blood or plasma concentrations over time following a known drug dose.

## Fundamental Pharmacokinetic Concepts

### Volume of Distribution

An oversimplified model of drug distribution throughout plasma and tissues is the dilution of a drug dose into a tank of water. The volume of distribution (Vd) is the apparent size of the tank required to explain a measured drug concentration from the tank water once the drug has had enough time to thoroughly mix within the tank (Fig. 4.1). The distribution volume is estimated using the simple relationship between dose (e.g., mg) and measured concentration (e.g., mg/L) as presented in Eq. 1.

Eq. 1

$$\text{Volume of distribution} = \frac{\text{Amount of dose (mg)}}{\text{Concentration (mg/L)}}$$

With an estimate of tank volume, drug concentration after any bolus dose can be calculated. Just as the tank has a volume regardless of whether there is drug in it, distribution volumes in people are an intrinsic property regardless of whether any drug has been given.

Human bodies are not water tanks. As soon as a drug is injected, it begins to be cleared from the body. To account

for this in the schematic presented in Fig. 4.1, a faucet is added to the tank to mimic drug elimination from the body (Fig. 4.2). Using Eq. 1, estimating the volume of distribution without accounting for elimination leads to volume of distribution estimates that become larger than initial volume. To refine the definition of distribution volume, the amount of drug that is present at a given time $t$ is divided by the concentrations at the same time.

Eq. 2

$$Vd = \frac{\text{Amount } (t)}{\text{Concentration } (t)}$$

If elimination occurs as a first-order process (i.e., elimination is proportional to the concentration at that time), the volume of distribution calculated by Eq. 2 will be constant (Figs. 4.2 and 4.3).

When a drug is administered intravenously, some drug stays in the vascular volume, but most of the drug distributes to peripheral tissues. This distribution is often represented as additional volumes of distribution (tanks) connected to a central tank (blood or plasma volume). Peripheral distribution volumes increase the total volume of distribution (Fig. 4.4).

The schematic in Fig. 4.4 presents a plasma volume and tissue volume. The peripheral tank represents distribution of drug in peripheral tissues. There may be more than one peripheral tank (volume) to best describe the entire drug disposition in the body. The size of the peripheral volumes represents a drug's solubility in tissue relative to blood or plasma. The more soluble a drug is in peripheral tissue relative to blood or plasma, the larger the peripheral volumes of distribution.

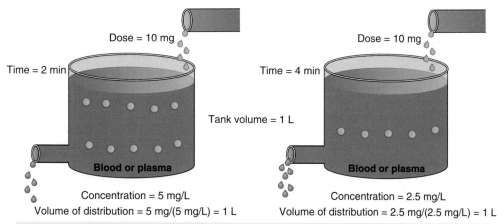

**Fig. 4.2** Schematic of a single-tank model of elimination as a first-order process. At 2 minutes *(left panel)* and 4 minutes *(right panel)* following a 10-mg drug bolus, tank concentrations are decreasing from 5 to 2.5 mg/mL. Accounting for elimination, estimates of the distribution volume at each time point are both 1 L. (From Miller RD, Cohen NH, Eriksson LI, et al, eds. *Miller's Anesthesia*. 8th ed. Philadelphia: Saunders Elsevier; 2014:Fig. 24.2.)

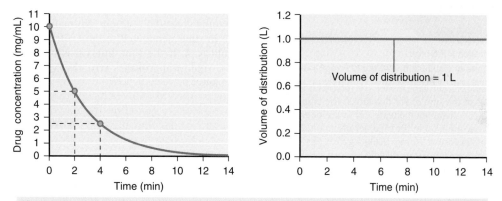

**Fig. 4.3** Simulation of concentration *(left)* and distribution volume *(right)* changes over time following a bolus dose for a single-tank (one-compartment) model. The distribution volume remains constant throughout. (From Miller RD, Cohen NH, Eriksson LI, et al, eds. *Miller's Anesthesia*. 8th ed. Philadelphia: Saunders Elsevier; 2014:Fig. 24.3.)

An important point illustrated in Fig. 4.4 is that drug not only distributes to the peripheral tank and thus increases the volume of distribution, but it also binds to tissue in that tank. This process further lowers the measurable concentration in the central tank. Thus, the total volume of distribution may even be larger than the two tanks added together. In fact, some anesthetics have huge distribution volumes (e.g., fentanyl has an apparent distribution volume of 4 L/kg) that are substantially larger than an individual's vascular volume (0.07 L/kg) or extracellular volume (0.2 L/kg).

With an additional tank, the volume of distribution no longer remains constant over time. As illustrated in Fig. 4.5, at time = 0, the volume of distribution is estimated as 4.3 L, the same as that of the model presented in Fig. 4.3, which has only one tank. The volume of distribution then increases to 48 L over the next 10 minutes. The

increase is due to the distribution of drug to the peripheral volume and elimination once drug is in the body. The amount of drug that moves to the peripheral tissue commonly surpasses the amount that is eliminated during the first few minutes after drug administration. As an example, consider a simulation of a propofol bolus that plots the accumulation of propofol in peripheral tissues and the amount eliminated over time (Fig. 4.6). During the first 4 minutes, the amount distributed to the peripheral tissue is larger than the amount eliminated from the body. Following 4 minutes, the amounts reverse.

### Clearance

Clearance describes the rate of drug removal from the plasma/blood. Two processes contribute to drug clearance: systemic (out of the tank) and intercompartmental (between the tanks) clearance (Fig. 4.7). Systemic clearance permanently removes drug from the body, either by eliminating the parent molecule or by transforming it into metabolites. Intercompartmental clearance moves drug between plasma and peripheral tissue tanks. By way of clarification, in this chapter the words *compartment* and *tank* are used interchangeably.

Clearance is defined in units of flow, that is, the volume completely cleared of drug per unit of time (e.g., L/min). Clearance is not to be confused with elimination rate (e.g., mg/min). To explain why elimination rates do

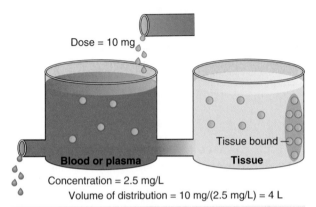

Dose = 10 mg

**Blood or plasma**

Tissue bound

**Tissue**

Concentration = 2.5 mg/L

Volume of distribution = 10 mg/(2.5 mg/L) = 4 L

**Fig. 4.4** Schematic of a two-tank model. The total volume of distribution consists of the sum of the two tanks. The blue dots in the ellipse in the peripheral volume represent tissue-bound drug. The measured concentration in the blood or plasma is 2.5 mg/mL just after a bolus dose of 10 mg. Using Fig. 4.1, this leads to a distribution volume of 4 L. (From Miller RD, Cohen NH, Eriksson LI, et al, eds. *Miller's Anesthesia*. 8th ed. Philadelphia: Saunders Elsevier; 2015:Fig. 24.4.)

not accurately characterize clearance, consider the simulation presented in Fig. 4.8. Using the volume of distribution, the total amount of drug can be calculated at every measured drug concentration. The concentration change in time window *A* is larger than that in time window *B* even though they are both 1 minute in duration. The elimination rates are 27 and 12 mg/min for time windows *A* and *B*, respectively. They are different and neither can be used as a parameter to predict drug concentrations when another dose of drug is administered. Because of this limitation with elimination rate, clearance was developed to provide a single number to describe the decay in drug concentration presented in Fig. 4.8.

For discussion purposes, assume that concentration is the power necessary to push drug out of the water tank. The higher the concentration, the larger the amount of drug eliminated. To standardize the elimination rate, the eliminated amount of drug is scaled to concentration. For example, the elimination rate in time window *A* (27 mg/min) scaled to the mean concentration during that time window (15 μg/mL) is 0.001807 mg/min/mg/L. Reducing the units gives 0.002 L/min. Normalizing the elimination rate in time window *B* to concentration gives the same result as *A*. If the time interval is narrowed so that the time window approaches zero, the definition of clearance becomes:

Eq. 3

$$\text{Clearance} = \frac{dA/dt}{C(t)}$$

where $dA/dt$ is the rate of drug elimination at given time $t$, and $C(t)$ is the corresponding concentration at

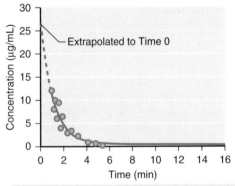

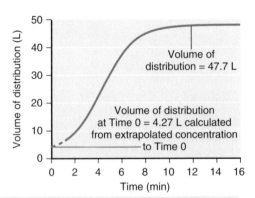

**Fig. 4.5** Simulation of concentration and apparent distribution volume changes over time following a bolus dose for a two-tank (two-compartment) model. On the left, the dots represent measured drug concentrations. The solid line represents a mathematical equation fit to the measured concentrations. The dotted line represents an extrapolation of the mathematical equation (i.e., pharmacokinetic model) to time 0. On the right, the apparent distribution volume is time dependent with the initial volume of distribution much smaller than the distribution volume at near steady state. The apparent distribution volume of time 0 is not a true reflection of the actual volume of distribution. (From Miller RD, Cohen NH, Eriksson LI, et al, eds. *Miller's Anesthesia*. 8th ed. Philadelphia: Saunders Elsevier; 2015:Fig. 24.5.)

time $t$. Rearranging Eq. 3, clearance can be expressed as follows:

$$\text{Eq. 4}$$

$$\text{Clearance} = \frac{Q\,(C_{\text{in}} - C_{\text{out}})}{C_{\text{in}}}$$

where $Q$ is the blood flow to metabolic organs, $C_{\text{in}}$ is the concentration of drug delivered to metabolic organs, and $C_{\text{out}}$ is the concentration of drug leaving metabolic organs. The fraction of inflowing drug extracted by the organ

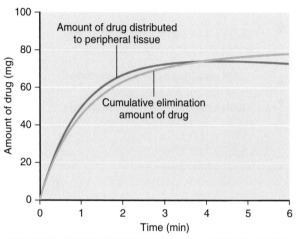

**Fig. 4.6** Simulation of propofol accumulation in the peripheral tissues *(blue line)* and the cumulative amount of propofol eliminated *(yellow line)* following a 2-mg/kg propofol bolus to a 77-kg (170-lb), 177-cm (5 ft 10 in) tall, 53-year-old man, using published pharmacokinetic model parameters.[1] Drug indicates propofol. (From Miller RD, Cohen NH, Eriksson LI, et al, eds. *Miller's Anesthesia*. 8th ed. Philadelphia: Saunders Elsevier; 2015:Fig. 24.6.)

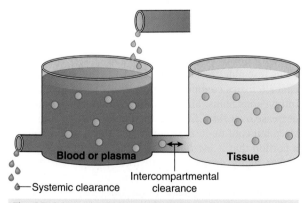

**Fig. 4.7** Schematic of a two-tank model illustrating two sources of drug removal from the central tank (blood or plasma): systemic and intercompartmental clearance. (From Miller RD, Cohen NH, Eriksson LI, et al, eds. *Miller's Anesthesia*. 8th ed. Philadelphia: Saunders Elsevier; 2015:Fig. 24.8.)

is $(C_{\text{in}} - C_{\text{out}})/C_{\text{in}}$ and is called the *extraction ratio* (ER). Clearance can be estimated as organ blood flow multiplied by the ER. Eq. 4 can be simplified as shown here:

$$\text{Eq. 5}$$

$$\text{Clearance} = Q \times \text{ER}$$

The total clearance is the sum of each clearance by metabolic organs such as the liver, kidney, and other tissues (Fig. 4.9).

Hepatic clearance has been well characterized. For example, the relationship between clearance, liver blood flow, and the extraction ratio is presented in Fig. 4.10.[2] For drugs with an extraction ratio of nearly 1 (e.g., propofol), a change in liver blood flow produces a nearly proportional change in clearance. For drugs with a low extraction ratio (e.g., alfentanil), clearance is nearly independent of the rate of liver blood flow. If nearly 100% of the drug is extracted by the liver, this implies that the liver has tremendous metabolic capacity for the drug. In this case, the rate-limiting step in metabolism is flow of drug to the liver, and such drugs are said to be "flow limited." Any reduction in liver blood flow, such as usually accompanies anesthesia, can be expected to reduce clearance. However, moderate changes in hepatic metabolic function per se will have little impact on clearance because hepatic metabolic capacity is overwhelmingly in excess of demand.

For many drugs (e.g., alfentanil), the extraction ratio is considerably less than 1. For these drugs, clearance is limited by the capacity of the liver to take up and metabolize drug. These drugs are said to be "capacity limited." Clearance will change in response to any change in the capacity of the liver to metabolize such drugs, as might be caused by liver disease or enzymatic induction. However, changes in liver blood flow, as might be caused by the anesthetic state itself, usually have little influence on clearance because the liver handles only a fraction of the drug that it sees anyway.

### Front-End Kinetics

Front-end kinetics refers to the description of intravenous drug behavior immediately following administration. How rapidly a drug moves from the blood into peripheral tissues directly influences the peak plasma drug concentration. With compartmental models, an important assumption is that an intravenous bolus instantly mixes in the central volume, with the peak concentration occurring at the moment of injection without elimination or distribution to peripheral tissues. For simulation purposes, the initial concentration and volume of distribution at time = 0 are extrapolated as if the circulation had been infinitely fast. This, of course, is not real. If drug is injected into an arm vein and that initial concentration is measured in a radial artery, drug appears in the arterial circulation 30 to 40 seconds after injection. The delay likely represents the time required for drug to pass through the venous volume of the upper part of the arm,

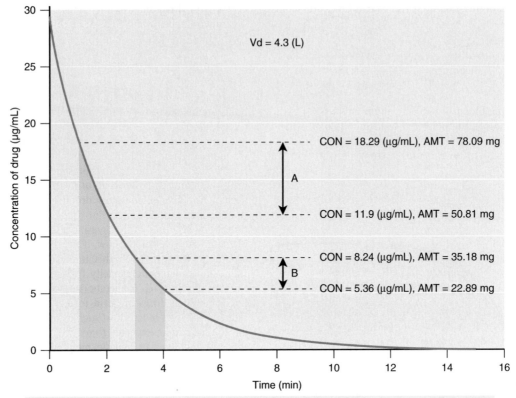

**Fig. 4.8** Simulation of drug concentration changes when a drug is administered to a single-tank model with linear elimination (see Fig. 4.2). The concentration changes for two time windows are labeled with diagonal lines from 1 to 2 minutes (time window *A*) and from 3 to 4 minutes (time window *B*), respectively. The concentrations *(CON)* at the beginning and end of each time window are used to calculate the amount *(AMT)* of drug that is eliminated (see text). *Vd*, Volume of distribution. (Modified from Miller RD, Cohen NH, Eriksson LI, et al, eds. *Miller's Anesthesia*. 8th ed. Philadelphia: Saunders Elsevier; 2015:Fig. 24.9.)

heart, great vessels, and peripheral arterial circulation. More sophisticated models (e.g., a recirculatory model)[3] account for this delay and are useful when characterizing the behavior of a drug immediately following bolus administration, such as with induction agents, when the speed of onset and duration of action are of interest.

### Compartmental Pharmacokinetic Models

Compartmental models have no physiologic correlate. They are built by using mathematical expressions fit to concentration over time data and then reparameterized in terms of *volumes and clearances*. The *one-compartment model* presented in Fig. 4.11 contains a single volume and a single clearance. Although used for several drugs, this model is perhaps oversimplified for anesthetic drugs. To better model anesthetic drugs, clinical pharmacologists have developed two or three compartment models that contain several tanks connected by pipes. As illustrated in Fig. 4.11, the volume to the right in the two-compartment model—and in the center of the three-compartment model—is the central volume. The other volumes are peripheral volumes. The sum of the all volumes is the

volume of distribution at steady state, Vdss. Clearance in which the central compartment is left for the outside is the *central* or *metabolic* clearance. Clearances between the central compartment and the peripheral compartments are the intercompartmental clearances.

### Multicompartment Models

Plasma concentrations over time after an intravenous bolus resemble the curve in Fig. 4.12. This curve has the characteristics common to most drugs when given as an intravenous bolus. First, the concentrations continuously decrease over time. Second, the rate of decline is initially steep but continuously becomes less steep, until we get to a portion that is *log-linear*.

For many drugs, three distinct phases can be distinguished, as illustrated for fentanyl in Fig. 4.12. A *rapid-distribution* phase (blue line) begins immediately after injection of the bolus. Very rapid movement of the drug from plasma to the rapidly equilibrating tissues characterizes this phase. Next, a second *slow-distribution* phase (red line) is characterized by movement of drug into more slowly equilibrating tissues

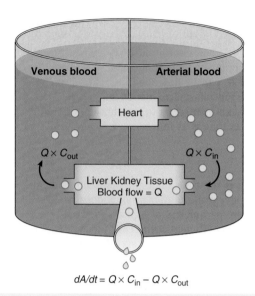

$$dA/dt = Q \times C_{in} - Q \times C_{out}$$

**Fig. 4.9** Schematic of drug extraction. $A$, Amount of drug; $C_{in}$ and $C_{out}$, drug concentrations presented to and leaving metabolic organs; $dA/dt$, drug elimination rate; $Q$, blood flow. (From Miller RD, Cohen NH, Eriksson LI, et al, eds. *Miller's Anesthesia*. 8th ed. Philadelphia: Saunders Elsevier; 2015:Fig. 24.10.)

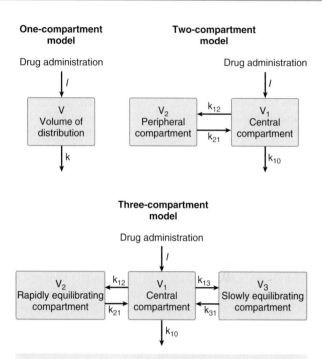

**Fig. 4.11** One-, two-, and three-compartment mammillary models. (From Miller RD, Cohen NH, Eriksson LI, et al, eds. *Miller's Anesthesia*. 8th ed. Philadelphia: Saunders Elsevier; 2015:Fig. 24.12.)

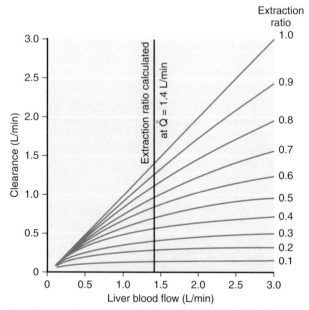

**Fig. 4.10** Relationship among liver blood flow ($Q$), clearance, and extraction ratio. For drugs with a high extraction ratio, clearance is nearly identical to liver blood flow. For drugs with a low extraction ratio, changes in liver blood flow have almost no effect on clearance.[2] (From Miller RD, Cohen NH, Eriksson LI, et al, eds. *Miller's Anesthesia*. 8th ed. Philadelphia: Saunders Elsevier; 2015:Fig. 24.11.)

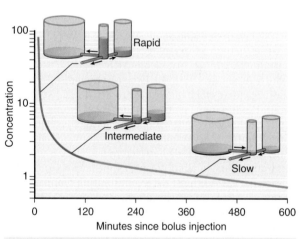

**Fig. 4.12** Hydraulic model of fentanyl pharmacokinetics. Drug is administered into the central tank, from which it can distribute into two peripheral tanks, or it may be eliminated. The volume of the tanks is proportional to the volumes of distribution. The cross-sectional area of the pipes is proportional to clearance.[4] (From Miller RD, Cohen NH, Eriksson LI, et al, eds. *Miller's Anesthesia*. 8th ed. Philadelphia: Saunders Elsevier; 2015:Fig. 24.13.)

and return of drug to plasma from the most rapidly equilibrating tissues. Third, the terminal phase (green line) is nearly a straight line when plotted on a semi-logarithmic graph. The terminal phase is often called the "elimination phase" because the primary mechanism for decreasing drug concentration during the terminal phase is elimination of drug from the body. The distinguishing characteristic of the terminal elimination phase is that the plasma concentration is lower than tissue concentrations and the relative proportion of drug in plasma and peripheral volumes of distribution remains constant. During this terminal phase, drug returns from the rapid- and slow-distribution volumes to plasma and is permanently removed from plasma by metabolism or excretion.

The presence of three distinct phases after bolus injection is a defining characteristic of a mammillary model with three compartments.[4] In this model, shown in Fig. 4.12, there are three tanks corresponding (from left to right) to the slowly equilibrating peripheral compartment, the central compartment (the plasma, into which drug is injected), and the rapidly equilibrating peripheral compartment. The horizontal pipes represent intercompartmental clearance or (for the pipe draining onto the page) metabolic clearance. The volumes of each tank correspond to the volumes of the compartments for fentanyl. The cross-sectional areas of the pipes correlate with fentanyl systemic and intercompartmental clearance. The height of water in each tank corresponds to drug concentration. By using this hydraulic model we can follow the processes that decrease drug concentration over time after bolus injection. Initially, drug flows from the central compartment to both peripheral compartments via intercompartmental clearance and completely out of the model via metabolic clearance. Because there are three places for drug to go, the concentration in the central compartment decreases very rapidly. At the transition between the blue line and the red line, there is a change in the role of the most rapidly equilibrating compartment. At this transition, the concentration in the central compartment falls below the concentration in the rapidly equilibrating compartment, and the direction of flow between them is reversed. After this transition (red line), drug in plasma has only two places to go: into the slowly equilibrating compartment or out the drain pipe. These processes are partly offset by the return of drug to plasma from the rapidly equilibrating compartment. The net effect is that once the rapidly equilibrating compartment has come to equilibration, the concentration in the central compartment falls far more slowly than before.

Once the concentration in the central compartment decreases below both the rapidly and slowly equilibrating compartments (green line), the only method of decreasing the plasma concentration is metabolic clearance, the drain pipe. Return of drug from both peripheral compartments to the central compartment greatly slows the rate of decrease in plasma drug concentration.

Curves that continuously decrease over time, with a continuously increasing slope (i.e., like the curve in Fig. 4.12), can be described by a sum of negative exponentials. In pharmacokinetics, one way of denoting this sum of exponentials is to say that the plasma concentration over time is as follows:

$$\text{Eq. 6}$$
$$C\,(t) = Ae^{-\alpha t} + Be^{-\beta t} + Ce^{-\gamma t}$$

where $t$ is the time since the bolus injection, $C\,(t)$ is the drug concentration after a bolus dose, and A, $\alpha$, B, $\beta$, C, and $\gamma$ are parameters of a pharmacokinetic model. A, B, and C are coefficients, whereas $\alpha$, $\beta$, and $\gamma$ are exponents. After a bolus injection, all six of the parameters in Eq. 6 will be greater than 0. Polyexponential equations are used mainly because they describe the plasma concentrations observed after bolus injection, except for the misspecification in the first few minutes, mentioned previously. Compartmental pharmacokinetic models are strictly empiric. These models have no anatomic correlate. They are based solely on fitting equations to measured plasma concentrations following a known dose. Kinetic models are transformed into models that characterize concentration changes over time in terms of volumes and clearances. Although more intuitive, they have no physiologic correlate.

Special significance is often ascribed to the smallest exponent. This exponent determines the slope of the final log-linear portion of the curve. When the medical literature refers to the half-life of a drug, unless otherwise stated, the half-life will be the terminal half-life. However, the terminal half-life for drugs with more than one exponential term is nearly uninterpretable. The terminal half-life sets an upper limit on the time required for the concentrations to decrease by 50% after drug administration. Usually, the time needed for a 50% decrease will be much faster than that upper limit.

Part of the continuing popularity of pharmacokinetic compartmental models is that they can be transformed from an unintuitive exponential form to a more intuitive compartmental form, as shown in Fig. 4.11. Microrate constants, expressed as $k_{ij}$, define the rate of drug transfer from compartment $i$ to compartment $j$. Compartment 0 is the compartment outside the model, so $k_{10}$ is the microrate constant for processes acting through metabolism or elimination that irreversibly remove drug from the central compartment (analogous to $k$ for a one-compartment model). The intercompartmental microrate constants ($k_{12}$, $k_{21}$, etc.) describe movement of drug between the central and peripheral compartments. Each peripheral compartment has at least two microrate constants, one for drug entry and one for drug exit. The microrate constants for the two- and three-compartment models can be seen in Fig. 4.11.

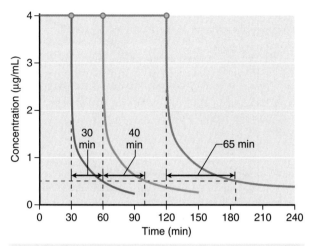

**Fig. 4.13** Simulation of decrement times for a target-controlled infusion set to maintain a target propofol concentration of 4 µg/mL for 30, 60, and 120 minutes. Once terminated, the time required to reach 0.5 µg/mL was 30, 40, and 65 minutes for each infusion, respectively. Simulations of the decrement times used a published pharmacokinetic model.[1] (From Miller RD, Cohen NH, Eriksson LI, et al, eds. *Miller's Anesthesia*. 8th ed. Philadelphia: Saunders Elsevier; 2015:Fig. 24.14.)

## Back-End Kinetics

Using estimates of distribution volume and clearance, back-end kinetics is a useful tool that describes the behavior of intravenous drugs when administered as continuous infusions. Back-end kinetics provides descriptors of how plasma drug concentrations decrease once a continuous infusion is terminated. An example is decrement time. It predicts the time required to reach a certain plasma concentration once an infusion is terminated. Decrement times are a function of infusion duration. Consider the example of decrement times for a set of continuous target-controlled infusions (Fig. 4.13). In this simulation, target-controlled infusion (TCI) of propofol is set to maintain a concentration of 4 µg/mL for 30, 60, and 120 minutes. Once the infusion is stopped, the time to reach 0.5 µg/mL is estimated. As illustrated, the longer the infusion, the longer the time required to reach 0.5 µg/mL. This example demonstrates how drugs accumulate in peripheral tissues with prolonged infusions. This accumulation prolongs the decrement time.

Another use of decrement times is as a tool to compare drugs within a drug class (e.g., opioids). As a comparator, plots of decrement times are presented as a function of infusion duration. When used this way, decrement times are determined as the time required to reach a target percentage of the concentration immediately after termination of a continuous infusion. Examples of 50% and 80% decrement times for selected opioids and sedatives are presented in Fig. 4.14. Of note, for shorter infusions, the decrement times are similar for both classes of anesthetic drugs. Once infusion duration exceeds 2 hours, the decrement times

vary substantially. A popular decrement time is the 50% decrement time, also known as the context-sensitive half-time.[5] The term *context-sensitive* refers to infusion duration. The term *half-time* refers to the 50% decrement time.

### Biophase

Biophase refers to the time delay between changes in plasma concentration and drug effect. Biophase accounts for the time required for drug to diffuse from the plasma to the site of action plus the time required, once drug is at the site of action, to elicit a drug effect. A simulation of various propofol bolus doses and their predicted effect on the electroencephalogram (EEG) bispectral index scale (BIS) is presented in Fig. 4.15. The time to peak effect for each dose is identical (approximately 1.5 minutes following the peak plasma concentration). The difference between each dose is the magnitude and duration of effect. A key principle is that when drug concentrations are in flux (i.e., during induction of anesthesia and emergence from anesthesia), changes in drug effect will lag behind changes in drug concentration. This lag between the plasma concentration and effect usually results in the phenomenon called *hysteresis*, in which two different plasma concentrations correspond to one drug effect or one plasma concentration corresponds to two drug effects. For example, Fig. 4.15 shows that the different concentrations at C and c correspond to the same BIS score.

To collapse the hysteresis between plasma concentration and effect and to match one plasma concentration to one drug effect, this lag is often modeled with an "effect site" compartment added to the central compartment. Kinetic microrate constants used to describe biophase include $k_{1e}$ and $k_{e0}$. The $k_{1e}$ describes drug movement from the central compartment to the effect site and $k_{e0}$ describes the elimination of drug from the effect site compartment. There are two important assumptions with the effect-site compartment: (1) The amount of drug that moves from the central compartment to the effect-site compartment is negligible and vice versa, and (2) there is no *volume* estimate to the effect-site compartment.

Typically, the relationship between plasma and the site of drug effect is modeled with an *effect-site* model, as shown in Fig. 4.16. The site of drug effect is connected to plasma by a first-order process. Eq. 7 relates effect-site concentration to plasma concentration:

Eq. 7

$$dCe = \frac{k_{e0} \times (Cp - Ce)}{dt}$$

where $Ce$ is the effect-site concentration, $Cp$ is the plasma drug concentration, and $k_{e0}$ is the rate constant for elimination of drug. The constant $k_{e0}$ describes the rate of rise and offset of drug effect (Fig. 4.17).

In summary, the conventional pharmacokinetic term *half-life* has little meaning to anesthesia providers, who

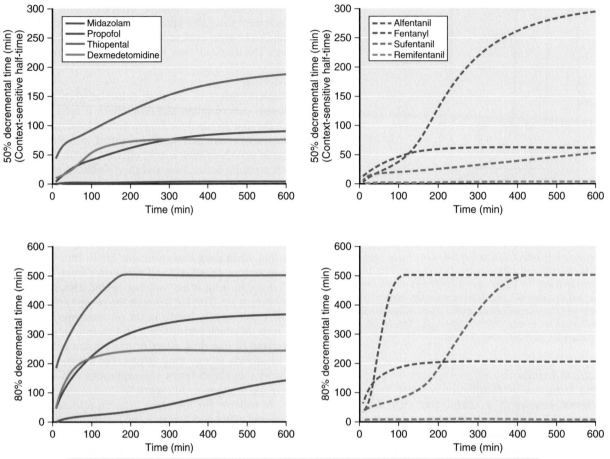

**Fig. 4.14** These graphs show 50% and 80% decrement times for selected sedatives *(left side)* and opioids *(right side)*. The vertical axis refers to the time required to reach the desired decrement time. The horizontal axis refers to infusion duration. Simulations of the decrement times used published pharmacokinetic models for each sedative and analgesic.[5-10] (From Miller RD, Cohen NH, Eriksson LI, et al, eds. *Miller's Anesthesia.* 8th ed. Philadelphia: Saunders Elsevier; 2015:Fig. 24.15.)

work with drugs whose clinical behavior is not well described by half-life. The pharmacokinetic principles discussed in this section (such as volume of distribution, clearance, elimination, front-end kinetics, back-end kinetics, context-sensitive half-time, and biophase) better illustrate how an anesthetic will behave.

## PHARMACODYNAMIC PRINCIPLES

Simply stated, pharmacokinetics describes what the body does to the drug, whereas pharmacodynamics describes what the drug does to the body. In particular, pharmacodynamics describes the relationship between drug concentration and pharmacologic effect.

Models used to describe the concentration-effect relationships are created in much the same way as pharmacokinetic models; they are based on observations and used to create a mathematical model. To create a

pharmacodynamic model, plasma drug levels and a selected drug effect are measured simultaneously. For example, consider the measured plasma concentrations of an intravenous anesthetic drug following a bolus dose and the associated changes on the EEG spectral edge frequency (a measure of anesthetic depth) from one individual, presented in Fig. 4.18. Shortly after the plasma concentration peaks, the spectral edge starts to decrease, reaches a nadir, and then returns back to baseline as the plasma concentrations drop to near 0.

Combining data from several individuals and plotting the measured concentrations versus the observed effect (modified to be a percentage of the maximal effect across all individuals) creates a hysteresis loop (Fig. 4.19). The ascending portion of the loop represents rising drug concentrations (see arrow). While rising, the increase in drug effect lags behind the increase in drug concentration. For the descending loop, the decrease drug effect lags behind the decrease in drug concentration.

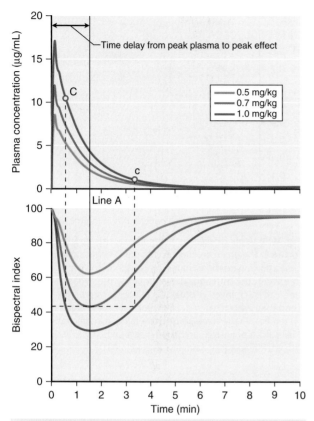

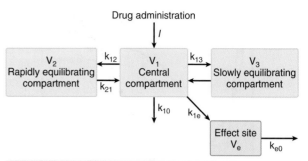

**Fig. 4.16** A three-compartment model with an added effect site to account for the delay in equilibration between the rise and fall in arterial drug concentrations and the onset and offset of drug effect. The effect site is assumed to have a negligible volume. (From Miller RD, Cohen NH, Eriksson LI, et al, eds. *Miller's Anesthesia*. 8th ed. Philadelphia: Saunders Elsevier; 2015:Fig. 24.17.)

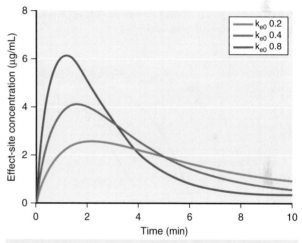

**Fig. 4.17** Effect of the $k_{e0}$ changes. As the $k_{e0}$ decreases, the time to peak effect is prolonged.[1,7,11] (From Miller RD, Cohen NH, Eriksson LI, et al, eds. *Miller's Anesthesia*. 8th ed. Philadelphia: Saunders Elsevier; 2015:Fig. 24.18.)

**Fig. 4.15** Demonstration of biophase. The top plot presents a simulation of three propofol doses and the resultant plasma concentrations. The bottom plot presents a simulation of the predicted effect on the bispectral index scale (BIS). These simulations assume linear kinetics: regardless of the dose, effects peak at the same time *(Line A)*, as do the plasma concentration. The time to peak effect is 1.5 minutes. Even the plasma concentrations of points *C* and *c* are different; however, the BIS scores of those two points are the same. This finding demonstrates the hysteresis between plasma concentration and BIS score. Simulations used published pharmacokinetic and pharmacodynamic models.[1,7] (From Miller RD, Cohen NH, Eriksson LI, et al, eds. *Miller's Anesthesia*. 8th ed. Philadelphia: Saunders Elsevier; 2015:Fig. 24.16.)

To create a pharmacodynamic model, the hysteresis loop is collapsed using modeling techniques that account for the lag time between plasma concentrations and the observed effect. These modeling techniques provide an estimate of the lag time, known as the $t_{1/2}k_{e0}$, and an estimate of the effect-site concentration (*Ce*) associated with a 50% probability of drug effect (*$C_{50}$*). Most concentration-effect relationships in anesthesia are described with a sigmoid curve. The standard equation for this relationship is the Hill equation, also known as the sigmoid $E_{max}$ relationship (Eq. 8):

Eq. 8

$$\text{Effect} = E_0 + (E_{max} - E_0)\ (C^{\gamma}/(C_{50}^{\gamma} + C^{\gamma}))$$

where $E_0$ is the baseline effect, $E_{max}$ is the maximal effect, $C$ is the drug concentration, and $\gamma$ represents the slope of the concentration-effect relationship; $\gamma$ is also known as the Hill coefficient. For values of $\gamma$ less than 1, the curve is hyperbolic, and for values greater than 1, the curve is sigmoid. Fig. 4.20 presents an example of this relationship: a fentanyl effect-site concentration-effect curve for analgesia. This example illustrates how $C_{50}$ and $\gamma$ characterize the concentration-effect relationship.

## Potency and Efficacy

Two important concepts are relevant to this relationship: potency and efficacy. Potency describes the amount of drug required to elicit an effect. The $C_{50}$ is a common parameter used to describe potency. For

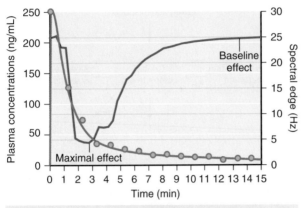

**Fig. 4.18** Schematic representation of drug plasma concentrations *(blue circles)* following a bolus and the associated changes in the electroencephalogram's spectral edge *(red line)* measured in one individual. Note that changes in spectral edge lag behind changes in plasma concentrations. (From Miller RD, Cohen NH, Eriksson LI, et al, eds. *Miller's Anesthesia.* 8th ed. Philadelphia: Saunders Elsevier; 2015:Fig. 24.19.)

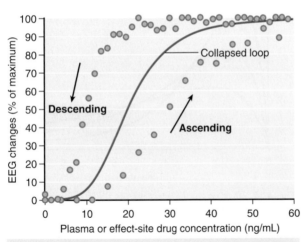

**Fig. 4.19** Schematic representation of plasma concentrations versus normalized spectral edge measurements (presented as a percentage of maximal effect) from several individuals *(blue circles)*. The black arrows indicate the ascending and descending arms of a hysteresis loop that coincide with increasing and decreasing drug concentrations. The red line represents the pharmacodynamic model developed from collapsing the hysteresis loop. EEG, electroencephalogram. (From Miller RD, Cohen NH, Eriksson LI, et al, eds. *Miller's Anesthesia.* 8th ed. Philadelphia: Saunders Elsevier; 2015:Fig. 24.20.)

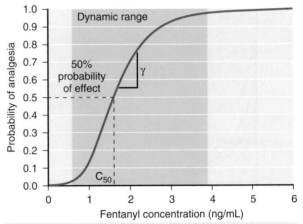

**Fig. 4.20** A pharmacodynamic model for the analgesic effect of fentanyl. The green area represents the dynamic range, the concentration range where changes in concentration lead to a change in effect. Concentrations above or below the dynamic range do not lead to changes in drug effect. The $C_{50}$ represents the concentration associated with 50% probability of analgesia. Gamma ($\gamma$) represents the slope of the curve in the dynamic range. (From Miller RD, Cohen NH, Eriksson LI, et al, eds. *Miller's Anesthesia.* 8th ed. Philadelphia: Saunders Elsevier; 2015:Fig. 24.21.)

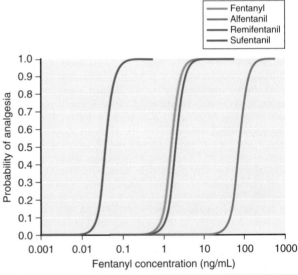

**Fig. 4.21** Pharmacodynamic models for fentanyl congeners. The $C_{50}$ for each drug is different, but the slope and maximal effect are similar.[12] (From Miller RD, Cohen NH, Eriksson LI, et al, eds. *Miller's Anesthesia.* 8th ed. Philadelphia: Saunders Elsevier; 2015:Fig. 24.22.)

drugs that have a concentration-versus-effect relationship that is shifted to the left (small $C_{50}$), the drug is considered to be more potent, and the reverse is true for drugs that have a concentration-versus-effect relationship shifted to the right. For example, as illustrated in Fig. 4.21, the analgesia $C_{50}$ for some of the fentanyl congeners ranges from small for sufentanil (0.04 ng/mL)

to large for alfentanil (75 ng/mL). Thus, sufentanil is more potent than alfentanil.

Efficacy is a measure of drug effectiveness once it occupies a receptor. Similar drugs that work through the same receptor may have varying degrees of effectiveness despite having the same receptor occupancy. For

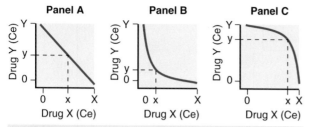

**Fig. 4.22** Drug interactions. For two drugs, *X* and *Y*, Panel A represents additive, Panel B represents synergistic, and Panel C represents antagonistic interactions. *Ce*, Effect-site concentration. (From Miller RD, Cohen NH, Eriksson LI, et al, eds. *Miller's Anesthesia*. 8th ed. Philadelphia: Saunders Elsevier; 2015:Fig. 24.26.)

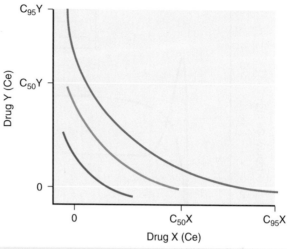

**Fig. 4.23** Schematic illustration of isoeffect (isobole) lines. The red, green, and blue lines represent the 50% and 95% isoboles for a synergistic interaction between drugs *X* and *Y*. Isoboles represent concentration pairs with an equivalent effect. A set of 5%, 50%, and 95% isoboles can be used to describe the dynamic range of the concentrations for drugs *X* and *Y* for a given effect. As with single concentration effect curves, the ideal dosing leads to concentration pairs that are near the 95% isobole. *Ce*, Effect-site concentration. (From Miller RD, Cohen NH, Eriksson LI, et al, eds. *Miller's Anesthesia*. 8th ed. Philadelphia: Saunders Elsevier; 2015:Fig. 24.27.)

example, with G protein–coupled receptors, some drugs may bind the receptor in such a way as to produce a more pronounced activation of second messengers, causing more of an effect than others. Drugs that achieve maximal effect are known as full agonists and those that have a less than maximal effect are known as partial agonists.

## Anesthetic Drug Interactions

An average clinical anesthetic rarely consists of one drug but rather a combination of drugs to achieve desired levels of hypnosis, analgesia, and muscle relaxation. Hypnotics, analgesics (also see Chapter 9), and muscle relaxants (also see Chapter 11) all interact with one another such that each drug, when administered in the presence of other drugs, rarely behaves as if it were administered alone. For example, when an analgesic is administered in the presence of a hypnotic, analgesia is more profound with the hypnotic than by itself, and hypnosis is more profound with the analgesic than by itself. Thus, anesthesia is the practice of applied drug interactions. This phenomenon is likely a function of each class of drug exerting an effect on different receptors.

Substantial studies have been performed exploring how anesthetic drugs interact with one another. As illustrated in Fig. 4.22, interactions have been characterized as antagonistic, additive, and synergistic. When drugs that have an additive interaction are coadministered, their overall effect is the sum of the two individual effects. With antagonistic interactions, the overall effect is less than if the drug combination was additive; with synergistic interactions, the overall effect is greater than if the drug combination was additive.

A term used to characterize the continuum of drug concentrations across various combinations of drug pairs (X in combination with Y) is the isobole. The isobole is an isoeffect line for a selected probability of effect. A common isobole is the 50% isobole line. It represents all possible combinations of two-drug effect-site concentrations that would lead to a 50% probability of a

given effect. Other isoboles are of more clinical interest. For example, the 95% isobole for loss of responsiveness represents the concentration pairs necessary to ensure a 95% probability of unresponsiveness. Similarly, the 5% isobole represents the concentration pairs having a low likelihood of that effect (i.e., most patients would be responsive). When formulating an anesthetic dosing regimen, dosing an anesthetic to achieve a probability of effect just above but not far beyond the 95% isobole is ideal (Fig. 4.23).

Several researchers have developed mathematical models that characterize anesthetic drug interactions in three dimensions. These models are known as response surface models and include effect-site concentrations for each drug as well as a probability estimate of the overall effect. Fig. 4.24 presents the propofol-remifentanil interaction for loss of responsiveness as published by Bouillon and associates.[13] The response surface presents the full range of remifentanil-propofol isoboles (0% to 100%) for loss of responsiveness. There are two common representations of the response surface model: the three-dimensional plot and the topographic plot. The topographic plot represents a top-down view of the response surface with drug concentrations on the vertical and horizontal axes. Drug effect is represented with selected isobole lines (i.e., 5%, 50%, and 95%).

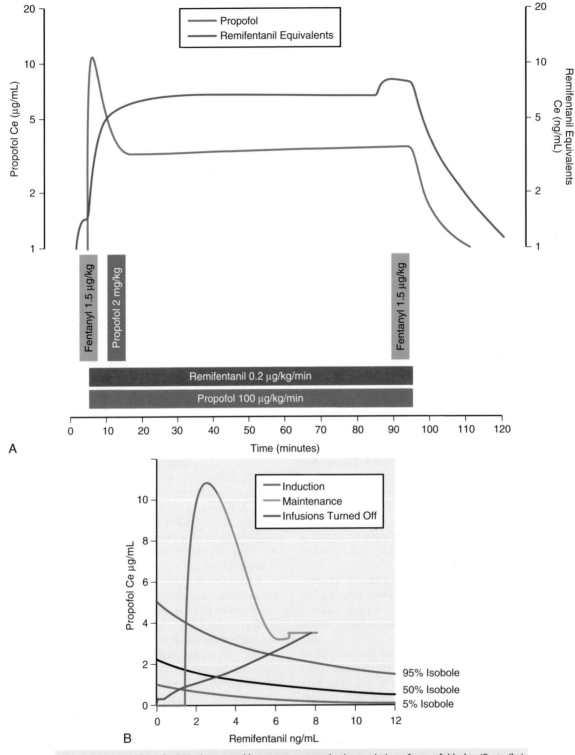

**Fig. 4.24** Simulation of a 90-minute total intravenous anesthetic consisting of propofol bolus (2 mg/kg) and infusion (100 μg/kg/min), remifentanil infusion (0.2 μg/kg/min), and intermittent fentanyl boluses (1.5 μg/kg). (A) Resultant effect-site concentrations (Ce) are presented. (B) Predictions of loss of responsiveness are presented on a topographic (top-down) view.

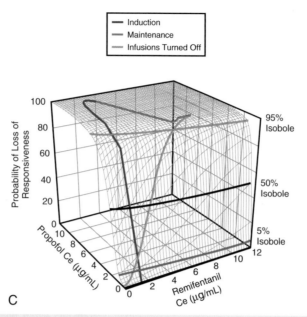

**Fig. 4.24, cont'd** (C) On a three-dimensional response surface plot, the green, black, and yellow lines represent the 5%, 50%, and 95% isoboles, respectively. Each isobole presents the propofol-remifentanil pairs that yield the same effect. The inward bow of the isoboles indicates that the interaction is synergistic. The isoboles are in close proximity to one another, indicating a steep transition from responsive to unresponsive. (From Miller RD, Cohen NH, Eriksson LI, et al, eds. *Miller's Anesthesia.* 8th ed. Philadelphia: Saunders Elsevier; 2015:Fig. 24.29. Author's representation based on data from Bouillon TW, Bruhn J, Radulescu L, et al. Pharmacodynamic interaction between propofol and remifentanil regarding hypnosis, tolerance of laryngoscopy, bispectral index, and electroencyphalographic apprpoximate entropy. *Anesthesiology.* 2004;100(6):1353–1372.

Response surface models have been developed for a variety of anesthetic effects to include responses to verbal and tactile stimuli, painful stimuli, hemodynamic or respiratory effects, and changes in electrical brain activity. For example, with airway instrumentation, response surface models have been developed for loss of response to placing a laryngeal mask airway,[14] laryngoscopy,[15,16] tracheal intubation,[17] and esophageal instrumentation[18] for selected combinations of anesthetic drugs. Although many response surface models exist, there are several gaps in available models covering all common combinations of anesthetic drugs and various forms of stimuli encountered in the perioperative environment.

## SPECIAL POPULATIONS

When formulating an anesthetic, many aspects of patient demographics and medical history need to be considered to determine the correct dose. Such factors include age; body habitus; gender; chronic exposure to opioids, benzodiazepines, or alcohol; presence of heart, lung, kidney, or liver disease; and the extent of blood loss or dehydration. Each of them can dramatically impact anesthetic drug kinetics and dynamics. How some patient characteristics (e.g., obesity) influence anesthetic drug behavior has been studied, whereas other patient characteristics remain difficult to assess (e.g., chronic opioid exposure). The findings are briefly summarized to characterize the pharmacokinetics and pharmacodynamics in a few unique special populations.

## Influence of Obesity on Anesthetic Drugs

Obesity is a worldwide epidemic, and overweight patients frequently undergo anesthesia and surgery. Therefore, anesthesia providers should be familiar with the pharmacologic alterations of anesthetics in obese individuals. In general, manufacturer dosing recommendations are scaled to kilograms of actual total body weight (TBW). However, anesthesia providers rarely use mg/kg dosing in obese patients for fear of administering an excessive dose (e.g., a 136-kg patient does not require twice as much drug as a patient of the same height who weighs 68 kg). Accordingly researchers have developed several weight scalars in an attempt to avoid excessive dosing or underdosing in this patient population. Some of these scalars include lean body mass (LBM), ideal body weight (IBW), and fat-free mass (FFM). Table 4.1 presents the formulas used to estimate these weight scalars. Table 4.2 presents samples of the resultant scaled weight for a lean individual and an obese individual. In general, the aim of weight scalars is to match dosing regimens for obese patients with what

**Table 4.1** Common Weight Scalars

| Scalar[a] | Equations |
|---|---|
| Ideal body weight | Male:<br>50 kg + 2.3 kg for each 2.54 cm (1 inch) over 152 cm (5 feet)<br>Female:<br>45.5 kg + 2.3 kg for each 2.54 cm (1 inch) over 152 cm (5 feet) |
| Lean body mass | Male:<br>$1.1 \times TBW - 128 \times (TBW/Ht)^2$<br>Female:<br>$1.07 \times TBW - 148 \times (TBW/Ht)^2$ |
| Fat-free mass[19] | Male:<br>$(9.27 \times 10^3 \times TBW)/(6.68 \times 10^3 + 216 \times BMI)$<br>Female:<br>$(9.27 \times 10^3 \times TBW)/(8.78 \times 10^3 + 244 \times BMI)$ |
| Pharmacokinetic mass[20,21] | $52/(1 + [196.4 \times e^{-0.025\,TBW} - 53.66]/100)$ (fentanyl only) |
| Modified fat-free mass[22,23] | $FFM + 0.4^b (TBW - FFM)$ |

[a]Superscript numbers in this column indicate references at the end of the chapter.
[b]The dose/kg using IBW, TBW, or FFM in an obese person are all less than the dose/kg using TBW in a nonobese patient.
BMI, Body mass index; FFM, fat-free mass; Ht, height in centimeters; IBW, ideal body weight; LBM, lean body mass; MFFM, modified fat-free mass; TBW, total body weight in kg.

**Table 4.2** Dosing Weights Based on Various Dosing Scalars

| Dosing Scalar | Dosing Weight, 176-cm (6-foot)- Tall Male | |
|---|---|---|
| | 68 kg BMI = 22 | 185 kg BMI = 60 |
| Total body weight (TBW) | 68 | 185 |
| Ideal body weight (IBW) | 72 | 72 |
| Lean body mass (LBM) | 56 | 62 |
| Fat-free mass (FFM) | 55 | 88 |
| Modified fat-free mass (MFFM) | 60 | 127 |

BMI, Body mass index (kg/m²).

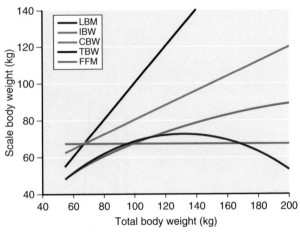

**Fig. 4.25** Scaled weights as a function of total body weight (TBW). Key points in this plot: IBW remains the same regardless of the TBW, and LBM starts to decline for weight increases above 127 kg. *CBW,* Corrected body weight; *FFM,* fat-free mass; *IBW,* ideal body weight; *LBM,* lean body mass (for a 40-year-old man, 176 cm tall). (From Miller RD, Cohen NH, Eriksson LI, et al, eds. *Miller's Anesthesia.* 8th ed. Philadelphia: Saunders Elsevier; 2015:Fig. 24.31.)

remifentanil, and fentanyl) in obese patients, including shortcomings of weight scalars when used in bolus and continuous infusion dosing.

### Propofol

The influence of obesity on propofol pharmacokinetics is not entirely clear (also see Chapter 8). Generally, in obese patients, the blood distributes more to nonadipose than to adipose tissues, resulting in higher plasma drug concentrations in obese patients with mg/kg dosing than in normal patients with less adipose mass. Furthermore, propofol clearance increases because of the increased liver volume and liver blood flow associated with obesity (and increased cardiac output). Changes to volumes of distribution likely influence concentration peaks with bolus dosing, whereas changes in clearance likely influence concentrations during and following infusions. Various weight scalars in propofol bolus and continuous infusion dosing have been studied.

### Dosing Scalars for Propofol

Simulations of an infusion using various weight scalars are presented in Fig. 4.26. The simulations predict propofol effect-site concentrations from a 60-minute infusion (167 µg/kg/min) in a 176-cm (6-foot)-tall obese (185 kg) and lean (68 kg) male patient. If dosed according to TBW, peak plasma concentrations in the lean and obese individuals are different. The other weight scalars lead to much smaller concentrations with the infusion.

is required for normal-size patients. These scaled weights are usually smaller than TBW in obese patients and thus help prevent excessive drug administration (Fig. 4.25). Scaled weights have been used in place of TBW for both bolus (mg/kg) and infusion (mg/kg/hr) dosing and also for target-controlled infusions (TCIs).

This section will discuss the pharmacologic alterations of select intravenous anesthetic drugs (propofol,

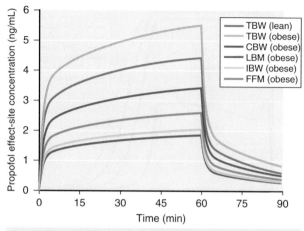

**Fig. 4.26** Simulations of propofol plasma concentrations that result from a 60-minute infusion (10 mg/kg/h [167 µg/kg/min]) to a 40-year-old man who is 176 cm tall. Simulations include the following dosing weights: total body weights (TBW) of 68 kg and 185 kg (body mass indices of 22 and 60, respectively) and scaled weights for the 185-kg weight to include Servin's corrected body weight (CBW), lean body mass (LBM), ideal body weight (IBW), and fat-free mass (FFM). Key points: At the 185-kg weight, when dosed to TBW, the infusion leads to high propofol concentrations, whereas when dosed to IBW or LBM, the infusion leads to low propofol concentrations. When the 185-kg individual is dosed using CBW, it best approximates the propofol concentrations that result from TBW in a lean individual. (From Miller RD, Cohen NH, Eriksson LI, et al, eds. *Miller's Anesthesia*. 8th ed. Philadelphia: Saunders Elsevier; 2014:Fig. 24.32.)

Of the many available dosing scalars, authors recommend LBM[24] for bolus dosing (i.e., during induction) and TBW or corrected body weight (CBW) for infusions.[17,25] For continuous infusions, other weight scalars are likely to result in inadequate dosing (most worrisome for LBM).

One concern with using TBW to dose continuous infusions (i.e., µg/kg/min) is drug accumulation. Prior investigations, however, do not support this assumption. Servin and colleagues[22] performed pharmacokinetic analyses of propofol administration to normal and obese patients using TBW and CBW. The CBW was defined as the IBW + 0.4 × (TBW − IBW).[24] They found similar concentrations at eye opening in both groups and absence of propofol accumulation in obese patients. However, some reports suggest that dosing infusions according to CBW may underdose morbidly obese patients.[25]

### Other Sedatives

Only limited information is available on the behavior of other sedatives (i.e., midazolam, ketamine, etomidate, and barbiturates) in obese patients (also see Chapter 8). Although not clinically validated in obese patients, bolus doses probably should be based on TBW, and use of other dosing scalars will lead to inadequate effect. In

contrast, continuous infusion rates should be dosed to IBW.[26]

### Opioids

#### Remifentanil

In obese patients, largely owing to its rapid metabolism by nonspecific esterases, the distribution volume and clearance of remifentanil are similar in lean and obese patients.[27] As with propofol, researchers have explored several scaled weights in an effort to optimize bolus dosing, continuous infusions, and TCIs.

#### Dosing Scalars

As described with propofol, simulation is used to predict remifentanil effect-site concentrations and analgesic effect for a variety of scaled weights in a 174-cm-tall obese (185 kg, BMI of 60) individual and lean (68 kg, BMI of 22) individual (Fig. 4.27). Several key points are illustrated in these simulations:

1. For an obese patient, dosing scaled to FFM or IBW resulted in almost identical remifentanil effect-site concentrations as in the lean patient dosed according to TBW. Unlike propofol, dosing remifentanil to CBW (red line, Fig. 4.27A) leads to higher plasma concentrations compared to levels achieved when dosing to TBW in a lean individual.
2. Dosing scaled to LBM in the obese individual resulted in lower effect-site concentrations than those in a lean individual dosed according to TBW.
3. Dosing the obese individual to TBW was excessive.
4. All dosing scalars, except LBM, provided effect-site concentrations associated with a high probability of analgesia.

As can be appreciated in Fig. 4.27, LBM has substantial shortcomings in morbidly obese patients.[29] First, dosing remifentanil to LBM leads to plasma concentrations with a low probability of effect compared to the other dosing scalars. Second, with excessive weight (BMI over 40), LBM actually becomes smaller with increasing TBW, making it impractical to use (see Fig. 4.25). A modified LBM,[24] FFM eliminates the extremely low dosing weight problem.[30] In this simulation, IBW also provides suitable effect-site concentrations, but this may not always be the case when using a weight scalar that is based only on patient height.

### Fentanyl

Despite widespread use in the clinical arena, relatively little work has explored how obesity affects fentanyl pharmacokinetics (also see Chapter 9). Published fentanyl pharmacokinetic models[31,32] tend to overestimate fentanyl concentrations as TBW increases.[22] Investigators have[20,21] explored ways to improve predictions using published models by modifying demographic data (e.g., either height or weight). Recommendations include use of a modified weight, called the *pharmacokinetic mass* to

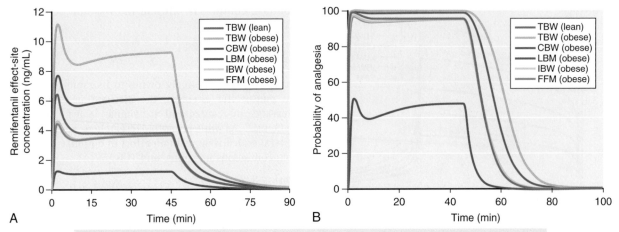

**Fig. 4.27** Simulations of remifentanil effect-site concentrations (A) and analgesic effect (B) that result from a 1-µg/kg bolus and a 60-minute infusion at a rate of 0.15 µg/kg/min to a 40-year-old man who is 176-cm tall. Simulations include the following dosing weights: total body weights (TBW) of 68 kg and 185 kg (body mass indices of 22 and 60, respectively) and scaled weights for the 185-kg weight to include Servin's corrected body weight (CBW), lean body mass (LBM), ideal body weight (IBW), and fat-free mass (FFM). Remifentanil effect-site concentrations and estimates of analgesic effect were estimated using published pharmacokinetic models.[6,28] Analgesia was defined as loss of response to 30 psi of pressure on the anterior tibia. (From Miller RD, Cohen NH, Eriksson LI, et al, eds. *Miller's Anesthesia.* 8th ed. Philadelphia: Saunders Elsevier; 2015:Fig. 24.34.)

improve the predictive performance of one of the many available fentanyl kinetic models.

### Other Opioids

Even less information regarding the impact of obesity on drug behavior is available for opioids other than remifentanil and fentanyl. Researchers have studied sufentanil in obese patients and found that its volume of distribution increases linearly with TBW[33] and clearance was similar between lean and obese individuals. They recommend bolus dosing using TBW and "prudently reduced" dosing for continuous infusions.

### Inhaled Anesthetics

A widely held perception of volatile anesthetics (also see Chapter 7) is that they accumulate more in obese than in lean patients and that this leads to prolonged emergence. This concept, however, has not been confirmed.[34] Two phenomena contribute to this observation: first, blood flow to adipose tissue *decreases* with increasing obesity,[35] and second, the time required to fill adipose tissue with volatile anesthetics is long.

## Influence of Increasing Age on Anesthetic Drug Pharmacology

Age is one of the most valuable covariates to consider when developing an anesthetic plan (also see Chapter 35). As with obesity, both remifentanil and propofol can serve as prototypes to understand how age influences anesthetic drug behavior. The influence of age on remifentanil and propofol are characterized in quantitative terms.[1,6,7,36]

With remifentanil, elderly patients require less drug to produce an opioid effect. The effectiveness of reduced doses in older patients is primarily a function of changes in pharmacodynamics but may involve pharmacokinetic changes as well.[6] Based on previously published pharmacokinetic and pharmacodynamic models built from measurements over a wide age range,[1,6,7,36] simulations can be performed to explore how age may influence dosing. For example, to achieve equipotent doses in 20- and 80-year-olds, the dose for the 80-year-old should be reduced by 55%. A similar analysis for propofol recommends that the dose for an 80-year-old should be reduced by 65% compared to that of a 20-year-old.

The mechanisms for these changes are not clear, especially for pharmacodynamic changes. One possible source of change in pharmacokinetic behavior may be due to decreased cardiac output. Decreased cardiac output in the elderly[27] results in slower circulation and drug mixing. This may lead to high peak concentrations[27,37] and decreased drug delivery to metabolic organs and reduced clearance. Many intravenous anesthetics (propofol, thiopental, and etomidate) have slower clearance and a smaller volume of distribution.[1,38-40] in the elderly. Beyond age-related changes in cardiac output, other comorbid conditions may reduce cardiovascular function as well.[41] Taking this into account, anesthesia providers often consider a patient's "physiologic" age instead of solely relying on chronologic age.[42,43] For some older patients, such as those with no significant coexisting disease, normal body habitus, and good exercise tolerance, a substantial reduction in dose may not be warranted.

## SUMMARY

This chapter reviewed basic principles of clinical pharmacology used to describe anesthetic drug behavior: pharmacokinetics, pharmacodynamics, and anesthetic drug interactions. These principles provide anesthesia practitioners with the information needed to make rational decisions about the selection and administration of anesthetics. From a practical aspect, these principles characterize the magnitude and time course of drug effect, but because of complex mathematics, they have limited clinical utility in everyday practice. Advances in computer simulation, however, have brought this capability to the point of real-time patient care. Perhaps one of the most important advances in our understanding of clinical pharmacology is the development of interaction models that describe how different classes of anesthetic drugs influence one another. This knowledge is especially relevant to anesthesia providers, given that they rarely use just one drug when providing an anesthetic.

## QUESTIONS OF THE DAY

1. In a multicompartment pharmacokinetic model (e.g., for fentanyl bolus administration), what are the three phases that can be distinguished?
2. How can a decrement time be used to compare drugs within a drug class? What is the definition of *context-sensitive half-time*? How does terminal elimination half-life differ from context-sensitive half-time?
3. What is the definition of *biophase*? What is the utility of an effect site compartment in describing anesthetic drug pharmacology?
4. What is the difference between antagonistic, additive, and synergistic anesthetic drug interactions? What is an isobole, and how can it be used to determine an appropriate anesthetic regimen?
5. How does obesity influence propofol pharmacokinetics? What weight scalar should be used for propofol bolus dose versus propofol infusion dose?
6. How does age influence the pharmacology of remifentanil? What are the mechanisms of these age-related changes?

## REFERENCES

1. Schnider TW, Minto CF, Gambus PL, et al. The influence of method of administration and covariates on the pharmacokinetics of propofol in adult volunteers. *Anesthesiology*. 1998;88(5):1170–1182.
2. Wilkinson GR, Shand DG. Commentary: a physiological approach to hepatic drug clearance. *Clin Pharmacol Ther*. 1975;18:377–390.
3. Krejcie TC, Avram MJ, Gentry WB, et al. A recirculatory model of the pulmonary uptake and pharmacokinetics of lidocaine based on analysis or arterial and mixed venous data from dogs. *J Pharmacokinet Biopharm*. 1997;25:169–190.
4. Youngs EJ, Shafer SL. Basic pharmacokinetic and pharmacodynamic principles. In: White PF, ed. *Textbook of Intravenous Anesthesia*. Baltimore: Williams & Wilkins; 1997.
5. Hughes MA, Glass PS, Jacobs JR. Context-sensitive half-time in multicompartment pharmacokinetic models for intravenous anesthetic drugs. *Anesthesiology*. 1992;76(3):334–341.
6. Minto CF, Schnider TW, Egan TD, et al. Influence of age and gender on the pharmacokinetics and pharmacodynamics of remifentanil. I. Model development. *Anesthesiology*. 1997;86(1):10–23.
7. Schnider TW, Minto CF, Shafer SL, et al. The influence of age on propofol pharmacodynamics. *Anesthesiology*. 1999;90(6):1502–1516.
8. Lee S, Kim BH, Lim K, et al. Pharmacokinetics and pharmacodynamics of intravenous dexmedetomidine in healthy Korean subjects. *J Clin Pharm Ther*. 2012;37:698–703.
9. Hudson RJ, Bergstrom RG, Thomson IR, et al. Pharmacokinetics of sufentanil in patients undergoing abdominal aortic surgery. *Anesthesiology*. 1989;70:426–431.
10. Scott JC, Stanski DR. Decreased fentanyl and alfentanil dose requirements with age. A simultaneous pharmacokinetic and pharmacodynamic evaluation. *J Pharmacol Exp Ther*. 1987;240(1):159–166.
11. Doufas AG, Bakhshandeh M, Bjorksten AR, et al. Induction speed is not a determinant of propofol pharmacodynamics. *Anesthesiology*. 2004;101:1112–1121.
12. Egan TD, Muir KT, Hermann DJ, et al. The electroencephalogram (EEG) and clinical measures of opioid potency: defining the EEG-clinical potency relationship ("fingerprint") with application to remifentanil. *Int J Pharm Med*. 2001;15(1):11–19.
13. Bouillon TW, Bruhn J, Radulescu L, et al. Pharmacodynamic interaction between propofol and remifentanil regarding hypnosis, tolerance of laryngoscopy, bispectral index, and electroencephalographic approximate entropy. *Anesthesiology*. 2004;100(6):1353–1372.
14. Heyse B, Proost JH, Schumacher PM, et al. Sevoflurane remifentanil interaction: comparison of different response surface models. *Anesthesiology*. 2012;116(2):311–323.
15. Kern SE, Xie G, White JL, Egan TD. A response surface analysis of propofol-remifentanil pharmacodynamic interaction in volunteers. *Anesthesiology*. 2004;100(6):1373–1381.
16. Manyam SC, Gupta DK, Johnson KB, et al. Opioid-volatile anesthetic synergy: a response surface model with remifentanil and sevoflurane as prototypes. *Anesthesiology*. 2006;105(2):267–278.
17. Mertens MJ, Engbers FH, Burm AG, Vuyk J. Predictive performance of computer-controlled infusion of remifentanil during propofol/remifentanil anaesthesia. *Br J Anaesth*. 2003;90(2):132–141.

18. LaPierre CD, Johnson KB, Randall BR, et al. An exploration of remifentanil-propofol combinations that lead to a loss of response to esophageal instrumentation, a loss of responsiveness, and/or onset of intolerable ventilatory depression. *Anesth Analg.* 2011; 113(3):490–499.

19. Janmahasatian S, Duffull SB, Ash S, et al. Quantification of lean bodyweight. *Clin Pharmacokinet.* 2005;44(10):1051–1065.

20. Shibutani K, Inchiosa Jr MA, Sawada K, Bairamian M. Accuracy of pharmacokinetic models for predicting plasma fentanyl concentrations in lean and obese surgical patients: derivation of dosing weight ("pharmacokinetic mass"). *Anesthesiology.* 2004;101(3):603–613.

21. Shibutani K, Inchiosa Jr MA, Sawada K, Bairamian M. Pharmacokinetic mass of fentanyl for postoperative analgesia in lean and obese patients. *Br J Anaesth.* 2005;95(3):377–383.

22. Servin F, Farinotti R, Haberer JP, Desmonts JM. Propofol infusion for maintenance of anesthesia in morbidly obese patients receiving nitrous oxide. A clinical and pharmacokinetic study. *Anesthesiology.* 1993;78(4):657–665.

23. Cortinez LI, Anderson BJ, Penna A, et al. Influence of obesity on propofol pharmacokinetics: derivation of a pharmacokinetic model. *Br J Anaesth.* 2010;105(4):448–456.

24. Albertin A, Poli D, La Colla L, et al. Predictive performance of "Servin's formula" during BIS-guided propofol-remifentanil target-controlled infusion in morbidly obese patients. *Br J Anaesth.* 2007;98(1):66–75.

25. Igarashi T, Nagata O, Iwakiri H, et al. [Two cases of intraoperative awareness during intravenous anesthesia with propofol in morbidly obese patients]. *Masui.* 2002;51(11):1243–1247.

26. Greenblatt DJ, Abernethy DR, Locniskar A, et al. Effect of age, gender, and obesity on midazolam kinetics. *Anesthesiology.* 1984;61(1):27–35.

27. Upton RN, Ludbrook GL, Grant C, Martinez AM. Cardiac output is a determinant of the initial concentrations of propofol after short-infusion administration. *Anesth Analg.* 1999;89(3):545–552.

28. Johnson KB, Syroid ND, Gupta DK, et al. An evaluation of remifentanil propofol response surfaces for loss of responsiveness, loss of response to surrogates of painful stimuli and laryngoscopy in patients undergoing elective surgery. *Anesth Analg.* 2008;106(2):471–479.

29. La Colla L, Albertin A, La Colla G, et al. No adjustment vs. adjustment formula as input weight for propofol target-controlled infusion in morbidly obese patients. *Eur J Anaesthesiol.* 2009;26(5):362–369.

30. La Colla L, Albertin A, La Colla G, et al. Predictive performance of the "Minto" remifentanil pharmacokinetic parameter set in morbidly obese patients ensuing from a new method for calculating lean body mass. *Clin Pharmacokinet.* 2010;49(2):131–139.

31. Anderson BJ, Holford NH. Mechanistic basis of using body size and maturation to predict clearance in humans. *Drug Metab Pharmacokinet.* 2009;24(1):25–36.

32. Duffull SB, Dooley MJ, Green B, et al. A standard weight descriptor for dose adjustment in the obese patient. *Clin Pharmacokinet.* 2004;43(16):1167–1178.

33. Schwartz AE, Matteo RS, Ornstein E, et al. Pharmacokinetics of sufentanil in obese patients. *Anesth Analg.* 1991; 73(6):790–793.

34. Cortinez LI, Gambús P, Trocóniz IF, et al. Obesity does not influence the onset and offset of sevoflurane effect as measured by the hysteresis between sevoflurane concentration and bispectral index. *Anesth Analg.* 2011;113(1):70–76.

35. Lesser GT, Deutsch S. Measurement of adipose tissue blood flow and perfusion in man by uptake of $^{85}$Kr. *J Appl Physiol.* 1967;23(5):621–630.

36. Minto CF, Schnider TW, Shafer SL. Pharmacokinetics and pharmacodynamics of remifentanil. II. Model application. *Anesthesiology.* 1997;86(1):24–33.

37. Krejcie TC, Avram MJ. What determines anesthetic induction dose? It's the front-end kinetics, doctor! *Anesth Analg.* 1999;89(3):541–544.

38. Arden JR, Holley FO, Stanski DR. Increased sensitivity to etomidate in the elderly: initial distribution versus altered brain response. *Anesthesiology.* 1986;65(1):19–27.

39. Homer TD, Stanski DR. The effect of increasing age on thiopental disposition and anesthetic requirement. *Anesthesiology.* 1985;62:714–724.

40. Stanski DR, Maitre PO. Population pharmacokinetics and pharmacodynamics of thiopental: the effect of age revisited. *Anesthesiology.* 1990;72(3):412–422.

41. Rodeheffer RJ, Gerstenblith G, Becker LC, et al. Exercise cardiac output is maintained with advancing age in healthy human subjects: cardiac dilatation and increased stroke volume compensate for a diminished heart rate. *Circulation.* 1984;69(2):203–213.

42. Avram MJ, Krejcie TC, Henthorn TK. The relationship of age to the pharmacokinetics of early drug distribution: the concurrent disposition of thiopental and indocyanine green. *Anesthesiology.* 1990;72(3):403–411.

43. Williams TF. Aging or disease? *Clin Pharmacol Ther.* 1987;42(6):663–665.

# 5 CLINICAL CARDIAC AND PULMONARY PHYSIOLOGY

## John Feiner

No specialty in medicine manages cardiac and pulmonary physiology as directly on a daily basis as anesthesiology.[1-3] An understanding of cardiorespiratory physiology prepares the anesthesia team to manage critical and common situations in anesthesia, including hypotension, arterial hypoxemia, hypercapnia, and high peak airway pressures.

## HEMODYNAMICS

### Arterial Blood Pressure

Systemic arterial blood pressure and mean arterial pressure (MAP) are commonly monitored by anesthesia providers via a blood pressure cuff or an indwelling arterial cannula. Although treatment of chronic systemic hypertension is sometimes necessary, acute hypotension is often a problem with many anesthetics. Hypotension varies from mild clinically insignificant reductions in MAP from general anesthesia or regional anesthesia to life-threatening emergencies. Hypotension can be of sufficient magnitude to jeopardize organ perfusion, causing injury and an adverse outcome. Organs of most immediate concern are the heart and brain, followed by the kidneys, liver, and lungs. All have typical injury patterns associated with prolonged "shock." Understanding the physiology behind hypotension is critical for diagnosis and treatment.

Intraoperative hemodynamic instability has long been thought to result in worse outcomes after surgery. In recent large retrospective studies, intraoperative hypotension of even 5 minutes' duration (systolic blood pressure [SBP] < 70 mm Hg, MAP < 50 mm Hg, diastolic blood pressure [DBP] < 30 mm Hg) is associated with increased postoperative morbidity and mortality risks.[4,5] In addition, the combination of hypotension, small volatile anesthetic concentrations, and low bispectral index scale (BIS) values have been associated with worse postoperative outcomes. Whether a change in anesthetic management will alter these risks needs future study.[6]

## Physiologic Approach to Hypotension

The logical treatment of acute hypotension categorizes MAP into its physiologic components:

$$MAP = SVR \times CO$$

where SVR is the systemic vascular resistance and CO is cardiac output.

Although most of our focus is on understanding MAP alone, the other pressures (e.g., SBP, DBP, and pulse pressure [PP = SBP – DBP]) also require attention. The pulse pressure is created by the addition of stroke volume (SV) on top of the DBP within the compliant vascular tree. The aorta is responsible for most of this compliance. Increased pulse pressure can occur with an increased SV but most often occurs because of the poor aortic compliance that accompanies aging (also see Chapter 35). Decreasing DBP can have more dramatic effects on SBP when vascular compliance is poor.

### Systemic Vascular Resistance

Most drugs administered during general anesthesia and neuraxial regional anesthesia (also see Chapter 17) decrease SVR. Several pathologic conditions can produce profound reductions in SVR, including sepsis, anaphylaxis, spinal shock, and reperfusion of ischemic organs. The calculation for SVR follows:

$$SVR = 80 \times (MAP - CVP)/CO$$

where CVP is the central venous pressure, and the factor 80 converts units into dyne/s/cm$^5$ from pressure in millimeters of mercury (mm Hg) and CO given in liters per minute (L/min).

Pulmonary artery (PA) catheterization can be used to obtain the measurements necessary for calculating SVR, but this monitor is not usually immediately available. Signs of adequate perfusion (e.g., warm extremities, good pulse oximeter plethysmograph waveform, and perfusion index*) may sometimes be present when hypotension is caused by low SVR. On the other hand, hypertension nearly always involves excessive vasoconstriction.

Resistance is inversely proportional to the fourth power of the radius. Individually, small vessels offer a very high resistance to flow. However, total SVR is decreased when there are many vessels arranged in parallel. Capillaries, despite being the smallest blood vessels, are not responsible for most of the SVR because there are so many in parallel. Most of the resistance to blood flow in the arterial side of the circulation is in the arterioles.

### Cardiac Output

As a cause of hypotension, decreased CO may be more difficult to treat than decreased SVR. Increased CO is not usually associated with systemic hypertension, and most

hyperdynamic states, such as sepsis and liver failure, are associated with decreased systemic blood pressure.

CO is defined as the amount of blood (in liters) pumped by the heart in 1 minute. Although the amount of blood pumped by the right side and left side of the heart can differ in the presence of certain congenital heart malformations, these amounts are usually the same. CO is the product of heart rate (HR) and SV, the net amount of blood ejected by the heart in one cycle:

$$CO = HR \times SV$$

CO can be measured clinically by thermodilution via a PA catheter and by transesophageal echocardiography (TEE). Less invasive devices to measure CO have been developed, including esophageal Doppler and pulse contour analysis. Because the normal CO changes according to body size, cardiac index (CO divided by body surface area) often is used.

### Heart Rate

Tachycardia and bradycardia can cause hypotension if CO is decreased. The electrocardiogram (ECG), pulse oximetry, or physical examination can identify the presence of bradycardia or tachycardia. The identification of a P wave on the ECG is essential for analyzing HR. Loss of sinus rhythm and atrial contraction results in decreased ventricular filling. Atrial contraction constitutes a significant percentage of preload, even more so in patients with a poorly compliant ventricle. A slow HR may result in enhanced ventricular filling and an increased SV, but an excessively slow HR results in an inadequate CO. Tachycardia may result in insufficient time for the left ventricle to fill and result in low CO and hypotension.

### Ejection Fraction and Stroke Volume

Ejection fraction (EF) is the percentage of ventricular blood volume that is pumped by the heart in a single contraction (SV/end-diastolic volume [EDV]). Unlike SV, the EF does not differ on the basis of body size, and an EF of 60% to 70% is considered normal. Hyperdynamic states such as sepsis and cirrhosis are reflected by an increased EF. Poor cardiac function is indicated by a small EF. Because CO can be maintained by increasing HR, the SV should be calculated to better assess cardiac function. However, with chronic dilated cardiomyopathy, the SV can improve despite the smaller EF.

### Preload

Preload refers to the amount the cardiac muscle is "stretched" before contraction. Preload is best defined clinically as the EDV of the heart, which can be measured directly with TEE. Filling pressures (e.g., left atrial [LA] pressure, pulmonary capillary wedge pressure [PCWP], pulmonary artery diastolic [PAD] pressure) can also assess preload. CVP measures filling pressures on the right side of the heart, which correlates with filling pressures on the left side of the heart in the absence of pulmonary disease and when cardiac function is normal. By using a balloon to stop flow in a PA, pressure equilibrates within the system so that

---

*Perfusion index is a measure of the pulsatile signal relative to the background absorption and is an important measure of signal strength.

PCWP is nearly equivalent to LA pressure and reflects the filling pressure of the left side of the heart. The relationship between pressure and volume of the heart in diastole is depicted by ventricular compliance curves (Fig. 5.1). With a poorly compliant heart, normal filling pressures may not produce an adequate EDV. Likewise, trying to fill a "stiff" left ventricle to a normal volume may increase intracardiac and pulmonary capillary pressures excessively.

### Frank-Starling Mechanism

The Frank-Starling mechanism is a physiologic description of the increased pumping action of the heart with increased filling. A larger preload results in increased contraction necessary to eject the added ventricular volume, resulting in a larger SV and similar EF. Reduced ventricular filling, as in hypovolemia, results in reduced SV. Small increases in preload may have dramatic effects ("volume responsiveness") on SV and CO (Fig. 5.2). At higher points on the curve, little additional benefit is derived from increases in preload.

### Causes of Low Preload

Causes of low preload include hypovolemia and venodilation. Hypovolemia may result from hemorrhage or fluid losses. Venodilation occurs with general anesthesia and may be even more prominent in the presence of neuraxial anesthesia (also see Chapter 17). Additional causes of decreased preload include tension pneumothorax and pericardial tamponade, which prevent ventricular filling due to increased pressure around the heart, even though blood volume and filling pressures are adequate.[7] Such conditions may manifest with systolic pressure variation (SPV), which describes changes in SBP with tidal breathing or ventilation that can be observed on an arterial blood pressure tracing.[8] The extreme form of this is pulsus paradoxus, a pulse that changes markedly during tidal breathing. In the setting of normal or increased CVP, the presence of cardiac tamponade may exist. Pulse pressure variation $((PP_{peak} - PP_{nadir})/PP_{average})$ is analogous to SPV but requires computer calculation. Both high SPV and pulse pressure variation (PPV) are also useful in identifying hypovolemia, and are more sensitive and specific indicators of intravascular volume responsiveness than filling pressures.

Pathologic problems on the right side of the heart may prevent filling of the left ventricle. Pulmonary embolism and other causes of pulmonary hypertension prevent the right side of the heart from pumping a sufficient volume to fill the left side of the heart. The interventricular septum may be shifted, further constricting filling of the left side of the heart.

### Contractility

Contractility, or the inotropic state of the heart, is a measure of the force of contraction independent of loading conditions (preload or afterload). It can be measured for research purposes by the rate at which pressure develops

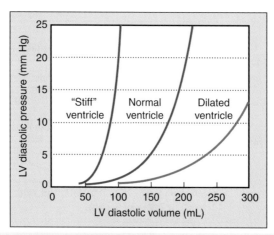

**Fig. 5.1** The pressure-volume relationship of the heart in diastole is shown in the compliance curves plotting left ventricular (LV) diastolic volume versus pressure. The "stiff" heart shows a steeper rise of pressure with increased volume than the normal heart. The dilated ventricle shows a much more compliant curve.

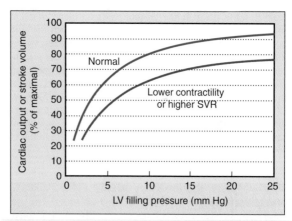

**Fig. 5.2** The cardiac function curve shows the typical relationship between preload, represented by left ventricular (LV) filling pressure, and cardiac function, reflected in cardiac output or stroke volume. Filling pressure can be measured as left atrial pressure or pulmonary capillary wedge pressure. At low preload, augmentation of filling results in significantly increased cardiac output. This is the steeper portion of the curve. At higher LV filling pressures, little improvement in function occurs with increased preload, and with overfilling, a decrement in function can occur because of impaired perfusion (not shown). Lower contractility or higher systemic vascular resistance (SVR) shifts the normal curve to the right and downward.

in the cardiac ventricles (dP/dT) or by systolic pressure-volume relationships (Fig. 5.3). Decreased myocardial contractility may be a cause of hypotension (Box 5.1).[9]

### Afterload

Afterload is the resistance to ejection of blood from the left ventricle with each contraction. Clinically, afterload is largely determined by SVR. When SVR is increased, the

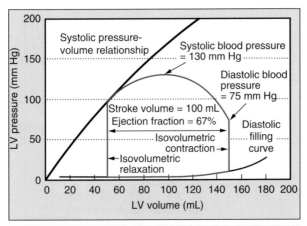

**Fig. 5.3** The closed loop *(red line)* shows a typical cardiac cycle. Diastolic filling occurs along the typical diastolic curve from a volume of 50 mL to an end-diastolic volume (EDV) of 150 mL. Isovolumetric contraction increases the pressure in the left ventricle (LV) until it reaches the pressure in the aorta (at diastolic blood pressure) and the aortic valve opens. The LV then ejects blood, and volume decreases. Pressure in the LV and aorta reaches a peak at some point during ejection (systolic blood pressure), and the pressure then drops until the point at which the aortic valve closes (roughly the dicrotic notch). The LV relaxes, without changing volume (isovolumetric relaxation). When the pressure decreases below left atrial pressure, the mitral valve opens, and diastolic filling begins. The plot shows a normal cycle, and the stroke volume (SV) is 100 mL, ejection fraction (EF) is SV/EDV = 67%, and blood pressure is 130/75 mm Hg. The systolic pressure-volume relationship *(black line)* can be constructed from a family of curves under different loading conditions (i.e., different preload) and reflects the inotropic state of the heart.

---

**Box 5.1** Conditions Associated With Decreased Myocardial Contractility As a Cause of Hypotension

Myocardial ischemia
Anesthetic drugs
Cardiomyopathy
Previous myocardial infarction
Valvular heart disease (decreased stroke volume independent of preload)

---

heart does not empty as completely, resulting in a lower SV, EF, and CO (see Fig. 5.2). High SVR also increases cardiac filling pressures. Low SVR improves SV and increases CO such that a low SVR is often associated with a higher CO (Fig. 5.4).

Low SVR decreases cardiac filling pressures. This finding may suggest that preload rather than afterload is the cause of hypotension. Low SVR allows more extensive emptying and a lower end-systolic volume (ESV), one of the hallmarks of low SVR on TEE. With the same venous return, the heart does not fill to the same EDV, resulting in lower left ventricular filling pressures (see Fig. 5.4). A similar process occurs when the SVR is increased. Such

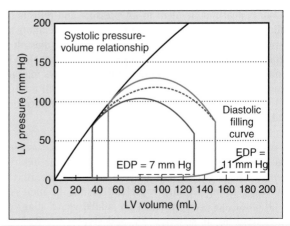

**Fig. 5.4** Changes in the cardiac cycle that can occur with vasodilatation are depicted. The cycle in green is the same cycle shown in Fig. 5.3. The red dashed line suggests the transition to the new cardiac cycle shown in blue. The systolic blood pressure has decreased to 105 mm Hg. The end-systolic volume has decreased, as has the end-diastolic volume. End-diastolic pressure (EDP) has decreased from 11 to 7 mm Hg in this example. The ejection fraction is slightly increased; however, the stroke volume may decrease, but with restoration of left ventricular (LV) filling pressures to the same level as before, the stroke volume will be higher.

stress-induced increases in cardiac filling pressures are more pronounced in patients with poor cardiac function.

## CARDIAC REFLEXES

The cardiovascular regulatory system consists of peripheral and central receptor systems that can detect various physiologic states, a central "integratory" system in the brainstem, and neurohumoral output to the heart and vascular system. A clinical understanding of cardiac reflexes is based on the concept that the cardiovascular system in the brainstem integrates the signal and provides a response through the autonomic nervous system.

### Autonomic Nervous System

The heart and vascular systems are controlled by the autonomic nervous system. Sympathetic and parasympathetic efferents innervate the sinoatrial and atrioventricular nodes. Sympathetic nervous system stimulation increases HR through activation of $\beta_1$-adrenergic receptors. Parasympathetic nervous system stimulation can profoundly slow HR through stimulation of muscarinic acetylcholine receptors in the sinoatrial and atrioventricular nodes, whereas parasympathetic nervous system suppression contributes to increased HR. Conduction through the atrioventricular node is increased and decreased by sympathetic and parasympathetic nervous system inner-vation, respectively. Sympathetic nervous system stimu-lation increases myocardial contractility. Parasympathetic nervous system stimulation may decrease myocardial contractility slightly, but it has its major effect through decreasing HR.

## Baroreceptors

Baroreceptors in the carotid sinus and aortic arch are acti-vated by increased systemic blood pressure that stimulates stretch receptors to send signals through the vagus and glossopharyngeal nerves to the central nervous system. The sensitivity of baroreceptors to systemic blood pres-sure changes varies and is significantly altered by long-standing essential hypertension. A typical response to acute hypertension is increased parasympathetic nervous system stimulation that decreases HR. Vagal stimulation and decreases in sympathetic nervous system activity also decrease myocardial contractility and cause reflex vaso-dilatation. This carotid sinus reflex can be used thera-peutically to produce vagal stimulation that may be an effective treatment for supraventricular tachycardia.

The atria and ventricles are innervated by a variety of sympathetic and parasympathetic receptor systems. Atrial stretch (i.e., Bainbridge reflex) can increase HR, which may help match CO to venous return.

Stimulation of the chemoreceptors in the carotid sinus has respiratory and cardiovascular effects. Arterial hypox-emia results in sympathetic nervous system stimulation, although more profound and prolonged arterial hypox-emia can result in bradycardia, possibly through central mechanisms. A variety of other reflexes include brady-cardia with ocular pressure (i.e., oculocardiac reflex) and bradycardia with stretch of abdominal viscera. The Cush-ing reflex includes bradycardia in response to increased intracranial pressure.

Many anesthetics blunt cardiac reflexes in a dose-dependent fashion, with the result that sympathetic ner-vous system responses to hypotension are reduced. The blunting of such reflexes represents an additional mecha-nism by which anesthetic drugs contribute to hypotension.

## CORONARY BLOOD FLOW

The coronary circulation is unique in that a larger per-centage of oxygen is extracted by the heart than in any other vascular bed, up to 60% to 70%, compared with the 25% extraction for the body as a whole. The consequence of this physiology is that the heart cannot increase oxy-gen extraction as a reserve mechanism. In cases of threat-ened oxygen supply, vasodilatation to increase blood flow is the primary compensatory mechanism of the heart.

Coronary reserve is the ability of the coronary cir-culation to increase flow more than the baseline state.

Endogenous regulators of coronary blood flow include adenosine, nitric oxide, and adrenergic stimulation. With coronary artery stenosis, compensatory vasodilatation downstream can maintain coronary blood flow until about 90% stenosis, when coronary reserve begins to become exhausted.

The perfusion pressure of a vascular bed is usually calculated as the difference between MAP and venous pressure. Instantaneous flow through the coronary arteries varies throughout the cardiac cycle, peaking during systole. The heart is fundamentally different from other organs, because the myocardial wall ten-sion developed during systole can completely stop blood flow in the subendocardium. The left ventricle is therefore perfused predominantly during diastole. The end-diastolic pressure in the left ventricle (LVEDP) may exceed CVP and represents the effective downstream pressure. Perfusion pressure to most of the left ventri-cle is therefore DBP minus LVEDP. The right ventricle, with its lower intramural pressure, is perfused during diastole and systole.

## PULMONARY CIRCULATION

The pulmonary circulation includes the right ventricle, pulmonary arteries, pulmonary capillary bed, and pul-monary veins, ending in the left atrium. The bronchial circulation supplies nutrients to lung tissue and empties into the pulmonary veins and left atrium. The pulmo-nary circulation differs substantially from the systemic circulation in its regulation, normal pressures (Table 5.1), and responses to drugs. Use of a PA catheter to measure pressures in the pulmonary circulation requires a funda-mental understanding of their normal values and their meaning. Pulmonary hypertension has idiopathic causes and may accompany several common diseases (e.g., cir-rhosis of the liver, sleep apnea). It is associated with sig-nificant anesthetic-related morbidity and mortality rates.

## Pulmonary Artery Pressure

Pulmonary artery pressure (PAP) is much lower than sys-temic pressure because of low pulmonary vascular resis-tance (PVR). Like the systemic circulation, the pulmonary circulation accepts the entire CO and must adapt its resis-tance to meet different conditions.

## Pulmonary Vascular Resistance

Determinants of PVR are different from SVR in the sys-temic circulation. During blood flow through the pul-monary circulation, resistance is thought to occur in the larger vessels, small arteries, and capillary bed. Vessels within the alveoli and the extra-alveolar vessels respond differently to forces within the lung.

| **Value** | **CVP** (mm Hg) | **PAS** (mm Hg) | **PAD** (mm Hg) | **PAM** (mm Hg) | **PCWP** (mm Hg) |
|---|---|---|---|---|---|
| Normal | 2-8 | 15-30 | 4-12 | 9-16 | 4-12 |
| High | >12 | >30 | >12 | >25 | >12 |
| Pathologic | >18 | >40 | >20 | >35 | >20 |

**Table 5.1** Normal Values for Pressures in the Venous and Pulmonary Arterial Systems

*CVP*, Central venous pressure; *PAD*, pulmonary artery diastolic pressure; *PAM*, pulmonary artery mean pressure; *PAS*, pulmonary artery systolic pressure; *PCWP*, pulmonary capillary wedge pressure.

The most useful physiologic model for describing changes in the pulmonary circulation is the *distention* of capillaries and the *recruitment* of new capillaries. The distention and recruitment of capillaries explain the changes in PVR in a variety of circumstances. Increased PAP causes distention and recruitment of capillaries, increasing the cross-sectional area and decreasing PVR. Increased CO also decreases PVR through distention and recruitment. The reciprocal changes between CO and PVR maintain pulmonary pressures fairly constant over a wide range of CO values.

Lung volumes have different effects on intra-alveolar and extra-alveolar vessels. With large lung volumes, intra-alveolar vessels can be compressed, whereas extra-alveolar vessels have lower resistance. The opposite is true at small lung volumes. Therefore, higher PVR occurs at large and small lung volumes. Increased PVR at small lung volumes helps to divert blood flow from collapsed alveoli, such as during one-lung ventilation.

Sympathetic nervous system stimulation can cause pulmonary vasoconstriction, but the effect is not large, in contrast to the systemic circulation, in which neurohumoral influence is the primary regulator of vascular tone. The pulmonary circulation has therefore been very difficult to treat with drugs. Nitric oxide is an important regulator of vascular tone and can be given by inhalation. Prostaglandins and phosphodiesterase inhibitors (e.g., sildenafil) are pulmonary vasodilators, but the pharmacologic responses that can be achieved in pulmonary hypertension are limited.

### Hypoxic Pulmonary Vasoconstriction

Hypoxic pulmonary vasoconstriction (HPV) is the pulmonary vascular response to a low alveolar oxygen partial pressure ($P_{AO_2}$). In many patients, HPV is an important adaptive response that improves gas exchange by diverting blood away from poorly ventilated areas, decreasing shunt fraction. Normal regions of the lung can easily accommodate the additional blood flow without increasing PAP. Global alveolar hypoxia, such as occurs with apnea or at high altitude, can cause significant HPV and increased PAP.

Anesthetic drugs such as the potent inhaled anesthetics can impair HPV, whereas commonly used intravenous drugs, such as propofol and opioids, demonstrate no inhibition of HPV. During surgical procedures requiring one-lung ventilation, HPV may play a role in the resolution of hypoxemia, although many other factors are also important, including acid-base status, CO, development of atelectasis, and concomitant drug administration.[10]

### Pulmonary Emboli

Pulmonary emboli obstruct blood vessels, increasing the overall resistance to blood through the pulmonary vascular system. Common forms of emboli are blood clots and air, but they also include amniotic fluid, carbon dioxide, and fat emboli.

### Arteriolar Thickening

Arteriolar thickening occurs in several clinical circumstances. It is associated with certain types of long-standing congenital heart disease. Primary pulmonary hypertension is an idiopathic disease associated with arteriolar hyperplasia. Similar changes are associated with cirrhosis of the liver (i.e., portopulmonary hypertension).

## Zones of the Lung

A useful concept in pulmonary hemodynamics is West's zones of the lung. Gravity determines the way pressures change in the vascular system relative to the measurement at the level of the heart. These differences are small compared with arterial pressures, but for venous pressure and PAP, these differences are clinically significant. Every 20 cm of change in height produces a 15-mm Hg pressure difference. This can create significant positional differences in PAP that affect blood flow in the lung in various positions, such as upright and lateral positions.

In zone 1, airway pressures exceed PAP and pulmonary venous pressures. Zone 1 therefore has no blood flow despite ventilation. Normally, zone 1 does not exist, but with positive-pressure ventilation or low PAP, as may occur under anesthesia or with blood loss, zone 1 may develop. In zone 2, airway pressure is more than pulmonary venous pressure, but it is not more than PAP. In zone 2, flow is proportional to the difference between PAP and airway pressure. In zone 3, PAP and venous pressure exceed airway pressure, and a normal blood flow pattern results (i.e., flow is proportional to the difference between PAP and venous pressure). Position can also be used therapeutically to decrease blood flow to abnormal areas of the lung, such as unilateral pneumonia, and thereby improve gas exchange. Blood flow through the collapsed lung during one-lung ventilation is also reduced by this physiologic effect.

## Pulmonary Edema

Intravascular fluid balance in the lung depends on hydrostatic driving forces. Excessive pulmonary capillary pressures cause fluid to leak into the interstitium and then into alveoli. Although the pulmonary lymphatic system is very effective in clearing fluid, it can be overwhelmed. Hydrostatic pulmonary edema is expected with high left ventricular filling pressures. Pulmonary edema occurs as PCWP exceeds 20 mm Hg, although patients may tolerate even higher pressures if these pressures persist chronically. Pulmonary edema can also occur with "capillary leak" from lung injury, such as acid aspiration of gastric contents, sepsis, or blood transfusion.

## PULMONARY GAS EXCHANGE

### Oxygen

Oxygen must pass from the environment to the tissues, where it is consumed during aerobic metabolism. Arterial hypoxemia is defined as a low partial pressure of oxygen in arterial blood ($Pa_{O_2}$). An arbitrary definition of arterial hypoxemia ($Pa_{O_2} < 60$ mm Hg) is commonly used but not necessary. Occasionally, arterial hypoxemia is used to describe a $Pa_{O_2}$ that is low relative to what might be expected based on the inspired oxygen concentration ($F_{IO_2}$). Arterial hypoxemia (which reflects pulmonary gas exchange) is distinguished from hypoxia, a more general term including tissue hypoxia, which also reflects circulatory factors.

Mild and even moderate arterial hypoxemia (e.g., at high altitude) can be well tolerated and is not usually associated with substantial injury or adverse outcomes. Anoxia, a nearly complete lack of oxygen, is potentially fatal and is often associated with permanent neurologic injury, depending on its duration. Arterial hypoxemia is most significant when anoxia is threatened, such as with apnea, and the difference between the two may be less than 1 minute.

#### Measurements of Oxygenation
Measurements of arterial blood oxygen levels include $Pa_{O_2}$, oxyhemoglobin saturation ($Sa_{O_2}$), and arterial oxygen content ($Ca_{O_2}$). $Pa_{O_2}$ and $Sa_{O_2}$ are related through the oxyhemoglobin dissociation curve (Fig. 5.5). Understanding the oxyhemoglobin dissociation curve is facilitated by the ability to measure continuous oxyhemoglobin saturation with pulse oximetry ($Sp_{O_2}$) and measurement of $Pa_{O_2}$ with arterial blood gas analysis.

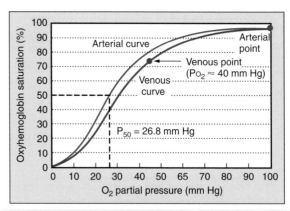

**Fig. 5.5** The oxyhemoglobin dissociation curve is S-shaped and relates oxygen partial pressure to the oxyhemoglobin saturation. A typical arterial curve is shown in red. The higher $Pco_2$ and the lower pH of venous blood cause a rightward shift of the curve and facilitate unloading of oxygen in the tissues (blue). Normal adult $P_{50}$, the $Po_2$ at which hemoglobin is 50% saturated, is shown (26.8 mm Hg). Normal $Pa_{O_2}$ of about 100 mm Hg results in an $Sa_{O_2}$ of about 98%. Normal $Pv_{O_2}$ is about 40 mm Hg, resulting in a saturation of about 75%.

| Table 5.2 | Events That Shift the Oxyhemoglobin Dissociation Curve | |
|---|---|---|
| **Left Shift** | **Right Shift** | |
| ($P_{50} < 26.8$ mm Hg) | ($P_{50} > 26.8$ mm Hg) | |
| Alkalosis | Acidosis | |
| Hypothermia | Hyperthermia | |
| Decreased 2,3-diphospho-glycerate (stored blood) | Increased 2,3-diphospho-glycerate (chronic arterial hypoxemia or anemia) | |

$P_{50}$, $Po_2$ value at which hemoglobin is 50% saturated with oxygen.

#### Oxyhemoglobin Dissociation Curve
Rightward and leftward shifts of the oxyhemoglobin dissociation curve provide significant homeostatic adaptations to changing oxygen availability. $P_{50}$, the $Po_2$ at which hemoglobin is 50% saturated with oxygen, is a measurement of the position of the oxyhemoglobin dissociation curve (see Fig. 5.5, Table 5.2). The normal $P_{50}$ value of adult hemoglobin is 26.8 mm Hg. Other points on the curve, such as the normal venous point and points for 80% and 90% oxygen saturations may also be clinically useful.

A rightward shift causes little change in conditions for loading oxygen (essentially the same $Sa_{O_2}$ at $Po_2$ of 100 mm Hg), but it allows larger amounts of oxygen to dissociate from hemoglobin in the tissues. This improves tissue oxygenation. Carbon dioxide and metabolic acid shift the oxyhemoglobin dissociation curve rightward, whereas alkalosis shifts it leftward. Fetal hemoglobin is

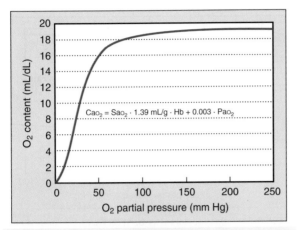

$$Ca_{O_2} = Sa_{O_2} \cdot 1.39 \text{ mL/g} \cdot Hb + 0.003 \cdot Pa_{O_2}$$

**Fig. 5.6** The relationship between $Pa_{O_2}$ and oxygen content is also sigmoidal, because most of the oxygen is bound to hemoglobin. Oxygen content at the plateau of the curve ($P_{O_2} > 100$ mm Hg) continues to rise because dissolved oxygen still contributes a small, but not negligible, quantity. *Hb*, Hemoglobin.

left shifted, an adaptation uniquely suited to placental physiology. Oxygen in arterial blood is bound to hemoglobin and dissolved in the plasma. The blood oxygen content is the sum of the two forms. Although amounts of dissolved oxygen are fairly trivial at normal $P_{O_2}$ levels, at high $F_{I_{O_2}}$ dissolved oxygen can be physiologically and clinically important. Although under normal conditions only a fraction (25%) of the oxygen on hemoglobin is used, all of the added dissolved oxygen added while giving supplemental oxygen can be used.

### Arterial Oxygen Content

$Ca_{O_2}$ is calculated based on $Sa_{O_2}$ and partial pressure plus the hemoglobin concentration (Fig. 5.6):

$$Ca_{O_2} = Sa_{O_2} (Hb \times 1.39) + 0.003 (Pa_{O_2})$$

In the equation, Hb is the hemoglobin level, 1.39 is the capacity of hemoglobin for oxygen (1.39 mL of $O_2$/g of Hb fully saturated), and 0.003 mL $O_2$/dL/mm Hg is the solubility of oxygen. For example, if Hb = 15 g/dL and $Pa_{O_2}$ = 100 mm Hg, resulting in nearly 100% saturation, the value of $Ca_{O_2}$ is calculated as follows:

$$Ca_{O_2} = 1.00 (15 \times 1.39) + 100 (0.003)$$
$$= 20.85 + 0.3$$
$$= 21.15 \text{ mL/dL}$$

Dissolved oxygen can continue to provide additional $Ca_{O_2}$, which can be clinically significant, with $F_{I_{O_2}}$ of 1.0 and with hyperbaric oxygen. The oxygen cascade depicts the passage of oxygen from the atmosphere to the tissues (Fig. 5.7).

### Multiwavelength Pulse Oximetry

Complete measurement of oxygen parameters are derived not just from analysis of arterial blood gases ($Pa_{O_2}$) but also from multiwavelength pulse oximetry. Oximetry provides measurement of methemoglobin (MetHb) and carboxyhemoglobin (COHb). Most blood gas machines are now combined with oximeters so that the $Sa_{O_2}$ provided is a true measured value, not calculated. This is called the *functional saturation*, which is the percent oxyhemoglobin saturation relative to hemoglobin available to bind oxygen. The *fractional saturation* is relative to all hemoglobin. Therefore, fractional saturation is the functional saturation minus MetHb and COHb. Newer pulse oximeters can now also measure MetHb and COHb.

### Determinants of Alveolar Oxygen Partial Pressure

The alveolar gas equation describes transfer of oxygen from the environment into the alveoli:

$$P_{A_{O_2}} = F_{I_{O_2}} \times (P_B - P_{H_2O}) - P_{C_{O_2}}/RQ$$

where $P_B$ is the barometric pressure, $P_{H_2O}$ is the vapor pressure of water (47 mm Hg at normal body temperature of 37° C), and RQ is the respiratory quotient (the ratio of carbon dioxide production to oxygen consumption). For example, while breathing 100% oxygen ($F_{I_{O_2}}$ = 1.0) at sea level ($P_B$ = 760 mm Hg) and the $P_{H_2O}$ = 47 mm Hg with $Pa_{CO_2}$ = 40 mm Hg, the alveolar $P_{O_2}$ ($P_{A_{O_2}}$) is calculated as follows. RQ is usually assumed to be approximately 0.8 on a normal diet.

$$P_{A_{O_2}} = 1.0 (760 - 47) - 40/0.8$$
$$= 713 - 50$$
$$= 663 \text{ mm Hg}$$

The alveolar gas equation describes the way in which inspired oxygen and ventilation determine $Pa_{O_2}$. It also describes the way in which supplemental oxygen improves oxygenation. One clinical consequence of this relationship is that supplemental oxygen can easily compensate for the adverse effects of hypoventilation (Fig. 5.8).

Low barometric pressure is a cause of arterial hypoxemia at high altitude. Modern anesthesia machines have safety mechanisms to prevent delivery of hypoxic gas mixtures. Nevertheless, death from delivery of gases other than oxygen is still occasionally reported because of errors in pipe connections made during construction or remodeling of operating rooms. Current anesthesia machines have multiple safety features to prevent delivery of hypoxic gas mixtures. Delivery of an inadequate $F_{I_{O_2}}$ may occur when oxygen tanks run out or with failure to recognize accidental disconnection of a self-inflating bag (Ambu) from its oxygen source.

Apnea is an important cause of arterial hypoxemia, and storage of oxygen in the lung is of prime importance in delaying the appearance of arterial hypoxemia in humans. Storage of oxygen on hemoglobin is secondary, because use of this oxygen requires significant oxyhemoglobin desaturation. In contrast to voluntary breath-holding, apnea during anesthesia or sedation occurs at functional residual capacity (FRC). This substantially

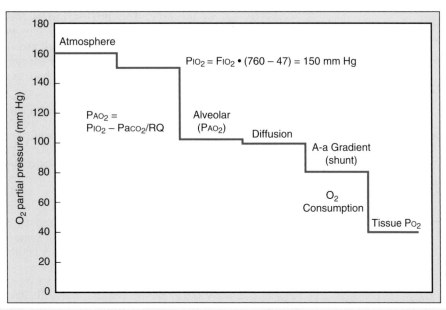

**Fig. 5.7** The oxygen cascade depicts the physiologic steps as oxygen travels from the atmosphere to the tissues. Oxygen starts at 21% in the atmosphere and is initially diluted with water vapor to about 150 mm Hg, $P_{IO_2}$. Alveolar $P_{O_2}$ ($P_{AO_2}$) is determined by the alveolar gas equation. Diffusion equilibrates $P_{O_2}$ between the alveolus and the capillary. The A-a (alveolar-to-arterial) gradient occurs with intrapulmonary shunt and ventilation to perfusion ($\dot{V}/\dot{Q}$) mismatch. Oxygen consumption then reduces $P_{O_2}$ to tissue levels (about 40 mm Hg).

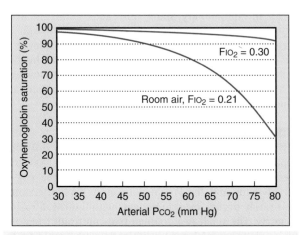

**Fig. 5.8** Hypoventilation decreases oxygenation, as determined by the alveolar gas equation. The blue curve shows what is expected for room air ($F_{IO_2} = 0.21$). High $Pa_{CO_2}$ further shifts the oxyhemoglobin dissociation curve to the right. However, as little as 30% oxygen can completely negate the effects of hypoventilation (red curve).

reduces the time to oxyhemoglobin desaturation compared with a breath-hold at total lung capacity.

The time can be estimated for $Sa_{O_2}$ to reach 90% when the FRC is 2.5 L and the $Pa_{O_2}$ is 100 mm Hg. Normal oxygen consumption is about 300 mL/min, although this is somewhat lower during anesthesia. It would take only about 30 seconds under these room air conditions to develop arterial hypoxemia. After breathing 100% oxygen, it might take 7 minutes to reach an $Sa_{O_2}$ of 90%. In reality, the time it takes to develop arterial hypoxemia after breathing 100% oxygen varies. Desaturation begins when sufficient numbers of alveoli have collapsed and intrapulmonary shunt develops, not simply when oxygen stores have become exhausted. In particular, obese patients develop arterial hypoxemia with apnea substantially faster than lean patients.

### Venous Admixture

Venous admixture describes physiologic causes of arterial hypoxemia for which $Pa_{O_2}$ is normal. The alveolar-to-arterial oxygen (A-a) gradient reflects venous admixture. Normal A-a gradients are 5 to 10 mm Hg, but they increase with age. For example, if the arterial $P_{O_2}$ while breathing 100% oxygen were measured as 310 mm Hg, the A-a gradient can be calculated from the previous example.

$$\begin{aligned} \text{A-a gradient} &= P_{AO_2} - Pa_{O_2} \\ &= 663 \text{ mm Hg} - 310 \text{ mm Hg} \\ &= 353 \text{ mm Hg} \end{aligned}$$

A picture of gas exchange can be accomplished mathematically by integrating all the effects of shunting, supplemental oxygen, and the oxyhemoglobin dissociation curve to create "isoshunt" diagrams (Fig. 5.9). Although calculating a shunt fraction may be the most exact way

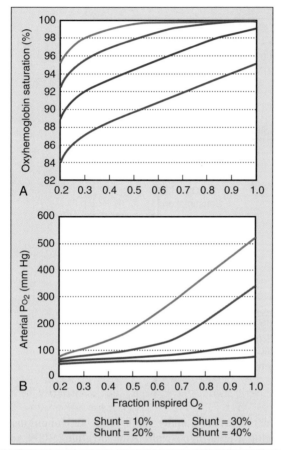

**Fig. 5.9** The effect of intrapulmonary shunting and $F_{IO_2}$ on $Pa_{O_2}$ (A) and $Sa_{O_2}$ (B) is shown graphically at shunt fractions from 10% (mild) to 40% (severe). Assumed values for these calculations are hemoglobin, 14 g/dL; $Pa_{CO_2}$, 40 mm Hg; arterial-to-venous oxygen content difference, 4 mL $O_2$/dL; and sea level atmospheric pressure, 760 mm Hg. Increased $F_{IO_2}$ still substantially improves oxygenation at high shunt fractions but is unable to fully correct it.

to quantitate problems in oxygenation, it requires information only available from a PA catheter and therefore is not always clinically useful. A-a gradients are clinically simpler and more useful to derive but do not represent a constant measurement of oxygenation with different $F_{IO_2}$ levels. A-a gradient is probably most useful in room air. The P/F ratio ($Pa_{O_2}/F_{IO_2}$) is a simple and useful measurement of oxygenation that remains more consistent at high $F_{IO_2}$ (Fig. 5.10).[11]

### Intrapulmonary Shunt
Intrapulmonary shunt is one of the most important causes of an increased A-a gradient and the development of arterial hypoxemia. In the presence of an intrapulmonary shunt, mixed venous blood is not exposed to alveolar gas, and it continues through the lungs to mix with oxygenated blood from normal areas

of the lung. This mixing lowers the $Pa_{O_2}$. Clinically, shunting occurs when alveoli are not ventilated, as with atelectasis, or when alveoli are filled with fluid, as with pneumonia or pulmonary edema. The quantitative effect of an intrapulmonary shunt is described by the shunt equation:

$$\dot{Q}s/\dot{Q}t = (Cc'o_2 - Cao_2)/(Cc'o_2 - C\bar{v}o_2)$$

In the equation, $\dot{Q}s/\dot{Q}t$ is the shunt flow relative to total flow (i.e., shunt fraction), C is the oxygen content, c′ is end-capillary blood (for a theoretical normal alveolus), a is arterial blood, and $\bar{v}$ is mixed venous blood.

### Ventilation-Perfusion Mismatch
Ventilation-perfusion ($\dot{V}/\dot{Q}$) mismatch is similar to intrapulmonary shunt ($\dot{V}/\dot{Q} = 0$), with some important distinctions. In $\dot{V}/\dot{Q}$ mismatch, disparity between the amount of ventilation and perfusion in various alveoli leads to areas of high $\dot{V}/\dot{Q}$ (i.e., well-ventilated alveoli) and areas of low $\dot{V}/\dot{Q}$ (i.e., poorly ventilated alveoli). Because of the shape of the oxyhemoglobin dissociation curve, the improved oxygenation in well-ventilated areas cannot compensate for the low $Po_2$ in the poorly ventilated areas, resulting in lower $Pa_{O_2}$ or arterial hypoxemia.

Clinically, in $\dot{V}/\dot{Q}$ mismatch, administering 100% oxygen can achieve a $Po_2$ on the plateau of the oxyhemoglobin dissociation curve even in poorly ventilated alveoli. Conversely, administering 100% oxygen in the presence of an intrapulmonary shunt only adds more dissolved oxygen in the normally perfused alveoli, although as seen in Fig. 5.9, this may result in more improvement in oxygenation than is often appreciated. Arterial hypoxemia remaining despite administration of 100% oxygen is always caused by the presence of an intrapulmonary shunt.

### Diffusion Impairment
Diffusion impairment is not equivalent to low diffusing capacity. For diffusion impairment to cause an A-a gradient, equilibrium has not occurred between the $Po_2$ in the alveolus and the $Po_2$ in pulmonary capillary blood. This rarely occurs, even in patients with limited diffusing capacity. The small A-a gradient that can result from diffusion impairment is easily eliminated with supplemental oxygen, making this a clinically unimportant problem. Clinically significant diffusion impairment can occur with exercise at extreme altitude, owing both to the smaller driving oxygen partial pressure and the limited time for equilibrium because of the rapid transit of blood through the pulmonary capillaries.

### Venous Oxygen Saturation
Low $S\bar{v}_{O_2}$ causes a subtle but important effect when intrapulmonary shunt is already present.[12] Shunt is a mixture of venous blood and blood from normal regions of the lungs. If the $S\bar{v}_{O_2}$ is lower, the resulting mixture must

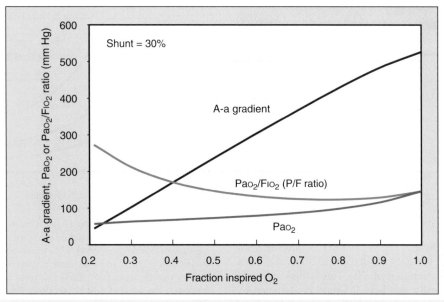

**Fig. 5.10** Despite a constant shunt fraction of 0.3 (30%), the A-a gradient is much higher at high $F_{IO_2}$, indicating problems in its usefulness as a measurement of oxygenation with different $F_{IO_2}$ values. The ratio of $Pa_{O_2}$ to $F_{IO_2}$ (the P/F ratio) is remarkably constant at high $F_{IO_2}$, making it a useful measurement of oxygenation when the gold standard, shunt fraction, is not available.

have a lower $Pa_{O_2}$. Low CO may lower $S\overline{v}_{O_2}$ significantly. This changes the way in which we interpret intrapulmonary shunt in different clinical conditions. For example, in sepsis, when the $S\overline{v}_{O_2}$ may be quite high, the shunt fraction may be higher than expected; high $S\overline{v}_{O_2}$ may be described as covering up a high shunt fraction.

## Carbon Dioxide

Carbon dioxide is produced in the tissues and removed from the lungs by ventilation. Carbon dioxide is carried in the blood as dissolved gas, as bicarbonate, and as a small amount bound to hemoglobin as carbaminohemoglobin. Unlike the oxyhemoglobin dissociation curve, the dissociation curve for carbon dioxide is essentially linear.

### Hypercapnia

Hypercapnia (i.e., high $Pa_{CO_2}$) may be a sign of respiratory difficulty or oversedation with opioids. Although hypercapnia itself may not be dangerous, $Pa_{CO_2}$ values greater than 80 mm Hg may cause $CO_2$ narcosis, possibly contributing to delayed awakening in the postanesthesia care unit. The greatest concern of hypercapnia is that it may indicate a risk of impending respiratory failure and apnea, in which arterial hypoxemia and anoxia can rapidly ensue. Although the presence of hypercapnia may be obvious if capnography is used, this monitor is not always available, and substantial hypercapnia may go unnoticed. Supplemental oxygen can prevent arterial hypoxemia despite severe hypercapnia, and an analysis

of arterial blood gases would not necessarily be performed if hypercapnia were not suspected (see Fig. 5.8).

The organ systems impacted by hypercapnia include the lungs (pulmonary vasoconstriction, right-shift of hemoglobin-oxygen dissociation curve), kidneys (renal bicarbonate resorption), central nervous system (somnolence, cerebral vasodilation), and heart (coronary artery vasodilation, decreased cardiac contractility).[13,14]

### Determinants of Arterial Carbon Dioxide Partial Pressure

$Pa_{CO_2}$ is a balance of production and removal. If removal exceeds production, $Pa_{CO_2}$ decreases. If production exceeds removal, $Pa_{CO_2}$ increases. The resulting $Pa_{CO_2}$ is expressed by an alveolar carbon dioxide equation:

$$Pa_{CO_2} = k \times \dot{V}_{CO_2} / \dot{V}_A$$

In the equation, k is a constant (0.863) that corrects units, $\dot{V}_{CO_2}$ is carbon dioxide production, and $\dot{V}_A$ is alveolar ventilation.

### Rebreathing

Because breathing circuits with rebreathing properties are frequently used in anesthesia, increased inspired $P_{CO_2}$ concentrations is a potential cause of hypercapnia. Exhausted carbon dioxide absorbents and malfunctioning expiratory valves on the anesthesia delivery circuit are possible causes of rebreathing in the operating room that are easily detected with capnography. Use of certain transport breathing circuits may be the most common cause of clinically significant rebreathing, which may be

**Box 5.2** Causes of Increased Carbon Dioxide Production

Fever
Malignant hyperthermia
Systemic absorption during laparoscopy procedures
(physiologically similar to increased production)
Thyroid storm
Tourniquet release
Administration of sodium bicarbonate

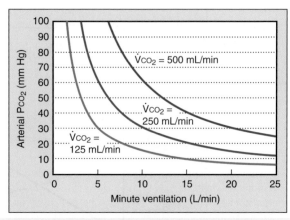

**Fig. 5.11** Carbon dioxide has a hyperbolic relationship with ventilation. The depicted curves are simulated with a normal resting carbon dioxide production (250 mL/min), low carbon dioxide production (125 mL/min, as during anesthesia), and increased carbon dioxide production (500 mL/min, as during moderate exercise). The value of physiologic dead space is assumed to be 30% in these calculations.

unrecognized because capnography is not routinely used during patient transport from the operating room.

### Increased Carbon Dioxide Production

Several important physiologic causes of increased carbon dioxide production may cause hypercapnia under anesthesia (Box 5.2). The anesthesia provider should not view $CO_2$ production in terms of cellular production but rather as the pulmonary excretion of $CO_2$. This is how it would be measured clinically and how it would be detected by the homeostatic mechanisms of the body. Other brief increases in $CO_2$ production may occur when administering sodium bicarbonate, which is converted into $CO_2$, or when releasing a tourniquet, where carbon dioxide has accumulated in the tissues of the leg and then returns to the circulation.

### Increased Dead Space

Dead space, or "wasted ventilation," refers to areas receiving ventilation that do not participate in gas exchange. Dead space is further categorized as anatomic, alveolar, and physiologic (total) dead space. Anatomic dead space represents areas of the tracheobronchial tree that are not involved in gas exchange. This includes equipment dead space, such as the endotracheal tube and tubing distal to the Y-connector of the anesthesia delivery circuit. Alveolar dead space represents alveoli that do not participate in gas exchange owing to lack of blood flow. Physiologic or total dead space represents the sum of anatomic and alveolar dead space. Most pathologically significant changes in dead space represent increases in alveolar dead space.

Dead space is increased in many clinical conditions. Emphysema and other end-stage lung diseases, such as cystic fibrosis, are often characterized by substantial dead space. Pulmonary embolism is a potential cause of significant increases in dead space. Physiologic processes that decrease PAP, such as hemorrhagic shock, can be expected to increase dead space (increased zone 1). Increased airway pressure and positive end-expiratory pressure (PEEP) can also increase dead space.

Quantitative estimates of dead space are described by the Bohr equation, which expresses the ratio of dead space ventilation ($\dot{V}_D$) relative to tidal ventilation ($\dot{V}_T$):

$$\dot{V}_D/\dot{V}_T = (Pa_{CO_2} - P\bar{E}_{CO_2})/Pa_{CO_2}$$

where $P\bar{E}_{CO_2}$ is the mixed-expired carbon dioxide.

For example, if the $Pa_{CO_2} = 40$ mm Hg and the $P\bar{E}_{CO_2} = 20$ mm Hg during controlled ventilation of the lungs, the $\dot{V}_D/\dot{V}_T$ can be calculated as follows:

$$\dot{V}_D/\dot{V}_T = (40 - 20)/40$$
$$= 20/40$$
$$= 0.5$$

Some physiologic dead space (25% to 30%) is considered normal because some anatomic dead space is always present. The $Pa_{CO_2} - P_{ET_{CO_2}}$ gradient is a useful indication of the presence of alveolar dead space. However, this gradient will change as $Pa_{CO_2}$ changes with hyperventilation or hypoventilation even when dead space is constant.

### Hypoventilation

Decreased minute ventilation is the most important and common cause of hypercapnia (Fig. 5.11). This may be due to decreased tidal volume, breathing frequency, or both. Alveolar ventilation ($\dot{V}_A$) combines minute ventilation and dead space ($\dot{V}_A = \dot{V}_T - \dot{V}_D$); however, it is more clinically useful to separate these processes. Ventilatory depressant effects of anesthetic drugs are a common cause of hypoventilation. Although increased minute ventilation can often completely compensate for elevated carbon dioxide production, rebreathing, or dead space, there is no physiologically useful compensation for inadequate minute ventilation.

If alveolar ventilation decreases by one half, $Pa_{CO_2}$ should double (see Fig. 5.11). This change occurs over several minutes as a new steady state develops. $CO_2$ changes during apnea are more complicated. During the first minute of apnea, $PaCO_2$ increases from a normal of 40 mm Hg to 46 mm Hg (the normal $PvCO2$).

This increase may be higher and more rapid in patients with smaller lung volumes or high arterial-to-venous carbon dioxide differences. After the first minute, $Paco_2$ increases more slowly as carbon dioxide production adds carbon dioxide to the blood, at about 3 mm Hg per minute.

### Differential Diagnosis of Increased Arterial Carbon Dioxide Partial Pressure

Increased $Paco_2$ values can be analyzed by assessing minute ventilation, capnography, and measuring an arterial blood gas value. Capnography can easily detect rebreathing. A clinical assessment of minute ventilation by physical examination and as measured by most mechanical ventilators should be adequate. Comparison of end-tidal $Pco_2$ with $Paco_2$ can identify abnormal alveolar dead space. Abnormal carbon dioxide production can be inferred. However, significant abnormalities of carbon dioxide physiology often are unrecognized when $Paco_2$ is normal, because increased minute ventilation can compensate for substantial increases in dead space and carbon dioxide production. Noticing the presence of increased dead space when minute ventilation is increased in volume and $Paco_2$ is 40 mm Hg is just as important as noticing abnormal dead space when the $Paco_2$ is 80 mm Hg and minute ventilation is normal.

## PULMONARY MECHANICS

Pulmonary mechanics concerns pressure, volume, and flow relationships in the lung and bronchial tree (Fig. 5.12). An understanding of pulmonary mechanics is essential for managing the ventilated patient. Pressures in the airway are routinely measured or sensed by the anesthesia provider delivering positive-pressure ventilation.

### Static Properties

The lung is made of elastic tissue that stretches under pressure (Fig. 5.13). Surface tension has a significant role in the compliance of the lung because of the air-fluid interface in the alveoli. Surfactant decreases surface tension and stabilizes small alveoli, which would otherwise tend to collapse.

The chest wall has its own compliance curve. At FRC, the chest wall tends to expand, but negative (subatmospheric) intrapleural pressure keeps the chest wall collapsed. The lungs tend to collapse, but they are held expanded due to the pressure difference from the airways to the intrapleural pressure. FRC is the natural balance point between the lungs tending to collapse and chest wall tending to expand.

### Dynamic Properties and Airway Resistance

Airway resistance is mainly determined by the radius of the airway, but turbulent gas flow may make resistance

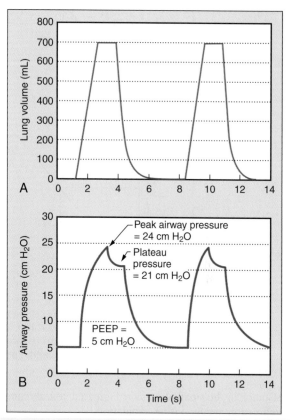

**Fig. 5.12** Lung volume is shown as a function of time (A) in a typical volume-controlled ventilator with constant flow rates. Lung volume increases at a constant rate during inspiration because of constant flow. Exhalation occurs with a passive relaxation curve. The lower panel (B) shows the development of pressure over time. Pressure is produced from a static compliance component (see Fig. 5.13) and a resistance component. If flow is held at the plateau, a plateau pressure is reached, where there is no resistive pressure component. In this example, peak airway pressure (PAP) is 24 cm $H_2O$, and positive end-expiratory pressure (PEEP) is 5 cm $H_2O$. Dynamic compliance is tidal volume (VT): (VT)/(PAP − PEEP) = 37 mL/cm $H_2O$. Plateau pressure (Pplat) is 21 cm $H_2O$, and static compliance is VT/(Pplat − PEEP) = 44 mL/cm $H_2O$.

worse. A number of clinical processes can affect airway resistance (Box 5.3). Resistance in small airways is physiologically different, because they have no cartilaginous structure or smooth muscle. Unlike capillaries, which have positive pressure inside to keep them open, small airways have zero (atmospheric) pressure during spontaneous ventilation. However, these airways are kept open by the same forces (i.e., pressure inside is greater than the pressure outside) that keep capillaries open. Negative pressure is transmitted from the intrapleural pressure through the structure of lung, and this pressure difference keeps small airways open. When a disease process, such as emphysema, makes pleural pressure less negative,

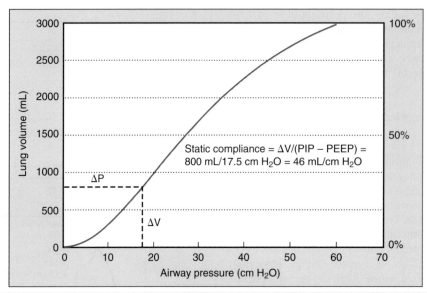

Static compliance = $\Delta V/(PIP - PEEP)$ = 800 mL/17.5 cm $H_2O$ = 46 mL/cm $H_2O$

**Fig. 5.13** A static compliance curve of a normal lung has a slight S shape. Slightly higher pressure can be required to open alveoli at low lung volumes (i.e., beginning of the curve), whereas higher distending pressures are needed as the lung is overdistended. Static compliance is measured as the change ($\Delta$) in volume divided by the change in pressure (inspiratory pressure [PIP] – positive end-expiratory pressure [PEEP]), which is 46 mL/cm $H_2O$ in this example.

resistance in the small airways is increased, and dynamic compression occurs during exhalation.

During positive-pressure ventilation, resistance in anesthesia breathing equipment or airways manifests as elevated airway pressures, because flow through resistance causes a pressure change. Distinguishing airway resistance effects from static compliant components is a useful first step in the differential diagnosis of high peak airway pressures. This is facilitated by anesthesia machines that are equipped to provide an inspiratory pause. During ventilation, airway pressure reaches a peak inspiratory pressure, but when ventilation is paused, the pressure component from gas flow and resistance disappears, and the airway pressure decreases toward a plateau pressure (see Fig. 5.12).

## CONTROL OF BREATHING

Anesthesia providers are in a unique position to observe ventilatory control mechanisms because most drugs administered for sedation and anesthesia depress breathing.

### Central Integration and Rhythm Generation

Specific areas of the brainstem are involved in generating the respiratory rhythm, processing afferent signal information, and changing the efferent output to the inspiratory and expiratory muscles.

---

**Box 5.3** Determinants of Airway Resistance

Radius of the airways
Smooth muscle tone
    Bronchospasm
    Inflammation of the airways (asthma, chronic bronchitis)
Foreign bodies
Compression of airways
Turbulent gas flow (helium a temporizing measure)
Anesthesia equipment

---

### Central Chemoreceptors

Superficial areas on the ventrolateral medullary surface respond to pH and $P_{CO_2}$. Carbon dioxide is in rapid equilibrium with carbonic acid and therefore immediately affects the local pH surrounding the central chemoreceptors. Although the signal is transduced by protons, not carbon dioxide directly, these chemoreceptors are described clinically as carbon dioxide responsive. The central chemoreceptors are protected from rapid changes in metabolic pH by the blood-brain barrier.

### Peripheral Chemoreceptors

Carotid bodies are the primary peripheral chemoreceptors in humans; aortic bodies have no significant role. Low $P_{O_2}$, high $P_{CO_2}$, and low pH stimulate the carotid bodies.[15] Unlike the central chemoreceptors, metabolic acids immediately affect peripheral chemoreceptors. Because of high

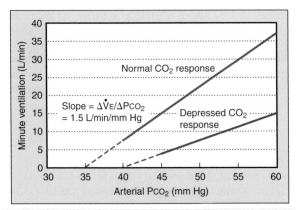

**Fig. 5.14** The hypercapnic ventilatory response (HCVR) is measured as the slope of the plot of $P_{CO_2}$ versus minute ventilation ($\dot{V}_E$). End-tidal $P_{CO_2}$ is usually substituted for $Pa_{CO_2}$ for clinical studies. The apneic threshold is the $P_{CO_2}$ at which ventilation is zero. It can be extrapolated from the curve, but it is difficult to measure in awake volunteers, although it is easy to observe in patients under general anesthesia. A depressed carbon dioxide response results from opioids, which lower the slope and raise the apneic threshold.

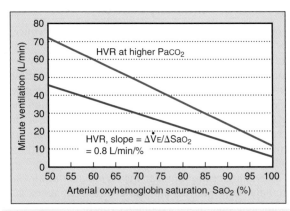

**Fig. 5.15** Hypoxic ventilatory response (HVR) expressed relative to $Sa_{O_2}$ is approximately linear, which is simpler than the curvilinear response expressed as a function of $Pa_{O_2}$. HVR is the slope of the linear plot. HVR is higher at higher carbon dioxide concentrations. Both absolute ventilation and the slope are shifted. Low $Pa_{CO_2}$ likewise lowers HVR.

blood flow, peripheral chemoreceptors are effectively at arterial, not venous, blood values.

## Hypercapnic Ventilatory Response

Ventilation increases dramatically as $Pa_{CO_2}$ is increased. In the presence of high $P_{O_2}$ values, most of this ventilatory response results from the central chemoreceptors, whereas in the presence of room air, about one third of the response results from peripheral chemoreceptor stimulation. The ventilatory response to carbon dioxide is moderately linear, although at $Pa_{CO_2}$ levels below resting values, minute ventilation does not tend to go to zero because of an "awake" drive to breathe (Fig. 5.14). At a high $Pa_{CO_2}$ value, minute ventilation is eventually limited by maximal minute ventilation.

Decreasing $Pa_{CO_2}$ during anesthesia, as produced by assisted ventilation, results in a point at which ventilation ceases, called the *apneic threshold*. As $CO_2$ rises, ventilation returns at the apneic threshold and then stabilizes at a $Pa_{CO_2}$ setpoint that is about 5 mm Hg higher.

The brainstem response to carbon dioxide is slow, requiring about 5 minutes to reach 90% of steady-state ventilation. When allowing the $Pa_{CO_2}$ to rise in an apneic patient, it may take a noticeably long time to stabilize minute ventilation, which is a direct consequence of the dynamics of the central ventilatory drive.

## Hypoxic Ventilatory Response

Ventilation increases as $Pa_{O_2}$ and $Sa_{O_2}$ decrease, reflecting stimulation of the peripheral chemoreceptors. The central response to hypoxemia actually results in decreased minute ventilation, called *hypoxic ventilatory decline* (HVD). The timing and combination of these effects mean that in prolonged arterial hypoxemia, ventilation rises to an initial peak, reflecting the rapid response of the peripheral chemoreceptors, and then decreases to an intermediate plateau in 15 to 20 minutes, reflecting the slower addition of HVD.

Although it is $P_{O_2}$ that affects the carotid body, it is easier to consider the hypoxic ventilatory response in terms of oxyhemoglobin desaturation because minute ventilation changes linearly with $Sa_{O_2}$ (Fig. 5.15). The effects of hypoxia and hypercapnia on the carotid body are synergistic. At high $Pa_{CO_2}$ levels, the response to hypoxia is much larger, whereas low $Pa_{CO_2}$ levels can dramatically decrease responsiveness. Unlike the hypercapnic ventilatory response, the response to hypoxia is rapid and takes only seconds to appear.

## Effects of Anesthesia

Opioids, sedative-hypnotics, and volatile anesthetics have dose-dependent depressant effects on ventilation and ventilatory control. Opioid receptors are present on neurons considered responsible for respiratory rhythm generation. Sedative-hypnotics work primarily on $\gamma$-aminobutyric acid A receptors ($GABA_A$), which provide inhibitory input in multiple neurons of the respiratory system. Volatile anesthetics decrease excitatory neurotransmission. All of these drugs exert most of their depressant effects in the central integratory area and therefore clinically appear to decrease the hypoxic and hypercapnic ventilatory responses similarly. Specific effects of drugs on peripheral chemoreceptors include the inhibitory effects of dopamine and the slight excitatory effects of dopaminergic blockers such as haloperidol.

## Disorders of Ventilatory Control

Neonates with a history of prematurity and of postconceptual age <60 weeks may have episodes of apnea after anesthesia. Likewise, sudden infant death syndrome may be a result of immature ventilatory control systems. Ondine's curse, originally described after surgery near the upper cervical spinal cord, results in profound hypoventilation during sleep and anesthesia due to abnormalities in the central integratory system that seem to blunt the hypoxic and hypercapnic ventilatory responses. Idiopathic varieties of Ondine's curse have occurred in children and are referred to as *primary central alveolar hypoventilation syndromes*. Morbidly obese patients and those with sleep apnea may exhibit abnormalities of ventilatory control.

Periodic breathing is commonly observed during drug-induced sedation. Mechanistically, this is most likely when peripheral chemoreceptors are activated by mild arterial hypoxemia. Continual overcorrection and undercorrection of the $Pa_{O_2}$ leads to oscillations of $Pa_{CO_2}$ and $Sa_{O_2}$. Periodic breathing is also common during sleep at higher altitudes.

## INTEGRATION OF THE HEART AND LUNGS

The interrelationship between the heart and lungs is suggested by the Fick equation, which relates oxygen consumption and oxygen needs at the tissue level:

$$\dot{V}_{O_2} = CO \times (Ca_{O_2} - C\bar{v}_{O_2})$$

where $\dot{V}_{O_2}$ is oxygen consumption, $Ca_{O_2}$ is the arterial oxygen content, and $C\bar{v}_{O_2}$ is the mixed venous oxygen content.

### Oxygen Delivery

Oxygen delivery ($Do_2$) is the total amount of oxygen supplied to tissues and is a function of CO and $Ca_{O_2}$:

$$Do_2 = CO \times Ca_{O_2}$$

$Do_2$ can be limited by decreases in CO or $Ca_{O_2}$. $Ca_{O_2}$ can be limited by anemia or hypoxemia.

### Oxygen Extraction

Different indices can be used to assess how much oxygen is removed from blood by tissues to meet their metabolic demand. Mixed venous oxygen saturation ($S\bar{v}_{O_2}$) is normally about 75%. If tissues extract more oxygen, $S\bar{v}_{O_2}$ decreases. However, with high $F_{I_{O_2}}$, $S\bar{v}_{O_2}$ may increase because of the added amount of dissolved oxygen, even though true extraction has not changed. The arteriovenous oxygen content difference ($Ca_{O_2} - C\bar{v}_{O_2}$) is independent of changes in $F_{I_{O_2}}$ and is therefore a useful measurement of the balance of oxygen supply and demand. On the other hand, the arteriovenous oxygen content difference decreases in anemia because extracting the same percentage of oxygen means extracting less total oxygen because of the lower hemoglobin concentration. The most reliable figure is the calculated oxygen extraction ratio:

$$O_2 \text{ extraction} = (Ca_{O_2} - C\bar{v}_{O_2})/Ca_{O_2}$$

### Anemia

An example of threatened oxygen supply is anemia. To adapt to anemia, the body can increase CO or extract more oxygen. The normal physiologic response is to increase CO and maintain $Do_2$. Increased HR and SV are responsible for this compensation. However, during anesthesia with a near-absent HR response, increased oxygen extraction is a more important mechanism of compensation.[16]

### Metabolic Demand

Increased oxygen consumption is usually met with a combination of increased CO and increased oxygen extraction. Whereas oxygen consumption is usually constant and relatively low under anesthesia, recovery from anesthesia may be associated with significant increases in metabolic demands. Shivering and early ambulation after outpatient surgery are stresses that may affect patients still recovering from anesthesia or after significant blood loss. Increased minute ventilation is required to meet increased oxygen needs and to eliminate the extra carbon dioxide produced.

## QUESTIONS OF THE DAY

1. What clinical conditions can lead to a low preload? How does systemic vascular resistance affect cardiac filling pressures?
2. What physiologic model can be used to describe changes in the pulmonary circulation? How do small and large lung volumes affect pulmonary vascular resistance?
3. How can the A-a gradient, PaO2 to FIO2 ratio, or isoshunt diagram be used to quantitate abnormalities of oxygenation? Which measurement of oxygenation depends the most on FIO2?
4. What are the determinants of arterial carbon dioxide partial pressure? What clinical conditions can cause hypercapnia during general anesthesia?
5. What is the physiologic basis for the hypercapnic ventilatory response and the hypoxic ventilatory response? What is the typical time course of these responses?

## REFERENCES

1. Berne RM, Levy MN. *Cardiovascular Physiology*. 8th ed. St. Louis: Mosby; 2001.
2. Nunn JF. *Nunn's Applied Respiratory Physiology*. 5th ed. Boston: Butterworth-Heinemann; 2000.
3. West JB. *Respiratory Physiology: The Essentials*. 8th ed. Philadelphia: Lippincott Williams & Wilkins; 2007.
4. Walsh M, Devereaux PJ, Garg AX, et al. Relationship between intraoperative mean arterial pressure and clinical outcomes after noncardiac surgery: toward an empirical definition of hypotension. *Anesthesiology*. 2013;119(3):507–515.
5. Monk TG, Bronsert MR, Henderson WG, et al. Association between intraoperative hypotension and hypertension and 30-day postoperative mortality in noncardiac surgery. *Anesthesiology*. 2015;123(2):307–319.
6. Willingham MD, Karren E, Shanks AM, et al. Concurrence of intraoperative hypotension, low minimum alveolar concentration, and low bispectral index is associated with postoperative death. *Anesthesiology*. 2015;123(4):775–785.
7. Gelman S. Venous function and central venous pressure. A physiologic story. *Anesthesiology*. 2008;108:735–748.
8. Michard F. Changes in arterial pressure during mechanical ventilation. *Anesthesiology*. 2005;103:419–428; quiz 449–445.
9. Topalian S, Ginsberg F, Parrillo JE. Cardiogenic shock. *Crit Care Med*. 2008;36:S66–S74.
10. Lumb AB, Slinger P. Hypoxic pulmonary vasoconstriction: physiology and anesthetic implications. *Anesthesiology*. 2015;122(4):932–946.
11. Feiner JR, Weiskopf RB: Evaluating Pulmonary Function: An Assessment of PaO2/FIO2. Crit Care Med. 2017;45:e40–48.
12. Shepherd SJ, Pearse RM. Role of central and mixed venous oxygen saturation measurement in perioperative care. *Anesthesiology*. 2009;111:649–656.
13. Weinberger SE, Schwartzstein RM, Weiss JW. Hypercapnia. *N Engl J Med*. 1989;321(18):1223–1231.
14. Crystal GJ. Carbon dioxide and the heart: physiology and clinical implications. *Anesth Analg*. 2015;121(3):610–623.
15. Weir EK, Lopez-Barneo J, Buckler KJ, et al. Acute oxygen-sensing mechanisms. *N Engl J Med*. 2005;353:2042–2055.
16. Weiskopf RB, Viele MK, Feiner J, Kelley S, Lieberman J, Noorani M, Leung JM, Fisher DM, Murray WR, Toy P, Moore MA: Human cardiovascular and metabolic response to acute, severe isovolemic anemia. JAMA. 1998;279:217–221.

II

# AUTONOMIC NERVOUS SYSTEM

Erica J. Stein and David B. Glick

The autonomic nervous system (ANS) is essential for survival and responsible for the body's involuntary activities such as cardiovascular, gastrointestinal, and thermoregulatory homeostasis. The ANS is divided into two major branches: the sympathetic nervous system (SNS), which controls the "fight or flight" responses, and the parasympathetic nervous system (PNS), which oversees the body's maintenance functions including digestion. Both disease states and the stress of surgery can lead to changes in the ANS that can have potentially deleterious effects. Thus, a primary goal of anesthetic management is to modulate the body's autonomic responses. Contemporary anesthesia providers have access to many pharmacologic drugs that can profoundly alter autonomic activity; thus, a thorough understanding of the anatomy and physiology of the ANS is essential.

## ANATOMY OF THE AUTONOMIC NERVOUS SYSTEM

### The Sympathetic Nervous System

The preganglionic fibers of the SNS originate from the thoracolumbar region (T1 to L2 or L3) of the spinal cord (Fig. 6.1). The cell bodies of these neurons lie in the spinal gray matter. The nerve fibers extend to paired ganglia, creating the sympathetic chains that lie immediately lateral to the vertebral column or extend to unpaired distal plexuses (e.g., the celiac and mesenteric plexuses). Preganglionic sympathetic fibers not only synapse at the ganglion of the level of their origin in the spinal cord but can also course up and down the paired ganglia. A sympathetic response, therefore, is not confined to the segment from which the stimulus originates, as discharge can be amplified and diffuse. The postganglionic neurons of the SNS then travel to the target organ. The sympathetic preganglionic fibers are relatively short because sympathetic ganglia are generally close to the central nervous system (CNS). In contrast, the postganglionic fibers run a long course before innervating effector organs (Fig. 6.2).

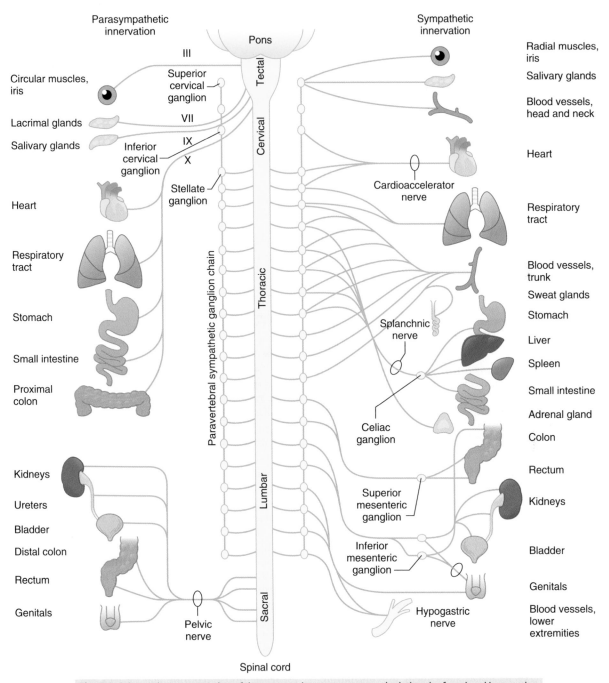

**Fig. 6.1** Schematic representation of the autonomic nervous system depicting the functional innervation of peripheral effector organs and the anatomic origin of peripheral autonomic nerves from the spinal cord. Although both paravertebral sympathetic ganglia chains are presented, the sympathetic innervation to the peripheral effector organs is shown only on the right side of the figure, whereas the parasympathetic innervation of peripheral effector organs is depicted on the left. The roman numerals on nerves originating in the tectal region of the brainstem refer to the cranial nerves that provide parasympathetic outflow to the effector organs of the head, neck, and trunk. (From Ruffolo R. Physiology and biochemistry of the peripheral autonomic nervous system. In Wingard L, Brody T, Larner J, et al, eds. *Human Pharmacology: Molecular to Clinical.* St. Louis: Mosby-Year Book; 1991:77.)

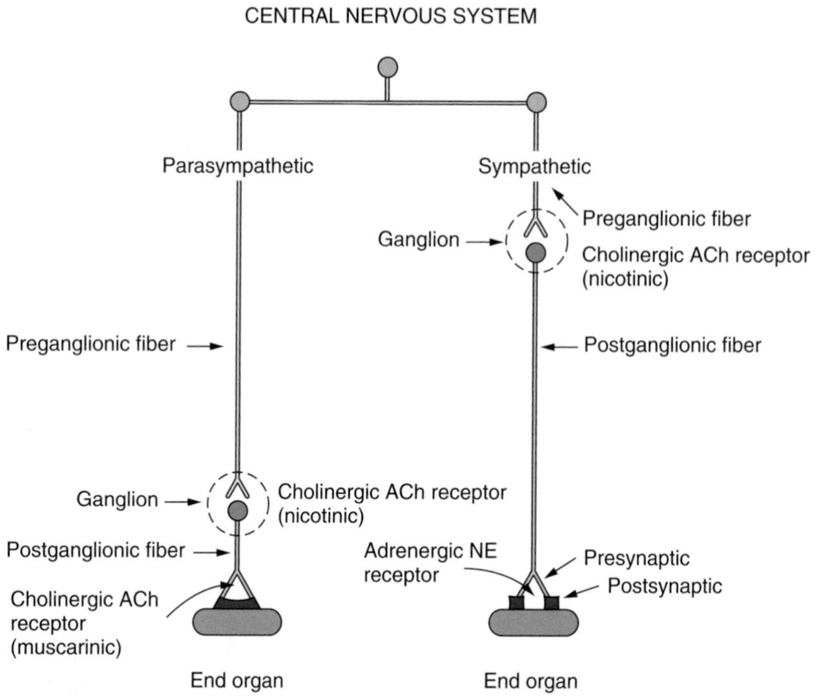

CENTRAL NERVOUS SYSTEM

**Fig. 6.2** Schematic diagram of the peripheral autonomic nervous system. Preganglionic fibers and postganglionic fibers of the parasympathetic nervous system release acetylcholine (ACh) as the neurotransmitter. Postganglionic fibers of the sympathetic nervous system release norepinephrine (NE) as the neurotransmitter (exceptions are fibers to sweat glands, which release ACh). (From Lawson NW, Wallfisch HK. Cardiovascular pharmacology: a new look at the pressors. In Stoelting RK, Barash J, eds. *Advances in Anesthesia*. Chicago: Year Book Medical Publishers; 1986:195-270.)

The neurotransmitter released at the terminal end of the preganglionic sympathetic neuron is acetylcholine (ACh), and the cholinergic receptor on the postganglionic neuron is a nicotinic receptor. Norepinephrine is the primary neurotransmitter released at the terminal end of the postganglionic neuron at the synapse with the target organ (Fig. 6.3). Other classic neurotransmitters of the SNS include epinephrine and dopamine. Additionally, co-transmitters, such as adenosine triphosphate (ATP) and neuropeptide Y, modulate sympathetic activity. Norepinephrine and epinephrine bind postsynaptically to adrenergic receptors, which include the $\alpha_1$-, $\beta_1$-, $\beta_2$-, and $\beta_3$-receptors. When norepinephrine binds to the $\alpha_2$-receptors, located presynaptically on the postganglionic sympathetic nerve terminal, subsequent norepinephrine release is decreased (negative feedback). Dopamine (D) binds to $D_1$ receptors postsynaptically or $D_2$ receptors presynaptically.

Sympathetic neurotransmitters are synthesized from tyrosine in the postganglionic sympathetic nerve ending (Fig. 6.4). The rate-limiting step is the transformation of tyrosine to dihydroxyphenylalanine (DOPA), which is catalyzed by the enzyme tyrosine hydroxylase. DOPA is then converted to dopamine and, once inside the storage vesicle at the nerve terminal, is $\beta$-hydroxylated to

norepinephrine. In the adrenal medulla, norepinephrine is methylated to epinephrine. The neurotransmitters are stored in vesicles until the postganglionic nerve is stimulated. Then the vesicles merge with the cell membrane and release their contents into the synapse (Fig. 6.5). In general, only 1% of the total stored norepinephrine is released with each depolarization; thus, there is a tremendous functional reserve. The released norepinephrine binds to the pre- and postsynaptic adrenergic receptors. The postsynaptic receptors then activate secondary messenger systems in the postsynaptic cell via G protein–linked activity. Norepinephrine is then released from these receptors and mostly taken up at the presynaptic nerve terminal and transported to storage vesicles for reuse. Norepinephrine that escapes this reuptake process and makes its way into the circulation is metabolized by either the monoamine oxidase (MAO) or catechol-O-methyltransferase (COMT) enzyme in the blood, liver, or kidney.

## The Parasympathetic Nervous System

The PNS arises from cranial nerves III, VII, IX, and X as well as from sacral segments S1-S4 (see Fig. 6.1). Unlike the ganglia of the SNS, the ganglia of the PNS are in

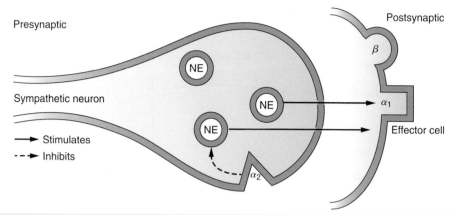

**Fig. 6.3** Schematic depiction of the postganglionic sympathetic nerve ending. Release of the neurotransmitter norepinephrine (NE) from the nerve ending results in stimulation of postsynaptic receptors, which are classified as $\alpha_1$, $\beta_1$, and $\beta_2$. Stimulation of presynaptic $\alpha_2$-receptors results in inhibition of NE release from the nerve ending. (Adapted from Ram CVS, Kaplan NM. Alpha- and beta-receptor blocking drugs in the treatment of hypertension. In Harvey WP, ed. *Current Problems in Cardiology.* Chicago: Year Book Medical Publishers; 1970.)

close proximity to (or even within) their target organs (see Fig. 6.2). Like the SNS, the preganglionic nerve terminals release ACh into the synapse, and the postganglionic cell binds the ACh via nicotinic receptors. The postganglionic nerve terminal then releases ACh into the synapse it shares with the target organ cell. The ACh receptors of the target organ are muscarinic receptors. Like the adrenergic receptors, muscarinic receptors are coupled to G proteins and secondary messenger systems. ACh is rapidly inactivated within the synapse by the cholinesterase enzyme. The effects of stimulating adrenergic and cholinergic receptors throughout the body are listed in Table 6.1.

## ADRENERGIC PHARMACOLOGY

### Endogenous Catecholamines

Table 6.2 summarizes the pharmacologic effects and therapeutic doses of catecholamines.

#### Norepinephrine

Norepinephrine, the primary adrenergic neurotransmitter, binds to $\alpha$- and $\beta$-receptors. It is used primarily for its $\alpha_1$-adrenergic effects that increase systemic vascular resistance. Like all the endogenous catecholamines, the half-life of norepinephrine is short (2.5 minutes), so it is usually given as a continuous infusion at rates of 3 µg/min or more and titrated to the desired effect. The increase in systemic resistance can lead to reflex bradycardia. Additionally, because norepinephrine vasoconstricts the pulmonary, renal, and mesenteric circulations, infusions must be carefully monitored to prevent injury to vital organs. Prolonged infusion of norepinephrine can

also cause ischemia in the fingers and toes because of the marked peripheral vasoconstriction.

#### Epinephrine

Like norepinephrine, epinephrine binds to $\alpha$- and $\beta$-adrenergic receptors. Exogenous epinephrine is used intravenously in life-threatening circumstances to treat cardiac arrest, circulatory collapse, and anaphylaxis. It is also commonly used locally to decrease the systemic absorption of local anesthetics and to reduce surgical blood loss. Among the therapeutic effects of epinephrine are positive inotropy, chronotropy, and enhanced conduction in the heart ($\beta_1$); smooth muscle relaxation in the vasculature and bronchial tree ($\beta_2$); and vasoconstriction ($\alpha_1$). The effects that predominate depend on the dose of epinephrine administered. Epinephrine also has endocrine and metabolic effects that include increasing the levels of blood glucose, lactate, and free fatty acids.

An intravenous dose of 1 mg can be given for cardiovascular collapse, asystole, ventricular fibrillation, pulseless electrical activity, or anaphylactic shock to constrict the peripheral vasculature and maintain myocardial and cerebral perfusion. In less acute circumstances, epinephrine can be given as a continuous infusion. The response of individual patients to epinephrine varies, so the infusion must be titrated to effect while the patient is monitored for signs of compromised renal, cerebral, or myocardial perfusion. In general, an infusion rate of 1 to 2 µg/min should primarily stimulate $\beta_2$-receptors and decrease airway resistance and vascular tone. A rate of 2 to 10 µg/min increases heart rate, contractility, and conduction through the atrioventricular node. When doses larger than 10 µg/min are given, the $\alpha_1$-adrenergic effects

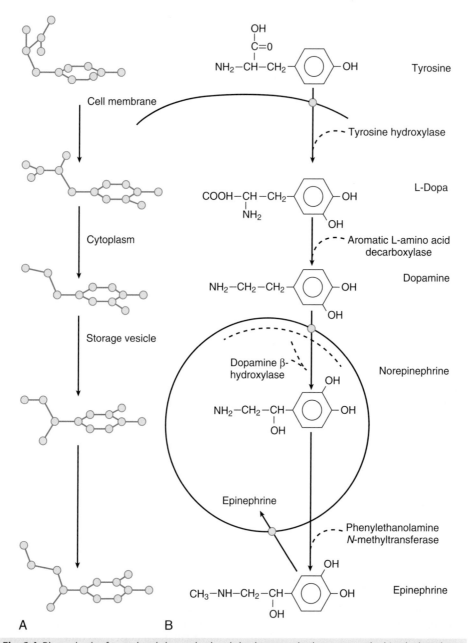

**Fig. 6.4** Biosynthesis of norepinephrine and epinephrine in sympathetic nerve terminal (and adrenal medulla). (A) Perspective view of molecules. (B) Enzymatic processes. (From Tollenaeré JP. *Atlas of the Three-Dimensional Structure of Drugs.* Amsterdam: Elsevier North-Holland; 1979, as modified by Vanhoutte PM. Adrenergic neuroeffector interaction in the blood vessel wall. *Fed Proc.* 1978;37:181.)

predominate, resulting in generalized vasoconstriction, which can lead to reflex bradycardia.

Epinephrine also can be administered as an aerosol to treat severe croup or airway edema. Bronchospasm is treated with epinephrine administered subcutaneously in doses of 300 µg every 20 minutes with a maximum of three doses. Epinephrine treats bronchospasm both via its direct effect as a bronchodilator and because it decreases

antigen-induced release of bronchospastic substances (as may occur during anaphylaxis) by stabilizing the mast cells that release these substances.

Because epinephrine decreases the refractory period of the myocardium, the risk of arrhythmias during halothane anesthesia is increased when epinephrine is given. The risk of arrhythmias seems to be less in children but increases with hypocapnia (also see Chapter 34).

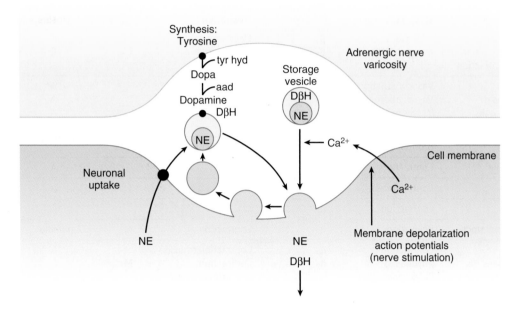

**Fig. 6.5** Release and reuptake of norepinephrine at sympathetic nerve terminals. *Solid circle,* Active carrier; *aad,* aromatic L-amino acid decarboxylase; *DβH,* dopamine β-hydroxylase; *Dopa,* L-dihydroxyphenylalanine; *NE,* norepinephrine; *tyr hyd,* tyrosine hydroxylase. (From Vanhoutte PM. Adrenergic neuroeffector interaction in the blood vessel wall. *Fed Proc.* 1978;37:181, as modified by Shepherd J, Vanhoutte P. Neurohumoral regulation. In Shepherd S, Vanhoutte P, eds. *The Human Cardiovascular System: Facts and Concepts.* New York: Raven Press; 1979:107.)

## Dopamine

In addition to binding to α- and β-receptors, dopamine binds to dopaminergic receptors. Besides its direct effects, dopamine acts indirectly by stimulating the release of norepinephrine from storage vesicles. Dopamine is unique in its ability to improve blood flow through the renal and mesenteric beds in shock-like states by binding to postjunctional $D_1$ receptors. Dopamine is rapidly metabolized by MAO and COMT and has a half-life of 1 minute, so it must be given as a continuous infusion. At doses between 0.5 and 2.0 μg/kg/min, $D_1$ receptors are stimulated and renal and mesenteric beds are dilated. When the infusion is increased to 2 to 10 μg/kg/min, the $\beta_1$-receptors are stimulated and cardiac contractility and output are increased. At doses of 10 μg/kg/min and higher, $\alpha_1$-receptor binding predominates and causes marked generalized constriction of the vasculature, negating any benefit to renal perfusion.

In the past, dopamine was frequently used to treat patients in shock. The belief was that infusions of dopamine, by improving renal blood flow, could protect the kidney and aid in diuresis. Subsequently, dopamine was not found to have a beneficial effect on renal function in shock states. Its routine use for patients in shock is questionable because it may increase mortality risk and the incidence of arrhythmic events.[1,2]

## Synthetic Catecholamines

### Isoproterenol

Isoproterenol (Isuprel) provides relatively pure and nonselective β-adrenergic stimulation. Its $\beta_1$-adrenergic stimulation is greater than its $\beta_2$-adrenergic effects. Its popularity has declined because of adverse effects such as tachycardia and arrhythmias. It is no longer part of the Advanced Cardiac Life Support protocols (also see Chapter 45), and its principal uses now are as a chronotropic drug after cardiac transplantation and to initiate atrial fibrillation or other arrhythmias during cardiac electrophysiology ablation procedures. With larger doses, isoproterenol may cause vasodilation due to $\beta_2$-adrenergic stimulation. Because isoproterenol is not taken up into the adrenergic nerve endings, its half-life is longer than that of the endogenous catecholamines.

### Dobutamine

Dobutamine, a synthetic analog of dopamine, has predominantly $\beta_1$-adrenergic effects. When compared with

| Table 6.1 | Responses Elicited in Effector Organs by Stimulation of Sympathetic and Parasympathetic Nerves | | | | |
|---|---|---|---|---|---|
| **Effector Organ** | **Adrenergic Response** | **Receptor Involved** | **Cholinergic Response** | **Receptor Involved** | **Dominant Response (A or C)** |
| Heart | Increase | $\beta_1$ | Decrease | $M_2$ | C |
| Rate of contraction | Increase | $\beta_1$ | Decrease | $M_2$ | C |
| Force of contraction | | | | | |
| Blood vessels | Vasoconstriction | $\alpha_1$ | | | A |
| Arteries (most) | Vasodilation | $\beta_2$ | | | A |
| Skeletal muscle | Vasoconstriction | $\alpha_2$ | | | A |
| Veins | | | | | |
| Bronchial tree | Bronchodilation | $\beta_2$ | Bronchoconstriction | $M_3$ | C |
| Splenic capsule | Contraction | $\alpha_1$ | | | A |
| Uterus | Contraction | $\alpha_1$ | Variable | | A |
| Vas deferens | Contraction | $\alpha_1$ | | | A |
| Gastrointestinal tract | Relaxation | $\alpha_2$ | Contraction | $M_3$ | C |
| Eye | Contraction | $\alpha_1$ | Contraction (miosis) | $M_3$ | A |
| Radial muscle, iris | (mydriasis) | $\beta_2$ | Contraction | $M_3$ | C |
| Circular muscle, iris | Relaxation | | (accommodation) | | C |
| Ciliary muscle | | | | | |
| Kidney | Renin secretion | $\beta_1$ | | | A |
| Urinary bladder | Relaxation | $\beta_2$ | Contraction | $M_3$ | C |
| Detrusor | Contraction | $\alpha_1$ | Relaxation | $M_3$ | A,C |
| Trigone and sphincter | | | | | |
| Ureter | Contraction | $\alpha_1$ | Relaxation | | A |
| Insulin release from pancreas | Decrease | $\alpha_2$ | | | A |
| Fat cells | Lipolysis | $\beta_1$ ($\beta_3$) | | | A |
| Liver glycogenolysis | Increase | $\alpha_1$ ($\beta_3$) | | | A |
| Hair follicles, smooth muscle | Contraction (piloerection) | $\alpha_1$ | | | A |
| Nasal secretion | Decrease | $\alpha_1$ | Increase | | C |
| Salivary glands | Increase secretion | $\alpha_1$ | Increase secretion | | C |
| Sweat glands | Increase secretion | $\alpha_1$ | Increase secretion | | C |

*A*, Adrenergic; *C*, cholinergic; *M*, muscarinic.
From Bylund DB. Introduction to the autonomic nervous system. In Wecker L, Crespo L, Dunaway G, et al, eds. *Brody's Human Pharmacology: Molecular to Clinical.* 5th ed. Philadelphia: Mosby; 2010:102.

isoproterenol, inotropy is more affected than chronotropy. It exerts less of a $\beta_2$-type effect than isoproterenol does and less of an $\alpha_1$-type effect than does norepinephrine. Unlike dopamine, endogenous norepinephrine is not released, and dobutamine does not act at dopaminergic receptors.

Dobutamine is potentially useful in patients with congestive heart failure (CHF) or myocardial infarction complicated by low cardiac output. Doses smaller than 20 µg/kg/min usually do not produce tachycardia. Because dobutamine directly stimulates $\beta_1$-receptors, it does not rely on endogenous norepinephrine stores for its effects and may still be useful in catecholamine-depleted states such as chronic CHF. However, prolonged treatment with dobutamine causes downregulation of $\beta$-adrenergic receptors. If given more than 3 days, tolerance and even tachyphylaxis may occur and can be avoided by intermittent infusions of dobutamine. However, there are no controlled trials demonstrating improved survival.[3]

**Table 6.2** Pharmacologic Effects and Therapeutic Doses of Catecholamines

| Catecholamine | Mean Arterial Pressure | Heart Rate | Cardiac Output | Systemic Vascular Resistance | Renal Blood Flow | Arrhythmogenicity | Preparation (mg/250 mL) | Intravenous Dose (µg / kg/min) |
|---|---|---|---|---|---|---|---|---|
| Dopamine | + | + | +++ | + | +++ | + | 200 (800 µg/mL) | 2-20 |
| Norepinephrine | +++ | − | − | +++ | − − − | + | 4 (16 µg/mL) | 0.01-0.1 |
| Epinephrine | + | ++ | ++ | ++ | − − | +++ | 1 (4 µg/mL) | 0.01-0.15 |
| Isoproterenol | − | +++ | +++ | − − | − | +++ | 1 (4 µg/mL) | 0.03-0.15 |
| Dobutamine | + | + | +++ | − | ++ | − | 250 (1000 µg/mL) | 2-20 |

+, Mild increase; + +, moderate increase; +++, marked increase; −, mild decrease; −−, moderate decrease; −−−, marked decrease.

## Fenoldopam

Fenoldopam is a selective $D_1$ agonist and potent vasodilator that enhances renal blood flow and diuresis. Because of mixed results in clinical trials, fenoldopam is no longer used for treatment of chronic hypertension or CHF. Instead, intravenous fenoldopam, at infusion rates of 0.1 to 0.8 µg/kg/min, has been approved for treatment of severe hypertension. Fenoldopam is an alternative to sodium nitroprusside with fewer side effects (e.g., no thiocyanate toxicity, rebound effect, or coronary steal) and improved renal function. Its peak effect takes 15 minutes.

## Noncatecholamine Sympathomimetic Amines

Most noncatecholamine sympathomimetic amines act at α- and β-receptors through both direct (binding of the drug by adrenergic receptors) and indirect (release of endogenous norepinephrine stores) activity. Mephentermine and metaraminol are rarely used currently, so the only widely used noncatecholamine sympathomimetic amine at this time is ephedrine.

## Ephedrine

Ephedrine increases arterial blood pressure and has a positive inotropic effect. Because it does not have detrimental effects on uterine blood flow in animal models, ephedrine became widely used as a pressor in hypotensive pregnant patients. However, phenylephrine is now the preferred treatment for hypotension in the parturient because of a decreased risk of fetal acidosis (also see Chapter 33). As a result of its $\beta_1$-adrenergic stimulating effects, ephedrine is helpful in treating moderate hypotension, particularly if accompanied by bradycardia. The usual dose is 2.5 to 10 mg given intravenously or 25 to 50 mg administered intramuscularly.

Tachyphylaxis to the indirect effects of ephedrine may develop as norepinephrine stores are depleted. In addition, although drugs with indirect activity are widely used as a first-line therapy for intraoperative hypotension, repeat doses of ephedrine administration in life-threatening events (instead of switching to epinephrine) may contribute to morbidity.[4]

## SELECTIVE α-ADRENERGIC RECEPTOR AGONISTS

### $\alpha_1$-Adrenergic Agonists

#### Phenylephrine

Phenylephrine (Neo-Synephrine), a selective $\alpha_1$-agonist, is frequently used for peripheral vasoconstriction when cardiac output is adequate (e.g., in the hypotension that may accompany spinal anesthesia). It is also used to maintain afterload in patients with aortic stenosis whose coronary perfusion is compromised by a decline in systemic vascular resistance. Given intravenously, phenylephrine has a rapid onset and relatively short duration of action (5 to 10 minutes). It may be given as a bolus of 40 to 100 µg or as an infusion starting at a rate of 10 to 20 µg/min. Larger doses, up to 1 mg, slow supraventricular tachycardia through reflex action. Phenylephrine is also a mydriatic and nasal decongestant. Applied topically, alone or in combination with local anesthetics, phenylephrine is used to prepare the nares for nasotracheal intubation.

### $\alpha_2$-Adrenergic Agonists

$\alpha_2$-Agonists are assuming greater importance as anesthetic adjuvants and analgesics. Their primary effect is sympatholytic. They reduce peripheral norepinephrine release by stimulation of prejunctional inhibitory $\alpha_2$-receptors. Traditionally, they have been used as antihypertensive drugs, but applications based on their sedative, anxiolytic, and analgesic properties are becoming increasingly common.

### Clonidine

Clonidine, the prototypical drug of this class, is a selective agonist for $\alpha_2$-adrenoreceptors. Its antihypertensive effects result from central and peripheral attenuation of sympathetic outflow. Clonidine withdrawal may precipitate a hypertensive crisis, so it should be continued throughout the perioperative period. A transdermal patch is available if a patient cannot take clonidine orally. If it is not continued perioperatively, arterial blood pressure should be monitored closely with ready ability to treat hypertension. Labetalol is used to treat clonidine withdrawal syndrome.

Although experience with $\alpha_2$-agonists as a sole anesthetic is limited (also see Chapter 8), these drugs can reduce the requirements for other intravenous or inhaled anesthetics as part of a general or regional anesthetic technique.[5] The results of a 2003 meta-analysis imply that perioperative use of clonidine and the other $\alpha_2$-agonists dexmedetomidine and mivazerol also decreased myocardial infarction and perioperative mortality rates in patients who had vascular surgery.[6] However, a more recent (2014) large randomized trial of perioperative clonidine did not show a reduction in death or nonfatal myocardial infarction within 30 days of noncardiac surgery.[7]

In addition to their use in the operative setting, $\alpha_2$-agonists provide effective analgesia for acute and chronic pain, particularly as adjuncts to local anesthetics and opioids. Epidural clonidine is indicated for the treatment of intractable pain, which is the basis for approval of parenteral clonidine in the United States as an orphan drug (also see Chapter 44). Clonidine also is used to treat patients with reflex sympathetic dystrophy and other neuropathic pain syndromes.

### Dexmedetomidine

Like clonidine, dexmedetomidine is highly selective for the $\alpha_2$-receptors. Its half-life of 2.3 hours and distribution half-life of less than 5 minutes make its clinical effect quite short. Unlike clonidine, dexmedetomidine is available as an intravenous solution in the United States. The usual dosing is an infusion of 0.3 to 0.7 μg/kg/h either with or without a 1-μg/kg initial dose given over 10 minutes.

In healthy volunteers, dexmedetomidine increases sedation, analgesia, and amnesia; it decreases heart rate, cardiac output, and circulating catecholamines in a dose-dependent fashion. The inhaled anesthetic-sparing, sedative, and analgesic effects demonstrated in preclinical and volunteer studies have been borne out in clinical practice. The relatively minor impact of $\alpha_2$-induced sedation on respiratory function combined with the short duration of action of dexmedetomidine has led to its use for awake fiberoptic endotracheal intubation.[8] Dexmedetomidine infusions for the perioperative management of obese patients with obstructive sleep apnea minimized the need for narcotics while providing adequate analgesia.[9]

## $\beta_2$-ADRENERGIC RECEPTOR AGONISTS

$\beta_2$-Agonists are used to treat reactive airway disease. With large doses the $\beta_2$-receptor selectivity can be lost, and severe side effects related to $\beta_1$-adrenergic stimulation are possible. Commonly used agonists include metaproterenol (Alupent, Metaprel), terbutaline (Brethine, Bricanyl), and albuterol (Proventil, Ventolin).

$\beta_2$-Agonists are also used to arrest premature labor (also see Chapter 33). Ritodrine (Yutopar) has been marketed for this purpose. Unfortunately, $\beta_1$-adrenergic adverse effects are common, particularly when the drug is given intravenously.

## $\alpha$-ADRENERGIC RECEPTOR ANTAGONISTS

$\alpha_1$-Antagonists have long been used as antihypertensive drugs, but their side effects, which include marked orthostatic hypotension and fluid retention, have made them less popular as other medications for controlling arterial blood pressure with more attractive side effect profiles have become available.

### Phenoxybenzamine

Phenoxybenzamine (Dibenzyline) is the prototypical $\alpha_1$-adrenergic antagonist (though it also has $\alpha_2$-antagonist effects). Because it irreversibly binds $\alpha_1$-receptors, new receptors must be synthesized before complete recovery. Phenoxybenzamine decreases peripheral resistance and increases cardiac output. Its primary adverse effect is orthostatic hypotension that can lead to syncope with rapid changes when patients move from the supine to standing positions. Nasal stuffiness is another effect. Phenoxybenzamine is most commonly used in the treatment of pheochromocytomas. It establishes a "chemical sympathectomy" preoperatively that makes arterial blood pressure less labile during surgical resection of these catecholamine-secreting tumors. When exogenous sympathomimetics are given after $\alpha_1$-blockade their vasoconstrictive effects are inhibited. Despite its irreversible binding to the receptor, the recommended treatment for a phenoxybenzamine overdose is an infusion of norepinephrine because some receptors remain free of the drug; vasopressin may also be effective in this setting.

### Prazosin

Prazosin (Minipress) is a potent selective $\alpha_1$-blocker that antagonizes the vasoconstrictor effects of norepinephrine and epinephrine. Orthostatic hypotension is a major problem with prazosin. Unlike other antihypertensive drugs, prazosin improves lipid profiles by lowering low-density lipid levels and raising the level of high-density lipids. The usual starting dose of prazosin is 0.5 to 1 mg given at bedtime because of the risk of orthostatic hypotension. Doxazosin (Cardura) and terazosin (Hytrin) have pharmacologic effects similar to those of prazosin but have longer pharmokinetic half-lives. Because of the high cost of phenoxybenzamine, these agents are being used with greater frequency for the preoperative preparation of patients with pheochromocytomas. However, because these agents provide competitive antagonism instead of permanent binding to the $\alpha$-receptors, modest intraoperative hypertensive episodes seem to be more common in these patients than in those who received phenoxybenzamine. Agents such as tamsulosin (Flomax) show selectivity for the $\alpha_{1A}$-receptor subtype and are effective in the treatment of benign prostatic hypertrophy without the hypotensive effects seen when the nonselective $\alpha_1$-blockers are used to treat this condition.

## Yohimbine

$\alpha_2$-Antagonists such as yohimbine increase the release of norepinephrine, but they have found little clinical utility in anesthesia.

## β-ADRENERGIC ANTAGONISTS

β-Adrenergic antagonists (i.e., β-blockers) are frequently taken by patients about to undergo surgery. Clinical indications for β-adrenergic blockade include ischemic heart disease, postinfarction management, arrhythmias, hypertrophic cardiomyopathy, hypertension, heart failure, migraine prophylaxis, thyrotoxicosis, and glaucoma. In patients with heart failure and reduced ejection fraction, β-blocker therapy has been shown to reverse ventricular remodeling and reduce mortality rate.[10] In the 1990s, a study by the Perioperative Ischemia Research Group demonstrated the value of initiating β-blockade perioperatively in patients at risk for coronary artery disease.[11] Study subjects given perioperative β-blockers had a markedly reduced all-cause 2-year mortality rate (68% survival rate in placebo group vs. 83% in atenolol-treated group). The presumed mechanism for this improved survival rate was a diminution of the surgical stress response by the β-blockers. These and other confirmatory findings led to tremendous political and administrative pressure to increase the use of β-blockers perioperatively. Subsequent studies, however, have questioned the value of perioperative β-blockade, including a large study of oral metoprolol started on the day of surgery and continuing for 30 days (POISE trial), which demonstrated increased

mortality rate in the β-blocker group.[12] A systematic review on perioperative β-blockade from the American College of Cardiology/American Heart Association (ACC/AHA) states that although perioperative continuation of β-blockade started 1 day or less before noncardiac surgery in high-risk patients prevents nonfatal myocardial infarctions, it increases the rate of death, hypotension, bradycardia, and stroke. In addition, there is insufficient data regarding continuation of β-blockade started 2 days or more before noncardiac surgery.[13] The 2014 ACC/AHA Guideline on Perioperative Cardiovascular Evaluation and Management of Patients Undergoing Noncardiac Surgery recommends that patients on chronic β-blocker therapy continue this therapy in the perioperative period, but β-blocker therapy should not be started on the day of surgery.[14] (Also see Chapter 13)

The most widely used β-adrenergic blockers in anesthetic practice are propranolol, metoprolol, labetalol, and esmolol because they are available as intravenous formulations and have well-characterized effects. The most important differences among these blockers are tied to cardioselectivity and duration of action. Nonselective β-blockers act at the $\beta_1$- and $\beta_2$-receptors. Cardioselective β-blockers have stronger affinity for $\beta_1$-adrenergic receptors than for $\beta_2$-adrenergic receptors. With $\beta_1$-receptor selective blockade, velocity of atrioventricular conduction, heart rate, and cardiac contractility decrease. The release of renin by the juxtaglomerular apparatus and lipolysis at adipocytes also decrease. With larger doses, the relative selectivity for $\beta_1$-receptors is lost and $\beta_2$-receptors are also blocked, with the potential for bronchoconstriction, peripheral vasoconstriction, and decreased glycogenolysis.

### Adverse Effects of β-Adrenergic Blockade

Life-threatening bradycardia, even asystole, may occur with β-adrenergic blockade, and decreased contractility may precipitate heart failure in patients with compromised cardiac function. In patients with bronchospastic lung disease, $\beta_2$-blockade may be fatal. Diabetes mellitus is a relative contraindication to the long-term use of β-adrenergic antagonists because warning signs of hypoglycemia (tachycardia and tremor) can be masked and because compensatory glycogenolysis is blunted. To avoid worsening of hypertension, use of β-blockers in patients with pheochromocytomas should be avoided unless α-receptors have already been blocked. Overdose of β-blocking drugs may be treated with atropine, but isoproterenol, dobutamine, or glucagon also may be required along with cardiac pacing to maintain an adequate rate of contraction.

Undesirable drug interactions are possible with β-blockers. The rate and contractility effects of verapamil are additive to those of β-blockers, so care must be taken when combining these drugs. Similarly, the combination of digoxin and β-blockers can have powerful effects on heart rate and conduction and should be used with special care.

## Specific β-Adrenergic Blockers

### Propranolol

Propranolol (Inderal, Ipran), the prototypical β-blocker, is a nonselective β-blocking drug. Because of its high lipid solubility, it is extensively metabolized in the liver, but metabolism varies greatly from patient to patient. Clearance of the drug can be affected by liver disease or altered hepatic blood flow. Propranolol is available in an intravenous form and was initially given as either a bolus or an infusion. Infusions of propranolol have largely been supplanted by the shorter-acting esmolol. For bolus administration, doses of 0.1 mg/kg may be given, but most practitioners initiate therapy with much smaller doses, typically 0.25 to 0.5 mg, and titrate to effect. Propranolol shifts the oxyhemoglobin dissociation curve to the right, which might account for its efficacy in vasospastic disorders.[15] Additionally, propranolol is commonly used in the treatment of hyperthyroidism to mitigate tachycardia that may result.

### Metoprolol

Metoprolol (Lopressor), a cardioselective β-adrenergic blocker, is approved for the treatment of angina pectoris and acute myocardial infarction. No dosing adjustments are necessary in patients with liver failure. The usual oral dose is 100 to 200 mg/day taken once or twice daily for hypertension and twice daily for angina pectoris. Intravenous doses of 2.5 to 5 mg may be administered every 2 to 5 minutes up to a total dose of 15 mg, with titration to heart rate and blood pressure.

### Labetalol

Labetalol (Trandate, Normodyne) acts as a competitive antagonist at the $\alpha_1$- and β-adrenergic receptors. Metabolized by the liver, its clearance is affected by hepatic perfusion. Labetalol may be given intravenously every 5 minutes in 5- to 10-mg doses or as an infusion of up to 2 mg/min. It can be effective in the treatment of patients with aortic dissection[16] and in hypertensive emergencies. Because vasodilation is not accompanied by tachycardia, labetalol has been given to cardiac patients postoperatively. It may be used to treat hypertension in pregnancy both on a long-term basis and in more acute situations.[17] Uterine blood flow is not affected, even with significant reductions in blood pressure[18] (also see Chapter 33).

### Esmolol

Because it is hydrolyzed by blood-borne esterases, esmolol (Brevibloc) has a uniquely short half-life of 9 to 10 minutes, which makes it particularly useful in anesthetic practice. It can be used when β-blockade of short duration is desired or in critically ill patients in whom the adverse effects of bradycardia, heart failure, or hypotension may require rapid withdrawal of the drug. Esmolol is cardioselective, and the peak effects of a loading dose are seen within 5 to 10 minutes and diminish within 20 to 30 minutes. It may be given as a bolus of 0.5 mg/kg or as an infusion. When used to treat supraventricular tachycardia a bolus of 500 μg/kg is given over 1 minute, followed by an infusion of 50 μg/kg/min for 4 minutes. If the heart rate is not controlled, a repeat loading dose followed by a 4-minute infusion of 100 μg/kg/min is given. If needed, this sequence is repeated with the infusion increased in 50-μg/kg/min increments up to 300 μg/kg/min. Esmolol is safe and effective for the treatment of intraoperative and postoperative hypertension and tachycardia. If continuous use is required, it may be replaced by a longer lasting cardioselective β-blocker such as metoprolol.

## CHOLINERGIC PHARMACOLOGY

In contrast to the rich selection of drugs to manipulate adrenergic responses, there is a relative paucity of drugs that affect cholinergic transmission. A small number of direct cholinergic agents are used topically for the treatment of glaucoma or to restore gastrointestinal or urinary function. The classes of drugs with relevance to the anesthesia provider are the anticholinergic agents (muscarinic antagonists) and the anticholinesterases.

## Muscarinic Antagonists

The muscarinic antagonists compete with neurally released ACh for access to muscarinic cholinoceptors and block ACh's effects. The results are faster heart rate, sedation, and dry mouth. With the exception of the quaternary ammonium compounds that do not readily cross the blood-brain barrier and have few actions on the CNS, there is no significant specificity of action among these drugs; they block all muscarinic effects with equal efficacy, although there are some quantitative differences in effect (Table 6.3).

In the era of ether anesthetics, a muscarinic antagonist was added to anesthetic premedication to decrease secretions and to prevent harmful vagal reflexes. This addition is less important with modern inhaled anesthetics. Preoperative use of these drugs continues in some pediatric and otorhinolaryngologic cases or when fiberoptic intubation is planned.

Atropine with its tertiary structure can cross the blood-brain barrier. Thus, large doses (1 to 2 mg) can affect the CNS. In contrast, because of the quaternary structure of the synthetic antimuscarinic drug glycopyrrolate (Robinul) it does not cross the blood-brain barrier. Glycopyrrolate has a longer duration of action than atropine and has largely

**Table 6.3**   Comparative Effects of Anticholinergics Administered Intramuscularly as Pharmacologic Premedication

| Effect | Atropine | Scopolamine | Glycopyrrolate |
|---|---|---|---|
| Antisialagogue effect | + | +++ | ++ |
| Sedative and amnesic effect | + | +++ | 0 |
| Increased gastric fluid pH | 0 | 0 | 0/+ |
| Central nervous system toxicity | + | ++ | 0 |
| Lower esophageal sphincter relaxation | ++ | ++ | ++ |
| Mydriasis and cycloplegia | + | +++ | 0 |
| Heart rate | ++ | 0/+ | + |

0, None; +, mild; ++, moderate; +++, marked.

replaced atropine for blocking the adverse muscarinic effects (bradycardia) of the anticholinesterase drugs that reverse neuromuscular blockade. Scopolamine also crosses the blood-brain barrier and can have profound CNS effects. The patch preparation of scopolamine is used prophylactically for postoperative nausea and vomiting, but it may be associated with adverse eye, bladder, skin, and psychological effects. The distortions of mentation (e.g., delusions or delirium) that can follow treatment with atropine or scopolamine are treated with physostigmine, an anticholinesterase that is able to cross the blood-brain barrier.

## Cholinesterase Inhibitors

Anticholinesterase drugs impair the inactivation of ACh by the cholinesterase enzyme and sustain cholinergic agonism at nicotinic and muscarinic receptors. These drugs are used to reverse neuromuscular blockade (see Chapter 11) and to treat myasthenia gravis. The most prominent side effect of these drugs is bradycardia. The commonly used cholinesterase inhibitors are physostigmine, neostigmine, pyridostigmine, and edrophonium. In addition to reversing the effects of neuromuscular blocking drugs by increasing the concentration of ACh at the

neuromuscular junction, cholinesterase inhibitors stimulate intestinal function or are applied topically to the eye as a miotic. One topical drug (echothiophate iodide) irreversibly binds cholinesterase and can interfere with the metabolism of succinylcholine (as the anticholinesterases impair the function of the pseudocholinesterase enzyme as well).

## QUESTIONS OF THE DAY

1. What are the cardiovascular, respiratory, endocrine, and metabolic effects of epinephrine? What are the expected cardiovascular effects of an intravenous epinephrine infusion as the dose increases?
2. How does the cardiovascular mechanism of action of phenylephrine differ from ephedrine?
3. What are the central nervous system, cardiovascular, and respiratory effects of dexmedetomidine infusion?
4. How does cardioselectivity and duration of action differ for the beta blockers available for intravenous use?
5. What are the most important differences in the side effect profile of the muscarinic antagonists atropine, glycopyrrolate, and scopolamine?

## REFERENCES

1. Holmes CL, Walley KR. Bad medicine: low-dose dopamine in the ICU. *Chest.* 2003;123:1266–1275.
2. DeBacker D, Aldecoa C, Nijimi H, et al. Dopamine versus norepinephrine in the treatment of septic shock: a meta-analysis. *Crit Care Med.* 2012; 40(3):725–730.
3. Krell MJ, Kline EM, Bates ER, et al. Intermittent, ambulatory dobutamine infusions in patients with severe congestive heart failure. *Am Heart J.* 1986;112:787–791.
4. Caplan RA, Ward RJ, Posner K, et al. Unexpected cardiac arrest during spinal anesthesia: a closed claims analysis of predisposing factors. *Anesthesiology.* 1988;68:5–11.
5. Maze M, Tranquilli W. Alpha-2 adrenergic agonists: defining the role in clinical anesthesia. *Anesthesiology.* 1991;74:581–605.
6. Wijeysundera DN, Naik JS, Beattie WS. Alpha-2 adrenergic agonists to prevent perioperative cardiovascular complications—a meta-analysis. *Am J Med.* 2003;114:742–752.
7. Devereaux PJ, Sessler DI, Leslie K, et al. Clonidine in patients undergoing noncardiac surgery. *N Engl J Med.* 2014;16:1504–1513.
8. Bergese SD, Khabiri B, Roberts WD, et al. Dexmedetomidine for conscious sedation in difficult awake fiberoptic intubation cases. *J Clin Anesth.* 2007;19:141–144.
9. Ramsay MA, Saha D, Hebeler RF. Tracheal resection in the morbidly obese patient: the role of dexmedetomidine. *J Clin Anesth.* 2006;18:452–454.
10. Florea VG, Cohn JN. The autonomic nervous system and heart failure. *Circ Res.* 2014;114:1815–1826.
11. Mangano DT, Layug EL, Wallace A, et al. Effect of atenolol on mortality and cardiovascular morbidity after noncardiac surgery. Multicenter Study of Perioperative Ischemia Research Group. *N Engl J Med.* 1996;335:1713–1720.
12. POISE Study Group. Effects of extended-release metoprolol succinate in patients undergoing non-cardiac surgery (POISE trial): a randomised controlled trial. *Lancet.* 2008;371:1839–1847.

13. Wijeysundera DN, Duncan D, Nkonde-Price C, et al. Perioperative beta blockade in noncardiac surgery: a systematic review for the 2014 ACC/AHA guideline on perioperative cardiovascular evaluation and management of patients undergoing noncardiac surgery. *J Am Coll Cardiol.* 2014;64:2406–2425.

14. Fleisher LA, Fleischmann KE, Auerbach AD, et al. ACC/AHA guideline on perioperative cardiovascular evaluation and management of patients undergoing noncardiac surgery: a report of the American College of Cardiology/American Heart Association Task Force on practice guidelines. *J Am Coll Cardiol.* 2014;64:e77–e137.

15. Pendleton RG, Newman DJ, Sherman SS, et al. Effect of propranolol upon the hemoglobin-oxygen dissociation curve. *J Pharmacol Exp Ther.* 1972;180:647–656.

16. DeSanctis RW, Doroghazi RM, Austen WG, et al. Aortic dissection. *N Engl J Med.* 1987;317:1060–1067.

17. Lavies NG, Meiklejohn BH, May AE, et al. Hypertensive and catecholamine response to tracheal intubations in patients with pregnancy-induced hypertension. *Br J Anaesth.* 1989;63:429–434.

18. Jouppila P, Kirkinen P, Koivula A, et al. Labetalol does not alter the placental and fetal blood flow or maternal prostanoids in pre-eclampsia. *Br J Obstet Gynaecol.* 1986;93:543–547.

# 7 INHALED ANESTHETICS

## Rachel Eshima McKay

## HISTORY

The discovery of inhaled anesthesia reflects the contributions of clinicians and scientists in the United States and England (Fig. 7.1).[1] The most commonly used inhaled anesthetics in modern anesthesia include volatile liquids (i.e., halothane, enflurane, isoflurane, desflurane, and sevoflurane) and a single gas (i.e., nitrous oxide) (Figs. 7.2 and 7.3). Halothane, enflurane, and isoflurane are no longer commonly used. Yet, none of these inhaled anesthetics meets all the criteria of an "ideal" inhaled anesthetic, and the chemical characteristics differ among the drugs (Table 7.1).

## THE FIRST INHALED ANESTHETICS

### Nitrous Oxide

Nitrous oxide gas was first synthesized in 1772 by the English chemist, author, and Unitarian minister Joseph Priestley. Twenty-seven years later, Sir Humphry Davy administered nitrous oxide for dental analgesia. Although he suspected that nitrous oxide might be used to relieve pain for surgery, it was not until it was used 42 years later by a 29-year-old dentist named Horace Wells who administered nitrous oxide to himself and found that it relieved his pain. Specifically, he noticed the hypnotic and analgesic effects of nitrous oxide at a public exhibition in Hartford, Connecticut, in 1842. The next day, Wells himself underwent a dental extraction by a fellow dentist. Wells felt only minimal pain with the extraction, and he subsequently learned the method of nitrous oxide synthesis to make it available to his own

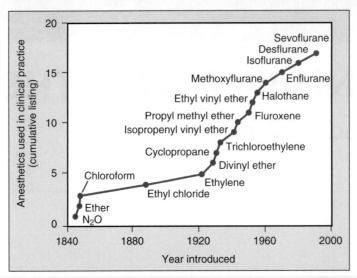

**Fig. 7.1** Anesthetics used in clinical practice. The history of anesthesia began with the introduction of nitrous oxide ($N_2O$), ether, and chloroform. After 1950, all introduced drugs, with the exception of ethyl vinyl ether, have contained fluorine. All anesthetics introduced beginning with halothane have been nonflammable. (From Eger EI. *Desflurane (Suprane): A Compendium and Reference.* Nutley, NJ: Anaquest; 1993:1-11, used with permission.)

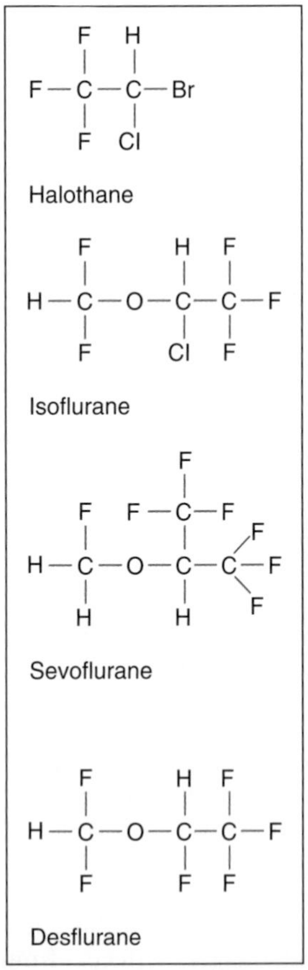

**Fig. 7.2** Molecular structures of potent volatile anesthetics. Halogenated volatile anesthetics are liquids at room temperature. Among the volatile anesthetics, halothane is an alkane derivative, whereas all the others are derivatives of methyl ethyl ether. Isoflurane is the chemical isomer of enflurane.

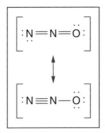

**Fig. 7.3** Molecular structure of nitrous oxide. Nitrous oxide is a linear molecule existing in two resonance structures. Dots denote nonbonding electrons.

patients. Two years later, he arranged to demonstrate painless dental surgery using nitrous oxide administration at the Massachusetts General Hospital. Not being completely successful, Wells was discredited as a result of this demonstration.

## Diethyl Ether

William Morton, a Boston dentist, noticed that diethyl ether, during "ether frolics" in which ether was breathed for its inebriating effects, had similar effects as nitrous oxide. Like Wells, Morton applied ether in his dental practice and then demonstrated its anesthetic properties at the Massachusetts General Hospital on October 16, 1846 ("ether day"). In contrast to Wells's debacle, Morton's demonstration was received with great enthusiasm. The results of successful ether anesthetics were soon published in the *Boston Medical and Surgical Journal.* Although Crawford Long administered diethyl ether to a patient in 1842, 4 years earlier than Morton, he did not

**Table 7.1**   Comparative Characteristics of Inhaled Anesthetics

| Characteristic | Isoflurane | Enflurane | Halothane | Desflurane | Sevoflurane | Nitrous Oxide |
|---|---|---|---|---|---|---|
| Partition coefficient | | | | | | |
| Blood-gas | 1.46 | 1.9 | 2.54 | 0.45 | 0.65 | 0.46 |
| Brain-blood | 1.6 | 1.5 | 1.9 | 1.3 | 1.7 | 1.1 |
| Muscle-blood | 2.9 | 1.7 | 3.4 | 2.0 | 3.1 | 1.2 |
| Fat-blood | 45 | 36 | 51 | 27 | 48 | 2.3 |
| MAC (age 30-55 years) % of 1 atmosphere | 1.15 | 1.63 | 0.76 | 6.0 | 1.85 | 104 |
| Vapor pressure at 20° C (mm Hg) | 240 | 172 | 244 | 669 | 160 | |
| Molecular weight (g) | 184.5 | 184.5 | 197.4 | 168 | 200 | 44 |
| Stable in hydrated $CO_2$ absorbent | Yes | Yes | No[a] | Yes | No[a] | Yes |
| Stable in dehydrated $CO_2$ absorbent | No | | No[ab] | No[b] | No[abc] | Yes |
| Percent metabolized | 0-0.2 | | 15-40 | 0-0.2 | 5-8 | |

[a]Compound A.
[b]Carbon monoxide.
[c]Severe exothermic reactions reported.
*MAC,* Minimum alveolar concentration.

publicize his work, and Morton therefore has traditionally been credited with the discovery of diethyl ether's capability to produce anesthesia.

## Chloroform

James Simpson, an obstetrician from Edinburgh, Scotland, developed chloroform, which did not share the protracted induction, flammability, and postoperative nausea seen with diethyl ether. Chloroform soon became popular as an inhaled anesthetic in England, although diethyl ether dominated medical practice in North America. Unfortunately, chloroform was associated with several unexplained intraoperative deaths of otherwise healthy patients and numerous cases of hepatotoxicity.

## INHALED ANESTHETICS BETWEEN 1920 AND 1940

Between 1920 and 1940, ethylene, cyclopropane, and divinyl ether were introduced into use as anesthetics, gaining acceptance over the older inhaled anesthetics (with the exception of nitrous oxide) by producing a faster, more pleasant induction of anesthesia and by allowing faster awakening at the conclusion of surgery. However, each had serious drawbacks. Many were flammable (i.e., diethyl ether, divinyl ether, ethylene, and cyclopropane), whereas others, halogenated entirely with chlorine, were toxic (i.e., chloroform, ethyl chloride, and trichloroethylene).

## FLUORINE CHEMISTRY AND MODERN INHALED ANESTHETICS

Techniques of fluorine chemistry, developed from efforts to produce the first atomic weapons, found a fortuitous, socially beneficial purpose in providing a method of synthesizing modern inhaled anesthetics.[2,3] Modern inhaled anesthetics are halogenated partly or entirely with fluorine (see Fig. 7.2). Fluorination provides greater stability and lesser toxicity.

## Halothane

Halothane was introduced into clinical practice in 1956 and became widely used. It had several advantages compared with the older anesthetics, including nonflammability, a pleasant odor, lesser organ toxicity, and pharmacokinetic properties allowing a much faster induction of anesthesia and emergence compared with ether. Unfortunately after 4 years of commercial use, reports of fulminant hepatic necrosis after halothane anesthesia began to appear in patients in which other causes of liver damage were not evident. The issue of unpredictable liver damage stimulated the search for other volatile anesthetics. Halothane also sensitizes the myocardium to the dysrhythmogenic effects of catecholamines.

## Methoxyflurane

Methoxyflurane was first introduced into clinical practice in 1960. Within the first decade of its introduction, reports of renal failure with methoxyflurane anesthesia appeared, leading to studies confirming a dose-related nephrotoxicity because of the inorganic fluoride that resulted from the metabolism of this anesthetic.

## Enflurane

Enflurane was introduced to clinical practice in 1972. Unlike halothane, it did not sensitize the heart to catecholamines and was not associated with hepatotoxicity. However, enflurane was metabolized to inorganic fluoride and could cause evidence of seizure activity on the electroencephalogram (EEG), especially when administered at high concentrations and in the presence of hypocapnia.

## Isoflurane

Isoflurane was introduced into clinical practice in 1980 and was widely used clinically. It was not associated with cardiac dysrhythmias. Because it is not metabolized as readily as halothane and enflurane, isoflurane was associated with less toxicity. Isoflurane allowed a more rapid onset of surgical anesthesia and faster awakening compared with its predecessors.

## Sevoflurane and Desflurane

Sevoflurane and desflurane are halogenated exclusively with fluorine and were first synthesized during the late 1960s and 1970s, respectively.[2,3] Both were expensive and difficult to synthesize and were therefore not immediately considered for commercial use. In the 1980s, their development was reconsidered in light of a new appreciation that a growing proportion of anesthetic practice was taking place in the outpatient setting and that drugs halogenated exclusively with fluorine were less soluble in blood and tissues, allowing faster awakening and recovery (see Fig. 7.1 and Table 7.1 and Box 7.1) (also see Chapter 37).

## MECHANISM OF ACTION

The question of how inhaled anesthetics produce the anesthetic state may be addressed at many levels of biologic organization, including their location of action within the central nervous system, the molecules with which they interact, and the nature of this biologic interaction. Answering these questions requires an ability to measure anesthetic

effects.[4] Although inhaled anesthetics have been used to provide surgical anesthesia for almost 160 years, there is no single, accepted definition of what constitutes the anesthetic state. For experimental purposes, an operational definition of immobility in response to surgical stimulation and amnesia for intraoperative events has proved useful.

## Measurable Characteristics

Measurable and universal characteristics of all inhaled anesthetics include production of *immobility* and *amnestic effects*. Immobility is measured by the minimum alveolar concentration (MAC) of anesthetic required to suppress movement to a surgical incision in 50% of patients (see Box 7.1).[2,5] However, the presence of amnesia or awareness

---

**Box 7.1** Factors That Increase or Decrease Anesthetic Requirements

**Factors Increasing MAC**
*Drugs*
  Amphetamine (acute use)
  Cocaine
  Ephedrine
  Ethanol (chronic use)

*Age*
  Highest at age 6 months

*Electrolytes*
  Hypernatremia
  Hyperthermia

*Red Hair*

**Factors Decreasing MAC**
*Drugs*
  Propofol
  Etomidate
  Barbiturates
  Benzodiazepines
  Ketamine
  $\alpha_2$-Agonists (clonidine, dexmedetomidine)
  Ethanol (acute use)
  Local anesthetics
  Opioids
  Amphetamines (chronic use)
  Lithium
  Verapamil

*Age*
  Elderly patients

*Electrolyte Disturbance*
  Hyponatremia

*Other Factors*
  Anemia (hemoglobin < 5 g/dL)
  Hypercarbia
  Hypothermia
  Hypoxia
  Pregnancy

*MAC,* Minimum alveolar concentration.

is difficult to assure (also see Chapters 20 and 47). Although *analgesia* is part of the anesthetic state, it also cannot be measured in an immobile patient who cannot remember. Surrogate measures of pain (i.e., increased heart rate or systemic arterial blood pressure) suggest that inhaled anesthetics do not suppress the perception of painful stimuli. Some inhaled anesthetics have hyperalgesic (pain-enhancing) effects in small concentrations. *Skeletal muscle relaxation* is a common, but not universal, central effect of inhaled anesthetics, as evidenced by nitrous oxide, which increases skeletal muscle tone.

### Immobility

Potent inhaled anesthetics produce immobility mostly by their actions on the spinal cord, as evidenced by determination of MAC in decerebrate animals.[6] Studies in rodents suggest that nitrous oxide activates descending noradrenergic pathways originating in the periaqueductal gray matter brainstem, which in turn inhibit nociceptive input in the dorsal horn of the spinal cord.[7,8]

### Amnestic Effects (Also See Chapter 47)

Supraspinal structures such as the amygdala, hippocampus, and cortex are considered highly probable targets for the amnestic effects of anesthetics.

### Central Nervous System Depression and Ion Channels

Inhaled anesthetics produce central nervous system depression by their actions on ion channels, which govern the electrical behavior of the nervous system.[4] Inhaled anesthetics probably produce anesthesia by enhancing the function of inhibitory ion channels and by blocking the function of excitatory ion channels. Enhancing the function of inhibitory ion channels leads to hyperpolarization of the neuron. Hyperpolarization results when chloride anions enter neurons through $\gamma$-aminobutyric acid A (GABA$_A$) receptors or glycine receptors or when there is an efflux of potassium cations out of neurons through potassium ion channels. Blocking the function of excitatory ion channels prevents depolarization of the neuron by preventing the passage of positive charges into the neuron (i.e., passage of sodium ions through *N*-methyl-D-aspartate [NMDA] receptors or sodium channels). Anesthetics may also affect the release of neurotransmitters, and this effect may be mediated in part by ion channels that regulate the release of neurotransmitters.

## PHYSICAL PROPERTIES

## Molecular Structure

Modern inhaled anesthetics, with the exception of nitrous oxide, are halogenated hydrocarbons (see Figs. 7.2 and 7.3). Halothane lacks the ether moiety present on isoflurane, sevoflurane, and desflurane, accounting for its capability to produce ventricular cardiac dysrhythmias.

Isoflurane and desflurane differ only by the substitution of one chlorine atom for fluorine. Fluorine substitution confers greater stability and resistance to metabolism.

## Vapor Pressure and Delivery

Nitrous oxide exists as a gas at ambient temperature, although it becomes a liquid at higher pressures. The remaining inhaled anesthetics are liquids at ambient temperatures.

### Variable-Bypass Vaporizers (Also See Chapter 15)

Halothane, sevoflurane, and isoflurane are delivered by variable-bypass vaporizers (Tec 4, 5, and 7; North American Draeger 19.n and 20.n). The variable-bypass vaporizer contains two streams of inflowing fresh gas—one contacting a reservoir (sump) of liquid anesthetic and the other bypassing the sump. The stream of gas traversing the sump becomes saturated with anesthetic as governed by the anesthetic's saturated vapor pressure. Because the volatile anesthetics produce clinically useful anesthesia at partial pressures far below that of their saturated vapor pressure, the gas exiting the sump must be diluted by gas that has not come into contact with anesthetic. The concentration of anesthetic in the gas exiting the vaporizer is determined by the relative flow (i.e., splitting ratio) of fresh gas through the sump channel versus the bypass channel. Control of anesthetic output concentration exiting the vaporizer occurs when the clinician adjusts the vaporizer dial or electronic control. Variable-bypass vaporizers are temperature compensated, maintaining constant output over a wide range of temperatures, and are calibrated for each individual anesthetic according to its differing vapor pressure (see Table 7.1). Tilting or overfilling of a vaporizer can potentially lead to delivery of an overdose of anesthetic if anesthetic vapor gets into the bypass channel.

The Datex-Ohmeda Aladin Cassette Vaporizer, used in the Datex-Ohmeda Anesthesia Delivery Unit (ADU) machines, is a single electronically controlled vaporizer with its bypass housed within the ADU and the sump located within interchangeable, magnetically coded cassettes for delivery of halothane, enflurane, isoflurane, sevoflurane, and desflurane. The Aladin utilizes variable bypass as a means of regulating output concentration, doing so via activity of a central processing unit (CPU). The CPU receives input from multiple sources, including the concentration setting, flowmeters, and internal pressure and temperature sensors, and in turn regulates a flow control valve at the outlet of the vaporizing chamber. If pressure in the cassette (sump) exceeds that in the bypass chamber, which would occur if room temperature exceeds 22.8° C during desflurane administration, a one-way check valve is designed to close, preventing retrograde flow of anesthetic saturated gas back into the ADU with subsequent anesthetic overdose.

## Heated Vaporizer

The vapor pressure of desflurane at sea level is 700 mm Hg at 20° C (near boiling state at room temperature), and delivery by a variable-bypass vaporizer can produce unpredictable concentrations. For this reason, a specially designed vaporizer (Tec 6, Datex-Ohmeda) that heats desflurane gas to 2 atm of pressure is used to accurately meter and deliver desflurane vapor corresponding to adjustments of the concentration dial by the anesthesia provider. In contrast to the variable-bypass vaporizers, the output concentration of desflurane from the Tec 6 is constant across a range of barometric pressures.[9] Therefore, at high altitudes, the partial pressure of desflurane will be lower at a given Tec 6 vaporizer setting and output (volume percent) concentration than at sea level, leading to underdosing of the anesthetic unless an adjustment is made accounting for the higher altitude: required vaporizer setting = (desired vaporizer setting at sea level × 760 mm Hg)/local barometric pressure (in mm Hg).[10] The converse (a greater output) can occur with variable-bypass vaporizers. However, the pharmacologically relevant quantitative parameter for anesthetic activity is partial pressure, not volume percent. Therefore, although a larger output of anesthesia from a vaporizer occurs at higher altitude for the same vaporizer setting, the delivered partial pressure, and anesthetic impact, will be similar in both locations as related to the vaporizer setting.

## Economic and Environmental Considerations

Fresh gas flow rate directly impacts the quantity of volatile liquid used, and consequently the cost of the anesthetic delivery. Higher fresh gas flows (at or above minute ventilation) minimize rebreathing and allow faster equilibration between inspired and central nervous system (CNS) partial pressures. However, use of nonrebreathing flows involve loss of anesthetic to the environment and should be used only for a limited period of minutes, usually at anesthetic induction, or in the circumstance of light sedation and imminent surgical stimulation. There is growing awareness and concern regarding the contribution of inhaled anesthetic release to overall greenhouse gas emission and climate change. Potential environmental impact appears to stem from the atmospheric lifetime gas, as well as unique infrared absorption spectrum, of each anesthetic. Atmospheric longevities of inhaled anesthetics differ substantially (nitrous oxide, desflurane, sevoflurane, and isoflurane having 114, 10, 3.6, and 1.2 estimated years, respectively). Individual infrared absorption spectra differ, with desflurane relatively possessing the greatest carbon dioxide equivalent impact when compared to sevoflurane with the lowest. Although impact of inhaled anesthetics to overall climate change remains a topic of controversy, several points warrant consideration. First, use of low fresh gas flows (0.5-1 L/min) will offset cost and release to the environment. Second,

development of systems to reclaim and reuse anesthetics hold promise to further limit environmental impact and save money.[11]

## Stability

Anesthetic degradation by metabolism or by an interaction with carbon dioxide absorbents (especially when desiccated) produces several potentially toxic compounds.[11]

### Metabolism and Degradation

Methoxyflurane produces inorganic fluoride, which was responsible for the sporadic incidence of nephrotoxicity (i.e., high-output renal failure) after prolonged anesthesia in the past. Compound A (i.e., fluoromethyl-2,2-difluoro-1-[trifluoromethyl] vinyl ether), produced from the breakdown of sevoflurane, and a similar compound produced from halothane are nephrotoxic in animals after prolonged exposure. In humans, prolonged anesthesia with sevoflurane and low fresh gas flows (1 L/min) results in compound A exposure adequate to produce transient proteinuria, enzymuria, and glycosuria, but there is no evidence of increased serum creatinine concentrations or long-term deleterious effects on renal function. Nevertheless, the package insert for sevoflurane recommends low fresh gas flow (<2 L/min) be restricted to less than 2 MAC hours (i.e., MAC concentration × duration of administration) of sevoflurane anesthesia.

### Carbon Dioxide Absorbents and Exothermic Reactions

Variables influencing the amount of volatile anesthetic degradation on exposure to carbon dioxide absorbents include the condition (i.e., hydration and temperature) and chemical makeup of the absorbent, fresh gas flow rates, minute ventilation, and, most important, the anesthetic itself.[12] Although desflurane and isoflurane are very stable in hydrated carbon dioxide absorbents up to temperatures of more than 60° C, full desiccation of conventional carbon dioxide absorbents containing sodium and potassium hydroxide causes degradation and carbon monoxide production from all volatile anesthetics regardless of temperatures (see Table 7.1). High fresh gas flow rates (especially those exceeding normal minute ventilation) accelerate the desiccation of absorbent, and the desiccation leads to accelerated degradation. Because degradation is an exothermic process, the absorbent temperature may increase dramatically.

The exothermic reaction that results from interaction of desiccated carbon dioxide absorbent and volatile anesthetics (especially sevoflurane) can produce extremely high temperatures inside the absorbent canister.[13,14] The temperature increase may lead to explosion and fire in the canister or anesthetic circuit. The remote risk of fire and explosion from exothermic reactions can be avoided entirely by employing measures that ensure maintenance of adequate hydration in the carbon dioxide absorbent (i.e., changing the absorbent regularly, turning fresh gas flow down or off on unattended anesthesia machines, limiting fresh gas flow rates during anesthesia, and when in doubt about the hydration of the absorbent, changing it). Commercially available carbon dioxide absorbents with decreased or absent monovalent bases (i.e., sodium hydroxide and potassium hydroxide) do not undergo extensive degradation on exposure to volatile anesthetics, regardless of the absorbent hydration status.

## RELATIVE POTENCY OF INHALED ANESTHETICS

The relative potency between inhaled anesthetics is most commonly described by the dose required to suppress movement in 50% of patients in response to surgical incision.[5] This dose (a single point on a dose-response curve) is designated the MAC. Because the standard deviation in the MAC is approximately 10%, 95% of patients should not move in response to incision at 1.2 MAC of the inhaled anesthetic, and 99% of patients should not move in response to incision at 1.3 MAC of the inhaled anesthetic. MAC is affected by several variables but is unaffected by gender or duration of surgery and anesthesia (see Box 7.1).[5]

MAC allows potencies to be compared among anesthetics (see Table 7.1); 1.15% isoflurane is equipotent with 6% desflurane in preventing movement in response to a surgical incision in patients of a similar age and body temperature. Remarkably, MAC values for different inhaled anesthetics are additive. For example, 0.5 MAC of nitrous oxide administered with 0.5 MAC of isoflurane has the same effect as 1 MAC of any inhaled anesthetic in preventing movement in response to incision (reflecting anesthetic-induced inhibition of reflex responses at the level of the spinal cord).[6] The concentration of anesthetic at the brain needed to prevent movement in response to a surgical incision is likely to be larger than the MAC.

The anesthetic dose required to produce amnesia probably has more variability than the MAC. The alveolar concentration of isoflurane preventing recall of a verbal stimulus was 0.20 MAC in 50% and 0.40 MAC in 95% of volunteers.[15] Assuming a standard normal distribution of dose response, the standard deviation in minimum concentration preventing recall is therefore approximately half the mean value (0.1 MAC). Referring to standard normal curves, we can calculate that the concentration needed by 1 in 100,000 subjects with the highest anesthetic requirement would be 4.27 standard deviations (SD) above the mean (i.e., greater than 0.627 MAC) to prevent recall of verbal stimulus. Extrapolation of this value to the context of surgery must be made with caution, however, because the dose required to prevent recall of painful as opposed to verbal stimulation may be considerably larger.[16] The ratio of concentration needed to prevent

> ### Box 7.2 Factors Determining Partial Pressure Gradients Necessary for Establishment of Anesthesia
>
> Transfer of inhaled anesthetic from anesthetic machine to alveoli
> Inspired partial pressure
> Alveolar ventilation
> Characteristics of anesthetic breathing system
> Transfer of inhaled anesthetic from alveoli to arterial blood
> Blood-gas partition coefficient
> Cardiac output
> Alveolar-to-venous partial pressure difference
> Transfer of inhaled anesthetic from arterial blood to brain
> Brain-blood partition coefficient
> Cerebral blood flow
> Arterial-to-venous partial pressure difference

motor response to surgical incision (reflected in MAC) to that required to suppress consciousness and prevent recall differs slightly between individual potent inhaled anesthetics and differs substantially between potent inhaled anesthetics collectively versus nitrous oxide. Volunteers given isoflurane did not exhibit recall given 0.45 MAC of isoflurane, whereas recall did occur with as much as 0.6 MAC of nitrous oxide.[17]

## PHARMACOKINETICS OF INHALED ANESTHETICS

Pharmacokinetics of inhaled anesthetics describes their uptake (absorption) from alveoli into the systemic circulation, distribution in the body, and eventual elimination by the lungs or metabolism principally in the liver (Box 7.2).[18] By controlling the inspired partial pressure (PI) (same as the concentration [%] when referring to the gas phase) of an inhaled anesthetic, a gradient is created such that the anesthetic is delivered from the anesthetic machine to its site of action, the brain. The primary objective of inhaled anesthesia is to achieve a constant and optimal brain partial pressure (Pbr) of the anesthetic.

The brain and all other tissues equilibrate with the partial pressure of the inhaled anesthetic delivered to them by the arterial blood (Pa). Likewise, the blood equilibrates with the alveolar partial pressure (PA) of the anesthetic:

$$PA \rightleftarrows Pa \rightleftarrows Pbr$$

alveolar partial pressure mirrors the brain partial pressure

Maintaining a constant and optimal PA becomes an indirect but useful method for controlling the Pbr. The PA of an inhaled anesthetic mirrors its Pbr and is the reason the PA is used as an index of anesthetic depth, a reflection of the rate of induction and recovery from anesthesia, and a measure of equal potency (see earlier discussion under "Relative Potency of Inhaled Anesthetics"). Understanding the factors that determine the PA and the Pbr allows the anesthesia provider to skillfully control and adjust the dose of inhaled anesthetic delivered to the brain.

## Factors That Determine the Alveolar Partial Pressure

The $P_A$ and ultimately the Pbr of an inhaled anesthetic are determined by input (delivery) into the alveoli minus uptake (loss) of the drug from the alveoli into the pulmonary arterial blood. Input of the inhaled anesthetic depends on the $P_I$, alveolar ventilation ($\dot{V}_A$), and characteristics of the anesthetic breathing system. Uptake of the inhaled anesthetic depends on the solubility, cardiac output (CO), and alveolar-to-venous partial pressure difference (PA – Pv). These six factors act simultaneously to determine the $P_A$. Metabolism and percutaneous loss of inhaled anesthetics do not significantly influence $P_A$ during induction and maintenance of anesthesia.

### Inspired Anesthetic Partial Pressure

A high $P_I$ is necessary during initial administration of an inhaled anesthetic. This initial high $P_I$ (i.e., input) offsets the impact of uptake into the blood and accelerates induction of anesthesia as reflected by the rate of increase in the $P_A$. This effect of the $P_I$ is known as the concentration effect. Clinically, the range of concentrations necessary to produce a concentration effect is probably possible only with nitrous oxide (Fig. 7.4).[19]

With time, as uptake into the blood decreases, the $P_I$ should be decreased to match the decreased anesthetic uptake. Decreasing the $P_I$ to match decreasing uptake with time is critical if the anesthesia provider is to achieve the goal of maintaining a constant and optimal Pbr. For example, if the $P_I$ were maintained constant with time (input constant), the $P_A$ (and depth of anesthesia as reflected by the Pbr) would progressively increase as uptake of the anesthetic into the blood diminished with time.

### Second Gas Effect

The second gas effect is a distinct phenomenon that occurs independently of the concentration effect. The ability of the large-volume uptake of one gas (first gas) to accelerate the rate of increase of the $P_A$ of a concurrently administered companion gas (second gas) is known as the second gas effect. For example, the initial large volume uptake of nitrous oxide accelerates the uptake of companion gases such as volatile anesthetics and oxygen. The transient increase (about 10%) in $Pao_2$ that accompanies the early phase of nitrous oxide administration reflects the second gas effect of nitrous oxide on oxygen. This increase in $Pao_2$ has been designated alveolar hyperoxygenation. Increased tracheal inflow of all inhaled gases (i.e., first and second gases) and concentration of the second gases in a smaller lung volume (i.e., concentrating effect) because of the high-volume uptake of the first gas

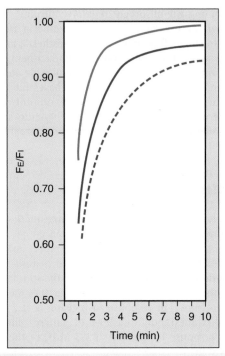

**Fig. 7.4** The impact of the inspired concentration (%) ($F_I$) on the rate of increase of the alveolar (end-tidal) concentration ($F_E$) is known as the concentration effect. The lines indicate concentrations of 85% (*green*), 50% (*blue*), and 10% (*dashed red*). (From Eger EI. Effect of inspired anesthetic concentration on the rate of rise of alveolar concentration. *Anesthesiology.* 1963;24:153-157, used with permission.)

are the explanations for the second gas effect. Although the second gas effect is based on proven pharmacokinetic principles, its clinical importance is doubtful.

### Alveolar Ventilation

Increased $\dot{V}_A$, like $P_I$, promotes input of inhaled anesthetics to offset uptake into the blood. The net effect is a more rapid rate of increase in the $P_A$ and induction of anesthesia. Predictably, hypoventilation has the opposite effect, acting to slow the induction of anesthesia.

Controlled ventilation of the lungs that results in hyperventilation and decreased venous return accelerates the rate of increase of the $P_A$ by virtue of increased input (i.e., increased $\dot{V}_A$) and decreased uptake (i.e., decreased CO). As a result, the risk of anesthetic overdose may be increased during controlled ventilation of the lungs, and it may be appropriate to decrease the $P_I$ of volatile anesthetics when ventilation of the lungs is changed from spontaneous to controlled to maintain the $P_A$ similar to that present during spontaneous ventilation.

Another effect of hyperventilation is decreased cerebral blood flow because of the associated decrease in the $Paco_2$. Conceivably, the impact of increased anesthetic input on the rate of increase of the $P_A$ would be offset by decreased delivery of anesthetic to the brain. Theoretically, coronary blood flow may remain unchanged, such that increased anesthetic input produces myocardial depression, and decreased cerebral blood flow prevents a concomitant onset of central nervous system depression.

## Anesthetic Breathing System (Also See Chapter 15)

Characteristics of the anesthetic breathing system that influence the rate of increase of the PA include the volume of the system, solubility of inhaled anesthetics in the rubber or plastic components of the system, and gas inflow from the anesthetic machine. The volume of the anesthetic breathing system acts as a buffer to slow attainment of the PA. High gas inflow from the anesthetic machine negates this buffer effect. Solubility of inhaled anesthetics in the components of the anesthetic breathing system initially slows the rate at which the PA increases. At the conclusion of an anesthetic, reversal of the partial pressure gradient in the anesthetic breathing system results in elution of the anesthetics that slows the rate at which the PA decreases.

## Solubility

The solubility of inhaled anesthetics in blood and tissues is denoted by partition coefficients (see Table 7.1). A partition coefficient is a distribution ratio describing how the inhaled anesthetic distributes itself between two phases at equilibrium (when the partial pressures are identical). For example, a blood-gas partition coefficient of 10 means that the concentration of the inhaled anesthetic is 10 in the blood and 1 in the alveolar gas when the partial pressures of that anesthetic in these two phases are identical. Partition coefficients are temperature dependent. For example, the solubility of a gas in a liquid is increased when the temperature of the liquid decreases. Unless otherwise stated, partition coefficients are given for 37° C.

## Blood-Gas Partition Coefficient

High blood solubility means that a large amount of inhaled anesthetic must be dissolved (i.e., undergo uptake) in the blood before equilibrium with the gas phase is reached. The blood can be considered a pharmacologically inactive reservoir, the size of which is determined by the solubility of the anesthetic in the blood. When the blood-gas partition coefficient is high, a large amount of anesthetic must be dissolved in the blood before the Pa equilibrates with the PA (Fig. 7.5).[18] Clinically, the impact of high blood solubility on the rate of increase of the PA can be offset to some extent by increasing the PI. When blood solubility is low, minimal amounts of the anesthetic have to be dissolved in the blood before equilibrium is reached such that the rate of increase of the PA and that of the Pa and Pbr are rapid (see Fig. 7.5).[20]

## Tissue-Blood Partition Coefficients

Tissue-blood partition coefficients determine the time necessary for equilibration of the tissue with the Pa

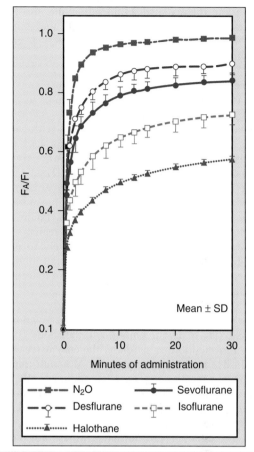

**Fig. 7.5** The blood-gas partition coefficient is the principal determinant of the rate at which the alveolar concentration (FA) increases toward a constant inspired concentration (FI). The rate of induction of anesthesia is paralleled by the rate of increase in the FA. Despite similar blood solubility (see Table 7.1), the rate of increase of FA is more rapid for nitrous oxide (*dashed brownish-gold line*) than for desflurane (*dashed purple line*) or sevoflurane (*solid blue line*), reflecting the impact of the concentration effect on nitrous oxide (see Fig. 7.4). Greater tissue solubility of desflurane and sevoflurane may also contribute to a slower rate of increase in the FA of these drugs compared with nitrous oxide. *SD*, Standard deviation. (From Yasuda N, Lockhart SH, Eger EI II, et al. Comparison of kinetics of sevoflurane and isoflurane in humans. *Anesth Analg*. 1991;72:316-324, used with permission.)

(see Table 7.1). This time can be predicted by calculating a time constant (i.e., amount of inhaled anesthetic that can be dissolved in the tissue divided by tissue blood flow) for each tissue. Brain-blood partition coefficients for a volatile anesthetic such as isoflurane result in time constants of about 3 to 4 minutes. Complete equilibration of any tissue, including the brain, with the Pa requires at least three time constants. This is the rationale for maintaining the PA of this volatile anesthetic constant for 10 to 15 minutes before assuming that the Pbr is similar. Time constants for less soluble anesthetics such as nitrous oxide, desflurane, and sevoflurane are about 2 minutes, and complete equilibration is achieved in approximately 6 minutes (i.e., three time constants).

### Anesthetic Transfer by Intertissue Diffusion

There is growing evidence that a portion of anesthetic uptake may occur not by blood flow to various tissues, but by direct transfer from tissues with lower to higher affinity for the anesthetic (i.e., from lean to adipose tissues), such as the interface between viscera and omental fat (see "Context-Sensitive Half-Time"). Larger people[21] and animals[22] with presumably greater lean-fat surface area interface show greater uptake of sevoflurane and isoflurane. Transfer to bulk fat by blood flow during an anesthetic of clinically realistic duration (less than 12 to 24 hours) is unlikely to explain these differences, given the relatively small blood flow received by the bulk fat compartment and its relatively large size.

### Nitrous Oxide and Methionine Synthase Inactivation

Nitrous oxide is unique among anesthetics by its inactivation of methionine synthase, the enzyme regulating vitamin $B_{12}$ and folate metabolism. Although impact of the enzyme inactivation may be subtle or subclinical in many patients, those with underlying critical illness or preexisting vitamin $B_{12}$ deficiency may suffer neurologic or hematologic sequelae. Homocysteine, which requires functional methionine synthase for conversion to methionine, is associated with increased risk of adverse coronary events when present in elevated concentration in the blood.[23] Patients receiving nitrous oxide during carotid endarterectomy showed significantly elevated homocysteine levels and frequency of myocardial ischemic episodes compared to patients not receiving nitrous oxide.[24]

### Nitrous Oxide Transfer to Closed Gas Spaces

The blood-gas partition coefficient of nitrous oxide (0.46) is 34 times greater than that of nitrogen (0.014). This differential solubility means that nitrous oxide can leave the blood to enter an air-filled cavity 34 times more rapidly than nitrogen can leave the cavity to enter the blood. As a result of this preferential transfer of nitrous oxide, the volume or pressure of the air-filled cavity increases. The entrance of nitrous oxide into an air-filled cavity surrounded by a compliant wall (e.g., intestinal gas, pneumothorax, pulmonary blebs, air embolism) causes the gas space to expand. Conversely, entrance of nitrous oxide into an air-filled cavity surrounded by a noncompliant wall (e.g., middle ear, cerebral ventricles, supratentorial subdural space) causes an increase in pressure.

The magnitude of volume or pressure increase in the air-filled cavity is influenced by the $P_A$ of nitrous oxide, blood flow to the air-filled cavity, and duration of nitrous oxide administration. In an animal model, inhalation of 75% nitrous oxide doubles the volume of a pneumothorax in 10 minutes.[25] The presence of a closed pneumothorax is a contraindication to the administration of nitrous oxide. Decreasing pulmonary compliance during administration of nitrous oxide to a patient with a history of chest trauma (i.e., rib fractures) may reflect nitrous oxide–induced expansion of a previously unrecognized pneumothorax. Likewise, air bubbles associated with venous air embolism expand rapidly when exposed to nitrous oxide. In contrast to the rapid expansion of a pneumothorax or air bubbles (i.e., venous air embolism), the increase in bowel gas volume produced by nitrous oxide is slow. The question of whether to administer nitrous oxide to patients undergoing intra-abdominal surgery is of little importance if the operation is short. Limiting the inhaled concentration of nitrous oxide to 50%, however, may be a prudent recommendation when bowel gas volume is increased (e.g., bowel obstruction) preoperatively. Following this guideline, bowel gas volume at most would double, even during prolonged operations.[25]

### Cardiac Output

The CO influences uptake into the pulmonary arterial blood and therefore $P_A$ by carrying away more or less anesthetic from the alveoli. A high CO (e.g., induced by anxiety) results in more rapid uptake, such that the rate of increase in the $P_A$ and the induction of anesthesia are slowed. A low CO (e.g., shock) speeds the rate of increase of the $P_A$ because there is less uptake into the blood to oppose input. A common clinical impression is that induction of anesthesia in patients in shock is rapid.

### Shunt

A right-to-left intracardiac or intrapulmonary shunt slows the rate of induction of anesthesia. This slowing reflects the dilutional effect of shunted blood containing no anesthetic on the partial pressure of anesthetic in blood coming from ventilated alveoli. A similar mechanism is responsible for the decrease in $Pa_{O_2}$ in the presence of a right-to-left shunt.

A left-to-right shunt (e.g., arteriovenous fistula, volatile anesthetic-induced increases in cutaneous blood flow) results in delivery to the lungs of venous blood containing a higher partial pressure of anesthetic than that present in venous blood that has passed through the tissues. As a result, a left-to-right tissue shunt offsets the dilutional effect of a right-to-left shunt on the $P_a$. The effect of a left-to-right shunt on the rate of increase in the $P_a$ is detectable only if there is the concomitant presence of a right-to-left shunt. Likewise, the dilutional effect of a right-to-left shunt is greatest in the absence of a left-to-right shunt. All factors considered, it seems unlikely that

**Table 7.2**  Body Tissue Compartments

| Compartment | Body Mass (% of 70-kg Adult Male) | Blood Flow (% Cardiac Output, 70-kg Adult Male) |
|---|---|---|
| Vessel-rich group | 10 | 75 |
| Muscle group | 50 | 19 |
| Fat group | 20 | 5 |
| Vessel-poor group | 20 | 1 |

**Box 7.3** Proposed Mechanisms of Circulatory Effects Produced by Inhaled Anesthetics

Direct myocardial depression
Inhibition of central nervous system and sympathetic nervous system outflow
Depression of transmission of impulses through autonomic ganglia
Attenuated carotid sinus reflex activity
Decreased formation of cyclic adenosine monophosphate
Inhibition of calcium reuptake by myocardial sarcoplasmic reticulum
Decreased influx of calcium ions through slow channels

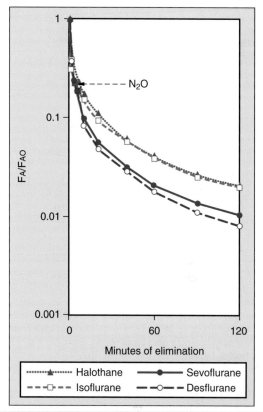

**Fig. 7.6** Elimination of inhaled anesthetics is reflected by the decrease in the alveolar concentration ($F_A$) compared with the concentration present at the conclusion of anesthesia ($F_{AO}$). Awakening from anesthesia is paralleled by these curves. (From Yasuda N, Lockhart SH, Eger EI II, et al. Comparison of kinetics of sevoflurane and isoflurane in humans. *Anesth Analg*. 1991;72:316-324, used with permission.)

the impact of a right-to-left shunt would be clinically apparent.

### Wasted Ventilation

Ventilation of nonperfused alveoli does not influence the rate of induction of anesthesia because a dilutional effect on the Pa is not produced. The principal effect of wasted ventilation is the production of a difference between the $P_A$ and Pa of the inhaled anesthetic. A similar mechanism is responsible for the difference often observed between the end-tidal $P_{CO_2}$ and $Pa_{CO_2}$.

### Alveolar-to-Venous Partial Pressure Differences

The $P_A - Pv$ reflects tissue uptake of inhaled anesthetics. Highly perfused tissues (i.e., brain, heart, kidneys, and liver) account for less than 10% of body mass but receive about 75% of the CO (Table 7.2). As a result, these highly perfused tissues equilibrate rapidly with the Pa. After three time constants (6 to 12 minutes for inhaled anesthetics), about 75% of the returning venous blood is at the same partial pressure as the $P_A$ (i.e., narrow $P_A - Pv$). For this reason, uptake of volatile anesthetics from the alveoli is greatly decreased after 6 to 12 minutes, as reflected by a narrowing of the $P_I - P_A$ difference. After this time, the inhaled concentrations of volatile anesthetics should be decreased to maintain a constant $P_A$ in the presence of decreased uptake.

Skeletal muscle and fat represent about 70% of the body mass but receive less than 25% of the CO (Box 7.3).

These tissues continue to act as inactive reservoirs for anesthetic uptake for several hours. Equilibration of fat with inhaled anesthetics in the arterial blood is probably never achieved.

### Recovery From Anesthesia

Recovery from anesthesia can be defined as the rate at which the $P_A$ decreases with time (Fig. 7.6).[20] In many respects, recovery is the inverse of induction of anesthesia. For example, $\dot{V}_A$, solubility, and CO determine the rate at which the $P_A$ decreases. After discontinuation of anesthetic administration, elimination of anesthetic occurs by ventilation of the lungs. As the alveolar partial pressure decreases, anesthetic is subsequently transferred from the tissues (including the brain) into the alveoli. Hypoventilation or use of fresh gas flows low enough to permit rebreathing of anesthetic will lead to transfer of anesthetic back into the tissues (including the brain), delaying patient recovery.

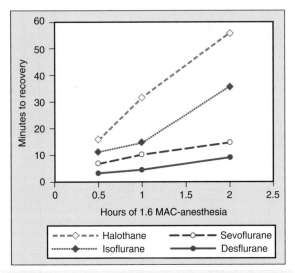

**Fig. 7.7** An increase in the duration of anesthesia during a constant dose of anesthetic (1.6 MAC) is associated with increases in the time to recovery (i.e., motor coordination in an animal model), with the greatest increases occurring with the most blood-soluble anesthetics. *MAC*, Minimum alveolar concentration. (From Eger EI II. *Desflurane (Suprane): A Compendium and Reference.* Nutley, NJ: Anaquest; 1993:1-11, used with permission.)

### How Does Recovery Differ From Induction of Anesthesia?
Recovery from anesthesia differs from induction of anesthesia with respect to the absence of a concentration effect on recovery (the $P_I$ cannot be less than zero), the variable tissue concentrations of anesthetics at the start of recovery, and the potential importance of metabolism on the rate of decrease in the $P_A$.

### Tissue Concentrations
Tissue concentrations of inhaled anesthetics serve as a reservoir to maintain the $P_A$ when the partial pressure gradient is reversed by decreasing the $P_I$ to or near zero at the conclusion of anesthesia. The impact of tissue storage depends on the duration of anesthesia and solubility of the anesthetics in various tissue compartments. For example, time to recovery is prolonged in proportion to the duration of anesthesia for a soluble anesthetic (e.g., isoflurane), whereas the impact of duration of administration on time to recovery is minimal with poorly soluble anesthetics (e.g., sevoflurane, desflurane) (Fig 7.7).[1] The variable concentrations of anesthetics in different tissues at the conclusion of anesthesia contrasts with induction of anesthesia, when all tissues initially have the same zero concentration of anesthetic.

### Metabolism
An important difference between induction of anesthesia and recovery from anesthesia is the potential impact of metabolism on the rate of decrease in the $P_A$ at the conclusion of anesthesia. In this regard, metabolism is a principal determinant of the rate of decrease in the $P_A$ of the highly lipid-soluble methoxyflurane. Metabolism and $\dot{V}_A$ are equally important in the rate of decrease in the $P_A$ of halothane, whereas the rate of decrease in the $P_A$ of less lipid-soluble isoflurane, desflurane, and sevoflurane principally results from $\dot{V}_A$.[26]

### Context-Sensitive Half-Time (Also See Chapter 4)
The pharmacokinetics of the elimination of inhaled anesthetics depends on the length of administration (the "context") and the solubility of the inhaled anesthetic in blood and tissues. As with intravenous anesthetics, it is possible to use computer simulations to determine context-sensitive decrement times for volatile anesthetics (the time required to decrease in anesthetic concentrations in the central nervous system to a fraction of that given from a starting point of interest). The kinetic modeling is based upon presence of each tissue compartment within the body (i.e., blood, vessel-rich group, muscle, fat), the relative size of each compartment, the proportional blood flow received by each compartment, and the solubility of each specific anesthetic in the tissue composing the compartment. During anesthetic administration, equilibration implies continued uptake of anesthetic until tissue concentration becomes almost as great as alveolar concentration. Equilibration of anesthetic concentration between the alveoli and a small (less than 10% body mass) compartment with high blood flow (i.e., heart, kidneys, brain) occurs within a relatively short period of time (10 to 15 minutes). Conversely, anesthetic equilibration in larger compartments with lesser proportional blood flow (i.e., skeletal muscle and bulk fat) occurs over a longer period of time (hours), as anesthetic uptake continues. The time needed for a 50% decrease in anesthetic concentrations of isoflurane, desflurane, and sevoflurane is less than 5 minutes and does not increase significantly with increasing duration of anesthesia.[27] Presumably, this is a reflection of the initial phase of elimination, which is primarily a function of $\dot{V}_A$. Determination of other decrement times ($\geq$80%) reveals larger differences between various inhaled anesthetics, especially as anesthetic duration becomes longer (Fig. 7.8). Simulation may underestimate the uptake of anesthesia, especially with more soluble anesthetics, because it does not account for anesthetic transferred from lean to fatty tissues by intertissue diffusion.

Elimination of all but small amounts of anesthetics (smaller than needed for patients to follow commands) must take place before a patient regains coordinated protective functions, such as the ability to swallow and breathe effectively. Surgical patients given longer anesthesia and a more soluble anesthetic (sevoflurane compared to desflurane) required a longer time interval between awakening and regaining the ability to swallow effectively.[22] Awake subjects given small concentrations of sevoflurane and isoflurane demonstrate pharyngeal

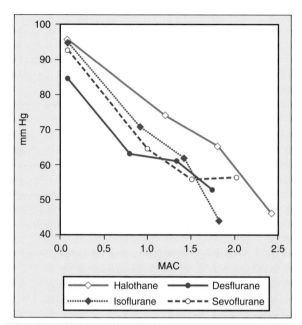

**Fig. 7.8** The effects of increasing concentrations (MAC) of halothane, isoflurane, desflurane, and sevoflurane on mean arterial pressure (mm Hg) when administered to healthy volunteers. *MAC*, Minimum alveolar concentration. (From Cahalan MK. *Hemodynamic Effects of Inhaled Anesthetics. Review Courses.* Cleveland: International Anesthesia Research Society; 1996:14-18, used with permission.)

discoordination[28] and diminished chemical ventilatory drive.[29]

Diffusion Hypoxia

Diffusion hypoxia may occur at the conclusion of nitrous oxide administration if patients are allowed to inhale room air. The initial high-volume outpouring of nitrous oxide from the blood into the alveoli when inhalation of this gas is discontinued can so dilute the $P_{AO_2}$ that the $Pa_{O_2}$ decreases. The occurrence of diffusion hypoxia is prevented by filling the patient's lungs with oxygen at the conclusion of nitrous oxide administration.

## Feasibility of Inhaled Anesthetic Use for Sedation in ICU

AnaConDa (Anaesthetic Conserving Device, Sedana Medical AB, Uppsala, Sweden) is a tool that facilitates delivery of inhaled anesthetic (isoflurane, sevoflurane) in the intensive care unit (ICU) (also see Chapter 41). Liquid anesthetic is delivered via syringe pump to a chamber that attaches to the breathing circuit, between the endotracheal tube and the Y-piece. The syringe delivers liquid anesthetic at a very slow rate to a porous plastic rod inside the chamber, where the liquid evaporates and mixes with fresh gas flowing from the inspiratory limb of the circuit. Exhaled gas is routed through a charcoal filter that absorbs and reclaims approximately 90% of the exhaled anesthetic. Subsequent inspiratory flow is routed through the charcoal filter, where absorbed anesthetic remixes with the fresh gas.

There is growing interest for the use of potent inhaled anesthetics outside the operating room for postsurgical patients in the ICU, and an increasing accumulation of evidence that doing so is feasible and possibly advantageous.[30,31] However, challenges to the use of inhaled anesthetic in the ICU setting include increased dead space and work of breathing due to the interposition of the anesthetic delivery device between the tracheal tube and circuit; loss of anesthetic to the environment during frequent tracheal tube suctioning; and questionable availability of appropriate equipment and caregivers with sufficient knowledge and technical expertise in the delivery of inhaled anesthetic.

## EFFECTS ON ORGAN SYSTEMS

### Circulatory Effects

Equipotent concentrations of inhaled anesthetics have similar circulatory effects, especially during the maintenance of anesthesia in human volunteers (see Box 7.3).[32] However, patients undergoing surgery may respond differently from healthy volunteers. For example, factors such as coexisting disease, extremes of age, nonoptimal intravascular volume status, presence of surgical stimulation, and concurrent drugs may alter, attenuate, or exaggerate the responses expected based on data obtained from healthy volunteers.

Responses During Maintenance of Anesthesia
Mean Arterial Pressure
Mean arterial pressure (MAP) decreases with increasing concentrations of desflurane, sevoflurane, isoflurane, halothane, and enflurane in a dose-dependent manner (see Fig. 7.8).[17,18] With the exception of halothane, the decrease in MAP primarily reflects a decrease in systemic vascular resistance (SVR) versus a decrease in CO (Figs. 7.9 and 7.10).[32,33] In contrast, halothane decreases MAP partly or entirely by decreasing CO, whereas SVR is relatively unchanged. These findings are supported by measurements of SVR in patients receiving desflurane, sevoflurane, and isoflurane while undergoing cardiopulmonary bypass perfusion. The dose-related decrease in SVR is minimized by substitution of nitrous oxide for a portion of the volatile drug (Fig. 7.11).[34] Nitrous oxide, in contrast to the other inhaled anesthetics, causes unchanged or mildly increased MAP (Box 7.4).

Heart Rate
Stepwise increases in the delivered concentrations of isoflurane, desflurane, and sevoflurane increase heart rates in patients and volunteers, although at different

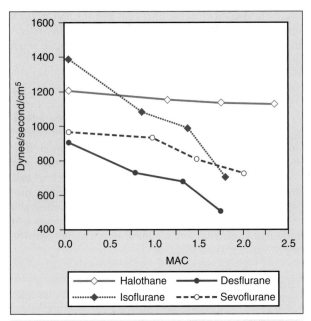

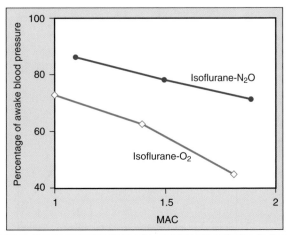

**Fig. 7.11** The substitution of nitrous oxide for a portion of isoflurane produces less decrease in systemic blood pressure than the same dose of volatile anesthetic alone. *MAC*, Minimum alveolar concentration. (From Eger EI II. *Isoflurane (Forane): A Compendium and Reference*. Madison, WI: Ohio Medical Products; 1985:1-110, used with permission.)

**Fig. 7.9** The effects of increasing concentrations (MAC) of halothane, isoflurane, desflurane, and sevoflurane on systemic vascular resistance (dynes/sec/cm$^5$) when administered to healthy volunteers. *MAC*, Minimum alveolar concentration. (From Cahalan MK. *Hemodynamic Effects of Inhaled Anesthetics. Review Courses*. Cleveland: International Anesthesia Research Society; 1996:14-18, used with permission.)

---

**Box 7.4** Evidence of a Sympathomimetic Effect of Nitrous Oxide Administered Alone or Added to Unchanging Concentrations of Volatile Anesthetics

---

Diaphoresis
Increased body temperature
Increased plasma concentrations of catecholamines
Increased right atrial pressure
Mydriasis
Vasoconstriction in the systemic and pulmonary circulations

---

concentrations (Fig. 7.12).[33] At concentrations as low as 0.25 MAC, isoflurane causes a linear, dose-dependent heart rate increase. Heart rate increases minimally with desflurane concentrations of less than 1 MAC. When desflurane concentrations are increased above 1 MAC, the heart rate accelerates in a linear, dose-dependent manner. In contrast to desflurane and isoflurane, heart rate in the presence of sevoflurane does not increase until the concentration exceeds 1.5 MAC.[35] However, induction with 8% sevoflurane (i.e., single-breath induction) causes tachycardia in both children and adult patients undergoing controlled hyperventilation. This tachycardia may result from sympathetic nervous system stimulation associated with epileptiform brain activity.[36]

The tendency for desflurane to stimulate the circulation (i.e., increase MAP and heart rate) is attenuated with administration of β-adrenergic blocker (esmolol), opioid (fentanyl), and passage of time (10 to 15 minutes) during maintenance of anesthesia (also see "Circulatory Effects With Rapid Concentration Increase"). The dose-related increase in heart rate seen with desflurane concentrations

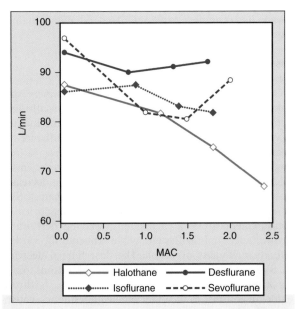

**Fig. 7.10** The effects of increasing concentrations (MAC) of halothane, isoflurane, desflurane, and sevoflurane on cardiac index (L/min) when administered to healthy volunteers. *MAC*, Minimum alveolar concentration. (From Cahalan MK. *Hemodynamic Effects of Inhaled Anesthetics. Review Courses*. Cleveland: International Anesthesia Research Society; 1996:14-18, used with permission.)

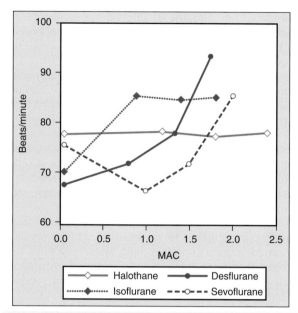

**Fig. 7.12** The effects of increasing concentrations (MAC) of halothane, isoflurane, desflurane, and sevoflurane on heart rate (beats/min) when administered to healthy volunteers. *MAC,* Minimum alveolar concentration. (From Cahalan MK. *Hemodynamic Effects of Inhaled Anesthetics. Review Courses.* Cleveland: International Anesthesia Research Society; 1996:14-18, used with permission.)

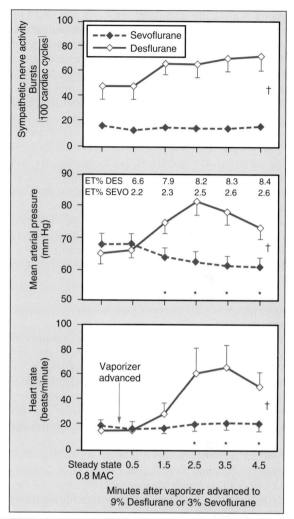

**Fig. 7.13** A rapid increase in the inspired concentration of sevoflurane from 0.8 MAC to 3% did not alter sympathetic nerve activity, mean arterial pressure, or heart rate. Conversely, a rapid increase in the inspired concentration of desflurane from 0.8 MAC to 9% significantly increased sympathetic nerve activity, mean arterial pressure, and heart rate (mean ± SE; *$p < 0.05$). *ET,* End-tidal; *MAC,* minimum alveolar concentration. (From Ebert TJ, Muzi M, Lopatka CW. Neurocirculatory responses to sevoflurane in humans: a comparison to desflurane. *Anesthesiology.* 1995;83:88-95, used with permission.)

more than 1 MAC is not attenuated by substitution of some of the desflurane by nitrous oxide. Isoflurane, sevoflurane, and desflurane, like halothane, diminish baroreceptor responses in a concentration-dependent manner. The transient increase in heart rate above 1 MAC seen with desflurane results from sympathetic nervous system stimulation rather than a reflex baroreceptor activity response to decreased MAP.[37]

### Cardiac Index

The cardiac index is minimally influenced by administration of desflurane, sevoflurane, or isoflurane over a wide range of concentrations in healthy young adults (see Fig. 7.10).[32] Transesophageal echocardiography data show that desflurane produces minor increases in the ejection fraction and left ventricular velocity of circumferential shortening compared with awake measurements.

### Circulatory Effects With Rapid Concentration Increase

At concentrations of less than 1 MAC, desflurane does not increase heart rate or MAP. However, abrupt increases in inspired desflurane concentrations above 1 MAC cause transient circulatory stimulation in the absence of opioids, adrenergic blockers, or other analgesic adjuncts (Fig. 7.13).[38] To a lesser extent, isoflurane has a similar capability to evoke increases in heart rate and blood pressure. Accompanying the hemodynamic stimulation seen with

abrupt increased concentrations of desflurane and isoflurane are increases in plasma epinephrine and norepinephrine concentrations and sympathetic nervous system activity. An abrupt increase in the inspired sevoflurane concentration from 1 MAC to 1.5 MAC is associated with a slight decrease in heart rate.

A stepwise increase in end-tidal desflurane concentration from 4% to 8% within 1 minute may result in a doubling of the heart rate and blood pressure above baseline. Administration of small doses of opioids, clonidine, or esmolol profoundly attenuates the heart rate and blood pressure responses to the stepwise increase in desflurane concentration. Repetition of the rapid increase in end-tidal desflurane concentration from 4% to 8% after 30 minutes results in minimal changes of the heart rate and MAP, suggesting that the receptors mediating these circulatory changes adapt to repeated stimulation. Circulatory stimulation is not seen with abrupt increases in the concentrations of sevoflurane, halothane, or enflurane up to 2 MAC (see Fig. 7.13).[38]

Sevoflurane and halothane are frequently given via inhalation to induce anesthesia because of their lack of pungency. Induction of anesthesia in children with halothane, but not sevoflurane, depresses myocardial contractility (also see Chapter 34). In adults, maintenance of anesthesia with 1 MAC of sevoflurane or halothane with 67% nitrous oxide decreases myocardial contractility. In adults, sevoflurane can transiently increase heart rate when controlled ventilation is used.

### Administration With Nitrous Oxide and Oxygen Versus 100% Oxygen

Desflurane, isoflurane, and sevoflurane, administered with nitrous oxide and oxygen, decrease the MAP, SVR, cardiac index, and left ventricular stroke work index (LVSWI) in a dose-dependent manner, whereas heart rate, pulmonary artery pressure, and central venous pressure increase, consistent with the findings in which each volatile anesthetic is administered in oxygen alone (see Fig. 7.11).[32,33] Direct comparison reveals a more pronounced diminution of MAP, SVR, cardiac index, and LVSWI and a more rapid heart rate and larger CO when desflurane is administered in oxygen rather than in nitrous oxide at roughly equivalent MAC multiples.[34]

### Myocardial Conduction and Dysrhythmogenicity

Isoflurane, sevoflurane, and desflurane do not predispose the heart to premature ventricular extrasystoles.[39] In contrast, halothane does sensitize the myocardium to premature ventricular extrasystoles, especially in the presence of catecholamines; this relationship is exaggerated with hypercarbia. Inhaled anesthetics probably suppress ventricular dysrhythmias during myocardial ischemia by prolonging the effective refractory period.

The choice of inhaled anesthetic influences the occurrence of reflex bradydysrhythmias that may result from vagal stimulation. Children anesthetized with sevoflurane, compared with halothane, exhibit fewer episodes of decreased heart rate or sinus node arrest in response to surgical traction on the ocular muscles (also see Chapters 31 and 34).

### QT Interval

Inhaled anesthetics prolong the QT interval on the electrocardiogram.[40] Although each anesthetic's relative tendency to prolong the QT interval has not been compared systematically, sevoflurane should be avoided in patients with known congenital long QT syndrome (LQTS). Although sevoflurane and propofol anesthetics cause QT interval prolongation in children, neither anesthetic increases transmural dispersion of repolarization, a measure of the heterogeneous rates of repolarization of myocardial cells during phases 2 and 3 of the action potential.[41] The clinical significance of QT prolongation with sevoflurane and other inhaled anesthetics in susceptible patients is unclear. In patients with LQTS, β-adrenergic blockade is the mainstay of therapy. Patients with known LQTS have been safely anesthetized with all modern inhaled anesthetics when concurrently receiving β-adrenergic blocking drugs. Numerous malignant intraoperative arrhythmias have occurred in patients undergoing anesthesia with halothane that were subsequently attributed to undiagnosed LQTS, and none of the patients had received β-blocking drugs.[40]

### Patients With Coronary Artery Disease (Also See Chapter 25)

Numerous studies in patients undergoing coronary artery bypass surgery or at risk for coronary artery disease have failed to demonstrate a difference in outcome between groups receiving inhaled (i.e., desflurane) versus intravenously administered (i.e., fentanyl or sufentanil) anesthetic techniques or between groups receiving one inhaled anesthetic versus another (i.e., desflurane vs. isoflurane or sevoflurane vs. isoflurane).[42] Concerns that isoflurane's capacity to dilate small-diameter coronary arteries might cause coronary steal, in which a patient with susceptible anatomy might develop regional myocardial ischemia as a result of coronary vasodilatation, were not valid. Volatile anesthetics instead exert a protective effect on the heart, limiting the area of myocardial injury and preserving function after exposure to ischemic insult.

### Anesthetic Preconditioning

The explanation for the protective benefits of volatile anesthetics against myocardial ischemia is called anesthetic preconditioning, and it is not explained by favorable alteration of myocardial oxygen supply-demand ratio. Evidence suggests that volatile anesthetics exert protective effects on the myocardium in the setting of compromised regional perfusion. In patients undergoing coronary artery bypass graft (CABG) surgery, maintenance with 0.2 to 1 MAC of desflurane or sevoflurane decreased the incidence of abnormally increased troponin levels compared with patients receiving propofol.[43] Sevoflurane administered for the entire duration of CABG surgery versus prebypass or postbypass administration resulted in a less frequent rate of postoperative myocardial infarction compared with sevoflurane administered only in the prebypass or postbypass period, and prebypass or postbypass administration resulted in a smaller risk of myocardial infarction compared with propofol anesthesia.[44]

### Mechanisms of Ischemic Preconditioning

Ischemic preconditioning is a fundamental protective mechanism present in all tissues in all species. In ischemic preconditioning, exposure to single or multiple brief episodes of ischemia can confer a protective effect on the myocardium against reversible or irreversible injury with a subsequent prolonged ischemic insult. There are two distinct periods after a brief ischemic episode during which the myocardium is protected. The first period occurs for 1 to 2 hours after the conditioning episode and then dissipates. In the second period, the benefit reappears 24 hours later and can last as long as 3 days. The opening of mitochondrial adenosine triphosphate (ATP)–sensitive potassium channels ($K_{ATP}$) is the crucial event that confers the protective activity, resulting from binding of various ligands to G protein–coupled receptors. Volatile anesthetics enhance ischemic preconditioning or provide direct myocardial protection, and the $K_{ATP}$ channels play a central role in their protective effects.[45]

## Ventilation Effects

Inhaled anesthetics increase the frequency of breathing and decrease tidal volume as anesthetic concentration increases. Although minute ventilation is relatively preserved, the decreased tidal volume leads to a relatively greater proportion of dead space ventilation relative to alveolar ventilation. Gas exchange becomes progressively less efficient at deeper levels of anesthesia, and $Pa_{CO_2}$ increases proportionally with anesthetic concentration (Fig. 7.14).[1] Effects are similar among potent anesthetics at given MAC multiples. Substitution of nitrous oxide (60%) for an equivalent portion of volatile anesthetic may attenuate the increase in $Pa_{CO_2}$ at deeper levels of anesthesia.

Volunteers and patients breathing desflurane (and other volatile anesthetics) show a dose-related blunting of carbon dioxide responsiveness, which leads to apnea in subjects receiving 1.7 MAC of desflurane in oxygen (Fig 7.15).[1] Compared with volunteers, the blunting of ventilation with inhaled anesthetics may be less pronounced in patients undergoing surgery, reflecting the stimulatory effect of surgery on breathing (Fig. 7.16).[1] Volatile anesthetics all blunt the ventilatory stimulation evoked by arterial hypoxemia.[46]

### Chest Wall Changes

Inhaled anesthetics contribute to conformational changes in the chest wall that may influence ventilatory mechanics. Cephalad displacement of the diaphragm and inward displacement of the rib cage occur from enhanced

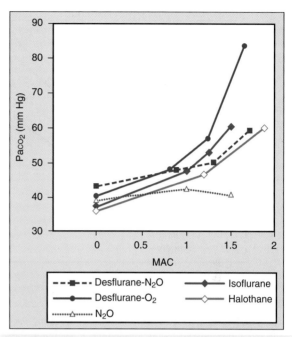

**Fig. 7.14** Inhaled anesthetics produce drug-specific and dose-dependent increases in $Pa_{CO_2}$. *MAC*, Minimum alveolar concentration. (From Eger EI II. *Desflurane (Suprane): A Compendium and Reference.* Nutley, NJ: Anaquest; 1993:1-119, used with permission.)

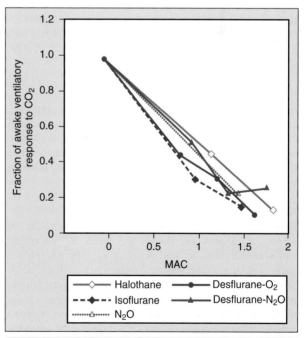

**Fig. 7.15** All inhaled anesthetics produce similar dose-dependent decreases in the ventilatory responses to carbon dioxide. *MAC*, Minimum alveolar concentration. (From Eger EI II. *Desflurane (Suprane): A Compendium and Reference.* Nutley, NJ: Anaquest; 1993:1-119, used with permission.)

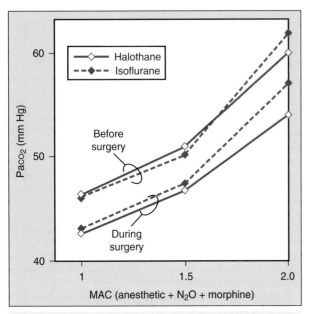

**Fig. 7.16** Impact of surgical stimulation on the resting $Paco_2$ (mm Hg) during administration of isoflurane or halothane. *MAC*, Minimum alveolar concentration. (From Eger EI II. *Desflurane (Suprane): A Compendium and Reference.* Nutley, NJ: Anaquest; 1993:1-119, used with permission.)

expiratory muscle activity, and the net result contributes to reduction in functional residual capacity. Atelectasis occurs preferentially in the dependent areas of the lung and occurs to a greater extent when spontaneous ventilation is permitted.

### Hypoxic Pulmonary Vasoconstriction
Inhaled anesthetics alter pulmonary blood flow, but inhibition of hypoxic pulmonary vasoconstriction is minimal. For example, arterial oxygenation is similar in patients undergoing one-lung ventilation with isoflurane versus desflurane anesthesia and sevoflurane versus propofol anesthesia.[47]

### Airway Resistance
In the absence of bronchoconstriction, bronchodilating effects of inhaled anesthetics are small. In volunteers, isoflurane, halothane, and sevoflurane, but not nitrous oxide and thiopental, decrease respiratory systemic resistance after tracheal intubation. In nonsmokers, airway resistance shows no change after tracheal intubation and desflurane anesthesia compared with a modest decrease with sevoflurane, whereas smokers show a mild, transient increase in airway resistance after tracheal intubation and desflurane anesthesia.[48] Some or all of the changes in airway resistance may be mediated by changes in gas density.

### Airway Irritant Effects
Inhaled anesthetics differ in their capacity to irritate airways (i.e., pungency). Sevoflurane, halothane, and nitrous oxide are nonpungent and cause minimal or no irritation over a broad range of concentrations. Desflurane and isoflurane are pungent, and they can irritate the airways in concentrations exceeding 1 MAC, particularly in the absence of intravenous medications (e.g., opioids, sedative-hypnotics) that decrease the perception of pungency.

Sevoflurane or halothane is selected most frequently when an inhaled induction of anesthesia is desired. However, desflurane and isoflurane may be administered to surgical patients by means of a laryngeal mask airway without a greater incidence of airway irritation (e.g., coughing, breath-holding, laryngospasm, arterial oxygen desaturation) compared with sevoflurane or propofol, because maintenance usually does not require a concentration in excess of 1 MAC (i.e., nonirritating concentrations).[49]

## Central Nervous System Effects

### Cerebral Blood Flow (Also See Chapter 30)
Nitrous oxide administered without volatile anesthetics causes cerebral vasodilatation and increases cerebral blood flow. The cerebral metabolic rate for oxygen ($CMRO_2$) increases modestly. Coadministration of opioids, barbiturates, or propofol (but not ketamine) counteracts these effects.[50] Inhaled anesthetics do not abolish cerebral vascular responsiveness to changes in $Paco_2$.[51]

Halothane, isoflurane, sevoflurane, and desflurane decrease $CMRO_2$. In normocapnic humans, these volatile anesthetics cause cerebral vasodilatation at concentrations above 0.6 MAC. There is a biphasic dose-dependent effect on cerebral blood flow. At 0.5 MAC, the decrease in $CMRO_2$ counteracts the vasodilatation such that cerebral blood flow does not change significantly. At concentrations in excess of 1 MAC, vasodilating effects predominate and cerebral blood flow increases, especially if systemic blood pressure is maintained at awake levels. The cerebral blood flow increase is relatively greater with halothane compared with isoflurane, sevoflurane, or desflurane.

### Intracranial Pressure (Also See Chapter 30)
Intracranial pressure increases with all of the volatile anesthetics at doses more than 1 MAC, and autoregulation (i.e., adaptive mechanism normalizing cerebral blood flow over a wide range of systemic arterial pressures in awake patients) is impaired at concentrations of less than 1 MAC. Patients undergoing craniotomy for supratentorial tumors who receive 1 MAC of isoflurane or desflurane show decreased cerebral perfusion pressure and an arteriovenous oxygen difference for oxygen but no change in intracranial pressure.[52] However, patients undergoing pituitary tumor

resection who receive 1 MAC of desflurane, isoflurane, or sevoflurane show small increases in intracranial pressure and decreased cerebral blood flow. Neurosurgical patients receiving 50% nitrous oxide plus 0.5 MAC of desflurane or isoflurane apparently have more brain relaxation than those receiving 1 MAC of desflurane or isoflurane without nitrous oxide. Inhaled anesthetics do not abolish cerebral vascular responsiveness to changes in $Pa_{CO_2}$.[51]

### Evoked Potentials

All volatile anesthetics and nitrous oxide depress the amplitude and increase the latency of somatosensory evoked potentials in a dose-dependent manner. Evoked potentials may be abolished at 1 MAC of volatile anesthetic alone or above 0.5 MAC administered with 50% nitrous oxide. Low concentrations of volatile anesthetics (0.2 to 0.3 MAC) can decrease the reliability of motor evoked potential monitoring, although the impact can be partially overcome by the use of multipulse stimuli.[53]

### Electroencephalographic Effects

Volatile anesthetics cause characteristic, dose-dependent changes in the EEG. Increasing depth of anesthesia from the awake state is characterized by increased amplitude and synchrony. Periods of electrical silence begin to occupy a greater proportion of the time as depth increases (i.e., burst suppression). This isoelectric pattern predominates on the EEG within the range of 1.5 to 2.0 MAC.

Sevoflurane and enflurane may be associated with epileptiform activity on the EEG, especially at higher concentrations or when controlled hyperventilation is instituted. Seizure-like activity has been reported in children during sevoflurane induction, but the clinical implications of these observations are not clear.[54]

## Neuromuscular Effects

Volatile anesthetics produce dose-related skeletal muscle relaxation and enhance the activity of neuromuscular blocking drugs (also see Chapter 11). Enhancement of the relaxant effect of rocuronium is more intense with anesthesia from desflurane than with sevoflurane or isoflurane, although all volatile anesthetics enhance skeletal muscle relaxation compared with intravenous anesthetics (e.g., propofol plus fentanyl). Elimination of volatile anesthetic enhances recovery from neuromuscular blockade. A decrease in the desflurane concentration to 0.25 MAC facilitates reversal of neuromuscular block after vecuronium administration more than an equipotent decrease in isoflurane concentration.

## Malignant Hyperthermia

Malignant hyperthermia (MH) continues to be a life-threatening complication of anesthesia. It is an inherited disorder of increased skeletal muscle metabolism that is triggered with the administration of a volatile anesthetic, especially halothane and/or succinylcholine. Although all potent inhaled volatile anesthetics also have the potential to trigger MH, studies with desflurane, sevoflurane, and possibly isoflurane suggest less risk than that of halothane. Males appear to be more susceptible to developing a clinical MH episode than females.([55,56]) The pediatric population accounts for 52.1% of all MH reactions([57,58]). Signs of MH are related to increased metabolism and include tachycardia, increased end-tidal carbon dioxide levels, muscle rigidity, and increased temperature.

More recent cases of MH are less severe due to improved diagnostic awareness, early detection through end-expired carbon dioxide, less use of potent anesthetic triggers, and the administration of drugs that attenuate fulminant episodes of MH.

The key aspects of management include discontinuation of volatile anesthetics and succinylcholine, immediate administration of intravenous dantrolene, and treatment of potentially life-threatening electrolyte abnormalities such as hyperkalemia. The Malignant Hyperthermia Association of the United States (MHAUS) provides detailed treatment recommendations on its website <http://www.mhaus.org/healthcare-professionals>. MHAUS also maintains a 24-hour hotline for emergency advice (1-800-644-9737 in USA; 001-209-417-3722 outside of USA).

## Hepatic Effects

Hepatic injury after anesthesia may be categorized as severe (immune mediated) or mild.[59]

### Immune-Mediated Liver Injury

Severe hepatic injury may follow anesthesia with halothane, isoflurane, sevoflurane, or desflurane. This severe form involves massive hepatic necrosis that can lead to death or necessitate liver transplantation. The mechanism for this severe injury is immunologic, requiring prior exposure to a volatile anesthetic. Halothane, isoflurane, and desflurane all undergo oxidative metabolism by cytochrome P-450 enzymes to produce trifluoroacetate. The trifluoroacetate can bind covalently to hepatocyte proteins. The trifluoroacetyl-hepatocyte moieties can act as haptens, which the body recognizes as foreign and to which the immune system forms antibodies. Subsequent exposure to any anesthetic capable of producing trifluoroacetate may provoke an immune response, leading to severe hepatic necrosis.[60] Sevoflurane is metabolized to hexafluoroisopropanol, a compound that does not have the equivalent antigenic behavior as trifluoroacetate.[61]

### Mild Liver Injury

A clinically mild form of liver injury may follow administration of halothane. The main characteristic of this more common entity is modest elevation of serum transaminase levels. This mild form of liver injury is thought to be mediated by reductive metabolism of halothane and may be more likely to occur after concomitant decreases in hepatic blood flow and associated reductions in oxygen delivery to the liver.

### History of Prior Anesthesia-Related Hepatic Dysfunction

Although volatile anesthetics are frequently not given in patients who have experienced unexplained symptoms of hepatic dysfunction after inhaled anesthesia on a previous occasion, volatile anesthetics are probably not harmful to patients with preexisting hepatic disease unrelated to anesthesia.

## Renal Effects

Methoxyflurane was the first nonflammable volatile anesthetic introduced to clinical practice. Its use was associated with renal injury. Subsequent investigation suggests that its extensive metabolism, specifically to inorganic fluoride and dichloroacetic acid from *O*-demethylation, is probably responsible for the injury. Yet, fluoride production from metabolism of other potent inhaled anesthetics, specifically sevoflurane, shows no association with renal injury.[62]

## QUESTIONS OF THE DAY

1. What physical properties of desflurane require its administration by a specially designed vaporizer? How is the output of a desflurane vaporizer affected by high altitudes?
2. Which inhaled anesthetics have the greatest impact on the environment in terms of "carbon dioxide equivalents" as well as atmospheric longevity?
3. How does the inhaled anesthetic dose required to produce amnesia compare to the dose required to prevent movement with the surgical incision? What is the standard deviation of MAC for surgical incision? What medications increase or decrease inhaled anesthetic requirements?
4. When administering an inhaled anesthetic, what six factors determine the alveolar partial pressure of the anesthetic?
5. During recovery from an inhaled anesthetic, what factors most influence the decrease in anesthetic partial pressure?
6. What are the circulatory effects of a rapid increase in the concentration of desflurane compared to isoflurane and sevoflurane? How can these effects be minimized?

## REFERENCES

1. Eger EI. *Desflurane (Suprane): A Compendium and Reference.* Nutley, NJ: Anaquest; 1993.
2. Eger EI II. *History of Modern Inhaled Anesthetics: The Pharmacology of Inhaled Anesthetics.* San Antonio, TX: Dannemiller Memorial Educational Foundation; 2000.
3. Eger II EI. New inhaled anesthetics. *Anesthesiology.* 1994;80:906–922.
4. Eger EI II, Koblin DD, Harris RA, et al. Hypothesis: inhaled anesthetics produce immobility and amnesia by different mechanisms at different sites. *Anesth Analg.* 1997;84:915–918.
5. Quasha AL, Eger EI II, Tinker JH, et al. Determination and application of MAC. *Anesthesiology.* 1980;53(4):315–334.
6. Rampil IJ. Anesthetic potency is not altered after hypothermic spinal cord transection in rats. *Anesthesiology.* 1994;80:606–610.
7. Guo TZ, Poree L, Golden W, et al. Antinociceptive response to nitrous oxide is mediated by supraspinal opiate and spinal alpha 2 adrenergic receptors in the rat. *Anesthesiology.* 1996;85(4):846–852.
8. Sawamura S, Kingery WS, Davies MF, et al. Antinociceptive action of nitrous oxide is mediated by stimulation of noradrenergic neurons in the brainstem and activation of [alpha]2B adrenoceptors. *J Neurosci.* 2000;20(24):9242–9251.
9. Weiskopf RB, Sampson D, Moore MA. The desflurane (Tec 6) vaporizer: design, design considerations and performance evaluation. *Br J Anaesth.* 1994;72(4):474–479.
10. Brockwell RC, Andrews JJ. Vaporizers (in delivery systems for inhaled anesthetics). In: Barash PG, Cullen BF, Stoelting RK, Cahallan M, eds. *Clinical Anesthesia.* 6th ed. Philadelphia: Lippincott Williams & Wilkins; 2009:667–669.
11. Carpenter RL, Eger EI II, Johnson BH, et al. The extent of metabolism of inhaled anesthetics in humans. *Anesthesiology.* 1986;65:201–205.
12. Wissing H, Kuhn I, Warnken U, et al. Carbon monoxide production from desflurane, enflurane, halothane, isoflurane, and sevoflurane with dry soda lime. *Anesthesiology.* 2001;95:1205–1212.
13. Laster MJ, Roth P, Eger EI II. Fires from the interaction of anesthetics with desiccated absorbent. *Anesth Analg.* 2004;99:769–774.
14. Wu J, Previte JP, Adler E, et al. Spontaneous ignition, explosion, and fire with sevoflurane and barium hydroxide lime. *Anesthesiology.* 2004;101:534–537.
15. Chortkoff BS, Bennett HL, Eger EI II. Subanesthetic concentrations of isoflurane suppress learning as defined by the category-example task. *Anesthesiology.* 1993;79(1):16–22.
16. Sonner JM, Gong D, Eger EI II. Naturally occurring variability in anesthetic potency among inbred mouse strains. *Anesth Analg.* 2000;91(3):720–726.
17. Dwyer R, Bennett HL, Eger EI II, et al. Effects of isoflurane and nitrous oxide in subanesthetic concentrations on memory and responsiveness in volunteers. *Anesthesiology.* 1992;77(5):888–898.
18. Eger EI II. Uptake of inhaled anesthetics: the alveolar to inspired anesthetic difference. In: Eger EI II, ed. *Anesthetic Uptake and Action.* Baltimore: Williams & Wilkins; 1974:77–96.
19. Eger EI. Effect of inspired anesthetic concentration on the rate of rise of alveolar concentration. *Anesthesiology.* 1963;24:153–157.
20. Yasuda N, Lockhart SH, Eger EI II, et al. Comparison of kinetics of sevoflurane and isoflurane in humans. *Anesth Analg.* 1992;72:316–324.
21. McKay RE, Malhotra A, Cakmakkaya OS, et al. Effect of increased body mass index and anaesthetic duration on recovery of protective airway reflexes after sevoflurane vs desflurane. *Br J Anaesth.* 2010;104:175–182.
22. Wahrenbrock EA, Eger EI II, Laravuso RB, et al. Anesthetic uptake–of mice and men (and whales). *Anesthesiology.* 1974;40(1):19–23.

23. Aronow WS, Ahn C. Increased plasma homocysteine is an independent predictor of new coronary events in older persons. *Am J Cardiol.* 2000;86(3):346–347.

24. Badner NH, Beattie WS, Freeman D, et al. Nitrous oxide-induced increased homocysteine concentrations are associated with increased postoperative myocardial ischemia in patients undergoing carotid endarterectomy. *Anesth Analg.* 2000;91(5):1073–1079.

25. Eger EI II, Saidman JL. Hazards of nitrous oxide anesthesia in bowel obstruction and pneumothorax. *Anesthesiology.* 1965;26:61–66.

26. Ryan S, Neilsen CJ. Global warming potential of inhaled anesthetics: application to clinical use. *Anesth Analg.* 2010;111:92–98.

27. Bailey JM. Context-sensitive half-times and other decrement times of inhaled anesthetics. *Anesth Analg.* 1997;85:681–686.

28. Sundman E, Witt H, Sandin R, et al. Pharyngeal function and airway protection during subhypnotic concentrations of propofol, isoflurane, and sevoflurane: volunteers examined by pharyngeal videoradiography and simultaneous manometry. *Anesthesiology.* 2001;95(5):1125–1132.

29. Dahan A, Teppema LJ. Influence of anaesthesia and analgesia on the control of breathing. *Br J Anaesth.* 2003;91:40–49.

30. Bellgardt M, Bomberg H, Herzog-Niescery J, et al. Survival after long-term isoflurane sedation as opposed to intravenous sedation in critically ill surgical patients: retrospective analysis. *Eur J Anaesthiol.* 2016;33(1):6–13.

31. Sackey PV, Martling CR, Granath F, Radell PJ. Prolonged isoflurane sedation of intensive care unit patients with the anesthetic conserving device. *Crit Care Med.* 2004;32(11):2241–2246.

32. Cahalan MK. *Hemodynamic Effects of Inhaled Anesthetics. Review Courses.* Cleveland: International Anesthesia Research Society; 1996.

33. Cahalan MK, Weiskopf RB, Eger EI II, et al. Hemodynamic effects of desflurane/nitrous oxide anesthesia in volunteers. *Anesth Analg.* 1991;73:157–164.

34. Eger EI. *Isoflurane (Forane): A Compendium and Reference.* Madison, WI: Ohio Medical Products; 1985.

35. Malan TP Jr, DiNardo JA, Isner RJ, et al. Cardiovascular effects of sevoflurane compared with those of isoflurane in volunteers. *Anesthesiology.* 1995;83:918–928.

36. Yli-Hankala A, Vakkuri AP, Sarkela M, et al. Epileptiform electroencephalogram during mask induction of anesthesia with sevoflurane. *Anesthesiology.* 1999;91:1596.

37. Ebert TJ, Perez F, Uhrich TD, et al. Desflurane-mediated sympathetic activation occurs in humans despite preventing hypotension and baroreceptor unloading. *Anesthesiology.* 1998;88:1227–1232.

38. Ebert TJ, Muzi M, Lopatka CW. Neurocirculatory responses to sevoflurane in humans: a comparison to desflurane. *Anesthesiology.* 1995;83:88–95.

39. Navarro R, Weiskopf RB, Moore MA, et al. Humans anesthetized with sevoflurane or isoflurane have similar arrhythmic response to epinephrine. *Anesthesiology.* 1994;80:545–549.

40. Booker PD, Whyte SD, Ladusans EJ. Long QT syndrome and anaesthesia. *Br J Anaesth.* 2003;90:349–366.

41. Whyte SD, Booker PD, Buckley DG. The effects of propofol and sevoflurane on the QT interval and transmural dispersion of repolarization in children. *Anesth Analg.* 2005;100:71–77.

42. Grundmann U, Muler M, Kleinschmidt S, et al. Cardiovascular effects of desflurane and isoflurane in patients with coronary artery disease. *Acta Anaesthesiol Scand.* 1996;40:1101–1107.

43. DeHert SG, Cromheecke S, ten Broecke PW, et al. Effects of propofol, desflurane, and sevoflurane on recovery of myocardial function after coronary surgery in elderly high-risk patients. *Anesthesiology.* 2003;99:314–323.

44. DeHert SG, Van der Linden PJ, Cromheecke S, et al. Cardioprotective properties of sevoflurane in patients undergoing coronary surgery and cardiopulmonary bypass are related to the modalities of its administration. *Anesthesiology.* 2004;101:299–310.

45. Zaugg M, Lucchinetti E, Spahn D, et al. Volatile anesthetics mimic cardiac preconditioning by priming the activation of the mitoKATP channels via multiple signaling pathways. *Anesthesiology.* 2002;97:4–14.

46. Sjögren D, Lindahl SG, Sollevi A. Ventilatory responses to acute and sustained hypoxia during isoflurane anesthesia. *Anesth Analg.* 1998;86:403–409.

47. Beck DH, Doepfmer UR, Sinemus C, et al. Effects of sevoflurane and propofol on pulmonary shunt fraction during one-lung ventilation for thoracic surgery. *Br J Anaesth.* 2001;86:38–43.

48. Goff MJ, Arain SR, Ficke DJ, et al. Absence of bronchodilation during desflurane anesthesia: a comparison to sevoflurane and thiopental. *Anesthesiology.* 2000;93:404–408.

49. Eshima R, Maurer A, King T, et al. A comparison of upper airway responses during desflurane and sevoflurane administration via a laryngeal mask airway. *Anesth Analg.* 2003;96:701–705.

50. Petersen KD, Landsfeldt U, Cold GE, et al. Intracranial pressure and cerebral hemodynamics in patients with cerebral tumors: a randomized prospective study of patients subjected to craniotomy in propofol-fentanyl, isoflurane-fentanyl, or sevoflurane-fentanyl anesthesia. *Anesthesiology.* 2003;98:329–336.

51. Mielck F, Stephen H, Buhre W, et al. Effects of 1 MAC desflurane on cerebral metabolism, blood flow and carbon dioxide reactivity in humans. *Br J Anaesth.* 1998;81:155–160.

52. Fraga M, Rama-Maceiras P, Rodino S, et al. The effects of isoflurane and desflurane on intracranial pressure, cerebral perfusion pressure, and cerebral arteriovenous oxygen content difference in normocapnic patients with supratentorial brain tumors. *Anesthesiology.* 2003;98:1085–1090.

53. Lotto ML, Banoub M, Schubert A. Effects of anesthetic agents and physiologic changes on intraoperative motor evoked potentials. *J Neurosurg Anesthesiol.* 2004;16:32–42.

54. Akeson J, Didricksson I. Convulsions on anaesthetic induction with sevoflurane in young children. *Acta Anaesthesiol Scand.* 2004;48:405–407.

55 Sumitani M, Uchida K, Yasunaga H, et al. Prevalence of malignant hyperthermia and relationship with anesthetics in Japan: data from the diagnosis procedure combination database. *Anesthesiology.* 2011;114:84–90.

56 Brady JE, Sun LS, Rosenberg H, et al. Prevalence of malignant hyperthermia due to anesthesia in New York state, 2001-2005. *Anesth Analg.* 2009;109:1162–1166.

57 Rosenberg H, Shutack JG. Variants of malignant hyperthermia. Special problems for the paediatric anesthesiologist. *Paediatr Anaesth.* 1996;6:87–93.

58 Rosenberg H, Davis M, James D, et al. Malignant hyperthermia. *Orphanet J Rare Dis.* 2007;2:21.

59. Martin JL. Volatile anesthetics and liver injury: a clinical update or what every anesthesiologist should know. *Can J Anesth.* 2005;52:125–129.

60. Njoku D, Laster MJ, Gong DH, et al. Biotransformation of halothane, enflurane, isoflurane and desflurane to trifluoroacetylated liver proteins: association between protein acetylation and hepatic injury. *Anesth Analg.* 1997;84:173–178.

61. Frink EJ, Ghantous H, Malan TP, et al. Plasma inorganic fluoride with sevoflurane anesthesia: correlation with indices of hepatic and renal function. *Anesth Analg.* 1992;74:231–235.

62. Kharasch ED. Adverse drug reactions with halogenated anesthetics. *Clin Pharmacol Ther.* 2008;84:158–162.

# 8 INTRAVENOUS ANESTHETICS

Michael P. Bokoch and Helge Eilers

Intravenous nonopioid anesthetics have an important role in modern anesthesia practice (Box 8.1).[1-7] They are widely used to facilitate a rapid induction of general anesthesia and provide sedation during monitored anesthesia care (MAC) and for patients in intensive care settings (also see Chapter 41). With the introduction of propofol, intravenous techniques are increasingly being used for maintenance of anesthesia. However, similar to inhaled anesthetics, the currently available intravenous drugs do not produce only desirable effects (hypnosis, amnesia, analgesia, immobility). Therefore, the concept of "balanced anesthesia" evolved by using smaller doses of multiple drugs rather than using larger doses with one or two drugs. The fundamental drugs used with "balanced anesthesia" include inhaled anesthetics, sedative/hypnotics, opioids, and neuromuscular blocking drugs (also see Chapters 7, 9, and 11).

The intravenous anesthetics used for induction of general anesthesia are lipophilic and preferentially partition into highly perfused lipid-rich tissues (brain, spinal cord),

---

**Box 8.1** Drugs Classified as Intravenous Anesthetics

Isopropylphenols
    Propofol
    Fospropofol
Barbiturates
    Thiopental
    Methohexital
Benzodiazepines
    Diazepam
    Midazolam
    Lorazepam
    Remimazolam
Phencyclidine
    Ketamine
Carboxylated imidazole
    Etomidate
$\alpha_2$-Adrenergic agonist
    Dexmedetomidine

which accounts for their rapid onset of action. Regardless of the extent and speed of their metabolism, termination of the effect of a single bolus dose is a result of redistribution of the drug into less perfused and inactive tissues such as skeletal muscles and fat. Thus, all drugs used for induction of anesthesia have a similar duration of action when administered as a single dose despite significant differences in their metabolism.

## PROPOFOL

Propofol is the most frequently administered anesthetic drug for induction of anesthesia.[2,3,6] In addition, propofol is used during maintenance of anesthesia and is a common selection for sedation in the operating room as well as in the intensive care unit (ICU). Increasingly, propofol is also utilized for sedation and short-duration general anesthesia in locations outside the operating room such as interventional radiology suites and the emergency room (also see Chapter 38).

### Physicochemical Characteristics

Propofol (2,6-diisopropylphenol) is an alkylphenol with hypnotic properties that is chemically distinct from other

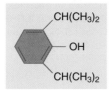

**Fig. 8.1** Chemical structure of 2,6-diisopropylphenol (propofol).

groups of intravenous anesthetics (Fig. 8.1). It is insoluble in aqueous solutions and formulated as an emulsion containing 10% soybean oil, 2.25% glycerol, and 1.2% lecithin (the major component of the egg yolk phosphatide fraction). Sterile technique is important because the available formulations support bacterial growth. Although either ethylenediaminetetraacetic acid (0.05 mg/mL), metabisulfite (0.25 mg/mL), or benzyl alcohol (1 mg/mL) is added to the emulsions by the different manufacturers as retardants of bacterial growth, solutions should be used as soon as possible or at least within 12 hours after opening the propofol vial. The solutions appear milky white and slightly viscous, their pH is approximately 7, and the propofol concentration is 1% (10 mg/mL). In some countries, a 2% formulation is available. Allergic reactions to propofol are rare, and there is no evidence for cross-reactivity in patients with immunoglobulin E confirmed allergy to egg, soy, or peanut.[8] The addition of metabisulfite in one of the formulations is of concern for patients with reactive airways (asthma) or sulfite allergies.

### Pharmacokinetics

Propofol is rapidly metabolized in the liver, and the resulting water-soluble compounds are presumed to be inactive and excreted through the kidneys (Table 8.1). Plasma clearance is rapid and exceeds hepatic blood flow, thus indicating the importance of extrahepatic metabolism, which has been confirmed during the anhepatic phase of liver transplantation. The lungs probably play a major role in this extrahepatic metabolism and likely account for the elimination of up to 30% of a bolus dose of propofol. The rapid plasma clearance explains the more complete recovery from propofol with less "hangover" than observed with thiopental. As with other intravenous drugs, the effects of

**Table 8.1**   Pharmacokinetic Data[a] for Intravenous Anesthetics

| Drug | Induction Dose (mg/kg IV) | Duration of Action (min) | $Vd_{ss}$ (L/kg) | $T_{1/2}\alpha$ (min) | Protein Binding (%) | Clearance (mL/kg/min) | $T_{1/2}\beta$ (h) |
|---|---|---|---|---|---|---|---|
| Propofol | 1-2.5 | 3-8 | 2-10 | 2-4 | 97 | 20-30 | 4-23 |
| Thiopental | 3-5 | 5-10 | 2.5 | 2-4 | 83 | 3.4 | 11 |
| Methohexital | 1-1.5 | 4-7 | 2.2 | 5-6 | 73 | 11 | 4 |
| Midazolam | 0.1-0.3 | 15-20 | 1.1-1.7 | 7-15 | 94 | 6.4-11 | 1.7-2.6 |
| Diazepam | 0.3-0.6 | 15-30 | 0.7-1.7 | 10-15 | 98 | 0.2-0.5 | 20-50 |
| Lorazepam | 0.03-0.1 | 60-120 | 0.8-1.3 | 3-10 | 98 | 0.8-1.8 | 11-22 |
| Ketamine | 1-2 | 5-10 | 3.1 | 11-16 | 12 | 12-17 | 2-4 |
| Etomidate | 0.2-0.3 | 3-8 | 2.5-4.5 | 2-4 | 77 | 18-25 | 2.9-5.3 |
| Dexmedetomidine | N/A | N/A | 2-3 | 6 | 94 | 10-30 | 2-3 |

[a]Data are for average adult patients. The duration of action reflects the duration after an average single IV dose.
*IV,* Intravenous; *N/A,* not applicable; $T_{1/2}\alpha$, distribution half-time; $T_{1/2}\beta$, elimination half-time; $Vd_{ss}$, volume of distribution at steady state.

propofol are terminated by redistribution from the plasma and highly perfused compartments (such as brain) to poorly perfused compartments (such as skeletal muscle). A patient usually awakens within 8 to 10 minutes after an induction dose of propofol, similar to the period of decline in plasma concentration after a single bolus dose (Fig. 8.2).[2,6]

### Continuous Intravenous Infusion

Propofol has two pharmacokinetic properties that make it ideal for use as a continuous intravenous infusion: (1) rapid metabolism and efficient clearance from plasma, and (2) slow redistribution from poorly perfused compartments back into the central compartment. One way to characterize an anesthetic infusion is the "context-sensitive half-time," a parameter that describes the time needed for the plasma levels of a drug to drop by 50% after stopping the infusion (Fig. 8.3).[9,10] This time depends on the duration for which an infusion has been run. The context-sensitive half-time of propofol is brief, even after a prolonged infusion, and recovery remains relatively prompt.

### Compartmental Model

The kinetics of propofol (and other intravenous anesthetics) after a single bolus and after continuous infusion is best described by a three-compartment model (also see Chapter 4). These mathematical models have been used as the basis for the development of systems for target-controlled infusions.[11]

## Pharmacodynamics

The presumed mechanism of action of propofol is through potentiation of the chloride current mediated through the γ-aminobutyric acid type A ($GABA_A$) receptor complex.[12]

### Central Nervous System

In the central nervous system (CNS), propofol primarily acts as a hypnotic and does not have any analgesic properties. It reduces the cerebral metabolic rate for oxygen ($CMRO_2$), which leads to decreased cerebral blood flow (CBF) through preserved flow-metabolism coupling. This results in decreases in cerebral blood volume, intracranial pressure (ICP), and intraocular pressure. The magnitude of these changes is comparable to those produced by thiopental. Although propofol can produce a desired decrease in ICP, the reduced CBF combined with the reduced mean arterial pressure caused by peripheral vasodilation can critically compromise cerebral perfusion (also see Chapter 30).

Propofol is probably neuroprotective during focal ischemia to the same extent as thiopental or isoflurane. When administered in large doses, propofol produces burst suppression in the electroencephalogram (EEG),[13] an end point that has been used for the administration of intravenous anesthetics for neuroprotection during neurosurgical procedures. Occasionally, excitatory effects such as twitching or spontaneous movement can be observed during induction of anesthesia with propofol. Although these effects may resemble seizure activity, propofol is actually an anticonvulsant and may be safely administered to patients with seizure disorders.[6] Although propofol may be toxic to developing neurons in animals and cell culture, no human study has demonstrated

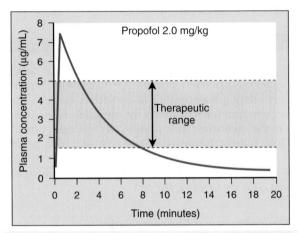

**Fig. 8.2** Time course of the propofol plasma concentration after a simulated single bolus injection of 2.0 mg/kg. The shape of this curve is similar for other induction drugs, although the slope and the absolute concentrations are different. (From Vuyk J, Sitsen E, Reekers M. Intravenous anesthetics. In: Miller RD, ed. *Miller's Anesthesia*. 8th ed. Philadelphia: Elsevier; 2015: 821-863. (Original chapter: Reves JG, Glass PSA. Chapter 9, Nonbarbiturate intravenous anesthetics. In: Miller RD, ed. *Miller's Anesthesia*. 3rd ed. New York, NY: Churchill Livingstone; 1990: 243-279.)

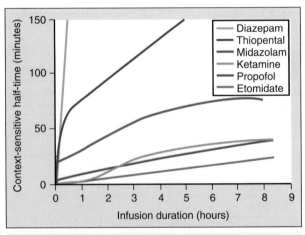

**Fig. 8.3** Context-sensitive half-time for the most commonly used intravenous anesthetics. Propofol, etomidate, and ketamine have the smallest increase in context-sensitive half-times, with prolonged infusions making these drugs more suitable for use as continuous infusions. (From Vuyk J, Sitsen E, Reekers M. Intravenous anesthetics. In: Miller RD, ed. *Miller's Anesthesia*. 8th ed. Philadelphia:Elsevier; 2015:821-863.)

long-term cognitive or memory problems in children who have received propofol anesthesia.[14]

### Cardiovascular System

Propofol produces a larger decrease in systemic arterial blood pressure than any other drug used for induction of anesthesia. Propofol causes profound vasodilation, whereas its direct myocardial depressant effect is not clear. Vasodilation occurs in both the arterial and venous circulation and leads to reductions in preload and afterload. The effect is worse with rapid injection, and is more pronounced in elderly patients, especially those with reduced intravascular fluid volume (also see Chapter 35). The degree of vasodilation may also be altered in patients with diabetes, hypertension, or obesity.[15] Propofol markedly inhibits the normal baroreflex response and produces only a small or no increase in heart rate, thus further exacerbating hypotension. Profound bradycardia and asystole after the administration of propofol can occur in healthy adults despite administration of prophylactic anticholinergic drugs.[16]

### Respiratory System

Propofol is a respiratory depressant and often produces apnea following a dose used to induce anesthesia. A maintenance infusion of propofol decreases minute ventilation via reductions in tidal volume and respiratory rate, with the effect on tidal volume being more pronounced. The ventilatory response to hypoxia and hypercapnia is also reduced. Propofol causes a more intense reduction in upper airway reflexes than does thiopental, which makes it well suited for instrumentation of the airway, such as placement of a laryngeal mask airway. Propofol increases collapsibility of the upper airway by inhibiting genioglossus and other muscles,[17] and airway obstruction may occur with sedative doses or during emergence from propofol anesthesia. When compared with thiopental, propofol decreases the incidence of wheezing after induction of anesthesia and tracheal intubation in healthy and asthmatic patients.[18]

### Other Effects

Unlike many other anesthetics, propofol has antiemetic activity. Similar to thiopental and unlike volatile anesthetics, propofol probably does not enhance neuromuscular blockade from neuromuscular blocking drugs. Yet, propofol often provides excellent clinical conditions for endotracheal intubation without the use of neuromuscular blocking drugs. Unexpected arrhythmias or electrocardiogram changes occurring during propofol anesthesia should prompt laboratory evaluation for possible metabolic acidosis, rhabdomyolysis, or hyperkalemia (propofol infusion syndrome).[19]

## Clinical Uses

Pain from injection of propofol is a common complaint that can lead to patient distress or dissatisfaction. The most effective and expedient means to reduce injection pain is selecting an antecubital vein (larger, faster venous flow rate) for injection.[20] Alternatively, if a hand vein is chosen, injecting a small dose of lidocaine (20 to 40 mg intravenously [IV]) and applying proximal venous occlusion for 15 to 60 seconds before injecting propofol is similarly effective. Other helpful and expedient techniques are premedication with a small dose of opioid,[20] pretreatment with larger doses of lidocaine (40 to 100 mg IV) without venous occlusion, and coadministration of lidocaine and propofol as an admixture.[21]

### Induction and Maintenance of General Anesthesia

Propofol (1 to 2.5 mg/kg IV) is the drug most commonly administered for induction of general anesthesia. The dose should be decreased in the elderly, especially those who have a reduced cardiovascular reserve, or after premedication with benzodiazepines or opioids. Children generally require larger doses (2.5 to 3.5 mg/kg IV). Obese patients require a larger total dose compared with nonobese patients of similar height and age, but boluses for morbidly obese patients should be calculated per kilogram of lean body weight rather than total body weight to avoid excess hypotension.[22] Generally, titration of the induction dose of propofol (i.e., rather than an arbitrary bolus dose) helps prevent severe hemodynamic changes. Propofol is also often used to maintain anesthesia as part of a balanced regimen in combination with volatile anesthetics, nitrous oxide, sedative-hypnotics, or opioids; or as part of a total intravenous anesthetic (TIVA) technique, usually in combination with opioids. Some clinical trials suggest a reduction in postoperative pain scores and opioid consumption for patients receiving propofol-based TIVA as compared with volatile anesthesia, but it is difficult to draw firm conclusions owing to small trial size and significant patient heterogeneity.[23] Therapeutic plasma concentrations for maintenance of anesthesia normally range between 3 and 8 µg/mL (typically requiring a continuous infusion rate between 100 and 200 µg/kg/min) when combined with nitrous oxide or opioids.

### Sedation

Propofol is a popular choice for sedation of mechanically ventilated patients in the ICU (also see Chapter 41) and for sedation during procedures in or outside the operating room. The required plasma concentration is 1 to 2 µg/mL, which normally requires a continuous infusion rate between 25 and 75 µg/kg/min. Because of its pronounced respiratory depressant effect and its narrow therapeutic range, propofol should be administered only by individuals trained in airway management. Spontaneous ventilation is usually preserved in children at quite rapid propofol infusion rates (200 to 250 µg/kg/min), making it a good choice for pediatric procedures such as magnetic resonance imaging scans[24] (also see Chapter 34).

Antiemetic

Subanesthetic bolus doses of propofol or a subanesthetic infusion can be used to treat postoperative nausea and vomiting (PONV) (10 to 20 mg IV, or 10 to 20 µg/kg/min as an infusion).[25,26] Propofol TIVA, as compared with volatile anesthetics, reduces PONV[27] but may not reduce unplanned admissions, postdischarge nausea and vomiting, or cost of anesthesia in the ambulatory setting.[28]

## FOSPROPOFOL

Propofol is the most commonly used intravenous anesthetic for induction and maintenance of anesthesia and probably also during MAC and conscious sedation. As mentioned earlier, the lipid emulsion formulation of propofol has several disadvantages including pain on injection, risk of bacterial contamination, and hypertriglyceridemia with prolonged infusion. Intense research has therefore focused on finding alternative formulations or related drugs to address some of these problems. Fospropofol, a water-soluble prodrug of propofol, was developed as an alternative and in 2008 was licensed by the Food and Drug Administration (FDA) as a sedating anesthetic for use during MAC.[29]

### Physicochemical Characteristics

Fospropofol, initially known under the name GPI 15715, is a water-soluble phosphate ester prodrug of propofol and is chemically described as 2,6-diisopropylphenoxymethyl phosphate disodium salt (Fig. 8.4). It is metabolized by alkaline phosphatase in a reaction producing propofol, phosphate, and formaldehyde. Aldehyde dehydrogenase in the liver and in erythrocytes rapidly metabolizes formaldehyde to produce formate, which is further metabolized by 10-formyltetrahydrofolate dehydrogenase.[29] The available fospropofol formulation is a sterile, aqueous, colorless, and clear solution that is supplied in a single-dose vial at a concentration of 35 mg/mL under the trade name Lusedra.

### Pharmacokinetics

Because fospropofol is a prodrug that requires metabolism to form the active compound propofol, the pharmacokinetics are complex. Onset and recovery are prolonged compared to propofol. Multicompartment models with two compartments for fospropofol and three for propofol have been used to describe the kinetics. In theory, a fospropofol bolus should yield lower peak plasma levels and a delayed time-to-peak compared with propofol. However, previous studies on pharmacokinetics/pharmacodynamics and tolerability of fospropofol were based on an inaccurate analytical

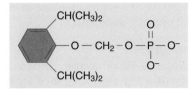

**Fig. 8.4** Structure of fospropofol.

assay, and, therefore, reliable data on the kinetics are lacking.[29] Six previously published studies were retracted in 2010.[30]

### Pharmacodynamics

The effect profile is similar to that of propofol. Given the kinetics previously described, fospropofol in theory should cause less hypotension[31] and less respiratory depression than propofol. However, these benefits have not yet been demonstrated in human studies.

### Clinical Uses

Fospropofol is currently approved for sedation during MAC. Given as a bolus (6.5 mg/kg IV), onset of sedation is slower (4 to 8 min) and duration of action is longer (5 to 18 min) than an equivalent dose of propofol.[32] Sedation can be maintained by redosing with 25% of the initial bolus as needed. These dosing guidelines are recommended only for patients weighing 60 to 90 kg, and dose reduction by 25% is recommended for elderly patients (age > 65) or those with American Society of Anesthesiologists (ASA) physical classification III or IV. Common side effects of fospropofol include a perineal burning sensation and pruritus.

Small trials have demonstrated safety and efficacy of fospropofol for sedation during colonoscopy, bronchoscopy, and minor surgical procedures.[32] Single studies have investigated fospropofol for TIVA during coronary artery bypass grafting[33] and for ICU sedation of mechanically ventilated patients.[34] Similar to propofol, airway compromise remains a major concern. Hence, fospropofol should be administered only by personnel trained in airway management.

## BARBITURATES

Before the introduction of propofol, the intravenous anesthetics most commonly used for induction of anesthesia were barbiturates (thiopental, methohexital).[2,4]

### Physicochemical Characteristics

Barbiturates are derived from barbituric acid (lacks hypnotic properties) through substitutions at the N1, C2, and

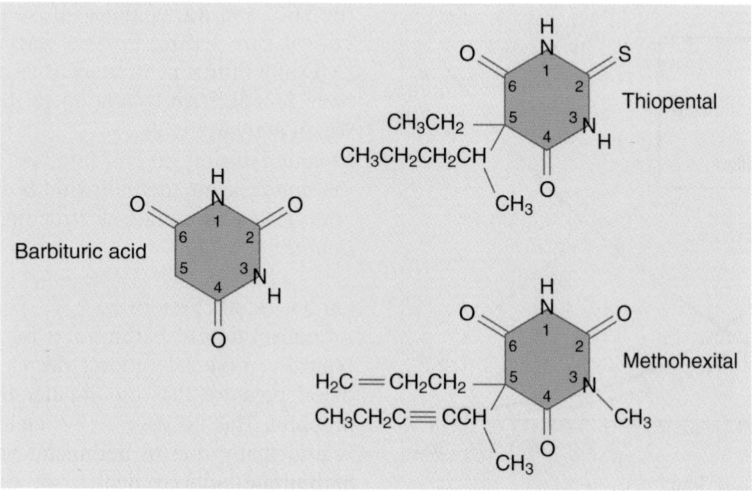

**Fig. 8.5** Structure of barbituric acid and its derivatives.

C5 positions (Fig. 8.5). Based on their substitution at position 2, barbiturates can be grouped into thiobarbiturates, substituted with a sulfur (thiopental), or oxybarbiturates, substituted with an oxygen (methohexital). Hypnotic, sedative, and anticonvulsant effects, as well as lipid solubility and onset time, are determined by the type and position of substitution.

Thiopental and methohexital are formulated as sodium salts mixed with anhydrous sodium carbonate. After reconstitution with water or normal saline, the solutions (2.5% thiopental and 1% methohexital) are alkaline with a pH higher than 10. Although this property prevents bacterial growth and helps increase the shelf life of the solution after reconstitution, it will lead to precipitation when mixed with acidic drug preparations such as neuromuscular blocking drugs. These precipitates can irreversibly block intravenous delivery lines if mixing occurs during administration. Furthermore, accidental injection into an artery or infiltration into paravenous tissue will cause extreme pain and may lead to severe tissue injury.

Several barbiturates, including thiopental and methohexital, have optical isomers with different potencies. However, the available formulations are racemic mixtures, and their potencies reflect the summation of the potencies of the individual isomers.

## Pharmacokinetics

Barbiturates, except for phenobarbital, undergo hepatic metabolism most importantly by oxidation, but also by N-dealkylation, desulfuration, and destruction of the barbituric acid ring structure. The resulting metabolites are inactive and excreted through urine and, after conjugation, through bile. In contrast, phenobarbital is mainly eliminated unchanged via renal excretion. Chronic administration of barbiturates or the administration of

other drugs that induce oxidative microsomal enzymes (enzyme induction) enhances barbiturate metabolism. Through stimulation of aminolevulinic acid synthetase, the production of porphyrins is increased. Therefore, barbiturates should not be administered to patients with acute intermittent porphyria.

Methohexital is cleared more rapidly by the liver than thiopental and thus has a shorter elimination half-time. This accounts for faster and more complete recovery after methohexital administration. Although thiopental is metabolized slowly and has a long elimination half-time, recovery after a single bolus administration is comparable to methohexital and propofol because it depends on redistribution to inactive tissue sites rather than metabolism (Fig. 8.6).[35] However, even single-bolus induction doses of thiopental can, in some cases, lead to psychomotor impairment that lasts up to several hours. If administered as repeated boluses or as a continuous infusion, especially when using larger doses to produce burst suppression on the EEG, recovery from the effects of thiopental will be markedly prolonged because of the long context-sensitive half-time (see Fig. 8.3).

## Pharmacodynamics

The mechanism of action for the effect of barbiturates in the CNS presumably involves both enhancement of inhibitory neurotransmission and inhibition of excitatory transmission. Although the effects on inhibitory transmission probably result from activation of the GABA_A receptor complex, the effects on excitatory transmission are less well understood. The pentameric GABA_A receptor can be composed of different combinations of subunits (see Benzodiazepines section), and the receptors may be found both at synapses and at extrasynaptic sites.[36] This diversity of location and composition may explain why

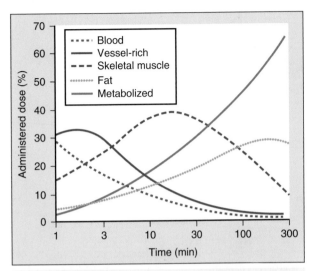

**Fig. 8.6** After rapid intravenous injection of thiopental, the percentage of the administered dose remaining in blood *(brown line)* rapidly decreases as the drug moves from blood to highly perfused vessel-rich tissues *(blue line)*, especially the brain. Subsequently, thiopental is redistributed to skeletal muscles *(red line)* and, to a lesser extent, to fat *(pink line)*. Ultimately, most of the administered dose of thiopental undergoes metabolism *(green line)*. (From Saidman LJ. Uptake, distribution, and elimination of barbiturates. In Eger EI, ed. *Anesthetic Uptake and Action.* Baltimore: Williams & Wilkins; 1974:264-284, used with permission.)

several different types of $GABA_A$-mediated currents are found in the CNS (fast versus slow, phasic versus tonic). Different intravenous anesthetics may have some selectivity for certain types of $GABA_A$ receptors.[37]

### Central Nervous System

Barbiturates produce dose-dependent CNS depression ranging from sedation to general anesthesia when administered in induction doses.[4] They do not have analgesic properties and may even reduce the pain threshold, and thus could be classified as anti-analgesics. Barbiturates are potent cerebral vasoconstrictors and produce predictable decreases in CBF, cerebral blood volume, and ICP. As a result, they decrease $CMRO_2$ in a dose-dependent manner up to the point where the EEG becomes a flat line. The ability of barbiturates to decrease ICP and $CMRO_2$ makes these drugs useful in the management of patients with space-occupying intracranial lesions[38] (also see Chapter 30). Furthermore, they may provide neuroprotection from focal cerebral ischemia (stroke, surgical retraction, temporary clips during aneurysm surgery) but probably not from global cerebral ischemia (cardiac arrest). Yet, the use of barbiturates to lower ICP after traumatic brain injury cannot be justified, as the associated hypotension may compromise cerebral perfusion pressure and worsen outcomes.[39] Most barbiturates decrease electrical activity on the EEG, and intravenous infusions may be useful in the critical care setting to treat refractory status epilepticus (typically third-line therapy after midazolam and propofol have failed).[40] An exception to this rule is methohexital, which activates epileptic foci, thus facilitating their identification during surgery targeted to ablate these sites. For the same reason, methohexital is also a popular choice for anesthesia to facilitate electroconvulsive therapy (also see Chapter 38).

### Cardiovascular System

Administration of barbiturates for induction of anesthesia typically produces modest decreases in systemic arterial blood pressure that are smaller than those produced by propofol. This decrease in systemic arterial blood pressure is principally due to peripheral vasodilation and reflects barbiturate-induced depression of the medullary vasomotor center and decreased sympathetic nervous system outflow from the CNS. Although barbiturates blunt the baroreceptor reflex, compensatory increases in heart rate limit the magnitude and duration of hypotension. Moreover, dilation of peripheral capacitance vessels leads to pooling of blood and decreased venous return, thus resulting in reduced cardiac output and systemic arterial blood pressure. Indeed, exaggerated decreases in blood pressure are likely to follow the administration of barbiturates to patients with hypovolemia, cardiac tamponade, cardiomyopathy, coronary artery disease, or cardiac valvular disease because these groups are less able to compensate for the effects of peripheral vasodilation. Hemodynamic effects are also more pronounced with larger doses and rapid injection. The negative inotropic effects of barbiturates, which are readily demonstrated in isolated heart preparations, are usually masked in vivo by baroreceptor reflex-mediated responses.

### Respiratory System

Barbiturates are respiratory depressants and lead to decreased minute ventilation via smaller tidal volumes and respiratory rates. Anesthetic induction doses of thiopental and methohexital typically induce transient apnea, which is more pronounced in the presence of other respiratory depressants. Barbiturates also decrease the ventilatory responses to hypercapnia and hypoxia. Resumption of spontaneous breathing after an anesthetic induction dose of a barbiturate is characterized by a slow breathing rate and decreased tidal volume. Suppression of laryngeal reflexes and cough reflexes is not as profound as after propofol administration, which makes barbiturates an inferior choice for airway instrumentation in the absence of neuromuscular blocking drugs. Furthermore, stimulation of the upper airway or trachea (secretions, laryngeal mask airway, direct laryngoscopy, tracheal intubation) during inadequate depression of airway reflexes may result in laryngospasm or bronchospasm. This phenomenon is not unique to barbiturates but is true in general when the dose of anesthetic is inadequate to suppress the airway reflexes.

## Side Effects

Accidental intra-arterial injection of barbiturates results in excruciating pain and intense vasoconstriction, often leading to severe tissue injury involving gangrene.[4] Aggressive therapy is directed at reversing the vasoconstriction to maintain perfusion and reduce the drug concentration by dilution. One approach to treatment is blockade of the sympathetic nervous system in the involved extremity (stellate ganglion block). Barbiturate crystal formation probably results in the occlusion of distal, small-diameter arterioles. Crystal formation in veins is less hazardous because of the ever-increasing diameter of veins. Accidental subcutaneous injection (extravasation) of barbiturates results in local tissue irritation, thus emphasizing the importance of using dilute concentrations (2.5% thiopental, 1% methohexital). If extravasation occurs, some recommend local injection of the tissues with 0.5% lidocaine (5 to 10 mL) in an attempt to dilute the barbiturate concentration.

Life-threatening allergic reactions to barbiturates are rare, with an estimated occurrence of 1 in 30,000 patients. However, barbiturate-induced histamine release is occasionally seen.

## Clinical Uses

The principal clinical uses of barbiturates are rapid intravenous induction of anesthesia, treatment of increased ICP, or to provide neuroprotection from focal cerebral ischemia.[4] A continuous intravenous infusion of a barbiturate such as thiopental is rarely used to maintain anesthesia because of its long context-sensitive half-time and prolonged recovery period (see Fig. 8.3).[10] Prolonged infusions to achieve "barbiturate coma" for neuroprotection may cause immune suppression, hypo- and hyperkalemia, and hypothermia.[38]

### Induction of Anesthesia

Administration of thiopental (3 to 5 mg/kg IV) or methohexital (1 to 1.5 mg/kg IV) produces unconsciousness in less than 30 seconds. Patients may experience a garlic or onion taste during induction of anesthesia. When used as an anesthetic for electroconvulsive therapy, methohexital may allow for longer seizure duration when compared with propofol.[41] With the introduction of sugammadex as a reversal drug for rocuronium neuromuscular blockade, methohexital plus rocuronium may become a more common anesthetic cocktail for electroconvulsive therapy (also see Chapter 11).

The utility of barbiturates can be illustrated by describing several different techniques for anesthesia induction.

After administering a barbiturate, it is common to give succinylcholine or a nondepolarizing neuromuscular blocking drug to produce skeletal muscle relaxation and facilitate tracheal intubation. In some situations, the anesthesia provider may choose a "rapid-sequence induction" of anesthesia, typically when a patient is at increased risk for aspiration of gastric contents. The classic drug regimen for rapid-sequence induction is a barbiturate, usually thiopental, followed by succinylcholine in rapid succession. Important advantages of this technique are avoidance of bag-mask ventilation and early tracheal intubation with a cuffed tube. Although thiopental was the traditional drug used for rapid-sequence induction, propofol is currently the more frequent choice.

For patients who are not at increased risk of aspirating gastric contents, intravenous barbiturates may be used to initiate a gradual induction. Small doses of thiopental (0.5 to 1.0 mg/kg IV) may improve patient acceptance of a face mask and negate any unpleasant memory of pungent volatile anesthetics. The induction can then be completed by delivering an inhaled agent such as sevoflurane. This type of slow induction helps titrate the anesthetic effect more carefully and avoids exaggerated hemodynamic responses. A gradual induction can also be accomplished by careful titration of intravenous anesthetics alone, but propofol is probably a more logical choice for this application because it has a shorter context-sensitive half-time (see Fig. 8.3).[10] Rectal administration of a barbiturate such as methohexital (20 to 30 mg/kg) may be used to facilitate induction of anesthesia in mentally challenged and uncooperative pediatric patients.

### Neuroprotection (Also See Chapter 30)

When used for neuroprotection, barbiturates have traditionally been titrated to achieve an isoelectric EEG, an end point that indicates maximal reduction of $CMRO_2$. More recent data demonstrating equal protection after smaller doses have challenged this practice.[4] One risk of using high-dose barbiturate therapy to decrease ICP or to provide protection against focal cerebral ischemia (cardiopulmonary bypass, carotid endarterectomy, thoracic aneurysm resection) is the associated hypotension, which can critically reduce cerebral perfusion pressure and may require the administration of vasoconstrictors to maintain systemic arterial blood pressure. In a large registry of patients undergoing repair of acute type A aortic dissection, there was no benefit from barbiturates for preventing permanent neurologic dysfunction,[42] and these drugs are unlikely to be of benefit during cardiac surgery.

## BENZODIAZEPINES

Benzodiazepines commonly used in the perioperative period include diazepam, midazolam, and lorazepam, as well as the selective benzodiazepine antagonist flumazenil.[1,5]

Benzodiazepines are unique among intravenous anesthetics in that their action can readily be terminated by administration of their selective antagonist flumazenil. Their most desired effects are anxiolysis and anterograde amnesia, which are extremely useful for premedication.

## Physicochemical Characteristics

The chemical structure of the benzodiazepines contains a benzene ring fused to a seven-member diazepine ring, hence their name (Fig. 8.7). The three benzodiazepines commonly used in the perioperative setting are all highly lipophilic, with midazolam having the highest lipid solubility. All three drugs are highly protein bound, mainly to serum albumin. Although they are used as parenteral formulations, all three drugs are absorbed after oral administration. Other possible routes of administration include intramuscular, intranasal, and sublingual. Exposure of the acidic midazolam preparation to the physiologic pH of blood causes a change in the ring structure that renders the drug more lipid soluble, thus speeding its passage across the blood-brain barrier and its onset of action.

## Pharmacokinetics

The highly lipid-soluble benzodiazepines rapidly enter the CNS, which accounts for their rapid onset of action, followed by redistribution to inactive tissue sites and subsequent termination of the drug effect (see Table 8.1). Metabolism of benzodiazepines occurs in the liver through microsomal oxidation (N-dealkylation and aliphatic hydroxylation) and glucuronide conjugation. Microsomal oxidation, the primary pathway for metabolism of midazolam and diazepam, is more susceptible to external factors such as age, diseases (hepatic cirrhosis), and the administration of other drugs that modulate the efficiency of the enzyme systems. Lorazepam is one of few benzodiazepines that does not undergo oxidative metabolism and is excreted after a single-step conjugation to glucuronic acid.

Diazepam undergoes hepatic metabolism to active metabolites (desmethyldiazepam and oxazepam) that may contribute to the prolonged effects of this drug. By contrast, midazolam is selectively metabolized by hepatic cytochrome P450 3A4 to a single dominant metabolite, 1-hydroxymidazolam. Whereas 1-hydroxymidazolam has sedative effects similar to the parent compound, it undergoes rapid glucuronidation and clearance.[2] This metabolite does not cause significant sedation in patients with normal hepatic and renal function unless midazolam is given as a prolonged infusion. Furthermore, the short duration of action of a single dose of midazolam is due to its lipid solubility and rapid redistribution as prevously described. Despite its prompt passage into the brain, midazolam is considered to have a slower effect-site equilibration time than propofol and thiopental. In this regard, intravenous doses of midazolam should be sufficiently spaced to permit the peak clinical effect to be recognized before a repeat dose is considered.

The elimination half-time of diazepam greatly exceeds that of midazolam, thus explaining why the CNS effects of diazepam are prolonged, especially in elderly patients. Of the three commonly used intravenous benzodiazepines, midazolam has the shortest context-sensitive half-time, making it the most suitable for continuous infusion (see Fig. 8.6).[10]

Recently, a new ultrashort-acting benzodiazepine named remimazolam (CNS-7056) has entered clinical trials. Remimazolam contains a carboxylic ester group that is rapidly hydrolyzed by tissue esterases, analogous to remifentanil (also see Chapter 9).[32] As compared to midazolam, remimazolam has a smaller volume of distribution, faster clearance, and clearance independent of body weight.[43] The metabolite of remimazolam has extremely low $GABA_A$ affinity (>400 times lower than CNS-7056) and is unlikely to yield clinically relevant sedation. The kinetic properties of remimazolam make it a promising intravenous anesthetic drug that may yield less prolonged sedation compared with midazolam, particularly in patients with liver disease or those taking cytochrome P450–inhibiting drugs.

## Pharmacodynamics

Benzodiazepines work through activation of the $GABA_A$ receptor complex and enhancement of GABA-mediated chloride currents, thereby leading to hyperpolarization

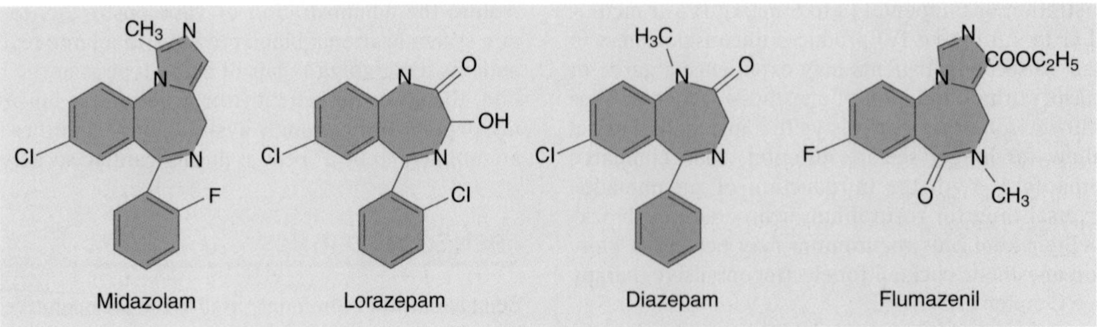

Midazolam    Lorazepam    Diazepam    Flumazenil

**Fig. 8.7** Chemical structure of the most commonly used benzodiazepines and their antagonist flumazenil.

of neurons and reduced excitability (Fig. 8.8).[44] There are specific binding sites for benzodiazepines on $GABA_A$ receptors, thus explaining why they were initially termed "benzodiazepine receptors." Consistent with its greater potency, midazolam has an affinity for $GABA_A$ receptors that is approximately twice that of diazepam.

$GABA_A$ receptors that are responsive to benzodiazepines occur almost exclusively on postsynaptic nerve endings in the CNS, with the greatest density found in the cerebral cortex. The anatomic distribution of $GABA_A$ receptors (restricted to the CNS) is consistent with the minimal effects of benzodiazepines outside the CNS. Indeed, the magnitude of depression of ventilation and the development of hypotension after the administration of benzodiazepines are lower than that observed when barbiturates are used for induction of anesthesia (Table 8.2).

### Spectrum of Effects

The wide spectrum of effects of benzodiazepines is similar for all drugs in this class, although potencies for individual effects may vary between drugs.[5] The most important effects of benzodiazepines are their sedative-hypnotic action and their amnestic properties (anterograde, but not retrograde, amnesia).[45] In addition, benzodiazepines function as anticonvulsants and are used to treat seizures. These effects are mediated through the α-subunits of the GABA receptor, whereas anxiolysis and muscle relaxation are mediated through the γ-subunits. The site of action for muscle relaxation is in the spinal cord, and this effect requires much larger doses.

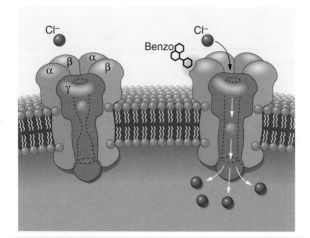

**Fig. 8.8** Schematic depiction of the γ-aminobutyric acid (GABA) type A receptor forming a chloride ion channel. Benzodiazepines (Benzo) attach selectively at the interface of α- and γ- subunits and are presumed to facilitate the action of the inhibitory neurotransmitter GABA. (From Mohler H, Richards JG. The benzodiazepine receptor: a pharmacological control element of brain function. *Eur J Anesthesiol Suppl.* 1988;2:15-24, used with permission.)

### Safety Profile

Benzodiazepines have a very favorable side effect profile. When administered alone, these drugs cause only minimal depression of ventilation and the cardiovascular system, making them relatively safe even in larger doses. Furthermore, the CNS effects can be reversed by the selective benzodiazepine antagonist, flumazenil, thus adding to the safety margin.

### Central Nervous System (Also See Chapter 30)

Like propofol and barbiturates, benzodiazepines decrease $CMRO_2$ and CBF, but to a lesser extent. In contrast to propofol and thiopental, midazolam is unable to produce an isoelectric EEG, thus emphasizing that there is a ceiling effect on reduction of $CMRO_2$ by benzodiazepines. Patients with decreased intracranial compliance demonstrate little or no change in ICP after the administration of midazolam. Benzodiazepines have not been shown to possess neuroprotective properties. They are potent anticonvulsants for the treatment of status epilepticus, alcohol withdrawal, and local anesthetic-induced seizures.

### Cardiovascular System

When used for induction of anesthesia, midazolam produces a larger decrease in arterial blood pressure than diazepam. These changes are most likely due to peripheral vasodilation inasmuch as cardiac output is not changed. Midazolam-induced hypotension is more likely in hypovolemic patients.

### Respiratory System

Benzodiazepines produce minimal depression of ventilation, although transient apnea may follow rapid intravenous administration of midazolam for induction of anesthesia, especially in the presence of opioid premedication. Benzodiazepines decrease the ventilatory response to carbon dioxide, but this effect is not usually significant if they are administered alone. More severe respiratory depression can occur when benzodiazepines are administered together with opioids.[1,46]

## Side Effects

Allergic reactions to benzodiazepines are extremely rare to nonexistent. Pain during intravenous injection and subsequent thrombophlebitis are most pronounced with diazepam and reflect the poor water solubility of this benzodiazepine. It is the organic solvent, propylene glycol, required to dissolve diazepam that is most likely responsible for pain during intramuscular or intravenous administration, as well as for the unpredictable absorption after intramuscular injection. Midazolam is more water soluble (but only at low pH), thus obviating the need for an organic solvent and decreasing the likelihood of exaggerated pain or erratic absorption after intramuscular injection or pain during intravenous administration.

**Table 8.2** Summary of the Pharmacodynamic Effects of Commonly Used Intravenous Anesthetics

| Dose/Effect | Propofol | Thiopental | Midazolam | Ketamine | Etomidate | Dexmedetomidine |
|---|---|---|---|---|---|---|
| Dose for induction of anesthesia (mg/kg IV) | 1.5-2.5 | 3-5 | 0.1-0.3 | 1-2 | 0.2-0.3 | |
| Systemic blood pressure | Decreased | Decreased | Unchanged to decreased | Increased [*] | Unchanged to decreased | Decreased [†] |
| Heart rate | Unchanged to decreased | Increased | Unchanged | Increased | Unchanged to increased | Decreased |
| Systemic vascular resistance | Decreased | Decreased | Unchanged to decreased | Increased | Unchanged to decreased | Decreased [†] |
| Ventilation | Decreased | Decreased | Unchanged | Unchanged | Unchanged to decreased | Unchanged to decreased |
| Respiratory rate | Decreased | Decreased | Unchanged to decreased | Unchanged | Unchanged to decreased | Unchanged |
| Response to carbon dioxide | Decreased | Decreased | Decreased | Unchanged | Decreased | Unchanged |
| Cerebral blood flow | Decreased | Decreased | Decreased | Increased to unchanged | Decreased | Decreased |
| Cerebral metabolic requirements for oxygen | Decreased | Decreased | Decreased | Increased to unchanged | Decreased | Unchanged |
| Intracranial pressure | Decreased | Decreased | Unchanged | Increased to unchanged | Decreased | Unchanged |
| Anticonvulsant | Yes | Yes | Yes | Yes? | No | No |
| Anxiolysis | No | No | Yes | No | No | Yes? |
| Analgesia | No | No | No | Yes | No | Yes? |
| Emergence delirium | No? | No | No | Yes | No | May reduce |
| Nausea and vomiting | Decreased | Unchanged | Decreased | Unchanged | Increased | Unchanged |
| Adrenocortical suppression | No | No | Yes? | No | Yes | No |
| Pain on injection | Yes | No | No | No | No | No |

[*]May cause direct myocardial depression and hypotension in critically ill or catecholamine-depleted patients.
[†]Bolus injection may increase systemic vascular resistance and blood pressure. *IV,* Intravenous.

## Clinical Uses

Benzodiazepines are used for (1) preoperative medication, (2) intravenous sedation, (3) intravenous induction of anesthesia, and (4) suppression of seizure activity. The slow onset and prolonged duration of action of lorazepam limit its usefulness for preoperative medication or induction of anesthesia, especially when rapid and sustained awakening at the end of surgery is desirable. Flumazenil (8 to 15 µg/kg IV) may be useful for treating patients experiencing delayed awakening, but its duration of action is brief (about 20 minutes) and resedation may occur.

Preoperative Medication and Sedation (Also See Chapter 13)
The amnestic, anxiolytic, and sedative effects of benzodiazepines are the basis for the use of these drugs for preoperative medication. Midazolam (1 to 2 mg IV) is effective for premedication, sedation during regional anesthesia, and brief therapeutic procedures.[5,47] Addition of midazolam to propofol sedation for colonoscopy may improve operating conditions without slowing recovery time or worsening cognitive impairment at discharge.[48] When compared with diazepam, midazolam produces a more rapid onset, with more intense amnesia and less postoperative sedation. Many patients who receive preoperative midazolam do not recall the operating room, and some have no memory of the preoperative holding area.[49] Both anesthesia providers and surgeons should be aware of this fact when providing information to patients and families prior to surgery. Although awareness during anesthesia is rare (also see Chapter 47), benzodiazepines seem

to be superior to ketamine and barbiturates for prevention of recall.[50] Midazolam is commonly used for oral premedication of children. For example, 0.5 mg/kg administered orally 30 minutes before induction of anesthesia provides reliable sedation and anxiolysis in children without producing delayed awakening.[51] Midazolam also lowers the incidence of PONV.[52] Despite these possible benefits, the routine use of premedication with benzodiazepines for elective surgery may not improve patient experience.[53]

The synergistic effects between benzodiazepines and other drugs, especially opioids and propofol, facilitate better sedation and analgesia. However, the combination of these drugs also exacerbates respiratory depression and may lead to airway obstruction or apnea.[46] These drugs may also increase the risk for aspiration of gastric contents by impairing pharyngeal function and the coordination between breathing and swallowing.[54] Benzodiazepine effects, as well as synergy with other respiratory depressants, are more pronounced in the elderly (also see Chapter 35) so smaller doses and careful titration may be necessary. Caution is advised when using benzodiazepines for sedation of critically ill, mechanically ventilated patients, as this drug class has been linked to longer duration of ICU stay and increased delirium compared with alternative regimens (propofol or dexmedetomidine).[55,56]

### Induction of Anesthesia
Although rarely used for this purpose, general anesthesia can be induced by the administration of midazolam (0.1 to 0.3 mg/kg IV). The onset of unconsciousness, however, is slower than after the administration of thiopental, propofol, or etomidate. Onset of unconsciousness is facilitated when a small dose of opioid (fentanyl, 50 to 100 µg IV) is injected 1 to 3 minutes before midazolam is administered. Despite the possible production of lesser circulatory effects, it is unlikely that the use of midazolam or diazepam for induction of anesthesia offers any advantages over barbiturates or propofol. Delayed awakening is a potential disadvantage after an induction dose of a benzodiazepine.

### Suppression of Seizure Activity
The efficacy of benzodiazepines as anticonvulsants owes to their ability to enhance the inhibitory effects of GABA, particularly in the limbic system. Indeed, diazepam (0.1 mg/kg IV) is often effective in abolishing seizure activity produced by local anesthetics or alcohol withdrawal. Lorazepam (0.1 mg/kg IV) is the intravenous benzodiazepine of choice for status epilepticus. Diazepam (0.2 mg/kg IV) may also be used. For prehospital treatment of status epilepticus, intramuscular (IM) administration of midazolam (10 mg IM for patients > 40 kg; 5 mg IM for patients 13 to 40 kg) is effective, can be performed more rapidly than intravenous therapy, and may decrease the need for hospitalization.[57]

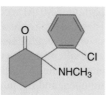

**Fig. 8.9** Chemical structure of ketamine.

## KETAMINE

Ketamine, a phencyclidine derivative that received FDA approval for clinical use in 1970, is different from most other intravenous anesthetics in that it produces significant analgesia.[2,3] The characteristic cataleptic state observed after an induction dose of ketamine is known as "dissociative anesthesia," wherein the patient's eyes remain open with a slow nystagmic gaze (cataleptic state).

### Physicochemical Characteristics

Ketamine is a partially water-soluble and highly lipid-soluble derivative of phencyclidine (Fig. 8.9). It is between 5 and 10 times more lipid soluble than thiopental. Of the two stereoisomers the S(+) form is more potent than the R(−) isomer. Only the racemic mixture of ketamine (10, 50, 100 mg/mL) is available in the United States.

After its initial introduction, ketamine was for a time established as a safe anesthetic. However, the popularity of ketamine has since declined, and its unpleasant psychomimetic side effects have limited its use in anesthesia. Still, the unique features of ketamine (potent analgesia with minimal respiratory depression) make it a very valuable alternative in certain settings. More recently it has become popular as an adjunct administered at subanalgesic doses to limit or reverse opioid tolerance and in the treatment of major depression.[58,59]

### Pharmacokinetics

The high lipid solubility of ketamine ensures a rapid onset of effect. Like other intravenous induction drugs, the effect of a single bolus injection is terminated by redistribution to inactive tissue sites. Metabolism occurs primarily in the liver and involves N-demethylation by the cytochrome P-450 system. Norketamine, the primary active metabolite, is less potent (one third to one fifth the potency of ketamine) and is subsequently hydroxylated and conjugated into water-soluble inactive metabolites that are excreted in urine. Ketamine is the only intravenous anesthetic that has low protein binding (12%) (see Table 8.1).

### Pharmacodynamics

The mechanism of action of ketamine is complex, but the major anesthetic effect is produced through inhibition of the $N$-methyl-D-aspartate (NMDA) receptor complex.[60] If ketamine is administered as the sole anesthetic, amnesia is not as complete as with the administration of a benzodiazepine. Reflexes are often preserved, but it cannot be assumed that patients are able to protect their upper airway. The eyes remain open, and the pupils are moderately dilated with a nystagmic gaze. Frequently, lacrimation and salivation are increased, and premedication with an anticholinergic drug may be indicated to limit this effect (see Table 8.2).

### Emergence Reactions

The unpleasant emergence reactions after ketamine administration are the main factor limiting its use. Such reactions may include vivid colorful dreams, hallucinations, out-of-body experiences, and increased and distorted visual, tactile, and auditory sensitivity. These reactions can be associated with fear and confusion. A euphoric state may also be induced, which explains the potential for abuse of the drug. Children usually have a lesser incidence of severe emergence reactions. Administration of a benzodiazepine in combination with ketamine may help limit the unpleasant emergence reactions and also increase amnesia.

### Central Nervous System (Also See Chapter 30)

In contrast to other intravenous anesthetics, ketamine is a cerebral vasodilator that increases CBF as well as $CMRO_2$. Thus, ketamine is usually avoided in patients with intracranial disease, especially increased ICP. Nevertheless, the undesirable effects on CBF may be blunted by controlled ventilation and the maintenance of normocapnia.[61] Despite the potential to produce myoclonic activity, ketamine is considered an anticonvulsant and may be considered for treatment of status epilepticus when more conventional drugs are ineffective.

### Cardiovascular System

Ketamine can produce significant, but transient increases in systemic arterial blood pressure, heart rate, and cardiac output, presumably by centrally mediated sympathetic stimulation. These effects, which are associated with increased cardiac work and myocardial oxygen consumption, are not always desirable and can be blunted by coadministration of benzodiazepines, opioids, or inhaled anesthetics. Though more controversial, ketamine is a direct myocardial depressant. This property is usually masked by its stimulation of the sympathetic nervous system, but it may become apparent in critically ill patients with limited ability to increase their sympathetic nervous system activity.

### Respiratory System

Ketamine does not produce significant respiratory depression. When used as a single drug, the respiratory response to hypercapnia is preserved and arterial blood gases remain stable. Transient hypoventilation and, in rare cases, a short period of apnea can follow rapid administration of large intravenous doses for induction of anesthesia. The ability to protect the upper airway in the presence of ketamine cannot be assumed despite the presence of active airway reflexes. Especially in children, the risk for laryngospasm because of increased salivation is increased and can be reduced by premedication with an anticholinergic drug. Ketamine relaxes bronchial smooth muscles and may be helpful in patients with reactive airways and in the management of patients experiencing bronchoconstriction.

## Clinical Uses

The unpleasant emergence reactions after the administration of ketamine have restricted its use as a general anesthetic.[62] Nevertheless, ketamine's unique properties, including profound analgesia, stimulation of the sympathetic nervous system, bronchodilation, and minimal respiratory depression, make it an important alternative to the other intravenous anesthetics and a desirable adjunct in many cases. Moreover, ketamine can be administered by multiple routes (intravenous, intramuscular, oral, rectal, epidural), thus making it a useful option for premedication in mentally challenged and uncooperative pediatric patients (also see Chapter 34).

### Induction and Maintenance of Anesthesia

Induction of anesthesia can be achieved with ketamine, 1 to 2 mg/kg IV or 4 to 6 mg/kg IM. Though not commonly used for maintenance of anesthesia, the short context-sensitive half-time makes ketamine a consideration for this purpose (see Fig. 8.3).[10] For example, general anesthesia can be achieved with the infusion of ketamine, 15 to 45 μg/kg/min, plus 50% to 70% nitrous oxide or by ketamine alone, 30 to 90 μg/kg/min.

### Analgesia

Small bolus doses of ketamine (0.2 to 0.8 mg/kg IV) may be useful during regional anesthesia when additional analgesia is needed (e.g., cesarean section under neuraxial anesthesia with an insufficient regional block). Ketamine provides effective analgesia without compromise of the airway. An infusion of a subanalgesic dose of ketamine (3 to 5 μg/kg/min) during general anesthesia and in the early postoperative period may be useful to produce analgesia or reduce opioid tolerance and opioid-induced hyperalgesia,[63] although not all studies examining the use of ketamine as an adjunct show the desired improvement in pain scores and recovery.[64] Because of the presence of NMDA receptors on peripheral nociceptors, local and topical application of ketamine appears to be a reasonable approach that might allow achievement of higher local tissue concentrations in an attempt to avoid undesired CNS effects. However, convincing evidence from controlled trials is lacking and so far support for this modality mainly comes from case reports.[65]

### Treatment of Major Depression

Ketamine has recently received increasing attention as a therapeutic option for treatment-resistant major depression. A single intravenous infusion of ketamine (0.5 mg/kg over 40 minutes) was shown to be superior to midazolam for reduction of depressive symptoms in less than 24 hours.[66] With optimization of dose, timing, and frequency of treatments, ketamine may prove useful for maintenance of antidepressant effects in treatment-resistant patients.[59]

## ETOMIDATE

Etomidate is an intravenous anesthetic with hypnotic but not analgesic properties and with minimal hemodynamic effects.[2,3,7] The pharmacokinetics of etomidate make it suitable for use as a continuous infusion, but it is not widely used mainly because of its endocrine side effects.

### Physicochemical Characteristics

Etomidate is a carboxylated imidazole derivative that has two optical isomers (Fig. 8.10). The available preparation contains only the active D(+) isomer, which has hypnotic properties. The drug is poorly soluble in water and is therefore supplied as a 2 mg/mL solution in 35% propylene glycol. The solution has a pH of 6.9 and thus does not cause problems with precipitation like thiopental does.

### Pharmacokinetics

An induction dose of etomidate produces rapid onset of anesthesia, and recovery depends on redistribution to inactive tissue sites (comparable to thiopental and propofol). Metabolism is primarily hepatic by ester hydrolysis to inactive metabolites, which are then excreted in urine (78%) and bile (22%). Less than 3% of an administered dose of etomidate is excreted unchanged in the urine. Clearance of etomidate is about five times that for thiopental, as reflected by a shorter elimination half-time (see Table 8.1). The duration of action is linearly related to the dose, with each 0.1 mg/kg providing about 100 seconds of unconsciousness. Because of its minimal effects on hemodynamics and short context-sensitive half-time, larger doses, repeated boluses, or continuous infusions can safely be administered (see Fig. 8.3).[10] Etomidate, like most other intravenous anesthetics, is highly protein bound (77%), primarily to albumin. Development of novel short-acting etomidate derivatives (e.g., ABP-700) is under way with the goal of finding an analog with limited adrenal side effects.[67]

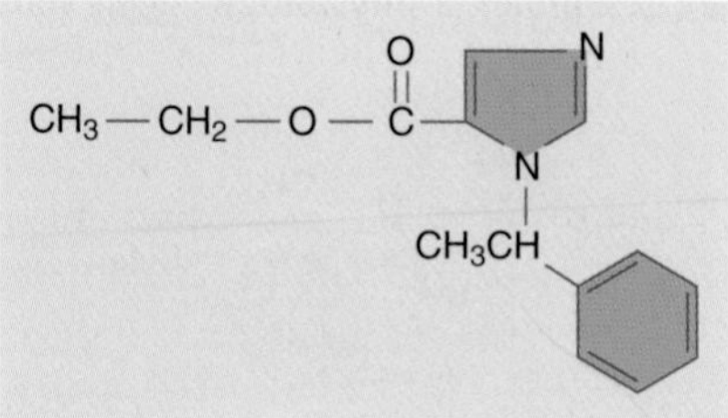

### Pharmacodynamics

Etomidate has GABA-like effects and seems to primarily act through potentiation of $GABA_A$-mediated chloride currents, like most other intravenous anesthetics.[7]

### Central Nervous System (Also See Chapter 30)

Etomidate is a potent cerebral vasoconstrictor, as reflected by decreases in CBF and ICP. These effects of etomidate are similar to those produced by comparable doses of thiopental. Despite its reduction of $CMRO_2$, etomidate failed to show neuroprotective properties in animal studies, and human studies are lacking. Excitatory spikes on the EEG are more frequent after etomidate than from thiopental. Similar to methohexital, etomidate may activate seizure foci, manifested as fast activity on the EEG. In addition, spontaneous movements characterized as myoclonus occur in more than 50% of patients receiving etomidate, and this myoclonic activity may be associated with seizure-like activity on the EEG.

### Cardiovascular System

A characteristic and desired feature of induction of anesthesia with etomidate is cardiovascular stability after bolus injection.[7] Arterial blood pressure decreases are modest or absent and principally reflect decreases in systemic vascular resistance. Any hypotensive effects of etomidate are probably exaggerated in the presence of hypovolemia. Etomidate produces minimal changes in heart rate and cardiac output. The depressive effects of etomidate on myocardial contractility are minimal at concentrations used for induction of anesthesia.

### Respiratory System

The depressant effects of etomidate on ventilation are less pronounced than those of barbiturates, although apnea may occasionally follow rapid intravenous injection. Depression of ventilation may be exaggerated when etomidate is combined with inhaled anesthetics or opioids.

### Endocrine System

Etomidate causes adrenocortical suppression by producing a dose-dependent inhibition of 11β-hydroxylase, an enzyme necessary for the conversion of cholesterol to cortisol (Fig. 8.11).[68] This suppression lasts at least 4 to 8

**Fig. 8.10** Chemical structure of etomidate.

hours after a single induction dose of etomidate, and relative adrenal insufficiency may last up to 24 to 48 hours.[69] This property has generated great controversy over the safety of etomidate for intubation of critically ill patients and as an induction drug for general anesthesia.[70]

## Clinical Uses

Etomidate is an alternative to propofol and barbiturates for the rapid intravenous induction of anesthesia, especially in patients with compromised myocardial contractility, coronary artery disease, or severe aortic stenosis.[71,72] After a standard induction dose (0.2 to 0.3 mg/kg IV), the onset of unconsciousness is comparable to that achieved by thiopental and propofol. There is a frequent incidence of pain during intravenous injection of etomidate, which may be followed by venous irritation. Involuntary myoclonic movements are common but may be masked by the concomitant administration of neuromuscular blocking drugs. Awakening after a single intravenous dose of etomidate is rapid, with little evidence of any residual depressant effects. Etomidate does not produce analgesia, and PONV may be more common than after the administration of thiopental or propofol. The principal limiting factor in the clinical use of etomidate for induction of anesthesia is its ability to transiently depress adrenocortical function.[68] Theoretically, this suppression may be either desirable if it reduces neurohormonal stresses during surgery and anesthesia, or undesirable if it prevents useful protective responses against perioperative stresses. Recent meta-analyses have challenged earlier findings

that etomidate increases mortality after a single dose for intubation of septic patients.[73-75] Etomidate remains a useful hypnotic for electroconvulsive therapy as it provides a longer seizure duration than propofol or methohexital (also see Chapter 38).[76]

## DEXMEDETOMIDINE

Dexmedetomidine is a highly selective $\alpha_2$-adrenergic agonist.[77] Recognition of the usefulness of $\alpha_2$-agonists was based on the observation that patients receiving chronic clonidine therapy have decreased anesthetic requirements. The effects of dexmedetomidine can be reversed with $\alpha_2$-antagonist drugs.

### Physicochemical Characteristics

Dexmedetomidine is the active S-enantiomer of medetomidine, a highly selective $\alpha_2$-adrenergic agonist and imidazole derivative that is used in veterinary medicine. Dexmedetomidine is water soluble and available as a parenteral formulation (Fig. 8.12).

### Pharmacokinetics

Dexmedetomidine undergoes rapid hepatic metabolism involving conjugation, N-methylation, and hydroxylation. Metabolites are excreted through urine and bile. Clearance is high, and the elimination half-time is short (see Table 8.1). However, there is a significant increase in the context-sensitive half-time from 4 minutes after a 10-minute infusion to 250 minutes after an 8-hour infusion.

### Pharmacodynamics

Dexmedetomidine produces its effects through activation of CNS $\alpha_2$-receptors.

#### Central Nervous System
Hypnosis presumably results from stimulation of $\alpha_2$-receptors in the locus ceruleus, and the analgesic effect originates at the level of the spinal cord. The sedative effect produced by dexmedetomidine has a different quality than that of other intravenous anesthetics in that it more resembles a physiologic sleep state through

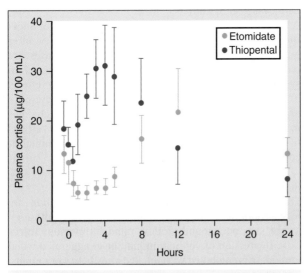

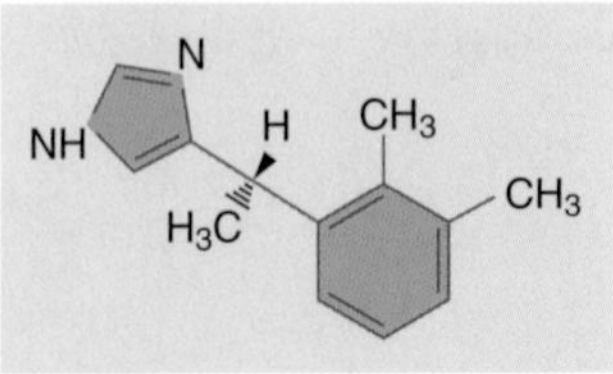

**Fig. 8.11** Etomidate, but not thiopental, is associated with decreases in the plasma concentrations of cortisol. $p < 0.005$ versus thiopental, mean ± SD (standard deviation). (From Fragen RT, Shanks CA, Molteni A, et al. Effects of etomidate on hormonal responses to surgical stress. *Anesthesiology*. 1984;61:652-656, used with permission.)

**Fig. 8.12** Chemical structure of dexmedetomidine.

activation of endogenous sleep pathways. Dexmedetomidine decreases CBF without significant changes in ICP and $CMRO_2$ (see Table 8.2). Tolerance and dependence can develop. Although changes in the EEG do occur, spikes from seizure foci are not suppressed making dexmedetomidine a useful drug for epilepsy surgery.[78] Evoked potentials monitored during spine surgery are not suppressed at usual infusion doses.[79]

### Cardiovascular System

Dexmedetomidine infusion produces moderate decreases in heart rate and systemic vascular resistance and, consequently, decreases in systemic arterial blood pressure. A bolus injection may produce transient *increases* in systemic arterial blood pressure and pronounced decreases in heart rate, an effect that is probably due to vasoconstriction mediated by peripheral $\alpha_2$-adrenergic receptors. Clinically useful initial doses (0.5 to 1 μg/kg IV over 10 minutes) increase systemic vascular resistance and mean arterial pressure, but probably do not significantly increase pulmonary vascular resistance.[80] Bradycardia or hypotension associated with dexmedetomidine infusion may require treatment. Increasing age and decreased baseline arterial blood pressure (mean arterial pressure < 70 mm Hg) are risk factors for hemodynamic instability during dexmedetomidine infusion.[81] Heart block, severe bradycardia, or asystole may result from unopposed vagal stimulation. The response to anticholinergic drugs is unchanged. When used as an adjunct to general anesthesia, dexmedetomidine reduces plasma catecholamine levels and may attenuate heart rate increases during emergence.[82,83]

### Respiratory System

The effects of dexmedetomidine on the respiratory system are a small to moderate decrease in tidal volume and minimal change in the respiratory rate. The ventilatory response to carbon dioxide is minimally impaired, but the response to hypoxia seems reduced to a similar degree as propofol.[84] Although the respiratory effects are mild, upper airway obstruction as a result of sedation is possible. In addition, dexmedetomidine has a synergistic sedative effect when combined with other sedative-hypnotics.

## Clinical Uses

Dexmedetomidine is principally used for the short-term sedation of tracheally intubated and mechanically ventilated patients in an intensive care setting.[77]

Although there is no evidence of benefit to mortality risk, dexmedetomidine may reduce the duration of mechanical ventilation, shorten length of ICU stay,[85] and improve sleep quality.[86] In the operating room, dexmedetomidine may be used as an adjunct to general anesthesia or to provide sedation during regional anesthesia or awake fiberoptic tracheal intubation.[87] When administered during general anesthesia, dexmedetomidine (0.5- to 1-μg/kg IV initial dose over a period of 10 to 15 minutes, followed by an infusion of 0.2 to 0.7 μg/kg/h) decreases the dose requirements for inhaled and intravenous anesthetics. Awakening and the transition to the postoperative setting may benefit from dexmedetomidine-produced sedative and analgesic effects without respiratory depression. Dexmedetomidine seems to decrease perioperative opioid consumption and improve pain scores,[88] but analgesic benefit has not been shown in all settings.[89]

Dexmedetomidine has been used extensively in children and has demonstrated efficacy in this population.[90] Specifically, it may be beneficial for prevention of emergence delirium after pediatric anesthesia[91] (also see Chapter 34). At the other extreme of age, dexmedetomidine may be superior to propofol for reducing delirium in elderly patients requiring sedation after cardiac or noncardiac surgery[92,93] (also see Chapter 35).

## QUESTIONS OF THE DAY

1. What are the expected cardiovascular and respiratory effects of propofol? What techniques can reduce injection pain with propofol?

2. What are the risks of high-dose barbiturate therapy to decrease intracranial pressure (ICP) or provide neuroprotection?

3. What are the respiratory effects of benzodiazepines when administered alone and when administered concurrently with opioids? How do benzodiazepines impact pharyngeal function?

4. How do the central nervous system (CNS) effects of ketamine differ from that of propofol or barbiturates? What are the potential benefits of ketamine as an analgesic drug?

5. What are the effects of dexmedetomidine on tidal volume and respiratory rate? What are the expected cardiovascular effects of dexmedetomidine infusion? What cardiovascular effects may be evident after a bolus injection of dexmedetomidine?

## REFERENCES

1. Olkkola KT, Ahonen J. Midazolam and other benzodiazepines. *Handb Exp Pharmacol.* 2008;182:335–360.
2. Vuyk J, Sitsen E, Reekers M. Intravenous anesthetics. In: Miller RD, ed. *Miller's Anesthesia.* 8th ed. Philadelphia: Elsevier; 2015:821–863.
3. Stoelting RK, Hillier SC. Nonbarbiturate intravenous anesthetic drugs. In: Stoelting RK, Hillier SC, eds. *Pharmacology and Physiology in Anesthetic Practice.* 4th ed. Philadelphia: Lippincott Williams & Wilkins; 2006:155–178.
4. Stoelting RK, Hillier SC. Barbiturates. In: Stoelting RK, Hillier SC, eds. *Pharmacology and Physiology in Anesthetic Practice.* 4th ed. Philadelphia: Lippincott Williams & Wilkins; 2006:127–139.
5. Stoelting RK, Hillier SC. Benzodiazepines. In: Stoelting RK, Hillier SC, eds. *Pharmacology and Physiology in Anesthetic Practice.* 4th ed. Philadelphia: Lippincott Williams & Wilkins; 2006:140–154.
6. Vanlersberghe C, Camu F. Propofol. *Handb Exp Pharmacol.* 2008;182:227–252.
7. Vanlersberghe C, Camu F. Etomidate and other non-barbiturates. *Handb Exp Pharmacol.* 2008;182:267–282.
8. Asserhøj LL, Mosbech H, Krøigaard M, et al. No evidence for contraindications to the use of propofol in adults allergic to egg, soy or peanut. *Br J Anaesth.* 2016;116(1):77–82.
9. Glass PS. Half-time or half-life: what matters for recovery from intravenous anesthesia? *Anesthesiology.* 2010;112:1266–1269.
10. Hughes MA, Glass PS, Jacobs JR. Context-sensitive half-time in multicompartment pharmacokinetic models for intravenous anesthetic drugs. *Anesthesiology.* 1992;76:334–341.
11. Short TG, Hannam JA, Laurent S, et al. Refining target-controlled infusion. *Anesth Analg.* 2016;122(1):90–97.
12. Franks NP. Molecular targets underlying general anaesthesia. *Br J Pharmacol.* 2006;147(suppl 1):S72–S81.
13. Purdon PL, Sampson A, Pavone KJ, Brown EN. Clinical electroencephalography for anesthesiologists: part I: background and basic signatures. *Anesthesiology.* 2015;123(4):937–960.
14. Bosnjak ZJ, Logan S, Liu Y, Bai X. Recent insights into molecular mechanisms of propofol-induced developmental neurotoxicity. *Anesth Analg.* 2016;123(5):1286–1296.
15. Kassam SI, Lu C, Buckley N, et al. The mechanisms of propofol-induced vascular relaxation and modulation by perivascular adipose tissue and endothelium. *Anesth Analg.* 2011;112(6):1339–1345.
16. Tramer MR, Moore RA, McQuay HJ. Propofol and bradycardia: causation, frequency and severity. *Br J Anaesth.* 1997;78:642–651.
17. Simons JC, Pierce E, Diaz-Gil D, et al. Effects of depth of propofol and sevoflurane anesthesia on upper airway collapsibility, respiratory genioglossus activation, and breathing in healthy volunteers. *Anesthesiology.* 2016;125(3):525–534.
18. Eames WO, Rooke GA, Wu RS, et al. Comparison of the effects of etomidate, propofol, and thiopental on respiratory resistance after tracheal intubation. *Anesthesiology.* 1996;84:1307–1311.
19. Krajčová A, Waldauf P, Anděl M, Duška F. Propofol infusion syndrome: a structured review of experimental studies and 153 published case reports. *Crit Care.* 2015;19:398.
20. Jalota L, Kalira V, George E, et al. Prevention of pain on injection of propofol: systematic review and meta-analysis. *BMJ.* 2011;342:d1110.
21. Euasobhon P, Dej-arkom S, Siriussawakul A, et al. Lidocaine for reducing propofol-induced pain on induction of anaesthesia in adults. *Cochrane Database Syst Rev.* 2016;(2):CD007874.
22. Ingrande J, Brodsky JB, Lemmens HJ. Lean body weight scalar for the anesthetic induction dose of propofol in morbidly obese subjects. *Anesth Analg.* 2011;113(1):57–62.
23. Peng K, Liu HY, Wu SR, et al. Does propofol anesthesia lead to less postoperative pain compared with inhalational anesthesia? *Anesth Analg.* 2016;123(4):846–858.
24. Heard C, Harutunians M, Houck J, et al. Propofol anesthesia for children undergoing magnetic resonance imaging. *Anesth Analg.* 2015;120(1):157–164.
25. Borgeat A, Wilder-Smith OH, Saiah M, Rifat K. Subhypnotic doses of propofol possess direct antiemetic properties. *Anesth Analg.* 1992;74(4):539–541.
26. Schulman SR, Rockett CB, Canada AT, Glass P. Long-term propofol infusion for refractory postoperative nausea—a case-report with quantitative propofol analysis. *Anesth Analg.* 1995;80(3):636–637.
27. Apfel CC, Korttila K, Abdalla M, et al. A factorial trial of six interventions for the prevention of postoperative nausea and vomiting. *N Engl J Med.* 2004;350(24):2441–2451.
28. Kumar G, Stendall C, Mistry R, et al. A comparison of total intravenous anaesthesia using propofol with sevoflurane or desflurane in ambulatory surgery: systematic review and meta-analysis. *Anaesthesia.* 2014;69(10):1138–1150.
29. Fechner J, Ihmsen H, Jeleazcov C, Schüttler J. Fospropofol disodium, a water-soluble prodrug of the intravenous anesthetic propofol (2,6-diisopropylphenol). *Expert Opin Investig Drugs.* 2009;18(10):1565–1571.
30. Struys MM, Fechner J, Schüttler J, Schwilden H. Erroneously published fospropofol pharmacokinetic-pharmacodynamic data and retraction of the affected publications. *Anesthesiology.* 2010;112(4):1056–1057.
31. Mcintosh MP, Iwasawa K, Rajewski RA, et al. Hemodynamic profile in rabbits of fospropofol disodium injection relative to propofol emulsion following rapid bolus injection. *J Pharm Sci.* 2012;101(9):3518–3525.
32. Ilic RG. Fospropofol and remimazolam. *Int Anesthesiol Clin.* 2015;53(2):76–90.
33. Fechner J, Ihmsen H, Schüttler J, Jeleazcov C. A randomized open-label phase I pilot study of the safety and efficacy of total intravenous anesthesia with fospropofol for coronary artery bypass graft surgery. *J Cardiothorac Vasc Anesth.* 2013;27(5):908–915.
34. Candiotti KA, Gan TJ, Young C, et al. A randomized, open-label study of the safety and tolerability of fospropofol for patients requiring intubation and mechanical ventilation in the intensive care unit. *Anesth Analg.* 2011;113(3):550–556.
35. Saidman L. Uptake, distribution, and elimination of barbiturates. In: Eger EI, ed. *Anesthetic Uptake and Action.* Baltimore: Williams & Wilkins; 1974:264–284.
36. Farrant M, Nusser Z. Variations on an inhibitory theme: phasic and tonic activation of GABAA receptors. *Nat Rev Neurosci.* 2005;6(3):215–229.
37. MacIver MB. Anesthetic agent-specific effects on synaptic inhibition. *Anesth Analg.* 2014;119(3):558–569.
38. Ellens N, Figueroa B, Clark J. The use of barbiturate-induced coma during cerebrovascular neurosurgery procedures: a review of the literature. *Brain Circ.* 2015;1(2):140–146.
39. Roberts I, Sydenham E. Barbiturates for acute traumatic brain injury. *Cochrane Database Syst Rev.* 2012;(12):CD000033.
40. Reznik ME, Berger K, Claassen J. Comparison of intravenous anesthetic agents for the treatment of refractory status epilepticus. *J Clin Med.* 2016;5(5):E54.
41. Lihua P, Su M, Ke W, Ziemann-Gimmel P. Different regimens of intravenous sedatives or hypnotics for electroconvulsive therapy (ECT) in adult patients with depression. *Cochrane Database Syst Rev.* 2014;(4):CD009763.

42. Krüger T, Hoffmann I, Blettner M, et al. GERAADA Investigators. Intraoperative neuroprotective drugs without beneficial effects? Results of the German Registry for Acute Aortic Dissection Type A (GERAADA). *Eur J Cardiothorac Surg.* 2013;44(5):939–946.

43. Antonik LJ, Goldwater DR, Kilpatrick GJ, et al. A placebo- and midazolam-controlled phase I single ascending-dose study evaluating the safety, pharmacokinetics, and pharmacodynamics of remimazolam (CNS 7056): part I. Safety, efficacy, and basic pharmacokinetics. *Anesth Analg.* 2012;115(2):274–283.

44. Mohler H, Richards JG. The benzodiazepine receptor: a pharmacological control element of brain function. *Eur J Anaesthesiol.* 1988;2:15–24.

45. Bulach R, Myles PS, Russnak M. Double-blind randomized controlled trial to determine extent of amnesia with midazolam given immediately before general anaesthesia. *Br J Anaesth.* 2005;94(3):300–305.

46. Bailey PL, Pace NL, Ashburn MA, et al. Frequent hypoxemia and apnea after sedation with midazolam and fentanyl. *Anesthesiology.* 1990;73:826–830.

47. Reves JG, Fragen RJ, Vinik HR, et al. Midazolam: pharmacology and uses. *Anesthesiology.* 1985;62:310–324.

48. Padmanabhan U, Leslie K, Eer AS, et al. Early cognitive impairment after sedation for colonoscopy: the effect of adding midazolam and/or fentanyl to propofol. *Anesth Analg.* 2009;109(5):1448–1455.

49. Chen Y, Cai A, Dexter F, et al. Amnesia of the operating room in the B-Unaware and BAG-RECALL Clinical Trials. *Anesth Analg.* 2016;122(4):1158–1168.

50. Messina AG, Wang M, Ward MJ, et al. Anaesthetic interventions for prevention of awareness during surgery. *Cochrane Database Syst Rev.* 2016;(10):CD007272.

51. Cote CJ, Cohen IT, Suresh S, et al. A comparison of three doses of a commercially prepared oral midazolam syrup in children. *Anesth Analg.* 2002;94:37–43.

52. Grant MC, Kim J, Page AJ, et al. The effect of intravenous midazolam on postoperative nausea and vomiting. *Anesth Analg.* 2016;122(3):656–663.

53. Maurice-Szamburski A, Auquier P, Viarre-Oreal V, et al. PremedX Study Investigators. Effect of sedative premedication on patient experience after general anesthesia: a randomized clinical trial. *JAMA.* 2015;313(9):916–925.

54. Cedborg AI, Sundman E, Boden K, et al. Effects of morphine and midazolam on pharyngeal function, airway protection, and coordination of breathing and swallowing in healthy adults. *Anesthesiology.* 2015;122(6):1253–1267.

55. Fraser GL, Devlin JW, Worby CP, et al. Benzodiazepine versus nonbenzodiazepine-based sedation for mechanically ventilated, critically ill adults: a systematic review and meta-analysis of randomized trials. *Crit Care Med.* 2013;41(9 suppl 1):S30–S38.

56. Zaal IJ, Devlin JW, Hazelbag M, et al. Benzodiazepine-associated delirium in critically ill adults. *Intensive Care Med.* 2015;41(12):2130–2137.

57. Prasad M, Krishnan PR, Sequeira R, Al-Roomi K. Anticonvulsant therapy for status epilepticus. *Cochrane Database Syst Rev.* 2014;(9). CD003723.

58. Peltoniemi MA, Hagelberg NM, Olkkola KT, Saari TI. Ketamine: a review of clinical pharmacokinetics and pharmacodynamics in anesthesia and pain therapy. *Clin Pharmacokinet.* 2016;55:1059–1077.

59. Singh JB, Fedgchin M, Daly EJ, et al. A double-blind, randomized, placebo-controlled, dose-frequency study of intravenous ketamine in patients with treatment-resistant depression. *Am J Psychiatry.* 2016;173(8):816–826.

60. Franks NP. General anaesthesia: from molecular targets to neuronal pathways of sleep and arousal. *Nat Rev Neurosci.* 2008;9:370–386.

61. Albanese J, Arnaud S, Rey M, et al. Ketamine decreases intracranial pressure and electroencephalographic activity in traumatic brain injury patients during propofol sedation. *Anesthesiology.* 1997;87:1328–1334.

62. Kohrs R, Durieux ME. Ketamine: teaching an old drug new tricks. *Anesth Analg.* 1998;87:1186–1193.

63. Gorlin AW, Rosenfeld DM, Ramakrishna H. Intravenous sub-anesthetic ketamine for perioperative analgesia. *J Anaesthesiol Clin Pharmacol.* 2016;32:160.

64. Grady MV, Mascha E, Sessler DI, Kurz A. The effect of perioperative intravenous lidocaine and ketamine on recovery after abdominal hysterectomy. *Anesth Analg.* 2012;115:1078–1084.

65. Sawynok J. Topical and peripheral ketamine as an analgesic. *Anesth Analg.* 2014;119:170–178.

66. Murrough JW, Iosifescu DV, Chang LC, et al. Antidepressant efficacy of ketamine in treatment-resistant major depression: a two-site randomized controlled trial. *Am J Psychiatry.* 2013;170(10):1134–1142.

67. Campagna JA, Pojasek K, Grayzel D, et al. Advancing novel anesthetics: pharmacodynamic and pharmacokinetic studies of cyclopropyl-methoxycarbonyl metomidate in dogs. *Anesthesiology.* 2014;121(6):1203–1216.

68. Fragen RJ, Shanks CA, Molteni A, et al. Effects of etomidate on hormonal responses to surgical stress. *Anesthesiology.* 1984;61:652–656.

69. Morel J, Salard M, Castelain C, et al. Haemodynamic consequences of etomidate administration in elective cardiac surgery: a randomized double-blinded study. *Br J Anaesth.* 2011;107(4):503–509.

70. Erdoes G, Basciani RM, Eberle B. Etomidate—a review of robust evidence for its use in various clinical scenarios. *Acta Anaesthesiol Scand.* 2014;58(4):380–389.

71. Haessler R, Madler C, Klasing S, et al. Propofol/fentanyl versus etomidate/fentanyl for the induction of anesthesia in patients with aortic insufficiency and coronary artery disease. *J Cardiothoracic Vasc Anesth.* 1992;6(2):173–180.

72. Bendel S, Ruokonen E, Pölönen P, Uusaro A. Propofol causes more hypotension than etomidate in patients with severe aortic stenosis: a double-blind, randomized study comparing propofol and etomidate. *Acta Anaesthesiol Scand.* 2007;51(3):284–289.

73. Gu WJ, Wang F, Tang L, Liu JC. Single-dose etomidate does not increase mortality in patients with sepsis: a systematic review and meta-analysis of randomized controlled trials and observational studies. *Chest.* 2015;147(2):335–346.

74. Bruder EA, Ball IM, Ridi S, et al. Single induction dose of etomidate versus other induction agents for endotracheal intubation in critically ill patients. *Cochrane Database Syst Rev.* 2015;(1):CD010225.

75. Chan CM, Mitchell AL, Shorr AF. Etomidate is associated with mortality and adrenal insufficiency in sepsis: a meta-analysis. *Crit Care Med.* 2012;40(11):2945–2953.

76. Avramov MN, Husain MM, White PF. The comparative effects of methohexital, propofol, and etomidate for electroconvulsive therapy. *Anesth Analg.* 1995;81(3):596–602.

77. Kamibayashi T, Maze M. Clinical uses of alpha2-adrenergic agonists. *Anesthesiology.* 2000;93:1345–1349.

78. Oda Y, Toriyama S, Tanaka K, et al. The effect of dexmedetomidine on electrocorticography in patients with temporal lobe epilepsy under sevoflurane anesthesia. *Anesth Analg.* 2007;105(5):1272–1277.

79. Rozet I, Metzner J, Brown M, et al. Dexmedetomidine does not affect evoked potentials during spine surgery. *Anesth Analg.* 2015;121(2):492–501.

80. Friesen RH, Nichols CS, Twite MD, et al. The hemodynamic response to dexmedetomidine loading dose in children with and without pulmonary hypertension. *Anesth Analg.* 2013;117(4):953–959.

81. Ice CJ, Personett HA, Frazee EN, et al. Risk factors for dexmedetomidine-associated hemodynamic instability in noncardiac intensive care unit patients. *Anesth Analg.* 2016;122(2):462–469.

82. Talke P, Chen R, Thomas B, et al. The hemodynamic and adrenergic effects of perioperative dexmedetomidine infusion after vascular surgery. *Anesth Analg.* 2000;90(4):834–839.

83. Li Y, Wang B, Zhang LL, et al. Dexmedetomidine combined with general anesthesia provides similar intraoperative stress response reduction when compared with a combined general and epidural anesthetic technique. *Anesth Analg.* 2016;122(4):1202–1210.

84. Lodenius Å, Ebberyd A, Hårdemark Cedborg A, et al. Sedation with dexmedetomidine or propofol impairs hypoxic control of breathing in healthy male volunteers: a nonblinded, randomized crossover study. *Anesthesiology.* 2016;125(4):700–715.

85. Chen K, Lu Z, Xin YC, et al. Alpha-2 agonists for long-term sedation during mechanical ventilation in critically ill patients. *Cochrane Database Syst Rev.* 2015;(1):CD010269.

86. Alexopoulou C, Kondili E, Diamantaki E, et al. Effects of dexmedetomidine on sleep quality in critically ill patients: a pilot study. *Anesthesiology.* 2014;121(4):801–807.

87. He XY, Cao JP, He Q, Shi XY. Dexmedetomidine for the management of awake fibreoptic intubation. *Cochrane Database Syst Rev.* 2014;(1):CD009798.

88. Blaudszun G, Lysakowski C, Elia N, Tramer MR. Effect of perioperative systemic alpha 2 agonists on postoperative morphine consumption and pain intensity systematic review and meta-analysis of randomized controlled trials. *Anesthesiology.* 2012;116(6):1312–1322.

89. Naik BI, Nemergut EC, Kazemi A, et al. The effect of dexmedetomidine on postoperative opioid consumption and pain after major spine surgery. *Anesth Analg.* 2016;122(5):1646–1653.

90. Mason KP, Lerman J. Dexmedetomidine in children. *Anesth Analg.* 2011;113(5):1129–1142.

91. Dahmani S, Delivet H, Hilly J. Emergence delirium in children. *Curr Opin Anaesthesiol.* 2014;27(3):309–315.

92. Djaiani G, Silverton N, Fedorko L, et al. Dexmedetomidine versus propofol sedation reduces delirium after cardiac surgery: a randomized controlled trial. *Anesthesiology.* 2016;124(2):362–368.

93. Su X, Meng ZT, Wu XH, et al. Dexmedetomidine for prevention of delirium in elderly patients after noncardiac surgery: a randomised, double-blind, placebo-controlled trial. *Lancet.* 2016;388(10054):1893–1902.

# 9 OPIOIDS

## Talmage D. Egan and Cynthia Newberry

Opioids play an indispensable role in the practice of anesthesiology, critical care, and pain management. A sound understanding of opioid pharmacology, including both basic science and clinical aspects, is critical for the safe and effective use of these important drugs. This chapter will focus almost exclusively on intravenous opioid receptor agonists used perioperatively.

## BASIC PHARMACOLOGY

### Structure-Activity

The opioids of clinical interest in anesthesiology share many structural features. Morphine is a benzylisoquinoline alkaloid (Fig. 9.1). Many commonly used semisynthetic opioids are created by simple modification of the morphine molecule. Codeine, for example, is the 3-methyl derivative of morphine. Similarly, hydromorphone, hydrocodone, and oxycodone are also synthesized by relatively simple modifications of morphine. More complex alterations of the morphine molecular skeleton result in mixed agonist-antagonists such as nalbuphine and even complete antagonists such as naloxone.

The fentanyl series of opioids are chemically related to meperidine. Meperidine is the first completely synthetic opioid and can be regarded as the prototype clinical phenylpiperidine (see Fig 9.1). Fentanyl is a simple modification of the basic phenylpiperidine structure. Other commonly used fentanyl congeners such as alfentanil and sufentanil are somewhat more complex versions of the same phenylpiperidine skeleton.

Opioids share many physicochemical features in common, although some individual drugs have unique features (Table 9.1). In general, opioids are highly soluble weak bases that are highly protein bound and largely ionized at physiologic pH. Opioid physicochemical properties influence their clinical behavior. For example, relatively unbound, un-ionized molecules such as alfentanil and remifentanil have a shorter latency to peak effect after bolus injection.

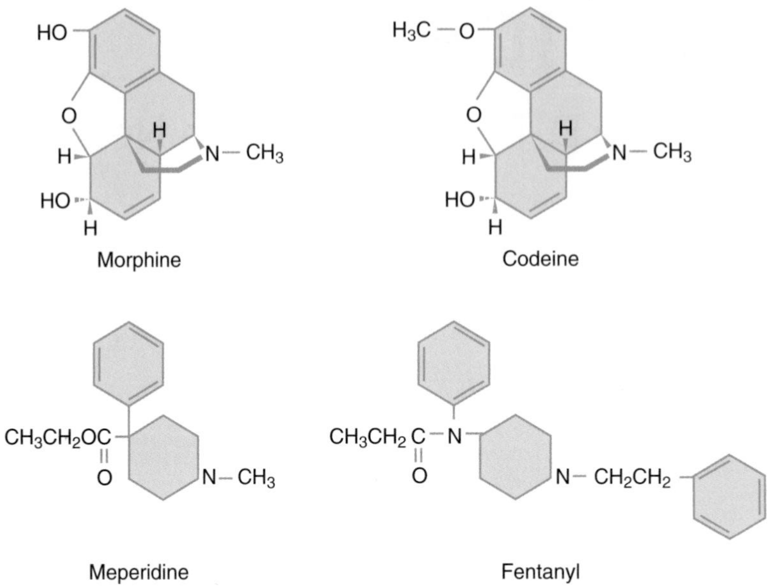

**Fig. 9.1** The molecular structures of morphine, codeine, meperidine, and fentanyl. Note that codeine is a simple modification of morphine (as are many other opiates); fentanyl and its congeners are more complex modifications of meperidine, a phenylpiperidine derivative.

**Table 9.1** Selected Opioid Physicochemical and Pharmacokinetic Parameters

| Parameter | Morphine | Fentanyl | Sufentanil | Alfentanil | Remifentanil |
|---|---|---|---|---|---|
| pKa | 8.0 | 8.4 | 8.0 | 6.5 | 7.1 |
| % un-ionized at pH 7.4 | 23 | <10 | 20 | 90 | 67 |
| Octanol-$H_2O$ partition coefficient | 1.4 | 813 | 1778 | 145 | 17.9 |
| % bound to plasma protein | 20-40 | 84 | 93 | 92 | 80 |
| Diffusible fraction (%) | 16.8 | 1.5 | 1.6 | 8.0 | 13.3 |
| Vdc (L/kg) | 0.1-0.4 | 0.4-1.0 | 0.2 | 0.1-0.3 | 0.06-0.08 |
| Vdss (L/kg) | 3-5 | 3-5 | 2.5-3.0 | 0.4-1.0 | 0.2-0.3 |
| Clearance (mL/min/kg) | 15-30 | 10-20 | 10-15 | 4-9 | 30-40 |
| Hepatic extraction ratio | 0.6-0.8 | 0.8-1.0 | 0.7-0.9 | 0.3-0.5 | NA |

*NA*, Not applicable; *Vdc*, volume of distribution of central compartment; *Vdss*, volume of distribution at steady state.
From Fukuda K. Opioid Analgesics. In Miller RD, ed. *Anesthesia*. 8th ed. Philadelphia, PA: Elsevier Saunders; 2015:887.

## Mechanism

Opioids produce their main pharmacologic effects by interacting with opioid receptors, which are typical of the G protein–coupled family of receptors widely found in biology (e.g., β-adrenergic, dopaminergic, among others). Expression of cloned opioid receptors in cultured cells has facilitated analysis of the intracellular signal transduction mechanisms activated by the opioid receptors.[1] Binding of opioid agonists with the receptors leads to activation of the G protein, producing effects that are primarily inhibitory (Fig. 9.2); these effects ultimately culminate in hyperpolarization of the cell and reduction of neuronal excitability.

Three classical opioid receptors have been identified using molecular biology techniques: μ, κ, and δ. More recently, a fourth opioid receptor, ORL1 (also known as NOP), has also been identified, although its function is

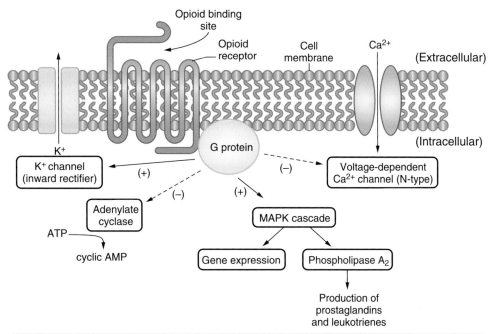

**Fig. 9.2** Opioid mechanisms of action. The endogenous ligand or drug binds to the opioid receptor and activates the G protein, resulting in multiple effects that are primarily inhibitory. The activities of adenylate cyclase and the voltage-dependent $Ca^{2+}$ channels are depressed. The inwardly rectifying $K^+$ channels and mitogen activated protein kinase (MAPK) cascade are activated. *AMP*, Adenosine monophosphate; *ATP*, adenosine triphosphate.

quite different from that of the classical opioid receptors. Each of these opioid receptors has a commonly employed experimental bioassay, associated endogenous ligand(s), a set of agonists and antagonists, and a spectrum of physiologic effects when the receptor is agonized (Table 9.2). Although the existence of opioid receptor subtypes (e.g., $\mu_1$ $\mu_2$) has been proposed, it is not clear from molecular biology techniques that distinct genes exist for them. Posttranslational modification of opioid receptors certainly occurs and may be responsible for conflicting data regarding opioid receptor subtypes.[2]

Opioids exert their therapeutic effects at multiple sites. They inhibit the release of substance P from primary sensory neurons in the dorsal horn of the spinal cord, mitigating the transfer of painful sensations to the brain. Opioid actions in the brainstem modulate nociceptive transmission in the dorsal horn of the spinal cord through descending inhibitory pathways. Opioids are thought to change the affective response to pain through actions in the forebrain; decerebration prevents opioid analgesic efficacy in rats.[3] Furthermore, morphine induces signal changes in "reward structures" in the human brain.[4]

Studies in genetically altered mice have yielded important information about opioid receptor function. In $\mu$ opioid receptor knockout mice, morphine-induced analgesia, reward effect, and withdrawal effect are absent.[5,6]

Importantly, $\mu$ receptor knockout mice also fail to exhibit respiratory depression in response to morphine.[7]

## Metabolism

The intravenously administered opioids in routine perioperative clinical use are transformed and excreted by many metabolic pathways. In general, opioids are metabolized by the hepatic microsomal system, although hepatic conjugation and subsequent excretion by the kidney are important for some opioids. For certain opioids, the specific metabolic pathway involved has important clinical implications in terms of active metabolites (e.g., morphine, meperidine) or an ultra short duration of action (e.g., remifentanil). For other opioids, genetic variation in the metabolic pathway can drastically alter the clinical effects (e.g., codeine). These nuances are addressed in a subsequent section focused on individual drugs.

## CLINICAL PHARMACOLOGY

### Pharmacokinetics

Pharmacokinetic differences are the primary basis for the rational selection and administration of opioids in perioperative anesthesia practice. Key pharmacokinetic behaviors are (1) the latency to peak effect-site concentration

| **Table 9.2** | A Summary of Selected Features of Opioid Receptors | | |
|---|---|---|---|
| **Feature** | **Mu (μ)** | **Delta (δ)** | **Kappa (κ)** |
| Tissue bioassay[a] | Guinea pig ileum | Mouse vas deferens | Rabbit vas deferens |
| Endogenous ligand | β-Endorphin | Leu-enkephalin | Dynorphin |
| | Endomorphin | Met-enkephalin | |
| Agonist prototype | Morphine | Deltorphin | Buprenorphine |
| | Fentanyl | | Pentazocine |
| Antagonist prototype | Naloxone | Naloxone | Naloxone |
| Supraspinal analgesia | Yes | Yes | Yes |
| Spinal analgesia | Yes | Yes | Yes |
| Ventilatory depression | Yes | No | No |
| Gastrointestinal effects | Yes | No | Yes |
| Sedation | Yes | No | Yes |

[a]Traditional experimental method to assess opioid receptor activity in vivo.
From Bailey PL, Egan TD, Stanley TH. Intravenous opioid anesthetics. In Miller RD, ed. *Anesthesia*. 5th ed. New York: Churchill Livingstone; 2000:312.

after bolus injection (i.e., bolus front-end kinetics), (2) the time to clinically relevant decay of concentration after bolus injection (i.e., bolus back-end kinetics), (3) the time to steady-state concentration after starting a continuous infusion (i.e., infusion front-end kinetics), and (4) the time to clinically relevant decay in concentration after stopping a continuous infusion (i.e., infusion back-end kinetics).

Applying opioid pharmacokinetic concepts to clinical anesthesiology requires recognition of several fundamental principles. First, a table of pharmacokinetic variables has limited clinical value (see Table 9.1). Understanding pharmacokinetic behavior is best achieved through computer simulation. Second, opioids administered by bolus injection or continuous infusion must be considered separately.[8] Third, pharmacokinetic information must be integrated with knowledge about the concentration-effect relationship and drug interactions (i.e., pharmacodynamics) in order to be clinically useful (also see Chapter 4).

The latency to peak effect and the offset of effect after bolus injection (i.e., bolus front-end kinetics and bolus back-end kinetics) of various intravenous opioids can be defined by predicting the time course of effect-site concentrations after a bolus is administered. Because the opioids differ in terms of potency (and thus the required dosages), for comparison purposes, the effect-site concentrations must be normalized to the percent of peak concentration for each drug. Considering morphine, fentanyl, sufentanil, alfentanil, and remifentanil as among the opioids most commonly used intraoperatively, pharmacokinetic simulation illustrates how opioids differ in terms of latency to peak effect after a bolus is administered (Fig. 9.3, top panel).[9-12]

The simulation of a bolus injection (see Fig. 9.3, top panel) has clinical implications. For example, when a rapid onset of opioid effect is desirable, morphine may not be a good choice. Similarly, when the clinical goal is a brief duration of opioid effect followed by rapid dissipation, remifentanil or alfentanil might be preferred. Note how remifentanil's concentration has declined very substantially before fentanyl's peak concentration has even been achieved. The simulation illustrates why the front-end kinetics of fentanyl make it a drug well suited for patient-controlled analgesia (PCA) (also see Chapters 39 and 40). In contrast to morphine, the peak effect of a fentanyl bolus is manifest before a typical PCA lockout period has elapsed, thus mitigating a "dose stacking" problem (also see Chapter 40).

The latency to peak effect is governed by the speed with which the plasma and effect site come to equilibrium (i.e., the ke0 parameter). Drugs with a more rapid equilibration have a higher "diffusible" fraction (i.e., the proportion of drug that is un-ionized and unbound) and high lipid solubility (see Table 9.1). However, a very large dose of even a slow onset opioid can produce an apparent rapid onset (because a supratherapeutic drug level in the effect site is reached even though the peak concentration comes later).

The time to steady-state after beginning a continuous infusion is also best examined by pharmacokinetic simulation. Using the same prototypes as with bolus administration, pharmacokinetic simulation (Fig. 9.3, middle panel) shows the time required to achieve steady-state effect-site concentrations (i.e., infusion front-end kinetics).

This simulation of simple, constant rate infusions has obvious clinical implications. First, the time required to

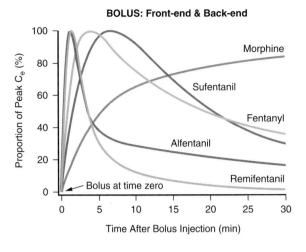

**BOLUS: Front-end & Back-end**

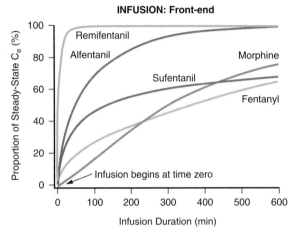

**INFUSION: Front-end**

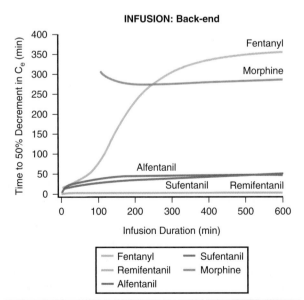

**INFUSION: Back-end**

| Fentanyl | Sufentanil |
| Remifentanil | Morphine |
| Alfentanil | |

**Fig. 9.3** Opioid pharmacokinetics. Simulations illustrating front-end and back-end pharmacokinetic behavior after administration by bolus injection or continuous infusions of morphine, fentanyl, alfentanil, sufentanil, and remifentanil using pharmacokinetic parameters from the literature (see text for details).[9-12,45]

reach a substantial fraction of the ultimate steady-state concentration is very long in the context of intraoperative use. To reach a near steady-state more quickly requires that a bolus be administered before the infusion is commenced (or increased). Remifentanil perhaps represents a partial exception to this general rule. Also, opioid concentrations will increase for many hours after an infusion is commenced; in other words, concentrations are typically increasing even though the infusion rate may have been the same for hours! That remifentanil achieves a near steady-state relatively quickly is certainly part of why it has emerged as a popular drug for total intravenous anesthesia (TIVA).

The time to offset of effect after stopping a steady-state infusion is best expressed by the context-sensitive half-time (CSHT) simulation.[13] Defined as the time required to achieve a 50% decrease in concentration after stopping a continuous, steady-state infusion, the CSHT is a means of normalizing the pharmacokinetic behavior of drugs so that rational comparisons can be made regarding the predicted offset of drug effect. The CSHT is thus focused on "infusion back-end" kinetics.

The bottom panel of Fig. 9.3 is a CSHT simulation for commonly used opioids. For most drugs, the CSHT changes with time. Thus, for brief infusions, the predicted back-end kinetics for the various drugs do not differ much (remifentanil is a notable exception to this general rule). As the infusion time lengthens, the CSHTs begin to differentiate, providing a rational basis for drug selection. Second, depending on the desired duration of opioid effect, either shorter-acting or longer-acting drugs can be chosen. Finally, the shapes of these curves differ depending on the degree of concentration decline required. In other words, the curves representing the time required to achieve a 20% or an 80% decrease in concentration (e.g., the 20% or 80% decrement time simulations) are quite different.[8] Thus, depending on the anesthesia technique applied, the CSHT simulations are not necessarily the clinically relevant simulations (i.e., a 50% decrease may not be the clinical goal). Also, CSHT simulation for morphine does not account for active metabolites (see later discussion of individual drugs under "Unique Features of Individual Opioids").

## Pharmacodynamics

In most respects, the μ-agonist opioids can be considered pharmacodynamic equals with important pharmacokinetic differences; that is, both the therapeutic and adverse effects are essentially the same. Their efficacy as analgesics and their propensity to produce ventilatory depression are indistinguishable from each other. Pharmacodynamic differences do exist with nonopioid receptor mechanisms such as histamine release.

Because the nervous system profoundly influences the function of the entire body, opioid μ-agonist

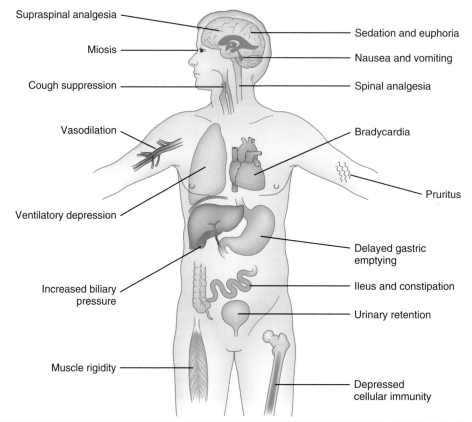

**Fig. 9.4** Opioid pharmacodynamics. A summary chart of selected effects of the fentanyl congeners (see text for details).

pharmacodynamic effects are observed in many organ systems. Fig. 9.4 summarizes the major pharmacodynamic effects of the fentanyl congeners. Depending on the clinical circumstances and clinical goals of treatment, some of these widespread effects can be viewed as therapeutic or adverse. For example, in some clinical settings the sedation produced by μ-agonists might be viewed as a goal of therapy. In others, drowsiness would clearly be thought of as an adverse effect.

Therapeutic Effects

The relief of pain is the primary therapeutic effect of opioid analgesics. Acting at spinal and brain μ-receptors, opioids provide analgesia both by attenuating the nociceptive traffic from the periphery and also by altering the affective response to painful stimulation centrally. μ-Agonists are most effective in treating "second pain" sensations carried by slowly conducting, unmyelinated C fibers; they are less effective in treating "first pain" sensations (carried by small, myelinated A-delta fibers) and neuropathic pain. A unique aspect of opioid-induced analgesia (in contrast to drugs like local anesthetics) is that other sensory modalities are not affected (e.g., touch, temperature, among others).

Perioperatively (certainly intraoperatively), the drowsiness produced by μ-agonists is also one of the targeted effects. The brain is the anatomic substrate for the sedative action of μ-agonists. With increasing doses, μ-agonists eventually produce drowsiness and sleep (the relief of pain no doubt contributes to the promotion of sleep in uncomfortable patients both pre- and postoperatively). With sufficient doses, the μ-agonists produce pronounced delta wave activity on the electroencephalogram, which resembles the pattern observed during natural sleep.

μ-Agonists can of course produce significant relief of pain by doses that do not produce sleep. This is the clinical basis for their use in the treatment of pain in ambulatory patients. Yet, the administration of additional doses eventually produces drowsiness (and, as a consequence, the inability to request additional doses) and is the essential scientific foundation for the safety of PCA devices (also see Chapter 40). However, even large doses of opioids do not reliably produce unresponsiveness and amnesia and thus opioids cannot be viewed as complete anesthetics when used alone.

Opioids also suppress the cough reflex via the cough centers in the medulla. Attenuation of the cough reflex presumably makes coughing and "bucking" against the indwelling endotracheal tube less likely.

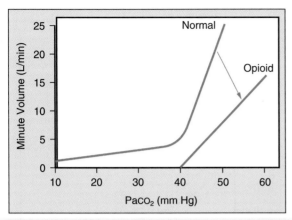

**Fig. 9.5** Opioid-induced ventilatory depression study methodology. The method characterizes the relationship between $Paco_2$ and minute volume. The curve labeled "Normal" represents the expected response of minute volume to rising $Paco_2$ levels in an awake human. Note the dramatic increase in minute volume as $CO_2$ tension rises. The curve labeled "Opioid" represents the blunted response of minute volume to rising $CO_2$ levels following administration of an opioid. Note that the slope of the curve decreases and the curve no longer has a "hockey stick" shape; this means that at physiologic $Paco_2$ levels, the patient receiving sufficient opioid may be apneic or severely hypoventilatory. (Adapted from Gross JB. When you breathe IN you inspire, when you DON'T breathe, you . . . expire: new insights regarding opioid-induced ventilatory depression. *Anesthesiology*. 2003;99:767-770, used with permission.)

## Adverse Effects

Depression of ventilation is the primary adverse effect associated with μ-agonist drugs. When the airway is secured and ventilation is controlled intraoperatively, opioid-induced depression of ventilation is of little consequence. However, opioid-induced respiratory depression in the postoperative period can lead to brain injury and death (also see Chapter 39).

μ-Agonists alter the ventilatory response to arterial carbon dioxide concentrations at the ventilatory control center in the medulla. The depression of ventilation is mediated by the μ-receptor; μ-receptor knockout mice do not exhibit respiratory depression from morphine.[14]

In unmedicated humans, increases in arterial carbon dioxide partial pressure markedly increase minute volume (Fig. 9.5). Under the influence of opioid analgesics, the curve is flattened and shifted to the right for a given carbon dioxide partial pressure and reflecting that the minute volume is smaller.[15] More importantly, the "hockey stick" shape of the normal curve is lost; that is, there may be a partial pressure of carbon dioxide below which the patient will not breathe (i.e., the "apneic threshold") in presence of opioids.

The clinical signs of depressed ventilation are quite subtle with moderate opioid doses. Postoperative patients receiving opioid analgesic therapy can be awake and alert and yet have a significantly decreased minute volume. Respiratory rate (often associated with a slightly increased tidal volume) also decreases. As the opioid concentration is increased, the respiratory rate and tidal volume progressively decrease, eventually culminating in an irregular ventilatory rhythm and then complete apnea.

Many factors can increase the risk of opioid-induced ventilatory depression. Clear risk factors include large opioid dose, advanced age, concomitant use of other central nervous system (CNS) depressants, and renal insufficiency (for morphine). Natural sleep also increases the ventilatory depressant effect of opioids.[16]

Opioids can alter cardiovascular physiology by a variety of different mechanisms. Compared to many other anesthetic drugs (e.g., propofol, volatile anesthetics), however, the cardiovascular effects of opioids, particularly the fentanyl congeners, are relatively minimal (morphine and meperidine are exceptions—see the following section on individual drugs).

The fentanyl congeners cause bradycardia by directly increasing vagal nerve tone in the brainstem, which experimentally can be blocked by microinjection of naloxone into the vagal nerve nucleus or by peripheral vagotomy.[17,18]

Opioids also produce vasodilation by depressing vasomotor centers in the brainstem and to a lesser extent by a direct effect on vessels. This action decreases both preload and afterload. Decreases in arterial blood pressure are more pronounced in patients with increased sympathetic tone such as patients with congestive heart failure or hypertension. Clinical doses of opioids do not appreciably alter myocardial contractility.

Opioids can induce muscle rigidity, usually from the rapid administration of large bolus doses of the fentanyl congeners. This rigidity can even make ventilation via a bag and mask during induction of anesthesia nearly impossible because of vocal cord rigidity and closure.[19] The appearance of rigidity tends to coincide with the onset of unresponsiveness.[20] Although the mechanism of opioid-induced muscle rigidity is unknown, it is not a direct action on muscle because it can be eliminated by the administration of neuromuscular blocking drugs.

Opioids also cause nausea and vomiting. Opioids stimulate the chemoreceptor trigger zone in the area postrema on the floor of the fourth ventricle in the brain. This can lead to nausea and vomiting, which are exacerbated by movement (this is perhaps why ambulatory surgery patients are more likely to be troubled by postoperative nausea and vomiting, PONV) (also see Chapter 37).

Pupillary constriction induced by μ-agonists can be a useful diagnostic sign indicating some ongoing opioid effect. Opioids stimulate the Edinger-Westphal nucleus of the oculomotor nerve to produce miosis. Even small doses of opioid elicit this response and very little tolerance to the effect develops. Thus, miosis is a useful, albeit nonspecific indicator of opioid exposure even in opioid-tolerant patients. Opioid-induced pupillary constriction is naloxone reversible.

Opioids have important effects on gastrointestinal physiology. Opioid receptors are located throughout the enteric plexus of the bowel. Stimulation of these receptors by opioids causes tonic contraction of gastrointestinal smooth muscle, thereby decreasing coordinated, peristaltic contractions. Clinically, this contraction results in delayed gastric emptying and presumably larger gastric volumes in patients receiving opioid therapy preoperatively. Postoperatively, patients can develop opioid-induced ileus that can potentially delay the resumption of proper nutrition and discharge from the hospital. An extension of this acute problem is the chronic constipation associated with long-term opioid therapy.

Similar effects are observed in the biliary system, which also has an abundance of μ-receptors. μ-Agonists can produce contraction of the gallbladder smooth muscle and spasm of the sphincter of Oddi, potentially causing a falsely positive cholangiogram during gallbladder and bile duct surgery. These effects are completely naloxone reversible and can be partially reversed by glucagon treatment.

Although the urologic effects are minimal, opioids can sometimes cause urinary retention by decreasing bladder detrusor tone and by increasing the tone of the urinary sphincter. These effects are in part centrally mediated, although peripheral effects are also likely given the widespread presence of opioid receptors in the genitourinary tract.[21,22] Although the urinary retention associated with opioid therapy is not typically pronounced, it can be troublesome in males, particularly when the opioid is administered intrathecally or epidurally.

Opioids depress cellular immunity. Morphine and the endogenous opioid β-endorphin, for example, inhibit the transcription of interleukin 2 in activated T cells, among other immunologic effects.[23] Individual opioids (and perhaps classes of opioids) may differ in terms of the exact nature and extent of their immunomodulatory effects. Although opioid-induced impairment of cellular immunity is not well understood, impaired wound healing, perioperative infections, and cancer recurrence are possible adverse outcomes.

## Drug Interactions

Drug interactions can be based on two mechanisms: pharmacokinetic (i.e., when one drug influences the concentration of the other) or pharmacodynamic (i.e., when one drug influences the effect of the other). In anesthesia practice, although unintended pharmacokinetic interactions

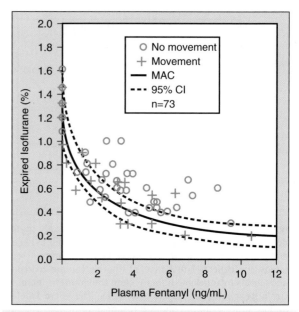

**Fig. 9.6** Volatile anesthetic minimum alveolar concentration (MAC) reduction by opioids: the prototype example of isoflurane and fentanyl. The solid curve is MAC; the dotted curves are the 95% confidence intervals (CIs) (see text for details). (Adapted from McEwan AI, Smith C, Dyar O, et al. Isoflurane minimum alveolar concentration reduction by fentanyl. *Anesthesiology.* 1993;78:864-869, used with permission.)

sometimes occur, pharmacodynamic interactions occur with virtually every anesthetic and are often produced by design.

The most common pharmacokinetic interaction in opioid clinical pharmacology is observed when intravenous opioids are combined with propofol. Perhaps because of the hemodynamic changes induced by propofol and their impact on pharmacokinetic processes, opioid concentrations may be larger when given in combination with a continuous propofol infusion.[24]

The most important pharmacodynamic drug interaction involving opioids is the synergistic interaction that occurs when opioids are combined with sedatives.[25] When combined with volatile anesthetics, opioids reduce the minimum alveolar concentration (MAC) of a volatile anesthetic (Fig. 9.6). Careful examination of "opioid-MAC reduction" data reveals several clinically critical concepts (see Fig. 9.6). First, opioids synergistically reduce MAC. Second, the MAC reduction is substantial (as much as 75% or more). Third, most of the MAC reduction occurs at moderate opioid levels (i.e., even modest opioid doses substantially reduce MAC). Fourth, reduction of MAC is not complete (i.e., opioids are not complete anesthetics). The addition of the opioid cannot completely eliminate the need for the other anesthetic. And fifth, there are an infinite number of hypnotic-opioid combinations that will achieve MAC (this implies that clinicians must choose the optimal combination based on the goals of the anesthetic and operation). All of these concepts also apply when opioids are used in combination with propofol for TIVA.[26]

## Special Populations

### Hepatic Failure

Even though the liver is the metabolic organ primarily responsible for the biotransformation of most opioids, liver failure is usually not severe enough to have a major impact on opioid pharmacokinetics. Of course, the anhepatic phase of orthotopic liver transplantation is a notable exception to this general rule (also see Chapter 36). With ongoing drug administration, concentrations of opioids that rely on hepatic metabolism increase when the patient has no liver. Even after partial liver resection, an increase in the ratio of morphine glucuronides to morphine occurs, indicating a decrease in the rate of morphine metabolism.[27] Because remifentanil's metabolism is completely unrelated to hepatic clearance mechanisms, its disposition is not affected during liver transplantation.[28]

Pharmacodynamic considerations can be important for opioid therapy in patients with severe liver disease. Patients with ongoing hepatic encephalopathy are especially vulnerable to the sedative effects of opioids. As a consequence, this drug class must be used with caution in this patient population.

### Kidney Failure

Renal failure has implications of major clinical importance with respect to morphine and meperidine (see the following discussion on individual drugs). For the fentanyl congeners, the clinical importance of kidney failure is much less marked. Remifentanil's metabolism is not impacted by kidney disease.[29]

Morphine is principally metabolized by conjugation in the liver; the resulting water-soluble glucuronides (i.e., morphine 3-glucuronide and morphine 6-glucuronide—M3G and M6G) are excreted via the kidney. The kidney also plays a role in the conjugation of morphine and may account for as much as half of its conversion to M3G and M6G.

M3G is inactive, but M6G is an analgesic with a potency rivaling morphine. Very large levels of M6G and life-threatening respiratory depression can develop in patients with renal failure (Fig. 9.7).[30] Consequently, morphine may not be a good choice in patients with severely altered renal clearance mechanisms.

The clinical pharmacology of meperidine is also significantly altered by renal failure. Normeperidine, the main metabolite, has analgesic and excitatory CNS effects that range from anxiety and tremulousness to myoclonus and frank seizures. Because the active metabolites are subject to renal excretion, CNS toxicity secondary to accumulation of normeperidine is especially a concern in patients with renal failure. This

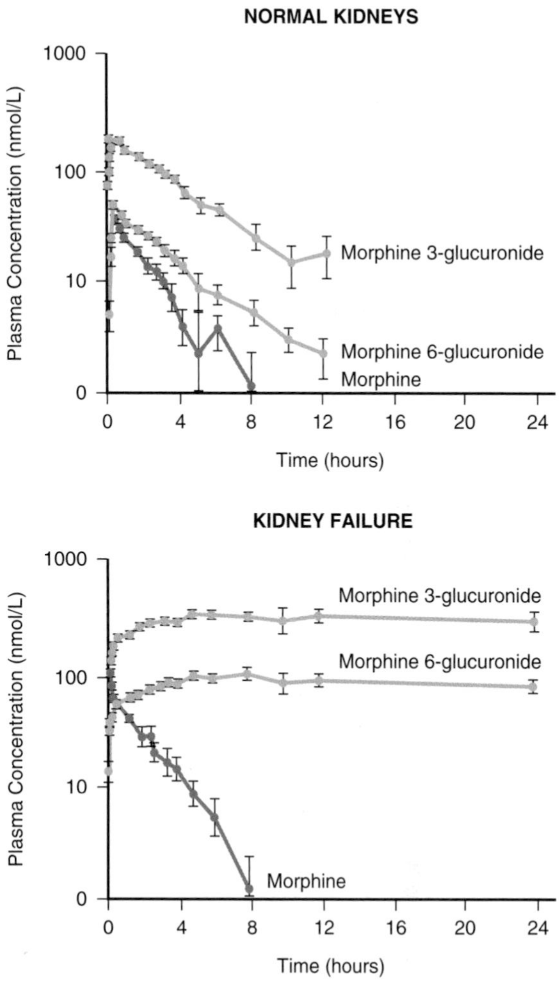

**Fig. 9.7** The pharmacokinetics of morphine and its metabolites in normal volunteers versus kidney failure patients. Note the significant accumulation of the metabolites in renal failure. (Adapted from Osborne R, Joel S, Grebenik K, et al. The pharmacokinetics of morphine and morphine glucuronides in kidney failure. *Clin Pharmacol Ther.* 1993;54:158-167, used with permission.)

shortcoming of meperidine has caused many hospital formularies to restrict its use or to remove it from the formulary altogether.

### Gender

Gender may have an important influence on opioid pharmacology. Morphine is more potent in women than in men and has a slower onset of action in women.[31] Some of these differences may be related to cyclic gonadal hormones and psychosocial factors.

### Age (Also See Chapter 35)

Advancing age is clearly an important factor influencing the clinical pharmacology of opioids. For example, fentanyl congeners are more potent in the older patient

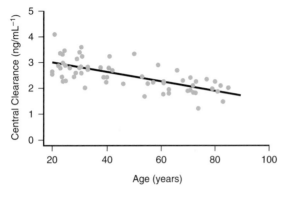

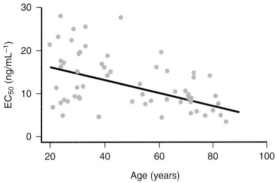

**Fig. 9.8** The influence of age on the clinical pharmacology of remifentanil. Although there is considerable variability, in general, older subjects have a lower central clearance and a higher potency (i.e., lower EC$_{50}$).[32]

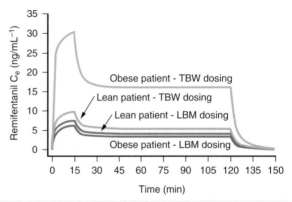

**Fig. 9.9** A pharmacokinetic simulation illustrating the consequences of calculating the remifentanil dosage based on total body weight (TBW) or lean body mass (LBM) in obese and lean patients (1 µg/kg bolus injection followed by an infusion of 0.5 µg/kg/min for 15 minutes and 0.25 µg/kg/min for an additional 105 minutes). Note that TBW-based dosing in an obese patient results in dramatically higher concentrations. (Adapted from Egan TD, Huizinga B, Gupta SK, et al. Remifentanil pharmacokinetics in obese versus lean patients. *Anesthesiology.* 1998;89:562-573, used with permission.)

(Fig. 9.8).[32,33] Decreases in clearance and central distribution volume also occur in older patients.

With advanced age, although pharmacokinetic changes also play a role, pharmacodynamic differences are primarily responsible for the decreased dose requirement in older patients (>65 years of age). Remifentanil doses should be decreased by at least 50% or more in elderly patients. Similar dosage reductions are also prudent for the other opioids as well.

### Obesity

Body weight is likely an important factor influencing the clinical pharmacology of opioids. Opioid pharmacokinetic variables, especially clearance, are more closely related to lean body mass (LBM) rather than to total body weight (TBW). In practical terms, this means that morbidly obese patients do require a larger dosage than lean patients in order to achieve the same target concentration, but not as much as would be suggested by their TBW.[34]

For example, as illustrated through pharmacokinetic simulation (Fig. 9.9), a TBW-based dosing scheme results in much larger remifentanil effect-site concentrations than a dosing calculation based on LBM.[35] In contrast, TBW and LBM dosing schemes result in similar concentrations for lean patients. These concepts likely apply to other opioids as well.

### Unique Features of Individual Opioids

#### Codeine

Codeine, although not commonly used intraoperatively, has special importance among opioids because of the well-characterized pharmacogenomic nuance associated with it. Codeine is actually a prodrug; morphine is the active compound. Codeine is metabolized (in part) by *O*-demethylation into morphine, a metabolic process mediated by the liver microsomal isoform CYP2D6.[36] Patients who lack CYP2D6 because of deletions, frame shift, or splice mutations (i.e., approximately 10% of the Caucasian population) or whose CYP2D6 is inhibited (e.g., patients taking quinidine) would not be expected to benefit from codeine even though they exhibit a normal response to morphine.[37,38]

#### Morphine

Morphine is the prototype opioid against which all newcomers are compared. There is no evidence that any synthetic opioid is more effective in controlling pain than nature's morphine. Were it not for the histamine release and the resulting hypotension associated with morphine, fentanyl may not have replaced morphine as the most commonly used opioid intraoperatively

Morphine has a slow onset time. Morphine's pKa renders it almost completely ionized at physiologic pH. This property and its low lipid solubility account for morphine's prolonged latency to peak effect; morphine penetrates the CNS slowly. This feature has both advantages and disadvantages associated with it. The prolonged latency to peak effect means that morphine is perhaps less likely to cause acute respiratory depression after bolus injection of typical analgesic doses compared to the more rapid-acting opioids. On the other hand, the slow onset time means that clinicians are perhaps more likely to inappropriately "stack" multiple morphine doses in a patient experiencing severe pain, thus creating the potential for a toxic "overshoot."[39]

Morphine's active metabolite, M6G, has important clinical implications. Although conversion to M6G accounts for only 10% of morphine's metabolism, M6G may contribute to morphine's analgesic effects even in patients with normal renal function, particularly with longer term use. Because of morphine's high hepatic extraction ratio, the bioavailability of orally administered morphine is significantly lower than after parenteral injection. The hepatic first pass effect on orally administered morphine results in high M6G levels. In fact, M6G may be the primary active compound when morphine is administered orally.[40] As noted in the earlier section, "Kidney Failure," M6G's accumulation to potentially toxic levels in dialysis patients is another important implication of this active metabolite.

## Fentanyl

Fentanyl may be the most important opioid used in modern anesthesia practice. As the original fentanyl congener, its clinical application is well entrenched and highly diverse. Fentanyl can be delivered in numerous ways. In addition to the intravenous route, fentanyl can be delivered by transdermal, transmucosal, transnasal, and transpulmonary routes.

Oral transmucosal delivery of fentanyl citrate (OTFC) results in the faster achievement of higher peak levels than when the same dose is swallowed.[41] Avoidance of the first pass effect results in substantially larger bioavailability. That OTFC is noninvasive and rapid in onset has made it a successful therapy for breakthrough pain in opioid-tolerant cancer patients, often in combination with a transdermal fentanyl patch (also see Chapter 40).

## Alfentanil

Alfentanil was the first opioid to be administered almost exclusively by continuous infusion. Because of its relatively short terminal half-life, alfentanil was originally predicted to have a rapid offset of effect after termination of a continuous infusion.[42] Subsequent advances in pharmacokinetic knowledge (i.e., the CSHT) proved this assertion to be false.[8] However, alfentanil is in fact a short-acting drug after a single bolus injection because of its high "diffusible fraction"; it reaches peak effect-site concentrations quickly and then begins to decline (see the previous discussion of "Pharmacokinetics"). Alfentanil illustrates how a drug can exhibit

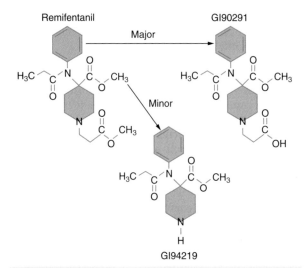

**Fig. 9.10** Remifentanil's metabolic pathway. De-esterification (i.e., ester hydrolysis) by nonspecific plasma and tissue esterases to an inactive acid metabolite (GI90291) accounts for the vast majority of remifentanil's metabolism. (Adapted from Egan TD, Huizinga B, Gupta SK, et al. Remifentanil pharmacokinetics in obese versus lean patients. *Anesthesiology.* 1998;89:562-573, used with permission.)

different pharmacokinetic profiles depending upon the method of administration (i.e., bolus versus continuous infusion). Alfentanil, more than fentanyl or sufentanil, displays unpredictable hepatic metabolism because of the significant interindividual variability of hepatic CYP3A4, the primary enzyme responsible for alfentanil biotransformation.

## Sufentanil

Sufentanil's distinguishing feature is that it is the most potent opioid commonly used in anesthesia practice. Because it is more intrinsically efficacious at the opioid receptor, the absolute doses used are much smaller compared to the other less potent drugs (e.g., 1000-fold less than morphine doses).

## Remifentanil

Remifentanil is a prototype example of how specific clinical goals can be achieved by designing molecules with specialized structure-activity (or structure-metabolism) relationships. By losing its μ-receptor agonist activity upon ester hydrolysis, a very short-acting opioid results (Fig. 9.10).[43] The perceived unmet need driving remifentanil's development was having an opioid with a rapid onset and offset so that the drug could be titrated up and down as necessary to meet the dynamic needs of the patient during the rapidly changing conditions of anesthesia and surgery.

Compared to the currently marketed fentanyl congeners, remifentanil's CSHT is short, on the order of about

5 minutes.[44] Pharmacodynamically, remifentanil exhibits a short latency to peak effect similar to alfentanil and a potency slightly less than fentanyl.[45]

Remifentanil's role in modern anesthesia practice is now relatively well established. Remifentanil is perhaps best suited for cases in which its responsive pharmacokinetic profile can be exploited to advantage (e.g., when rapid recovery is desirable; when the anesthetic requirement rapidly fluctuates; when opioid titration is unpredictable or difficult or when there is a substantial danger to opioid overdose; or when a "large dose" opioid technique is advantageous but the patient is not going to be mechanically ventilated postoperatively).[46] Remifentanil's most common clinical application is the provision of TIVA in combination with propofol. It is also commonly administered by an intravenous bolus when only a very brief pulse of opioid effect followed by rapid recovery is desired (e.g., in preparation for local anesthetic injection during monitored anesthesia care) (see Chapter 37).

## Opioid Agonist-Antagonists and Pure Antagonists

Opioid agonist-antagonists act as partial agonists at the μ-receptor, while having competitive antagonist properties at the same receptors. These drugs serve as analgesics with more limited ventilatory depression and a lesser potential for dependence as they demonstrate a "ceiling effect," producing less analgesia compared to pure agonists. The lower abuse potential was the primary perceived unmet need underlying the development of these drugs. Drugs in this category are used for the treatment of chronic pain, as well as the treatment of opioid addiction (also see Chapter 40). These drugs cause some degree of competitive antagonism when administered in the presence of ongoing full agonist activity (e.g., when administered after morphine and other pure agonists).

Pure opioid antagonists, of which naloxone is the prototype, are complete competitive antagonists of the opioid receptor that are devoid of any agonist activity. These pure antagonists are used in the management of acute opioid overdose and chronic abuse.

### Tramadol

Tramadol is a centrally acting analgesic with moderate μ-receptor affinity and weak κ- and δ-receptor affinity. Notably, tramadol also has antagonist activity at the 5-hydroxytryptamine (5-HT) and nicotinic acetylcholine (NA) receptors. While providing analgesia through both opioid and serotonin receptor pathways, tramadol carries less risk of respiratory depression. However, when combined with serotonin reuptake inhibitors or other serotonergic medications, it carries the risk of serotonin syndrome and also of CNS excitability and seizures.[47]

### Buprenorphine

Buprenorphine is an opioid agonist-antagonist with a high affinity for the μ-receptor. It can be administered sublingually, transdermally, or parenterally but undergoes extensive first pass hepatic metabolism with oral administration. Although moderate doses can be used to treat chronic pain, higher doses used in the treatment of chronic pain can antagonize the effects of other opioids, making the treatment of acute on chronic pain difficult. Because it binds opioid receptors with such high affinity and its elimination half-life is in the range of 20 to 72 hours, large-dose opioid full agonists are required to overcome its effects.[48]

### Nalbuphine

Also an opioid agonist-antagonist, nalbuphine has a potency and duration of action similar to morphine. It can be used as a sole drug for sedation with minimal respiratory depression, as well as a drug to reverse ventilatory depression in opioid overdose while maintaining some analgesia.[49]

### Naloxone/Naltrexone

Naloxone is an injectable μ-antagonist that reverses both the therapeutic and adverse effects of μ-agonists.[50] Naloxone's most common indication is the emergency reversal of opioid-induced ventilatory depression after acute overdose. Its important role in this regard has merited naloxone's inclusion on the World Health Organization's "List of Essential Medicines." Naloxone is sometimes used in much smaller doses during emergence from anesthesia to restore adequate ventilatory effort and thereby expedite extubation of the trachea. The treatment of opioid-induced pruritus (requiring only small doses) is another common therapeutic application.

Although naloxone is very effective in reversing the ventilatory depression associated with opioids, it has numerous untoward effects, including acute withdrawal syndrome, nausea, vomiting, tachycardia, hypertension, seizures, and pulmonary edema, among others.[51] Recognizing that naloxone's duration of action is shorter than that of most of the μ-agonists is a key point in determining the dosing schedule; repeated doses may be necessary to sustain its effects.

In response to the opioid abuse epidemic in the United States, new delivery systems have been developed that are intended for emergency use by laypersons in the event of opioid overdose; these include nasal spray and auto-injector preparations.[52,53]

Naltrexone, a longer acting opioid μ-antagonist available in oral, injectable, and implantable forms, is used in the long-term management of opioid addicts in combination with other nonpharmacologic therapies.[54]

## CLINICAL APPLICATION

Opioids play a vital role in virtually every area of anesthesia practice. In the treatment of postoperative pain (also see Chapter 40), opioids are of prime importance, whereas in most other settings in perioperative medicine opioids are therapeutic adjuncts used in combination with other drugs.

### Common Clinical Indications

Postoperative analgesia is the longest standing indication for opioid therapy in anesthesia practice. In the modern era, opioid administration via PCA devices is perhaps the most common mode of delivery (also see Chapter 40). In recent years, opioids are increasingly combined postoperatively with various other analgesics, such as nonsteroidal antiinflammatory drugs (NSAIDs), to increase efficacy and safety.

Internationally, the most common clinical indication for opioids in anesthesia practice is their use for what has come to be known as *balanced anesthesia*. This perhaps misguided term connotes the use of multiple drugs (e.g., volatile anesthetics, neuromuscular blockers, sedative-hypnotics, and opioids) in smaller doses to produce the state of anesthesia. With this technique, the opioids are primarily used for their ability to decrease MAC. A basic assumption underlying this balanced anesthesia approach is that the drugs used in combination mitigate the disadvantages of the individual drugs (i.e., the volatile anesthetics) used in larger doses as single drug therapy.

"Large-dose opioid anesthesia," a technique originally described for morphine in the early days of open heart surgery[55] and later associated with the fentanyl congeners,[56] is another common application of opioids in clinical anesthesia. The original scientific underpinning of this approach was that large doses of opioids enabled the clinician to reduce the concentration of volatile anesthetic to a minimum, thereby avoiding the direct myocardial depression and other untoward hemodynamic effects in patients whose cardiovascular systems were already compromised. In addition, fentanyl often produces a relative bradycardia that could be helpful in patients with myocardial ischemia. Although the general concept is still applied, currently the opioid doses used are smaller. Opioids are also administered for their possible beneficial effects in terms of cardioprotection (i.e., preconditioning).

TIVA is a more recently developed and increasingly popular indication for opioids in anesthesia practice. This technique relies entirely upon intravenous drugs for the provision of general anesthesia. Most commonly, continuous infusions of remifentanil or alfentanil are combined with a propofol infusion. Both the opioid and the sedative are often delivered by target-controlled infusion (TCI) enabled pumps. A clear advantage of this technique, perhaps among others, is the enhanced patient well-being in the early postoperative period, including less nausea and vomiting and often a feeling of euphoria.[57]

### Rational Drug Selection and Administration

In articulating a scientific foundation for rational opioid selection, pharmacokinetic considerations are extremely important. Indeed, the μ-agonists (opioids) can be considered pharmacodynamic equals with important pharmacokinetic differences.[58] Thus, rational selection of one opioid μ-agonist over another requires the clinician to identify the desired temporal profile of drug effect and then choose an opioid that best enables the clinician to achieve it (within obvious constraints such as pharmacoeconomic concerns).

In selecting the appropriate opioid, among the key questions to address are How quickly must the desired opioid effect be achieved? How long must the opioid effect be maintained? How critical is it that the opioid-induced ventilatory depression or sedation dissipate quickly (e.g., will the patient be mechanically ventilated postoperatively)? Is the capability to increase and decrease the level of opioid effect quickly during the anesthetic critical? Will there be significant pain postoperatively that will require opioid treatment? All of these questions relate to the optimal temporal profile of opioid effect. The answers to these questions are addressed through the application of pharmacokinetic concepts.

For example, when a brief pulse of opioid effect followed by rapid recovery is desired (e.g., to provide analgesia for a retrobulbar block), a bolus of remifentanil or alfentanil might be preferred. When long-lasting opioid effect is desired, such as when there will be significant postoperative pain or when the trachea will remain intubated, a fentanyl infusion is a prudent choice. If the patient should be awake and alert shortly after the procedure is finished (e.g., a craniotomy in which the surgeons hope to perform a neurologic examination in the operating room immediately postoperatively), a remifentanil infusion might be advantageous.

The formulation of a rational administration strategy also requires the proper application of pharmacokinetic principles. An important goal of any dosing scheme is to reach and maintain a steady-state level of opioid effect. Nowadays, in order to achieve a steady-state concentration in the site of action, opioids are frequently administered by continuous infusion. This is increasingly accomplished through the use of TCI technology, which requires that the clinician be familiar with the appropriate pharmacokinetic model for the opioid of interest. When these systems are not available, the clinician must remember that infusions must be preceded by a bolus in order to come to a near steady-state in a timely fashion.

## EMERGING DEVELOPMENTS

### Opioids and Cancer Recurrence

The influence of opioid therapy on cancer recurrence is controversial. As the immunosuppressive effects of opioids (particularly morphine) and their impact on angiogenesis have been demonstrated in animal and in vitro studies, concern over the influence of these drugs on cancer recurrence and survival has emerged. Some early retrospective data comparing cancer recurrence rates in patients receiving standard postoperative opioid analgesia with those receiving alternative techniques (e.g., epidural pain management) suggested a more frequent rate of cancer recurrence in the opioid therapy group; other studies found conflicting results. A retrospective review of more than 34,000 breast cancer patients from 1996 to 2008 demonstrated no association between opioid therapy and cancer recurrence.[59] Similarly, a retrospective review of 819 hepatocellular carcinoma patients who received either postoperative intravenous fentanyl or postoperative epidural with morphine found no effect on recurrence-free survival.[60]

However, other studies have suggested some improved outcomes with opioid-sparing techniques. A review of 984 non–small cell lung cancer patients from 2006 to 2011 found improved survival and longer disease-free survival in opioid-sparing pain management strategies.[61] Thus, the role of perioperative opioid therapy in cancer recurrence remains controversial; ongoing trials will further refine anesthesia-related clinical decision making in the treatment of oncologic patients.

### Opioid Abuse Epidemic

Deaths related to the abuse and diversion of prescription opioids have skyrocketed in the United States and elsewhere (also see Chapter 44).[62] In addition to fatalities, this pervasive pattern of prescription and illicit opioid abuse has resulted in a huge surge in admissions to opioid abuse treatment facilities.[63] The trend may be due at least in part to opioid prescribing practices for chronic pain conditions that may predispose some patients to addiction.[64,65]

The epidemic has reached such a crisis level that federal and state government authorities in the USA have enacted legislation and set aside funding to support research, prevention, and treatment of the problem.[66,67] State-approved pharmacy-based naloxone dispensing (without a physician's prescription) for patients filling opioid prescriptions is a notable example of the efforts supported by such legislation.[68] In addition, professional societies and the Centers for Disease Control and Prevention (CDC) have produced new guidelines for opioid prescribing.[69] This is currently an area of intense public discussion and medical investigation.

## QUESTIONS OF THE DAY

1. A patient requires postoperative patient-controlled analgesia (PCA). From a pharmacokinetic perspective, what are the relative advantages of fentanyl compared to morphine for use in PCA?
2. What pharmacokinetic parameter is most suitable for describing the offset time of a continuous opioid infusion?
3. What are the effects of opioids on minute ventilation and ventilatory response to carbon dioxide?
4. How does renal failure affect the pharmacokinetics of morphine and meperidine?
5. A patient with postoperative respiratory depression from morphine is given intravenous naloxone. What are the potential side effects of naloxone?
6. What key questions should be addressed when selecting an opioid for intraoperative use?

## REFERENCES

1. Minami M, Satoh M. Molecular biology of the opioid receptors: structures, functions and distributions. *Neurosci Res.* 1995;23:121–145.
2. Pan L, Xu J, Yu R, et al. Identification and characterization of six new alternatively spliced variants of the human mu opioid receptor gene. *Oprm. Neuroscience.* 2005;133:209–220.
3. Matthies BK, Franklin KB. Formalin pain is expressed in decerebrate rats but not attenuated by morphine. *Pain.* 1992;51:199–206.
4. Becerra L, Harter K, Gonzalez RG, Borsook D. Functional magnetic resonance imaging measures of the effects of morphine on central nervous system circuitry in opioid-naive healthy volunteers. *Anesth Analg.* 2006;103:208–216.
5. Matthes HW, Maldonado R, Simonin F, et al. Loss of morphine-induced analgesia, reward effect and withdrawal symptoms in mice lacking the mu-opioid-receptor gene. *Nature.* 1996;383:819–823.
6. Sora I, Takahashi N, Funada M, et al. Opiate receptor knockout mice define mu receptor roles in endogenous nociceptive responses and morphine-induced analgesia. *Proc Natl Acad Sci U S A.* 1997;94:1544–1549.
7. Dahan A, Sarton E, Teppema L, et al. Anesthetic potency and influence of morphine and sevoflurane on respiration in mu-opioid receptor knockout mice. *Anesthesiology.* 2001;94:824–832.
8. Shafer SL, Varvel JR. Pharmacokinetics, pharmacodynamics, and rational opioid selection. *Anesthesiology.* 1991;74:53–63.
9. Lotsch J, Skarke C, Schmidt H, et al. Pharmacokinetic modeling to predict morphine and morphine-6-glucuronide plasma concentrations in healthy young volunteers. *Clin Pharmacol Ther.* 2002;72:151–162.

10. Lotsch J, Skarke C, Schmidt H, et al. The transfer half-life of morphine-6-glucuronide from plasma to effect site assessed by pupil size measurement in healthy volunteers. *Anesthesiology.* 2001;95:1329–1338.

11. Gepts E, Shafer SL, Camu F, et al. Linearity of pharmacokinetics and model estimation of sufentanil. *Anesthesiology.* 1995;83:1194–1204.

12. Scott JC, Cooke JE, Stanski DR. Electroencephalographic quantitation of opioid effect: comparative pharmacodynamics of fentanyl and sufentanil. *Anesthesiology.* 1991;74:34–42.

13. Hughes MA, Glass PS, Jacobs JR. Context-sensitive half-time in multicompartment pharmacokinetic models for intravenous anesthetic drugs [see comments]. *Anesthesiology.* 1992;76:334–341.

14. Romberg R, Sarton E, Teppema L, et al. Comparison of morphine-6-glucuronide and morphine on respiratory depressant and antinociceptive responses in wild type and mu-opioid receptor deficient mice. *Br J Anaesth.* 2003;91:862–870.

15. Gross JB. When you breathe IN you inspire, when you DON'T breathe, you... expire: new insights regarding opioid-induced ventilatory depression. *Anesthesiology.* 2003;99:767–770.

16. Forrest Jr WH, Bellville JW. The effect of sleep plus morphine on the respiratory response to carbon dioxide. *Anesthesiology.* 1964;25:137–141.

17. Laubie M, Schmitt H, Vincent M. Vagal bradycardia produced by microinjections of morphine-like drugs into the nucleus ambiguus in anaesthetized dogs. *Eur J Pharmacol.* 1979;59:287–291.

18. Reitan JA, Stengert KB, Wymore ML, Martucci RW. Central vagal control of fentanyl-induced bradycardia during halothane anesthesia. *Anesth Analg.* 1978;57:31–36.

19. Bennett JA, Abrams JT, Van Riper DF, Horrow JC. Difficult or impossible ventilation after sufentanil-induced anesthesia is caused primarily by vocal cord closure. *Anesthesiology.* 1997;87:1070–1074.

20. Streisand JB, Bailey PL, LeMaire L, et al. Fentanyl-induced rigidity and unconsciousness in human volunteers. Incidence, duration, and plasma concentrations. *Anesthesiology.* 1993;78:629–634.

21. Dray A, Metsch R. Inhibition of urinary bladder contractions by a spinal action of morphine and other opioids. *J Pharmacol Exp Ther.* 1984;231:254–260.

22. Dray A, Metsch R. Spinal opioid receptors and inhibition of urinary bladder motility in vivo. *Neurosci Lett.* 1984;47:81–84.

23. Borner C, Warnick B, Smida M, et al. Mechanisms of opioid-mediated inhibition of human T cell receptor signaling. *J Immunol.* 2009;183:882–889.

24. Bouillon T, Bruhn J, Radu-Radulescu L, et al. Non-steady state analysis of the pharmacokinetic interaction between propofol and remifentanil. *Anesthesiology.* 2002;97:1350–1362.

25. McEwan AI, Smith C, Dyar O, et al. Isoflurane minimum alveolar concentration reduction by fentanyl. *Anesthesiology.* 1993;78:864–869.

26. Vuyk J, Lim T, Engbers FH, et al. The pharmacodynamic interaction of propofol and alfentanil during lower abdominal surgery in women. *Anesthesiology.* 1995;83:8–22.

27. Rudin A, Lundberg JF, Hammarlund-Udenaes M, et al. Morphine metabolism after major liver surgery. *Anesth Analg.* 2007;104:1409–1414.

28. Dershwitz M, Hoke JF, Rosow CE, et al. Pharmacokinetics and pharmacodynamics of remifentanil in volunteer subjects with severe liver disease. *Anesthesiology.* 1996;84:812–820.

29. Hoke JF, Shlugman D, Dershwitz M, et al. Pharmacokinetics and pharmacodynamics of remifentanil in persons with renal failure compared with healthy volunteers. *Anesthesiology.* 1997;87:533–541.

30. Osborne R, Joel S, Grebenik K, et al. The pharmacokinetics of morphine and morphine glucuronides in kidney failure. *Clin Pharmacol Ther.* 1993;54:158–167.

31. Sarton E, Olofsen E, Romberg R, et al. Sex differences in morphine analgesia: an experimental study in healthy volunteers. *Anesthesiology.* 2000;93:1245–1254; discussion 6A.

32. Minto CF, Schnider TW, Egan TD, et al. Influence of age and gender on the pharmacokinetics and pharmacodynamics of remifentanil. I. Model development. *Anesthesiology.* 1997;86:10–23.

33. Scott JC, Stanski DR. Decreased fentanyl and alfentanil dose requirements with age. A simultaneous pharmacokinetic and pharmacodynamic evaluation. *J Pharmacol Exp Ther.* 1987;240:159–166.

34. Bouillon T, Shafer SL. Does size matter? *Anesthesiology.* 1998;89:557–560.

35. Egan TD, Huizinga B, Gupta SK, et al. Remifentanil pharmacokinetics in obese versus lean patients. *Anesthesiology.* 1998;89:562–573.

36. Poulsen L, Brosen K, Arendt-Nielsen L, et al. Codeine and morphine in extensive and poor metabolizers of sparteine: pharmacokinetics, analgesic effect and side effects. *Eur J Clin Pharmacol.* 1996;51:289–295.

37. Caraco Y, Sheller J, Wood AJ. Pharmacogenetic determination of the effects of codeine and prediction of drug interactions. *J Pharmacol Exp Ther.* 1996;278:1165–1174.

38. Eckhardt K, Li S, Ammon S, et al. Same incidence of adverse drug events after codeine administration irrespective of the genetically determined differences in morphine formation. *Pain.* 1998;76:27–33.

39. Lotsch J, Dudziak R, Freynhagen R, et al. Fatal respiratory depression after multiple intravenous morphine injections. *Clin Pharmacokinet.* 2006;45:1051–1060.

40. Osborne R, Joel S, Trew D, Slevin M. Morphine and metabolite behavior after different routes of morphine administration: demonstration of the importance of the active metabolite morphine-6-glucuronide. *Clin Pharmacol Ther.* 1990;47:12–19.

41. Streisand JB, Varvel JR, Stanski DR, et al. Absorption and bioavailability of oral transmucosal fentanyl citrate. *Anesthesiology.* 1991;75:223–229.

42. Stanski DR, Hug Jr CC. Alfentanil—a kinetically predictable narcotic analgesic. *Anesthesiology.* 1982;57:435–438.

43. Egan TD. Remifentanil pharmacokinetics and pharmacodynamics. A preliminary appraisal. *Clin Pharmacokinet.* 1995;29:80–94.

44. Egan TD, Lemmens HJ, Fiset P, et al. The pharmacokinetics of the new short-acting opioid remifentanil (GI87084B) in healthy adult male volunteers. *Anesthesiology.* 1993;79:881–892.

45. Egan TD, Minto CF, Hermann DJ, et al. Remifentanil versus alfentanil: comparative pharmacokinetics and pharmacodynamics in healthy adult male volunteers [published erratum appears in Anesthesiology. 1996;85(3):695], Anesthesiology. 1996;84:821–833.

46. Egan TD. The clinical pharmacology of remifentanil: a brief review. *J Anesth.* 1998;12:195–204.

47. Grond S, Sablotzki A. Clinical pharmacology of tramadol. *Clin Pharmacokinet.* 2004;43:879–923.

48. Chen KY, Chen L, Mao J. Buprenorphine-naloxone therapy in pain management. *Anesthesiology.* 2014;120:1262–1274.

49. Errick JK, Heel RC. Nalbuphine. A preliminary review of its pharmacological properties and therapeutic efficacy. *Drugs.* 1983;26:191–211.

50. Jasinski DR, Martin WR, Haertzen CA. The human pharmacology and abuse potential of N-allylnoroxymorphone (naloxone). *J Pharmacol Exp Ther.* 1967;157:420–426.

51. Jasinski DR, Martin WR, Sapira JD. Antagonism of the subjective, behavioral, pupillary, and respiratory depressant effects of cyclazocine by naloxone. *Clin Pharmacol Ther.* 1968;9:215–222.

52. Edwards ET, Edwards ES, Davis E, et al. Comparative usability study of a novel auto-injector and an intranasal system for naloxone delivery. *Pain Ther.* 2015;4:89–105.

53. Krieter P, Chiang N, Gyaw S, et al. Pharmacokinetic properties and human use characteristics of an FDA approved intranasal naloxone product for the treatment of opioid overdose. *J Clin Pharmacol.* 2016;56(10):1243–1253.

54. Kunoe N, Lobmaier P, Ngo H, Hulse G. Injectable and implantable sustained release naltrexone in the treatment of opioid addiction. *Br J Clin Pharmacol.* 2014;77:264–271.

55. Lowenstein E, Hallowell P, Levine FH, et al. Cardiovascular response to large doses of intravenous morphine in man. *N Engl J Med.* 1969;281:1389–1393.

56. Lunn JK, Stanley TH, Eisele J, et al. High dose fentanyl anesthesia for coronary artery surgery: plasma fentanyl concentrations and influence of nitrous oxide on cardiovascular responses. *Anesth Analg.* 1979;58:390–395.

57. Hofer CK, Zollinger A, Buchi S, et al. Patient well-being after general anaesthesia: a prospective, randomized, controlled multi-centre trial comparing intravenous and inhalation anaesthesia. *Br J Anaesth.* 2003;91:631–637.

58. Mather LE. Pharmacokinetic and pharmacodynamic profiles of opioid analgesics: a sameness amongst equals? *Pain.* 1990;43:3–6.

59. Cronin-Fenton DP, Heide-Jorgensen U, Ahern TP, et al. Opioids and breast cancer recurrence: a Danish population-based cohort study. *Cancer.* 2015;121:3507–3514.

60. Cao L, Chang Y, Lin W, et al. Long-term survival after resection of hepatocellular carcinoma: a potential risk associated with the choice of postoperative analgesia. *Anesth Analg.* 2014;118:1309–1316.

61. Wang K, Qu X, Wang Y, et al. Effect of mu agonists on long-term survival and recurrence in nonsmall cell lung cancer patients. *Medicine (Baltimore).* 2015;94(33):e1333.

62. Rudd RA, Aleshire N, Zibbell JE, Gladden RM. Increases in drug and opioid overdose deaths—United States, 2000-2014. *MMWR Morb Mortal Wkly Rep.* 2016;64:1378–1382.

63. Brady KT, McCauley JL, Back SE. Prescription opioid misuse, abuse, and treatment in the United States: an update. *Am J Psychiatry.* 2016;173:18–26.

64. Johnson SR. The opioid abuse epidemic: how healthcare helped create a crisis. *Mod Healthcare.* 2016;46(7):8–9.

65. Weisberg DF, Becker WC, Fiellin DA, Stannard C. Prescription opioid misuse in the United States and the United Kingdom: cautionary lessons. *Int J Drug Policy.* 2014;25:1124–1130.

66. Kharasch ED, Brunt LM. Perioperative opioids and public health. *Anesthesiology.* 2016;124:960–965.

67. Office of the Press Secretary. The White House. President Obama proposes $1.1 billion in new funding to address the prescription opioid abuse and heroin use epidemic. *J Pain Palliat Care Pharmacother.* 2016;30(2):134–137.

68. Bachyrycz A, Shrestha S, Bleske BE, et al. Opioid overdose prevention through pharmacy-based naloxone prescription program: innovations in healthcare delivery. *Subst Abus. Epub.* 2016 May 10.

69. Frieden TR, Houry D. Reducing the risks of relief—the CDC Opioid-Prescribing Guideline. *N Engl J Med.* 2016;374:1501–1504.

# 10 LOCAL ANESTHETICS

## Charles B. Berde, Anjali Koka, and Kenneth Drasner

Local anesthesia can be defined as loss of sensation in a discrete region of the body caused by disruption of impulse generation or propagation. Local anesthesia can be produced by various chemical and physical means. However, in routine clinical practice, local anesthesia is produced by several compounds whose mechanism of action is similar, although they have different durations of action, and from which recovery is normally spontaneous, predictable, and complete.

## HISTORY

Clinical use of local anesthetics began with cocaine in the 1880s.[1] The topically applied local anesthetic benzocaine and the injectable drugs procaine, tetracaine, and chloroprocaine were subsequently developed as adaptations of cocaine's structure as an amino ester (Figs. 10.1 and 10.2).

In 1948, lidocaine was introduced as the first member of a new class of local anesthetics, the amino amides. Advantages of the amino amides over the earlier amino esters included more stability and a reduced frequency of allergic reactions. Because of these favorable properties, lidocaine became the template for the development of a series of amino-amide anesthetics (see Fig. 10.2).

Along with lidocaine, most amino-amide local anesthetics are derived from the aromatic amine xylidine, including mepivacaine, bupivacaine, ropivacaine, and levobupivacaine. Ropivacaine and levobupivacaine share an additional distinctive characteristic: they are single enantiomers rather than racemic mixtures. They are products of a developmental strategy that takes advantage of the differential stereoselectivity of neuronal and cardiac sodium ion channels in an effort to reduce the potential for cardiac toxicity (see "Adverse Effects"). Almost all of the amides undergo biotransformation in the liver, whereas the esters undergo hydrolysis in plasma.

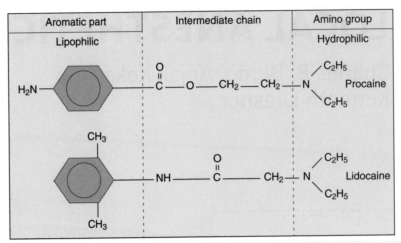

**Fig. 10.1** Local anesthetics have three portions: (1) lipophilic, (2) hydrophilic, and a connecting (3) hydrocarbon chain. This figure illustrates creative ways of altering this basic structure for desired pharmacologic characteristics (duration of action, cardiovascular).

## NERVE CONDUCTION

Under normal or resting circumstances, the neural membrane is characterized by a negative potential of roughly −90 mV (the potential inside the nerve fiber is negative relative to the extracellular fluid). This negative potential is created by energy-dependent outward transport of sodium and inward transport of potassium ions, combined with greater membrane permeability to potassium ions relative to sodium ions. With excitation of the nerve, there is an increase in the membrane permeability to sodium ions, causing a decrease in the transmembrane potential. If a critical potential is reached (i.e., threshold potential), there is a rapid and self-sustaining influx of sodium ions resulting in a propagating wave of depolarization, the action potential, after which the resting membrane potential is reestablished.

Nerve fibers can be classified according to fiber diameter, presence (type A and B) or absence (type C) of myelin, and function (Table 10.1). The nerve fiber diameter influences conduction velocity; a larger diameter correlates with more rapid nerve conduction. The presence of myelin also increases conduction velocity. This effect results from insulation of the axolemma from the surrounding media, forcing current to flow through periodic interruptions in the myelin sheath (i.e., nodes of Ranvier) (Fig. 10.3).

## LOCAL ANESTHETIC ACTIONS ON SODIUM CHANNELS

Local anesthetics act on a wide range of molecular targets, but they exert their predominant desired clinical effects by blocking sodium ion flux through voltage-gated sodium channels. Voltage-gated sodium channels are complex transmembrane proteins comprising large alpha subunits and much smaller beta subunits[2] (Fig. 10.4).

The alpha subunits have four homologous domains arranged in a square, each composed of six transmembrane helices, and the pore lies in the center of these four domains. Beta subunits modulate electrophysiologic properties of the channel and they also have prominent roles in channel localization, binding to adhesion molecules, and connection to intracellular cytoskeletons. There are nine major subtypes of sodium channel alpha subunits in mammalian tissues and four major subtypes of beta subunits.

Different sodium channel subtypes are expressed in different tissues, at diverse developmental stages, and in a range of disease states. Sodium channel subtypes are an active area of investigation around human diseases with spontaneous pain and pain insensitivity, as targets of new analgesics, and in other areas of medicine, including cardiology and neurology.[2,3] Sodium channel subtypes will be discussed briefly again later in this chapter (see "When Local Anesthesia Fails" and "Future Local Anesthetics").

From an electrophysiologic standpoint, local anesthetics block conduction of impulses by decreasing the rate of depolarization in response to excitation, preventing achievement of the threshold potential. They do not alter the resting transmembrane potential, and they have little effect on the threshold potential.

Sodium channels cycle between resting, open, and inactive conformations. During excitation, the sodium channel moves from a resting closed state to an open activated state, with an increase in the inward flux of sodium ions and consequent depolarization. The channel transitions to an inactive state and must undergo further

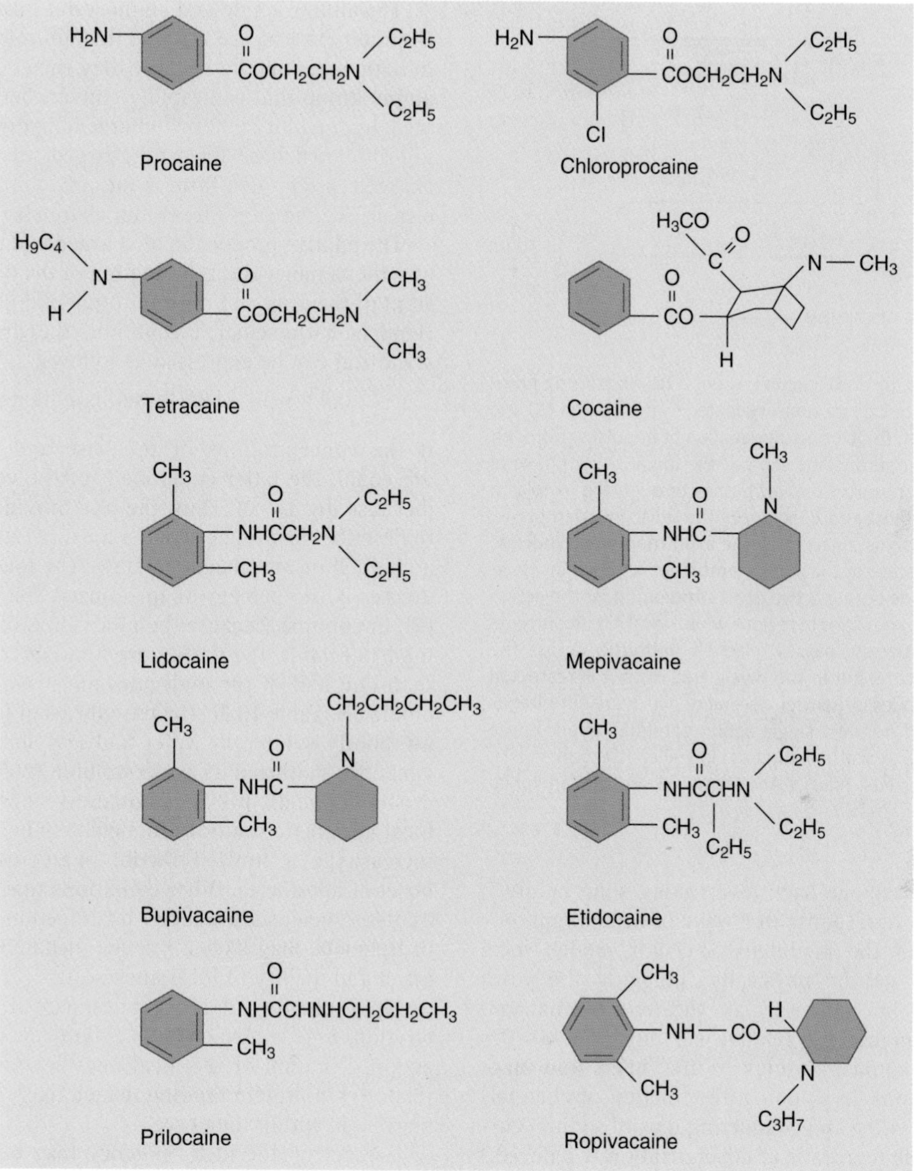

**Fig. 10.2** Chemical structures of ester (i.e., procaine, chloroprocaine, tetracaine, and cocaine) and amide (i.e., lidocaine, mepivacaine, bupivacaine, etidocaine, prilocaine, and ropivacaine) local anesthetics.

**Table 10.1** Classification of Nerve Fibers

| Type | Fiber Subtype | Diameter (μm) | Conduction Velocity (m/sec) | Function |
|------|---------------|---------------|------------------------------|----------|
| A (myelinated) | Alpha | 12-20 | 80-120 | Proprioception, large motor |
| | Beta | 5-15 | 35-80 | Small motor, touch, pressure |
| | Gamma | 3-8 | 10-35 | Muscle tone |
| | Delta | 2-5 | 5-25 | Pain, temperature, touch |
| B (myelinated) | | 3 | 5-15 | Preganglionic autonomic |
| C (unmyelinated) | | 0.3-1.5 | 0.5-2.5 | Dull pain, temperature, touch |

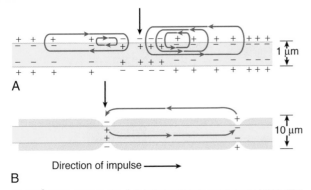

A

B

Direction of impulse ⟶

**Fig. 10.3** Pattern of "local circuit currents" flowing during propagation of an impulse in a nonmyelinated C fiber's axon (A) and a myelinated axon (B). During propagation of impulses, from left to right, current entering the axon at the initial rising phase of the impulse *(large vertical arrows)* passes through the axoplasm (local circuit current) and depolarizes the adjacent membrane. Plus and minus signs adjacent to the axon membrane indicate the polarization state of the axon membrane: negative inside at rest, positive inside during active depolarization under the action potential, and less negative in regions where local circuit currents flow. This ionic current passes relatively uniformly across the nonmyelinated axon, but in the myelinated axon it is restricted to entry at the nodes of Ranvier, several of which are simultaneously depolarized during a single action potential. (From Berde CB, Strichartz GR. Local anesthetics. In Miller RD, Cohen NH, Eriksson LI, et al, eds. *Miller's Anesthesia.* 8th ed. Philadelphia: Saunders Elsevier; 2015.)

conformational change back to a resting state before it can again open in response to a wave of depolarization.

According to the modulated receptor model, local anesthetics act not by physically "plugging the pore" of the channel but rather by an allosteric mechanism; that is, by changing the relative stability and kinetics of cycling of channels through resting, open, and inactive conformations. In so doing, the fraction of channels accessible to opening and conducting inward sodium currents in response to a wave of depolarization is reduced.[4] This mechanism provides nerve blocks that are either a "use-dependent" or "frequency-dependent" type of block; that is, the block intensifies with more frequent rates of nerve firing.

## pH, Net Charge, and Lipid Solubility

The predominant binding site for local anesthetics on sodium channels is near the cytoplasmic side of the plasma membrane. A major structural requirement for a molecule to be an effective local anesthetic is sufficient solubility and rapid diffusion in both hydrophilic environments (extracellular fluid, cytosol, and the head-group region of membrane phospholipids) and in the hydrophobic environment of the lipid bilayers in plasma membranes.

The amino-amide and amino-ester local anesthetics in common clinical use achieve this aim of good solubility in both water and fat because they each contain a tertiary amine group that can rapidly convert between a protonated hydrochloride form (charged, hydrophilic) and an unprotonated base form (uncharged, hydrophobic). The charged, protonated form is the predominant active species at binding sites on sodium channels (Fig. 10.5).[5]

The relative proportion of charged and uncharged local anesthetic molecules is a function of the dissociation constant of the drug and the environmental pH. Recalling the Henderson-Hasselbalch equation, the dissociation constant ($Ka$) can be expressed as follows:

$$pKa = pH - \log ([base]/[conjugate\ acid])$$

If the concentrations of the base and conjugate acid are equal, the latter component of the equation cancels (because log 1 = 0). Thus, the pKa provides a useful way to describe the propensity of a local anesthetic to exist in a charged or an uncharged state. The lower the pKa, the greater is the percent of un-ionized fraction at a given pH. In contrast, because the pKa values of the commonly used injectable anesthetics are between 7.6 and 8.9, less than one half of the molecules are un-ionized at physiologic pH (Table 10.2). The base forms of local anesthetics are poorly soluble in water and less stable, so they are generally marketed as water-soluble hydrochloride salts at slightly acidic pH. Bicarbonate is sometimes added to local anesthetic solutions immediately before injection to increase the un-ionized fraction in an effort to hasten the onset of anesthesia. Other conditions that lower pH, such as tissue acidosis produced by infection, inflammation, or ischemia, may likewise have a negative impact on the onset and quality of local anesthesia.

Lipid solubility of a local anesthetic affects tissue penetration, time course of uptake, potency, and duration of action. Duration of the local anesthetic action also correlates with protein binding, which likely serves to retain anesthetic within the nerve.

Degrees of anesthetic potency may be altered by the in vitro or in vivo system in which these effects are determined. For example, tetracaine is approximately 20 times more potent than bupivacaine when assessed in isolated nerve, but these drugs are nearly equipotent when assessed in vivo. Even when assessed in vivo, comparisons among local anesthetics may vary based on the specific site of application (spinal versus peripheral block) because of secondary effects such as the inherent vasoactive properties of the anesthetic.

## DIFFERENTIAL LOCAL ANESTHETIC BLOCKADE

From a clinical viewpoint and from electrophysiologic measurements, local anesthesia is not an all-or-none

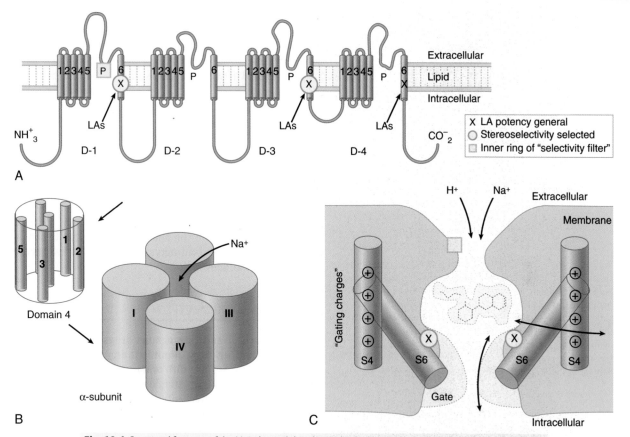

**Fig. 10.4** Structural features of the Na⁺ channel that determine local anesthetic (LA) interactions. (A) Consensus arrangement of the single peptide of the Na⁺ channel α-subunit in a plasma membrane. Four domains with homologous sequences (D-1 through D-4) each contain six α-helical segments that span the membrane (S1 to S6). Each domain folds within itself to form one cylindrical bundle of segments, and these bundles converge to form the functional channel's quaternary structure (B). Activation gating leading to channel opening results from primary movement of the positively charged S4 segments in response to membrane depolarization (see panel C). Fast inactivation of the channel follows binding to the cytoplasmic end of the channel of part of the small loop that connects D-3 to D-4. Ions travel through an open channel along a pore defined at its narrowest dimension by the P region formed by partial membrane penetration of the four extracellular loops of protein connecting S5 and S6 in each domain. Intentional, directed mutations of different amino acids on the channel indicate residues that are involved in LA binding in the inner vestibule of the channel (X on S6 segments), at the interior regions of the ion-discriminating "selectivity filter (square on the P region), and also are known to influence stereoselectivity for phasic inhibition (circle, also on S6 segments). (C) Schematic cross section of the channel speculating on the manner in which S6 segments, forming a "gate," may realign during activation to open the channel and allow entry and departure of a bupivacaine molecule by the "hydrophilic" pathway. The closed (inactivated) channel has a more intimate association with the LA molecule, whose favored pathway for dissociation is no longer between S6 segments (the former pore) but now, much more slowly, laterally between segments and then through the membrane, the "hydrophobic" pathway. Na⁺ ions entering the pore will compete with the LA for a site in the channel, and H⁺ ions, which pass very slowly through the pore, can enter and leave from the extracellular opening, thereby protonating and deprotonating a bound LA molecule and thus regulating its rate of dissociation from the channel. (From Berde CB, Strichartz GR. Local anesthetics. In Miller RD, Cohen NH, Eriksson LI, et al, eds. *Miller's Anesthesia*. 8th ed. Philadelphia: Saunders Elsevier; 2015.)

phenomenon: patients experience gradations in the intensity of sensory and motor blockade that vary over time following local anesthetic injections. Clinically apparent "numbness" generally correlates with intraneural concentrations of local anesthetics but also reflects complex integration and processing of inputs in the spinal dorsal horn and at supraspinal sites in the somatosensory pathway. When compound action potentials are recorded in peripheral nerves exposed to local anesthetics in varying concentrations and lengths of nerve exposed, conduction

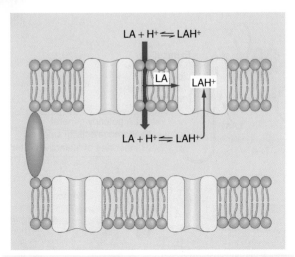

$$LA + H^+ \rightleftharpoons LAH^+$$

Fig. 10.5 During diffusion of local anesthetic across the nerve sheath and membrane to receptor sites within the inner vestibule of the sodium channel, only the uncharged base (LA) can penetrate the lipid membrane. After reaching the axoplasm, ionization occurs, and the charged cationic form (LAH⁺) attaches to the receptor. Anesthetic may also reach the channel laterally (i.e., hydrophobic pathway). (From Covino BG, Scott DB, Lambert DH. *Handbook of Spinal Anesthesia and Analgesia.* Philadelphia: WB Saunders; 1994:7, used with permission.)

blockade is facilitated either by increasing the concentration of local anesthetic or by increasing the length of nerve exposed to more dilute concentrations. At the limit of short lengths of nerve exposed to local anesthetic, conduction blockade requires exposure of at least three successive nodes of Ranvier to prevent the action potential from "skipping over" the region of local anesthetic exposure.

Historically, the term *differential blockade* in clinical textbooks referred to the observation that infusions of dilute concentrations of local anesthetic could produce analgesia and signs of autonomic blockade with relative sparing of motor strength. This clinical trend is not readily explained by the electrophysiologic observations of action potential blockade in large and small fibers perfused to steady state.[6] The mechanisms underlying this divergence between clinical experience and experimental data are poorly understood, but they may be related to the anatomic and geographic arrangement of nerve fibers, variability in the longitudinal spread required for neural blockade, effects on other ion channels, and inherent impulse activity.

## SPREAD OF LOCAL ANESTHESIA AFTER INJECTION

When local anesthetics are deposited around a peripheral nerve, they must cross a series of diffusion barriers to access sodium channels in nerve axons (Fig. 10.6).

With large nerve trunks, they diffuse from the outer surface (mantle) toward the center (core) of the nerve along a concentration gradient (Fig. 10.7).[7] As a result, nerve fibers located in the mantle of the mixed nerve are blocked first. These mantle fibers are generally distributed to more proximal anatomic structures, whereas distal structures are innervated by fibers near the core. This anatomic arrangement accounts for the initial development of proximal anesthesia with subsequent distal involvement as local anesthetic diffuses to reach more central core nerve fibers. Skeletal muscle weakness may precede sensory blockade if the motor nerve fibers are more superficial. The sequence of onset and recovery from conduction blockade of sympathetic, sensory, and motor nerve fibers in a mixed peripheral nerve depends as much or more on the anatomic location of the nerve fibers within the mixed nerve as on their intrinsic sensitivity to local anesthetics.

## PHARMACOKINETICS

For most oral and intravenous drugs, systemic uptake carries the drug from administration site to effect site. Local anesthetics are different: when drug is deposited near the target site, systemic absorption competes with drug entry into effect sites in nerves. Thus, rapid and efficient systemic uptake from an injection site diminishes, rather than increases, efficacy in nerve blockade. This principle is illustrated in Fig. 10.8. High plasma concentrations of local anesthetics after absorption from injection sites (or unintended intravascular injection) are undesirable and are the origin of their potential toxicity. Peak plasma concentrations achieved are determined by the rate of systemic uptake and, to a lesser extent, the rate of clearance of the local anesthetic. Uptake is affected by several factors related to the physiochemical properties of the local anesthetic and local tissue blood flow. Uptake tends to be delayed for local anesthetics with high lipophilicity and protein binding.

### Local Anesthetic Vasoactivity

Anesthetics differ in their tendencies to cause either vasoconstriction or vasodilation of blood vessels. These effects vary with site of injection, concentration, and balance of local direct actions on vascular smooth muscle versus indirect actions via blockade of sympathetic efferent fibers. Such differences may be clinically important. For example, the less frequent incidence of systemic toxicity of S (–) ropivacaine compared with the R (+) enantiomer in part may result from its vasoconstrictive activity (see "Adverse Effects"). The variable effect of vasoconstrictors added to local anesthetic solutions used for spinal anesthesia is another example. In contrast to lidocaine or

**Table 10.2**   Comparative Pharmacology and Common Current Use of Local Anesthetics

| Classification and Compounds | pKa | % Nonionized at pH 7.4 | Potency[a] | Max. Dose (mg) for Infiltration[b] | Duration After Infiltration (min) | Topical | Local | IV | Periph | Epi | Spinal |
|---|---|---|---|---|---|---|---|---|---|---|---|
| **Esters** | | | | | | | | | | | |
| Procaine | 8.9 | 3 | 1 | 500 | 45-60 | No | Yes | No | Yes | No | Yes |
| Chloroprocaine | 8.7 | 5 | 2 | 600 | 30-60 | No | Yes | Yes | Yes | Yes | Yes[c] |
| Tetracaine | 8.5 | 7 | 8 | Yes | Yes[d] | No | No | No | Yes | | |
| **Amides** | | | | | | | | | | | |
| Lidocaine | 7.9 | 24 | 2 | 300 | 60-120 | Yes | Yes | Yes | Yes | Yes | Yes[c] |
| Mepivacaine | 7.6 | 39 | 2 | 300 | 90-180 | No | Yes | No | Yes | Yes | Yes[c] |
| Prilocaine | 7.9 | 24 | 2 | 400 | 60-120 | Yes[e] | Yes | Yes | Yes | Yes | Yes[c] |
| Bupivacaine, levobupivacaine | 8.1 | 17 | 8 | 150 | 240-480 | No | Yes | No | Yes | Yes | Yes |
| Ropivacaine | 8.1 | 17 | 6 | 200 | 240-480 | No | Yes | No | Yes | Yes | Yes |

[a]Relative potencies vary based on experimental model or route of administration.
[b]Dosage should take into account the site of injection, use of a vasoconstrictor, and patient-related factors.
[c]Use of procaine, lidocaine, mepivacaine, prilocaine, and chloroprocaine for spinal anesthesia is somewhat controversial; indications are evolving (see text).
[d]Used in combination with another local anesthetic to increase duration.
[e]Formulated with lidocaine as eutectic mixture.
*Epi,* Epidural; *IV,* intravenous; *Periph,* peripheral.

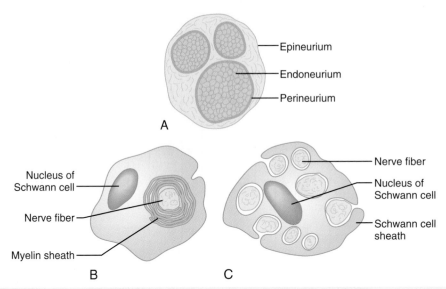

**Fig. 10.6** Transverse sections of a peripheral nerve (A) showing the outermost epineurium; the inner perineurium, which collects nerve axons in fascicles; and the endoneurium, which surrounds each my-elinated fiber. Each myelinated axon (B) is encased in the multiple membranous wrappings of myelin formed by one Schwann cell, each of which stretches longitudinally more than approximately 100 times the diameter of the axon. The narrow span of axon between these myelinated segments, the node of Ranvier, contains the ion channels that support action potentials. Nonmyelinated fibers (C) are enclosed in bundles of 5 to 10 axons by a chain of Schwann cells that tightly embrace each axon with but one layer of membrane. (From Berde CB, Strichartz GR: Local anesthetics. In Miller RD, Cohen NH, Eriksson LI, et al, eds. *Miller's Anesthesia.* 8th ed. Philadelphia: Saunders Elsevier; 2015.)

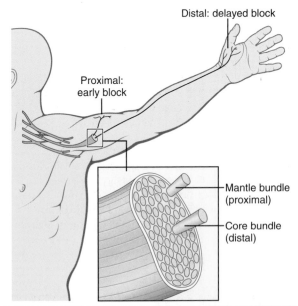

**Fig. 10.7** Local anesthetics deposited around a peripheral nerve diffuse along a concentration gradient to block nerve fibers on the outer surface (mantle) before more centrally located (core) fibers. This accounts for early manifestations of anesthesia in more proximal areas of the extremity.

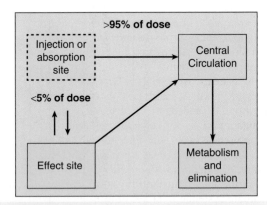

**Fig. 10.8** Heuristic model of local anesthetic uptake and distribution. Systemic uptake of local anesthetics from the perineural injection compartment competes with drug entry into nerves. Vasoconstrictors delay systemic uptake from the perineural injection compartment, reducing peak blood concentrations of local anesthetics, and maintaining a higher concentration gradient favoring drug entry into nerves over the first 30 minutes after injection.

bupivacaine, there is some evidence that tetracaine produces a significant increase in spinal cord blood flow. Consequently, prolongation of spinal anesthesia by epinephrine or other vasoconstrictors is more pronounced with tetracaine than with other commonly used spinal anesthetics.

## Metabolism

The amino-ester local anesthetics undergo hydrolysis by plasma esterases, whereas the amino-amide local anesthetics undergo metabolism by hepatic microsomal enzymes. The lungs are also capable of extracting local anesthetics such as lidocaine, bupivacaine, and prilocaine from the circulation. The rate of this metabolism and first-pass pulmonary extraction may influence toxicity (see "Systemic Toxicity"). In this regard, the relatively rapid hydrolysis of the ester local anesthetic chloroprocaine makes it less likely to produce sustained plasma concentrations than other local anesthetics, particularly the amino amides. However, patients with atypical plasma cholinesterase levels may be at increased risk of developing excessive plasma concentrations of chloroprocaine or other ester local anesthetics owing to absent or limited plasma hydrolysis. Hepatic metabolism of lidocaine is extensive, and clearance of this local anesthetic from plasma parallels hepatic blood flow. Liver disease or decreases in hepatic blood flow, as occur with congestive heart failure or general anesthesia, can decrease the rate of metabolism of lidocaine. Less than 5% of injected local anesthetics are excreted unchanged in the urine.

## Additives

Epinephrine is the most common additive in local anesthetic solutions. In a typical concentration of 5 µg/mL (1:200,000), epinephrine produces local vasoconstriction, which slows the rate of tissue absorption and therefore reduces peak systemic concentrations, decreasing the odds of systemic toxicity (see later discussion). Depending on injection site and the local anesthetic to which epinephrine is added, epinephrine may result in some prolongation of sensory or motor block. Epinephrine can also be used as a marker for detection of intravascular injection, based on effects on heart rate, arterial blood pressure, or symptoms. However, systemic absorption of epinephrine may contribute to cardiac dysrhythmias or accentuate systemic hypertension in vulnerable patients. Epinephrine should be avoided when performing peripheral nerve blocks in areas that may lack collateral flow (e.g., digital blocks). In contrast, epinephrine-induced vasoconstriction decreases local bleeding and may provide added benefit when combined with local anesthetics used for infiltration anesthesia.

Several other additives have been studied in efforts to prolong analgesia from peripheral nerve blocks, including the $\alpha_2$-agonist clonidine and the glucocorticoid dexamethasone. Both of these additives cause meaningful prolongations from some blocks more than others, as well as meaningful prolongation of sensory block and

clinical analgesia from systemic as well as local perineural administration.[8]

Traditionally, anesthesia providers have exercised considerable freedom in mixing their own additives and combinations. There is a growing recognition that this practice sometimes produces drug administration errors. In addition, although some additives have undergone proper preclinical testing to ensure absence of local tissue toxicities on nerve and muscle, others have not (see "Local Tissue Toxicity"). New additives that lack sufficient preclinical safety data and a regulatory evaluation process probably should not be used clinically.

## ADVERSE EFFECTS

Important adverse effects of local anesthetics, although rare, may occur from systemic absorption, local tissue toxicity, allergic reactions, and drug-specific effects.

### Systemic Toxicity

Systemic toxicity of local anesthetics results from excessive plasma concentrations of these drugs, most often from accidental intravascular injection during performance of peripheral nerve blocks. Less often, excessive plasma concentrations result from absorption of local anesthetics from tissue injection sites. The magnitude of local anesthetic systemic absorption depends on the dose injected, the specific site of injection, and the inclusion of a vasoconstrictor in the local anesthetic solution. Systemic absorption of local anesthetic is maximal after injection for intercostal nerve blocks and caudal anesthesia, intermediate after epidural anesthesia, and least after brachial plexus blocks (Fig. 10.9).[9]

Clinically significant systemic toxicity results from effects on the central nervous system and cardiovascular system. Establishment of maximal acceptable local anesthetic doses for performance of regional anesthesia is an attempt to limit plasma concentrations that can result from systemic absorption of these drugs (see Table 10.2). However, standard dosage recommendations are not entirely evidence-based and are inconsistent, and they fail to take into account the specific injection-site and patient-related factors.[10] Nonetheless, dosage recommendations represent a starting point for dose adjustments based on clinical circumstances and evolving evidence.

#### Central Nervous System Toxicity

Increasing plasma concentrations of local anesthetics classically produce circumoral numbness, facial tingling, restlessness, vertigo, tinnitus, and slurred speech, culminating in tonic-clonic seizures, though marked variation from this pattern is quite common.[11] Local anesthetics are neuronal depressants, and onset of seizures likely reflect selective

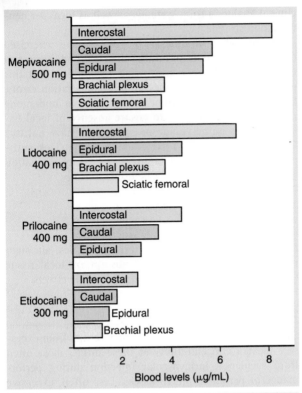

**Fig. 10.9** Peak plasma concentrations of local anesthetics resulting during performance of various types of regional anesthetic procedures. (From Covino BD, Vassals HG. *Local Anesthetics: Mechanism of Action in Clinical Use.* Orlando, FL: Grune & Stratton; 1976:97, used with permission.)

depression of cortical inhibitory neurons, leaving excitatory pathways unopposed. However, larger doses may affect inhibitory and excitatory pathways, resulting in central nervous system depression and even coma. These effects generally parallel anesthetic potency. Arterial hypoxemia and metabolic acidosis can occur rapidly during seizure activity, and hypoxemia and acidosis both can enhance the central nervous system toxicity of the local anesthetics.

Treatment of central nervous system toxic reactions begins with prompt intervention with administration of supplemental oxygen and assisting ventilation as indicated to prevent hypoxemia and hypercarbia. Benzodiazepines (i.e., midazolam, lorazepam, diazepam) are generally the drugs of first choice to terminate seizures because of their efficacy and relative hemodynamic stability. Propofol, although more immediately accessible, should be used with caution for seizure suppression as it can compromise cardiac function.

Cardiovascular System Toxicity

The cardiovascular system is generally more resistant to the toxic effects of local anesthetics than the central nervous system. Nevertheless, high plasma concentrations of

local anesthetics can produce profound hypotension due to relaxation of arteriolar vascular smooth muscle and direct myocardial depression. The cardiac toxicity, in part, reflects the ability of local anesthetics to block cardiac sodium ion channels as well as other ion channels. As a result, cardiac automaticity and conduction of cardiac impulses are impaired, manifesting on the electrocardiogram as prolongation of the PR interval and widening of the QRS complex. Local anesthetics may profoundly depress myocardial contractility to varying degrees. For example, the ratio of the dose required to produce cardiovascular collapse compared with that producing seizures for lidocaine is about twice that for bupivacaine.[12] Such findings support the concept that bupivacaine is more likely to cause cardiac toxicity, which has been the driving force for development of single-enantiomer anesthetics, such as ropivacaine and levobupivacaine.

### Lipid Resuscitation[13-15]

Intravenous infusions of lipid emulsions have become a standard treatment of local anesthetic systemic toxicity (LAST) (also see Chapter 18). The mechanism by which lipid is effective is not clear but is likely related to its ability to extract bupivacaine (or other lipophilic drugs) from aqueous plasma or tissue targets, thus reducing their effective free concentration ("lipid sink"). Accordingly, solutions of lipid emulsion should be stocked and readily accessible in any area where major conduction blockade is performed, as well as locations where overdoses from any lipophilic drug might be treated. A more detailed discussion of this topic and guidelines for administration of lipid emulsions (20%), checklists, and treatment protocols can be found in a publication by the American Society of Regional Anesthesia and Pain Medicine (ASRA) Task Force on Local Anesthetic Systemic Toxicity.[10,16,17]

According to the ASRA guidelines, an intravenous bolus dose of lipid emulsion starts with a bolus of 1.5 mL/kg (100 mg in adults) followed by a continuous infusion at 0.25 mL/kg/min. Although lipid rescue is important and should be used, it is not 100% effective and not a substitute for following dosing guidelines and safe practice regarding patient monitoring, fractionated dosing, and observation for early warning signs of systemic toxicity.

ASRA guidelines recommend additional modifications of standard advanced cardiac life support (ACLS) protocols, including avoidance of vasopressin, calcium channel blockers, β-adrenergic blockers, or other local anesthetics (lidocaine, amiodarone). Incremental dosing of epinephrine should be decreased to less than 1 μg/kg.[10]

### Local Tissue Toxicity

Local anesthetics are in general well tolerated in terms of their local tissue effects. Nevertheless, all currently available local anesthetics have intrinsic toxicities to nerve and muscle that occasionally become clinically apparent. These incidences of toxicities increase with local tissue concentration[18] and duration of exposure, and these risks may be exacerbated by factors that increase nerve vulnerability and predispose to nerve ischemia, including preexisting nerve dysfunction, metabolic and inflammatory conditions, increased tissue pressure, and systemic hypotension. Intraneural concentrations can rise steadily during prolonged perineural infusions. For these reasons, for prolonged perineural infusions, we recommend use of relatively dilute local anesthetic concentrations, generally no more than 0.2% for bupivacaine or ropivacaine.

## Allergic Reactions

Allergic reactions to local anesthetics are rare, despite the frequent use of these drugs. Less than 1% of all adverse reactions to local anesthetics are caused by allergic mechanisms. Most adverse responses attributed to allergic reactions are instead due to additives or manifestations of systemic toxicity from excessive plasma concentrations of the local anesthetic. Hypotension associated with syncope may be vagally mediated, whereas tachycardia and palpitations may occur from systemic absorption of epinephrine.

### Cross-Sensitivity

The amino-ester local anesthetics, which produce metabolites related to para-aminobenzoic acid, are more likely to evoke hypersensitivity reactions than the amino amides. Allergic reactions may also be caused by methylparaben or similar compounds that resemble para-aminobenzoic acid, which are used as preservatives in commercial formulations of ester and amide local anesthetics. Although patients known to be allergic to amino-ester local anesthetics can receive amino-amide local anesthetics, this recommendation should be cautiously accepted because it assumes that the local anesthetic was responsible for evoking the initial allergic reaction, rather than a common preservative.

### Documentation

Documentation of an allergy to local anesthetics is based principally on clinical history (e.g., rash, laryngeal edema, hypotension, bronchospasm). However, increases of serum tryptase, a marker of mast cell degranulation, may have some value with respect to confirmation, and intradermal testing may help establish the local anesthetic as the offending antigen if other drugs (e.g., sedative-hypnotics, opioids) have been administered concurrently.

## SPECIFIC LOCAL ANESTHETICS

### Amino Esters

#### Procaine

The earliest injectable local anesthetic, procaine, enjoyed extensive use during the first half of the past century,

primarily as a spinal anesthetic. Its instability and the considerable potential for hypersensitivity reactions resulted in limited use after the introduction of lidocaine. Concerns regarding transient neurologic symptoms (TNS) associated with spinal lidocaine (see "Lidocaine") have renewed interest in procaine as a spinal anesthetic. However, limited data suggest that procaine offers only a small advantage with respect to TNS, and spinal procaine is associated with a significantly greater incidence of nausea.[19]

#### Tetracaine

Tetracaine is still commonly used for spinal anesthesia. As such, it has a long duration of action, particularly if used with a vasoconstrictor, although this combination results in a surprisingly high risk of TNS.[20] Tetracaine is available as a 1% solution or as Niphanoid crystals; the crystal form is preferable because of the relative instability of the anesthetic in solution. Tetracaine is rarely used for epidural anesthesia or peripheral nerve blocks because of its slow onset, profound motor blockade, and potential toxicity when administered at high doses. Although it is an ester, its rate of metabolism is one fourth that of procaine and one tenth that of chloroprocaine.

#### Chloroprocaine

Chloroprocaine initially gained popularity as an epidural anesthetic, particularly in obstetrics, because its rapid hydrolysis virtually eliminated concern about systemic toxicity and fetal exposure to the local anesthetic. Unfortunately, neurotoxic injury, presumed to occur from accidental intrathecal injection of large doses intended for the epidural space, tempered enthusiasm for neuraxial administration of chloroprocaine. This toxicity was thought to be caused by the preservative, sodium bisulfite, contained in the commercial formulation.[21] However, subsequent studies do not demonstrate neurotoxicity from intrathecal bisulfite; instead it was found not to be neurotoxic and may even have neuroprotective effects.[22] In any event, a formulation of chloroprocaine devoid of preservatives and antioxidants is available.

Chloroprocaine produces epidural anesthesia of a relatively short duration. Epidural administration of chloroprocaine is sometimes avoided because it impairs the anesthetic or analgesic action of epidural bupivacaine and of opioids used concurrently or sequentially.[23] Chloroprocaine has been reevaluated as a spinal anesthetic,[24-26] reflecting clinical concerns related to the possible toxicity of lidocaine placed in the subarachnoid space,[27] and the small doses required for spinal anesthesia would not be predicted to produce toxicity. These initial reports have been encouraging, and the off-label use of chloroprocaine for this purpose is now common. Despite the controversy, chloroprocaine solutions used for spinal anesthesia should be bisulfite-free, and the intrathecal dose should not exceed 60 mg.

Because of its rapid plasma clearance, chloroprocaine has two unique roles in pediatric regional anesthesia: (1) as a continuous epidural infusion in neonates and very young infants, and (2) for repeat loading doses in patients receiving postoperative epidural or peripheral perineural infusions, in the setting where a repeat loading dose with the more commonly used amino-amide local anesthetics would result in stepwise increase of blood concentrations into a toxic range.

## Amino Amides

### Lidocaine

Lidocaine is the most commonly used local anesthetic. It is used for local, topical, and regional intravenous block, peripheral nerve block, and spinal and epidural anesthesia. Although recent issues have led to restricted use of lidocaine for spinal anesthesia, this local anesthetic remains popular for all other applications, including epidural anesthesia.

Potential neurotoxicity (i.e., cauda equina syndrome) when lidocaine is administered for spinal anesthesia has emerged as a concern, especially when used with a continuous spinal technique.[28] Most of the initial injuries resulted from neurotoxic concentrations of anesthetic in the caudal region of the subarachnoid space achieved by the combination of maldistribution and relatively large doses of anesthetic administered through small-gauge spinal catheters.[29] However, even doses of lidocaine routinely used for single-injection spinal anesthesia (75 to 100 mg) have been associated with neurotoxicity.[27]

TNS is a syndrome of pain and dysesthesia that may occur in up to one third of patients receiving intrathecal doses of lidocaine (but rarely occurs with bupivacaine).[20,30,31] These symptoms were initially called transient radicular irritation, but this term was later abandoned in favor of TNS because of the lack of certainty regarding their cause. In addition to the use of intrathecal lidocaine, cofactors that contribute to the occurrence of TNS include the lithotomy position,[20,30] positioning for knee arthroscopy,[30] and outpatient status.[20] In contrast, local anesthetic concentration, the presence of glucose, concomitant administration of epinephrine, and technique-related factors such as the size or type of needle do not alter the incidence of TNS with lidocaine.[20]

Symptoms of TNS generally manifest within the first 12 to 24 hours after surgery, most often resolve within 3 days, and rarely persist beyond a week. Although self-limited, the pain can be quite severe, often exceeding that induced by the surgical procedure, and on rare occasions requiring rehospitalization for pain control. Nonsteroidal antiinflammatory drugs are often fairly effective and

should be used as first-line treatment. TNS is not associated with sensory loss, motor weakness, or bowel and bladder dysfunction. The cause and significance of these symptoms remain to be established, but discrepancies between factors affecting TNS and experimental animal toxicity cast doubt that TNS and persistent neurologic deficits (e.g., cauda equina syndrome) are mediated by the same mechanism.

### Mepivacaine

Mepivacaine was the first in the series of pipecholyl xylidines, combining the piperidine ring of cocaine with the xylidine ring of lidocaine (see Fig. 10.2). This resulted in an anesthetic with characteristics very similar to lidocaine, although with less vasodilation, and a slightly longer duration of action. The clinical use of mepivacaine parallels lidocaine, with the exception that it is relatively ineffective as a topical local anesthetic. Mepivacaine's lower incidence of TNS makes it an attractive alternative to lidocaine for short-duration spinal anesthesia.

### Prilocaine

Prilocaine was introduced into clinical practice with the anticipation that its rapid metabolism and infrequent acute toxicity (central nervous system toxicity about 40% less than lidocaine) would make it a useful drug. Unfortunately, administration of large doses (>600 mg) may result in clinically significant accumulation of the metabolite ortho-toluidine, an oxidizing compound capable of converting hemoglobin to methemoglobin. Prilocaine-induced methemoglobinemia spontaneously subsides and can be reversed by the administration of methylene blue (1 to 2 mg/kg given intravenously over a 5-minute period). Nevertheless, the capacity to induce dose-related methemoglobinemia has limited the clinical acceptance of prilocaine.

Similar to other anesthetics, prilocaine has recently received attention as a spinal anesthetic, owing to dissatisfaction with spinal lidocaine. Available data, albeit limited, suggest prilocaine has a duration of action similar to lidocaine with a lower incidence of TNS. Prilocaine is not currently approved for use in the United States, nor is there any formulation available that would be appropriate for intrathecal administration.

### Bupivacaine

Bupivacaine is a congener of mepivacaine, with a butyl rather than a methyl group on the piperidine ring, a modification that imparts a longer duration of action. This characteristic, combined with its high-quality sensory anesthesia relative to motor blockade, has established bupivacaine as the most commonly used local anesthetic for epidural anesthesia during labor and for postoperative pain management. Bupivacaine is also commonly used for peripheral nerve block, and it has a relatively unblemished record as a spinal anesthetic.

Refractory cardiac arrest has been associated with the use of 0.75% bupivacaine when accidentally injected intravenously during attempted epidural anesthesia,[32] and this concentration is no longer recommended for epidural anesthesia. The most likely mechanism for bupivacaine's cardiotoxicity relates to the nature of its interaction with cardiac sodium ion channels.[33] When electrophysiologic differences between anesthetics are compared, lidocaine enters the sodium ion channel quickly and leaves quickly. In contrast, recovery from bupivacaine blockade during diastole is relatively prolonged, making it far more potent with respect to depressing the maximum upstroke velocity of the cardiac action potential ($V_{max}$) in ventricular cardiac muscle. As a result, bupivacaine has been labeled a "fast-in, slow-out" local anesthetic. This characteristic likely creates conditions favorable for unidirectional block and reentry. Other mechanisms may contribute to bupivacaine's cardiotoxicity, including disruption of atrioventricular nodal conduction, depression of myocardial contractility, and indirect effects mediated by the central nervous system.[34] This potential for cardiotoxicity places important limitations on the total dose of bupivacaine, and it underscores the vital role of fractional dosing and methods to detect inadvertent intravascular injection when large doses of local anesthetic (especially bupivacaine) are given for regional block. The recent identification of lipid emulsion as a therapeutic intervention for bupivacaine cardiotoxicity does not diminish the critical importance of these preventive measures. Cardiotoxicity is of no concern when small doses are administered for spinal anesthesia.

## Single Enantiomers

Concerns for bupivacaine cardiotoxicity have focused attention on the stereoisomers of bupivacaine and on its homolog, ropivacaine.

### Stereochemistry

Isomers are different compounds that have the same molecular formula. Subsets of isomers that have atoms connected by the same sequence of bonds but that have different spatial orientations are called stereoisomers. Enantiomers are a particular class of stereoisomers that exist as mirror images. The term *chiral* is derived from the Greek *cheir,* meaning "hand," because the forms can be considered nonsuperimposable mirror images. Enantiomers have identical physical properties except for the direction of the rotation of the plane of polarized light. This property is used to classify the enantiomer as dextrorotatory (+) if the rotation is to the right or clockwise and as levorotatory (−) if it is to the left or counterclockwise. A racemic mixture is a mixture of equal parts of enantiomers and is optically inactive because the rotation caused by the molecules of one isomer is canceled by the opposite rotation of its enantiomer. Chiral compounds can also be classified on the basis of absolute configuration, generally designated as R (rectus) or S (sinister). Enantiomers may differ with respect to specific biologic activity. For example, the S (−) enantiomer of bupivacaine has inherently less cardiotoxicity than its R (+) mirror image.

### Ropivacaine

Ropivacaine (levopropivacaine) is the S (−) enantiomer of the homolog of mepivacaine and bupivacaine with a propyl tail on the piperidine ring. In addition to a more favorable interaction with cardiac sodium ion channels. It has a more likely propensity to produce vasoconstriction, which may contribute to its reduced cardiotoxicity.

Motor blockade is less pronounced, and electrophysiologic studies raise the possibility that C fibers are preferentially blocked, together suggesting that ropivacaine may more easily produce a differential block. However, as expected from its lower lipid solubility, ropivacaine is less potent than bupivacaine. The question of potency is critical to any comparison of these anesthetics; if more drug needs to be administered to achieve a desired effect, the apparent benefits with respect to cardiotoxicity (or differential block) may not exist when more appropriate equipotent dose comparisons are made. Ropivacaine likely offers some advantage with respect to cardiotoxicity, but any benefit over bupivacaine with respect to differential block is marginal, at best.

### Levobupivacaine

Levobupivacaine is the single S (−) enantiomer of bupivacaine. Similar to ropivacaine, cardiotoxicity is reduced, but there is no advantage over bupivacaine with respect to differential blockade. As with ropivacaine, the clinically significant advantage of this compound over the racemic mixture is restricted to situations in which relatively high doses of anesthetic are administered.

## Topical Local Anesthetics

Local anesthetics are commonly administered on mucosal surfaces,[35] on cut skin to facilitate laceration repair,[36] and on intact skin, especially for needle procedures in children. Systemic absorption through mucosal surfaces is relatively rapid and efficient. Systemic toxicity is a recognized problem with excessive dosing of local anesthetic sprays and gels from the oral, nasal, or tracheobronchial mucosa, particularly in infants and children.

The keratinized layer of the skin provides an effective barrier to diffusion of topical anesthetics, making it relatively more difficult to achieve anesthesia of intact skin by topical application. This limitation can be overcome by using relatively high concentrations of local anesthetic (e.g., 5% lidocaine as in LMX or tetracaine 4% gel as in Ametop). A combination of 2.5% lidocaine and 2.5% prilocaine cream (i.e., eutectic mixture of local anesthetics [EMLA]) is widely used on intact skin.[37,38] This mixture has a lower melting point than either component, and it exists as an oil at room temperature that is capable of overcoming the barrier of the skin. EMLA cream is particularly useful in children (also see Chapter 34) for the prevention or attenuation of pain associated with venipuncture or placement of an intravenous catheter, although it may take up to an hour before adequate topical anesthesia is produced. Another product, Synera, uses a heating element to accelerate onset of skin analgesia from a lidocaine-tetracaine patch.

## Tumescent Local Anesthesia

A variety of plastic and cosmetic surgical procedures are commonly performed by a technique known as tumescent local anesthesia, which involves subcutaneous infusion of large volumes of very dilute local anesthetic.[39-41] The total lidocaine doses used in this approach are very large, such as eightfold larger than recommended doses for infiltration or peripheral nerve blockade. Nevertheless, there is a pharmacokinetic basis for this approach. When recommended dose guidelines and techniques are followed, plasma lidocaine concentrations remain in a safe range, though plasma concentrations commonly peak more than 12 hours after injection. Several case series support the general safety of this approach when recommended guidelines are followed. Conversely, adverse events have occurred when guidelines were not followed. In particular, additional dosing of other local anesthetics over the next day has resulted in toxic reactions. Any health facility using this technique should have resources and protocols for treatment of LAST.

## Systemic Local Anesthetics for Acute and Chronic Pain

Local anesthetics and related sodium channel blockers such as mexiletine can be administered as systemic analgesics as well as for local anesthesia. There is evidence for effectiveness as adjuvant analgesics for postoperative pain[42] as well as for several types of neuropathic pain.[43] For some patients with neuropathic pain, brief intravenous lidocaine infusions may produce a remarkable, though poorly understood, extended duration of pain relief (e.g., for days or weeks) that far outlasts any apparent pharmacologic duration of lidocaine.[18,44]

## WHEN LOCAL ANESTHESIA FAILS

Anesthesia providers and all clinicians should strive to improve the reliability of clinical use of local anesthetics. Historically, a common cause of failed local anesthesia has been technical failure; that is, needle placement and injection of the solution not sufficiently close to the intended site of action. The widespread use of ultrasound guidance has clearly improved technical success of many forms of regional anesthesia, especially involving peripheral nerve and plexus blocks (also see Chapter 18). Although multiple studies indicate that ultrasound facilitates more successful rates of regional anesthesia with much smaller volumes of local anesthetics, the median effective dose or volume (i.e., effectiveness for 50% of subjects) is not a relevant variable for clinical practice; what is more relevant is an $ED_{95}$ (an effective dose preventing movement in 95% of subjects).[45] Long-established techniques, such as thoracic epidural anesthesia, have significant technical failure rates when inserted using solely "blind" techniques such as loss of resistance. There is a growing appreciation for more extensive roles for more objective approaches for confirmation of needle and catheter placement for many forms of regional anesthesia in addition to ultrasound, such as Tsui's nerve stimulation approach for epidural catheter placement,[46] transduction of epidural space pressure waves, and selective use of fluoroscopy[47] (also see Chapters 17 and 18).

Aside from technical failure in needle location, local anesthesia can fail for a range of other reasons. Clinicians can make erroneous assumptions about the relevant neuroanatomy of pain arising from a surgical procedure, leading to coverage of an inadequate subset of the nerves innervating a surgical site.

In addition, there is an underappreciation of biologic sources of variation in local anesthetic responsiveness. For example, some patients with Ehlers-Danlos syndrome type III show relative resistance to local anesthetics.[48]

Local anesthetics commonly have diminished effectiveness in sites of infection or inflammation. Inflammation-induced local anesthetic resistance probably results from both pharmacokinetic factors (local acidosis, edema, hyperemia) that reduce drug entry into nerves, as well as pharmacodynamic factors, including peripheral and central sensitization.[49]

Rapidly developing tolerance (tachyphylaxis) can occur in some patients with repeated dosing or prolonged infusion. Animal studies[50] and clinical observations[51] associate tachyphylaxis with the development of hyperalgesia. Tachyphylaxis can be diminished or prevented by coadministration of antihyperalgesic drugs or other analgesics with central actions.[52]

Patients with long-standing chronic pain and hyperalgesia often appear to require larger volumes or concentrations, or both, of local anesthetics to achieve adequate analgesia, as well as coadministration of other analgesic or antihyperalgesic drugs. Although psychological factors may influence a patient's ability to tolerate surgery with regional anesthesia, clinicians should avoid "blaming the patient" for insufficient degrees of sensory block or analgesia due to a variety of technical or biologic factors that influence block effectiveness.

There are other possible effects of chronic pain and its treatment on peripheral nerves and sodium channels. Nerve injury and inflammation change the expression of different sodium channel subtypes. Although the alpha subunit of the sodium channel composes the "pore," beta subunits are also differentially expressed following nerve injury or inflammation and these beta subunits modulate channel electrophysiology and thereby may alter local anesthetic responsiveness. A 2016 study reported that chronic, but not acute, opioid exposure caused impaired local anesthetic responsiveness in the rat sciatic nerve.[53]

## FUTURE LOCAL ANESTHETICS

Local anesthetics play a central role in modern anesthetic practice. However, despite major advances in pharmacology and techniques for administration over the past century, this class of compounds has a relatively narrow therapeutic index with respect to their potential for neurotoxicity and for adverse cardiovascular and central nervous system effects. Another class of molecules that block sodium channels by a different site and mechanism are called the *site 1 sodium channel blockers*. They appear devoid of neurotoxicity and myotoxicity in some preliminary studies.[54,55] These observations suggest that sodium channel blockade and local tissue toxicity to nerve and muscle may not be mediated by a common mechanism. Site 1 blockers also appear to have minimal cardiotoxicity,[56] probably owing to their much weaker affinity for the predominant sodium channel subtype in the myocardium, Nav1.5.

Regional anesthesia has assumed growing importance in postoperative analgesia as well as intraoperatively (also see Chapters 17, 18, and 40). Opioid sparing per se is recognized as a beneficial consequence of using regional anesthesia and analgesia. Available local anesthetics typically provide less than 12 hours of analgesia following a single injection. Although analgesia can be prolonged using continuous catheter approaches, these infusions involve additional potential for dislodgement, additional postoperative care and expense, and some risks. Therefore, there have been several approaches to producing prolonged local anesthesia for wound infiltration or peripheral nerve blockade via a single injection. Controlled release of bupivacaine has been achieved

from microparticles, liposomes, hydrogels, and other vehicles. One liposomal bupivacaine product, Exparel, is now on the market in the United States with approval for wound infiltration. In clinical trials, outcomes have been mixed.[57,58]

Our group* is actively investigating the site 1 sodium channel blockers in animals[59] and in early clinical trials.[60] Site 1 blockers show profound synergism with existing local anesthetics and marked prolongation by epinephrine.

Another limitation of existing local anesthetics is the absence of modality selectivity. For example, in epidural analgesia for labor, it would be very desirable to have intense analgesia, avoidance of weakness and hypotension, and preservation of sufficient sensation to feel an urge to push (also see Chapter 33). Recent research has approached sensory-selective blockade by two predominant strategies: (1) targeting local anesthetic entry preferentially into small sensory nerve fibers[61] and (2) developing drugs that bind preferentially to subtypes of sodium channels located predominantly in small sensory fibers.

## CONCLUSIONS

Local anesthetics are used widely in anesthesiology and many areas of medicine. They have some risks and side effects, but they can be used with very good safety and clinical effectiveness by attention to safe dosing guidelines, early recognition of intravascular injection, and optimal technique. Local anesthetics are not a "solved problem," and current research may lead to improvements in regional anesthesia and postoperative care in the future.

## QUESTIONS OF THE DAY

1. What is the site of action of local anesthetics? How do local anesthetics block impulse conduction from an electrophysiologic perspective?
2. What is the typical pattern of local anesthetic spread after injection near a peripheral nerve? What are the expected clinical manifestations of this pattern of spread?
3. What are the potential advantages to the use of epinephrine as a local anesthetic additive? In what situations should epinephrine be avoided as an additive?

---

*Disclosure—Charles B. Berde, his collaborators, and Boston Children's Hospital have licensed the site 1 blocker neosaxitoxin for commercial development, with a potential for future milestone payments and royalties.

4. What are the central nervous system and cardiovascular manifestations of local anesthetic toxicity?
5. What is the initial dose of intravenous lipid emulsion for treatment of local anesthetic systemic toxicity (LAST)? What are the recommended modifications to advanced cardiac life support in a patient with LAST?
6. Besides technical failure in local anesthesia injection, what factors can explain the inability to achieve satisfactory local anesthetic block for a given patient?

## REFERENCES

1. Drasner K. Local anesthetic systemic toxicity: a historical perspective. *Reg Anesth Pain Med*. 2010;35:162–166.
2. Catterall WA. Voltage-gated sodium channels at 60: structure, function and pathophysiology. *J Physiol*. 2012;590:2577–2589.
3. Dib-Hajj SD, Cummins TR, Black JA, Waxman SG. Sodium channels in normal and pathological pain. *Annu Rev Neurosci*. 2010;33:325–347.
4. Wang GK, Strichartz GR. State-dependent inhibition of sodium channels by local anesthetics: a 40-year evolution. *Biochem (Mosc) Suppl Ser A Membr Cell Biol*. 2012;6:120–127.
5. Covino BG, Scott DB, Lambert DH. *Handbook of Spinal Anaesthesia and Analgesia*. Philadelphia: WB Saunders; 1994:7.
6. Gissen AJ, Covino BG, Gregus J. Differential sensitivities of mammalian nerve fibers to local anesthetic agents. *Anesthesiology*. 1980;53:467–474.
7. Winnie AP, Tay CH, Patel KP, et al. Pharmacokinetics of local anesthetics during plexus blocks. *Anesth Analg*. 1977;56:852–861.
8. Kirksey MA, Haskins SC, Cheng J, Liu SS. Local anesthetic peripheral nerve block adjuvants for prolongation of analgesia: a systematic qualitative review. *PLoS One*. 2015;10:e0137312.
9. Covino BG, Vassallo HG. *Local Anesthetics: Mechanisms of Action and Clinical Use*. Philadelphia: Grune & Stratton; 1976.
10. Rosenberg PH, Veering BT, Urmey WF. Maximum recommended doses of local anesthetics: a multifactorial concept. *Reg Anesth Pain Med*. 2004;29:564–575. discussion 524.
11. Neal JM, Bernards CM, Butterworth JF, et al. ASRA practice advisory on local anesthetic systemic toxicity. *Reg Anesth Pain Med*. 2010;35:152–161.
12. de Jong RH, Ronfeld RA, DeRosa RA. Cardiovascular effects of convulsant and supraconvulsant doses of amide local anesthetics. *Anesth Analg*. 1982;61:3–9.
13. Weinberg G, Ripper R, Feinstein DL, Hoffman W. Lipid emulsion infusion rescues dogs from bupivacaine-induced cardiac toxicity. *Reg Anesth Pain Med*. 2003;28:198–202.
14. Spence AG. Lipid reversal of central nervous system symptoms of bupivacaine toxicity. *Anesthesiology*. 2007;107:516–517.
15. Rosenblatt MA, Abel M, Fischer GW, et al. Successful use of a 20% lipid emulsion to resuscitate a patient after a presumed bupivacaine-related cardiac arrest. *Anesthesiology*. 2006;105:217–218.
16. American Society of Regional Anesthesia and Pain Medicine. Checklist for Treatment of Local Anesthetic Toxicity. www.asra.com/content/documents/asra_last_checklist.
17. Weinberg G. LipidRescue Resuscitation. www.lipidrescue.org.
18. Lambert LA, Lambert DH, Strichartz GR. Irreversible conduction block in isolated nerve by high concentrations of local anesthetics. *Anesthesiology*. 1994;80:1082–1093.
19. Hodgson PS, Liu SS, Batra MS, et al. Procaine compared with lidocaine for incidence of transient neurologic symptoms. *Reg Anesth Pain Med*. 2000;25:218–222.
20. Freedman JM, Li DK, Drasner K, et al. Transient neurologic symptoms after spinal anesthesia: an epidemiologic study of 1,863 patients. *Anesthesiology*. 1998;89:633–641.
21. Gissen A, Datta S, Lambert D. The chloroprocaine controversy. II. Is chloroprocaine neurotoxic? *Reg Anesth*. 1984;9:135–144.
22. Taniguchi M, Bollen AW, Drasner K. Sodium bisulfite: scapegoat for chloroprocaine neurotoxicity? *Anesthesiology*. 2004;100:85–91.
23. Eisenach JC, Schlairet TJ, Dobson CE 2nd, Hood DH. Effect of prior anesthetic solution on epidural morphine analgesia. *Anesth Analg*. 1991;73:119–123.
24. Casati A, Fanelli G, Danelli G, et al. Spinal anesthesia with lidocaine or preservative-free 2-chloroprocaine for outpatient knee arthroscopy: a prospective, randomized, double-blind comparison. *Anesth Analg*. 2007;104:959–964.
25. Drasner K. Chloroprocaine spinal anesthesia: back to the future? *Anesth Analg*. 2005;100:549–552.
26. Kouri ME, Kopacz DJ. Spinal 2-chloroprocaine: a comparison with lidocaine in volunteers. *Anesth Analg*. 2004;98:75–80. table of contents.
27. Drasner K. Lidocaine spinal anesthesia: a vanishing therapeutic index? *Anesthesiology*. 1997;87:469–472.
28. Drasner K. Local anesthetic neurotoxicity: clinical injury and strategies that may minimize risk. *Reg Anesth Pain Med*. 2002;27:576–580.
29. Rigler ML, Drasner K. Distribution of catheter-injected local anesthetic in a model of the subarachnoid space. *Anesthesiology*. 1991;75:684–692.
30. Hampl KF, Schneider MC, Ummenhofer W, Drewe J. Transient neurologic symptoms after spinal anesthesia. *Anesth Analg*. 1995;81:1148–1153.
31. Pollock JE, Neal JM, Stephenson CA, Wiley CE. Prospective study of the incidence of transient radicular irritation in patients undergoing spinal anesthesia. *Anesthesiology*. 1996;84:1361–1367.
32. Albright GA. Cardiac arrest following regional anesthesia with etidocaine or bupivacaine. *Anesthesiology*. 1979;51:285–287.
33. Clarkson CW, Hondeghem LM. Mechanism for bupivacaine depression of cardiac conduction: fast block of sodium channels during the action potential with slow recovery from block during diastole. *Anesthesiology*. 1985;62:396–405.
34. Bernards CM, Artu AA. Hexamethonium and midazolam terminate dysrhythmias and hypertension caused by intracerebroventricular bupivacaine in rabbits. *Anesthesiology*. 1991;74:89–96.
35. Roberts MH, Gildersleve CD. Lignocaine topicalization of the pediatric airway. *Paediatr Anaesth*. 2016;26:337–344.
36. Smith GA, Strausbaugh SD, Harbeck-Weber C, et al. New non-cocaine-containing topical anesthetics compared with tetracaine-adrenaline-cocaine during repair of lacerations. *Pediatrics*. 1997;100:825–830.
37. Butler-O'Hara M, LeMoine C, Guillet R. Analgesia for neonatal circumcision: a randomized controlled trial of EMLA cream versus dorsal penile nerve block. *Pediatrics*. 1998;101:E5.
38. Eichenfield LF, Funk A, Fallon-Friedlander S, Cunningham BB. A clinical study to evaluate the efficacy of ELA-Max (4% liposomal lidocaine) as compared with eutectic mixture of local anesthetics cream for pain reduction of venipuncture in children. *Pediatrics*. 2002;109:1093–1099.

39. Nordstrom H, Stange K. Plasma lidocaine levels and risks after liposuction with tumescent anaesthesia. *Acta Anaesthesiol Scand.* 2005;49:1487–1490.

40. Housman TS, Lawrence N, Mellen BG, et al. The safety of liposuction: results of a national survey. *Dermatol Surg.* 2002;28:971–978.

41. Grazer FM, de Jong RH. Fatal outcomes from liposuction: census survey of cosmetic surgeons. *Plast Reconstr Surg.* 2000;105:436–446. discussion 447–448.

42. Kranke P, Jokinen J, Pace NL, et al. Continuous intravenous perioperative lidocaine infusion for postoperative pain and recovery. *Cochrane Database Syst Rev.* 2015. CD009642.

43. Challapalli V, Tremont-Lukats IW, McNicol ED, et al. Systemic administration of local anesthetic agents to relieve neuropathic pain. *Cochrane Database Syst Rev.* 2005. CD003345.

44. Araujo MC, Sinnott CJ, Strichartz GR. Multiple phases of relief from experimental mechanical allodynia by systemic lidocaine: responses to early and late infusions. *Pain.* 2003;103:21–29.

45. Fisher D. What if half of your patients moved (or remembered or did something else bad) at incision? *Anesthesiology.* 2007;107:1–2.

46. Tsui BC, Wagner A, Cave D, Kearney R. Thoracic and lumbar epidural analgesia via the caudal approach using electrical stimulation guidance in pediatric patients: a review of 289 patients. *Anesthesiology.* 2004;100:683–689.

47. Taenzer AH, Clark Ct, Kovarik WD. Experience with 724 epidurograms for epidural catheter placement in pediatric anesthesia. *Reg Anesth Pain Med.* 2010;35:432–435.

48. Arendt-Nielsen L, Kaalund S, Bjerring P, Hogsaa B. Insufficient effect of local analgesics in Ehlers Danlos type III patients (connective tissue disorder). *Acta Anaesthesiol Scand.* 1990;34:358–361.

49. Cairns BE, Gambarota G, Dunning PS, et al. Activation of peripheral excitatory amino acid receptors decreases the duration of local anesthesia. *Anesthesiology.* 2003;98:521–529.

50. Lee KC, Wilder RT, Smith RL, Berde CB. Thermal hyperalgesia accelerates and MK-801 prevents the development of tachyphylaxis to rat sciatic nerve blockade. *Anesthesiology.* 1994;81:1284–1293.

51. Bromage PR, Pettigrew RT, Crowell DE. Tachyphylaxis in epidural analgesia: I. Augmentation and decay of local anesthesia. *J Clin Pharmacol J New Drugs.* 1969;9:30–38.

52. Lund C, Mogensen T, Hjortso NC, Kehlet H. Systemic morphine enhances spread of sensory analgesia during postoperative epidural bupivacaine infusion. *Lancet.* 1985;2:1156–1157.

53. Liu Q, Gold MS. Opioid-induced loss of local anesthetic potency in the rat sciatic nerve. *Anesthesiology.* 2016;125(4):755–764.

54. Sakura S, Bollen AW, Ciriales R, Drasner K. Local anesthetic neurotoxicity does not result from blockade of voltage-gated sodium channels. *Anesth Analg.* 1995;81:338–346.

55. Epstein-Barash H, Shichor I, Kwon AH, et al. Prolonged duration local anesthesia with minimal toxicity. *Proc Natl Acad Sci U S A.* 2009;106:7125–7130.

56. Wylie MC, Johnson VM, Carpino E, et al. Respiratory, neuromuscular, and cardiovascular effects of neosaxitoxin in isoflurane-anesthetized sheep. *Reg Anesth Pain Med.* 2012;37:152–158.

57. Hadley RM, Dine AP. Where is the evidence? A critical review of bias in the reporting of clinical data for exparel: a liposomal bupivacaine formulation. *J Clin Res Bioeth.* 2014;5:189.

58. Noviasky J, Pierce DP, Whalen K, et al. Bupivacaine liposomal versus bupivacaine: comparative review. *Hosp Pharm.* 2014;49:539–543.

59. Templin JS, Wylie MC, Kim JD, et al. Neosaxitoxin in rat sciatic block: improved therapeutic index using combinations with bupivacaine, with and without epinephrine. *Anesthesiology.* 2015;123:886–898.

60. Lobo K, Donado C, Cornelissen L, et al. A phase 1, dose-escalation, double-blind, block-randomized, controlled trial of safety and efficacy of neosaxitoxin alone and in combination with 0.2% bupivacaine, with and without epinephrine, for cutaneous anesthesia. *Anesthesiology.* 2015;123:873–885.

61. Binshtok AM, Bean BP, Woolf CJ. Inhibition of nociceptors by TRPV1-mediated entry of impermeant sodium channel blockers. *Nature.* 2007;449:607–610.

# 11 NEUROMUSCULAR BLOCKING DRUGS

Ronald D. Miller

Neuromuscular blocking drugs (NMBDs) interrupt transmission of nerve impulses at the neuromuscular junction (NMJ) and thereby produce paresis or paralysis of skeletal muscles. On the basis of electrophysiologic differences in their mechanisms of action and duration of action, these drugs can be classified as depolarizing NMBDs (mimic the actions of acetylcholine [ACh]) and nondepolarizing NMBDs (interfere with the actions of ACh), the latter of which are further subdivided into long-, intermediate-, and short-acting drugs (Box 11.1). Succinylcholine (SCh) is the only depolarizing NMBD used clinically. It is also the only NMBD that has both a rapid onset and ultrashort duration of action. Among the nondepolarizing NMBDs, rocuronium's rapid onset time most closely resembles that of SCh.

---

**Box 11.1** Classification of Neuromuscular Blocking Drugs

**Depolarizing (Rapid Onset and Ultrashort-Acting)**
Succinylcholine

**Nondepolarizing**
Long-acting
    Pancuronium
Intermediate-acting
    Vecuronium
    Rocuronium
    Atracurium
    Cisatracurium
Short-acting
    Mivacurium

---

## CLINICAL USES

The principal clinical uses of NMBDs are to produce skeletal muscle relaxation for facilitation of tracheal intubation and to provide optimal surgical working conditions. NMBDs may also be administered during cardiopulmonary resuscitation (also see Chapter 45) and to patients in emergency departments (also see Chapter 42) and intensive care units (also see Chapter 41) to facilitate mechanical ventilation of the patient's lungs. Of prime importance is to recognize that NMBDs lack analgesic or anesthetic effects and should not be used to render an inadequately anesthetized patient paralyzed. An inadequately anesthetized but paralyzed patient is a major risk for awareness during general anesthesia (see Chapter 47). Ventilation of the lungs must be mechanically provided whenever significant skeletal muscle weakness is produced by NMBDs. Clinically, intraoperative clinical evaluation of neuromuscular blockade is typically provided by visually monitoring the mechanical response (twitch response) produced by electrical stimulation of a peripheral nerve (usually a branch of the ulnar or facial nerve) delivered from a peripheral nerve stimulator (see the section, "Monitoring the Effects of Nondepolarizing Neuromuscular Blocking Drugs"). This chapter places increased emphasis on the value of monitoring by use of a peripheral nerve stimulator when NMBDs are given. Also, neostigmine has been the standard "reversal" drug for a nondepolarizing neuromuscular blockade; sugammadex is a relatively new reversal drug that has a unique mechanism of action and specifically reverses a rocuronium- and vecuronium-induced neuromuscular blockade.

### Choice of Neuromuscular Blocking Drug

The choice of NMBD is influenced by its speed of onset, duration of action, route of elimination, and associated side effects, such as drug-induced changes in systemic arterial blood pressure, heart rate, or both. Rapid onset and brief duration of skeletal muscle paralysis, characteristic of SCh, are useful when tracheal intubation is the reason for administering an NMBD. Because of its rapid onset time, rocuronium is often used to facilitate tracheal intubation, but its duration of action is much longer than that of SCh. However, an approved indication for sugammadex is reversal of a profound neuromuscular blockade specifically from rocuronium or vecuronium. For example, if rocuronium were given to facilitate endotracheal intubation, but the trachea could not be intubated, sugammadex could reverse a profound neuromuscular blockade. Although SCh can be given intermittently, nondepolarizing NMBDs are usually selected when longer periods of neuromuscular blockade (e.g., more than 15 to 45 minutes) are needed. When rapid onset of skeletal muscle paralysis is not necessary, skeletal muscle relaxation can be induced by the administration of other long- or intermediate-acting nondepolarizing NMBDs to facilitate tracheal intubation.

### Hypersensitivity Reactions

The overall incidence of life-threatening anesthetic-related hypersensitivity reactions ranges between 1/10,000 and 1/20,000 procedures and varies widely between countries.[1] Although antibiotics are likely the most common cause, NMBDs are the triggering drugs in 11% to 35% of these reactions. Rocuronium and SCh are the most common offenders. Even though it does not release histamine, rocuronium was identified as producing an increased risk for hypersensitivity reactions in France and Norway, with no confirmation from other countries. More recently, a follow-up study from Norway of 83 cases of anaphylaxis during general anesthesia revealed that 77% of these reactions were mediated by immunoglobulin E and 93% were associated with NMBDs, with SCh being the most common drug.[2] In an analysis of all allergic drugs used in anesthesia at the Mayo Clinic,[3] antibiotics were the most common cause, with NMBDs being second at 11% of the reactions. There may be cross-sensitivity among all NMBDs because of the presence of a common antigenic component, the quaternary ammonium group. Anaphylactic reactions after the first exposure to an NMBD may reflect sensitization from previous contact with cosmetics or soaps that also contain antigenic quaternary ammonium groups. Sugammadex (see the section, "Antagonism of Nondepolarizing Neuromuscular Blocking Drugs" later in this chapter) was recently approved by the Food and Drug Administration (FDA). The delay in sugammadex's approval was partly because of hypersensitivity concerns. The conclusion was that the most common signs of occasional cases of hypersensitivity were nausea and urticaria. However, sugammadex has been approved in Europe and other countries for several years. Treatment of a life-threatening hypersensitivity reaction requires immediate therapy including cardiopulmonary resuscitation and epinephrine (see Chapter 45 for details).

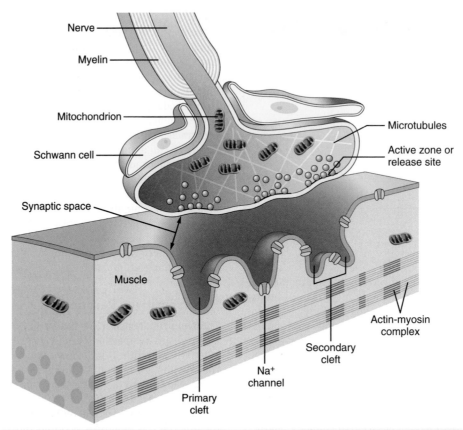

**Fig. 11.1** Adult neuromuscular junction with the three cells that constitute the synapse: the motor neuron (i.e., nerve terminal), muscle fiber, and Schwann cell. The motor neuron from the ventral horn of the spinal cord innervates the muscle. Each fiber receives only one synapse. The motor nerve loses its myelin and terminates on the muscle fiber. The nerve terminal, covered by a Schwann cell, has vesicles clustered about the membrane thickenings, which are the active zones, toward its synaptic side and mitochondria and microtubules toward its other side. A synaptic gutter, made up of a primary and many secondary clefts, separates the nerve from the muscle. The muscle surface is corrugated, and dense areas on the shoulders of each fold contain acetylcholine receptors. Sodium channels are present at the clefts and throughout the muscle membrane. (From Martyn JAJ. Neuromuscular physiology and pharmacology. In Miller RD, ed. *Miller's Anesthesia*. 8th ed. Philadelphia: Elsevier Saunders; 2015.)

## NEUROMUSCULAR JUNCTION

The anatomy of the NMJ consists of a prejunctional motor nerve ending separated from the highly folded postjunctional membrane of the skeletal muscle by a synaptic cleft (Fig. 11.1).[4] Nicotinic acetylcholine receptors (nAChRs) are located at pre- and postjunctional sites. Neuromuscular transmission is initiated by arrival of an impulse at the motor nerve terminal with an associated influx of calcium ions and resultant release of the ligand ACh. ACh binds to AChRs (the ligand-gated channel) on postjunctional membranes and thereby causes a change in membrane permeability to ions, principally potassium and sodium. This change in permeability and movement of ions causes a decrease in the transmembrane potential from about –90 mV to –45 mV (threshold potential), at

which point a propagated action potential spreads over the surfaces of skeletal muscle fibers and leads to muscular contraction. ACh is rapidly hydrolyzed (within 15 ms) by the enzyme acetylcholinesterase (true cholinesterase), thus restoring membrane permeability (repolarization) and preventing sustained depolarization. Acetylcholinesterase is primarily located in the folds of the end-plate region, which places it in close proximity to the site of action of ACh.

### Prejunctional Receptors and Release of Acetylcholine

ACh is synthesized in the motor nerve terminal, and the protein synapsin anchors the ACh vesicle to the release site of the terminal. Some of the ACh is then released,

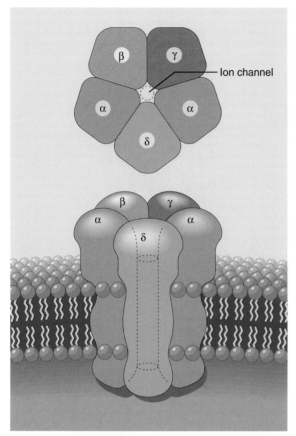

**Fig. 11.2** The postjunctional nicotinic cholinergic receptor consists of five subunits (α, α, β, γ, δ) arranged to form an ion channel. (From Taylor P. Are neuromuscular blocking agents more efficacious in pairs? *Anesthesiology*. 1985;63:1-3, used with permission.)

The two α-subunits are the binding sites for ACh and are the sites occupied by NMBDs. For example, occupation of one or both α-subunits by a nondepolarizing NMBD causes the ion channel to remain closed, and ion flow to produce depolarization cannot occur. SCh attaches to α-sites and causes the ion channel to remain open (mimics ACh), thereby resulting in prolonged depolarization. Large doses of nondepolarizing NMBDs (large molecules) may also act to occlude the channel and in this way prevent the normal flow of ions. Neuromuscular blockade secondary to occlusion of the channels is resistant to drug-enhanced antagonism with anticholinesterase drugs. The lipid environment around cholinergic receptors can be altered by drugs such as volatile anesthetics, thus changing the properties of the ion channels. This probably accounts for the augmentation of neuromuscular blockade by volatile anesthetics.

## Extrajunctional Receptors

Postjunctional receptors are confined to the area of the end plate precisely opposite the prejunctional receptors, whereas extrajunctional receptors (the ε-unit is replaced by γ-subunits) are present throughout skeletal muscles. Extrajunctional receptor synthesis is normally suppressed by neural activity. Prolonged inactivity, sepsis, and denervation or trauma (burn injury) to skeletal muscles may be associated with a proliferation of extrajunctional receptors. When activated, extrajunctional receptors stay open longer and permit more ions to flow, which in part explains the exaggerated hyperkalemic response when SCh is administered to patients with denervation or burn injury. Proliferation of these receptors also accounts for the resistance or tolerance to nondepolarizing NMBDs, as can occur with burns or prolonged (several days) immobilization (also see discussion under the section, "Hyperkalemia").[5,6]

## STRUCTURE-ACTIVITY RELATIONSHIPS

NMBDs are quaternary ammonium compounds that have at least one positively charged nitrogen atom that binds to the α-subunit of postsynaptic cholinergic receptors (Fig. 11.3). In addition, these drugs have structural similarities to the endogenous neurotransmitter ACh. For example, SCh is two molecules of ACh linked by methyl groups. The long, slender, flexible structure of ACh allows it to bind to and activate cholinergic receptors. The bulky rigid molecules that are characteristic of nondepolarizing NMBDs, though containing portions similar to ACh, do not activate cholinergic receptors.

Nondepolarizing NMBDs are either aminosteroid compounds (pancuronium, vecuronium, rocuronium) or benzylisoquinolinium compounds (atracurium, cisatracurium, mivacurium). Pancuronium is the bisquaternary

and the rest is held in reserve for response to a stimulus. Presynaptic receptors, aided by calcium, facilitate replenishment of the motor nerve terminal, which can be stimulated by SCh and neostigmine and depressed by small doses of nondepolarizing NMBDs. Inhibition of these presynaptic nAChRs explains the fade in response to high-frequency repetitive stimulation such as tetanic or even train-of-four (TOF) stimulation.[4]

## Postjunctional Receptors

Postjunctional receptors are glycoproteins consisting of five subunits (Fig. 11.2).[4] The subunits of the receptor are arranged such that a channel is formed that allows the flow of ions along a concentration gradient across cell membranes. This flow of ions is the basis of normal neuromuscular transmission. Extrajunctional receptors retain the two α-subunits but may have an altered γ- or δ-subunit by the substitution of an ε-unit.

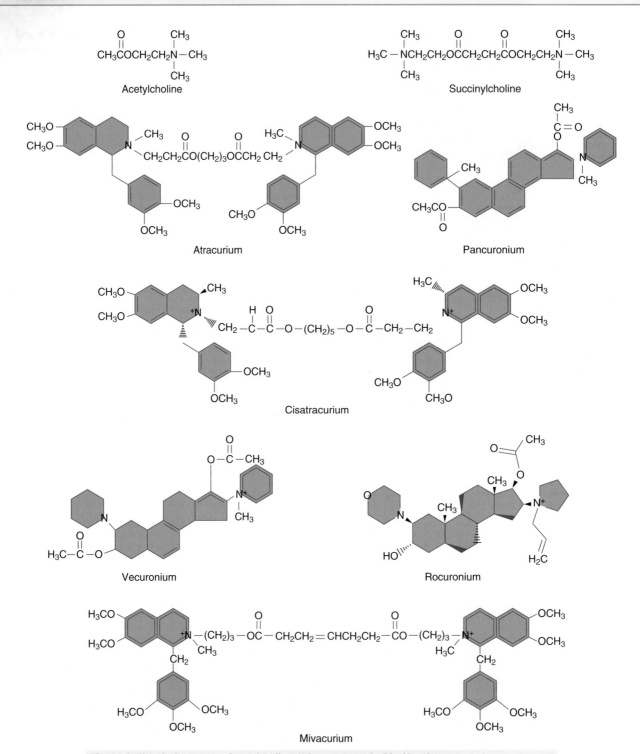

**Fig. 11.3** Chemical structure of acetylcholine and neuromuscular blocking drugs.

aminosteroid NMBD most closely related to ACh structurally. The ACh-like fragments of pancuronium give the steroidal molecule its high degree of neuromuscular blocking activity. Vecuronium and rocuronium are monoquaternary analogs of pancuronium. Aminosteroid NMBDs lack hormonal activity. Benzylisoquinolinium derivatives are more likely than aminosteroid derivatives to evoke the release of histamine, presumably reflecting the presence of a tertiary amine.

## DEPOLARIZING NEUROMUSCULAR BLOCKING DRUGS

SCh is the only depolarizing NMBD used clinically. Furthermore, it is the only NMBD with both a rapid onset and ultrashort duration of action. Typically, doses of 0.5 to 1.5 mg/kg are administered intravenously and produce a rapid onset of skeletal muscle paralysis (30 to 60 seconds) that lasts 5 to 10 minutes because of its unique breakdown (Fig. 11.4). These characteristics make SCh ideal for providing rapid skeletal muscle paralysis to facilitate tracheal intubation. SCh has been used clinically for more than 60 years. Despite consistent industrial efforts, no drug has been developed that is better than SCh for tracheal intubation.[7] Although an intravenous dose of 0.5 mg/kg may be adequate, 1.0 to 1.5 mg/kg is commonly administered to facilitate tracheal intubation. If a subparalyzing dose of a nondepolarizing NMBD (pretreatment with 5% to 10% of its 95% effective dose [ED$_{95}$]) is administered 2 to 4 minutes before injection of SCh to blunt fasciculations, the dose of SCh should be increased by about 70%. Although ideal for facilitating tracheal intubation, SCh has many adverse effects (Box 11.2). As an alternative, the intermediate-acting nondepolarizing NMBD rocuronium has an onset time as rapid as SCh in doses ranging from 1.0 to 1.2 mg/kg.

### Characteristics of Blockade

SCh mimics the action of ACh and produces a sustained depolarization of the postjunctional membrane. Skeletal muscle paralysis occurs because a depolarized postjunctional membrane and inactivated sodium channels cannot respond to subsequent release of ACh (hence, the designation depolarizing neuromuscular blockade). Depolarizing neuromuscular blockade is also referred to as *phase I blockade*. Phase II blockade is present when the postjunctional membrane has become repolarized but still does not respond normally to ACh (desensitization neuromuscular blockade). The mechanism of phase II blockade is unknown but may reflect the development of nonexcitable areas around the end plates that become repolarized but nevertheless prevent the spread of impulses initiated by the action of ACh. With the initial

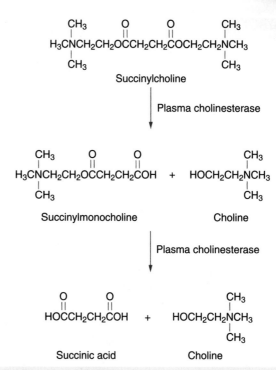

**Fig. 11.4** The brief duration of action of succinylcholine is due to its rapid hydrolysis in plasma by cholinesterase enzyme to inactive metabolites (succinylmonocholine has 1/20 and 1/80 the activity of succinylcholine at the neuromuscular junction).

| **Box 11.2** Adverse Side Effects of Succinylcholine |
| --- |
| Cardiac dysrhythmias |
|     Sinus bradycardia |
|     Junctional rhythm |
|     Sinus arrest |
| Fasciculations |
| Hyperkalemia |
| Myalgia |
| Myoglobinuria |
| Increased intraocular pressure |
| Increased intragastric pressure |
| Trismus |

dose of SCh, subtle signs of a phase II blockade begin to appear (fade to tetanic stimulation).[8] Phase II blockade, which resembles the blockade produced by nondepolarizing NMBDs, predominates when the intravenous dose of SCh exceeds 3 to 5 mg/kg (Table 11.1).

The sustained depolarization produced by the initial administration of SCh is initially manifested as transient generalized skeletal muscle contractions known as *fasciculations*. Furthermore, the sustained opening of sodium channels produced by SCh is associated with leakage of potassium from the interior of cells sufficient to increase plasma concentrations of potassium by about

**Table 11.1** Comparison of Depolarizing (Succinylcholine) and Nondepolarizing (Rocuronium) Neuromuscular Blocking Drugs

| | Succinylcholine | | |
|---|---|---|---|
| Feature | Phase I | Phase II | Rocuronium |
| Administration of rocuronium | Antagonize | Augment | Augment |
| Administration of succinylcholine | Augment | Augment | Antagonize |
| Administration of neostigmine | Augment | Antagonize | Antagonize |
| Fasciculations | Yes | | No |
| Response to single electrical stimulation (single twitch) | Decreased | Decreased | Decreased |
| Train-of-four ratio | >0.7 | <0.3 | <0.3 |
| Response to continuous (tetanus) electrical stimulation | Sustained | Unsustained | Unsustained |
| Post-tetanic facilitation | No | Yes | Yes |

**Table 11.2** Variants of Plasma Cholinesterase and Duration of Action of Succinylcholine

| Variants of Plasma Cholinesterase | Type of Buty butyrylcholinesterase/ TG lcholinesterase | Incidence | Dibucaine Number (% Inhibition of Enzyme Activity) | Duration of Succinylcholine-Induced Neuromuscular Blockade (min) |
|---|---|---|---|---|
| Homozygous, typical (usual, U) | UU | Normal | 70-80 | 5-10 |
| Heterozygous | UA | 1/480 | 50-60 | 20 |
| Homozygous, atypical (A) | AA | 1/3200 | 20-30 | 60-180 |

0.1 to 0.4 mEq/L. With proliferation of extrajunctional nAChRs and damaged muscle membranes, many more channels will leak potassium and thereby lead to acute hyperkalemia.

## Metabolism

Hydrolysis of SCh to inactive metabolites is accomplished by plasma cholinesterase (pseudocholinesterase) produced in the liver (see Fig. 11.4). Plasma cholinesterase has an enormous capacity to hydrolyze SCh at a rapid rate (ACh is metabolized even more rapidly by acetylcholinesterase) such that only a small fraction of the original intravenous dose reaches the NMJ. Because plasma cholinesterase is not present at the NMJ, the neuromuscular blockade produced by SCh is terminated by its diffusion away from the NMJ into extracellular fluid. Therefore, plasma cholinesterase influences the duration of action of SCh by controlling the amount of SCh that is hydrolyzed before reaching the NMJ. Liver disease must be severe before decreases in the synthesis of plasma cholinesterase are sufficient to prolong the effects of SCh. Potent anticholinesterases, as used in the treatment of myasthenia gravis, and certain chemotherapeutic drugs (nitrogen mustard, cyclophosphamide) may so decrease plasma cholinesterase activity that prolonged skeletal muscle paralysis follows the administration of SCh.

### Atypical Plasma Cholinesterase

Atypical plasma cholinesterase lacks the ability to hydrolyze ester bonds in drugs such as SCh and mivacurium. The presence of this atypical enzyme is often recognized only after an otherwise healthy patient experiences prolonged skeletal muscle paralysis (>1hour) after the administration of a conventional dose of SCh or mivacurium. Subsequent determination of the dibucaine number permits diagnosis of the presence of atypical plasma cholinesterase. Dibucaine is an amide local anesthetic that inhibits normal plasma activity by about 80%, whereas the activity of atypical enzyme is inhibited by about 20% (Table 11.2). The dibucaine number reflects the quality of plasma cholinesterase (ability to metabolize SCh and mivacurium) and not the quantity of enzyme that is circulating in plasma. For example, decreases in plasma

**Table 11.3**   Autonomic Nervous System and Histamine-Releasing Effects of Neuromuscular Blocking Drugs

| Drug[a] | Nicotinic Receptors at Autonomic Ganglia | Cardiac Postganglionic Muscarinic Receptors | Histamine Release |
|---|---|---|---|
| Succinylcholine | Modest stimulation | Modest stimulation | Minimal |
| Pancuronium | None | Modest blockade | None |
| Vecuronium | None | None | None |
| Rocuronium | None | None | None |
| Atracurium | None | None | Slight[b] |
| Cisatracurium | None | None | None |
| Mivacurium | None | None | Slight[b] |

[a]At 95% effective dose ($ED_{95}$).
[b]Occurs only with doses estimated to be 2 to 3 × $ED_{95}$.

cholinesterase activity because of liver disease or anticholinesterases are often associated with a normal dibucaine number.

## Adverse Side Effects

Adverse side effects after the administration of SCh are numerous and may limit or even contraindicate the use of this NMBD in certain patients (see Box 11.2). After 60 years of use, SCh continues to cause serious complications.[9,10] SCh usually should not be given to patients 24 to 72 hours after major burns, trauma, and extensive denervation of skeletal muscles because it may result in acute hyperkalemia and cardiac arrest.[5,6] Administration of SCh to apparently healthy boys with unrecognized muscular dystrophy has resulted in acute hyperkalemia and cardiac arrest. For this reason, the FDA has issued a warning against the use of SCh in children, except for emergency control of the airway.

### Cardiac Dysrhythmias

Sinus bradycardia, junctional rhythm, and even sinus arrest may follow the administration of SCh. These responses reflect the action of SCh at cardiac postganglionic muscarinic receptors, where this drug mimics the normal effects of ACh (Table 11.3). Cardiac dysrhythmias are most likely to occur when a second intravenous dose of SCh is administered about 5 minutes after the first dose. Intravenous administration of atropine 1 to 3 minutes before SCh decreases the likelihood of these cardiac responses. Yet, atropine administered intramuscularly with the preoperative medication does not reliably protect against SCh-induced decreases in heart rate. The effects of SCh at autonomic nervous system ganglia also mimic the actions of the neurotransmitter ACh and may be manifested as ganglionic stimulation with associated increases in systemic blood pressure and heart rate (see Table 11.3).

### Hyperkalemia

Administration of SCh can rapidly result in massive hyperkalemia, serious cardiac arrythmias, and even cardiac arrest.[5,6] In some patients, potassium levels can exceed 10 mEq/L. The classic conditions that lead to hyperkalemia after SCh include burns, trauma, and spinal cord or other major neurologic damage. Any time prolonged skeletal muscle inactivity (critical care) or extensive muscle damage exists, patients may be susceptible to hyperkalemia 48 hours after injury, and this is dependent on the development of extrajunctional, atypical receptors as previously described.[4-6] When muscle has returned to its normal state, hyperkalemia will not occur. However, the judgment as to the "normal" state of the muscle is a clinically difficult estimation. In addition, extrajunctional receptors and hyperkalemia will develop in any patient who is immobile (critical care patients) for several days if SCh is given. For example, cardiac arrest has occurred when SCh has been used for emergency endotracheal intubation in the intensive care unit. The use of SCh for urgent tracheal intubation is contraindicated or not allowed in many intensive care units. The duration of susceptibility to the hyperkalemic effects of SCh is unknown, but the risk is probably decreased 3 to 6 months after denervation injury. All factors considered, it might be prudent to avoid administration of SCh to any patient more than 24 hours after a burn injury, extensive trauma, or spinal cord transection or who may become an intensive care patient.

Even though they may have increased potassium levels, patients with renal failure are not susceptible to an exaggerated release of potassium, and SCh can be safely administered to these patients, unless they have uremic neuropathy.

### Myalgia

Postoperative skeletal muscle myalgia, manifested particularly in the muscles of the neck, back, and abdomen, may follow the administration of SCh. Myalgia localized to neck muscles may be described as a "sore throat" by the patient and incorrectly attributed to the previous presence of a tracheal tube. Young adults undergoing minor surgical procedures that permit early ambulation seem most likely to complain of myalgia. Unsynchronized contractions of skeletal muscle fibers (fasciculations) associated with generalized depolarization lead to myalgia. Prevention of fasciculations by prior administration of subparalyzing doses of a nondepolarizing NMBD (pretreatment) or lidocaine will decrease the incidence but not totally prevent myalgia.[11] Magnesium will prevent fasciculations but not myalgia. Nonsteroidal antiinflammatory drugs are effective in treating the myalgia.

### Increased Intraocular Pressure

SCh causes a maximum increase in intraocular pressure 2 to 4 minutes after its administration. This increase in intraocular pressure is transient and lasts only 5 to 10 minutes. The mechanism by which SCh increases intraocular pressure is unknown, although contraction of extraocular muscles with associated compression of the globe may be involved. The concern that contraction of extraocular muscles could cause extrusion of intraocular contents in the presence of an open eye injury has resulted in the common clinical practice of avoiding the administration of SCh to these patients. This theory has never been substantiated and is challenged by the report of patients with an open eye injury in whom intravenous administration of SCh did not cause extrusion of globe contents.[12] Furthermore, there is evidence that contraction of extraocular muscles does not contribute to the increase in intraocular pressure that accompanies the administration of SCh.[13]

### Increased Intracranial Pressure

Increases in intracranial pressure after the administration of SCh can occur but are of little or no concern.

### Increased Intragastric Pressure

SCh causes unpredictable increases in intragastric pressure. When intragastric pressure does increase, it seems to be related to the intensity of fasciculations, thus emphasizing the potential value of preventing this skeletal muscle activity by prior administration of a subparalyzing dose of a nondepolarizing NMBD. An unproven hypothesis is that this increased intragastric pressure may cause passage of gastric fluid and contents into the esophagus and pharynx, with a subsequent risk for pulmonary aspiration.

### Trismus

Incomplete jaw relaxation with masseter jaw rigidity after a halothane-SCh sequence is not uncommon in children (occurs in about 4.4% of patients) and is considered a normal response. In extreme cases this response may be so severe that the ability to mechanically open the patient's mouth is limited. The difficulty lies in separating the normal response to SCh from the masseter rigidity that may be associated with malignant hyperthermia. Because SCh is not recommended for use in children, except for emergency airway control, trismus is less of an issue.

## NONDEPOLARIZING NEUROMUSCULAR BLOCKING DRUGS

Nondepolarizing NMBDs are classified clinically as long-, intermediate-, and short-acting (see Box 11.1). These drugs act by competing with ACh for α-subunits at the postjunctional nicotinic cholinergic receptors and preventing changes in ion permeability (see Fig. 11.2). As a result, depolarization cannot occur (hence, the designation *nondepolarizing neuromuscular blockade*), and skeletal muscle paralysis develops. Differences in onset, duration of action, rate of recovery, metabolism, and clearance influence the clinical decision to select one drug versus another (Table 11.4). For example, rocuronium has the most rapid onset time and minimal cardiovascular effects; cisatracurium is not dependent on the kidney for its elimination. Do these characteristics make rocuronium the choice for facilitating endotracheal intubation and cisatracurium for kidney transplantation? Yet, only vecuronium and, more important, rocuronium are antagonized by sugammadex (described later). These are a few of the variables that influence the choice of NMBD to be used for individual clinical situations.

### Pharmacokinetics

Nondepolarizing NMBDs, because of their quaternary ammonium groups, are highly ionized, water-soluble compounds at physiologic pH and possess limited lipid solubility. As a result, these drugs cannot easily cross lipid membrane barriers, such as the blood-brain barrier, renal tubular epithelium, gastrointestinal epithelium, or placenta. Therefore, nondepolarizing NMBDs do not produce central nervous system effects, renal tubular reabsorption is minimal, oral administration is ineffective, and maternal administration does not adversely affect the fetus. Redistribution of nondepolarizing NMBDs also exerts a role in the pharmacokinetics of these drugs.

Many of the variable pharmacologic responses of patients to nondepolarizing NMBDs can be explained by differences in pharmacokinetics, which can be changed by many factors, such as hypovolemia, hypothermia, and the presence of hepatic or renal disease (or both). Renal and hepatic elimination is aided by access to a large fraction of the administered drug because of the high degree of ionization, which maintains high plasma concentrations of nondepolarizing NMBDs and also prevents renal reabsorption of excreted drug.

**Table 11.4**   Comparative Pharmacology of Nondepolarizing Neuromuscular Blocking Drugs

| Drug | ED$_{95}$ (mg/kg) | Onset to Maximum Twitch Depression (min) | Duration to Return to ≥25%[a] | Intubating Dose (mg/kg) | Continuous Infusion (mg/kg/min) | Renal Excretion (% Unchanged) | Hepatic Degrada-tion (%) | Biliary Excretion (% Un-changed) | Hydrolysis in Plasma |
|---|---|---|---|---|---|---|---|---|---|
| Pancuro-nium | 0.07 | 3-5 | 60-90 | 0.1 | | 80 | 10 | 5-10 | No |
| Vecuro-nium | 0.05 | 3-5 | 20-35 | 0.08-0.1 | 1 | 15-25 | 20-30 | 40-75 | No |
| Rocuro-nium | 0.3 | 1-2 | 20-35 | 0.6-1.2 | | 10-25 | 10-20 | 50-70 | No |
| Atracu-rium | 0.2 | 3-5 | 20-35 | 0.4-0.5 | 6-8 | NS | NS | NA | Enzymatic, spontane-ous |
| Cisatracu-rium | 0.05 | 3-5 | 20-35 | 0.1 | 1-1.5 | NS | NS | NS | Spontane-ous |
| Mivacu-rium | 0.08 | 2-3 | 12-20 | 0.25 | 5-6 | NS | NS | NS | Enzymatic |

[a]Control twitch height (minutes).
*ED$_{95}$*, 95% effective dose; *NS*, not significant.

Renal disease markedly alters the pharmacokinetics of only the long-acting nondepolarizing NMBDs, such as pancuronium. The intermediate-acting NMBDs are eliminated by the liver (rocuronium), by metabolism by plasma cholinesterase (mivacurium), by Hofmann elimination (atracurium or cisatracurium), or by a combination of these mechanisms. The new reversal drug sugammadex is not recommended in patients with "severe" renal impairment.

## Pharmacodynamic Responses

Enhancement of neuromuscular blockade by volatile anesthetics reflects a pharmacodynamic action as manifested by decreased plasma concentrations of nondepolarizing NMBDs required to produce a given degree of neuromuscular blockade in the presence of volatile anesthetics. In addition to volatile anesthetics, other drugs, such as aminoglycoside antibiotics, local anesthetics, cardiac antiarrhythmic drugs, dantrolene, magnesium, lithium, and tamoxifen (an antiestrogenic drug), may enhance the neuromuscular blockade produced by nondepolarizing NMBDs. A few drugs may diminish the effects of a nondepolarizing NMBD, including calcium, corticosteroids, and anticonvulsant (phenytoin) drugs. Some neuromuscular diseases can be associated with altered pharmacodynamic responses (myasthenia gravis, Duchenne muscular dystrophy). Burn injury causes resistance to the effects of nondepolarizing NMBDs, as reflected by the need to establish a higher plasma concentration of drug to achieve the same pharmacologic effect as in patients without a burn injury. There is resistance to the effects of nondepolarizing NMBDs in skeletal muscles affected by a cerebrovascular accident, perhaps reflecting proliferation of extrajunctional receptors that respond to ACh.

## Cardiovascular Effects

Nondepolarizing NMBDs may exert minor cardiovascular effects through drug-induced release of histamine, effects on cardiac muscarinic receptors, or effects on nicotinic receptors at autonomic ganglia (see Table 11.4). Transient hypotension can occur with atracurium and mivacurium but usually with large doses (>0.4 and 0.15 mg/kg, respectively). The relative magnitude of the circulatory effects varies from patient to patient and depends on factors such as underlying autonomic nervous system activity, blood volume status, preoperative medication, drugs administered for maintenance of anesthesia, and concurrent drug therapy.

## Critical Care Medicine and Critical Illness Myopathy and Polyneuropathy[14,15]

Currently, NMBDs are not used as often as in the past. Yet a small fraction of patients with asthma (receiving corticosteroids) or acutely injured patients with multiple organ system failure (including sepsis) who require mechanical ventilation of the lungs for prolonged periods (usually more than 6 days) may manifest prolonged skeletal muscle weakness on recovery that is augmented by the skeletal muscle paralysis produced by NMBDs. These patients exhibit moderate to severe quadriparesis with or without areflexia, but they usually retain normal sensory function. The time course of the weakness is unpredictable, and in some patients the weakness may progress and persist for weeks or months. The pathophysiology of this myopathy is not well understood. Therefore, NMBDs should be given for 2 days or less and only after the use of analgesics, sedatives, and adjustments to ventilator settings have been maximally used. Although myopathy occurs autonomously, administration of NMBDs can augment the severity of this condition. SCh probably should not be used to facilitate endotracheal intubation in critically ill patients because of reports of cardiac arrest, presumably caused by acute hyperkalemia. In fact, SCh is not allowed for use in many critical care units.

## LONG-ACTING NONDEPOLARIZING NEUROMUSCULAR BLOCKING DRUG

### Pancuronium

Pancuronium is a bisquaternary aminosteroid nondepolarizing NMBD with an $ED_{95}$ of 70 μg/kg; it has an onset of action of 3 to 5 minutes and a duration of action of 60 to 90 minutes (see Table 11.4 and Fig. 11.3). An estimated 80% of a single dose of pancuronium is eliminated unchanged in urine. In the presence of renal failure, plasma clearance of pancuronium is decreased 30% to 50%, thus resulting in a prolonged duration of action. An estimated 10% to 40% of pancuronium undergoes hepatic deacetylation to inactive metabolites, with the exception of 3-desacetylpancuronium, which is approximately 50% as potent as pancuronium at the NMJ.

#### Cardiovascular Effects

Pancuronium typically produces a modest 10% to 15% increase in heart rate, mean arterial pressure, and cardiac output. The increase in heart rate reflects pancuronium-induced selective blockade of cardiac muscarinic receptors (atropine-like effect), principally in the sinoatrial node. Histamine release and autonomic ganglion blockade are not produced by pancuronium.

## INTERMEDIATE-ACTING NONDEPOLARIZING NEUROMUSCULAR BLOCKING DRUGS

Rocuronium, vecuronium, atracurium, and cisatracurium are classified as intermediate-acting nondepolarizing NMBDs. In contrast to the long-acting nondepolarizing NMBD pancuronium, these drugs possess efficient clearance mechanisms that create a shorter duration of action.

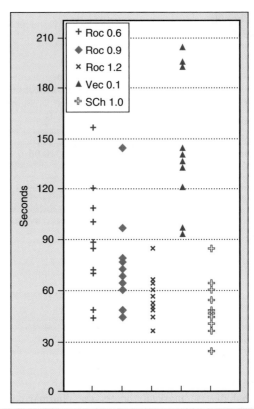

**Fig. 11.5** The onset of maximum twitch depression is similar after the intravenous administration of rocuronium (Roc) at doses of 0.9 mg/kg and 1.2 mg/kg; succinylcholine (Sch) at 1.0 mg/kg; and vecuronium (Vec) at 0.1 mg/kg. (From Magorian TT, Flannery KB, Miller RD. Comparison of rocuronium, succinylcholine, and vecuronium for rapid-sequence induction of anesthesia in adult patients. *Anesthesiology.* 1993;79:913-918, used with permission.)

When compared with pancuronium, these drugs have (1) a similar onset of maximum neuromuscular blockade, with the exception of rocuronium, which is unique because of its rapid onset, which can (with large doses) parallel that of SCh; (2) approximately one third the duration of action (hence the designation *intermediate acting*); (3) a 30% to 50% more rapid rate of recovery; and (4) minimal to absent cardiovascular effects except for atracurium. Neostigmine or sugammadex (only rocuronium and vecuronium) antagonism of the neuromuscular blockade produced by intermediate-acting nondepolarizing NMBDs is facilitated by the concomitant spontaneous recovery that occurs after rapid clearance of the drug.

### Vecuronium

Vecuronium is a monoquaternary aminosteroid nondepolarizing NMBD with an $ED_{95}$ of 50 μg/kg that produces an onset of action of 3 to 5 minutes and a duration of action of 20 to 35 minutes (see Fig. 11.3 and Table 11.4). This drug undergoes both hepatic and renal excretion. Metabolites are pharmacologically inactive, with the exception of 3-desacetylvecuronium, which is approximately 50% to 70% as potent as the parent compound. The increased lipid solubility of vecuronium as compared with pancuronium also facilitates biliary excretion of vecuronium. The effect of renal failure on the duration of action of vecuronium is small, but repeated or large doses may result in prolonged neuromuscular blockade. Vecuronium is typically devoid of circulatory effects, emphasizing its lack of vagolytic effects (pancuronium) or histamine release (atracurium).

## Rocuronium

Rocuronium is a monoquaternary aminosteroid nondepolarizing NMBD with an $ED_{95}$ of 0.3 mg/kg that has an onset of action of 1 to 2 minutes and a duration of action of 20 to 35 minutes (see Table 11.4 and Fig. 11.3). The lack of potency of rocuronium in comparison to vecuronium is an important factor in determining the rapid onset of neuromuscular blockade produced by this NMBD. Conceptually, when a large number of molecules are administered, the result is a larger number of molecules that are available to diffuse to the NMJ. Thus, a rapid onset of action is more likely to be achieved with a less potent drug such as rocuronium. The onset of maximum single twitch depression after the intravenous administration of rocuronium at 3 to 4 × $ED_{95}$ (1.2 mg/kg) resembles the onset of action of SCh after the intravenous administration of 1 mg/kg (Fig. 11.5).[16] However, the large doses of rocuronium (3 to 4 × $ED_{95}$) needed to mimic the onset time of SCh produce a duration of action resembling that of pancuronium.[17]

Clearance of rocuronium is largely as an unchanged drug in bile, with deacetylation not occurring. Renal excretion of the drug may account for as much as 30% of a dose, and administration of this drug to patients in renal failure could result in a longer duration of action, especially with repeated doses or prolonged intravenous infusion.

## Atracurium

Atracurium is a bisquaternary benzylisoquinolinium nondepolarizing NMBD (mixture of 10 stereoisomers) with an $ED_{95}$ of 0.2 mg/kg that produces an onset of action of 3 to 5 minutes and a duration of action of 20 to 35 minutes (see Table 11.4 and Fig. 11.3). Clearance of this drug is by a chemical mechanism (spontaneous nonenzymatic degradation at normal body temperature and pH known as Hofmann elimination) and a biologic mechanism (ester hydrolysis by nonspecific plasma esterases). Laudanosine is the major metabolite of both pathways. This metabolite is not active at the NMJ but may, in high, nonclinical concentrations, cause central nervous system stimulation.

The two routes of metabolism occur simultaneously and are independent of hepatic and renal function, as well as plasma cholinesterase activity. As such, the duration of atracurium-induced neuromuscular blockade is similar in normal patients and those with absent or impaired renal or hepatic function or those with atypical plasma cholinesterase (emphasizes that ester hydrolysis of atracurium is unrelated to the plasma cholinesterase responsible for the hydrolysis of SCh and mivacurium). Ester hydrolysis accounts for an estimated two thirds of degraded atracurium. Hofmann elimination (also known as *exhaustive methylation*) accounts for the remaining breakdown of atracurium.

### Cardiovascular Effects

Because of histamine release with larger doses, atracurium can cause hypotension and tachycardia. However, doses smaller than 2 × $ED_{95}$ rarely cause cardiovascular effects.

## Cisatracurium

Cisatracurium is a benzylisoquinolinium nondepolarizing NMBD with an $ED_{95}$ of 50 µg/kg that has an onset of action of 3 to 5 minutes and a duration of action of 20 to 35 minutes (see Table 11.4 and Fig. 11.3).[18] Structurally, cisatracurium is an isolated form of 1 of the 10 stereoisomers of atracurium. This drug principally undergoes degradation by Hofmann elimination. In contrast to atracurium, nonspecific plasma esterases do not seem to be involved in the clearance of cisatracurium. The organ-independent clearance of cisatracurium means that this nondepolarizing NMBD, like atracurium, can be administered to patients with renal or hepatic failure without a change in its duration of action. Cisatracurium is often used in patients undergoing renal transplantation. Cisatracurium, in contrast to atracurium, is devoid of histamine-releasing effects, so cardiovascular changes do not accompany the rapid intravenous administration of even large doses of cisatracurium.

## SHORT-ACTING NONDEPOLARIZING NEUROMUSCULAR BLOCKING DRUG

### Mivacurium

Mivacurium is a benzylisoquinolinium nondepolarizing NMBD with an $ED_{95}$ of 80 µg/kg that has an onset of action of 2 to 3 minutes and a duration of action of 12 to 20 minutes (see Table 11.4 and Fig. 11.3). As such, the duration of action of mivacurium is approximately twice that of SCh and 30% to 40% that of the intermediate-acting nondepolarizing NMBDs. Mivacurium consists of three stereoisomers, with the two most active isomers undergoing hydrolysis by plasma cholinesterase at a rate equivalent to 88% that of SCh. Hydrolysis of these two isomers is responsible for the short duration of action of mivacurium. As with SCh, hydrolysis of mivacurium is decreased and its duration of action increased in patients with atypical plasma cholinesterase (see Table 11.2). Mivacurium is currently not being marketed in the United States and not available for delivering anesthetic care.

## MONITORING THE EFFECTS OF NONDEPOLARIZING NEUROMUSCULAR BLOCKING DRUGS

Evaluation of the mechanically evoked responses produced by electrical stimulation delivered from a peripheral nerve stimulator is the most reliable method to monitor the pharmacologic effects of NMBDs. Use of a peripheral nerve stimulator permits titration of the NMBD to produce the desired pharmacologic effect, and at the conclusion of surgery the responses evoked by the nerve stimulator are used to judge spontaneous recovery from an NMBD-induced neuromuscular blockade, which is facilitated by the administration of anticholinesterase drugs (e.g., neostigmine or sugammadex) (see the discussion under "Antagonism of Nondepolarizing Neuromuscular Blocking Drugs").

Routine monitoring of neuromuscular function and blockade is strongly recommended by all experts in the field[19] and supported by large epidemiologic studies[20] and various safety organizations such as the Anesthesia Patient Safety Foundation (APSF). Yet monitoring of the neuromuscular blockade from NMBDs surprisingly is not routinely used during administration of anesthesia. Most surveys have found that only 30% to 70% of anesthesiologists in the United States and Europe use peripheral nerve stimulation as a monitor. Yet such monitoring allows NMBDs to be given in a more efficacious manner. Monitoring also provides a more precise guide for NMBD requirements intraoperatively and for the

effective antagonism by neostigmine or sugammadex. More recently, complications in the postanesthesia care unit (PACU) have been documented to be less frequent when monitoring is used.

Even though not consistently done, monitoring the effects of NMBDs should be routinely performed.[21] As with many other monitors (e.g., pulse oximetry, see Chapter 20), perhaps using objective monitoring (i.e., peripheral nerve stimulation) will become mandatory. No matter which pattern of peripheral nerve stimulation is used, clinical care will be improved if such monitoring is used. Despite the presence of studies designed to establish the relative efficacy of different types of stimulation,[22] the type of stimulation being used is of secondary importance. Nevertheless, the well-informed clinician should have some basic knowledge of the various types of stimulation proposed and used. Furthermore, the various types of stimulation have varying sensitivity with the degree of neuromuscular blockade detected (Table 11.5). Conceptually, the question that can be asked is, "How many receptors can be still occupied and have a normal response to that particular pattern of stimulation?" When the pattern of stimulation requires more receptors to be unoccupied in order to have a normal response, then that approach will be more sensitive in detecting residual neuromuscular blockade. Now the technical aspects of monitoring of neuromuscular blockade will be described.

Most often, superficial electrodes or subcutaneous needles (must have a metal hub) are placed over the ulnar nerve at the wrist or elbow or the facial nerve on the lateral aspect of the face, and a supramaximal electrical stimulus is delivered from the peripheral nerve stimulator.[23,24] The adductor pollicis muscle is innervated solely by the ulnar nerve, which accounts for the popularity of placing stimulating electrodes from the peripheral nerve stimulator over the ulnar nerve. Facial nerve stimulation and observation of the orbicularis oculi muscle, though difficult to quantitate, may be a consideration when mechanically evoked

| **Table 11.5** | Choice of Anticholinesterase Drug | | | |
|---|---|---|---|---|
| **TOF Visible Twitches** | **Estimated TOF Fade** | **Anticholinesterase Drug and Dose (mg/kg IV)** | **Anticholinergic Drug and Dose (μg/kg IV)[a]** |
| None[b] | | Not recommended | Not recommended |
| ≤2 | ++++ | Neostigmine 0.07 | Glycopyrrolate 7 or atropine 15 |
| 3-4 | +++ | Neostigmine 0.04 | Glycopyrrolate 7 or atropine 15 |
| 4 | ++ | Edrophonium 0.5 | Atropine 7 |
| 4 | 0 | Edrophonium 0.25 | Atropine 7 |

[a]Administered simultaneously with an anticholinesterase drug.
[b]Postpone drug-assisted antagonism until some evoked response is visible.
++++, Marked; +++, moderate; ++, minimal; 0, none; IV, intravenous; TOF, train-of-four.
Modified from Bevan DR, Donati F, Kopman AF. Reversal of neuromuscular blockade. *Anesthesiology.* 1992;77:785-792, used with permission.

responses to stimulation of the ulnar nerve are not visible because of positioning of the upper extremities.[25] Another consideration is the observation that monitoring the response of the orbicularis oculi muscle to facial nerve stimulation more closely reflects the onset of neuromuscular blockade at the larynx than does the response of the adductor pollicis to ulnar nerve stimulation (Fig. 11.6).[26] Moreover, the onset of neuromuscular blockade after the administration of nondepolarizing NMBDs is more rapid but less intense at the laryngeal muscles (vocal cords) than at the peripheral muscles (adductor pollicis) (see Fig. 11.5).[25] In this regard, the period of laryngeal paralysis may be dissipating before a maximum effect is reached at the adductor pollicis. In contrast, the onset of neuromuscular blockade at the laryngeal muscles and at the muscles innervated by the ulnar nerve is similar when SCh is administered. Thus, monitoring the twitch response at the adductor pollicis is more likely to parallel the intensity of the drug-induced effect at the laryngeal adductors when SCh is administered.

## Patterns of Stimulation

Mechanically evoked responses used for monitoring the effects of NMBDs include the single twitch response, TOF ratio, double burst stimulation, tetanus, and post-tetanic stimulation (Figs. 11.6 to 11.10).[23,24] These mechanically evoked responses are evaluated visually, manually by touch (tactile), or by recording. The depth of neuromuscular blockade may be defined as the percentage of a predetermined inhibition of twitch response from control height (ED$_{95}$, dose necessary to depress the twitch

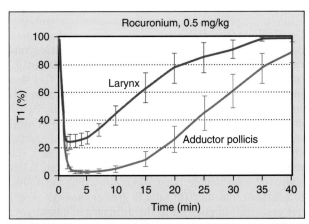

**Fig. 11.6** The effects of rocuronium (in terms of maximum depression of the single twitch [T1] response) are less intense and the duration of action is less at the adductor muscles of the larynx than at the adductor pollicis. (From Meistelman C, Plaud B, Donati F. Rocuronium [ORG 9426] neuromuscular blockade at the adductor muscles of the larynx and adductor pollicis in humans. *Can J Anaesth.* 1992;39:665-669, used with permission.)

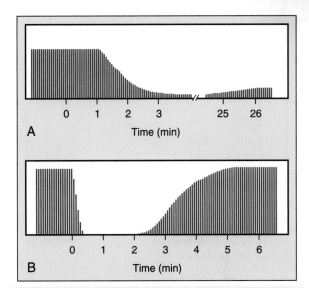

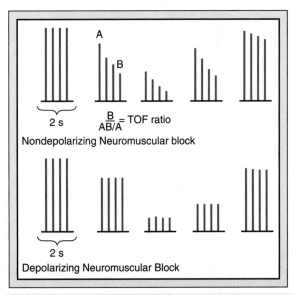

**Fig. 11.7** Schematic illustration of the onset and recovery from the neuromuscular blocking effects of a nondepolarizing (A) or a depolarizing (B) neuromuscular blocking drug ("0 time" indicates injection of the neuromuscular blocking drug) as depicted by the mechanically evoked single twitch response to repeated electrical stimulation of the nerve. (Modified from Viby-Mogensen J. Clinical assessment of neuromuscular transmission. *Br J Anaesth.* 1982;54:209-223, used with permission.)

**Fig. 11.8** Schematic illustration of the mechanically evoked response to train-of-four (TOF) electrical stimulation of the nerve after injection of a nondepolarizing neuromuscular blocking drug (upper panel) or a depolarizing (succinylcholine) neuromuscular blocking drug (lower panel). The TOF ratio, given by the relation of the first response (upper panel) to the fourth (lower panel), is less than 1 (fades) only in the presence of (upper panel) effects at the neuromuscular junction produced by a nondepolarizing neuromuscular blocking drug. (Modified from Viby-Mogensen J. Clinical assessment of neuromuscular transmission. *Br J Anaesth.* 1982;54:209-223, used with permission.)

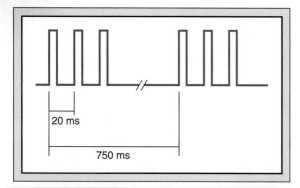

**Fig. 11.9** Schematic illustration of the stimulation pattern of double burst stimulation (three electrical impulses at 50 Hz separated by 750 ms). (From Bevan DR, Donati F, Kopman AF. Reversal of neuromuscular blockade. *Anesthesiology.* 1992;77:785-792, used with permission.)

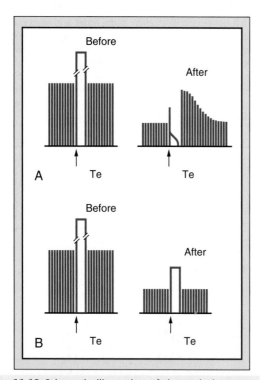

**Fig. 11.10** Schematic illustration of the evoked response to tetanic (Te) stimulation (50 Hz for 5 seconds) before and after the intravenous injection of a nondepolarizing neuromuscular blocking drug (A) or a depolarizing (succinylcholine) neuromuscular blocking drug (B). (Modified from Viby-Mogensen J. Clinical assessment of neuromuscular transmission. *Br J Anaesth.* 1982;54:209-223, used with permission.)

response 95%) and the duration of drug effect as the time from drug administration until the twitch response recovers to a percentage of control height (see Table 11.4).

The response to peripheral nerve stimulation can be used to answer the following questions:

1. Is the neuromuscular blockade adequate for surgery?
2. Is the neuromuscular blockade excessive?
3. Can this neuromuscular blockade be antagonized?

Depression of the twitch response greater than 90% or elimination of two to three twitches of the TOF correlates with acceptable skeletal muscle relaxation for performance of intra-abdominal surgery in the presence of an adequate concentration of volatile anesthetic. If all twitches from TOF stimulation are absent, more NMBD should not be given until some twitch is present. If some of the twitches from TOF stimulation are present, antagonism is likely to be successful (see the section, "Antagonism of Nondepolarizing Neuromuscular Blocking Drugs").

### Train-of-Four Stimulation

TOF stimulation (four electrical stimulations at 2 Hz delivered every 0.5 second) is based on the concept that ACh is depleted by successive stimulations. Only four twitches are necessary because subsequent stimulation fails to further alter the release of additional ACh. In the presence of effects produced at the NMJ by nondepolarizing NMBDs, the height of the fourth twitch is lower than that of the first twitch, thereby allowing calculation of a TOF ratio (fade) (see Fig. 11.8).[23] Recovery of the TOF ratio to greater than 0.7 correlates with complete return to control height of a single twitch response. In the presence of effects produced at the NMJ by SCh, the TOF ratio remains near 1.0 because the height of all four twitch responses is decreased by a similar amount (phase I blockade) (see Fig. 11.8).[23] A TOF ratio of less than 0.3 in the presence of SCh reflects phase II blockade (see Table 11.1).

### Double Burst Stimulation

Accurate estimation of the TOF ratio is not reliable clinically by either visual or manual assessment. Difficulty in estimating the TOF ratio may be due to the fact that the two middle twitch responses interfere with comparison of the first and last twitch response. In this regard, double burst stimulation (two bursts of three electrical stimulations separated by 750 ms) is perceived by the observer as two separate twitches (see Fig. 11.9).[24] The observer's ability to detect a TOF ratio less than 0.3 is improved with double burst stimulation, but the ability to conclude that the TOF ratio is greater than 0.7 is still not ensured.[27] In contrast to the difficulty in quantifying the TOF ratio, determination of the number of electrically evoked twitch responses to TOF stimulation is more likely to be reproducible. For example, the fourth twitch can be observed when the first twitch is equivalent to 30% to 40% of control twitch height, which corresponds to a TOF ratio of about 0.35. Counting the number of visible TOF responses may be helpful in predicting the ease with which neuromuscular blockade can be antagonized

**Table 11.6**   Clinical Tests of Neuromuscular Transmission

| Test | Normal Function | % of Receptors Occupied[a] | Comment |
|---|---|---|---|
| Tidal volume | 5 mL/kg | 80 | Insensitive |
| Train-of-four | No fade | 70 | Somewhat uncomfortable |
| Vital capacity | At least 20 mL/kg | 70 | Requires patient cooperation |
| Sustained tetanus (50 Hz) | No fade | 60 | Uncomfortable |
| Double burst stimulation | No fade | 60 | Uncomfortable |
| Head lift | 180 degrees for 5 s | 50 | Requires patient cooperation |
| Handgrips | Sustained for 5 s | 50 | Requires patient cooperation |

[a]Approximate percentage of receptors occupied when the response returns to its normal value.
Modified from Naguib M, Lien CA. Pharmacology of muscle relaxants and their antagonists. In Miller RD, ed. *Miller's Anesthesia*. 6th ed. Philadelphia: Churchill Livingstone; 2005; and from Viby-Morgensen J, Claudius C. Neuromuscular monitoring. In Miller RD, ed. *Miller's Anesthesia*. 8th ed. Philadelphia: Elsevier Saunders; 2015.

with an anticholinesterase drug (see Table 11.6) (see the section, "Antagonism of Nondepolarizing Neuromuscular Blocking Drugs").[24]

### Tetanus

Tetanus (continuous or tetanic electrical stimulation for 5 seconds at about 50 Hz) is an intense stimulus for the release of ACh at the NMJ. In the presence of effects produced at the NMJ by nondepolarizing NMBDs, the response to tetanus is not sustained (fades), whereas in the presence of SCh-induced effects at the NMJ, the response to tetanus is greatly decreased but does not fade with a phase I blockade (see Fig. 11.10).[23] A sustained response to tetanus is present when the TOF ratio is greater than 0.7. At the cessation of tetanus, there is an increase in the immediately available stores of ACh such that the subsequent twitch responses are transiently enhanced (post-tetanic facilitation) (see Fig. 11.10).[23,25,26]

## ANTAGONISM OF NONDEPOLARIZING NEUROMUSCULAR BLOCKING DRUGS

For decades, antagonism of the effects of nondepolarizing NMBDs has been achieved by the intravenous administration of an anticholinesterase drug (usually neostigmine, but possibly and rarely edrophonium or pyridostigmine) on a routine basis. Now both neostigmine and sugammadex are available. Some principles are the same for both reversal drugs. Even if all tests of the adequacy of normal neuromuscular function are normal, 50% of the receptors at the NMJ may still be occupied by an NMBD. Patients will likely need more available receptors for adequate skeletal muscle strength. The unresolved question is if the response to peripheral nerve stimulation is normal, should one still give a small dose of neostigmine (e.g., 1.0 mg/70 kg) or sugammadex (e.g., 2 mg/kg)? An excellent rule to follow is, "When in doubt, it is better to have as many receptors free of the effects of NMBDs as possible" (see Tables 11.5 and 11.6).[23,24] Unequivocal clinical confirmation (sustained head lift or leg lift, or both, for 5 seconds, tongue depressor test, or a TOF > 0.9) provides assurance of adequate recovery (spontaneous and drug assisted) from the effects of NMBDs.

## ADVERSE OUTCOMES FROM INADEQUATE ANTAGONISM OF NEUROMUSCULAR BLOCKADE

The time starting with the extubation of the trachea, transport to the PACU, and the first 30 minutes in the PACU can be one of the most dangerous times in the perioperative period. Inadequately antagonized or residual neuromuscular blockade can impair the integrity of the airway[28] and cause critical respiratory events in the PACU.[29] Analysis of large numbers of patients indicate that residual neuromuscular blockade is usually a component of adverse outcomes and even death. Specifically, residual neuromuscular blockade contributes to airway obstruction, inadequate ventilation, and hypoxia and has an incidence of 0.8% to 6.9%.[29] Other factors contributing to adverse effects in the PACU include obesity, opioids, emergency surgery, long duration of surgery, and abdominal surgery.[29] Clearly, clinicians should do everything possible to assure that residual neuromuscular blockade does not persist into the postoperative period by careful monitoring,[30,31] close observation, and alertness that such a blockade might exist.[32] The importance of residual neuromuscular blockade is increasingly recognized by scholarly analysis of this topic.[31-33]

### Anticholinesterase Drugs (Neostigmine)

Anticholinesterase drugs are typically administered during the time when spontaneous recovery from the neuromuscular blockade is occurring so that the effect of the pharmacologic antagonist adds to the rate of spontaneous recovery from the nondepolarizing NMBD. Neostigmine is the most common anticholinesterase drug currently used. The rapid spontaneous recovery rate characteristic of intermediate-acting NMBDs is an advantage over a long-acting NMBD such as pancuronium. For example, the incidence of weakness in the postoperative period despite administration of neostigmine is more frequent in patients receiving pancuronium than an intermediate- or short-acting NMBD.

Anticholinesterase drugs, such as neostigmine, accelerate the already established pattern of spontaneous recovery at the NMJ by inhibiting the activity of acetylcholinesterase and thereby leading to the accumulation of ACh at nicotinic neuromuscular and muscarinic sites. Increased amounts of ACh in the region of the NMJ improve the chance that two ACh molecules will bind to the α-subunits of the nicotinic cholinergic receptors (see Fig. 11.2). This action alters the balance of the competition between ACh and a nondepolarizing NMBD in favor of the neurotransmitter (ACh) and restores neuromuscular transmission. In addition, neostigmine may generate antidromic action potentials and repetitive firing of motor nerve endings (presynaptic effects).

The quaternary ammonium structure of anticholinesterase drugs greatly limits their entrance into the central nervous system such that selective antagonism of the peripheral nicotinic effects of nondepolarizing NMBDs at the NMJ is possible. For example, the peripheral cardiac muscarinic effects of neostigmine (bradycardia) are prevented by the prior or simultaneous intravenous administration of atropine or glycopyrrolate. In fact, either atropine or glycopyrrolate must be given when neostigmine is given.

## Factors Influencing the Success of Antagonism of Neuromuscular Blocking Drugs

Factors influencing the success of antagonism of NMBDs include (1) the intensity of the neuromuscular blockade at the time that the pharmacologic antagonist is administered, (2) the choice of antagonist drug, (3) the dose of antagonist drug, (4) the rate of spontaneous recovery from the NMBD, and (5) the concentration of the inhaled anesthetic.

Although sugammadex is an exciting, relatively new antagonist of vecuronium and rocuronium, for over 50 years neostigmine has been the most commonly administered antagonist for nearly all nondepolarizing NMBDs. First, neostigmine will be described. The greater the spontaneous recovery, as judged by the response to peripheral nerve stimulation, the more rapidly complete recovery will occur from neostigmine administration. Although large doses of neostigmine will result in more rapid antagonism, the maximum dose should be limited to 60 to 70 μg/kg. Antagonism will be more rapid in the presence of an NMBD with rapid elimination (atracurium instead of pancuronium). The rate of antagonism can also be hastened by reducing the concentration of the volatile anesthetic.

## Evaluation of the Adequacy of Antagonism

Adequacy of recovery (spontaneous and drug assisted) from the neuromuscular blocking effects produced by nondepolarizing NMBDs should be determined by the result of multiple tests of skeletal muscle strength (see Table 11.6).[30-33] Even though a TOF ratio of at least 0.9 has been recommended, visual estimation of the TOF is neither accurate nor reliable. In the absence of an accurately measured TOF ratio, a sustained response to tetanus or the ability to maintain head lift for 5 to 10 seconds usually indicates a TOF ratio greater than 0.9. Grip strength is also a useful indicator of recovery from the effects of NMBDs. Although a TOF ratio higher than 0.7 or its equivalent provides evidence of the patient's ability to sustain adequate ventilation, the pharyngeal musculature may still be weak and upper airway obstruction remains a risk. Furthermore, diplopia, dysphagia, an increased risk of aspiration of gastric contents, and a decreased ventilatory response to hypoxia in the presence of a TOF ratio more than 0.9 emphasize the value of more sensitive clinical methods for assessing neuromuscular function, such as sustained head lift or leg lift (or both) for 5 seconds or an evaluation of masseter muscle strength (tongue depressor test).[33]

Allowing spontaneous recovery from NMBDs without the aid of drug-assisted antagonism (i.e., administration of neostigmine or sugammadex) is not recommended unless there is compelling clinical evidence that significant residual neuromuscular blockade does not persist.

When the initial response to an anticholinesterase drug (i.e., neostigmine) seems inadequate, the following questions should be answered before additional antagonist drug is administered:

1. Has sufficient time elapsed for neostigmine or sugammadex to antagonize the nondepolarizing NMBD (15 to 30 minutes with neostigmine and more rapidly with sugammadex)?
2. Is the neuromuscular block too intense to be antagonized?
3. Is acid-base and electrolyte status normal?
4. Is body temperature normal?
5. Is the patient taking any drugs that could interfere with antagonism?
6. Has clearance of the nondepolarizing NMBD from plasma been decreased by renal or hepatic dysfunction (or by both)?

Answers to these questions will often provide the reason for failure of anticholinesterase drugs, such as neostigmine, to adequately antagonize nondepolarizing neuromuscular blockade.

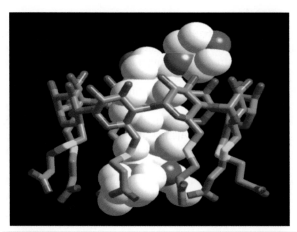

**Fig. 11.11** The sugammadex-rocuronium complex. The white central structure is rocuronium. The green, red, and a bit of yellow tubular structure is sugammadex. A simple explanation is that sugammadex "encircles" rocuronium and transports it away from the neuromuscular junction. In the literature it is stated that sugammadex "encapsulates rocuronium." That complex leaves the neuromuscular junction to be excreted. The neuromuscular junction can then restore its normal function. (From Bom A, Bradley M, Cameron K, et al. A novel concept of reversing neuromuscular block: chemical encapsulation of rocuronium bromide by a cyclodextrin-based synthetic host. *Angew Chem Int Ed Engl.* 41:266-270, 2002.)

## A New Antagonist of Neuromuscular Blocking Drugs[34]

A γ-cyclodextrin (sugammadex) (Fig. 11.11) is a relatively new antagonist, which antagonizes steroidal NMBDs, especially rocuronium and vecuronium, by encapsulating and inactivating them. Sugammadex transports rocuronium or vecuronium away from the NMJ. This mechanism of action is totally different from that of neostigmine in that no action on any cholinesterase takes place. Sugammadex has no action itself at the NMJ. The rate that it reliably reverses even a profound neuromuscular block is rapid (2 to 3 minutes) and complete. Furthermore, no cardiovascular effects occur; therefore, no other drug such as atropine is needed. Large doses of sugammadex can be given alone without cardiovascular effects. It could have significant impact in three major ways. First, a rocuronium-sugammadex combination can be used for a rapid sequence induction of anesthesia and recovery more rapid than with SCh. Second, it can allow more profound neuromuscular blocks to be induced intraoperatively without fear of inadequate reversal. Last, as indicated earlier, the incidence of residual neuromuscular blockade should be reduced or possibly eliminated.[35-37]

Sugammadex has been approved for use in Europe and successfully used in thousands of patients. It was approved in many other countries in 2010. As of December 2015, it has been approved in the United States. Many years ago, it was this author's original belief that sugammadex would completely replace neostigmine. Although sugammadex is growing in popularity, neostigmine is still commonly used as a routine antagonist of a rocuronium or possibly vecuronium neuromuscular blockade. Sugammadex has been much more expensive than neostigmine. Ironically, as reported in a "Letter to the Editor" in the August 2015 issue of the AANA, neostigmine may undergo additional review, which could alter its presentation and cost.

In certain clinical situations specific doses of sugammadex are recommended: (1) sugammadex, 2 mg/kg, if two of the four twitches from TOF stimulation appear; and (2) sugammadex, 4 mg/kg, should be given if one or two post-tetanic counts (PTC) occur and there is no recovery of the twitch response from TOF stimulation. These recommendations apply to either vecuronium or rocuronium. The last recommendation is for only rocuronium. If rocuronium, 1.2 mg/kg, has been given for a rapid sequence induction of anesthesia, the neuromuscular blockade can be terminated by giving sugammadex, 16 mg/kg. This approach may be necessary with extreme airway problems. Of prime importance is that nearly all of the FDA instructions or recommendations assume that adequate monitoring of neuromuscular function is being performed.

A common concept is to allow as much spontaneous recovery from neuromuscular blockade as possible before giving neostigmine. The ability of neostigmine to antagonize a profound neuromuscular blockade has always been questionable. Clearly the proper use of sugammadex should allow more clinical use of profound neuromuscular blockade and with a resultant successful reversal. One possibility is that laparoscopic surgery procedures may benefit from continuous profound neuromuscular blockade, especially when closing the surgical wound. Sugammadex can reverse a profound neuromuscular blockade.[37,38] Understandably, surgeons would prefer a profound neuromuscular block for the entire surgical procedure.[39] However, patient outcome is not clearly better. For example, Staehr-Rye and associates[38] found that deep neuromuscular blockade was only marginally better than moderate block for laparosopic cholecystectomy.

Anesthesia for electroconvulsive therapy is commonly achieved by the administration of thiopental and SCh. The use of rocuronium and sugammadex for electroconvulsive therapy may be associated with fewer cardiac arrhythmias and muscle pain.

## SUMMARY

NMBDs are vital components of anesthetic care and airway management. When these drugs were introduced over 50 years ago, we were taught to either give small doses or even avoid paralysis if possible. We now have much safer drugs, better antagonist drugs and monitoring devices, and more knowledge. We even have evidence that proper use of NMBDs can add a measure of safety if properly used.[33] The principles in this chapter represent contemporary use of NMBDs and their antagonists.[34]

## QUESTIONS OF THE DAY

1. What is the normal sequence of neuromuscular transmission, beginning with the arrival of an impulse at the motor nerve terminal?

2. What mechanism is responsible for the termination of succinylcholine (SCh) neuromuscular blockade? How does this compare to the termination of acetylcholine's (ACh's) s actions at the neuromuscular junction?

3. What are the potential adverse effects of SCh? Which effects are potentially life threatening?

4. What are the train-of-four (TOF), double burst, and tetanus patterns of peripheral nerve stimulation? How can the results of peripheral nerve stimulation be used to determine if neuromuscular blockade is adequate for surgery?

5. How can TOF monitoring be used to determine whether a nondepolarizing neuromuscular block can be antagonized with neostigmine? How can the adequacy of antagonism be evaluated?

6. What is the mechanism of sugammadex antagonism of steroidal neuromuscular blockade? What are the clinical advantages and disadvantages of sugammadex compared to neostigmine?

## REFERENCES

1. McNeill O, Kerridge RK, Boyle MJ. Review of procedures for investigation of anaesthesia-associated anaphylaxis in Newcastle, Australia. *Anaesth Intensive Care.* 2008;36:201–207.

2. Harboe T, Guttormsen AB, Irgens A, et al. Anaphylaxis during anesthesia in Norway: a 6-year single-center follow-up study. *Anesthesiology.* 2005;102:897–903.

3. Gurrieri C, Weingarten TN, Martin DP. Allergic reactions during anesthesia at a large United States referral center. *Anesth Analg.* 2011;113:1202–1212.

4. Fagerlund MJ, Eriksson LI. Current concepts in neuromuscular transmission. *Br J Anaesth.* 2009;103:108–114.

5. Gronert GA. Succinylcholine-induced hyperkalemia and beyond. *Anesthesiology.* 1975;2009(111):1372–1377.

6. Martyn JAJ, Richtsfeld M. Succinylcholine-induced hyperkalemia in acquired pathologic states: etiologic factors and molecular mechanisms. *Anesthesiology.* 2006;104:158–169.

7. Miller R. Will succinylcholine ever disappear? *Anesth Analg.* 2004;98:1674–1675.

8. Naguib M, Lien CA, Aker J, et al. Posttetanic potentiation and fade in the response to tetanic and train-of-four stimulation during succinylcholine-induced block. *Anesth Analg.* 2004;98:1686–1691.

9. Baumann A, Studnicska D, Audibert G, et al. Refractory anaphylactic cardiac arrest after succinylcholine administration. *Anesth Analg.* 2009;109:137–140.

10. Holak EJ, Connelly JF, Pagel PS. Suxamethonium-induced hyperkalaemia 6 weeks after chemoradiotherapy in a patient with rectal carcinoma. *Br J Anaesth.* 2007;98:766–768.

11. Schreiber JU, Lysakowski C, Fuchs-Buder T, et al. Prevention of succinylcholine-induced fasciculation and myalgia: a meta-analysis of randomized trials. *Anesthesiology.* 2005;103:877–884.

12. Libonati MM, Leahy JJ, Ellison N. The use of succinylcholine in open eye surgery. *Anesthesiology.* 1985;62:637–640.

13. Kelly RE, Dinner M, Turner LS, et al. Succinylcholine increases intraocular pressure in the human eye with the extraocular muscles detached. *Anesthesiology.* 1993;79:948–952.

14. Farhan H, Moreno-Duarte I, Latronico N, et al. Acquired muscle weakness in the surgical intensive care unit: nosology, epidemiology, diagnosis, and prevention. *Anesthesiology.* 2016;124:207–234.

15. Appleton R, Kinsella J. Intensive care unit-acquired weakness. *Contin Educ Anaesth Crit Care Pain.* 2012;12:62–65.

16. Magorian T, Flannery KB, Miller RD. Comparison of rocuronium, succinylcholine and vecuronium for rapid sequence induction of anesthesia. *Anesthesiology.* 1993;79:913–918.

17. Sluga M, Ummenhofer W, Studer W, et al. Rocuronium versus succinylcholine for rapid sequence induction of anesthesia and endotracheal intubation: a prospective, randomized trial in emergent cases. *Anesth Analg.* 2005;101:1356–1361.

18. Mellinghoff H, Radbruch L, Diefenbach C, et al. A comparison of cisatracurium and atracurium: onset of neuromuscular block after bolus injection and recovery after subsequent infusion. *Anesth Analg.* 1996;83:1072–1075.

19. Brull SJ, Prielipp RC. Reversal of neuromuscular blockade. *Anesthesiology.* 2015;122:1183–1184.

20. McLean DJ, Diaz-Gil D, Farhan HN, et al. Dose-dependent association between intermediate-acting neuromuscular-blocking agents and postoperative respiratory complications. *Anesthesiology.* 2015;122:1201–1216.

21. Eriksson LI. Evidence-based practice and neuromuscular monitoring: it's time for routine quantitative assessment. *Anesthesiology.* 2003;98:1037–1039.

22. Claudius C, Skovgaard LT, Viby-Mogensen J. Is the performance of acceleromyography improved with preload and normalization? *Anesthesiology.* 2009;110:1261–1270.

23. Viby-Mogensen J. Clinical assessment of neuromuscular transmission. *Br J Anaesth.* 1982;54:209–223.

24. Bevan DR, Donati F, Kopman AF. Reversal of neuromuscular blockade. *Anesthesiology.* 1992;77:785–792.

25. Sayson SC, Mongan PD. Onset of action of mivacurium chloride: a comparison of neuromuscular blockade monitoring at the adductor pollicis and the orbicularis oculi. *Anesthesiology.* 1994;81:35–42.

26. Meistelman C, Plaud B, Donati F. Rocuronium (ORG 9426) neuromuscular blockade at the adductor muscles of the larynx and adductor pollicis in humans. *Can J Anaesth.* 1992;39:665–669.

27. Kopman AF, Yee PS, Neuman GG. Relationship of the train-of-four fade to the clinical signs and symptoms of residual paralysis in awake volunteers. *Anesthesiology.* 1997;86:765–771.

28. Herbstreit F, Peters J, Eikermann M. Impaired upper airway integrity by residual neuromuscular blockade: increased airway collapsibility and blunted genioglossus muscle activity in response to negative pharyngeal pressure. *Anesthesiology.* 2009;110:1253–1260.

29. Murphy GS, Szokol JW, Marymont JH, et al. Residual neuromuscular blockade and critical respiratory events in the postanesthesia care unit. *Anesth Analg.* 2008;107:130–137.

30. Brull SJ, Naguib M, Miller RD. Residual neuromuscular block: rediscovering the obvious. *Anesth Analg.* 2008;107:11–14.

31. Murphy GS, Szokol JW, Marymont JH, et al. Intraoperative acceleromyographic monitoring reduces the risk of residual neuromuscular blockade and adverse respiratory events in the postanesthesia care unit. *Anesthesiology.* 2008;109:389–398.

32. Kopman AF. Residual neuromuscular block and adverse respiratory events. *Anesth Analg.* 2008;107:1756.

33. Srivastava A, Hunter JM. Reversal of neuromuscular block. *Br J Anaesth.* 2009;103:115–129.

34. Caldwell JE, Miller RD. Clinical implications of sugammadex. *Anaesthesia.* 2009;64:66–72.

35. Hammaguchi S, Tezuka N, Nagao M. Rocuronium and sugammadex under TOF monitoring on mECT. *J Anesth.* 2015;29:815.

36. Bruekmann B, Sasaki N, Grobara P, et al. Effects of sugammadex on incidence of postoperative residual neuromuscular blockade: a randomized, controlled study. *Br J Anaesth.* 2015;115:743–751.

37. Kim HJ, Lee K, Park WK, et al. Deep neuromuscular block improves the surgical conditions for laryngeal microsurgery. *Br J Anaesth.* 2015;115:867–872.

38. Staehr-Rye AM, Rassmussen LS, Rosenberg J, et al. Surgical space conditions during low-pressure laparoscopic cholecystectomy with deep versus moderate neuromuscular blockade. *Anesth Analg.* 2014;119:1084–1091.

39. Donati F, Brull SJ. More muscle relaxation does not necessarily mean better surgeons or "the problem of muscle relaxation in surgery." *Anesth Analg.* 2014;119:1019–1021.

II

# 12 ANESTHETIC NEUROTOXICITY*

## Mary Ellen McCann and Sulpicio G. Soriano, II

A major concern within the specialty of anesthesiology for many years has been the impact of general anesthesia and sedative drugs on neurodevelopment and cognition across the life span. Although definitive conclusions cannot be made, anesthesia providers should follow the progress of our knowledge regarding longer-term effects of anesthesia on the brain. For sure, neuronal cell death and neurocognitive impairments after general anesthesia have been unequivocally demonstrated in laboratory animal models.[1] This public health concern has prompted the Food and Drug Administration to issue a Drug Safety Communication "warning that repeated or lengthy use of general anesthetic and sedation drugs during surgeries or procedures in children younger than 3 years of age or in pregnant women during their third trimester may affect the development of children's brains"[2] (also see Chapter 34). However, this is not a new concern. In 1953, Eckenhoff warned about an abnormal incidence of postoperative personality changes in children.[3] Since then, preclinical reports on juvenile animal models unequivocally demonstrate a causal effect of general anesthesia on subsequent neurotoxic and neurocognitive dysfunction.[4] In addition, in 1955 Bedford wrote about behavioral changes in the elderly after general anesthesia.[5] Laboratory reports from several groups have found that anesthetic drugs induce histologic, biochemical, and neurocognitive deficits in mature rodents.[6]

Anesthetic drugs are potent modulators of the central nervous system (CNS) and reversibly render patients insensate to painful procedures and surgery.[7] Although the exact molecular mechanisms that produce immobility, analgesia, and amnesia are unknown, most anesthetic and sedative drugs are either γ-aminobutyric acid (GABA) receptor agonists, N-methyl-D-aspartate (NMDA) glutamate receptor antagonists, or a combination of the

*This work was supported by the National Institutes of Health grant 1-R01 HD06 1136-01A1 (MEM) and the Boston Children's Hospital Endowed Chair in Pediatric Neuroanesthesia (SGS).

two. General anesthesia and sedation can be achieved by inhaled or intravenous administration of specific drugs. Both GABA agonists and NMDA antagonists have been implicated in causing anesthetic-induced developmental neurotoxicity (AIDN). Both the short-term and the long-term neurocognitive effects of general anesthesia should be considered.

## ANESTHETIC DRUGS AS A CAUSE FOR NEURODEGENERATION AND LONG-TERM NEUROCOGNITIVE DEFICITS

### Basic Science of Anesthetic-Induced Developmental Neurotoxicity

Determining the root cause of the neurotoxic effect of CNS depressant drugs on the developing brain is complicated by the myriad of molecular targets and the still unknown mechanistic pathway to achieve general anesthesia.[8] AIDN has been demonstrated in laboratory models, both in vivo and in vitro, by exposure to most anesthetic and sedative drugs commonly administered to pediatric patients (also see Chapter 34). A comparable pattern of neurodegeneration and impaired neurocognitive development has been described with the perinatal administration of alcohol and anticonvulsant drugs.[9,10] AIDN was first described more than 40 years ago in fetal and postnatal rats exposed to halothane,[11] but its impact was not fully publicized to both the scientific and lay community until a 1999 report that emphasized that ketamine increased neurodegeneration in neonatal rat pups.[12] Subsequently, it was found that the combination of commonly used anesthetic drugs—isoflurane, nitrous oxide, and midazolam—not only induced neuroapoptosis but resulted in deficits in hippocampal synaptic function and learning behavior.[13] Although the anesthetic mechanisms of NMDA antagonists (ketamine and nitrous oxide) and GABA agonists (isoflurane, sevoflurane, desflurane, propofol, and midazolam) are divergent, preclinical reports clearly demonstrate neurodegenerative and neurocognitive changes in animal models.

Anesthesia removes sensory input and suppresses normal neural traffic, which in turn diminishes the trophic support required for neurogenesis and context-dependent modulation of neuroplasticity. However, several reports have described neuronal cell death mechanisms such as excitotoxicity, mitochondrial dysfunction, aberrant cell cycle reentry, trophic factor dysregulation, and disruption of cytoskeletal assembly.[14-18] Although GABA acts as an inhibitory drug in the mature brain, it is an excitatory agent during early stages of brain development, owing to the preponderance of the immature Na/K/2Cl transporter protein NKCC1, which produces a chloride influx leading to neuron depolarization. Therefore, GABA remains excitatory until the GABA receptors are switched to the normal inhibitory mode when the mature chloride transporter, KCC2, is expressed, which actively transports chloride out of the neural cell.[19]

### Age-Dependent Vulnerability of Anesthetic

Neural development progresses through several steps that include neurogenesis, neuronal morphogenesis, and synaptogenesis.[20] Neurogenesis starts with the creation of progenitor cells, which proliferate and differentiate into neurons or glial cells. Then oligodendrocytes and astrocytes appear, which serve as supporting cells for neurons. This proliferative (cell cycle) stage produces an overabundance of progenitor cells that develop into neural and glial cells.[21] These cells can exit the cell cycle at different times to assume specific functions. A subpopulation remains undifferentiated and remains in the cell cycle. As neurons undergo terminal differentiation into a postmitotic state, they can no longer replicate. Dendrites and axons extend from the cell body to form functional synapses with other neurons. Most neurons (up to 70%) are eliminated during normal development by early elimination and programmed cell death (apoptosis), both normal components of neurodevelopment.[22] CNS neural development is regulated by early elimination during the embryonal stage and programmed cell death after birth. Redundant neural progenitor cells and neurons that do not migrate properly or make synapses are physiologically pruned by apoptosis.[23]

Critical periods of plasticity during brain development are modulated by environmental cues and have been implicated in perceptual development in vision and speech.[24,25] Likewise, the perioperative environment can influence brain development. Anesthetic drugs are powerful modulators of neuronal circuits and have an impact on the constant flux of CNS development and remodeling in both health and disease states.[26] Because neurogenesis is ongoing throughout life, from the fetus to the elderly, these neural progenitor cells are vulnerable to the toxic effects of anesthetic drugs. Exposure to isoflurane produces neuronal cell death in brain regions where neural progenitor cells reside.[27] Therefore, susceptibility to AIDN extends from the fetal period to late adulthood.

Brain growth spurt in most species is likely the time of maximal susceptibility to AIDN. This time corresponds with the time of maximal synaptogenesis. The growth spurt of human brains occurs in the last trimester of gestation until about 3 to 4 years of age, which is the time that children are most vulnerable to the negative effects of general anesthesia (also see Chapter 34). There is controversy about this though. Yet, neuroinformatic mapping of the development of corticospinal tracts across species demonstrates that 7-day-old rat pups are neurodevelopmentally closer to 20- to 22-week-old human fetuses.[28] This is also the time of maximal susceptibility to fetal alcohol syndrome, which involves fetal exposure to alcohol, which is both a GABA agonist as well as an NMDA antagonist.

The timing of maximal brain growth during development is species dependent. Rodents are altricial species and much of their neurodevelopment occurs postnatally. This time period occurs from about postnatal day 6 through postnatal day 21. Simian species including humans are usually considered precocial and typically have a longer gestation because offspring are born at a relatively advanced stage of development. Rhesus monkeys are susceptible to anesthetic-induced neuroapoptosis when exposed as fetuses or up to day 6 of life.[29-32] However, AIDN has not been demonstrated when the exposure occurs on day 35 postnatally.[14] Five-day-old rhesus monkeys given equivalent human concentrations (0.5%-1.5%) of isoflurane for 4 to 6 hours, either with or without nitrous oxide, developed extensive neuroapoptosis found in the temporal, frontal, and hippocampal areas of the brain.[31] However, ketamine given in very large doses for a prolonged duration causes both an increased level of neuroapoptosis, and later, learning deficits in exposed rhesus monkeys.[32,33]

The time of exposure during development results in contrasting patterns of neural fate. Exposure of anesthetics to pregnant rats results in increased apoptotic cells in the brains of the fetuses.[34] Administration of anesthetics to neonatal rodents leads to increased apoptosis and stunted axonal growth and dendritic arborization. In contrast, anesthetic exposure in juvenile rat models does not increase apoptosis but leads to enhanced dendritic formation and synaptic density.[35,36] It is of concern that similar altered dendritic morphologic appearance has been observed in psychiatric and neurologic disorders.[37]

## Characterization of AIDN

### Pathologic Apoptosis

Accelerated apoptosis is the hallmark of AIDN (Table 12.1).[12,13] Although an essential process in controlling neural development, the apoptotic pathway is also activated by cellular stress.[38] Such stresses include glucocorticoids, heat, radiation, starvation, infection, hypoxia, pain, and anesthetics. Apoptosis is almost always executed by caspase enzymes, which are cysteine dependent aspartate proteases that either initiate the apoptotic process (caspases 2, 8, 9, and 10) or affect the process (caspases 3, and 7). The two main pathways are the extrinsic and intrinsic pathways. The extrinsic pathway is mediated by death receptors on the cell membrane wall whereas the intrinsic pathway is dependent on mitochondrial activation.

The extrinsic pathway involves the Fas ligand to the Fas cell wall receptor, which then becomes the Fas-associated death domain, or FADD. This joins with either procaspase 8 or 10 to become a death-inducing signaling complex (DISC). This activates the effector caspase 3 to induce cell death. The extrinsic pathway can also be induced by the tumor necrosis factor–related apoptosis-inducing ligand (TRAIL), which also causes activation of FADD, DISC formation, and apoptosis.

The intrinsic pathway involves the mitochondria, which under stress release proapoptotic proteins such as cytochrome $c$, procaspases, Smac/Diablo, endonuclease G, adenylate kinase-2, and apoptosis-inducing factor (AIF). AIF can induce apoptosis without caspase activation, which differs from other proteins. These proapoptotic proteins are released from the space between the inner and outer mitochondrial layers by increased permeability of the outer mitochondrial wall. The Bcl-2 cytosolic proteins are made up of proapoptotic and prosurvival components. The mitochondrial outer wall permeability is induced by the Bax proteins (Bcl-2 proapoptotic) and leads to the release of cytochrome $c$ as well as other proteins that activate caspase 9. Exposure to volatile anesthetics impairs mitochondrial function, which in turn activitates the intrinsic apoptotic pathway.[15,39] Reactive oxygen species (ROS) scavengers and restoration of mitochondrial integrity mitigate this response.[40,41]

### Impeded Neurogenesis

Anesthetics affect neurogenesis in animals in an age-dependent manner. Isoflurane causes loss of neural stem cells and reduced neurogenesis in neonatal but not adult rats, where it causes a brief increase in neurogenesis.[42] Likewise propofol decreases hippocampal cell proliferation in young rats but not in adults. Exposure to isoflurane impairs growth and delayed maturation of astrocytes in young animals. Inflammation caused by general anesthetics may also cause a decrease in neurogenesis in animals. Based on both in vivo and in vitro evidence, general anesthetics may decrease both the pool of neural stem cells and their capacity for self-renewal, especially in juveniles and adults.[27,43]

### Altered Dendritic Development

Dendritic spines are small protrusions of the neurons that typically receive input from a single synapse of an axon

| Table 12.1 | Key Features of Anesthetic-Induced Developmental Neurotoxicity (AIDN) |
|---|---|
| **Feature** | **Comment (see text for details)** |
| Pathologic apoptosis | The hallmark of AIDN Can be induced by extrinsic or intrinsic pathways. |
| Impeded neurogenesis | Effect of anesthetics on neurogenesis is age-dependent |
| Altered dendritic development | Anesthetics affect dendritic morphogenesis in age-dependent manner |
| Aberrant glial development | Isoflurane can interfere with release of trophic factors by astrocytes |

and are essential components of synaptogenesis. Exposure to ketamine and isoflurane decreases synapse and spine density in very young infant rats.[44-46] However, in slightly older rats (age postnatal days 15, 16, and 20), exposure to propofol, midazolam, isoflurane, sevoflurane, desflurane, and ketamine leads to an increase in dendritic spine formation.[35,36] The implications of a decrease in dendritic spine formation at a very young age and an increase in slightly older animals are unclear. However, the impact of the vulnerability of specific developmental stages on AIDN is clear. Motor skill learning by subjecting rats to running on a rotarod enhances dendritic development. Exposure to ketamine and xylazine at postnatal day 14 resulted in a reduction of dendritic spine formation.[47] Taken together, the impact of anesthetics on dendritic morphogenesis clearly differs with the age at which exposure occurs.

### Aberrant Glial Development

The glial cells within the CNS form the scaffolding, which guides the migration and synaptogenesis of the neurons during development. Astrocytes are impaired during neural development by exposure to isoflurane.[48] This anesthetic interferes with the release of brain-derived neurotrophic factor (BDNF) by astrocytes, which in turn deprive the developing neurons of trophic support for axonal outgrowth. Isoflurane also induces apoptosis of oligodendrocytes in fetuses and neonate rhesus monkeys.[30,31]

### Anesthetic Effects on Spinal Cord

General anesthetic exposure (isoflurane, nitrous oxide) in very young rat pups causes an increase in apoptosis in the spinal cord with a preponderance of injury in the ventral horns.[49] However, no motor functional disabilities were detected in exposed rats that were allowed to mature. Postnatal day 3 rat pups that received an intrathecal injection of ketamine had increased apoptosis and microglial activation on histologic examination of their spinal cords and deranged spinal function at adulthood.[50] Intrathecal morphine produced analgesia, but no histologic or functional changes on the spinal cord.[51] Exposure to a local anesthetic (bupivacaine) in the same population did not cause an increased level of apoptosis.[52]

### Neuroinflammation

Activation of neuroinflammatory cascades may influence the development of postoperative cognitive dysfunction[53] (also see Chapter 35). Surgical trauma clearly activates neuroinflammation.[54,55] Therefore, the administration of anesthetic and analgesic drugs during surgery and painful procedures should minimize this response. However, sevoflurane increases markers of neuroinflammation in young but not adult mice.[56] It is unclear if the impact of surgical trauma and anesthetic exposure are additive in inducing neuroinflammation.

### Alzheimer-Related Neuropathology

Preclinical reports demonstrate expression of biologic precursors of Alzheimer disease.[57] Experimental surgery on mice increased β-amyloid accumulation in the hippocampus. Furthermore, exposure to isoflurane leads to increased β-amyloid levels in cell culture and rodent brains.[58,59] Neuroinflammation and Alzheimer disease neuropathology is a potent combination that could diminish neurocognitive function.[60]

### Neurocognitive Function

Decrements in neurocognitive function clearly occur after fetal and neonatal exposure to anesthetic drugs in rodents.[13,61,62] Standard behavioral measures in rodents include the Morris water navigation test, radial arm maze, startle, prepulse inhibition of the startle reflex, and odor recognition testing. Behavioral tests were also described in rhesus monkeys exposed to ketamine or sevoflurane with operant test battery or human intruder paradigm, respectively.[33,63] The operant test battery is a measure of motivation and recognition memory, whereas the human intruder paradigm is a test for emotional reactivity. Both reports demonstrated a diminution of performance at an older age after neonatal exposure to these drugs.

Exposure to anesthetic drugs also adversely impacts neurobehavioral assessments of elderly rats. Six- and 20-month-old rats anesthetized with isoflurane and nitrous oxide equally developed persistent deficits in the radial arm maze test.[64] However, propofol did not result in impaired radial arm maze test results in a similar experimental paradigm.[65] These reports clearly demonstrate that exposure to anesthetic drugs can lead to neurobehavioral functional consequence at a later age (also see Chapter 35).

## Relevant Anesthetic Durations and Concentrations

The duration of exposure may be more relevant than the concentration of exposure, although both are important. Almost all the animal studies involved an anesthetic exposure of at least 4 hours with some trials exposing primates to 24 hours of continuous anesthesia. Exposures of less than 1 hour regardless of the animal studied did not cause increased neuroapoptosis. Exposure to volatile anesthetics of 0.25% to 0.5% minimum alveolar concentration (MAC) for 6 hours increased caspase 3 marker levels, indicating an increase in cell death or apoptosis in rat pups. There is inconsistency about the relative neurotoxic potential of individual volatile anesthetics. Whether desflurane induces more neuroapoptosis than sevoflurane or halothane is not clear. Also, whether anesthetics given in combinations are more neurotoxic than solitary anesthetics is not known. Although nitrous oxide in combination with isoflurane is more neurotoxic than isoflurane alone, it may be because the total MAC exposure is higher when given in combination rather than a synergistic effect.

## Anesthetic and Sedative Drugs

GABAergic general anesthetics act on the $GABA_A$ receptor. Although GABA is inhibitory in the mature brain, it is an excitatory agent during early stages of brain development.[66,67] The immature Na/K/2Cl transporter protein NKCC1 produces a chloride influx leading to neuron depolarization. As a consequence GABA remains excitatory until the GABA neurons switch to the normal inhibitory mode when the mature chloride transporter, KCC2, is expressed, which actively transports chloride out of the neural cell.[68] This switch begins around the 15th postnatal week in term human infants but is not complete until about 1 year of age.

The N-methyl-D-aspartate glutamate receptor (NMDAR) is found in neurons and is activated when glutamate, glycine, or D-serine binds to it. It is critical for synaptic plasticity, which is needed for learning and memory. Structurally the NMDAR is a protein composed of four subunits—two GluN1 (formerly called NR1) and two GluN2 (formerlly called NR2). The GluN1 subunit binds the coagonist glycine, and the GluN2 subunit binds glutamate. Ketamine, which is a noncompetitive NMDAR antagonist, has been associated with AIDN in animals and causes an upregulation of the GluN1 subunit.[69]

In general, opioids do not increase neuroapoptosis but under some experimental conditions, repeated morphine administration over 7 days is associated with increased apoptosis in the sensory cortex and amygdala of neonatal rats.[70] However, a single dose of morphine given to postnatal day 7 rat pups did not increase neuroapoptosis.[71] Furthermore, daily administration of morphine for 9 consecutive days did not alter dendritic morphologic appearance. These areas of the brain are not the areas of the brain that are affected by volatile and intravenous anesthetics, which preferentially affect the learning and memory areas (hippocampus) of developing brains.

## Alleviation of AIDN

Several molecular mechanisms for anesthetic-induced apoptosis have been elucidated. This finding has led to studies designed to determine whether there are clinically available neuroprotective strategies that can ameliorate the negative effects of general anesthetics on developing young children. Several nonspecific drugs, which have neuroprotective properties (lithium, melatonin, estrogen, erythropoietin, estradiol, and dexmedetomidine), alleviate AIDN. Dexmedetomidine mitigates isoflurane-induced neuroapoptosis and behavioral impairment.[72] However, large doses of dexmedetomidine can induce neuroapoptosis.[73] The neuroprotective effect of dexmedetomidine probably induces cell survival signaling pathways at clinical doses.[74] Finally, an enhanced and stimulating environment mitigates neurobehavioral deficits after neonatal exposure to sevoflurane.[56,75]

## CLINICAL EVIDENCE FOR NEUROTOXICITY

Taken together, three factors appear to induce AIDN in laboratory models: (1) susceptibility during a critical period of development, (2) large dose of the anesthetic, and (3) prolonged duration of exposure. Extrapolation of these laboratory data to the human neonate is problematic. A rat brain develops over a matter of weeks, whereas a human brain develops over years. Six hours of anesthesia in a neonatal rat pup may equate to weeks in a human neonate. With the exception of sedation in intensive care patients, this extreme condition is not common in clinical practice. Therefore, uncovering the effect of an equivalent exposure on the neurologic outcome in a human neonate is difficult. Prolonged and repetitive exposure and exposure at a young age to general anesthesia causes the most neuroapoptosis and later developmental delays in animals. Children who need frequent examinations under anesthesia or radiation treatments for cancer theoretically are at increased risk for the neurotoxic effects of general anesthesia.

The implication that general anesthesia may be harmful to children is limited to retrospective epidemiologic analyses (also see Chapter 34). This evidence may be confounded by the effects of surgery and the effects of the underlying comorbid conditions. Although control for obvious confounders has been attempted, the retrospective nature of these investigations makes it impossible to control for all the known and unknown confounders. There have been several epidemiologic studies originating from the Mayo Clinic. The population in Olmsted County, Minnesota, is stable, and researchers there have access to both their medical records as well as the school records of this population. A retrospective cohort study of over 5000 children born from 1976 through 1982 found more reading, written language, and math learning disabilities in the 593 patients who were exposed to anesthesia before the age of 4 years.[76] Risk factors included more than one anesthetic exposure and general anesthesia lasting longer than 2 hours. A similar study was done using a matched cohort of 8530 children from Olmsted County, which found that the 64 children less than 2 years of age who had more than one anesthetic exposure were almost twice as likely to have speech and language disabilities as the children who had a single or no anesthetic exposure.[77] An analysis of these retrospective studies disclosed that halothane (no longer a commonly used inhaled anesthetic) was the chief anesthetic used, most of the cases were performed before pulse oximetry was commonly used, and the records used were handwritten so that there may have been some informational bias.

A database of over 200,000 children was developed using the New York State Medicaid billing codes. Initial studies from this database revealed that children undergoing inguinal hernia repair at less than 1 year of age had almost a threefold increase in diagnoses relating to developmental and behavioral issues.[78] When this group was controlled for gender and birth weight there was still a nearly twofold increase in these issues. However, a follow-up study matching exposed twins with nonanesthetic exposed twin siblings found that there was no association between general anesthesia receipt and later neurologic and developmental problems.[79] A small retrospective cohort paper was published of children who received anesthesia before the age of 4 years.[80] Fifty-three exposed children were matched with the same number of control children. All the children underwent cranial magnetic resonance imaging studies as well as neurocognitive examinations. They found that the previously exposed children scored significantly lower in listening comprehension and performance intelligence quotient (IQ). Exposure did not lead to gross elimination of gray matter in regions previously identified as vulnerable in animals. Decreased performance IQ and language comprehension, however, were associated with lower gray matter density in the occipital cortex and cerebellum. The general conclusion is that there is a more frequent risk to children who have had two or more anesthetic exposures. However, a 2012 prospectively followed cohort study from Australia of 2608 children exposed to a wide variety of general anesthetics and surgical procedures before the age of 3 years found that even a single exposure to general anesthesia was related to decreased performance on receptive and expressive language and cognitive testing performed at age 10 years.[81] Another prospective evaluation compared a smaller group of children exposed to anesthesia before 1 year of age to a similar number of age- and gender-matched children who had not received anesthesia. The study revealed that the anesthetized children had deficits in measures of long-term recognition memory, but no differences in familiarity, IQ, and Child Behavior Checklist scores.[62]

Large database clinical investigations from Canada and Sweden reveal that exposure to surgery and anesthesia at an age older than 2 to 4 years increased the odds ratio of cognitive deficits, though not to the extent of previously published retrospective reports from smaller populations.[82-84] Scrutiny of these large datasets reveals a lower percentage in academic achievement scores for toddlers undergoing ear, nose, and throat surgery. This finding suggests that early derangements in hearing and speech may have an impact on subsequent cognitive domains as assessed by school performance.

Other studies have cast doubt on the association between exposure to general anesthesia at a young age and later school problems. A study from the Netherlands evaluating the educational achievements of 1143 identical twin pairs found that twin pairs in which any member of the twin pair was exposed to general anesthesia had lesser educational achievements than unexposed twin pairs.[85] However, the educational achievements of discordant twin pairs (one twin exposed, one twin nonexposed) were similar to each other, meaning that the receipt of general anesthesia did not appear to be a relevant factor. Similarly, a large cohort study of 2689 children born in Denmark between 1986 and 1990 who underwent inguinal herniorrhaphy as infants were matched to control subjects who were randomly selected from an age-matched sample representing 5% of the population.[86] This study found no statistically significant differences between the exposed and nonexposed children after adjusting for known confounders.

Two published large prospective cohort studies support the contention that there is no impact of anesthetic exposure on subsequent neurocognitive domains in children. The GAS study is the only prospective randomized controlled trial to date comparing the effects of general anesthesia with regional anesthesia for inguinal hernia surgery in early infancy.[87] This interim analysis found no evidence that 1 hour of sevoflurane anesthesia in infancy increases the risk of adverse neurodevelopmental outcome at 2 years of age compared with awake-regional anesthesia. The primary outcome, which is a 5-year assessment, is under way. The PANDA study prospectively examined the impact of inguinal hernia surgery in infants younger than 36 months of age. An extensive battery of neurocognitive tests was used to compare each anesthetized infant to a sibling who had no anesthesia exposure.[88] When compared to a sibling cohort naïve to surgery and general anesthesia, there was no significant difference in the tested neurocognitive domains. Both negative studies only examined the impact of short exposures to general anesthesia and surgery. These findings are consistent with the lack of AIDN after exposures of short duration in laboratory animals. Furthermore, the neurocognitive assessments in all the clinical reports were performed in childhood and adolescence, not at adulthood. Therefore, the relationship between prolonged exposure to anesthetic drugs and neurocognitive performance in later stages of the life span needs to be addressed in future investigations.

On the other end of the age spectrum, elderly patients are at increased risk of developing postoperative cognitive dysfunction after surgery and anesthesia[89] (also see Chapter 35).

## INTRAOPERATIVE COURSE AND NEUROCOGNITIVE OUTCOMES

Yet, anesthetic drugs are not clinically administered in a vacuum. The developing CNS is an exquisitely sensitive internal milieu. Because critical periods of plasticity during brain development are modulated by the environment,[24,25] the perioperative environment has the potential to influence brain development. Anesthetic drugs are powerful modulators of neuronal circuits and have an impact on the constant flux of CNS development and remodeling in both health and disease states.[26] Therefore, nonphysiologic exposure to various drugs and stressors (painful stimuli, maternal deprivation, hypoglycemia, hypoxia, and ischemia) during these critical periods of development may lead to neuronal injury and altered neuroplasticity.[90] Are there other confounding variables involved in this process? Deterioration in long-term neurodevelopmental outcomes occurs in neonates undergoing surgery, which could cause congenital anomalies. The potential contribution of previously unknown genetic syndromes that are associated with both infant surgery-requiring lesions and developmental delay should be considered.

In anesthetized or sedated patients undergoing surgery or painful procedures, respectively, hemodynamic and metabolic changes may influence the neurocognitive outcomes of patients exposed to general anesthesia. These influences could work in concert with the neurotoxic potential of general anesthetics or independently to cause poor neurocognitive outcomes. Some of the factors that are implicated in causing poor outcomes in babies receiving neonatal intensive care may be important to infants undergoing general anesthesia (also see Chapter 34). These factors include perioperative blood pressure, carbon dioxide tensions, hyperoxia or hypoxia, temperature, and serum glucose levels (Table 12.2). Furthermore, cognitive decline that occurs with aging (also see Chapter 35) will have an impact on cognitive function in the elderly.[91]

## Arterial Blood Pressure

Determining the optimal arterial blood pressure management for very young infants is complicated by the many definitions for hypotension in the neonate and young infant. Two commonly used definitions are a mean

| Table 12.2 | Intraoperative Factors Influencing Neurocognitive Outcomes |
|---|---|
| **Factor** | **Comment (see text for details)** |
| Arterial blood pressure | Interpatient variability in lower limits of cerebral autoregulation |
| Carbon dioxide tension | Hypocapnia causes cerebral vasoconstriction |
| Hyperoxia or hypoxia | Hyperoxia produces reactive oxygen species<br>Hypoxia can cause cerebral ischemia |
| Temperature | Mild hypothermia is protective in neonate with prior ischemic injury<br>Hyperthermia with prior ischemic injury is associated with neurocognitive disability |
| Serum glucose | Extremes of hypoglycemia and hyperglycemia are associated with adverse outcomes |

arterial blood pressure (MAP) below the 5th or 10th percentile for age or a MAP less than the infant's gestational age in weeks for infants who were born premature. Furthermore, normal arterial blood pressures for very young infants rapidly increase during the first 6 weeks of life and thereafter are fairly constant for the first year of life. Maintaining arterial blood pressure within the limits of cerebral autoregulation is optimal for cerebral protection, although sustaining adequate cerebral perfusion less than the limits of cerebral autoregulation is sometimes necessary. The lower limits of cerebral autoregulation in neonates is likely variable and not precisely known. Furthermore, a wide range of interinfant variability likely exists. The lower limits of cerebral autoregulation for some infants is indeed close to the definition of hypotension using the infant's age in gestational weeks. Yet, some premature infants have cerebral autoregulation at a MAP level considerably lower than their gestational age in weeks.[92] A study of children younger than 2 years undergoing sevoflurane anesthesia found that in infants less than 6 months of age, the lower limit of autoregulation occurred at 38 mm Hg or a 20% decrease from baseline awake MAP.[93] In contrast, in infants older than 6 months the lower limit of autoregulation did not occur until arterial blood pressure had decreased to 40% of the normal arterial blood pressure. A follow-up study on this group of children using near-infrared spectroscopy and Doppler flow technology showed that the lower limits of autoregulation occurred at a MAP of 45 mm Hg but that patients were not at risk for cerebral ischemia until the MAP was less than 35 mm Hg. So, infants have less cerebral autoregulatory reserve and may be at risk for inadequate cerebral perfusion following a decrease in arterial blood pressure after induction of general anesthesia. Inadequate perfusion from hypotension can lead to partial asphyxia. Partial ischemia often causes damage in the watershed areas between major cerebral blood vessels and is most often caused by sharp decreases in arterial blood pressure.[94] Most general anesthetics cause some degree of hypotension, which can be ameliorated by surgical stimulation. Prolonged inductions of anesthesia or surgical preparation times may lead to protracted periods of hypotension in neonates.

## Hypocapnia and the Brain

The partial arterial carbon dioxide pressure ($Paco_2$) is an important modulator of the cerebral blood flow (CBF) with its main effect on cerebral arteries[95] (also see Chapter 30). Hypocapnia results in vasoconstriction of cerebral vessels leading to decreases in CBF. Hypocapnia-induced vasoconstriction may alter neuronal nuclear membranes and increase nuclear $Ca^{2+}$ influx through ischemia-induced tissue hypoxia and free radical generation, through alterations in the NMDAR, or by changes in cerebral energy metabolism, leading to apoptotic cell death. Hypocapnia, which leads to cerebral alkalosis, not only decreases cerebral perfusion but decreases the ability of hemoglobin to release oxygen. Premature infants may be particularly susceptible to the effects of hypocapnia. In general, it is recommended to keep the end-tidal $CO_2$ levels above 35 mm Hg in infants and children undergoing general anesthesia.

## Oxygen Management

Excessive administered oxygen delivered during general anesthesia can lead to an increased production of ROS causing cell stress and apoptosis. Ordinarily there is a balance between ROS and cell antioxidants. This balance is easily overwhelmed in young infants because their antioxidant defenses are not well developed at birth. During the last stages of fetal development there is an increase in endogenous production of antioxidants as well as an increase in maternal-fetal transfer of antioxidants in order to prepare the fetus for the relatively hyperoxic environment after birth compared with the relatively hypoxic fetal environment. Premature infants are at greater risk than term infants from oxygen damage because they are deficient in both of the previous factors. The antioxidant enzymes involved include superoxide dismutase, catalase, and glutathione peroxidase. These enzymes convert reactive superoxide radicals to hydrogen peroxide and then to water. Hyperoxia in young animals leads to neuroapoptosis presumably by oxidative stress and a decrease in neurotrophin activities. Oxygen can trigger inflammatory cytokines, which further cause cell stress.

Hypoxia and anoxia can cause brain ischemia. Neurons begin to lose their electrochemical gradients and there is an influx of calcium into the cytosol as a result of glutamate release from synaptic vesicles. This leads to early necrotic cell death. This is heralded by nuclear swelling, mitochondrial collapse, and inflammation. A proportion of neurons that are stressed by ischemia will not die immediately but will go on to die an apoptotic death sometime after the ischemic stress is eliminated.

## Temperature

Temperature maintenance during anesthesia is one of the challenges of pediatric anesthesia (also see Chapters 20 and 34). Infants have a large skin surface area/body mass ratio and a high basal metabolic rate, which accelerate radiant and evaporative heat loss. In addition, reduced vasoconstriction and decreased subcutaneous fat increase their radiant and conductive heat losses during procedures. Infants who are hypothermic at the conclusion of anesthesia may not have the energy stores to both rewarm themselves and spontaneously ventilate, necessitating postoperative ventilation in these infants. However, mild hypothermia (core temperature 32° C to 34° C) is neuroprotective in neonates who have suffered prior hypoxic ischemic injury. Hyperthermia in these same neonates was associated with more neurocognitive disabilities when these children underwent testing at age 18 months.

## CONCLUSION

Accumulating evidence from laboratory investigations definitively demonstrates that anesthetic and sedative drugs are potent modulators of CNS development and function throughout the life span, which in turn can lead to neuroapoptosis, altered dendritic formation, synaptogenesis, and subsequent neurocognitive deficits.[96] Yet, evidence from retrospective clinical reports in pediatric and elderly surgical populations is inconclusive.

Because anesthetic and sedative drugs are important in the management of surgical patients, the problem of AIDN must be eventually addressed. In the meantime, anesthesia providers should be sensitive to the possibility that brain development in younger years and its decline in older patients can be an issue for perioperative care.

## QUESTIONS OF THE DAY

1. What pathologic process is the hallmark of anesthetic-induced developmental neurotoxicity (AIDN)?
2. What anesthetic medications have been associated with AIDN in animal models?
3. In laboratory models, what factors are most important in the development of AIDN?
4. What is the clinical evidence for neurotoxicity in children who have received general anesthesia?
5. What intraoperative factors may have an influence on neurocognitive outcomes in a child receiving general anesthesia?

## REFERENCES

1. Lin EP, Soriano SG, Loepke AW. Anesthetic neurotoxicity. *Anesthesiol Clin.* 2014;32:133–155.
2. Rappaport B, Mellon RD, Simone A, Woodcock J. Defining safe use of anesthesia in children. *N Engl J Med.* 2011;364:1387–1390.
3. Eckenhoff JE. Relationship of anesthesia to postoperative personality changes in children. *Am J Dis Child.* 1953;86:587–591.
4. Stratmann G. Review article: neurotoxicity of anesthetic drugs in the developing brain. *Anesth Analg.* 2011;113: 1170–1179.
5. Bedford PD. Adverse cerebral effects of anaesthesia on old people. *Lancet.* 1955;269:259–263.
6. Terrando N, Eriksson LI, Eckenhoff RG. Perioperative neurotoxicity in the elderly: summary of the 4th International Workshop. *Anesth Analg.* 2015;120:649–652.
7. Rudolph U, Antkowiak B. Molecular and neuronal substrates for general anaesthetics. *Nat Rev Neurosci.* 2004;5:709–720.
8. Franks NP. General anaesthesia: from molecular targets to neuronal pathways of sleep and arousal. *Nat Rev Neurosci.* 2008;9:370–386.
9. Ikonomidou C, Bittigau P, Ishimaru MJ, et al. Ethanol-induced apoptotic neurodegeneration and fetal alcohol syndrome. *Science.* 2000;287:1056–1060.
10. Bittigau P, Sifringer M, Genz K, et al. Antiepileptic drugs and apoptotic neurodegeneration in the developing brain. *Proc Natl Acad Sci U S A.* 2002;99(23):15089–15094.
11. Quimby KL, Katz J, Bowman RE. Behavioral consequences in rats from chronic exposure to 10 ppm halothane during early development. *Anesth Analg.* 1975;54:628–633.
12. Ikonomidou C, Bosch F, Miksa M, et al. Blockade of NMDA receptors and apoptotic neurodegeneration in the developing brain. *Science.* 1999;283:70–74.
13. Jevtovic-Todorovic V, Hartman RE, Izumi Y, et al. Early exposure to common anesthetic agents causes widespread neurodegeneration in the developing rat brain and persistent learning deficits. *J Neurosci.* 2003;23:876–882.
14. Slikker Jr W, Paule MG, Wright LK, et al. Systems biology approaches for toxicology. *J Appl Toxicol.* 2007;27:201–217.
15. Sanchez V, Feinstein SD, Lunardi N, et al. General anesthesia causes long-term impairment of mitochondrial morphogenesis and synaptic transmission in developing rat brain. *Anesthesiology.* 2011;115:992–1002.
16. Boscolo A, Milanovic D, Starr JA, et al. Early exposure to general anesthesia disturbs mitochondrial fission and fusion in the developing rat brain. *Anesthesiology.* 2013;118:1086–1097.
17. Soriano SG, Liu Q, Li J, et al. Ketamine activates cell cycle signaling and apoptosis in the neonatal rat brain. *Anesthesiology.* 2010;112:1155–1163.
18. Head BP, Patel HH, Niesman IR, et al. Inhibition of p75 neurotrophin receptor attenuates isoflurane-mediated neuronal apoptosis in the neonatal central nervous system. *Anesthesiology.* 2009;110:813–825.
19. Ben-Ari Y. Excitatory actions of GABA during development: the nature of the nurture. *Nat Rev Neurosci.* 2002;3:728–739.
20. Tau GZ, Peterson BS. Normal development of brain circuits. *Neuropsychopharmacology.* 2010;35:147–168.
21. Ohnuma S, Harris WA. Neurogenesis and the cell cycle. *Neuron.* 2003;40:199–208.
22. de la Rosa EJ, de Pablo F. Cell death in early neural development: beyond the neurotrophic theory. *Trends Neurosci.* 2000;23:454–458.
23. Buss RR, Sun W, Oppenheim RW. Adaptive roles of programmed cell death during nervous system development. *Annu Rev Neurosci.* 2006;29:1–35.
24. Hensch TK. Critical period plasticity in local cortical circuits. *Nat Rev Neurosci.* 2005;6:877–888.
25. Werker JF, Hensch TK. Critical periods in speech perception: new directions. *Annu Rev Psychol.* 2015;66:173–196.
26. Vutskits L. General anesthesia: a gateway to modulate synapse formation and neural plasticity? *Anesth Analg.* 2012;115:1174–1182.
27. Hofacer RD, Deng M, Ward CG, et al. Cell-age specific vulnerability of neurons to anesthetic toxicity. *Ann Neurol.* 2013;73:695–704.
28. Clancy B, Kersh B, Hyde J, et al. Web-based method for translating neurodevelopment from laboratory species to humans. *Neuroinformatics.* 2007;5:79–94.
29. Brambrink AM, Evers AS, Avidan MS, et al. Ketamine-induced neuroapoptosis in the fetal and neonatal rhesus macaque brain. *Anesthesiology.* 2012;116:372–384.
30. Brambrink AM, Back SA, Riddle A, et al. Isoflurane-induced apoptosis of oligodendrocytes in the neonatal primate brain. *Ann Neurol.* 2012;72:525–535.
31. Creeley CE, Dikranian KT, Dissen GA, et al. Isoflurane-induced apoptosis of neurons and oligodendrocytes in the fetal rhesus macaque brain. *Anesthesiology.* 2014;120:626–638.
32. Slikker W, Zou X, Hotchkiss CE, et al. Ketamine-induced neuronal cell death in the perinatal rhesus monkey. *Toxicol Sci.* 2007;98:145–158.
33. Paule MG, Li M, Allen RR, et al. Ketamine anesthesia during the first week of life can cause long-lasting cognitive deficits in rhesus monkeys. *Neurotoxicol Teratol.* 2011;33:220–230.
34. Wang S, Peretich K, Zhao Y, et al. Anesthesia-induced neurodegeneration in fetal rat brains. *Pediatr Res.* 2009;66: 435–440.
35. De Roo M, Klauser P, Briner A, et al. Anesthetics rapidly promote synaptogenesis during a critical period of brain development. *PLoS One.* 2009;4:e7043.
36. Briner A, De Roo M, Dayer A, et al. Volatile anesthetics rapidly increase dendritic spine density in the rat medial prefrontal cortex during synaptogenesis. *Anesthesiology.* 2010;112:546–556.
37. Penzes P, Cahill ME, Jones KA, et al. Dendritic spine pathology in neuropsychiatric disorders. *Nat Neurosci.* 2011;14:285–293.
38. Blomgren K, Leist M, Groc L. Pathological apoptosis in the developing brain. *Apoptosis.* 2007;12:993–1010.
39. Amrock LG, Starner ML, Murphy KL, Baxter MG. Long-term effects of single or multiple neonatal sevoflurane exposures on rat hippocampal ultrastructure. *Anesthesiology.* 2015;122:87–95.
40. Boscolo A, Starr JA, Sanchez V, et al. The abolishment of anesthesia-induced cognitive impairment by timely protection of mitochondria in the developing rat brain: the importance of free oxygen radicals and mitochondrial integrity. *Neurobiol Dis.* 2012;45:1031–1041.
41. Boscolo A, Ori C, Bennett J, et al. Mitochondrial protectant pramipexole prevents sex-specific long-term cognitive impairment from early anaesthesia exposure in rats. *Br J Anaesth.* 2013;110(suppl 1):i47–i52.
42. Stratmann G, Sall JW, May LD, et al. Isoflurane differentially affects neurogenesis and long-term neurocognitive function in 60-day-old and 7-day-old rats. *Anesthesiology.* 2009;110:834–848.
43. Culley DJ, Boyd JD, Palanisamy A, et al. Isoflurane decreases self-renewal capacity of rat cultured neural stem cells. *Anesthesiology.* 2011;115:754–763.
44. Vutskits L, Gascon E, Potter G, et al. Low concentrations of ketamine initiate dendritic atrophy of differentiated GABAergic neurons in culture. *Toxicology.* 2007;234:216–226.
45. Vutskits L, Gascon E, Tassonyi E, Kiss JZ. Effect of ketamine on dendritic arbor development and survival of immature GABAergic neurons in vitro. *Toxicol Sci.* 2006;91:540–549.

46. Vutskits L, Gascon E, Tassonyi E, Kiss JZ. Clinically relevant concentrations of propofol but not midazolam alter in vitro dendritic development of isolated gamma-aminobutyric acid-positive interneurons. *Anesthesiology.* 2005;102:970–976.

47. Huang L, Yang G. Repeated exposure to ketamine-xylazine during early development impairs motor learning-dependent dendritic spine plasticity in adulthood. *Anesthesiology.* 2015;122:821–831.

48. Ryu YK, Khan S, Smith SC, Mintz CD. Isoflurane impairs the capacity of astrocytes to support neuronal development in a mouse dissociated coculture model. *J Neurosurg Anesthesiol.* 2014;26:363–368.

49. Sanders RD, Xu J, Shu Y, et al. General anesthetics induce apoptotic neurodegeneration in the neonatal rat spinal cord. *Anesth Analg.* 2008;106:1708–1711.

50. Walker SM, Westin BD, Deumens R, et al. Effects of intrathecal ketamine in the neonatal rat: evaluation of apoptosis and long-term functional outcome. *Anesthesiology.* 2010;113: 147–159.

51. Westin BD, Walker SM, Deumens R, et al. Validation of a preclinical spinal safety model: effects of intrathecal morphine in the neonatal rat. *Anesthesiology.* 2010;113:183–199.

52. Yahalom B, Athiraman U, Soriano SG, et al. Spinal anesthesia in infant rats: development of a model and assessment of neurologic outcomes. *Anesthesiology.* 2011;114:1325–1335.

53. Vacas S, Degos V, Feng X, Maze M. The neuroinflammatory response of postoperative cognitive decline. *Br Med Bull.* 2013;106:161–178.

54. Terrando N, Monaco C, Ma D, et al. Tumor necrosis factor-alpha triggers a cytokine cascade yielding postoperative cognitive decline. *Proc Natl Acad Sci U S A.* 2010;107:20518–20522.

55. Cibelli M, Fidalgo AR, Terrando N, et al. Role of interleukin-1beta in postoperative cognitive dysfunction. *Ann Neurol.* 2010;68:360–368.

56. Shen X, Dong Y, Xu Z, et al. Selective anesthesia-induced neuroinflammation in developing mouse brain and cognitive impairment. *Anesthesiology.* 2013;118:502–515.

57. Xu Z, Dong Y, Wang H, et al. Age-dependent postoperative cognitive impairment and Alzheimer-related neuropathology in mice. *Sci Rep.* 2014; 4:3766.

58. Xie Z, Dong Y, Maeda U, et al. Isoflurane-induced apoptosis: a potential pathogenic link between delirium and dementia. *J Gerontol A Biol Sci Med Sci.* 2006;61:1300–1306.

59. Xie Z, Culley DJ, Dong Y, et al. The common inhalation anesthetic isoflurane induces caspase activation and increases amyloid beta-protein level in vivo. *Ann Neurol.* 2008;64:618–627.

60. Tang JX, Mardini F, Janik LS, et al. Modulation of murine Alzheimer pathogenesis and behavior by surgery. *Ann Surg.* 2013;257:439–448.

61. Palanisamy A, Baxter MG, Keel PK, et al. Rats exposed to isoflurane in utero during early gestation are behaviorally abnormal as adults. *Anesthesiology.* 2011;114:521–528.

62. Stratmann G, Lee J, Sall JW, et al. Effect of general anesthesia in infancy on long-term recognition memory in humans and rats. *Neuropsychopharmacology.* 2014;39:2275–2287.

63. Raper J, Alvarado MC, Murphy KL, Baxter MG. Multiple anesthetic exposure in infant monkeys alters emotional reactivity to an acute stressor. *Anesthesiology.* 2015;123:1084–1092.

64. Culley DJ, Baxter MG, Yukhananov R, Crosby G. Long-term impairment of acquisition of a spatial memory task following isoflurane-nitrous oxide anesthesia in rats. *Anesthesiology.* 2004;100:309–314.

65. Jagodic MM, Pathirathna S, Joksovic PM, et al. Upregulation of the T-type calcium current in small rat sensory neurons after chronic constrictive injury of the sciatic nerve. *J Neurophysiol.* 2008;99:3151–3156.

66. Zhang LL, Pathak HR, Coulter DA, et al. Shift of intracellular chloride concentration in ganglion and amacrine cells of developing mouse retina. *J Neurophysiol.* 2006;95:2404–2416.

67. Dzhala VI, Talos DM, Sdrulla DA, et al. NKCC1 transporter facilitates seizures in the developing brain. *Nat Med.* 2005;11:1205–1213.

68. Edwards DA, Shah HP, Cao W, et al. Bumetanide alleviates epileptogenic and neurotoxic effects of sevoflurane in neonatal rat brain. *Anesthesiology.* 2010;112:567–575.

69. Wang C, Sadovova N, Hotchkiss C, et al. Blockade of N-methyl-D-aspartate receptors by ketamine produces loss of postnatal day 3 monkey frontal cortical neurons in culture. *Toxicol Sci.* 2006;91:192–201.

70. Bajic D, Commons KG, Soriano SG. Morphine-enhanced apoptosis in selective brain regions of neonatal rats. *Int J Dev Neurosci.* 2013;31:258–266.

71. Massa H, Lacoh CM, Vutskits L. Effects of morphine on the differentiation and survival of developing pyramidal neurons during the brain growth spurt. *Toxicol Sci.* 2012;130: 168–179.

72. Sanders RD, Xu J, Shu Y, et al. Dexmedetomidine attenuates isoflurane-induced neurocognitive impairment in neonatal rats. *Anesthesiology.* 2009;110: 1077–1085.

73. Pancaro C, Segal BS, Sikes RW, et al. Dexmedetomidine and ketamine show distinct patterns of cell degeneration and apoptosis in the developing rat neonatal brain. *J Matern Fetal Neonatal Med.* 2016;29(23):3827–3833.

74. Sanders RD, Sun P, Patel S, et al. Dexmedetomidine provides cortical neuroprotection: impact on anaesthetic-induced neuroapoptosis in the rat developing brain. *Acta Anaesthesiol Scand.* 2010;54:710–716.

75. Shih J, May LD, Gonzalez HE, et al. Delayed environmental enrichment reverses sevoflurane-induced memory impairment in rats. *Anesthesiology.* 2012;116:586–602.

76. Wilder RT, Flick RP, Sprung J, et al. Early exposure to anesthesia and learning disabilities in a population-based birth cohort. *Anesthesiology.* 2009;110:796–804.

77. Flick RP, Katusic SK, Colligan RC, et al. Cognitive and behavioral outcomes after early exposure to anesthesia and surgery. *Pediatrics.* 2011;128:e1053–e1061.

78. DiMaggio C, Sun LS, Kakavouli A, et al. A retrospective cohort study of the association of anesthesia and hernia repair surgery with behavioral and developmental disorders in young children. *J Neurosurg Anesthesiol.* 2009;21:286–291.

79. Dimaggio C, Sun L, Li G. Early childhood exposure to anesthesia and risk of developmental and behavioral disorders in a sibling birth cohort. *Anesth Analg.* 2011;113:1143–1151.

80. Backeljauw B, Holland SK, Altaye M, Loepke AW. Cognition and brain structure following early childhood surgery with anesthesia. *Pediatrics.* 2015;136(1):e1–e12.

81. Ing C, DiMaggio C, Whitehouse A, et al. Long-term differences in language and cognitive function after childhood exposure to anesthesia. *Pediatrics.* 2012;130:e476–e485.

82. O'Leary JD, Janus M, Duku E, et al. A population-based study evaluating the association between surgery in early life and child development at primary school entry. *Anesthesiology.* 2016;125:272–279.

83. Graham MR, Brownell M, Chateau DG, et al. Neurodevelopmental assessment in kindergarten in children exposed to general anesthesia before the age of 4 years: a retrospective matched cohort study. *Anesthesiology.* 2016;125(4):667–677.

84. Glatz P, Sandin RH, Pedersen NL, et al. Association of anesthesia and surgery during childhood with long-term academic performance. *JAMA Pediatr.* 2017;171(1):e163470.

85. Bartels M, Althoff RR, Boomsma DI. Anesthesia and cognitive performance in children: no evidence for a causal relationship. *Twin Res Hum Genet.* 2009;12:246–253.

86. Hansen TG, Pedersen JK, Henneberg SW, et al. Academic performance in adolescence after inguinal hernia repair in infancy: a nationwide cohort study. *Anesthesiology.* 2011;114(5):1076–1085.

87. Davidson AJ, Disma N, de Graaff JC, et al. GAS consortium. Neurodevelopmental outcome at 2 years of age after general anaesthesia and awake-regional anaesthesia in infancy (GAS): an international multicentre, randomised controlled trial. *Lancet.* 2015;387(10015):239–250.

88. Sun LS, Li G, Miller TL, et al. Association between a single general anesthesia exposure before age 36 months and neurocognitive outcomes in later childhood. *JAMA.* 2016;315:2312–2320.

89. Berger M, Nadler JW, Browndyke J, et al. Postoperative cognitive dysfunction: minding the gaps in our knowledge of a common postoperative complication in the elderly. *Anesthesiol Clin.* 2015;33(3):517–550.

90. McCann ME, Soriano SG. Perioperative central nervous system injury in neonates. *Br J Anaesth.* 2012;109(suppl 1):i60–i67.

91. Hovens IB, Schoemaker RG, van der Zee EA, et al. Thinking through postoperative cognitive dysfunction: how to bridge the gap between clinical and pre-clinical perspectives. *Brain Behav Immun.* 2012;26:1169–1179.

92. Cayabyab R, McLean CW, Seri I. Definition of hypotension and assessment of hemodynamics in the preterm neonate. *J Perinatol.* 2009;29(suppl 2):S58–S62.

93. Vavilala MS, Lee LA, Lee M, et al. Cerebral autoregulation in children during sevoflurane anaesthesia. *Br J Anaesth.* 2003;90:636–641.

94. Torvik A. The pathogenesis of watershed infarcts in the brain. *Stroke.* 1984;15:221–223.

95. Meng L, Gelb AW. Regulation of cerebral autoregulation by carbon dioxide. *Anesthesiology.* 2015;122:196–205.

96. Xie Z, Vutskits L. Lasting impact of general anaesthesia on the brain: mechanisms and relevance. *Nat Rev Neurosci.* 2016;17(11):705–717.

# PREOPERATIVE PREPARATION AND INTRAOPERATIVE MANAGEMENT

**Section III**

# 13 PREOPERATIVE EVALUATION AND MEDICATION

## Rebecca M. Gerlach and Bobbie Jean Sweitzer

## PREOPERATIVE ASSESSMENT: OVERVIEW

The specialty of anesthesia is continually expanding in scope, particularly in the area of perioperative medicine. The role of an anesthesiologist today encompasses not only the intraoperative period but also preoperative risk assessment and implementation of perioperative risk reduction strategies for improving surgical outcomes. The preoperative evaluation is the cornerstone of safe and effective anesthesia care. Whether performed in a specific preoperative medicine clinic or immediately before anesthesia, the goal of the medical history and physical examination is the same: to formulate an anesthetic plan to minimize risk and maximize the quality of recovery. Testing or consultation with other physicians may be indicated in advance of surgery to diagnose disease based on identified risk factors or to optimize treatment. Medical records and previous anesthetic records often reveal details about past diagnoses or complications and are always reviewed during assessment. The American Society of Anesthesiologists (ASA) Practice Advisory for Preanesthesia Evaluation provides guidance for the preanesthesia history and physical examination and for the selection and timing of preoperative tests.[1]

### History and Physical Examination

A preanesthesia history includes the planned procedure, presenting illness, comorbid conditions, detailed review of systems, past anesthetic history with review of complications, assessment of allergies and medications, documentation of substance use or abuse, and the last oral intake if done on the day of surgery. Severity of disease, efficacy of treatment, and impact on daily function is explored to determine if an alteration in anesthesia plan is appropriate. The preanesthesia history is a comprehensive assessment of the patient's current state of health and ability to perform daily functions, aspects of which are combined to assign an ASA Physical Status (ASA

**Table 13.1** American Society of Anesthesiologists Physical Status Classification System

| ASA PS Classification[a] | Definition | Examples, including, but not limited to |
|---|---|---|
| ASA I | A normal healthy patient | Healthy, nonsmoking, no or minimal alcohol use |
| ASA II | A patient with mild systemic disease | Mild diseases only without substantive functional limitations. Examples include (but are not limited to) current smoker, social alcohol drinker, pregnancy, obesity (30 < BMI < 40), well-controlled DM/HTN, mild lung disease |
| ASA III | A patient with severe systemic disease | Substantive functional limitations; One or more moderate to severe diseases. Examples include (but are not limited to) poorly controlled DM or HTN, COPD, morbid obesity (BMI ≥ 40), active hepatitis, alcohol dependence or abuse, implanted pacemaker, moderate reduction of ejection fraction, ESRD undergoing regularly scheduled dialysis, premature infant PCA < 60 weeks, history (>3 months) of MI, CVA, TIA, or CAD/stents. |
| ASA IV | A patient with severe systemic disease that is a constant threat to life | Examples include (but are not limited to) recent (<3 months) MI, CVA, TIA, or CAD/stents, ongoing cardiac ischemia or severe valve dysfunction, severe reduction of ejection fraction, sepsis, DIC, ARDS, or ESRD not undergoing regularly scheduled dialysis |
| ASA V | A moribund patient who is not expected to survive without the operation | Examples include (but are not limited to) ruptured abdominal/thoracic aneurysm, massive trauma, intracranial bleed with mass effect, ischemic bowel in the face of significant cardiac pathology or multiple organ/system dysfunction |
| ASA VI | A declared brain-dead patient whose organs are being removed for donor purposes | |

[a]The addition of "E" denotes emergency surgery. (An emergency is defined as existing when delay in treatment of the patient would lead to a significant increase in the threat to life or body part).
*ARDS*, Acute respiratory disease syndrome; *ASA*, American Society of Anesthesiologists; *ASA PS*, ASA physical status; *BMI*, body mass index; *CAD*, coronary artery disease; *COPD*, chronic obstructive pulmonary disease; *CVA*, cerebral vascular accident; *DIC*, disseminated intravascular coagulopathy; *DM*, diabetes mellitus; *ESRD*, end-stage renal disease; *HTN*, hypertension; *MI*, myocardial infarction; *PCA*, postconceptual age; *TIA*, transient ischemic attack.
From American Society of Anesthesiologists. ASA Physical Status Classification System. www.asahq.org.

PS) score (Table 13.1). Assessment of functional capacity, or cardiorespiratory fitness, directs further investigations. The ability to achieve a moderate level of activity without symptoms, denoted by a metabolic equivalent of task score (METS) of 4 or more predicts a low risk of perioperative complications (Box 13.1).[2] An inability to exercise indicates either lack of cardiorespiratory reserve or may result from neuromuscular or pulmonary disease, anemia, or general deconditioning, all of which indicate elevated risk.

Clinical predictors of difficult airway management identified through screening questions may prompt alterations in care (Table 13.2; also see Chapter 16). A personal or family history of malignant hyperthermia or pseudocholinesterase deficiency (also see Chapter 11) is noted so appropriate precautions are taken.

A preanesthesia physical examination begins with general inspection of the patient, such as dependent functional status (e.g., walker or wheelchair aids) or altered

**Box 13.1** Metabolic Equivalents of Functional Capacity

**METs—Levels of Exercise**
1—Eating, working at computer, dressing
2—Walking downstairs or in your house, cooking
3—Walking 1-2 blocks
4—Raking leaves, gardening
5—Climbing 1-2 flights of stairs, dancing, bicycling
6—Playing golf, carrying clubs
7—Playing singles tennis
8—Rapidly climbing stairs, jogging slowly
9—Jumping rope slowly, moderate cycling
10—Swimming quickly, running or jogging briskly
11—Skiing cross country, playing full-court basketball
12—Running rapidly for moderate to long distances

*MET*, Metabolic equivalent. 1 MET = consumption of 3.5 mL $O_2$/min/kg of body weight.
From Jette M, Sidney K, Blümchen G. Metabolic equivalents (METS) in exercise testing, exercise prescription, and evaluation of functional capacity. *Clin Cardiol*. 1990;13:555-565.

| Table 13.2 | Preoperative Patient Characteristics Associated With Possible Difficult Airway Management |
|---|---|

| Difficult Mask Ventilation[a] | Difficult Direct Laryngoscopy |
|---|---|
| Age > 55 years | Reported history of difficult intubation, aspiration pneumonia after intubation, dental or oral trauma following intubation |
| Obstructive sleep apnea (OSA) or snoring | OSA or snoring |
| Previous head/neck radiation, surgery, or trauma | Previous head/neck radiation, surgery, or trauma |
| Lack of teeth | Congenital disease: Down syndrome, Treacher-Collins syndrome, Pierre Robin syndrome |
| A beard | Inflammatory/arthritic disease: rheumatoid arthritis, ankylosing spondylitis, scleroderma |
| Body mass index (BMI) > 26 kg/m$^2$ | Obesity Cervical spine disease or previous surgery |

[a]Data from Langeron O, Masso E, Huraux C, et al. Prediction of difficult mask ventilation. *Anesthesiology*. 2000;92:1229-1236.

| Table 13.3 | Components of the Airway Examination |
|---|---|

| Airway Examination Component | Nonreassuring Findings |
|---|---|
| Length of upper incisors | Relatively long |
| Relationship of maxillary and mandibular incisors during normal jaw closure | Prominent "overbite" (maxillary incisors anterior to mandibular incisors) |
| Relationship of maxillary and mandibular incisors during voluntary protrusion of mandible (ability to prognath; upper lip bite test) | Inability to bring mandibular incisors anterior to (in front of) maxillary incisors; unable to bite the upper lip |
| Interincisor distance | Less than 3 cm |
| Visibility of uvula | Not visible when tongue is protruded with patient in sitting position (e.g., Mallampati class II) |
| Compliance of the mandibular/oral space | Highly arched or very narrow; radiation or surgical changes; stiff, indurated, occupied by mass or nonresilient |
| Thyromental distance | <3 fingerbreadths or <6 cm |
| Length of neck | Short |
| Thickness of neck | Thick |
| Range of motion of head and neck | Cannot touch tip of chin to chest or extend neck |

Modified from Apfelbaum JL, Hagberg CA, Caplan RA, et al. Practice guidelines for management of the difficult airway: an updated report by the American Society of Anesthesiologists Task Force on Management of the Difficult Airway. *Anesthesiology*. 2013;118:251.

respiratory status (e.g., oxygen or accessory muscle use, cyanosis). Altered mental status is important to identify. Examination includes assessment of the airway (Table 13.3)[3] including Mallampati classification (Fig. 13.1); vital signs including oxygen saturation; and measurement of height and weight. Inspection of the pulse for rate and rhythm, auscultation for murmurs, and examination for peripheral edema are done. Auscultation for abnormal breath sounds is important. Findings divergent from a patient's baseline may indicate new or evolving disease.

## Investigations and Testing

Preoperative investigations are indicated for evaluating existing medical conditions or disease diagnosis when an abnormal result will have an impact on management of the patient or direct further testing (Box 13.2). Performing a battery of *screening* or *routine* preoperative tests is seldom helpful, yet this unnecessary practice persists among some physicians based on "practice tradition, belief that other physicians want tests done, medicolegal worries, concerns about surgical delays or cancellation, and lack of awareness of evidence or guidelines."[4] Yet routine (not

disease-indicated) preoperative testing rarely results in changes in management or benefit to the patient.[5] Mandatory preoperative testing is not cost-conscious medical care, as testing is expensive and follow-up of results is time-consuming for limited clinical utility.[6] Preoperative tests may be indicated based on disease-based criteria, as summarized in Table 13.4, provided that abnormal results will have an impact on patient management. Also, testing for selected patients may be indicated based on the planned procedure or patient status (Table 13.5).

For most patients undergoing ambulatory or low-risk surgery, no preoperative testing is required (also see Chapter 37). For patients having ambulatory surgery with stable or nonsevere disease, there is no increase in adverse perioperative events or differences in outcome in those who have no preoperative tests.[7] Additionally, for cataract surgery (also see Chapter 31), eliminating preoperative medical testing does not change outcomes and provides a significant cost savings.[8] Investigations

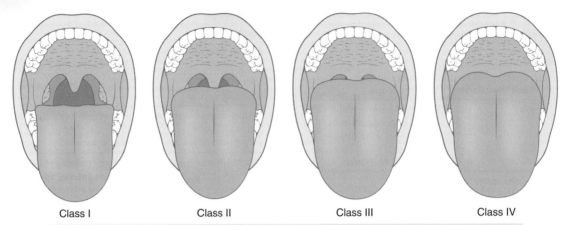

| Class I | Class II | Class III | Class IV |

**Fig. 13.1** The Mallampati airway classification is a clinical instrument used to assess the ease of obtaining an airway. Class I, visualization of the soft palate, fauces, uvula, and both anterior and posterior pillars. Class II, visualization of the soft palate, fauces, and uvula. Class III, visualization of the soft palate and the base of the uvula. Class IV (difficult), the soft palate is not visible at all.

---

**Box 13.2** Appropriate Indications for Preoperative Testing

Preoperative testing is recommended when an abnormal result is suspected based on clinical risk factors and this result will:
- Establish a new diagnosis
- Direct further preoperative testing or consultation
- Inform preoperative medication use
- Alter intraoperative monitoring or management
- Influence choice of surgical approach or anesthetic technique
- Influence decision to postpone or cancel surgery
- Change postoperative disposition
- Establish perioperative risk profile for communication with other physicians and patient

---

are indicated only when clinical evaluation of the patient reveals new or worsening symptoms that warrant testing even in the absence of an upcoming procedure. Eliciting a history of increased dyspnea on exertion, new-onset chest pain, or syncope is of greater benefit than routinely ordering electrocardiogram (ECG) or chest radiographs. In choosing preoperative investigations, both the disease-based indications and risk profile of the proposed surgical procedure are considered to ensure only indicated tests are ordered and unnecessary testing avoided.

Although commonly ordered, routine preoperative ECG does not add value to the care of surgical patients, particularly if ordered for those of advanced age[5,9] (also see Chapter 35). Recommendations for age-based testing were derived from the frequent incidence of abnormalities found on ECGs of elderly patients. The specificity of an ECG abnormality in predicting postoperative cardiac adverse events is only 26%, and a normal ECG does not exclude cardiac disease.[10] The

ASA Practice Advisory for Preanesthesia Evaluation advises that age alone, in the absence of other clinical risk factors, may not be an indication for an ECG (Box 13.3).[1] ECG may be useful for suspected electrolyte abnormalities, active cardiac symptoms, suspected or known pulmonary hypertension, and arrhythmias (see Table 13.4 for more details). See Table 13.5 for recommendations from the American College of Cardiology/American Heart Association (ACC/AHA) regarding preoperative ECG.

Routine pregnancy testing, particularly of adolescents, is a controversial issue. Some practices and facilities provide patients with information about the potential risks of anesthesia and surgery on pregnancy but allow them to decline testing. Other practices mandate that all females of childbearing age undergo a urine pregnancy test on the day of surgery (also see Chapter 34). The ASA Practice Advisory for Preoperative Evaluation states that "the literature is inadequate to inform patients or physicians on whether anesthesia causes harmful effects on early pregnancy" and recommends that pregnancy testing be offered to women if the test result will alter management.[1] If proceeding with testing, rapid reliable results are obtained from urine screening and the test is best performed on the day of surgery rather than in advance unless the history suggests pregnancy.

## Consultations

Forming a comprehensive preoperative management plan for a patient with complex or undifferentiated comorbid conditions is often best accomplished in collaboration with consultant specialists. The purpose of consultation is to seek specific advice regarding the diagnosis

**Table 13.4**   Preoperative Diagnostic Testing Recommendations[a]

| Test | Clinical Scenario |
|---|---|
| Albumin | Anasarca; liver disease; malnutrition; malabsorption |
| β-hCG | Suspected pregnancy |
| CBC | Alcohol abuse; anemia; dyspnea; hepatic or renal disease; malignancy; malnutrition; personal history of bleeding; poor exercise tolerance; recent chemotherapy or radiation therapy |
| Creatinine | Renal disease; poorly controlled diabetes |
| Chest radiograph | Active, acute or chronic significant pulmonary symptoms such as cough or dyspnea; abnormal unexplained physical findings on chest examination; decompensated heart failure; malignancy within the thorax; radiation therapy[b] |
| Electrocardiogram | Alcohol abuse; active cardiac condition (new or worsening chest pain or dyspnea, palpitations, tachycardia, irregular rhythm, unexplained bradycardia, undiagnosed murmur, $S_3$, decompensated heart failure); implanted cardioverter-defibrillator (ICD); obstructive sleep apnea; pacemaker; pulmonary hypertension; radiation therapy[b]; severe obesity; syncope; use of amiodarone or digoxin |
| Electrolytes | Alcohol abuse; cardiovascular, hepatic, renal, or thyroid disease; diabetes; malnutrition; use of digoxin or diuretics |
| Glucose and/or HbA$_{1c}$ | Diabetes; severe obesity; use of steroids |
| LFTs | Alcohol abuse; hepatic disease; recent hepatitis exposure; undiagnosed bleeding disorder |
| Platelet count | Alcohol abuse; hepatic disease; bleeding disorder (personal or family history); hematologic malignancy; recent chemotherapy or radiation therapy; thrombocytopenia |
| PT | Alcohol abuse; hepatic disease; malnutrition; bleeding disorder (personal or family history); use of warfarin |
| PTT | Bleeding disorder (personal or family history); undiagnosed hypercoagulable state; use of unfractionated heparin |
| TSH, $T_3$, $T_4$ | Goiter; thyroid disease; unexplained dyspnea, fatigue, palpitations, tachycardia |
| Urinalysis | Urinary tract infection (suspected) |

[a]These tests are only indicated to either establish a diagnosis, predict risk, or alter treatments in situations when it will impact perioperative management. This is less likely to be useful for low-risk procedures or in patients with chronic, stable conditions.
[b]Only with radiation therapy to chest, breasts, lungs, thorax.
*β-hCG*, β-Human chorionic gonadotropin [assay] (pregnancy test); *CBC*, complete blood count; *HbA1c*, glycated hemoglobin; *LFTs*, liver function tests (albumin, bilirubin, alanine, and aspartate aminotransferases); *PT*, prothrombin time; *PTT*, partial thromboplastin time; *S3*, third heart sound; $T_3$, triiodothyronine; $T_4$, thyroxine; *TSH*, thyroid-stimulating hormone.

or management of a condition in order to aid safe anesthetic planning, not for *preoperative clearance,* which is seldom helpful. A summary of the patient's medical history and relevant diagnostic testing along with a specific question or goal for consultation improves utility. Close coordination and good communication among the preoperative anesthesiologist, surgeon, and consultant are vitally important for improving perioperative outcomes and avoiding adverse events.

Preoperative consultations may be sought for the following:

(1) Diagnosis, evaluation, and improvement of a new or poorly controlled condition, or
(2) Creation of a clinical risk profile that the patient and perioperative team use to make management decisions.

## ANESTHETIC IMPLICATIONS OF COMMON COMORBID CONDITIONS

### Hypertension

The severity and duration of hypertension (HTN) correlate with the degree of end-organ damage, morbidity, and mortality risks. Ischemic heart disease, heart failure, renal insufficiency, and cerebrovascular disease are common in hypertensive patients. Severe preinduction of anesthesia hypertension (systolic blood pressure [BP] > 200 mm Hg) is an independent risk factor for postoperative myocardial infarction (MI).[11] Hypertensive patients are more likely to have arrhythmias, labile intraoperative BP, and myocardial ischemia. However, in patients with BP less than 180/110 mm Hg, there is little

**Table 13.5** Recommendations for Patient-Specific Baseline Testing Before Anesthesia[a]

| Procedure/Patient Type | Test |
|---|---|
| Injection of contrast dye | Creatinine[b] |
| Potential for significant blood loss | Hemoglobin/hematocrit[b] |
| Likelihood of transfusion requirement | Type and screen |
| Possibility of pregnancy | Pregnancy test[c] |
| End-stage renal disease | Potassium level[d] |
| Diabetes | Glucose level determination on day of surgery[d] |

[a]Not to establish a diagnosis or to guide *preoperative* management.
[b]Results from laboratory tests within 3 months of surgery are acceptable unless major abnormalities are present or the patient's condition has changed.
[c]A routine pregnancy test before surgery is not recommended before the day of surgery. A careful history and local practice determine whether a pregnancy test is indicated.
[d]No absolute level of either potassium or glucose has been determined to preclude surgery and anesthesia. The benefits of the procedure must be balanced against the risk of proceeding in a patient with abnormal results.

---

**Box 13.3** Recommendations for Preoperative Resting 12-Lead Electrocardiogram

**Class IIa**
- Preoperative resting 12-lead electrocardiogram (ECG) is reasonable for patients with known coronary heart disease, significant arrhythmia, peripheral arterial disease, cerebrovascular disease, or other significant structural heart disease, except for those undergoing low-risk surgery

**Class IIb**
- Preoperative resting 12-lead ECG may be considered for asymptomatic patients without known coronary heart disease, except for those undergoing low-risk surgery

**Class III: No Benefit**
- Routine preoperative resting 12-lead ECG is not useful for asymptomatic patients undergoing low-risk surgical procedures

From Fleisher LA, Fleischmann KE, Auerbach AD, et al. 2014 ACC/AHA guideline on perioperative cardiovascular evaluation and management of patients undergoing noncardiac surgery: a report of the American College of Cardiology/American Heart Association Task Force on practice guidelines. *J Am Coll Cardiol.* 2014;64:e77-137.

evidence that delaying surgery improves patient outcome.[12] A true baseline BP is best established by taking several consecutive measurements in a low-stress environment, rather than immediately before induction in the operating room. Maintaining BP within 20% of the patient's baseline is recommended for adequate organ perfusion. If significant end-organ damage is present, or intraoperative hypotensive techniques are planned, risk is minimized by excellent BP control through titration of medications in advance of surgery.[12] This requires weeks of therapy for slow regression of vascular changes, as sudden decreases in BP may result in myocardial ischemia or cerebrovascular events.

## Coronary Artery Disease

Coronary artery disease (CAD) varies from a mild, stable disease with little impact on perioperative outcome to a severe disease accounting for significant complications during anesthesia and surgery. The history and the physical examination, especially a determination of functional status, form the foundation for the cardiac assessment. The goal is to identify those patients likely to benefit from further medical therapy or rarely coronary revascularization before surgery. The ACC/AHA Guideline on Perioperative Cardiovascular Evaluation and Management of Patients Undergoing Noncardiac Surgery guides evaluation for CAD and appropriate testing to identify patients at risk of major adverse cardiovascular events (MACE).[9]

Not all patients with suspected CAD require stress testing or angiography. In patients with stable symptoms (e.g., excluding patients with symptomatic heart failure, significant arrhythmias, severe valvular heart disease, new-onset angina, or an acute coronary syndrome), a moderate or greater functional capacity (≥4 METS) excludes the need for further cardiac investigation.[9] Patients at low risk (<1%) of MACE based on combined clinical and surgical risk do *not* require additional testing.[9] Fig. 13.2 details an algorithm for assessment for CAD. Risk of MACE is easily calculated through online tools established by the American College of Surgeons National Surgical Quality Improvement Program (ACS NSQIP).[13] These assessment tools were developed through data analysis from over 1.4 million patients at multiple institutions and incorporate patient factors and Current Procedural Terminology (CPT) codes to estimate risk of specific adverse outcomes. Alternatively, the Revised Cardiac Risk Index (RCRI) is a validated tool for assessing risk of MACE and incorporates six criteria: (1) presence of ischemic heart disease, (2) history of heart failure, (3) history of cerebrovascular disease, (4) diabetes mellitus treated with insulin, (5) creatinine level of 2 mg/dL or more, and (6) intrathoracic, intra-abdominal, or suprainguinal vascular procedures.[14] The presence of 0, 1, 2, or 3 of these factors is associated with 0.5%, 1.3%, 4%, and 9% risk of MACE, respectively.[14] Therefore, the presence of 2 or more RCRI criteria constitutes increased risk. Patients with increased risk of MACE (>1%) who cannot function at 4 METs of exertion may benefit from pharmacologic stress testing but only if the results will have an impact on perioperative care.[9]

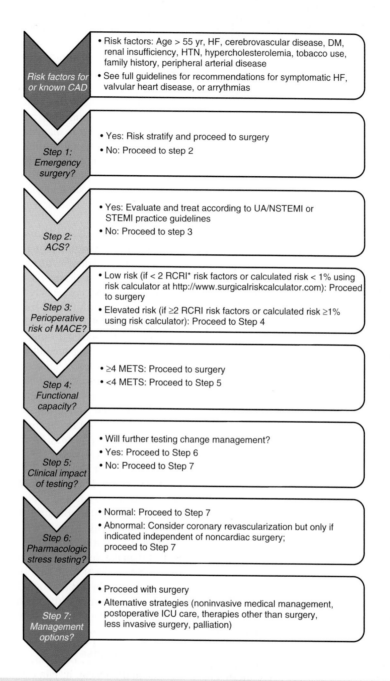

**Fig. 13.2** Simplified algorithm for cardiovascular evaluation of patients for noncardiac surgery. *ACS,* Acute coronary syndrome; *CAD,* coronary artery disease; *Cr,* serum creatinine; *DM,* diabetes mellitus; *HF,* heart failure; *ICU,* intensive care unit; *MACE,* major adverse cardiac event; *METS,* metabolic equivalent of task score; *NSTEMI,* non–ST-segment elevation myocardial infarction; *STEMI,* ST-segment elevation MI; *UA,* unstable angina. *Revised Cardiac Risk Index (RCRI) = ischemic disease, HF, DM, Cr > 2, cerebrovascular disease or higher risk surgery (intrathoracic, intra-abdominal, or vascular). (Modified from Fleisher LA, Fleischmann KE, Auerbach AD, et al. 2014 ACC/AHA guideline on perioperative cardiovascular evaluation and management of patients undergoing noncardiac surgery: a report of the American College of Cardiology/American Heart Association Task Force on practice guidelines. *J Am Coll Cardiol.* 2014;64:e77-137.)

**Box 13.4** Recommendations for Perioperative Management of Antiplatelet Drugs in Patients With Coronary Stents

- Premature discontinuation of thienopyridine (e.g., clopidogrel or ticlopidine) therapy has potentially catastrophic consequences. Health care providers should discuss strategies for periprocedural antiplatelet therapy with the patient's cardiologist prior to discontinuation.
- Elective procedures requiring discontinuation of thienopyridine therapy should be deferred until 1 month after placement of bare metal stents (BMS).
- Elective procedures requiring discontinuation of thienopyridine therapy should be deferred until 6 months after placement of a drug-eluting stent (DES) if placed for stable coronary artery disease, or until 12 months after DES if placed for acute coronary syndrome (ACS) or in other high risk situations (e.g., multiple stents, small stents, recent in-stent stenosis).
- Proceeding with urgent surgery within 3 to 6 months following DES placement may be considered if the risk with delayed surgery is greater than the stent thrombosis risk.
- Patients with either a BMS or DES should continue aspirin if at all possible throughout the procedure. The recommended daily dose is 81 mg (range 75-100 mg) as the bleeding risk is lower and with comparable ischemic protection.

Levine GN, Bates ER, Bittl JA, et al. 2016 ACC/AHA Guideline Focused Update on Duration of Dual Antiplatelet Therapy in Patients With Coronary Artery Disease. A Report of the American College of Cardiology/American Heart Association Task Force on Clinical Practice Guidelines 68(10): 1082-1115.

Contrary to what might be expected, coronary revascularization with percutaneous coronary intervention (PCI) or coronary artery bypass grafting (CABG) before noncardiac surgery does not benefit most patients with CAD. The only randomized prospective study of preoperative revascularization versus medical management failed to show a difference in outcome.[15] Noncardiac surgery soon after revascularization is actually associated with higher rates of morbidity and mortality.[15] Only those patients with unstable or severe disease who would undergo revascularization even in the absence of noncardiac surgery are likely to benefit from preoperative revascularization. The management of antiplatelet agents is complex in patients having preoperative PCI, especially with drug-eluting stents (DES), as they require months, if not a lifetime, of antiplatelet therapy to prevent catastrophic stent restenosis or acute thrombosis. The type of stent, DES or bare metal stent (BMS), must be identified and managed in collaboration with a cardiologist according to published recommendations, which were updated in 2016 by the ACC/AHA (Box 13.4).[16,16a] Prescribed antiplatelet therapy should not be interrupted during the high-risk period without consultation with a cardiologist familiar with coronary stents and an in-depth discussion with the patient regarding the risks of terminating these drugs, especially for elective procedures.[16] If at all possible, aspirin is continued throughout the perioperative period and the thienopyridine (typically clopidogrel) restarted as soon as possible. Evidence supports continuation of aspirin for high-risk patients (secondary prevention or after coronary stenting) during most procedures despite the small risk of bleeding complications.[17] See Fig. 13.3 for details regarding antiplatelet agents in specific situations. In the event of stent thrombosis, PCI can be performed safely even in the immediate postoperative period, so high-risk patients are best managed in facilities with immediate access to interventional cardiology.[12]

Further medical therapy with β-adrenergic blockade or statin therapy in patients with CAD may reduce MACE. See Box 13.5 for a summary of these recommendations.

## Heart Failure

Heart failure is a significant risk factor for perioperative adverse events. Patients with symptomatic heart failure are at a significantly increased risk of perioperative death than patients with CAD, especially those with left ventricular ejection fraction (LVEF) of less than 30%.[9] Heart failure may be caused by systolic dysfunction (decreased ejection fraction from abnormal contractility), diastolic dysfunction (increased filling pressures with abnormal relaxation but normal contractility and ejection fraction), or a combination of the two. Symptoms and signs of heart failure include complaints of shortness of breath, fatigue, orthopnea, paroxysmal nocturnal dyspnea, rales/crackles, or third heart sound. Assessment of left ventricular function by echocardiography may be indicated in patients with a change in physical status (Box 13.6).[9] Diastolic dysfunction accounts for up to half of all cases of heart failure, but there is little science to guide care in the perioperative period. Advanced age and hypertension are associated with diastolic dysfunction. Because decompensated heart failure is a high-risk cardiac condition, elective surgery should be postponed until it is controlled.

Based on the New York Heart Association Functional Classification,[18] patients with class IV failure (symptoms at rest) need evaluation by a cardiologist before undergoing anesthesia. Minor procedures with monitored anesthesia care (MAC) may proceed as long as the patient's condition is stable.

## Valvular Disease

Cardiac murmurs can be clinically unimportant or a sign of valvular abnormalities. Functional murmurs from turbulent flow across the aortic or pulmonary outflow tracts are found with high-output states (hyperthyroidism, pregnancy, anemia). Elderly patients and those with risk factors for CAD, a history of rheumatic fever, excessive intravascular volume, pulmonary disease, cardiomegaly, or an abnormal ECG and a murmur are more likely to have valvular disease. Diastolic murmurs are always pathologic and require evaluation. If significant valvular disease is suspected, evaluation with

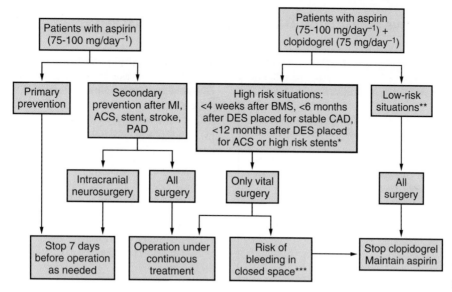

MI, Myocardial infarction; *ACS,* acute coronary syndrome; *PAD,* peripheral arterial disease; *PCI,* percutaneous coronary intervention; *BMS,* bare metal stent; *DES,* drug-eluting stent.

*High-risk stents: long (>36 mm), proximal, overlapping, or multiple stents, stents in chronic total occlusions, or in small vessels or bifurcated lesions.

**Examples of low-risk situations: >1 month after BMS, stroke, uncomplicated MI, PCI without stenting.

***Risk of bleeding in closed space: intracranial neurosurgery, intra-medullary canal surgery, posterior eye chamber ophthalmic surgery. In these situations, the risk/benefit ratio of upholding vs. withdrawing aspirin must be evaluated for each case individually; in case of aspirin upholding, early postoperative re-institution is important.

**Fig. 13.3** Algorithm for perioperative management of patients taking antiplatelet therapy. (From Chassot PG, Delabays A, Spahn DR. Perioperative antiplatelet therapy: the case for continuing therapy in patients at risk of myocardial infarction. *Br J Anaesth.* 2007;99:316-328. Modified to reflect updates in Levine GN, Bates ER, Bittl JA, et al. 2016 ACC/AHA Guideline focused update on duration of dual antiplatelet therapy in patients with coronary artery disease. A report of the American College of Cardiology/American Heart Association Task Force on clinical practice guidelines. 2016;68[10]: 1082-1115.)

---

**Box 13.5** Perioperative Risk Reduction with β-Adrenergic Blockade and Statins: Recommendations

**β-Adrenergic Blockade**

*Class I*

- β-Adrenergic blockers should be continued in patients undergoing surgery who have been on β-adrenergic blockers chronically.

*Class IIa*

- It is reasonable for the management of β-adrenergic blockers after surgery to be guided by clinical circumstances, independent of when the agent was started.

*Class IIb*

- In patients with intermediate- or high-risk myocardial ischemia noted in preoperative risk stratification tests, it may be reasonable to begin perioperative β-adrenergic blockers.
- In patients with three or more Revised Cardiac Risk Index (RCRI) risk factors (e.g., diabetes mellitus, HF, CAD, renal insufficiency, cerebrovascular accident), it may be reasonable to begin β-adrenergic blockers before surgery.
- In patients with a compelling long-term indication for β-adrenergic blocker therapy but no other RCRI risk factors, initiating β-adrenergic blockers in the perioperative setting as an approach is of uncertain benefit to reduce perioperative risk.

- In patients in whom β-adrenergic blocker therapy is initiated, it may be reasonable to begin perioperative β-adrenergic blockers long enough in advance to assess safety and tolerability, preferably more than 1 day before surgery.

*Class III: Harm*

- β-Adrenergic blocker therapy should not be started on the day of surgery.

**Statins**

*Class I*

- Statins should be continued in patients currently taking statins and scheduled for noncardiac surgery.

*Class IIa*

- Perioperative initiation of statin use is reasonable in patients undergoing vascular surgery.

*Class IIb*

- Perioperative initiation of statins may be considered in patients with clinical indications according to guideline-directed medical therapy who are undergoing elevated-risk procedures.

*CAD,* Coronary artery disease; *HF,* heart failure.
From Fleisher LA, Fleischmann KE, Auerbach AD, et al. 2014 ACC/AHA guideline on perioperative cardiovascular evaluation and management of patients undergoing noncardiac surgery: a report of the American College of Cardiology/American Heart Association Task Force on practice guidelines. *J Am Coll Cardiol.* 2014;64:e77-e137.

**Box 13.6** Assessment of Left Ventricular Function: Recommendations

**Class IIa**
- It is reasonable for patients with dyspnea of unknown origin to undergo preoperative evaluation of left ventricular (LV) function.
- It is reasonable for patients with heart failure with worsening dyspnea or other change in clinical status to undergo preoperative evaluation of LV function.

**Class IIb**
- Reassessment of LV function in clinically stable patients with previously documented LV dysfunction may be considered if there has been no assessment within a year.

**Class III: No benefit**
- Routine preoperative evaluation of LV function is not recommended.

From Fleisher LA, Fleischmann KE, Auerbach AD, et al. 2014 ACC/AHA guideline on perioperative cardiovascular evaluation and management of patients undergoing noncardiac surgery: a report of the American College of Cardiology/American Heart Association Task Force on practice guidelines. *J Am Coll Cardiol.* 2014;64:e77-e137.

**Box 13.7** Valvular Heart Disease: Perioperative Recommendations for Aortic and Mitral Valve Disease

**Class I**
1. It is recommended that patients with clinically suspected moderate or greater degrees of valvular stenosis or regurgitation undergo preoperative echocardiography if there has been either (1) no prior echocardiography within 1 year or (2) a significant change in clinical status or physical examination since last evaluation.
2. For adults who meet standard indications for valvular intervention (replacement and repair) on the basis of symptoms and severity of stenosis or regurgitation, valvular intervention before elective noncardiac surgery is effective in reducing perioperative risk.

**Class IIa**
1. Elevated-risk elective noncardiac surgery with appropriate intraoperative and postoperative hemodynamic monitoring is reasonable to perform in patients with asymptomatic severe aortic stenosis.
2. Elevated-risk elective noncardiac surgery with appropriate intraoperative and postoperative hemodynamic monitoring is reasonable in adults with asymptomatic severe mitral regurgitation.
3. Elevated-risk elective noncardiac surgery with appropriate intraoperative and postoperative hemodynamic monitoring is reasonable in adults with asymptomatic severe aortic regurgitation (AR) and a normal LVEF.

**Class IIb**
1. Elevated-risk elective noncardiac surgery using appropriate intraoperative and postoperative hemodynamic monitoring may be reasonable in asymptomatic patients with severe mitral stenosis if valve morphologic appearance is not favorable for percutaneous mitral balloon commissurotomy.

*LVEF,* Left ventricular ejection fraction.
From Nishimura RA, Otto CM, Bonow RO, et al. 2014 AHA/ACC guideline for the management of patients with valvular heart disease: a report of the American College of Cardiology/American Heart Association Task Force on Practice Guidelines. *Circulation.* 2014;129:e521-e643.

echocardiography is recommended if general or spinal anesthesia is planned. In patients found to have a severe valvular lesion (regurgitation or stenosis) for which intervention would be indicated, preoperative repair should be considered prior to nonurgent surgery (Box 13.7).[19]

Antibiotic prophylaxis to prevent infective endocarditis is no longer recommended for patients with valvular abnormalities in native hearts (Box 13.8).[20] Patients with previous cardiac transplant and valvular disease, or with a prosthetic valve, do require prophylaxis but only for certain dental procedures or manipulation of infected tissue. Recommendations for infective endocarditis prophylaxis are contained in Box 13.8.

## Cardiac Implantable Electronic Devices

Pacemakers and implantable cardioverter-defibrillators (ICDs) are types of cardiac implantable electronic devices (CIEDs). They can be affected by electromagnetic interference (EMI) commonly encountered during procedures, such as from monopolar cautery, external radiation, magnetism, or other electrical stimulation. A CIED may sense EMI and interpret it (1) as an underlying heart rate and inappropriately hold pacing (called *oversensing*) while the patient is bradycardic or (2) as an arrhythmia and deliver an inappropriate defibrillation for the perceived abnormality. Oversensing may cause hemodynamic instability in a pacer-dependent patient (whose underlying heart rate is very slow or absent) during periods of continuous EMI (e.g., prolonged periods of cautery, magnetic resonance imaging). Inappropriate defibrillation may result in unexpected patient movement at a critical moment, such as during ocular surgery or neurosurgery, causing serious patient harm. If occurring during ventricular repolarization (R-on-T wave), defibrillation can actually cause ventricular fibrillation. For these reasons, if EMI is anticipated, the CIED requires preoperative management (e.g., deactivation of the ICD or placement of the pacemaker in asynchronous mode). Consultation with the device manufacturer or cardiologist may be needed and contact information is usually recorded on a wallet card carried by the patient.

Sometimes, the use of a magnet is appropriate to temporarily alter CIED function. In general, a magnet will cause a pacemaker to pace in an asynchronous mode at a set rate (e.g., it will ignore all external stimuli and continue to pace regardless of EMI or a patient's underlying rate). A magnet will generally cause an ICD to suspend antitachyarrhythmia features.

**Box 13.8** Recommendations for Endocarditis Prophylaxis in Cardiac Conditions Associated With the Highest Risk of Adverse Outcome

**Class IIa**

1. Prophylaxis against infective endocarditis is reasonable for the following patients *at highest risk* for adverse outcomes from infective endocarditis who undergo dental procedures that involve manipulation of either gingival tissue or the periapical region of teeth or perforation of the oral mucosa:
   - Patients with prosthetic cardiac valves or prosthetic material used for cardiac valve repair.
   - Patients with previous infective endocarditis.
   - Patients with CHD.
   - Unrepaired cyanotic CHD, including palliative shunts and conduits.
   - Completely repaired congenital heart defect repaired with prosthetic material or device, whether placed by surgery or by catheter intervention, during the first 6 months after the procedure.
   - Repaired CHD with residual defects at the site or adjacent to the site of a prosthetic patch or prosthetic device (both of which inhibit endothelialization).
   - Cardiac transplant recipients with valve regurgitation due to a structurally abnormal valve.

**Class III**

1. Prophylaxis against infective endocarditis is not recommended for nondental procedures (such as transesophageal echocardiogram, esophagogastroduodenoscopy, or colonoscopy) in the absence of active infection.

*CHD,* Congenital heart disease.
Modified from Nishimura RA, Carabello BA, Faxon DP, et al. ACC/AHA 2008 guideline update on valvular heart disease: focused update on infective endocarditis: a report of the American College of Cardiology/American Heart Association Task Force on Practice Guidelines: endorsed by the Society of Cardiovascular Anesthesiologists, Society for Cardiovascular Angiography and Interventions, and Society of Thoracic Surgeons. *Circulation.* 2008;118:887-896.

These rules do not always apply for certain devices, so preoperative interrogation by the electrophysiology service is recommended to verify magnet function and reprogram the CIED if needed. An important exception is for a CIED that functions as both a patient's pacemaker *and* ICD. In this case, a magnet will *only* deactivate the ICD and will *not* affect the pacing function, so these devices require reprogramming if EMI is anticipated in a pacemaker-dependent patient.[21] ICDs are deactivated with either a magnet or reprogramming only after arrival to a facility with devices for monitoring and external cardioversion. If a CIED is reprogrammed, the device must be re-interrogated and re-enabled before the patient leaves a monitored setting. Methods to avoid EMI interference include use of bipolar (vs. monopolar) cautery when possible and placement of the Bovie return pad to avoid current transmission across the CIED. Generally, procedures below the umbilicus will not cause EMI with a CIED.

**Table 13.6**   Positive Predictive Factors of Postoperative Pulmonary Complications[a]

| Risk Factor | Odds Ratio |
| --- | --- |
| **Potential Patient-Related Risk Factor** | |
| Advanced age | 2.09-3.04 |
| ASA class $\geq$ II | 2.55-4.87 |
| CHF | 2.93 |
| Functionally dependent | 1.65-2.51 |
| COPD | 1.79 |
| Weight loss | 1.62 |
| Impaired sensorium | 1.39 |
| Cigarette use | 1.26 |
| Alcohol use | 1.21 |
| **Potential Procedure-Related Risk Factor** | |
| Aortic aneurysm repair | 6.90 |
| Thoracic surgery | 4.24 |
| Abdominal surgery | 3.01 |
| Upper abdominal surgery | 2.91 |
| Neurosurgery | 2.53 |
| Prolonged surgery | 2.26 |
| Head and neck surgery | 2.21 |
| Emergency surgery | 2.21 |
| Vascular surgery | 2.10 |
| General anesthesia | 1.83 |
| Perioperative transfusion | 1.47 |
| **Laboratory Tests** | |
| Albumin level < 35 g/L | 2.53 |
| Chest radiography | 4.81 |

[a]At least fair to good evidence to support the particular risk factor.
*ASA,* American Society of Anesthesiologists; *CHF,* congestive heart failure; *COPD,* chronic obstructive pulmonary disease.
Modified from Smetana GW, Lawrence VA, Cornell JE. American College of Physicians: preoperative pulmonary risk stratification for noncardiothoracic surgery: systematic review for the American College of Physicians. *Ann Intern Med.* 2006;144:581-595.

## Pulmonary Disease

Pulmonary disease increases both pulmonary and nonpulmonary perioperative complications. Predictors of postoperative pulmonary complications (PPC) include advanced age, heart failure, chronic obstructive pulmonary disease (COPD), smoking, general health status (including impaired sensorium and functional dependency), and obstructive sleep apnea (OSA) (Table 13.6).[22] Well-controlled asthma does not increase perioperative complications, whereas

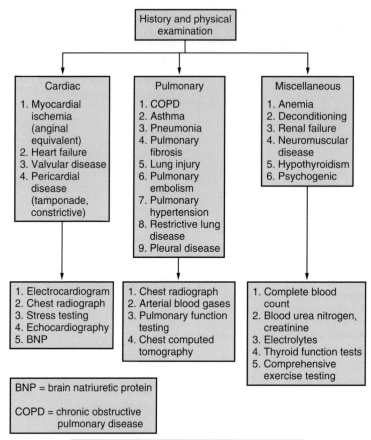

**Fig. 13.4** Guideline for the evaluation of dyspnea.

patients with poorly controlled asthma (as evidenced by wheezing at the time of anesthetic induction) are at risk for complications. Unlike asthma, increasing COPD severity increases the risk of pulmonary complications; however, there is no degree of severity that absolutely precludes surgery. The risks with COPD are less than those with heart failure, advanced age, or poor general health.

The value of routine and often expensive preoperative testing is appropriately and increasingly questioned. Surprisingly, routine pulmonary function tests, chest radiography, or analysis of arterial blood gases do not predict pulmonary risk and offer little more information than can be determined by clinical evaluation. PPC rates are reduced by maximizing airflow in obstructive disease, treating infections and heart failure, and using lung expansion maneuvers such as coughing, deep breathing, incentive spirometry, positive end-expiratory pressure (PEEP), and continuous positive airway pressure (CPAP). "Prehabilitation" before surgery through regulated exercise to increase the functional capacity of patients may be an effective means of improving recovery and decreasing complications.[23]

A history of dyspnea is commonly caused by COPD or asthma. However, there are many other pulmonary and nonpulmonary causes of dyspnea from which these must be differentiated. Myocardial ischemia, heart failure, restrictive lung disease, anemia, and neuromuscular disorders can cause dyspnea. See Fig. 13.4 for a suggested diagnostic plan for delineating dyspnea.

## Obstructive Sleep Apnea

Obstructive sleep apnea (OSA) is caused by intermittent airway obstruction (also see Chapter 50) and is a risk factor for perioperative complications.[24] Patients with OSA have increased rates of diabetes, hypertension, atrial fibrillation, bradyarrhythmias, ventricular ectopy, stroke, heart failure, pulmonary hypertension, dilated cardiomyopathy, and CAD.[22] Ventilation via a mask, direct laryngoscopy, endotracheal intubation, and fiberoptic visualization of the airway are more difficult in patients with OSA.[24] Such patients are likely to have perioperative airway obstruction, hypoxemia, atelectasis, myocardial ischemia, pneumonia, and prolonged hospitalizations.[25]

Snoring, daytime sleepiness, hypertension, obesity, and a family history of OSA are risk factors for OSA.[26] The

STOP-BANG questionnaire was developed and validated in an anesthesia preoperative clinic to screen for OSA (Fig. 13.5).[26] Patients who use CPAP devices should bring them for their procedures. The ASA and the Society of Ambulatory Anesthesia (SAMBA) have published recommendations for the perioperative care of patients with OSA, which includes preoperative diagnosis and treatment of OSA if possible and appropriateness of ambulatory surgery.[27,28]

## Obesity

Extreme obesity is defined by a body mass index (BMI) of 40 or more. Obese patients may have OSA, heart failure, diabetes, hypertension, pulmonary hypertension, difficult airways, decreased arterial oxygenation, and increased gastric volume. Special equipment is needed to care for obese patients: oversized BP cuffs, airway management devices, and large procedure tables and gurneys to support excessive weight.

## Diabetes Mellitus

Patients with poorly controlled diabetes are at risk for perioperative complications for multiple reasons. End-organ damage from chronic hyperglycemia results in renal insufficiency, strokes, peripheral neuropathies, visual impairment, and cardiovascular disease. Poorly controlled diabetes, as assessed by elevated glycosylated hemoglobin (HbA$_{1c}$ ≥ 7%), contributes to surgical site infections, bloodstream infections, other morbidity, and death.[29] Increased HbA$_{1c}$ preoperatively predicts perioperative glucose levels.[30] Targeting control in the short-term perioperative period likely will not have a substantial impact on outcomes in diabetics having surgery; however, optimal preoperative control of blood sugar should be a goal before elective higher risk surgeries. Diabetic ketoacidosis and hypoglycemia (glucose < 70 g/dL) are the only conditions that absolutely warrant perioperative intervention. The goals of glucose control are to prevent hypoglycemia during fasting and to avoid extreme hyperglycemia and ketosis.

## Renal Disease

Renal disease is associated with hypertension, cardiovascular disease, excessive intravascular volume, electrolyte disturbances, metabolic acidosis, and often a need to alter the types and amounts of anesthetic drugs administered. Hemodialysis should be performed the day before elective surgery to avoid complications related to hyper- or hypovolemia and major electrolyte abnormalities. Many patients with renal insufficiency are chronically hyperkalemic and tolerate slight increases in serum potassium concentrations without consequence. A serum potassium concentration less than 6 mEq/dL obtained immediately prior to surgery is acceptable.

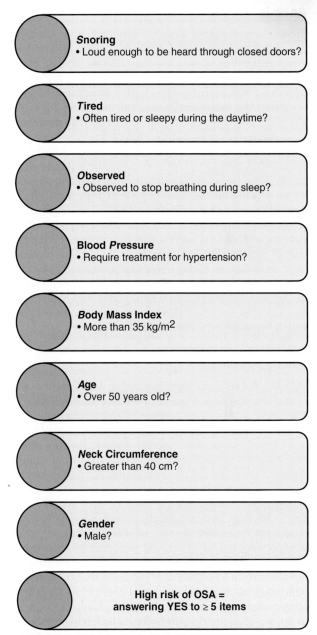

**Snoring**
• Loud enough to be heard through closed doors?

**Tired**
• Often tired or sleepy during the daytime?

**Observed**
• Observed to stop breathing during sleep?

**Blood Pressure**
• Require treatment for hypertension?

**Body Mass Index**
• More than 35 kg/m$^2$

**Age**
• Over 50 years old?

**Neck Circumference**
• Greater than 40 cm?

**Gender**
• Male?

**High risk of OSA = answering YES to ≥ 5 items**

Fig. 13.5 STOP-BANG screening questionnaire for obstructive sleep apnea (OSA). (From Chung F, Yegneswaran B, Liao P, et al. STOP Questionnaire. A tool to screen patients for obstructive sleep apnea. *Anesthesiology.* 2008;108:812-821.)

Radiocontrast media transiently decrease glomerular filtration rate (GFR) in almost all patients, but patients with diabetes or renal insufficiency are at significantly increased risk of developing contrast-induced nephropathy. Simple hydration with nonhyperchloremic solution and maintenance of adequate mean arterial BP reduce injury.[31]

## Anemia

Preoperative anemia is a common finding and is strongly associated with the need for blood transfusion (also see Chapter 24). Both anemia and transfusions increase morbidity and mortality risks.[32] An evaluation of the cause of anemia is indicated before elective procedures. Simply reviewing the mean corpuscular volume (MCV) for classification as micro-, normo-, or macrocytic will guide the need for further testing. Iron studies and screening for occult blood loss in microcytic anemia is especially helpful, as this common cause of anemia may be improved with preoperative iron supplementation. Erythropoietin administration is indicated in certain patients (e.g., renal insufficiency, anemia of chronic disease, refusal of transfusion) if significant blood loss is anticipated.[33] For asymptomatic patients with chronic anemia and no history of CAD who may be planning low-risk procedures, the minimal physiologic perturbations during a well-conducted anesthetic are unlikely to pose enough risk to warrant transfusion unless the hemoglobin is less than 6 g/dL[33] (also see Chapter 24). Patients with sickle cell disease are managed in concert with a hematologist familiar with the disease.

## Elderly Patients

Elderly patients (also see Chapter 35) have declines in organ function and respond differently to medications. They have an increased number of comorbid conditions including arthritis, hypertension, heart disease, diabetes, renal insufficiency, and vascular disease. Patients older than 85 years with a history of hospital admission within the previous 6 months are at high risk for postoperative admission after ambulatory surgery.[34] Yet, the rate of perioperative complications among the very elderly (>85 years old) does not exclude them from having surgical procedures[35] (also see Chapter 35). Discharge planning in advance may lessen the costs of perioperative elder care. Preoperative clinics can be designed to offer multidisciplinary care and postdischarge planning that coordinates with surgical, nursing, and social service departments. Many elderly patients have or desire advance directives or do-not-resuscitate (DNR) orders, which require special discussion. Automatically suspending or enforcing DNR orders while in the operating room does not fully respect a patient's right to autonomy and informed consent regarding anesthesia and surgery. Several options for modification of DNR orders exist and they should be discussed with the patient in advance (Fig. 13.6 and Box 13.9).

## FORMULATION OF AN ANESTHETIC PLAN

### Risk Assessment and Informed Consent

There are several important factors to consider when formulating an anesthetic plan, which may make certain choices more advisable than others (Box 13.10).

Risk assessment is useful to compare outcomes, control costs, allocate compensation, and assist in the difficult decisions to recommend canceling or postponing a procedure when the risks are too severe or likely. A simple and robust risk assessment tool used commonly is the ASA PS classification system (see Table 13.1); however, additional procedure-related risk must also be considered (Fig. 13.7). The ACS NSQIP surgical risk calculator provides a more complete estimate of patient and procedural risk.[13] Assessment of risk is important in order to inform patients during the consent process (Box 13.11).

Informed consent must be obtained for all nonemergency procedures and is a legal requirement in all jurisdictions of the United States and is extensively used internationally. At a minimum, informed consent involves the indications for the treatment in terms a layperson can understand and elucidation of alternatives. Many anesthesiologists perform preoperative evaluation and obtain informed consent moments before a patient will undergo a major, potentially life-threatening or disfiguring procedure. The effects of extensive disclosure are stressful at a time when patients and families may be ill prepared to rationally consider the implications. Informed consent should contain a discussion of risks that are common but minor, as well as rare but serious complications (see Box 13.11). Throughout the preoperative discussion, a professional and reassuring interaction will assist in allaying patient anxiety.

## Medications

Instructions to patients to continue or discontinue medications are a critical part of a perioperative plan, as medications can be beneficial or detrimental during surgery, or the sudden cessation of therapy may be harmful. Patient comorbid conditions and the nature of the procedure are considered when managing medications. A summary of recommendations for perioperative administration of medications is in Table 13.7. Several drug classes deserve special mention.

Generally, cardiac medications and antihypertensive drugs are continued preoperatively. Angiotensin-converting enzyme inhibitors (ACEIs), angiotensin receptor blockers (ARBs), diuretics, and anticoagulants may be beneficial even on the day of surgery. Decisions about these drugs depend on the intravascular volume, hemodynamic status, the degree of cardiac dysfunction, the adequacy of arterial BP control of the patient, and any anticipated anesthetic or intravascular volume concerns. The best approach for patients with severe disease is to continue all cardiac medications. A similar approach is likely beneficial for patients who do not require general anesthesia or who are undergoing low- to intermediate-risk procedures. If ACEIs and ARBs are continued, doses of drugs used to induce anesthesia and other anesthetics may be altered. The potential for hypotension must be balanced against

_____ Option 1 - Full Resuscitation

I, _____ , desire that full resuscitation measures be employed during my anesthesia and in the postanesthesia care unit, regardless of the situation.

_____ Option 2 - Limited Resuscitation: Procedure-directed

During my anesthesia and in the postanesthesia care unit, I, _____ , refuse the following procedures:

_____

_____

_____ Option 3 - Limited Resuscitation: Goal-directed

I, _____ , desire attempts to resuscitate me during my anesthesia and in the postanesthesia care unit only if, in the clinical judgement of the attending anesthesiologist and surgeon, the adverse clinical events are believed to be both temporary and reversible.

_____ Option 4 - Limited Resuscitation: Goal-directed

I, _____ , desire attempts to resuscitate me during my anesthesia and in the postanesthesia care unit only if, in the clinical judgement of the attending anesthesiologist and surgeon, such resuscitation efforts will support the following goals and values of mine: _____

_____

| | |
|---|---|
| Patient or surrogate signature | Date |
| Physician signature | Date |
| Witness signature | Date |

**Fig. 13.6** Anesthesia care for the patient with an existing do-not-resuscitate (DNR) order. (From Truog RD, Waisel DB. Do-not-resuscitate orders: from the ward to the operating room; from procedures to goals. _Int Anesthesiol Clin._ 2001;39:53-65.)

---

**Box 13.9** Do-Not-Resuscitate (DNR) Orders in the Perioperative Period

The administration of anesthesia necessarily involves some practices and procedures that might be viewed as "resuscitation" in other settings. Prior to procedures requiring anesthetic care, any existing directives to limit the use of resuscitation procedures (that is, do-not-resuscitate orders and/or advance directives) should, when possible, be reviewed with the patient or designated surrogate. As a result of this review, the status of these directives should be clarified or modified based on the preferences of the patient. One of the three following alternatives may provide for a satisfactory outcome in many cases.

A. _Full Attempt at Resuscitation:_ The patient or designated surrogate may request the full suspension of existing directives during the anesthetic and immediate postoperative period, thereby consenting to the use of any resuscitation procedures that may be appropriate to treat clinical events that occur during this time.

B. _Limited Attempt at Resuscitation Defined With Regard to Specific Procedures:_ The patient or designated surrogate may elect to continue to refuse certain specific resuscitation procedures (e.g., chest compressions, defibrillation, or tracheal intubation). The anesthesiologist should inform the patient or designated surrogate about which procedures are (1) essential to the success of the anesthesia and the proposed procedure and (2) which procedures are not essential and may be refused.

C. _Limited Attempt at Resuscitation Defined With Regard to the Patient's Goals and Values:_ The patient or designated surrogate may allow the anesthesiologist and surgical/procedural team to use clinical judgment in determining which resuscitation procedures are appropriate in the context of the situation and the patient's stated goals and values. For example, some patients may want full resuscitation procedures to be used to manage adverse clinical events that are believed to be quickly and easily reversible but to refrain from treatment for conditions that are likely to result in permanent sequelae, such as neurologic impairment or unwanted dependence upon life-sustaining technology.

From American Society of Anesthesiologists. Ethical Guidelines for the Anesthesia Care of Patients With Do-Not-Resuscitate Orders or Other Directives That Limit Treatment. October 16, 2013. www.asahq.org.

**Box 13.10** Considerations That Influence the Choice of Anesthetic Technique

**Patient Factors**
- Coexisting diseases
- Risk of aspiration
- Age of the patient
- Patient cooperation
- Anticipated ease of airway management
- Coagulation status
- Previous response to anesthesia
- Preference of the patient

**Procedural Factors**
- Site of the surgery
- Operative technique (e.g., laparoscopic versus open approach)
- Position of the patient during surgery
- Duration of surgery

**Logistical Factors**
- Postoperative disposition
- Postoperative analgesic plan
- Equipment availability (e.g., ultrasound)

**Box 13.11** Commonly Disclosed Risks of Anesthesia

**With General Anesthesia**
**Frequently occurring, minimal impact**
- Oral or dental damage
- Sore throat
- Hoarseness
- Postoperative nausea/vomiting
- Drowsiness/confusion
- Urinary retention

**Infrequently occurring, severe impact**
- Awareness
- Visual loss
- Aspiration
- Organ failure
- Malignant hyperthermia
- Drug reactions
- Failure to wake up/recover
- Death

**With Regional Anesthesia**
**Frequently occurring, minimal impact**
- Prolonged numbness/weakness
- Post–dural puncture headache
- Failure of technique

**Infrequently occurring, severe impact**
- Bleeding
- Infection
- Nerve damage/paralysis
- Persistent numbness/weakness
- Seizures
- Coma
- Death

Modified from O'Leary CE. Informed consent: principles and practice. *ASA Monitor.* 2010;74:20-21.

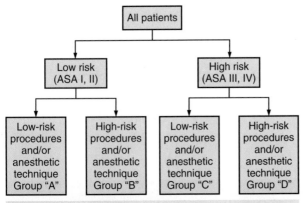

**Fig. 13.7** Example of a risk classification incorporating both patient comorbid conditions and surgical severity. ASA, American Society of Anesthesiologists. (From Pasternak LR. Risk assessment in ambulatory surgery: challenges and new trends. *Can J Anaesth.* 2004;51[S1]:R1-R5.)

the positive therapeutic impact of continuing these drugs perioperatively.[36]

It is recommended (class I indication) that β-blockers be continued in patients who take them to treat angina, symptomatic arrhythmias, or hypertension (see Box 13.5).[37] Minimizing risk for high-risk patients scheduled for elective surgery may entail postponing surgery to optimize β-adrenergic blockers and statin therapy (see Box 13.5). Statins reduce length of hospital stay and risk of stroke, renal dysfunction, MI, and even death.[38,39] Terminating statin administration is associated with an increased risk.[40]

Aspirin is commonly used to decrease vascular events in patients with known or suspected vascular disease, diabetes, renal insufficiency, or simply advanced age. Traditionally, aspirin was withdrawn in the perioperative period because of concern of bleeding, but this practice has come under scrutiny. A meta-analysis of almost 50,000 patients undergoing a variety of noncardiac surgeries (30% taking aspirin perioperatively) found that aspirin increased bleeding complications by a factor of 1.5, but not the severity of bleeding, except in patients undergoing intracranial surgery and possibly transurethral resection of the prostate.[17] However, acute coronary syndromes in at-risk patients are more common after aspirin cessation, and uncertainty remains over best-practice recommendations.[17,41] Aspirin is withheld for 5 to 7 days before elective surgery in patients without guideline-based indications for aspirin therapy.[41] For most minor, superficial procedures such as cataract extraction, endoscopies, and peripheral procedures, the risk of withdrawing aspirin in at-risk patients is more than the risk of bleeding, so aspirin is continued. Aspirin is discontinued if taken only for primary prevention (no history of stents, strokes, MI) (see Fig. 13.3 and Table 13.7).[42] Aspirin administration should be continued if taken for secondary prevention (history of stents or vascular disease), except for procedures with a risk of bleeding in closed spaces (e.g., intracranial, intraspinal).[41]

**Table 13.7**   Preanesthesia Medication Instructions

| Continue on Day of Surgery | Discontinue on Day of Surgery Unless Otherwise Indicated |
|---|---|
| Antidepressant, antianxiety, and psychiatric medications (including monoamine oxidase inhibitors[a]) | |
| Antihypertensives<br>• Generally to be continued | Antihypertensives<br>• May consider discontinuing angiotensin-converting enzyme inhibitors or angiotensin receptor blockers 12-24 h before surgery if taken only for hypertension; especially with lengthy procedures, significant blood loss or fluid shifts, use of general anesthesia, multiple antihypertensive medications, well-controlled blood pressure |
| Aspirin[b]<br>• Patients with known vascular disease<br>• Patients with previous cardiac stents<br>• Before cataract surgery<br>• Before vascular surgery<br>• Taken for secondary prophylaxis (vascular disease of any type) | Aspirin[b]<br>• Discontinue 5-7 days before surgery<br>  • If risk of bleeding > risk of thrombosis<br>  • For surgeries with serious consequences from bleeding<br>  • If taken only for primary prophylaxis (no known vascular disease) |
| Asthma medications | |
| Autoimmune medications<br>• Methotrexate (if no risk of renal failure) | Autoimmune medications<br>• Methotrexate (if risk of renal failure)<br>• Entanercept (Enbrel), infliximab (Remicade), adalimumab (Humira): check with prescriber (typically *not* stopped for inflammatory bowel disease) |
| β-Blockers | |
| Birth control pills | Birth control pills (if high risk of thrombosis) |
| Clopidogrel (Plavix)[a]<br>• Patients with drug-eluting stents for <6 months<br>• Patients with bare metal stents for <1 month<br>• Before cataract surgery | Clopidogrel (Plavix)[a]<br>• Patients not included in group recommended for continuation<br>• Patients with drug-eluting stents for 3-6 months if risk of delaying surgery is greater than risk of stent thrombosis |
| Diuretics<br>• Triamterene, hydrochlorothiazide | Diuretics<br>• Potent loop diuretics |
| Eye drops | |
| Estrogen compounds<br>• When used for birth control or cancer therapy (unless high risk of thrombosis) | Estrogen compounds<br>• When used to control menopause symptoms or for osteoporosis |
| Gastrointestinal reflux medications<br>• Histamine antagonists, proton-pump inhibitors, gastric motility agents | Gastrointestinal reflux medications<br>• Particulate antacids (e.g., Tums) |
| | Herbals and nonvitamin supplements<br>• 7-14 days before surgery |
| Insulin<br>• *Type 1 diabetes*: take ~ one third of intermediate to long-acting (NPH, Lente)<br>• *Type 2 diabetes*: take up to one half long-acting (NPH) or combination (70/30) preparations<br>• Glargine (Lantus): decrease only if dose is ≥1 unit/kg<br>• With insulin pump delivery, continue lowest nighttime basal rate<br>• Discontinue if blood sugar level <100 | Hypoglycemic agents, oral<br>Insulin<br>• Regular insulin (*exception*: with insulin pump, continue lowest basal rate—generally nighttime dose) |

*Continued*

| Table 13.7 | Preanesthesia Medication Instructions—cont'd |
| --- | --- |

| Continue on Day of Surgery | Discontinue on Day of Surgery Unless Otherwise Indicated |
| --- | --- |
| Opioid medications for pain or addiction | |
| Seizure medications | |
| | Nonsteroidal antiinflammatory drugs<br>• Discontinue for 5 half-lives of the drug[c] |
| Statins | |
| | Topical creams and ointments |
| Steroids (oral or inhaled) | |
| Thyroid medications | |
| | Vitamins, minerals, iron |
| | Viagra or similar medications<br>• Discontinue 24 h before surgery |
| Warfarin<br>• Cataract surgery | Warfarin[d]<br>• Discontinue 5 days before surgery if normal INR (international normalized ratio) is required |

[a]See text for details.

[b]Except when the risk or consequences of bleeding are severe (generally only with intracranial or posterior eye procedures). If regional anesthesia considered, see Table 13.8.

[c]See Table 13.8.

[d]Bridging may be necessary; see text and Table 13.9 for details.

The management of antiplatelet agents (e.g., aspirin, nonsteroidal antiinflammatory drugs [NSAIDs], clopidogrel) and anticoagulants (e.g., heparin, low-molecular-weight heparin [LMWH], dabigatran, rivaroxiban) in patients having regional or neuraxial anesthesia is complex. The American Society of Regional Anesthesia (ASRA) stratifies recommendations for management by the bleeding complication risk of the procedure: low risk (e.g., peripheral nerve blocks); intermediate risk (e.g., paravertebral blocks); and high risk (e.g., epidural instrumentation, intrathecal catheter).[43] Peripheral regional anesthesia in patients taking aspirin is safe and endorsed by the ASRA; however, the decision to continue aspirin during intermediate- or high-risk procedures requires shared assessment and risk stratification.[43] NSAIDs are held for five half-lives of the drug for high-risk procedures only.[43] Clopidogrel is discontinued 7 days before a planned neuraxial procedure.[43] LMWH is discontinued 12 (for prophylactic dosing) to 24 hours (for therapeutic dosing) before procedures with a risk of bleeding or a planned neuraxial procedure[43] (also see Chapter 17). Warfarin may increase bleeding except during minor procedures such as cataract surgery and is held 5 days before surgery if a normal international normalized ratio (INR) is required.[43] Table 13.8 details current recommendations for commonly encountered medications (for complete recommendations, the reader is referred to the ASRA guidelines).[43]

Bridging anticoagulation with LMWH while longer acting anticoagulants are not given may be indicated for patients at high risk (>10% annual risk) of arterial thromboembolism (e.g., stroke) or recurrent venous thromboembolism. Table 13.9 details an approach to risk stratification, although there are additional high-risk patient features that may not fall directly into these categories.[44] For patients at low risk, bridging anticoagulation is not recommended.[45]

Type 1 diabetics have an absolute insulin deficiency and require insulin to prevent ketoacidosis even if they are not hyperglycemic. Type 2 diabetics are often insulin-resistant and prone to extreme hyperglycemia. Both type 1 and 2 diabetics should discontinue intermittent short-acting insulin (also see Chapter 29). Patients with insulin pumps continue with their lowest basal rate, which is typically a nighttime rate. Type 1 diabetics take a small amount (usually one third to one half) of their usual intermediate- to long-acting morning insulin (e.g., Lente or NPH) the day of surgery to avoid ketoacidosis. Type 2 diabetics take none or up to half a dose of intermediate- to long-acting (e.g., Lente or NPH) or a combination (70/30 preparations) insulin on the day of surgery. Ultra-long-acting insulin such as glargine insulin is taken as scheduled.

Metformin is held on the day of surgery but will not cause hypoglycemia if continued during fasting periods

**Table 13.8** Management Recommendations for Selected Antiplatelet/Anticoagulant Medications Before Regional or Neuraxial Procedures

| Drug | When to Stop | | | When to Restart |
| | High-Risk Procedure | Intermediate-Risk Procedure | Low-Risk Procedure | |
| --- | --- | --- | --- | --- |
| Aspirin and combination | Primary prophylaxis: 6 days OR seconday prophylaxis: shared assessment and risk stratification[a] | Shared assessment and risk stratification[a] | No | 24 hours |
| NSAIDs | 5 half-lives | No | No | 24 hours |
| Diclofenac | 1 day | | | |
| Ketorolac | 1 day | | | |
| Ibuprofen | 1 day | | | |
| Indomethacin | 2 days | | | |
| Naproxen | 4 days | | | |
| Meloxicam | 4 days | | | |
| **Antiplatelets** | | | | |
| Dipyridamole | 2 days | No | No | N/A |
| Clopidogrel | 7 days | 7 days | No | 12-24 hours |
| **Anticoagulants** | | | | |
| Warfarin | 5 days, normal INR | 5 days, normal INR | No OR shared assessment and risk stratification[a] | 24 hours |
| IV heparin infusion | 4 hours | 4 hours | 4 hours | 2 hours[b] |
| Subcutaneous heparin, bid and tid | 8-10 hours | 8-10 hours | 8-10 hours | 2 hours |
| LMWH: prophylactic | 12 hours | 12 hours | 12 hours | 4 hours after low-risk OR 12-24 hours after intermediate- to high-risk procedures |
| LMWH: therapeutic | 24 hours | 24 hours | 24 hours | |
| Dabigatran | 4-5 days OR 6 days (impaired renal function) | 4-5 days OR 6 days (impaired renal function) | Shared assessment and risk stratification[a] | 24 hours |
| Rivaroxaban | 3 days | 3 days | | |
| Apixaban | 3-5 days | 3-5 days | | |
| Fibrinolytic agents | 48 hours | 48 hours | 48 hours | 48 hours |

[a]Case-by-case analysis of risks and benefits of continued therapy recommended.
[b]If an intermediate- or high-risk procedure was bloody, then a 24-hour interval should be observed.
*bid*, Twice a day; *INR*, international normalized ratio; *IV*, intravenous; *LMWH*, low-molecular-weight heparin; *tid*, three times a day.
Modified from Narouze S, Benzon HT, Provenzano DA, et al. Interventional spine and pain procedures in patients on antiplatelet and anticoagulant medications: guidelines from the American Society of Regional Anesthesia and Pain Medicine, the European Society of Regional Anaesthesia and Pain Therapy, the American Academy of Pain Medicine, the International Neuromodulation Society, the North American Neuromodulation Society, and the World Institute of Pain. *Reg Anesth Pain Med.* 2015;40:182-212.

| Table 13.9 | Risk Stratification for Perioperative Thromboembolism: Assessment of Need for Perioperative Bridging Anticoagulation |
|---|---|

| | Indication for Anticoagulation Bridging Therapy | | |
|---|---|---|---|
| **Risk Stratum** | **Mechanical Heart Valve** | **Atrial Fibrillation** | **Venous Thromboembolism** |
| High[a] | • Any mitral valve prosthesis<br>• Any caged-ball or tilting disc aortic valve prosthesis<br>• Recent (within 6 months) stroke or TIA | • CHADS$_2$ score of 5 or 6<br>• Recent (within 3 months) stroke or TIA<br>• Rheumatic valvular heart disease | • Recent (within 3 months) VTE<br>• Severe thrombophilia (e.g., deficiency of protein C, protein S, or antithrombin; antiphospholipid antibodies; multiple abnormalities) |
| Moderate | • Bileaflet aortic valve prosthesis and one or more of the following risk factors: AF, prior stroke or TIA, HTN, DM, heart failure, age >75 yr | • CHADS$_2$ score of 3 or 4 | • VTE in past 3-12 months<br>• Nonsevere thrombophilia (e.g., heterozygous factor V$_{Leiden}$ or prothrombin gene mutation)<br>• Recurrent VTE<br>• Active cancer (treated within 6 months or palliative) |
| Low | • Bileaflet aortic valve prosthesis without AF and no other risk factors for stroke | • CHADS$_2$ score of 0 to 2 (assuming no prior stroke or TIA) | • VTE >12 months and no other risk factors |

[a]High-risk patients may also include those with prior stroke or TIA occurring >3 months before the planned surgery and a CHADS$_2$ score <5, those with prior VTE during temporary interruption of anticoagulation, or those undergoing certain types of surgeries associated with an increased risk of stroke or other thromboembolism (e.g., cardiac valve replacement, carotid endarterectomy, major vascular surgery).

*AF*, Atrial fibrillation; *CHADS$_2$*, congestive heart failure, hypertension, age ≥75 years, diabetes mellitus, and stroke or TIA (2 points for stroke or TIA); *DM*, diabetes mellitus; *HTN*, hypertension; *TIA*, transient ischemic attack; *VTE*, venous thromboembolism.

From Douketis JD, Spyropoulos AC, Spencer FA, et al. Perioperative management of antithrombotic therapy: Antithrombotic Therapy and Prevention of Thrombosis, 9th ed: American College of Chest Physicians Evidence-Based Clinical Practice Guidelines. *Chest.* 2012;141(2 Suppl):e326S-e350S.

of 1 to 2 days. There is no risk of lactic acidosis with metformin in patients with a functioning liver and kidneys, and surgery does not need to be delayed in patients who take metformin on the day of surgery.[46] Sulfonylurea drugs with very long half-lives (e.g., chlorpropamide) can cause hypoglycemia in fasting patients. Newer oral drugs (acarbose, pioglitazone) used as single-agent therapy do not cause hypoglycemia during fasting. However, to avoid confusion, all oral hypoglycemic drugs are generally withheld on the day of surgery.

Patients taking steroids regularly take their usual dose on the day of surgery. Stress-associated adrenal insufficiency in some patients may require additional steroids perioperatively. A normal daily adrenal output of cortisol (30 mg) is equivalent to 5 to 7.5 mg of prednisone. The hypothalamic-pituitary axis (HPA) is not suppressed with less than 5 mg/day of prednisone or its equivalent. The HPA is suppressed with more than 20 mg/day of prednisone or its equivalent when taken for more than 3 weeks. The risk of adrenal insufficiency may remain up to 1 year after use of high-dose steroids. Supplementation with steroids depends on the amount of stress, duration, and severity of the procedure and the regular daily dose of steroid (Table 13.10). Infections, psychosis,

poor wound healing, and hyperglycemia increase with high doses of perioperative steroids, which are rarely necessary.[47]

Herbals and supplements are discontinued 7 to 14 days before surgery. The exception is valerian, a central nervous system depressant, which may cause a benzodiazepine-like withdrawal when discontinued. If possible, intake of valerian should be tapered before a planned anesthetic. Mandatory discontinuation of these medications, or cancellation of anesthesia when these medications have been continued, is not supported by available data.

Historically, monoamine oxidase inhibitors (MAOIs) were discontinued for 3 weeks before surgery because of their long duration of action and potential for extremely exaggerated response to sympathomimetics. However, discontinuation of MAOIs may produce severe depression or result in suicide, so the safest alternative is to continue MAOIs and adjust the anesthetic plan. Other drugs associated with withdrawal are continued perioperatively, including anxiolytics, opioids, and nicotine-replacement therapies.

Patients with a history of severe postoperative nausea and vomiting (PONV) can be offered a prescription for a scopolamine patch to be placed 2 to 4 hours

**Table 13.10**   Recommendations for Perioperative Glucocorticoid Coverage

| Surgical Stress | Hydrocortisone-Equivalent | Preoperative | Intraoperative | Postoperative Days 1 and 2 |
|---|---|---|---|---|
| Minor (e.g., inguinal herniorrhaphy) | 25 mg/day for 1 day, then usual daily dose | None[a] | None[a] | Usual daily dose[a,b] |
| Moderate (e.g., colectomy, total joint replacement, lower extremity revascularization) | 50-75 mg/day for 1-2 days, then usual daily dose | 50 mg[a] hydrocortisone | 20 mg[a] hydrocortisone every 8 h | 20 mg[a] hydrocortisone every 8 h |
| Major (e.g., pancreatoduodenectomy, esophagectomy) | 100-150 mg/day for 2-3 days, then usual daily dose | 50 mg[a] hydrocortisone | 50 mg[a] hydrocortisone every 8 h | 50 mg[a] hydrocortisone every 8 h |

[a]If postoperative complications occur, continued glucocorticoid administration will be necessary commensurate with the level of stress.
[b]If the postoperative course is uncomplicated, the patient can resume the usual steroid dose on postoperative day 1.
From Salem M, Tainsh RE, Bromberg J, et al. Perioperative glucocorticoid coverage. A reassessment 42 years after emergence of a problem. *Ann Surg.* 1994;219:416-425.

**Table 13.11**   Guidelines for Food and Fluid Intake Before Elective Surgery[a] in Healthy Patients[b]

| Food or Fluid Intake | Minimum Fasting Period | Examples |
|---|---|---|
| Clear liquids | 2 h | Water, fruit juices without pulp, sports drinks, carbonated beverages, tea, and coffee (no dairy) |
| Breast milk | 4 h | |
| Infant formula | 6 h | |
| Nonhuman milk | 6 h | Cow, goat, or soy milk |
| Light meal | 6 h | Toast, clear liquids, nonalcoholic beverages |
| Full meal | >8 h | Fried or fatty foods, meat, alcoholic beverages |

[a]These guidelines apply to any patient undergoing general anesthesia, regional anesthesia, or monitored anesthesia care. They are not intended for patients undergoing procedures under local anesthesia only, when impairment of upper airway reflexes is not anticipated.
[b]These guidelines may not apply to, or may need to be modified for, (1) patients with coexisting diseases or conditions that can affect gastric emptying or fluid volume (e.g., pregnancy, obesity, diabetes, hiatal hernia, gastroesophageal reflux disease, ileus or bowel obstruction, emergency care, enteral tube feeding) and (2) patients in whom airway management might be difficult.
Modified from American Society of Anesthesiologists Committee. Practice guidelines for preoperative fasting and the use of pharmacologic agents to reduce the risk of pulmonary aspiration: application to healthy patients undergoing elective procedures: an updated report by the American Society of Anesthesiologists Committee on Standards and Practice Parameters. *Anesthesiology.* 2011;114:495-511.

preoperatively. Patients with angle-closure glaucoma should not be given scopolamine. Premedication to alter gastric contents may be beneficial in patients at risk for aspiration. H$_2$ antagonists (ranitidine, famotidine), proton pump inhibitors (omeprazole), and antacids (sodium citrate) increase gastric fluid pH, whereas prokinetics (metoclopramide) stimulate gastric emptying.

## Fasting Guidelines

In preparation for elective surgery, current ASA practice guidelines recommend that healthy patients may consume clear liquids (e.g., water, juice without pulp, coffee or tea without cream or milk) until 2 hours before anesthesia; breast milk until 4 hours before anesthesia; nonhuman milk, infant formula, or a light meal until 6 hours before anesthesia; and no fatty food or alcoholic beverages for at least 8 hours before anesthesia (Table 13.11).[48] In the past, patients were restricted from all intake (nothing by mouth, or nil per os [NPO]) after midnight before anesthesia and this may still be advisable for patients with delayed gastric emptying (e.g., gastroparesis, diabetes, ileus, or bowel obstruction), but for healthy patients, carbohydrate-rich fluids until 2 to 3 hours before surgery is part of Enhanced Recovery After Surgery (ERAS) protocols, as this improves early return of bowel function.[49]

## CONCLUSION

Thorough preoperative evaluation and tailored preanesthetic medication instructions decrease complications and improve outcomes during and after procedures requiring anesthesia. Innovation in best practice for preoperative preparation requires ongoing research and willingness to modify systems of care. Anesthesiologists play a key role in perioperative outcomes by identification and modification of risk throughout the perioperative period.

## QUESTIONS OF THE DAY

1. What principles should guide the anesthesia provider when deciding whether to obtain preoperative diagnostic testing before elective surgery? What is the difference between routine and disease-indicated preoperative testing?

2. A patient presents for preoperative evaluation with blood pressure of 180/110 mm Hg. What perioperative risks are increased for this patient? What additional factors should be evaluated before deciding whether to proceed with surgery?

3. What are the intraoperative risks in a patient with a cardiac implantable electronic device (CIED) (implanted cardioverter-defibrillator or pacemaker)? Is there a consistent response of a CIED to magnet placement? Under what circumstances should a CIED be reprogrammed prior to surgery?

4. A patient is receiving clopidogrel (Plavix) after drug-eluting coronary stent placement. How many months after stent placement can clopidogrel be discontinued prior to elective surgery with a risk of bleeding? Would the time period be different if the patient had received a bare metal stent instead?

5. A patient with chronic atrial fibrillation is receiving prophylactic warfarin therapy. How should the anesthesia provider decide whether the patient should receive anticoagulation bridging therapy before elective surgery?

6. What are the ASA recommended preoperative fasting guidelines for liquids and solid food? Under what circumstances might a patient benefit from a strict "nothing by mouth after midnight" fasting period?

## REFERENCES

1. Apfelbaum JL, Connis RT, Nickinovich DG, et al. Practice advisory for preanesthesia evaluation: an updated report by the American Society of Anesthesiologists Task Force on Preanesthesia Evaluation. *Anesthesiology.* 2012;116:522–538.

2. Jette M, Sidney K, Blümchen G. Metabolic equivalents (METS) in exercise testing, exercise prescription, and evaluation of functional capacity. *Clin Cardiol.* 1990;13:555–565.

3. Apfelbaum JL, Hagberg CA, Caplan RA, et al. Practice guidelines for management of the difficult airway: an updated report by the American Society of Anesthesiologists Task Force on Management of the Difficult Airway. *Anesthesiology.* 2013;118:251.

4. Brown SR, Brown J. Why do physicians order unnecessary preoperative tests? A qualitative study. *Fam Med.* 2011;43(5):338–343.

5. van Klei WA, Bryson GL, Yang H, et al. The value of routine preoperative electrocardiography in predicting myocardial infarction after noncardiac surgery. *Ann Surg.* 2007;246:165–170.

6. Finegan BA, Rashiq S, McAlister FA, O'Connor P. Selective ordering of preoperative investigations by anesthesiologists reduces the number and cost of tests. *Can J Anaesth.* 2005;52:575–580.

7. Chung F, Yuan H, Yin L, et al. Elimination of preoperative testing in ambulatory surgery. *Anesth Analg.* 2009;108:467.

8. Keay L, Lindsley K, Tielsch J, et al. Routine preoperative medical testing for cataract surgery. *Cochrane Database Syst Rev.* 2012;(3): CD007293.

9. Fleisher LA, Fleischmann KE, Auerbach AD, et al. 2014 ACC/AHA guideline on perioperative cardiovascular evaluation and management of patients undergoing noncardiac surgery: a report of the American College of Cardiology/American Heart Association Task Force on practice guidelines. *J Am Coll Cardiol.* 2014;64:e77–e137.

10. Liu LL, Dzankic S, Leung JM. Preoperative electrocardiogram abnormalities do not predict postoperative cardiac complications in geriatric surgical patients. *J Am Geriatr Soc.* 2002;50:1186–1191.

11. Wax DB, Porter SB, Lin H-M, et al. Association of preanesthesia hypertension with adverse outcomes. *J Cardiothorac Vasc Anesth.* 2010;24:927–930.

12. Howell SJ, Sear JW, Foëx P. Hypertension, hypertensive heart disease and perioperative cardiac risk. *Br J Anaesth.* 2004;92:570–583.

13. Bilimoria KY, Liu Y, Paruch JL, et al. Development and evaluation of the universal ACS NSQIP surgical risk calculator: a decision aid and informed consent tool for patients and surgeons. *J Am Coll Surg.* 2013;217:833–842. e1-e3. See also http://www.riskcalculator.facs.org. or surgicalriskcalculator.com/miorcardiacarrest.com.

14. Lee TH, Marcantonio ER, Mangione CM, et al. Derivation and prospective validation of a simple index for prediction of cardiac risk of major noncardiac surgery. *Circulation.* 1999;100:1043–1049.

15. McFalls EO, Ward HB, Moritz TE, et al. Coronary-artery revascularization before elective major vascular surgery. *N Engl J Med.* 2004;351:2795–2804.

16. Grines CL, Bonow RO, Casey DE, et al. Prevention of premature discontinuation of dual antiplatelet therapy in patients with coronary artery stents: a science advisory from the American Heart Association, American College of Cardiology, Society for Cardiovascular Angiography and Interventions, American College of Surgeons, and American Dental Association, with representation from the American College of Physicians. *Circulation.* 2007;115:813–818.

16a. Levine GN, Bates ER, Bittl JA, et al. ACC/AHA Guideline Focused Update on Duration of Dual Antiplatelet Therapy in Patients With Coronary Artery Disease. A Report of the American College of Cardiology/American Heart Association Task Force on Clinical Practice Guidelines 2016; 68(10):1082–1115.

17. Burger W, Chemnitius JM, Kneissl GD, Rücker G. Low-dose aspirin for secondary cardiovascular prevention—cardiovascular risks after its perioperative withdrawal versus bleeding risks with its continuation—review and meta-analysis. *J Intern Med.* 2005;257: 399–414.

18. American Heart Association. About Heart Failure: classes of Heart Failure. April 6, 2015 http://www.heart.org/HEARTORG/Conditions/HeartFailure/AboutHeartFailure.

19. Nishimura RA, Otto CM, Bonow RO, et al. 2014 AHA/ACC guideline for the management of patients with valvular heart disease: a report of the American College of Cardiology/American Heart Association Task Force on Practice Guidelines. *Circulation.* 2014;129:e521–e643.

20. Nishimura RA, Carabello BA, Faxon DP, et al. ACC/AHA 2008 guideline update on valvular heart disease: focused update on infective endocarditis: a report of the American College of Cardiology/American Heart Association Task Force on Practice Guidelines: endorsed by the Society of Cardiovascular Anesthesiologists, Society for Cardiovascular Angiography and Interventions, and Society of Thoracic Surgeons. *Circulation.* 2008;118:887–896.

21. Crossley GH, Poole JE, Rozner MA, et al. The Heart Rhythm Society (HRS)/American Society of Anesthesiologists (ASA) Expert Consensus Statement on the perioperative management of patients with implantable defibrillators, pacemakers and arrhythmia monitors: facilities and patient management this document was developed as a joint project with the American Society of Anesthesiologists (ASA), and in collaboration with the American Heart Association (AHA), and the Society of Thoracic Surgeons (STS). *Heart Rhythm.* 2011;8:1114–1154.

22. Smetana GW, Lawrence VA, Cornell JE. American College of Physicians: preoperative pulmonary risk stratification for noncardiothoracic surgery: systematic review for the American College of Physicians. *Ann Intern Med.* 2006;144:581–595.

23. Mayo NE, Feldman L, Scott S, et al. Impact of preoperative change in physical function on postoperative recovery: argument supporting prehabilitation for colorectal surgery. *Surgery.* 2011;150:505–514.

24. Liao P, Yegneswaran B, Vairavanathan S, et al. Postoperative complications in patients with obstructive sleep apnea: a retrospective matched cohort study. *Can J Anaesth.* 2009;56:819–828.

25. Hwang D, Shakir N, Limann B, et al. Association of sleep-disordered breathing with postoperative complications. *Chest.* 2008;133:1128–1134.

26. Chung F, Yegneswaran B, Liao P, et al. STOP questionnaire: a tool to screen patients for obstructive sleep apnea. *Anesthesiology.* 2008;108:812–821.

27. American Society of Anesthesiologists Task Force on Perioperative Management of patients with obstructive sleep apnea. Practice guidelines for the perioperative management of patients with obstructive sleep apnea: an updated report by the American Society of Anesthesiologists Task Force on Perioperative Management of patients with obstructive sleep apnea. *Anesthesiology.* 2014;120(2):268–286.

28. Joshi GP, Ankichetty SP, Gan TJ, Chung F. Society for Ambulatory Anesthesia consensus statement on preoperative selection of adult patients with obstructive sleep apnea scheduled for ambulatory surgery. *Anesth Analg.* 2012;115(5):1060–1068.

29. Lipshutz AK, Gropper MA. Perioperative glycemic control. *Anesthesiology.* 2009;110:408–421.

30. Moitra VK, Greenberg J, Arunajadai S, Sweitzer B. The relationship between glycosylated hemoglobin and perioperative glucose control in patients with diabetes. *Can J Anaesth.* 2010;57:322–329.

31. Zarbock A, Milles K. Novel therapy for renal protection. *Curr Opin Anaesthesiol.* 2015;28:431–438.

32. Lasocki S, Krauspe R, von Heymann C, et al. PREPARE: the prevalence of perioperative anaemia and need for patient blood management in elective orthopaedic surgery: a multicentre, observational study. *Eur J Anaesthesiol.* 2015;32:160–167.

33. American Society of Anesthesiologists Task Force on Perioperative Blood Management. Practice guidelines for perioperative blood management: an updated report by the American Society of Anesthesiologists Task Force on Perioperative Blood Management. *Anesthesiology.* 2015;122(2):241–275.

34. Fleisher LA, Pasternak LR, Herbert R, Anderson GF. Inpatient hospital admission and death after outpatient surgery in elderly patients: importance of patient and system characteristics and location of care. *Arch Surg.* 2004;139:67–72.

35. Polanczyk CSA, Marcantonio E, Goldman L, et al. Impact of age on perioperative complications and length of stay in patients undergoing noncardiac surgery. *Ann Intern Med.* 2001;134:637–643.

36. Rosenman DJ, McDonald FS, Ebbert JO, et al. Clinical consequences of withholding versus administering renin-angiotensin-aldosterone system antagonists in the preoperative period. *J Hosp Med.* 2008;3:319–325.

37. Wijeysundera DN, Duncan D, Nkonde-Price C, et al. Perioperative beta blockade in noncardiac surgery: a systematic review for the 2014 ACC/AHA Guideline on Perioperative Cardiovascular Evaluation and Management of Patients Undergoing Noncardiac Surgery: a report of the American College of Cardiology/American Heart Association Task Force on Practice Guidelines. *Circulation.* 2014;130:2246–2264.

38. Ouattara A, Benhaoua H, Le Manach Y, et al. Perioperative statin therapy is associated with a significant and dose-dependent reduction of adverse cardiovascular outcomes after coronary artery bypass graft surgery. *J Cardiothorac Vasc Anesth.* 2009;23:633–638.

39. Kapoor AS, Kanji H, Buckingham J, et al. Strength of evidence for perioperative use of statins to reduce cardiovascular risk: systematic review of controlled studies. *BMJ.* 2006;333:1149.

40. Le Manach Y, Godet G, Coriat P, et al. The impact of postoperative discontinuation or continuation of chronic statin therapy on cardiac outcome after major vascular surgery. *Anesth Analg.* 2007;104:1326–1333.

41. Gerstein NS, Carey MC, Cigarroa JE, Schulman PM. Perioperative aspirin management after POISE-2: some answers, but questions remain. *Anesth Analg.* 2015;120:570–575.

42. Chassot PG, Delabays A, Spahn DR. Perioperative antiplatelet therapy: the case for continuing therapy in patients at risk of myocardial infarction. *Br J Anaesth.* 2007;99:316–328.

43. Narouze S, Benzon HT, Provenzano DA, et al. Interventional spine and pain procedures in patients on antiplatelet and anticoagulant medications: guidelines from the American Society of Regional Anesthesia and Pain Medicine, the European Society of Regional Anaesthesia and Pain Therapy, the American Academy of Pain Medicine, the International Neuromodulation Society, the North American Neuromodulation Society, and the World Institute of Pain. *Reg Anesth Pain Med.* 2015;40:182–212.

44. Douketis JD, Spyropoulos AC, Spencer FA, et al. Perioperative management of antithrombotic therapy: antithrombotic Therapy and Prevention of Thrombosis, 9th ed: American College of Chest Physicians Evidence-Based Clinical Practice Guidelines. *Chest.* 2012;141(2 suppl):e326S–e350S.

45. Langeron O, Masso E, Huraux C, et al. Prediction of difficult mask ventilation. *Anesthesiology.* 2000;92: 1229–1236.

46. Salpeter SR, Greyber E, Pasternak GA, Salpeter EE. Risk of fatal and nonfatal lactic acidosis with metformin use in type 2 diabetes mellitus. *Cochrane Database Syst Rev.* 2010;(4): CD002967.

47. Salem M, Tainsh RE, Bromberg J, et al. Perioperative glucocorticoid coverage. A reassessment 42 years after emergence of a problem. *Ann Surg.* 1994;219:416–425.

48. American Society of Anesthesiologists Committee. Practice guidelines for preoperative fasting and the use of pharmacologic agents to reduce the risk of pulmonary aspiration: application to healthy patients undergoing elective procedures: an updated report by the American Society of Anesthesiologists Committee on Standards and Practice Parameters. *Anesthesiology.* 2011;114(3):495–511.

49. Miller TE, Roche AM, Mythen M. Fluid management and goal-directed therapy as an adjunct to Enhanced Recovery After Surgery (ERAS). *Can J Anaesth.* 2015;62:158–168.

# 14 CHOICE OF ANESTHETIC TECHNIQUE

## Elizabeth L. Whitlock and Manuel C. Pardo, Jr.

The decision-making process regarding anesthetic technique begins with the preoperative evaluation (see Chapter 13). The three most important factors include type of surgical procedure, the patient's coexisting diseases, and patient preferences. The ultimate responsibility for anesthetic choice lies with the anesthesia provider. Often, there is no single best choice. The anesthesia provider must have the ability to implement a range of anesthetic plans and be prepared to address unexpected events that may necessitate a sudden change in plan.

## TYPES OF ANESTHESIA

Choices for anesthesia include (1) general anesthesia, (2) regional anesthesia, and (3) monitored anesthesia care (MAC).

Although there is some debate about the clinical definition of general anesthesia, the components include immobility, amnesia, analgesia, and lack of patient harm.[1] The American Society of Anesthesiologists (ASA) defines general anesthesia as "a drug-induced loss of consciousness during which patients are not arousable, even by painful stimulation."[2] Modern approaches to general anesthesia involve administration of a combination of medications, such as hypnotic drugs (see Chapters 7 and 8), neuromuscular blocking drugs (see Chapter 11), and analgesic drugs (see Chapter 9).

Regional anesthesia includes neuraxial (spinal, epidural, caudal) anesthesia (see Chapter 17) as well as peripheral nerve blocks (see Chapter 18). With a cooperative patient, regional anesthesia may ensure the appropriate immobility and analgesia required for surgery, without exposing the patient to the risks of general anesthesia.

The editors and publisher would like to thank Dr. Ronald D. Miller for contributing to this chapter in the previous edition of this work. It has served as the foundation for the current chapter.

**Table 14.1** Continuum of Depth of Sedation

| Function | Minimal Sedation (Anxiolysis) | Moderate Sedation (Conscious Sedation) | Deep Sedation | General Anesthesia |
|---|---|---|---|---|
| Response (stimulation type) | Normal (verbal stimulus) | Purposeful (verbal or tactile stimulus) | Purposeful (repeated or painful stimulus) | None (even with painful stimulus) |
| Ability to maintain airway and spontaneous ventilation | Not affected | Airway maintained without intervention; ventilation adequate | Airway intervention may be required; ventilation may be inadequate | Airway intervention often required; ventilation frequently inadequate |
| Cardiovascular function | Not affected | Usually maintained | Usually maintained | May be impaired |

From Continuum of Depth of Sedation: Definition of General Anesthesia and Levels of Sedation/Analgesia (approved by the ASA House of Delegates on October 13, 1999, and last amended on October 15, 2014).

The phrase *monitored anesthesia care* was created by the ASA in the 1980s to replace the term *standby anesthesia* and to facilitate professional fee billing. The original description of MAC referred to the anesthesiologist providing anesthesia services to a patient receiving local anesthesia or no anesthesia at all.[3] The ASA currently defines MAC as "a specific anesthesia service in which an anesthesiologist has been requested to participate in the care of a patient undergoing a diagnostic or therapeutic procedure." The ASA has also described a continuum of depth of sedation that includes progressive levels of sedation (Table 14.1). These definitions are used by regulatory bodies such as The Joint Commission to create standards for administration of sedation by nonanesthesiologist personnel. The term MAC is not part of the description of the sedation continuum, as the level of consciousness may change during a procedure and even progress to an "unplanned" general anesthetic. The preoperative evaluation, monitoring, and other anesthesia care standards apply equally to the patient receiving MAC.

## CHOOSING AN APPROPRIATE ANESTHETIC TECHNIQUE

Factors identified in the preoperative evaluation can indicate that general anesthesia may be the most appropriate anesthetic choice (Box 14.1). If general anesthesia is chosen, the anesthesia provider must then determine a plan for airway management, induction of anesthesia, maintenance of anesthesia, and immediate postoperative care. If general anesthesia is not chosen, other anesthetic options include regional anesthesia or MAC.

Certain patient or procedure characteristics may preclude safe regional anesthesia (Box 14.2). Depending on the level of sedation required, a regional technique may allow surgical anesthesia with complete preservation of upper airway reflexes, even in the patient at risk for aspiration of gastric contents. Regional anesthesia cannot provide surgical

**Box 14.1** Clinical Settings Appropriate for General Anesthesia

A requirement for systemic neuromuscular blockade
A requirement for establishment of a secure airway
    Due to surgical procedures that may compromise native airway integrity, oxygenation, or ventilation
    Due to level of consciousness required to provide immobility, analgesia, or anxiolysis
Patient or procedural characteristics that are not appropriate for monitored anesthesia care
    Uncooperative patient or patient refusal
    Surgical pain not amenable to local or topical anesthesia
Patient or procedural characteristics that are not suitable for regional anesthetic
Preferences of the patient, anesthesia provider, and/or surgeon

**Box 14.2** Situations in Which Regional Anesthesia May Not Be Appropriate

Preferences and experience of the patient, anesthesia provider, and surgeon
The need for an immediate postoperative neurologic examination in the anatomic area impacted by the regional anesthetic
Coagulopathy
Preexisting neurologic disease (e.g., multiple sclerosis, neurofibromatosis)
Infected or abnormal skin at the planned cutaneous puncture site

**Specific Considerations for Neuraxial Anesthesia**
Hypovolemia increases the risk for significant hypotension
Coagulopathy (including anticoagulant and antiplatelet medication therapy) increases risk of epidural hematoma
Increased intracranial pressure may result in cerebral herniation with intentional or inadvertent dural puncture

analgesia for all procedures. The most important factor is the planned location of the surgical incision (Fig. 14.1).

If the analgesic requirements for the planned procedure can be met with local or topical anesthesia, or if the

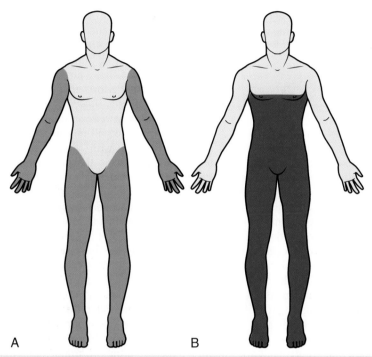

**Fig. 14.1** Anatomic regions potentially amenable to peripheral nerve or neuraxial block. (A) Peripheral nerve block: green areas indicate where complete surgical analgesia can typically be provided. (B) Neuraxial block: blue areas indicate where complete surgical analgesia can typically be provided.

planned procedure is not associated with pain (e.g., diagnostic radiology procedure such as magnetic resonance imaging), MAC may be the most appropriate choice. However, the anesthesia provider must be prepared to convert to general anesthesia if it becomes apparent that appropriate analgesia and immobility cannot be achieved by other means. The anesthetic risks associated with MAC are not necessarily different from general or regional anesthesia. An ASA Closed Claims study of patient injury documented a comparable incidence of injury severity with MAC compared to general anesthesia.[4] In patients receiving MAC, respiratory depression from sedative drugs (e.g., propofol, benzodiazepines, opioids) is an important mechanism of injury.

Anesthetic techniques can be combined to meet patient or surgical goals. For example, a patient with subarachnoid hemorrhage who requires diagnostic cerebral angiography may initially receive MAC. If the imaging reveals a cerebral aneurysm requiring endovascular coiling, the anesthesia provider may be asked to convert to general anesthesia to provide patient immobility and control of ventilation during the procedure.

Neuraxial and peripheral nerve blockade may be combined with general anesthesia to provide long-lasting postoperative analgesia following a surgical procedure that may not be amenable to regional anesthesia alone (also see Chapter 40). A 2013 systematic review documented that, in a broad range of surgical procedures, use of local infiltration or peripheral nerve block in addition to general anesthesia improved postoperative pain scores and decreased opiate consumption.[5] This result may be directly due to analgesia provided by the technique or by "preventive analgesia," which is defined as analgesia lasting longer than 5.5 half-lives of an analgesic drug. Even use of a peripheral nerve block in addition to a single-shot spinal block improves postoperative analgesia for many surgeries of the lower extremity.[5]

The addition of a regional technique to general anesthesia may reduce intraoperative blood loss and, in some situations, the rate of perioperative transfusion.[6] Addition of neuraxial or peripheral nerve blockade to general anesthesia also reduces rates of postoperative chronic pain.[7] A meta-analysis of systematic reviews did not find a mortality rate benefit for the addition of neuraxial anesthesia to general anesthesia.[8] The same meta-analysis suggested that neuraxial anesthesia was associated with lower 30-day mortality rates compared to general anesthesia alone in patients with an intermediate risk of cardiac complications. However, most of the studies reviewed were performed in the 1970s to 1990s, and management of cardiovascular disease has evolved significantly in subsequent decades.[8]

There is increasing emphasis on improving patient outcomes not just in the immediate term (e.g., intraoperatively) but facilitating in-hospital recovery, mitigating risks for development of postoperative chronic pain, and improving long-term survival.

Fig. 14.2 provides a summary of the decision-making process in choosing an appropriate anesthetic for an individual patient.

## PRACTICAL ASPECTS OF ANESTHESIA CHOICE

### General Anesthesia

The choice of general anesthesia includes planning for induction of anesthesia, airway management, maintenance of anesthesia, and postoperative care. Induction of anesthesia can be accomplished via the inhaled or intravenous route of anesthetic administration. Both choices may benefit from verbal or pharmacologic (e.g., benzodiazepine) anxiolysis. Preoxygenation–also called *denitrogenation*–is the deliberate replacement of nitrogen in the patient's functional residual capacity (FRC) with oxygen. Eight vital capacity breaths of 100% oxygen over 60 seconds, or tidal volume breathing of 100% oxygen for 3 minutes, replaces roughly 80% of the FRC with oxygen. This provides a crucial margin of safety during periods of apnea or upper airway obstruction that can occur with induction of general anesthesia. Thus, adequate preoxygenation can delay or eliminate the onset of hypoxemia during the time period between the intravenous induction of anesthesia and the start of controlled ventilation.

An inhaled induction of anesthesia is often chosen for pediatric patients in whom preinduction placement of an intravenous catheter is impractical (also see Chapter 34). Also, it may be indicated in the patient who is anticipated to have a difficult airway to manage, because spontaneous respiratory efforts are preserved with an inhaled induction of anesthesia. However, inhaled anesthetics ablate protective airway reflexes and pharyngeal muscular tone, so this method will not be suitable for all patients in whom difficulties with airway management are anticipated. Sevoflurane is the most commonly used anesthetic for inhaled induction of anesthesia because of its low pungency, high potency (permitting delivery of high-inspired oxygen concentration), and rapidity of onset. To further hasten onset, a technique called *priming* can be used. This involves filling the breathing circuit with 8% sevoflurane by emptying the reservoir bag, opening the adjustable pressure-limiting valve, and using a high fresh gas flow (e.g., 8 L/min) for 1 minute before applying the face mask to the patient. This approach to inhaled induction of anesthesia can produce loss of consciousness within 1 minute.

Intravenous induction of anesthesia is the most common technique in the adult patient. Pharmacologic options include propofol, thiopental, etomidate, ketamine, and a benzodiazepine-opioid combination (also see Chapters 8 and 9). After the patient loses consciousness, ventilation via a mask is initiated. The anesthesia provider may then choose to administer an inhaled anesthetic to increase the

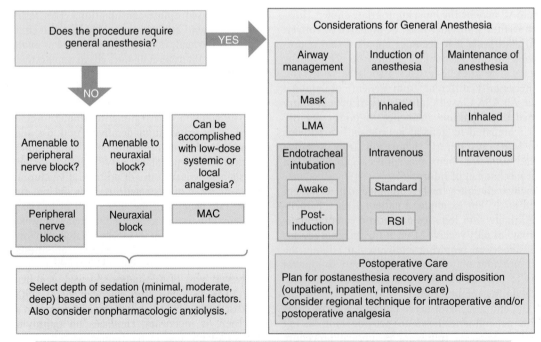

**Fig. 14.2** Decision-making process for anesthetic choice. An approach to determining anesthetic plan based on surgical procedure, patient's coexisting diseases, and patient preferences. *GA,* General anesthesia; *LMA,* laryngeal mask airway; *MAC,* monitored anesthesia care; *RSI,* rapid sequence induction.

depth of anesthesia prior to airway instrumentation. If tracheal intubation is planned, a neuromuscular blocking drug is usually given to facilitate direct laryngoscopy (also see Chapter 11).

Sometimes an intravenous rapid sequence induction (RSI) is indicated. RSI is performed in patients at increased risk for aspiration of gastric contents (e.g., clinically significant gastroesophageal reflux disease, delayed gastric emptying, unknown fasting state, or a known full stomach). The goal of RSI is to minimize the time between onset of unconsciousness and tracheal intubation and reduce the risk of regurgitation by applying cricoid pressure. The sequence of events involves (1) preoxygenation; (2) intravenous administration of a hypnotic (e.g., propofol); (3) immediate administration a of a rapid-onset neuromuscular blocking drug (e.g., succinylcholine 1.0-1.5 mg/kg or rocuronium 1.0-1.2 mg/kg); (4) application of cricoid pressure (using force of 30 newtons, approximately 7 pounds); (5) avoidance of ventilation via a mask or (6) tracheal intubation; and (7) release of cricoid pressure after confirmation of correct endotracheal tube placement. Though ventilation via a mask is generally avoided with RSI, the use of positive pressure less than 20 cm $H_2O$ (called *modified* RSI) should minimize the risk of gastric insufflation and may be needed if the patient develops hypoxemia prior to tracheal intubation. Although RSI with cricoid pressure has been used for several decades and is a standard of care approach, a recent meta-analysis did not demonstrate a measurable impact of cricoid pressure on clinical outcomes during RSI.[9]

Airway management techniques (e.g., direct laryngoscopy, supraglottic airway placement) are implemented after the intravenous or inhaled induction of anesthesia. However, if the anesthesia provider anticipates difficulty with ventilation via a mask or tracheal intubation then tracheal intubation should be initiated prior to induction of anesthesia (i.e., awake intubation) (also see Chapter 16).

After induction of anesthesia and appropriate airway management, anesthesia is maintained typically by administration of a combination of anesthetic drugs, each titrated to achieve the desired anesthetic goal while minimizing side effects. For example, although high concentrations of inhaled anesthetics can produce skeletal muscle relaxation, the risks of cardiac depression and vasodilation increase. Neuromuscular blocking drugs can facilitate surgical exposure once adequate hypnosis and analgesia are achieved. Thus, the anesthesia provider selects medications that target specific anesthetic requirements while minimizing the cumulative risk of undesired effects. Individual patients and particular surgical procedures may present special considerations that influence the choice of anesthesia maintenance strategy.

Potent inhaled anesthetics (also see Chapter 7) represent the mainstay of drugs used to maintain anesthesia in most clinical situations. They are easily titratable, reduce the autonomic response to noxious stimulation, and at clinically relevant doses can often provide sufficient muscle relaxation to facilitate surgical exposure. Another inhaled anesthetic, nitrous oxide, can provide both hypnosis and analgesia at clincially relevant doses but cannot be used as a sole drug for general anesthesia because it lacks the potency of the volatile inhaled anesthetics (also see Chapter 47) as a processed electroencephalogram (EEG) monitor.[10] However, inhaled anesthetics increase the risk for postoperative nausea and vomiting. Emergence from hypnosis provided by volatile anesthetics can be associated with airway hyperreactivity and coughing, although those side effects can be mitigated by coadministration of other drugs. Another inhaled anesthetic, nitrous oxide, can provide both hypnosis and analgesia at clinically relevant doses but cannot be used as a sole agent for general anesthesia because it but lacks the potency of the newer inhaled anesthetics. The minimum alveolar concentration required to prevent movement to surgical stimulation is greater than the concentration that can be delivered at atmospheric pressure, so it cannot be used alone to provide reliable hypnosis. Substitution of nitrous oxide for a portion of the inhaled anesthetic dose can reduce the cardiovascular effects observed with potent inhaled anesthetics while maintaining the same anesthetic depth. Nitrous oxide also provides analgesia and is rapidly titratable because of its low blood-gas partition coefficient. The concern that use of nitrous oxide may increase rates of perioperative cardiac complications after noncardiac surgery could not be documented in a large 2015 trial.[11]

Intravenous hypnotic drugs can also be used for maintenance of anesthesia (also see Chapter 8). Propofol reduces the incidence of postoperative nausea and vomiting and may have more favorable emergence characteristics with less coughing and laryngospasm risk compared to inhaled anesthetics alone. However, depth of hypnosis cannot be reliably measured in the absence of EEG or auditory evoked potential monitoring. For certain surgical procedures, intravenous maintenance of anesthesia is most appropriate. For example, laryngeal surgery with intraoperative jet ventilation is accomplished without an endotracheal tube, making delivery of inhaled anesthetics difficult. Patients undergoing scoliosis surgery often require somatosensory and motor evoked potential monitoring. The inhaled anesthetics produce a decrease in amplitude and increase in latency of both somatosensory and motor evoked potential signals. Therefore, a combination of propofol, ketamine, and opioid infusions is commonly administered for maintenance of anesthesia in these patients.[12]

The postoperative disposition of the patient also influences anesthetic choice for maintenance and emergence from anesthesia. For example, if the patient will receive postoperative mechanical ventilation in the intensive care unit, the use of short-acting anesthetic drugs is less important, and prolonged neuromuscular blockade is not likely to be a significant clinical issue. Patients undergoing outpatient surgery require special attention to the prevention of postoperative and postdischarge nausea and vomiting (also see Chapter 37). This may involve selection of a less emetogenic anesthetic maintenance drug (e.g., propofol) as well as administration of multiple antiemetic drugs (also see Chapter 39).

## Regional Anesthesia

Superficial and deep operations on the extremities—particularly the distal extremities—may be amenable to peripheral nerve block (see Chapter 18). Because surgical anesthesia may be achieved without sedation, this technique is particularly attractive in patients for whom systemic disease (e.g., severe pulmonary disease, cardiovascular disease, or renal failure) may present a significant challenge during general anesthesia. Unlike neuraxial anesthesia, the localized sympathectomy resulting from peripheral nerve block rarely results in systemic hypotension. However, peripheral nerve blockade as the primary anesthetic technique requires patient cooperation and may be inappropriate in patients with dementia, acute intoxication, or other conditions associated with altered mental status. Peripheral nerve blockade may be difficult to accomplish or may result in an inadequate, "patchy" block. If surgical anesthesia is not achieved with a peripheral nerve block, the anesthesia provider is faced with the options of supplementing the block with local anesthesia, administering intravenous analgesics and hypnotics, postponing surgery and reattempting the block at a later time, or converting to general anesthesia.

Neuraxial anesthesia can provide excellent operating conditions in the lower extremities and lower abdomen. Higher levels of neuraxial blockade (e.g., midthoracic to high thoracic) with surgical anesthesia concentrations of local anesthetic (e.g., epidural 2% lidocaine) result in more profound sympathectomy and increased risk of hypotension, which may require infusion of vasoactive medications to maintain hemodynamic stability. However, analgesic concentrations of local anesthetic (e.g., epidural 0.1% ropivacaine) are commonly given via thoracic epidural catheter to provide postoperative analgesia after open thoracic surgery. The smaller concentration of local anesthetic required for analgesia (as opposed to surgical anesthesia) results in decreased incidence of hypotension.

Postoperative disposition of the patient also influences medication choice or type of regional anesthesia. Patients undergoing ambulatory surgery who receive spinal anesthesia may have prolonged recovery time if they receive long-acting local anesthetics, because they must be able to ambulate prior to discharge. Ambulatory surgical patients undergoing procedures associated with significant postoperative pain may benefit from a long-lasting peripheral nerve block or nerve catheter placement.[13]

## Monitored Anesthesia Care

Pharmacologic sedation using opioids or hypnotic medications is often provided as a component of MAC (also see Chapters 8 and 9). Nonpharmacologic approaches such as video or audio distraction or verbal reassurance can also complement a MAC technique. The ASA depth of sedation continuum can be used to choose the level of sedation that is most appropriate for the patient undergoing MAC. Local or topical anesthesia administered by the surgeon is commonly used during MAC to provide adequate analgesia for the procedure. The anesthesia provider must track the total dose of local anesthetic and be alert for signs of local anesthetic toxicity (also see Chapter 10). The injection of local anesthetic near sensitive areas (e.g., face, eyes) may initially require a deeper level of sedation until the injection is complete. The most dangerous anesthetic risk during MAC is respiratory depression from excessive sedation. The manifestations of respiratory depression include upper airway obstruction, hypoventilation, and hypoxemia. During MAC, end-tidal capnography can be accomplished with a nasal cannula that has a dedicated sampling line attached. However, capnography monitoring is less reliable in this setting, and the absence of increased end-tidal $CO_2$ does not guarantee the adequacy of ventilation. The medications typically used for sedation during MAC (benzodiazepines, opioids, propofol) produce dose-dependent respiratory depression. Ketamine and dexmedetomidine are less likely to cause hypoventilation but have other potential side effects and may have synergistic sedative effects with other hypnotic medications (also see Chapter 8).

The anesthesia provider may choose to administer sedation to improve patient comfort during a procedure performed under regional anesthesia, although the term MAC would not be used if the primary anesthetic was a regional technique. Depth of hypnosis has recently come under scrutiny as a possible contributor to postoperative outcomes. A randomized clinical trial of light versus deep sedation in elderly hip fracture surgical patients receiving spinal anesthesia showed a short-term reduction in postoperative delirium and a reduction in 1-year mortality rate in the sickest patients for the light-sedation group (i.e., deep sedation was associated with increased risk of complications).[14]

## ENVIRONMENTAL IMPACT

Anesthetic choice has important implications for environmental impact and cost of care. The potent inhaled anesthetics and nitrous oxide are ozone-depleting, and nitrous oxide is an important greenhouse gas. In 2006, the anesthetic use of nitrous oxide was responsible for 3% of total nitrous oxide emissions in the United States. Nitrous oxide is estimated to be the single largest ozone-depleting potential (ODP)-weighted emission for the rest of the 21st century. Of halogenated anesthetics, desflurane is the worst offender, with a global warming potential almost 4000 times that of carbon dioxide.[15,16] The environmental impact of inhaled anesthetics can be minimized by use of total intravenous anesthesia, low-flow anesthesia, or closed-circuit anesthesia.

## QUESTIONS OF THE DAY

1. What are the most important factors in determining whether general anesthesia is an appropriate choice for a patient undergoing a surgical procedure?

2. What are the potential benefits of the addition of a regional anesthesia technique to general anesthesia?

3. What are the advantages and disadvantages of volatile anesthetics versus intravenous anesthetics for maintenance of anesthesia?

4. What is the most dangerous anesthetic risk for a patient undergoing monitored anesthesia care? What steps can be taken to diagnose and prevent anesthetic complications during monitored anesthesia care?

## REFERENCES

1. Urban BW, Bleckwenn M. Concepts and correlations relevant to general anaesthesia. *Br J Anaesth.* 2002;89(1):3–16.

2. American Society of Anesthesiologists. Continuum of Depth of Sedation: Definition of General Anesthesia and Levels of Sedation/Analgesia. Amended October 15, 2014. http://www.asahq.org/~/media/Sites/ASAHQ/Files/Public/Resources/standards-guidelines/continuum-of-depth-of-sedation-definition-of-general-anesthesia-and-levels-of-sedation-analgesia.pdf. Accessed May 3, 2016.

3. Cohen NA, McMichael JP. What's New in … Definitions of monitored anesthesia care. *American Society of Anesthesiologists Newsletter.* 2004;68(6):22–26.

4. Bhananker SM, Posner KL, Cheney FW, et al. Injury and liability associated with monitored anesthesia care: a closed claims analysis. *Anesthesiology.* 2006;104(2):228–234.

5. Barreveld A, Witte J, Chahal H, et al. Preventive analgesia by local anesthetics: the reduction of postoperative pain by peripheral nerve blocks and intravenous drugs. *Anesth Analg.* 2013;116:1141–1161.

6. Guay J. The effect of neuraxial blocks on surgical blood loss and blood transfusion requirements: a meta-analysis. *J Clin Anesth.* 2006;18:124–128.

7. Andreae MH, Andreae DA. Regional anaesthesia to prevent chronic pain after surgery: a Cochrane systematic review and meta-analysis. *Br J Anaesth.* 2013;111:711–720.

8. Guay J, Choi PT, Suresh S, et al. Neuraxial anesthesia for the prevention of postoperative mortality and major morbidity: an overview of Cochrane Systematic Reviews. *Anesth Analg.* 2014;119:716–725.

9. Algie CM, Mahar RK, Tan HB, et al. Effectiveness and risks of cricoid pressure during rapid sequence induction for endotracheal intubation. *Cochrane Database Syst Rev.* 2015;(11):CD011656.

10. Mashour GA, Shanks A, Tremper KK, et al. Prevention of intraoperative awareness with explicit recall in an unselected surgical population: a randomized comparative effectiveness trial. *Anesthesiology.* 2012;117(4):717–725.

11. Leslie K, Myles PS, Kasza J, et al. Nitrous oxide and serious long-term morbidity and mortality in the Evaluation of Nitrous Oxide in the Gas Mixture for Anaesthesia (ENIGMA)-II Trial. *Anesthesiology.* 2015;123(6):1267–1280.

12. Glover CD, Carling NP. Neuromonitoring for scoliosis surgery. *Anesthesiol Clin.* 2014;32(1):101–114.

13. Ilfeld BM. Continuous peripheral nerve blocks: a review of the published evidence. *Anesth Analg.* 2011;113(4):904–925.

14. Brown CHt, Azman AS, Gottschalk A, et al. Sedation depth during spinal anesthesia and survival in elderly patients undergoing hip fracture repair. *Anesth Analg.* 2014;118:977–980.

15. Ryan SM, Nielsen CJ. Global warming potential of inhaled anesthetics: application to clinical use. *Anesth Analg.* 2010;111:92–98.

16. Ishizawa Y. Special article: general anesthetic gases and the global environment. *Anesth Analg.* 2011;112:213–217.

III

# 15 ANESTHESIA DELIVERY SYSTEMS

Patricia Roth

An anesthesia delivery system consists of the anesthesia workstation (anesthesia machine) and anesthetic breathing system (circuit), which permit delivery of known concentrations of inhaled anesthetics and oxygen to the patient, as well as removal of the patient's carbon dioxide. Carbon dioxide can be removed either by washout (delivered gas flow greater than 5 L/min from the anesthesia machine) or by chemical neutralization.

## ANESTHESIA WORKSTATION

The anesthesia machine has evolved from a simple pneumatic device to a complex integrated computer-controlled multicomponent workstation (Figs. 15.1 and 15.2).[1] The components within the anesthesia workstation function in harmony to deliver known concentrations of inhaled anesthetics to the patient. The multiple components of the anesthesia workstation include what was previously recognized as the anesthesia machine (the pressure-regulating and gas-mixing components), vaporizers, anesthesia breathing circuit, ventilator, scavenging system, and respiratory and physiologic monitoring systems (electrocardiogram, arterial blood pressure, temperature, pulse oximeter, and inhaled and exhaled concentrations of oxygen, carbon dioxide, anesthetic gases, and vapors) (Box 15.1).[1] Alarm systems to signal apnea or disconnection of the anesthetic breathing system from the patient are included. The alarms present on the workstation including pulse oximeter and capnograph must be active and audible to the anesthesia provider. Most anesthesia machines are powered by both electric and pneumatic power.

The anesthesia workstation ultimately provides delivery of medical gases and the vapors of volatile anesthetics at known concentrations to the common gas outlet. These gases enter the anesthetic breathing system to be delivered to the patient by spontaneous or mechanical ventilation. Exhaled gases either exit the system via the

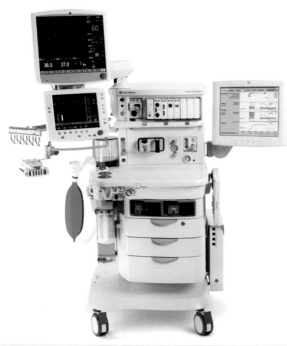

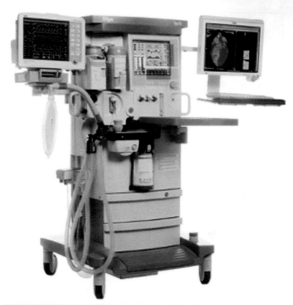

**Fig. 15.2** Dräger Apollo Anesthesia Workstation. (Courtesy of Dräger, Lübeck, Germany.)

**Fig. 15.1** GE Aisys Anesthesia Delivery System. (Courtesy of GE Healthcare, Little Chalfont, UK.)

scavenging system or are returned to the patient after passing through a $CO_2$ absorbent.

## Fail-Safe Valve

Anesthesia machines are equipped with a fail-safe valve designed to prevent the delivery of hypoxic gas mixtures from the machine in the event of failure of the oxygen supply. This valve shuts off or proportionally decreases the flow of all gases when the pressure in the oxygen delivery line decreases to less than 30 psi. This safety measure is designed to protect against unrecognized exhaustion of oxygen delivery from a cylinder attached to the anesthesia machine or from a central source. This valve, however, does not prevent the delivery of 100% nitrous oxide when the oxygen flow is zero but gas pressure in the circuit of the anesthesia machine is maintained. In this situation, an oxygen analyzer is necessary to detect the delivery of a hypoxic gas mixture. Far superior to the fail-safe valve or an oxygen analyzer is the continuous presence of a vigilant anesthesia provider.

## Compressed Gases

Gases used in the administration of anesthesia (oxygen, nitrous oxide, air) are most often delivered to the anesthesia machine from a central supply source located in the hospital (Fig. 15.3).[2] Hospital-supplied gases enter the operating room from a central source through

> **Box 15.1** Common Features of Anesthesia Machines
>
> - Inlet of hospital pipeline for compressed gases (oxygen, nitrous oxide, and air)
> - Inlet of compressed gas cylinders
> - Pressure regulators to reduce pipeline and cylinder pressure to safe and consistent levels
> - Fail-safe device
> - Flowmeters to control the amount of gases delivered to the breathing limb
> - Vaporizers for adding volatile anesthetic gas to the carrier gas
> - Common gas line through which compressed gases mixed with a volatile agent enter the breathing limb
> - Breathing limb, including an oxygen analyzer, inspiratory one-way valve, circle system, gas sampling line, spirometer to measure the respiratory rate and volume, expiratory one-way valve, adjustable pressure-limiting valve, carbon dioxide absorbent, reservoir bag, mechanical ventilator, and scavenging system

pipelines to color-coded wall outlets (green for oxygen, blue for nitrous oxide, and yellow for air). Color-coded pressure hoses are connected to the wall outlets by fittings that are noninterchangeable (diameter index safety system [DISS] or quick connects), which are designed to prevent misconnections of pipeline gases. Oxygen or air from a central supply source may also be used to pneumatically drive the ventilator on the anesthesia machine.

Gas enters the anesthesia machine through pipeline inlet connections that are gas specific (threaded noninterchangeable connections) to minimize the possibility

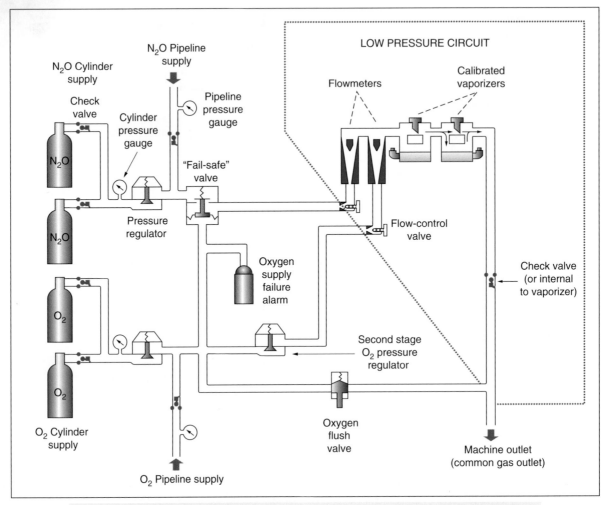

**Fig. 15.3** Schematic diagram of the internal circuitry of an anesthesia machine. Oxygen and nitrous oxide enter the anesthesia machine through a central supply line (most common); alternatively (infrequently), they are provided from gas cylinders attached to pin-indexed yokes on the machine. Check valves prevent transfilling of gas cylinders or flow of gas from cylinders into the central supply line. Pressure regulators decrease pressure in the tubing from the gas cylinders to about 50 psi. The fail-safe valve prevents flow of nitrous oxide if the pressure in the oxygen supply circuit decreases to less than 30 psi. Needle valves control gas flow to rotameters (flowmeters). Agent-specific vaporizers provide a reliable means to deliver preselected concentrations of a volatile anesthetic. An interlock system allows only one vaporizer to be in the "on" (delivery) setting at a time. After mixing in the manifold of the anesthesia machine, the total fresh gas flow enters the common outlet for delivery to the patient through the anesthetic breathing system (circuit). (Modified from American Society of Anesthesiologists. *Check-Out. A Guide for Preoperative Inspection of an Anesthetic Machine.* Park Ridge, IL: American Society of Anesthesiologists; 1987:1-14, used with permission.)

of a misconnection. The gas must be delivered from the central supply source at an appropriate pressure (about 50 psi) for the flowmeters on the anesthesia machine to function properly.

Anesthesia machines are also equipped with cylinders of oxygen and nitrous oxide for use should the central gas supply fail (see Fig. 15.3).[2] Color-coded cylinders are attached to the anesthesia machine by a hanger yoke assembly, which consists of two metal pins that correspond to holes in the valve casing of the gas cylinder (pin indexed safety system [PISS]) (Table 15.1). This design makes it impossible to attach an oxygen cylinder to any yoke on the anesthesia machine other than that designed for oxygen. Otherwise, a cylinder containing nitrous oxide could be attached to the oxygen yoke, which would result in the delivery of nitrous oxide when the oxygen flowmeter was activated. Color-coded pressure gauges (green for oxygen,

**Table 15.1**  Characteristics of Compressed Gases Stored in E Size Cylinders Attached to the Anesthesia Machine

| Characteristic | Oxygen | Nitrous Oxide | Carbon Dioxide | Air |
|---|---|---|---|---|
| Cylinder color | Green[a] | Blue | Gray | Yellow[a] |
| Physical state in cylinder | Gas | Liquid and gas | Liquid and gas | Gas |
| Cylinder contents (L) | 625 | 1590 | 1590 | 625 |
| Cylinder weight empty (kg) | 5.90 | 5.90 | 5.90 | 5.90 |
| Cylinder weight full (kg) | 6.76 | 8.80 | 8.90 | |
| Cylinder pressure full (psi) | 2000 | 750 | 838 | 1800 |

[a]The World Health Organization specifies that cylinders containing oxygen for medical use be painted white, but manufacturers in the United States use green. Likewise, the international color for air is white and black, whereas cylinders in the United States are color-coded yellow.

blue for nitrous oxide) on the anesthesia machine indicate the pressure of the gas in the corresponding gas cylinder (see Table 15.1).

### Calculation of Cylinder Contents

The pressure in an oxygen cylinder is directly proportional to the volume of oxygen in the cylinder. For example, a full E size oxygen cylinder contains about 625 L of oxygen at a pressure of 2000 psi and half this volume when the pressure is 1000 psi. Therefore, how long a given flow rate of oxygen can be maintained before the cylinder is empty can be calculated. In contrast to oxygen, the pressure gauge for nitrous oxide does not indicate the amount of gas remaining in the cylinder because the pressure in the gas cylinder remains at 750 psi as long as any liquid nitrous oxide is present. When nitrous oxide leaves the cylinder as a vapor, additional liquid is vaporized to maintain an unchanging pressure in the cylinder. After all the liquid nitrous oxide is vaporized, the pressure begins to decrease, and it can be assumed that about 75% of the contents of the gas cylinder have been exhausted. Because a full nitrous oxide cylinder (E size) contains about 1590 L, approximately 400 L of nitrous oxide remains when the pressure gauge begins to decrease from its previously constant value of 750 psi. Vaporization of a liquefied gas (nitrous oxide), as well as expansion of a compressed gas (oxygen), absorbs heat, which is extracted from the metal cylinder and the surrounding atmosphere. For this reason, atmospheric water vapor often accumulates as frost on gas cylinders and in valves, particularly during high gas flow from these tanks. Internal icing does not occur because compressed gases are free of water vapor.

### Flowmeters

Flowmeters on the anesthesia machine precisely control and measure gas flow to the common gas inlet (see Fig. 15.3).[2]

Measurement of the flow of gases is based on the principle that flow past a resistance is proportional to pressure. Typically, gas flow enters the bottom of a vertically positioned and tapered (the cross-sectional area increases upward from site of gas entry) glass flow tube. Gas flow into the flowmeter tube raises a bobbin or ball-shaped float. The float comes to rest when gravity is balanced by the decrease in pressure caused by the float. The upper end of the bobbin or the equator of the ball indicates the gas flow in milliliters or liters per minute. Proportionality between pressure and flow is determined by the shape of the tube (resistance) and the physical properties (density and viscosity) of the gas. The flowmeters are initially calibrated for the indicated gas at the factory. Because few gases have the same density and viscosity, flowmeters are not interchangeable with other gases. The scale accompanying an oxygen flowmeter is green, whereas the scale for the nitrous oxide flowmeter is blue.

Gas flow exits the flowmeters and passes into a manifold (mixing chamber) located at the top of the flowmeters (see Fig. 15.3).[2] The oxygen flowmeter should be the last in the sequence of flowmeters, and thus oxygen should be the last gas added to the manifold. This arrangement reduces the possibility that leaks in the apparatus proximal to oxygen inflow can diminish the delivered oxygen concentration, whereas leaks distal to that point result in loss of volume without a qualitative change in the mixture. Nevertheless, an oxygen flowmeter tube leak can produce a hypoxic mixture regardless of the flowmeter tube arrangement (Fig. 15.4).[3] Indeed, flowmeter tube leaks are a hazard, reflecting the fragile construction of this component of the anesthesia machine. Subtle cracks may be overlooked and result in errors in delivered flow.

Gases mix in the manifold and flow to an outlet port on the anesthesia machine, where they are directed into either a vaporizer or an anesthetic breathing system (see Fig. 15.3).[2] For emergency purposes, provision is made for delivery of a large volume of oxygen (35 to 75 L/

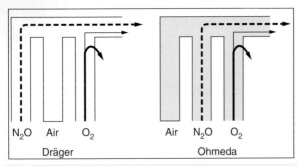

**Fig. 15.4** Oxygen flow tube leak. An oxygen flow tube leak can produce a hypoxic mixture regardless of the flow tube arrangement. (From Brockwell RC. Inhaled anesthetic delivery systems. In Miller RD, ed. *Miller's Anesthesia*. 7th ed. Philadelphia: Churchill Livingstone; 2010:680, used with permission.)

min) to the outlet port through an oxygen flush valve that bypasses the flowmeters and manifold. The oxygen flush valve allows direct communication between the oxygen high-pressure circuit and the low-pressure circuit (see Fig. 15.3).[2] Activation of the oxygen flush valve during a mechanically delivered inspiration from the anesthesia machine ventilator permits the transmission of high airway pressure to the patient's lungs, with the possibility of barotrauma.

## VAPORIZERS

Volatile anesthetics are liquids at room temperature and atmospheric pressure. Vaporization, which is the conversion of a liquid to a vapor, takes place in a closed container, referred to as a *vaporizer*. The vapor concentration resulting from vaporization of a volatile liquid anesthetic must be delivered to the patient with the same accuracy and predictability as other gases (oxygen, nitrous oxide).

### Physics of Vaporization

The molecules that make up a liquid are in constant random motion. In a vaporizer containing a volatile liquid anesthetic, there is an asymmetric arrangement of intermolecular forces applied to the molecules at the liquid-oxygen interface. The result of this asymmetric arrangement is a net attractive force pulling the surface molecules into the liquid phase. This force must be overcome if surface molecules are to enter the gas phase, where their relatively sparse density constitutes a vapor. The energy necessary for molecules to escape from the liquid is supplied as heat. The heat of vaporization of a liquid is the number of calories required at a specific temperature to convert 1 g of a liquid into a vapor. The heat of vaporization necessary for molecules to leave the liquid phase is greater when the temperature of the liquid decreases.

Vaporization in the closed confines of a vaporizer ceases when equilibrium is reached between the liquid and vapor phases such that the number of molecules leaving the liquid phase is the same as the number reentering. The molecules in the vapor phase collide with each other and the walls of the container, thereby creating pressure. This pressure is termed vapor pressure and is unique for each volatile anesthetic. Furthermore, vapor pressure is temperature dependent such that a decrease in the temperature of the liquid is associated with a lower vapor pressure and fewer molecules in the vapor phase. Cooling of the liquid anesthetic reflects a loss of heat (heat of vaporization) necessary to provide energy for vaporization. This cooling is undesirable because it lowers the vapor pressure and limits the attainable vapor concentration.

### Vaporizer Classification and Design

Vaporizers are classified as agent-specific, variable-bypass, flow-over, temperature-compensated (equipped with an automatic temperature-compensating device that helps maintain a constant vaporizer output over a wide range of temperatures), and out of circuit (Fig. 15.5).[1] These contemporary vaporizers are unsuitable for the controlled vaporization of desflurane, which has a vapor pressure near 1 atm (664 mm Hg) at 20° C. For this reason, a desflurane vaporizer is electrically heated to 23° C to 25° C and pressurized with a backpressure regulator to 1500 mm Hg to create an environment in which the anesthetic has relatively lower, but predictable, volatility.

Variable bypass describes dividing (splitting) the total fresh gas flow through the vaporizer into two portions. The first portion of the fresh gas flow (20% or less) passes into the vaporizing chamber of the vaporizer, where it becomes saturated (flow-over) with the vapor of the liquid anesthetic. The second portion of the fresh gas flow passes through the bypass chamber of the vaporizer. Both portions of the fresh gas flow mix at the patient outlet side of the anesthesia machine. The proportion of fresh gas flow diverted through the vaporizing chamber, and thus the concentration of volatile anesthetic delivered to the patient, is determined by the concentration control dial. The scale on the concentration control dial is in volume percent for the specific anesthetic drug. A temperature-sensitive bimetallic strip or an expansion element influences proportioning of total gas flow between the vaporizing and bypass chambers as the vaporizer temperature changes (temperature compensated) (see Fig. 15.5).[1] For example, as the temperature of the liquid anesthetic in the vaporizer chamber decreases, the temperature-sensing elements allow increased gas inflow into this chamber to offset the effect of decreased anesthetic liquid vapor pressure.

Vaporizers are often constructed of metals with high thermal conductivity (copper, bronze) to further minimize heat loss. As a result, vaporizer output is nearly linear

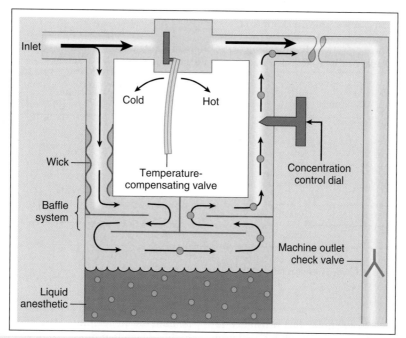

**Fig. 15.5** Simplified schematic of the Ohmeda Tec-type vaporizer. Rotation of the concentration control dial diverts a portion of the total fresh gas flow through the vaporizing chamber, where wicks saturated with liquid anesthetic ensure a large gas-liquid interface for efficient vaporization. A temperature-compensating valve diverts more or less fresh gas flow through the vaporizing chamber to offset the effects of changes in temperature on the vapor pressure of the liquid anesthetic (temperature-compensated vaporizer). Gases saturated with the vapor of the liquid anesthetic join gases that have passed through the bypass chamber for delivery to the machine outlet check valve. When the concentration control dial is in the off position, no fresh gas inflow enters the vaporizing chamber.

between 20° C and 35° C.[3] Designation of vaporizers as agent specific and out of circuit emphasizes that these devices are calibrated to accommodate a single volatile anesthetic and are isolated from the anesthetic breathing system.

Tipping of vaporizers can cause liquid anesthetic to spill from the vaporizing chamber into the bypass chamber, with a resultant increased vapor concentration exiting from the vaporizer. Nevertheless, the likelihood of tipping is minimized because vaporizers are secured to the anesthesia machine and there is little need to move them. Leaks associated with vaporizers are most often due to a loose filler cap.

Commonly, two to three anesthetic-specific vaporizers are present on the anesthesia machine. A safety interlock mechanism ensures that only one vaporizer at a time can be turned on. Turning on a vaporizer requires depression of a release button on the concentration dial, followed by counterclockwise rotation of the dial. This prevents accidental movement of the dial from the off to the on position. The location of the filler port on the lower portion of the vaporizer minimizes the likelihood of overfilling of the vaporizing chamber (>125 mL) with liquid anesthetic. A window near the filler port permits visual verification of the level of liquid anesthetic in the vaporizing chamber. Use of an anesthetic-specific keyed filler device prevents placement of a liquid anesthetic into the vaporizing chamber that is different from the anesthetic for which the vaporizer was calibrated. This is uniquely important for desflurane because its vapor pressure is near 1 atm and accidental placement of desflurane in a contemporary vaporizer could result in an anesthetic overdose.[4] As with anesthesia machines, periodic maintenance (usually every 12 months) is recommended by the manufacturers of vaporizers.

## ANESTHETIC BREATHING SYSTEMS

The function of anesthetic breathing systems is to deliver oxygen and anesthetic gases to the patient and to eliminate carbon dioxide. Conceptually, the anesthetic breathing system is a tubular extension of the patient's upper airway. Anesthetic breathing systems can add considerable resistance to inhalation because peak flows as high as 60 L/min are reached during spontaneous inspiration. This resistance is influenced by unidirectional valves and connectors. The components of the breathing system, particularly the tracheal tube connector, should have

**Table 15.2** Classification of Anesthetic Breathing Systems

| System | Gas Reservoir Bag | Rebreathing of Exhaled Gases | Chemical Neutralization of Carbon Dioxide | Unidirectional Valves | Fresh Gas Inflow Rate[a] |
|---|---|---|---|---|---|
| **Open** | | | | | |
| Insufflation | No | No | No | None | Unknown |
| Open drop | No | No | No | None | Unknown |
| **Semiopen** | | | | | |
| Mapleson A, B, C, D | Yes | No[b] | No | One | High |
| Bain | Yes | No[b] | No | One | High |
| Mapleson E | No | No[b] | No | None | High |
| Mapleson F (Jackson-Rees) | Yes | No[b] | No | One | High |
| **Semiclosed circle** | Yes | Partial | Yes | Three | Moderate |
| **Closed circle** | Yes | Total | Yes | Three | Low |

[a]High, greater than 6 L/min; moderate, 3 to 6 L/min; low, 0.3 to 0.5 L/min.
[b]No rebreathing of exhaled gases only when fresh gas inflow is adequate.

the largest possible lumen to minimize this resistance to breathing. Right-angle connectors should be replaced with curved connectors to minimize resistance. Substituting controlled ventilation of the patient's lungs for spontaneous breathing can offset the increased resistance to inhalation imparted by anesthetic breathing systems.

Anesthetic breathing systems are classified as open, semiopen, semiclosed, and closed according to the presence or absence of (1) a gas reservoir bag in the circuit, (2) rebreathing of exhaled gases, (3) means to chemically neutralize exhaled carbon dioxide, and (4) unidirectional valves (Table 15.2). The most commonly used anesthetic breathing systems are the (1) Mapleson F (Jackson-Rees) system, (2) Bain circuit, and (3) circle system.

## Mapleson Breathing Systems

In 1954, Mapleson analyzed and described five different arrangements of fresh gas inflow tubing, reservoir tubing, face mask, reservoir bag, and an expiratory valve to administer anesthetic gases (Fig. 15.6).[5] These five different semiopen anesthetic breathing systems are designated Mapleson A to E. The Mapleson F system, which is a Jackson-Rees modification of the Mapleson D system, was added later. The Bain circuit is a modification of the Mapleson D system (Fig. 15.7).[6]

### Flow Characteristics
The Mapleson systems are characterized by the absence of valves to direct gases to or from the patient and the absence of chemical carbon dioxide neutralization. Because of no clear separation of inspired and expired gases, rebreathing occurs when inspiratory flow exceeds the fresh gas flow. The composition of the inspired mixture depends on how much rebreathing takes place. The

amount of rebreathing associated with each system is highly dependent on the fresh gas flow rate. The optimal fresh gas flow may be difficult to determine. The fresh gas flow should be adjusted when changing from spontaneous and controlled ventilation. Monitoring end-tidal $CO_2$ is the best method to determine the optimal fresh gas flow. The performance of these circuits is best understood by studying the gas disposition at end exhalation during spontaneous and controlled ventilation (Fig. 15.8).[7]

## Mapleson F (Jackson-Rees) System

The Mapleson F (Jackson-Rees) system is a T-piece arrangement with a reservoir bag and an adjustable pressure-limiting overflow valve on the distal end of the gas reservoir bag (see Fig. 15.6).[5] The degree of rebreathing when using this anesthetic breathing system is influenced by the method of ventilation (spontaneous versus controlled) and adjustment of the pressure-limiting overflow valve (venting). Fresh gas flow equal to two to three times the patient's minute ventilation is recommended to prevent rebreathing of exhaled gases.

### Flow Characteristics
During spontaneous ventilation, exhaled gases pass down the expiratory limb and mix with fresh gases (see Fig. 15.8).[7] The expiratory pause allows the fresh gas to push the exhaled gases down the expiratory limb. With the next inspiration, the inhaled gas mixture comes from the fresh gas flow and from the expiratory limb, including the reservoir bag.

### Clinical Uses
The Mapleson F system is commonly used for controlled ventilation during transport of tracheally intubated patients. Because there are no moving parts except the

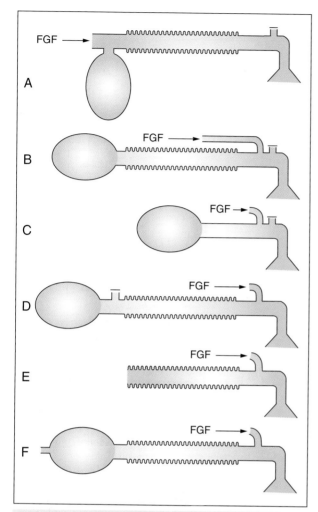

Fig. 15.6 Anesthetic breathing systems classified as semi-open Mapleson A through F. *FGF*, Fresh gas flow. (Modified from Willis BA, Pender JW, Mapleson WW. Rebreathing in a T-piece: volunteer and theoretical studies of Jackson-Rees modification of Ayre's T-piece during spontaneous respiration. *Br J Anaesth.* 1975;47:1239-1246, used with permission.)

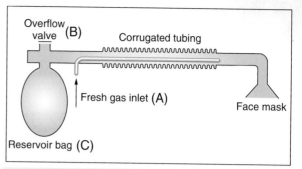

Fig. 15.7 Schematic diagram of the Bain system showing fresh gas flow (FGF) entering a narrow tube within the larger corrugated expiratory limb (A). The only valve in the system (B) is an adjustable pressure-limiting (overflow) valve located near the FGF inlet and reservoir bag (C). (Modified from Bain JA, Spoerel WE. A streamlined anaesthetic system. *Can Anaesth Soc J.* 1972;19:426-435, used with permission.)

pressure-limiting overflow valve, circuit dead space and resistance are minimal. This is ideal for pediatric anesthesia (see Chapter 34). The Mapleson F system may be used for both spontaneous and controlled ventilation. It is inexpensive, can be used with a face mask or endotracheal tube, is lightweight, and can be repositioned easily. Pollution of the atmosphere with anesthetic gases when using this system can be decreased by adapting it to scavenging systems.

### Disadvantages

Disadvantages of the Mapleson F system include (1) the need for high fresh gas inflow to prevent rebreathing, (2) the possibility of high airway pressure and barotrauma should the overflow valve become occluded, and (3) the lack of humidification. Lack of humidification can be

offset by allowing the fresh gas to pass through an in-line heated humidifier.

## Bain System

The Bain circuit is a coaxial version of the Mapleson D system in which the fresh gas supply tube runs coaxially inside the corrugated expiratory tubing (see Fig. 15.7).[6] The fresh gas tube enters the circuit near the reservoir bag, but the fresh gas is actually delivered at the patient end of the circuit. The exhaled gases are vented through the overflow valve near the reservoir bag. The Bain circuit may be used for both spontaneous and controlled ventilation. Prevention of rebreathing during spontaneous ventilation requires a fresh gas flow of 200 to 300 mL/kg/min and a flow of only 70 mL/kg/min during controlled ventilation.

### Advantages

Advantages of the Bain circuit include (1) warming of the fresh gas inflow by the surrounding exhaled gases in the corrugated expiratory tube, (2) conservation of moisture as a result of partial rebreathing, and (3) ease of scavenging waste anesthetic gases from the overflow valve. It is lightweight, easily sterilized, reusable, and useful when access to the patient is limited, such as during head and neck surgery.

### Disadvantages

Hazards of the Bain circuit include unrecognized disconnection or kinking of the inner fresh gas tube. The outer expiratory tube should be transparent to allow inspection of the inner tube.

## Circle System

The circle system is the most popular anesthetic breathing system in the United States. It is so named because its

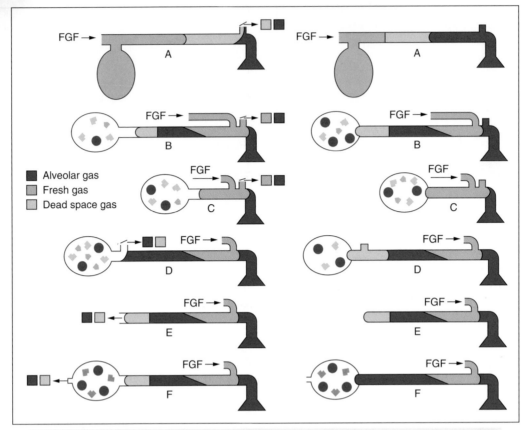

**Fig. 15.8** Gas disposition at end exhalation during spontaneous ventilation *(left)* or controlled ventilation *(right)* of the lungs in semiopen Mapleson A through F anesthetic breathing systems. The relative efficiency of different Mapleson systems for preventing rebreathing during spontaneous ventilation is A > DF > C > B. The relative efficiency of different Mapleson systems for preventing rebreathing during controlled ventilation is DF > B > C > A. *FGF,* Fresh gas flow. (Modified from Sykes MK. Rebreathing circuits. A review. *Br J Anaesth.* 1968;40:666-674, used with permission.)

essential components are arranged in a circular manner (Fig. 15.9).[3] The circle system prevents rebreathing of carbon dioxide by chemical neutralization of carbon dioxide with carbon dioxide absorbents.

### Classification

A circle system can be classified as semiopen, semiclosed, or closed, depending on the amount of fresh gas inflow (see Table 15.2). In a semiopen system, very high fresh gas flow is used to eliminate rebreathing of gases. A semiclosed system is associated with rebreathing of gases and is the most commonly used approach. In a closed system, the inflow gas exactly matches that being consumed by the patient. Rebreathing of exhaled gases in the semiclosed and closed circle systems results in (1) some conservation of airway moisture and body heat and (2) decreased pollution of the surrounding atmosphere with anesthetic gases when the fresh gas inflow rate is set at less than the patient's minute ventilation.

### Disadvantages

Disadvantages of the circle system include (1) increased resistance to breathing because of the presence of unidirectional valves and carbon dioxide absorbent, (2) bulkiness with loss of portability, and (3) enhanced opportunity for malfunction because of the complexity of the apparatus.

### Impact of Rebreathing

Rebreathing of exhaled gases in a semiclosed circle system influences the inhaled anesthetic concentrations of these gases. For example, when uptake of the anesthetic gas is high, as during induction of anesthesia, rebreathing of exhaled gases depleted of anesthetic greatly dilutes the concentration of anesthetic in the fresh gas inflow. This dilutional effect of uptake is offset clinically by increasing the delivered concentration of anesthetic. As uptake of anesthetic diminishes, the impact of dilution on the inspired concentration produced by rebreathing of exhaled gases is lessened.

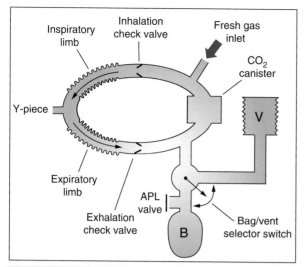

**Fig. 15.9** Schematic diagram of the components of a circle absorption anesthetic breathing system. Rotation of the bag/vent selector switch permits substitution of an anesthesia machine ventilator (V) for the reservoir bag (B). The volume of the reservoir bag is determined by the fresh gas inflow and adjustment of the adjustable pressure-limiting (APL) valve. (From Brockwell RC, Andrews JJ. Delivery systems for inhaled anesthetics. In Barash PG, Cullen BF, Stoelting RK, eds. *Clinical Anesthesia*. Philadelphia: Lippincott Williams & Wilkins; 2006:557-594, used with permission.)

## Components

The circle system consists of (1) a fresh gas inlet, (2) inspiratory and expiratory unidirectional check valves, (3) inspiratory and expiratory corrugated tubing, (4) a Y-piece connector, (5) an adjustable pressure-limiting (APL) valve, also referred to as an overflow or pop-off valve, (6) a reservoir bag, (7) a canister containing carbon dioxide absorbent, (8) a bag/vent selector switch, and (9) a mechanical anesthesia ventilator (see Fig. 15.9).[3]

### Fresh Gas Inlet and Unidirectional Valves

Fresh gas enters the circle system through a connection from the common gas outlet of the anesthesia machine. Two unidirectional valves are situated in different limbs of the corrugated tubing such that one functions for inhalation and the other for exhalation. These valves (1) permit positive-pressure breathing and (2) prevent the rebreathing of exhaled gases until they have passed through the carbon dioxide absorbent canister and have had their oxygen content replenished. Rebreathing and hypercapnia can occur if the unidirectional valves stick in the open position, and total occlusion of the circuit can occur if they are stuck in the closed position. If the expiratory valve is stuck in the closed position, breath stacking and barotrauma can occur. If the unidirectional valves are functioning properly, the only dead space in the circle system is between the Y-piece and the patient.

### Corrugated Tubing

The inspiratory and expiratory corrugated tubes serve as conduits for delivery of gases to and from the patient. Their large bore provides minimal resistance, and the corrugations provide flexibility, resist kinking, and promote turbulent instead of laminar flow. During positive-pressure ventilation, some of the delivered gas distends the corrugated tubing and some is compressed within the circuit, which leads to a smaller delivered tidal volume.

### Y-Piece Connector

A Y-piece connector at the patient end of the circuit has (1) a curved elbow, (2) an outer diameter of 22 mm to fit inside a face mask, and (3) an inner diameter of 15 mm to fit onto an endotracheal tube connector.

### Adjustable Pressure-Limiting Valve

When the bag/vent selector switch is set to "bag," the APL (overflow or pop-off) valve (1) allows venting of excess gas from the breathing system into the waste gas scavenging system and (2) can be adjusted to allow the anesthesia provider to provide assisted or controlled ventilation of the patient's lungs by manual compression of the gas reservoir bag. The APL valve should be fully open during spontaneous ventilation so that circuit pressure remains negligible throughout inspiration and expiration.

### Reservoir Bag

When the bag/vent selector switch is set to "bag," the gas reservoir bag maintains an available reserve volume of gas to satisfy the patient's spontaneous inspiratory flow rate (up to 60 L/min), which greatly exceeds conventional fresh gas flows (commonly 3 to 5 L/min) from the anesthesia machine. The bag also serves as a safety device because its distensibility limits pressure in the breathing circuit to less than 60 cm $H_2O$, even when the APL valve is closed.

## Closed Anesthetic Breathing System

In a closed anesthetic breathing system, there is total rebreathing of exhaled gases after absorption of carbon dioxide, and the APL valve or relief valve of the ventilator is closed. A closed system is present when the fresh gas inflow into the circle system (150 to 500 mL/min) satisfies the patient's metabolic oxygen requirements (150 to 250 mL/min during anesthesia) and replaces anesthetic gases lost by virtue of tissue uptake. If sidestream gas analyzers are used, the analyzed gas exiting the analyzer must be returned to the breathing system to maintain a closed system.

### Advantages

Advantages of a closed circle anesthetic breathing system over a semiclosed circle anesthetic breathing system include (1) maximal humidification and warming of inhaled gases, (2) less pollution of the surrounding atmosphere with anesthetic gases, and (3) economy in the use of anesthetics.

### Disadvantages

A disadvantage of a closed circle anesthetic breathing system is an inability to rapidly change the delivered concentration of anesthetic gases and oxygen because of the low fresh gas inflow.

### Dangers of Closed Anesthetic Breathing System

The principal dangers of a closed anesthetic breathing system are delivery of (1) unpredictable and possibly insufficient concentrations of oxygen and (2) unknown and possibly excessive concentrations of potent anesthetic gases.

#### Unpredictable Concentrations of Oxygen

Unpredictable and possibly insufficient delivered concentrations of oxygen when using a closed anesthetic breathing system are more likely if nitrous oxide is included in the fresh gas inflow. For example, decreased tissue uptake of nitrous oxide with time in the presence of unchanged uptake of oxygen can result in a decreased concentration of oxygen in the alveoli (Box 15.2). Therefore, the use of an oxygen analyzer placed on the inspiratory or expiratory limb of the circle system is mandatory when nitrous oxide is delivered through a closed anesthetic breathing system.

#### Unknown Concentrations of Potent Anesthetic Gases

Exhaled gases, devoid of carbon dioxide, form a major part of the inhaled gases when a closed anesthetic breathing system is used. This means that the composition of the inhaled gases is influenced by the concentration present in the exhaled gases. The concentration of anesthetic in exhaled gases reflects tissue uptake of anesthetic. Initially, tissue uptake is maximal, and the concentration of anesthetic in the exhaled gases is minimal. Subsequent rebreathing of these exhaled gases dilutes the inhaled concentration of anesthetic delivered to the patient. Therefore, high inflow concentrations of anesthetic are necessary to offset maximal tissue uptake. Conversely, only small amounts of anesthetic need to be added to the inflow gases when tissue uptake has decreased. The unknown impact of tissue uptake on the concentration of anesthetic in exhaled gases makes it difficult to estimate the inhaled concentration delivered to the patient through a closed anesthetic breathing system. This disadvantage can be partially offset by administering higher fresh gas inflow (3 L/min) for about 15 minutes before instituting the use of a closed anesthetic breathing system. This approach permits elimination of nitrogen from the lungs and corresponds to the time of greatest tissue uptake of anesthetic.

## ANESTHESIA MACHINE VENTILATORS

When the bag/vent selector switch is set to "vent," the gas reservoir bag and APL valve are eliminated from the circle anesthetic system, and the patient's ventilation is delivered from the mechanical anesthesia ventilator. Anesthesia ventilators are powered by compressed gas, electricity, or both. Most conventional anesthesia machine ventilators are pneumatically driven by oxygen or air that is pressurized and, during the inspiratory phase, routed to the space inside the ventilator casing between the compressible bellows and the rigid casing. Pressurized air or oxygen entering this space forces the bellows to empty its contents into the patient's lungs through the inspiratory limb of the breathing circuit. This pressurized air or oxygen also causes the ventilator relief valve to close, thereby preventing inspiratory anesthetic gas from escaping into the scavenging system.

Oxygen is preferable to air as the ventilator driving gas because if there is a leak in the bellows, the fraction of inspired oxygen will be increased. If there is a leak in the bellows in a ventilator driven by 50 psi oxygen or air, peak inspiratory pressures will rise. During exhalation, the driving gas is either vented into the room or directed to the scavenging system, and the bellows refills as the patient exhales. Some newer anesthesia machines have mechanically driven piston-type ventilators. The piston operates much like the plunger of a syringe to deliver the desired tidal volume or airway pressure to the patient.

### Bellows

Ventilators with bellows that rise during exhalation (standing or ascending bellows) are preferred because the

---

**Box 15.2** Alveolar Gas Concentration With a Closed Circle Anesthetic Breathing System

**Example 1**

Gas inflow is nitrous oxide, 300 mL/min, and oxygen, 300 mL/min, for 15 minutes. Nitrous oxide uptake by tissues at the time is 200 mL/min, and oxygen consumption is 250 mL/min. Alveolar gas after tissue uptake consists of 100 mL nitrous oxide and 50 mL oxygen. The alveolar concentration of oxygen ($F_{AO_2}$) is

$F_{AO_2}$ = 50 mL oxygen/(100 mL nitrous oxide + 50 mL oxygen) × 100 = 33%

**Example 2**

Gas inflow as in Example 1, but the duration of administration is 1 hour. At this time, tissue uptake of nitrous oxide has decreased to 100 mL/min, but oxygen consumption remains unchanged at 250 mL/min. Alveolar gas after tissue uptake consists of 200 mL nitrous oxide and 50 mL oxygen. The alveolar concentration of oxygen ($F_{AO_2}$) is

$F_{AO_2}$ = 50 mL oxygen/(200 mL nitrous oxide + 50 mL oxygen) × 100 = 20%

---

bellows will not rise (fill) if there is a leak in the anesthesia breathing system or the system becomes accidentally disconnected (Fig. 15.10).[8] Ventilators with bellows that descend during exhalation (hanging or descending bellows) are potentially dangerous because the bellows will continue to rise and fall during a disconnection. Whenever a ventilator is used, a disconnect alarm must be activated and audible.

## Humidity and Heat Exchange in the Breathing Circuit

The upper respiratory tract (especially the nose) functions as the principal heat and moisture exchanger (HME) to bring inspired gas to body temperature and 100% relative humidity in its passage to the alveoli. Water is removed from medical gases (cylinders or piped) to prevent corrosion and condensation. Tracheal intubation or

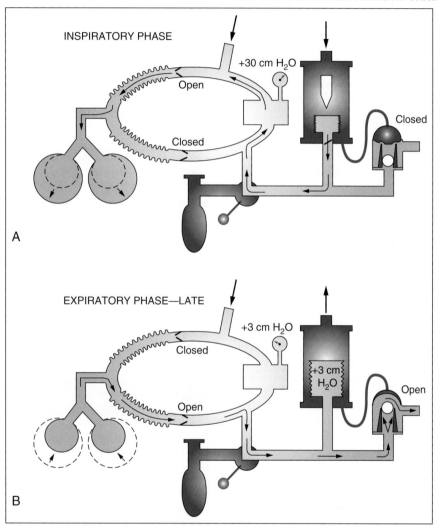

**Fig. 15.10** Inspiratory (A) and expiratory (B) phases of gas flow in a traditional circle system with an ascending bellows anesthesia ventilator. The bellows physically separates the driving gas circuit from the patient's gas circuit. The driving gas circuit is located outside the bellows, and the patient's gas circuit is inside the bellows. During the inspiratory phase (A), the driving gas enters the bellows chamber and causes the pressure within it to increase. This increased pressure causes the ventilator's relief valve to close, thus preventing anesthetic gas from escaping into the scavenging system, and the bellows to compress, thereby delivering the anesthetic gas within the bellows to the patient's lungs. During the expiratory phase (B), the driving gas exits the bellows chamber. The pressure within the bellows chamber and the pilot line decline to zero, which causes the mushroom portion of the ventilator's relief valve to open. Gas exhaled by the patient fills the bellows before any scavenging occurs because a weighted ball is incorporated into the base of the ventilator's relief valve. Scavenging occurs solely during the expiratory phase because the ventilator's relief valve is open only during expiration. (From Andrews JJ. *The Circle System. A Collection of 30 Color Illustrations.* Washington, DC: Library of Congress; 1998, used with permission.)

the use of a laryngeal mask airway bypasses the upper airway and thus leaves the tracheobronchial mucosa the burden of heating and humidifying inspired gases. Humidification of inspired gases by the lower respiratory tract in intubated patients can lead to dehydration of the mucosa, impaired ciliary function, impaired surfactant function, inspissation of secretions, atelectasis, and a rise in the alveolar-to-arterial gradient. Breathing of dry and room-temperature gases in intubated patients is associated with water and heat loss from the patient. Heat loss is more important than water loss, and the most important reason to provide heated humidification in intubated patients is to decrease heat loss and associated decreases in body temperature, especially in infants and children, who are rendered poikilothermic by general anesthesia.

## Humidification

Humidification is a form of vaporization in which water vapor (moisture) is added to the gases delivered by the anesthetic breathing system to minimize water and heat loss. The water formed and the heat generated by chemical neutralization of carbon dioxide help humidify and heat the gases in the breathing circuit. Humidifiers used for anesthesia and in the intensive care unit include (1) HME humidifiers, (2) heated water vaporizers and humidifiers, and (3) nebulizers.

### Heat and Moisture Exchanger Humidifiers

HME humidifiers are devices that, when placed between the endotracheal tube and Y-piece of the circle system, conserve some of the exhaled water and heat and return it to the inspired gases. They contain a porous hydrophobic or hygroscopic membrane that traps exhaled humidified gases and returns them to the patient on inspiration. Bacterial and viral filters can be incorporated in HME humidifiers to convert them into heat and moisture exchanging filters (HMEFs).

### Advantages

The advantages of HME humidifiers over other types of humidifiers are that they are (1) simple and easy to use, (2) lightweight, (3) not dependent on an external power source, (4) disposable, and (5) low cost.

### Disadvantages

The disadvantages of HME humidifiers are that they (1) are not as effective as heated water vaporizers and humidifiers in maintaining patient temperature, (2) add resistance and increase the work of breathing and therefore should be used with caution in spontaneously ventilating patients, (3) can become clogged with patient secretions or blood, and (4) can increase dead space, which can cause significant rebreathing in pediatric patients. Special low-volume HMEs are available for pediatric patients.

### Heated Water Vaporizers and Humidifiers

Heated water vaporizers and humidifiers are used to deliver a relative humidity higher than that delivered by HME humidifiers. Heated water vaporizers are more frequently used in pediatric anesthesia and intensive care unit patients. Risks from heated water vaporizers and humidifiers include (1) thermal injury, (2) nosocomial infection, (3) increased work of breathing, and (4) increased risk of malfunction due to the complexity of these systems.

### Nebulizers

Nebulizers produce a mist of microdroplets of water suspended in a gaseous medium. The quantity of water droplets delivered is not limited by the temperature of the carrier gas. In addition to water, nebulizers can deliver medications to peripheral airways.

## POLLUTION OF THE ATMOSPHERE WITH ANESTHETIC GASES

Chronic exposure to low concentrations of inhaled anesthetics may pose a health hazard to operating room personnel. The Occupational Safety and Health Administration (OSHA) presently has no required exposure limits regulating nitrous oxide and volatile anesthetics. In the operating room, OSHA recommends that the concentration of nitrous oxide not exceed 25 ppm and exposure concentrations of volatile anesthetics not exceed 2 ppm. Recommendations regarding waste anesthetic gases have been made by the American Society of Anesthesiologists (Box 15.3).[9]

Control of pollution of the atmosphere with anesthetic gases requires (1) scavenging of waste anesthetic gases,

---

**Box 15.3** Recommendations of the American Society of Anesthesiologists Task Force on Waste Anesthetic Gases

- Waste anesthetic gases should be scavenged.
- Appropriate work practices should be used to minimize exposure to waste anesthetic gases.
- Personnel working in areas where waste anesthetic gases may be present should be educated regarding (1) current studies on the health effects of exposure to waste anesthetic gases, (2) appropriate work practices to minimize exposure, and (3) machine checkout and maintenance procedures.
- There is insufficient evidence to recommend routine monitoring of trace concentrations of waste anesthetic gases in the operating room and postanesthesia care unit.
- There is insufficient evidence to recommend routine medical surveillance of personnel exposed to trace concentrations of waste anesthetic gases, although each institution should have a mechanism for employees to report suspected work-related health problems.

From McGregor DG, Baden JM, Bannister C, et al. *Waste Anesthetic Gases: Information for the Management in Anesthetizing Areas and the Postanesthesia Care Unit (PACU).* Park Ridge, IL: American Society of Anesthesiologists; 1999.

(2) periodic preventive maintenance of anesthesia equipment, (3) attention to the anesthetic technique, and (4) adequate ventilation of the operating rooms.

## Scavenging Systems

Scavenging is the collection and subsequent removal of vented gases from the operating room. The excess gas comes from either the APL valve if the bag/vent selector switch is set to "bag" or from the ventilator relief valve if the bag/vent selector switch is set to "vent." All excess gas from the patient exits the breathing system through these valves. In addition, when the bag/vent selector switch is set to "vent," some anesthetic breathing systems direct the drive gas inside the bellows canister to the scavenging system. The amount of delivered gas used to anesthetize a patient commonly far exceeds the patient's needs. The anesthesia provider must be certain that the scavenging system is operational and adjusted properly to ensure adequate scavenging. If sidestream gas analyzers are used, the analyzed gas exiting the analyzer must be directed to the scavenging system or returned to the breathing system.

Scavenging systems may be characterized as active or passive. An active system, is connected to the hospital's vacuum system, and gases are drawn from the machine by a vacuum. A passive system is connected to the hospital's ventilation duct, and waste gases flow out of the machine on their own.

Many anesthesia machines provide scavenging with a waste gas receiver mounted on the side of the anesthesia machine. Advantages of this system include (1) a needle valve that allows the clinician to manually adjust the amount of vacuum flow through the scavenging system, (2) a needle valve that can be adjusted such that the 3-L reservoir bag will be slightly inflated and appear to "breathe" with the patient, and (3) unlike other active scavenging systems, a waste gas receiver that does not require a strong vacuum to operate.

### Hazards

Hazards of scavenging systems include (1) obstruction of the scavenging pathways, which can result in excessive positive pressure in the breathing circuit and possible barotrauma, and (2) excessive vacuum applied to the scavenging system, which can cause negative pressures in the breathing system. Scavenging systems contain two relief valves to minimize these hazards. If gas accumulates in the scavenging system and cannot leave the anesthesia machine properly, the positive-pressure scavenge relief valve opens when the pressure reaches 10 cm $H_2O$ to allow the gas to escape into the room. If negative pressure is applied to the scavenging system, the negative-pressure scavenge relief valve opens and allows room air to be drawn in (instead of drawing gas from the patient). Additionally, if the amount of fresh gas flow exceeds the capacity of the scavenging system, the excess waste anesthetic gas exits the scavenging system through the positive-pressure relief valve and pollutes the operating room.

## Periodic Preventive Maintenance of Anesthesia Equipment

High-pressure leakage of nitrous oxide can occur as a result of faulty yokes attaching the nitrous oxide tank to the anesthesia machine or faulty connections from the central nitrous oxide gas supply to the anesthesia machine. Low-pressure leakage of anesthetic gases can occur because of leaks inside the anesthesia machine and leaks between the machine and patient. Periodic preventive maintenance of the anesthesia machine by qualified service representatives is recommended.

## Anesthetic Technique

Anesthetic techniques that can lead to operating room pollution include (1) poorly fitting face masks, (2) flushing the anesthetic delivery circuit, (3) filling anesthetic vaporizers, (4) the use of uncuffed endotracheal tubes, (5) failure to turn off the nitrous oxide flow or vaporizers at the end of the anesthetic, and (6) the use of semiopen breathing circuits such as the Jackson-Rees, which are difficult to scavenge.

## Adequate Room Ventilation

The air in the operating room should be exchanged at least 15 times per hour by the operating room ventilation system. This rate should be checked periodically by the hospital's clinical engineering department.

## ELIMINATION OF CARBON DIOXIDE

Open and semiopen breathing systems eliminate carbon dioxide by venting all exhaled gases to the atmosphere. Semiclosed and closed breathing systems eliminate carbon dioxide by chemical neutralization. Chemical neutralization is accomplished by directing the exhaled gases through a carbon dioxide absorber, which consists of a canister containing carbon dioxide absorbent granules. Gas flow through the absorber during exhalation is usually from top to bottom. A space below the canister at the base of the absorber allows the collection of dust and water.

### Carbon Dioxide Absorbents

All carbon dioxide absorbents use calcium hydroxide $(Ca[OH]_2)$ as the neutralizing base for carbon dioxide produced during respiration. Water is an essential ingredient common to all carbon dioxide absorbents, and is necessary for efficient and safe carbon dioxide absorption.

| Table 15.3 | Comparison of Carbon Dioxide Absorbents | | | |
|---|---|---|---|---|
| **Feature** | | **Soda Lime** | **Amsorb Plus** | **Litholyme** |
| Contents | | | | |
| $Ca(OH)_2$ (%) | | 76-81 | >80 | >75 |
| Water (%) | | 14-19 | 13-18 | 12-19 |
| NaOH (%) | | 4 | 0 | 0 |
| KOH (%) | | 1 | 0 | 0 |
| $CaCl_2$ (%) | | 0 | 4 | 0 |
| LiCl (%) | | 0 | 0 | 3 |
| Mesh size | | 4-8 | 4-8 | 4-10 |
| Generation of compound A with sevoflurane | | Yes | No | No |
| Generation of carbon monoxide with inhaled anesthetics | | Yes | No | No |
| Risk of exothermic reactions and fire in the presence of sevoflurane | | No | No | No |

Carbon dioxide absorbents also contain catalysts that are responsible for the differences in absorptive properties and safety profiles between individual absorbents.

Traditional Carbon Dioxide Absorbents: Soda Lime
Soda lime granules consist of calcium hydroxide, water, and small amounts of the strong bases sodium hydroxide (NaOH) and potassium hydroxide (KOH) that serve as catalysts for carbon dioxide absorption (Table 15.3). Soda lime granules fragment easily and produce alkaline dust, which can lead to bronchospasm if inhaled. Silica is added to the granules to provide hardness and minimize alkaline dust formation.

Neutralization of carbon dioxide with soda lime begins with reaction of carbon dioxide with water present in the soda lime granules and the subsequent formation of carbonic acid. Carbonic acid then reacts with the hydroxides present in the soda lime granules to form carbonates (with bicarbonates as intermediates), water, and heat (Box 15.4).

The water formed from the neutralization of carbon dioxide, the water present in the soda lime granules, and the water condensed from the patient's exhaled gases leach the alkaline bases from the soda lime granules and produce a slurry containing NaOH and KOH in the bottom of the canister. These monovalent bases can be corrosive to the skin.

The strong base NaOH and KOH catalysts in soda lime can lead to degradation of sevoflurane to compound A and degradation of inhaled anesthetics to clinically significant concentrations of carbon monoxide.

New-Generation Carbon Dioxide Absorbents: Amsorb Plus and Litholyme
Amsorb Plus and Litholyme are new-generation carbon dioxide absorbents that consist of calcium hydroxide and water, but unlike soda lime, they do not contain the strong bases NaOH or KOH. Instead they contain catalysts that are chemically inert and do not degrade sevoflurane

**Box 15.4** Chemical Neutralization of Carbon Dioxide

**Soda Lime**
$CO_2 + H_2O \rightarrow H_2CO_3$
$H_2CO_3 + 2NaOH$ (or $KOH$) $\rightarrow Na_2CO_3$ (or $K_2CO_3$) $+ 2H_2O +$ Heat
$Na_2CO3$ (or $K_2CO_3$) $+ Ca(OH)_2 \rightarrow CaCO_3 + 2NaOH$ (or $KOH$)
$H_2CO_3 + Ca(OH)_2 \rightarrow CaCO_3 + 2H_2O +$ Heat

**Amsorb Plus and Litholyme**
$CO_2 + H_2O \rightarrow H_2CO_3$
$H_2CO_3 + Ca(OH)_2 \rightarrow CaCO_3 + 2H_2O +$ Heat

to compound A or degrade inhaled anesthetics to carbon monoxide.

Neutralization of carbon dioxide with Amsorb Plus or Litholyme begins with reaction of carbon dioxide with water present in the granules and the subsequent formation of carbonic acid. Carbonic acid then reacts with the calcium hydroxide present in the granules to form calcium carbonate, water, and heat (see Box 15.4).

Heat of Neutralization
The water formed by the neutralization of carbon dioxide with soda lime, Amsorb Plus, and Litholyme is useful for humidifying the gases and for dissipating some of the heat generated in these exothermic reactions. The heat generated during the neutralization of carbon dioxide can be detected by warmness of the canister. Failure of the canister to become warm should alert the anesthesia provider to the possibility that chemical neutralization of carbon dioxide is not taking place.

## Efficiency of Carbon Dioxide Neutralization

The efficiency of carbon dioxide neutralization is influenced by the size of the carbon dioxide granules and the presence or absence of channeling in the carbon dioxide canister.

## Absorbent Granule Size

The optimal absorbent granule size represents a compromise between absorptive efficiency and resistance to airflow through the carbon dioxide absorbent canister. Absorbent efficiency increases as absorbent granule size decreases because the total surface area coming in contact with carbon dioxide increases. The smaller the absorbent granules, however, the smaller the interstices through which gas must flow and the greater the resistance to flow.

Absorbent granule size is designated as mesh size, which refers to the number of openings per linear inch in a sieve through which the granular particles can pass. The granular size of carbon dioxide absorbents in anesthesia practice is between 4 and 10 mesh, a size at which absorbent efficiency is maximal with minimal resistance. A 4-mesh screen means that there are 4 quarter-inch openings per linear inch. A 10-mesh screen has 10 tenth-inch openings per linear inch.

## Channeling

Channeling is the preferential passage of exhaled gases through the carbon dioxide absorber canister via pathways of low resistance such that the bulk of the carbon dioxide absorbent granules are bypassed. Channeling resulting from loose packing of absorbent granules can be minimized by gently shaking the canister before use to ensure firm packing of the absorbent granules. Carbon dioxide absorbent canisters are designed to facilitate uniform dispersion of exhaled gas flow through the absorbent granules.

## Absorptive Capacity

Absorptive capacity is determined by the maximum amount of carbon dioxide that can be absorbed by 100 g of carbon dioxide absorbent. Channeling of exhaled gases through the absorbent granules can substantially decrease their efficiency. Carbon dioxide absorbent canister design also influences the absorptive capacity of the carbon dioxide absorbent.

## Indicators

Carbon dioxide absorbents contain a pH-sensitive indicator dye that changes color when the carbon dioxide absorbent granules are exhausted. When the absorptive components of the granules are exhausted, carbonic acid accumulates and produces a change in the pH and thus in the indicator dye color.

The indicator dye in soda lime changes granule color from white to purple when exhausted. However, over time, exhausted soda lime granules may revert to their original white color even though absorptive capacity does not recover with time. On reuse, the dye quickly produces the purple color change again.

In contrast, Amsorb Plus and Litholyme each contain an indicator dye that changes granule color from white to purple when exhausted and, once changed, does not revert to its original color.

## Degradation of Inhaled Anesthetics

Soda lime, either moist and containing a normal water complement or dry, degrades sevoflurane to nephrotoxic compounds (compound A). Desiccated soda lime may degrade desflurane, enflurane, or isoflurane to carbon monoxide. In contrast, Amsorb Plus and Litholyme, either desiccated or moist, do not degrade inhaled anesthetics.

### Generation of Compound A

Degradation of sevoflurane by soda lime can result in the production of compound A, which is a dose- and time-dependent nephrotoxin. Production of compound A with soda lime increases with (1) low fresh gas flows, (2) higher concentrations of sevoflurane, and (3) higher absorbent temperatures. To date, no clinically significant renal toxicity has been associated with the use of sevoflurane.[10] In contrast, Amsorb Plus and Litholyme do not degrade sevoflurane to compound A.

### Generation of Carbon Monoxide

Carbon monoxide (CO) is an odorless, colorless, gas that is poisonous because it displaces oxygen from hemoglobin in blood and thereby leads to the formation of carboxyhemoglobin. Degradation of inhaled anesthetics by desiccated soda lime can lead to significant concentrations of carbon monoxide that can produce carboxyhemoglobin concentrations reaching 30% or higher.[11] Production of carbon monoxide and carboxyhemoglobin increases with (1) the inhaled anesthetic used (desflurane = enflurane > isoflurane >> halothane = sevoflurane), (2) low fresh gas flows, (3) higher concentrations of inhaled anesthetics, (4) higher absorbent temperatures, and most important, (5) the degree of dryness of the absorbent (desiccation).

Desiccation of soda lime increases the degradation of inhaled anesthetics to carbon monoxide. Desiccation requires a prolonged period (usually 48 hours) of high dry gas flow between cases. Desiccation is worsened if the breathing bag is left off the circuit. In this circumstance the inspiratory valve produces resistance to forward flow and the fresh gas takes the retrograde path of least resistance through the bottom to the top of the absorbent canister and out the 22 mm breathing bag mount. Accordingly, most instances of increased blood concentrations of carboxyhemoglobin occur in patients anesthetized on a Monday after continuous flow of oxygen (flowmeter accidentally left on) through the soda lime carbon dioxide absorbent over the weekend. In contrast, Amsorb Plus and Litholyme do not degrade inhaled anesthetics to carbon monoxide.

### Fire and Extreme Heat in the Breathing System

Desiccation of the carbon dioxide absorbent Baralyme (no longer clinically available) can lead to fire within the circle system with sevoflurane use.[12] A poorly characterized chemical reaction between sevoflurane and Baralyme can produce sufficient heat and combustible degradation products to lead to the spontaneous generation of fires within the carbon dioxide absorber canister and breathing circuit. Cases of extreme heat without fire associated with desiccated soda lime have been reported in Europe. To avoid this problem, anesthesia providers should make every effort to not use desiccated carbon dioxide absorbents.

### Recommendations Regarding Safe Use of Carbon Dioxide Absorbents

The Anesthesia Patient Safety Foundation (see Chapter 1) has published suggested steps regarding the selection of carbon dioxide absorbents and steps to take should desiccation of the carbon dioxide absorbent be a potential risk (Box 15.5).[13]

## CHECKING ANESTHESIA MACHINE AND CIRCLE SYSTEM FUNCTION

Improperly checking anesthesia equipment prior to use can lead to patient injury and has also been associated with an increased risk of severe morbidity and mortality related to anesthesia care.[14,15] In 1993 a preanesthesia checkout (PAC) was developed by the Food and Drug Administration and widely accepted to be an important step in the process of preparing to deliver anesthesia care.[16] Since that time anesthesia delivery systems have evolved to the point that one checkout procedure is not applicable to all anesthesia delivery systems currently on the market.

### ASA 2008 Recommendations for Preanesthesia Checkout Procedures

In 2008 the American Society of Anesthesiologists developed new Recommendations for Pre-Anesthesia Checkout Procedures in order to provide guidelines applicable to all anesthesia delivery systems so that individual departments could develop a PAC specific to the anesthesia delivery systems currently used at their facilities that could be performed consistently and expeditiously. Specifically, for newer anesthesia delivery systems that incorporate automated checkout features, items that are not evaluated by the automated checkout need to be identified, and supplemental manual checkout procedures included as needed. This information is available on the ASA website in the Clinical Information Section (Box 15.6).[17]

A complete anesthesia machine and circle system function checkout procedure should be performed each day before the first case (see Box 15.6, items 1-15).[17] An abbreviated checkout should be performed before each subsequent use that day (see Box 15.6, items 2, 4, 7, 11-15).[17] The most important preoperative checks are (1) verification that an auxiliary oxygen cylinder and self-inflating manual ventilation device (Ambu bag) are available and functioning, (2) a leak check of the machine's low-pressure system, (3) calibration of the oxygen monitor, and (4) a positive-pressure leak check of the breathing system.

#### Verification That Auxiliary Oxygen Cylinder and Manual Ventilation Device Are Available and Functioning

Failure to ventilate is a major cause of morbidity and death related to anesthesia care. Because equipment failure with resulting inability to ventilate the patient can occur at any time, a self-inflating manual ventilation device (e.g., Ambu bag) should be present at every anesthetizing location for every case and should be checked for proper function. In addition, a source of oxygen separate from the anesthesia machine and pipeline supply, specifically an oxygen cylinder with regulator and a means to open the cylinder valve, should be immediately available and checked (see Box 15.6, item 1).[17]

#### Leak Check of the Machine's Low-Pressure System

A leak check of the machine's low-pressure system is performed to confirm the integrity of the anesthesia machine

**Box 15.6** American Society of Anesthesiologists 2008 Recommendations for Preanesthesia Checkout Procedures

**To Be Completed Daily**

Item 1: Verify that auxiliary oxygen cylinder and self-inflating manual ventilation device are available and functioning.

Item 2: Verify that patient suction is adequate to clear the airway.

Item 3: Turn on anesthesia delivery system and confirm that AC power is available.

Item 4: Verify availability of required monitors, including alarms.

Item 5: Verify that pressure is adequate on the spare oxygen cylinder mounted on the anesthesia machine.

Item 6: Verify that the piped gas pressures are ≥50 psig.

Item 7: Verify that vaporizers are adequately filled and, if applicable, that the filler ports are tightly closed.

Item 8: Verify that there are no leaks in the gas supply lines between the flowmeters and the common gas outlet.

Item 9: Test scavenging system function.

Item 10: Calibrate, or verify calibration of, the oxygen monitor and check the low oxygen alarm.

Item 11: Verify that carbon dioxide absorbent is not exhausted.

Item 12: Perform breathing system pressure and leak testing.

Item 13: Verify that gas flows properly through the breathing circuit during both inspiration and exhalation.

Item 14: Document completion of checkout procedures.

Item 15: Confirm ventilator settings and evaluate readiness to deliver anesthesia care. (ANESTHESIA TIME OUT)

**To Be Completed Before Each Procedure**

Item 2: Verify that patient suction is adequate to clear the airway.

Item 4: Verify availability of required monitors, including alarms.

Item 7: Verify that vaporizers are adequately filled and, if applicable, that the filler ports are tightly closed.

Item 11: Verify that carbon dioxide absorbent is not exhausted.

Item 12: Perform breathing system pressure and leak testing.

Item 13: Verify that gas flows properly through the breathing circuit during both inspiration and exhalation.

Item 14: Document completion of checkout procedures.

Item 15: Confirm ventilator settings and evaluate readiness to deliver anesthesia care. (ANESTHESIA TIME OUT)

From American Society of Anesthesiologists Committee on Equipment and Facilities. *Recommendations for Pre-Anesthesia Checkout Procedures.* 2008. https://www.asahq.org/resources/clinical-information/2008-asa-recommendations-for-pre-anesthesia-checkout.

from the flowmeters to the common gas outlet (see Box 15.6, item 8).[17] It evaluates the portion of the anesthesia machine that is downstream from all safety devices, except the oxygen monitor. The low-pressure circuit is the most vulnerable part of the anesthesia machine because the components located within this area are the ones most subject to breakage and leaks. (Fig. 15.11).[18] The machine's low-pressure system must be checked because leaks in this circuit can lead to hypoxia or patient awareness, or both.

The leak test of the low-pressure system for some anesthesia machine designs varies, and the anesthesia provider must refer to the operator's manual for instructions. Newer anesthesia machines use automated checks of the machine's low-pressure system, but internal vaporizer leaks may not be detected unless each vaporizer is turned on individually during the low-pressure system self-test.

### Calibration of the Oxygen Monitor

The oxygen monitor is the only machine safety device that detects problems downstream from the flowmeters (see Box 15.6, item 10).[17] The other machine safety devices (the fail-safe valve, the oxygen supply failure alarm, and the proportioning system) are all upstream from the flowmeters.

### Positive-Pressure Leak Check of the Breathing System

A positive-pressure leak check of the breathing system must be performed before every procedure (see Box 15.6, item 12).[17] This test does not check the integrity of the unidirectional valves because a breathing system will pass the leak check even if the unidirectional valves are incompetent or stuck shut (see Box 15.6, item 13).[17]

## QUESTIONS OF THE DAY

1. What features of the anesthesia workstation are designed to prevent delivery of a hypoxic gas mixture?

2. A tracheally intubated patient who is receiving 10 L/min oxygen via Jackson-Reese breathing circuit requires transport from the operating room to the intensive care unit. The oxygen E-cylinder has pressure of 1000 psi. How many minutes of oxygen remain in the cylinder?

3. What are the advantages and disadvantages of the Mapleson F (Jackson-Rees) breathing system compared to a simple face mask or nasal cannula? Under what circumstances would use of a Jackson-Rees system lead to rebreathing of carbon dioxide?

4. What are the advantages and potential dangers of a closed anesthetic breathing system?

5. What gases are removed by the anesthesia workstation scavenging system? What are the potential hazards of the scavenging system, and how can they be prevented?

6. What are the advantages of Amsorb Plus or Litholyme versus soda lime for carbon dioxide removal in a circle breathing system?

7. What are the most important components of the ASA Recommended Preanesthesia Checkout Procedure? For the anesthesia delivery system in your institution, which (if any) of these items are performed by the automated machine check function?

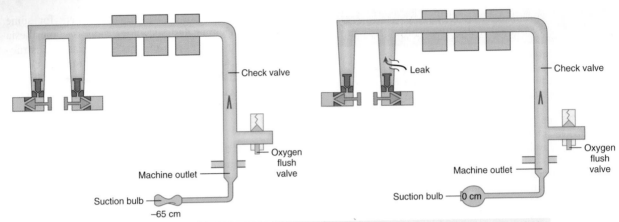

**Fig. 15.11** Food and Drug Administration negative-pressure leak test. Left, A negative-pressure leak-testing device is attached directly to the machine outlet. Squeezing the bulb creates a vacuum in the low-pressure circuit and opens the check valve. Right, When a leak is present in the low-pressure circuit, room air is entrained through the leak and the suction bulb inflates. (From Andrews JJ. Understanding anesthesia machines. In 1988 Review Course Lectures. Cleveland, OH: International Anesthesia Research Society; 1988:78, reprinted with permission.)

## REFERENCES

1. Brockwell RC, Andrews JJ. Delivery systems for inhaled anesthetics. In: Barash PG, Cullen BF, Stoelting RK, eds. *Clinical Anesthesia*. Philadelphia: Lippincott Williams & Wilkins; 2006:557–594.
2. American Society of Anesthesiologists. *Check-Out: A Guide for Preoperative Inspection of an Anesthetic Machine*. Park Ridge, IL: American Society of Anesthesiologists; 1987:1–14.
3. Brockwell RC, Andrews JJ. Inhaled anesthetic delivery systems. In: Miller RD, ed. *Miller's Anesthesia*. 7th ed. Philadelphia: Churchill Livingstone; 2010:667–718.
4. Andrews JJ, Johnston RV, Kramer GC. Consequences of misfilling contemporary vaporizers with desflurane. *Can J Anaesth*. 1993;40:71–74.
5. Willis BA, Pender JW, Mapleson WW. Rebreathing in a T-piece: volunteer and theoretical studies of Jackson-Rees modification of Ayre's T-piece during spontaneous respiration. *Br J Anaesth*. 1975;47:1239–1246.
6. Bain JA, Spoerel WE. A streamlined anaesthetic system. *Can Anaesth Soc J*. 1972;19:426–435.
7. Sykes MK. Rebreathing circuits: a review. *Br J Anaesth*. 1968;40:666–674.
8. Andrews JJ. *The Circle System. A Collection of 30 Color Illustrations*. Washington, DC: Library of Congress; 1998.
9. McGregor DG, Baden JM, Bannister C, et al. *Waste Anesthetic Gases: Information for the Management in Anesthetizing Areas and the Postanesthesia Care Unit (PACU)*. Park Ridge, IL: American Society of Anesthesiologists; 1999.
10. Kharasch ED, Frink EJ, Artru A, et al. Long-duration low-flow sevoflurane and isoflurane effects on postoperative renal and hepatic function. *Anesth Analg*. 2001;93:1511–1520.
11. Baxter PJ, Garton K, Kharasch ED. Mechanistic aspects of carbon monoxide formation from volatile anesthetics. *Anesthesiology*. 1998;89:929–941.
12. Lester M, Roth P, Eger EI. Fires from the interaction of anesthetics with desiccated absorbent. *Anesth Analg*. 2004;99:769–774.
13. Olympio MA. Carbon dioxide absorbent desiccation safety conference convened by APSF. *Anesth Pat Saf Found Newsletter*. 2005. Summer:25-29 (www.apsf.org).
14. Cooper JB, Newbower RS, Kitz RJ. An analysis of major errors and equipment failures in anesthesia management: considerations for prevention and detection. *Anesthesiology*. 1984;60:34–42.
15. Arbous MS, Meursing AE, van Kleef JW, de Lange JJ. Impact of anesthesia management characteristics on severe morbidity and mortality. *Anesthesiology*. 2005;102:257–268.
16. Food and Drug Administration. *Anesthesia Apparatus Checkout Recommendations*. Rockville, MD: Food and Drug Administration; 1993.
17. American Society of Anesthesiologists Committee on Equipment and Facilities. *Recommendations for Pre-Anesthesia Checkout Procedures*; 2008. http://www.asahq.org/clinical/fda.htm.
18. Andrews JJ. *Understanding Anesthesia Machines*. Cleveland, OH: International Anesthesia Research Society Review Course Lectures; 1988.

# 16 AIRWAY MANAGEMENT

## Kerry Klinger and Andrew Infosino

Expertise in airway management is critical for administering anesthesia safely. Difficult airway management is defined as the clinical situation in which conventionally trained anesthesia personnel experience difficulty with ventilation via a face mask or endotracheal intubation or both.[1] Difficult or failed airway management is a major factor in anesthesia-related morbidity (dental damage, aspiration of gastric contents, airway trauma, unanticipated surgical airway, anoxic brain injury, cardiopulmonary arrest) and fatality.[1,2] Competence in airway management requires (1) knowledge of the anatomy and physiology of the airway, (2) ability to evaluate the patient's history that is relevant to airway management, (3) physical examination of anatomic features correlating with difficult airway management, (4) skill with the many devices for airway management, and (5) appropriate application of the American Society of Anesthesiologists (ASA) algorithm for difficult airway management (Fig. 16.1).[1]

The editors and publisher would like to thank Dr. Robin A. Stackhouse for contributing to this chapter in the previous edition of this work. It has served as the foundation for the current chapter.

## DIFFICULT AIRWAY ALGORITHM

1. Assess the likelihood and clinical impact of basic management problems:
   - Difficulty with patient cooperation or consent
   - Difficult mask ventilation
   - Difficult supraglottic airway placement
   - Difficult laryngoscopy
   - Difficult intubation
   - Difficult surgical airway access

2. Actively pursue opportunities to deliver supplemental oxygen throughout the process of difficult airway management.

3. Consider the relative merits and feasibility of basic management choices:
   - Awake intubation *vs.* intubation after induction of general anesthesia
   - Non-invasive technique *vs.* invasive techniques for the initial approach to intubation
   - Video-assisted laryngoscopy as an initial approach to intubation
   - Preservation *vs.* ablation of spontaneous ventilation

4. Develop primary and alternative strategies:

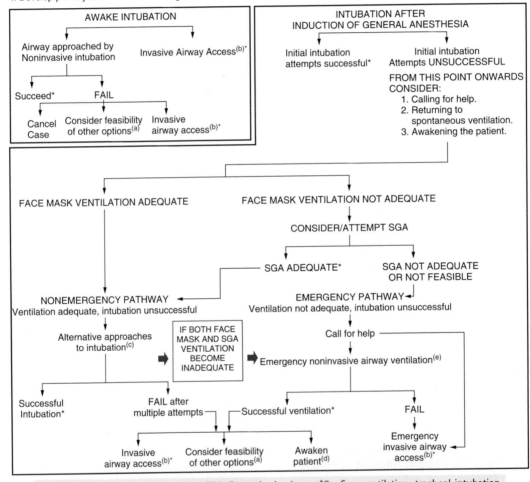

**Fig. 16.1** Difficult airway algorithm. *SGA,* Supraglottic airway. *Confirm ventilation, tracheal intubation, or SGA placement with exhaled $CO_2$. [a]Other options include (but not limited to): surgery utilizing face mask or supraglottic airway (SGA) anesthesia (e.g., LMA, ILMA, laryngeal tube), local anesthesia infiltration or regional nerve blockade. Pursuit of these options usually implies that mask ventilation will not be problematic. Therefore, these options may be limited value if this step in the algorithm has been reached via the Emergency Pathway. [b]Invasive airway access include surgical or percutaneous airway, jet ventilation, and retrograde intubation. [c]Alternative difficult intubation approaches include (but or note limited to): video assisted laryngoscopy, alternative laryngoscopy blades, SGA (e.g. LMA, ILMA) as an intubation conduit (with and without fiberoptic guidance), fiberoptic intubation, intubation stylet or tube changer, light wand, and blind oral or nasal intubation. [d]Consider re-preparation of the patient for awake intubation or cancelling surgery. [e]Emergency non-invasive airway ventilation consists of a SGA. (From Apfelbaum JL, Hagberg CA, Caplan RA, et al. Practice guidelines for management of the difficult airway: an updated report by the American Society of Anesthesiologists Task Force on Management of the Difficult Airway. *Anesthesiology.* 2013;118(2):251-270, used with permission.)

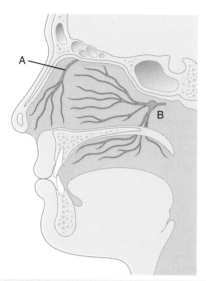

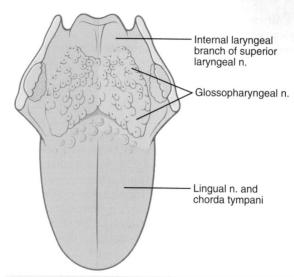

**Fig. 16.2** Innervation of the nasal cavity. A diagram of the lateral wall of the nasal cavity illustrates its sensory nerve supply. The anterior ethmoidal nerve, a branch of the ophthalmic division of the trigeminal nerve, supplies the anterior third of the septum and lateral wall (*A*). The maxillary division of the trigeminal nerve via the sphenopalatine ganglion supplies the posterior two thirds of the septum and the lateral wall (*B*). (From Ovassapian A. *Fiberoptic Airway Endoscopy in Anesthesia and Critical Care.* New York: Raven Press; 1990:57-79, used with permission.)

**Fig. 16.3** Sensory innervation of the tongue. (From Stackhouse RA. Fiberoptic airway management. *Anesthesiol Clin North Am.* 2002;20:933-951.)

## ANATOMY AND PHYSIOLOGY OF THE UPPER AIRWAY

### Nose

Air is warmed and humidified as it passes through the nares during normal breathing. Resistance to airflow through the nasal passages is twice that through the mouth and accounts for approximately 50% to 75% of total airway resistance.[3] The majority of the sensory innervation of the nasal cavity is derived from the ethmoidal branch of the ophthalmic nerve and branches of the maxillary division of the trigeminal nerve from the sphenopalatine ganglion (Fig. 16.2).[3,4]

### Mouth and Pharynx

Branches of the maxillary division of the trigeminal nerve that innervate the mouth include the greater and lesser palatine nerves and the lingual nerve. The greater and lesser palatine nerves provide most of the sensation to the hard palate, soft palate, and the tonsils, and the lingual nerve provides sensation to the anterior two thirds of the tongue. The posterior third of the tongue, the soft palate, and the oropharynx are innervated by the glossopharyngeal nerve (cranial nerve IX) (Figs. 16.3 and 16.4).[5]

The pharynx connects the nasal and oral cavities to the larynx and esophagus. The pharynx is composed of the

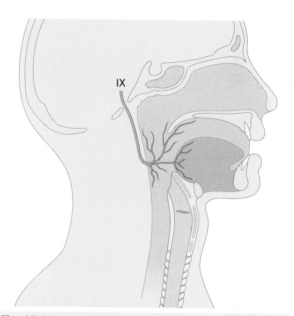

**Fig. 16.4** Sensory distribution of the glossopharyngeal nerve (cranial nerve IX). (From Patil VU, Stehling LC, Zauder HL. *Fiberoptic Endoscopy in Anesthesia.* St. Louis: Mosby; 1983.)

nasopharynx, oropharynx, and hypopharynx. The nasopharynx is separated from the oropharynx by the soft palate. The epiglottis demarcates the border between the oropharynx and the hypopharynx. The internal branch of the superior laryngeal nerve, which is a branch of cranial nerve X (vagus), provides sensory innervation to the hypopharynx, including the base of the tongue, posterior surface of the epiglottis, aryepiglottic folds, and arytenoids (Fig. 16.5).[6]

Airway resistance may be increased by prominent lymphoid tissue in the nasopharynx. The tongue is the predominant cause of airway resistance in the oropharynx. Obstruction by the tongue is increased by relaxation of the genioglossus muscle during anesthesia.

## Larynx

The adult larynx is located at the level of the third to sixth cervical vertebrae.[7] One of its primary functions is to protect the distal airways by closing when stimulated to prevent aspiration. This protective mechanism, when exaggerated, becomes laryngospasm. The larynx is composed of a cartilaginous framework connected by fascia, muscles, and ligaments. There are three unpaired and three paired cartilages. The unpaired

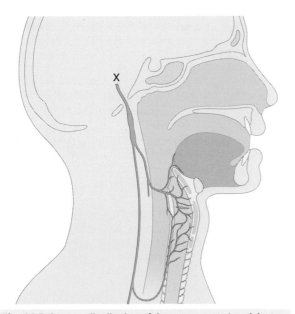

**Fig. 16.5** Sensory distribution of the vagus nerve (cranial nerve X). (From Patil VU, Stehling LC, Zauder HL. *Fiberoptic Endoscopy in Anesthesia.* St. Louis: Mosby; 1983.)

cartilages are the epiglottis, thyroid, and cricoid, and the paired cartilages are the arytenoids, corniculates, and cuneiforms. The cricoid cartilage is shaped like a signet ring, wider in the cephalocaudal dimension posteriorly, and is the only cartilage that is a full ring structure. The vocal cords are formed by the thyroarytenoid ligaments and are the narrowest portion of the adult airway. An understanding of the motor and sensory innervation of the laryngeal structures is important for performing anesthesia of the upper airway (Table 16.1).

## Trachea

The trachea extends from the larynx to the carina, which overlies the fifth thoracic vertebra. An adult trachea is 10 to 15 cm long and supported by 16 to 20 horseshoe-shaped cartilages. The sensory innervation of the trachea is from the recurrent laryngeal nerve, a branch of cranial nerve X (vagus).

## AIRWAY ASSESSMENT

### History and Anatomic Examination

A comprehensive assessment of the airway should consist of a history of the patient's airway experiences, review of previous anesthetic and medical records, physical examination, and additional evaluations when necessary.[1] The airway history should be evaluated to determine whether there are any medical, surgical, or anesthetic factors that have implications for airway management, including the risk of aspiration of gastric contents.[1,8] Various congenital and acquired disease states have a correlation with difficult airway management (Tables 16.2 and 16.3). Patients who have had a previous problem with airway management should have been informed of the problem. Patients' difficult airway specifics can be documented by a written letter, an alert or note in the medical record, a notification bracelet such as the medical alert system or equivalent device, or by discussion with the patient's surgeon,

| **Table 16.1** | Motor and Sensory Innervation of Larynx | |
|---|---|---|
| **Nerve** | **Sensory** | **Motor** |
| Superior laryngeal, internal division | Epiglottis<br>Base of tongue<br>Supraglottic mucosa<br>Thyroepiglottic joint<br>Cricothyroid joint | None |
| Superior laryngeal, external division | Anterior subglottic mucosa | Cricothyroid membrane |
| Recurrent laryngeal | Subglottic mucosa<br>Muscle spindles | Thyroarytenoid membrane<br>Lateral cricoarytenoid membrane. Interarytenoid membrane<br>Posterior cricoarytenoid membrane |

primary care physician, family member, or patient representative. The previous anesthetic record should contain a description of the airway difficulties (i.e., difficult laryngeal mask, supraglottic airway or intubation, or both), what airway management techniques were used, and whether they were successful.[1]

### Physical Examination Findings

Physical examination of the airway should evaluate multiple features to detect predictors of a difficult airway (Table 16.4). Physical examination features and other bedside tests have a low sensitivity and specificity for any single test and its implications for difficult airway management.[9,10] Combining tests and other risk factors correlates with some improvement in the accuracy of predicting a difficult airway.[10,11] Examination of the oropharyngeal space, submandibular space and compliance, and cervical spine mobility as well as evaluation of patients' body habitus can help to identify increased risk of difficult airway management. Recognition of patients who may be a difficult laryngoscopy and intubation as well as difficult mask, supraglottic airway placement, or surgical airway can highlight the need for further evaluation and preparation.[1]

### Oropharyngeal Space

The Mallampati test is used to evaluate the oropharyngeal space and its predicted effect on ease of direct laryngoscopy and endotracheal intubation.[12] There is a correlation between a modified Mallampati score of 3 and 4 with difficult laryngoscopy. The airway is classified according to what structures are visible. For the modified Mallampati score, the observer should be at eye level with the patient holding the head in a neutral position, opening the mouth maximally, and protruding the tongue without phonating (Fig. 16.6).[13]

Class I: The soft palate, fauces, uvula, and tonsillar pillars are visible.
Class II: The soft palate, fauces, and uvula are visible.
Class III: The soft palate and base of the uvula are visible.
Class IV: The soft palate is not visible.

In conjunction with the Mallampati examination, the interincisor gap, the size and position of the maxillary and mandibular teeth, and the conformation of the palate can be assessed.[1] An interincisor gap of less than 3 to 4.5 cm correlates with difficulty achieving a line of view on direct laryngoscopy.[11] Maxillary prominence or a receding mandible also correlate with a poor laryngoscopic view. Overbite results in a reduction in the effective interincisor gap when the patient's head and neck are optimally positioned for direct laryngoscopy. A narrow or highly arched palate is another airway examination finding that is associated with a potential difficult airway.[1]

The submandibular space is the area into which the soft tissues of the pharynx must be displaced to obtain a line of vision during direct laryngoscopy. Anything that limits the submandibular space or compliance of the tissue will decrease the amount of anterior displacement that can be achieved. Micrognathia limits the pharyngeal space (tongue positioned more posterior) and the space in which the soft tissues need to be displaced. This causes the glottic structures to be anterior to the line of vision during direct laryngoscopy.

The extent of an individuals' ability to prognath the mandible is another correlate of the visualization of glottic structures on direct laryngoscopy. The upper lip bite test (ULBT) classification system is as follows (class III is associated with a difficult intubation):[11]

Class I: Lower incisors can bite above the vermilion border of the upper lip.
Class II: Lower incisors cannot reach vermilion border.
Class III: Lower incisors cannot bite upper lip.[14]

Ludwig's angina, tumors or masses, radiation scarring, burns, and previous neck surgery are conditions that can decrease submandibular compliance.[1]

### Thyromental/Sternomental Distance

A thyromental distance (mentum to thyroid cartilage) less than 6 to 7 cm correlates with a poor laryngoscopic view. This is typically seen in patients with a receding mandible or a short neck, which creates a more acute angle between the oral and pharyngeal axes and limits the ability to bring them into alignment. This distance is often estimated in fingerbreadths. Three ordinary fingerbreadths approximate this distance. If the sternomental distance is used, it should measure more than 12.5 to 13.5 cm.[9,11]

| Table 16.2 | Congenital Syndromes Associated With Difficult Endotracheal Intubation |
|---|---|
| **Syndrome** | **Description** |
| Trisomy 21 | Large tongue, small mouth make laryngoscopy difficult<br>Small subglottic diameter possible<br>Laryngospasm is common |
| Goldenhar (oculoauriculovertebral anomalies) | Mandibular hypoplasia and cervical spine abnormality make laryngoscopy difficult |
| Klippel-Feil | Neck rigidity because of cervical vertebral fusion |
| Pierre Robin | Small mouth, large tongue, mandibular anomaly |
| Treacher Collins (mandibular dysostosis) | Laryngoscopy is difficult |
| Turner | High likelihood of difficult endotracheal intubation |

**Table 16.3** Pathologic States That Influence Airway Management

| Pathologic State | Difficulty |
|---|---|
| Epiglottitis (infectious) | Laryngoscopy may worsen obstruction |
| Abscess (submandibular, retropharyngeal, Ludwig's angina) | Distortion of the airway renders face mask ventilation or endotracheal intubation extremely difficult |
| Croup, bronchitis, pneumonia | Airway irritability with a tendency for cough, laryngospasm, bronchospasm |
| Papillomatosis | Airway obstruction |
| Tetanus | Trismus renders oral endotracheal intubation impossible |
| Traumatic foreign body | Airway obstruction |
| Cervical spine injury | Neck manipulation may traumatize the spinal cord |
| Basilar skull fracture | Nasotracheal intubation attempts may result in intracranial tube placement |
| Maxillary or mandibular injury | Airway obstruction, difficult face mask ventilation and endotracheal intubation<br>Cricothyroidotomy may be necessary with combined injuries |
| Laryngeal fracture | Airway obstruction may worsen during instrumentation<br>Endotracheal tube may be misplaced outside the larynx and worsen the injury |
| Laryngeal edema (after intubation) | Irritable airway<br>Narrowed laryngeal inlet |
| Soft tissue neck injury (edema, bleeding, subcutaneous emphysema) | Anatomic distortion of the upper airway<br>Airway obstruction |
| Neoplastic upper airway tumors (pharynx, larynx) | Inspiratory obstruction with spontaneous ventilation |
| Lower airway tumors (trachea, bronchi, mediastinum) | Airway obstruction may not be relieved by endotracheal intubation<br>Lower airway is distorted |
| Radiation therapy | Fibrosis may distort the airway or make manipulation difficult |
| Inflammatory rheumatoid arthritis | Mandibular hypoplasia, temporomandibular joint arthritis, immobile cervical vertebrae, laryngeal rotation, and cricoarytenoid arthritis make endotracheal intubation difficult |
| Ankylosing spondylitis | Fusion of the cervical spine may render direct laryngoscopy impossible |
| Temporomandibular joint syndrome | Severe impairment of mouth opening |
| Scleroderma | Tight skin and temporomandibular joint involvement make mouth opening difficult |
| Sarcoidosis | Airway obstruction (lymphoid tissue) |
| Angioedema | Obstructive swelling renders ventilation and endotracheal intubation difficult |
| Endocrine or metabolic acromegaly | Large tongue<br>Bony overgrowths |
| Diabetes mellitus | May have decreased mobility of the atlanto-occipital joint |
| Hypothyroidism | Large tongue and abnormal soft tissue (myxedema) make ventilation and endotracheal intubation difficult |
| Thyromegaly | Goiter may produce extrinsic airway compression or deviation |
| Obesity | Upper airway obstruction with loss of consciousness<br>Tissue mass makes successful face mask ventilation difficult |

**Table 16.4** Components of the Preoperative Airway Physical Examination

| Airway Examination Component | Nonreassuring Findings |
| --- | --- |
| Length of upper incisors | Relatively long |
| Relationship of the maxillary and mandibular incisors during normal jaw closure | Prominent overbite (maxillary incisors anterior to the mandibular incisors) |
| Relationship of the maxillary and mandibular incisors during voluntary protrusion of the mandible | Patient cannot bring the mandibular incisors anterior to (in front of) the maxillary incisors |
| Interincisor distance | Less than 3 cm |
| Visibility of the uvula | Not visible when the tongue is protruded with the patient in a sitting position (Mallampati class higher than II) |
| Shape of the palate | Highly arched or very narrow |
| Compliance of the mandibular space | Stiff, indurated, occupied by a mass, or nonresilient |
| Thyromental distance | Less than three fingerbreadths |
| Length of the neck | Short |
| Thickness of the neck | Thick |
| Range of motion of the head and neck | Patient cannot touch the tip of the chin to the chest or cannot extend the neck |

### Atlanto-Occipital Extension/Cervical Spine Mobility

Extension of the head on the atlanto-occipital joint is important for aligning the oral and pharyngeal axes to obtain a line of vision during direct laryngoscopy (Fig. 16.7). Flexion of the lower neck, by elevating the head approximately 10 cm, aligns the laryngeal and pharyngeal axes. These maneuvers place the head in the "sniffing" position and bring the three axes into optimal alignment. Atlanto-occipital extension is quantified by the angle traversed by the occlusal surface of the maxillary teeth when the head is fully extended from the neutral position. More than 30% limitation of atlanto-occipital joint extension from a norm of 35 degrees, or less than 80 degrees of extension/flexion, is associated with an increased incidence of difficult endotracheal intubation.[15,16]

### Body Habitus/Other Examination Findings

Obesity, with a body mass index (BMI) greater than 30, is associated with an increased incidence of difficult airway management.[9,17] Proper positioning with a wedge-shaped bolster behind the patient's back results in a more optimal sniffing position. However, the problem of decreased functional residual capacity (FRC) with subsequent decreased time to arterial oxygen desaturation still persists. Other factors that are associated with difficult airway include increased neck circumference and the presence of a beard.[17,18]

### Cricothyroid Membrane

Assessing the ease of performing invasive airway procedures before airway instrumentation has been advocated and is especially important with predicted difficult

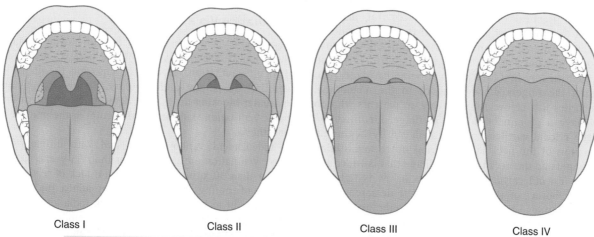

Class I    Class II    Class III    Class IV

**Fig. 16.6** Mallampati classification. (From Samsoon GLT, Young JRB. Difficult tracheal intubation: a retrospective study. *Anaesthesia.* 1987;42:487-490, used with permission.)

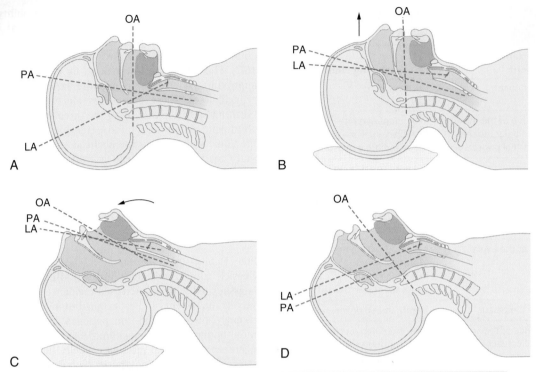

**Fig. 16.7** Schematic diagram showing alignment of the oral axis (OA), pharyngeal axis (PA), and laryngeal axis (LA) in four different head positions. Each head position is accompanied by an inset that magnifies the upper airway (the oral cavity, pharynx, and larynx) and superimposes, as a variously bent bold dotted line, the continuity of these three axes with the upper airway. (A) The head is in a neutral position with a marked degree of nonalignment of the OA, PA, and LA. (B) The head is resting on a large pad that flexes the neck on the chest and the LA with the PA. (C) The head is resting on a pad (which flexes the neck on the chest) with concomitant extension of the head on the neck, which brings all three axes into alignment (sniffing position). (D) Extension of the head on the neck without concomitant elevation of the head.

airway management.[1,19] When routine airway management techniques have failed, ventilation is not adequate, and endotracheal intubation is unsuccessful, invasive airway control through the cricothyroid membrane is indicated; therefore, correctly identifying the cricothyroid membrane can be crucial (see Fig. 16.1).[1] It can be identified by first locating the thyroid cartilage, then sliding the fingers down the neck to the membrane, which lies just below. Alternatively, in patients who do not have a prominent thyroid cartilage, identification of the cricoid cartilage can be achieved by beginning palpation of the neck at the sternal notch and sliding the fingers up the neck until a cartilage that is wider and higher (cricoid cartilage) than those below is felt. The superior border of the cricoid cartilage demarcates the inferior border of the cricothyroid membrane. Predictors of difficulty identifying the cricothyroid membrane include female sex, age less than 8 years, presence of large neck circumference, a displaced airway, and overlying neck malformation.[18]

## AIRWAY MANAGEMENT TECHNIQUES

### Ventilation Via a Face Mask

Ventilation via a face mask is a vital airway management tool. Prospectively identifying patients at risk for difficult ventilation via a mask, ensuring the ability to ventilate the patient's lungs before administering neuromuscular blocking drugs, and developing proficient face mask ventilation skills are fundamental to the practice of anesthesia.

Independent variables associated with difficult face mask ventilation are (1) age older than 55 years, (2) BMI higher than 30 kg/m$^2$, (3) a beard, (4) lack of teeth, (5) a history of snoring or obstructive sleep apnea, (6) Mallampati class III to IV, (7) history of neck radiation, (8) male sex, (9) limited ability to protrude the mandible, and (10) history of an airway mass or tumor.[19,20] In addition, difficult ventilation via mask can develop after multiple laryngoscopy attempts. The incidence of difficult face mask

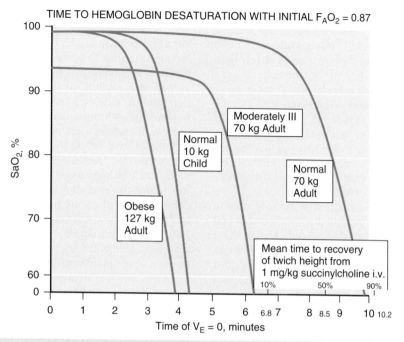

TIME TO HEMOGLOBIN DESATURATION WITH INITIAL $F_AO_2 = 0.87$

**Fig. 16.8** The oxygen saturation ($SaO_2$) versus time of apnea of various types of patients. The time to reach an oxygen saturation of 80% was 8.7 minutes in a healthy 70-kg adult, but was 3.1 minutes in an obese patient. $F_AO_2$, alveolar fraction of oxygen; $V_E$, minute ventilation. (From Benumof JL, Dagg R, Benumof R. Critical hemoglobin desaturation will occur before return to an unparalyzed state following 1 mg/kg intravenous succinylcholine. *Anesthesiology.* 1997;87(4):979-982.)

ventilation ranges from 0.9% to 7.8%[18,20] and may be due to one or more of the following problems: inadequate mask or supraglottic airway seal, excessive gas leak, or excessive resistance to the ingress or egress of gas.[1] Severe adverse outcomes related to difficult ventilation via a mask include inability to oxygenate, ventilate, prevent aspiration of gastric contents, or a combination of these factors, which can result in hypoxic brain damage or death.[2,20]

### Face Mask Characteristics

Face masks are available in a variety of sizes. A properly sized face mask should have the top of mask fit over the bridge of the nose, with the upper border aligned with the pupils and the bottom of the mask should sit between the lower lip and the chin. Most face masks come with a hooked rim around the 15- to 22-mm fitting that attaches to the anesthesia breathing circuit. This rim allows straps to be used to hold the face mask in place when a patient is breathing spontaneously or to improve the seal during face mask ventilation.

Prior to induction of anesthesia, breathing 100% $O_2$ allows for a longer duration of apnea without desaturation by increasing oxygen reserves (denitrogenation). A healthy adult, who is not obese, can be apneic for approximately 9 minutes before significant desaturation occurs. This time is primarily dependent on oxygen consumption and the FRC. Obesity, pregnancy, and other conditions

that significantly decrease FRC or factors that increase oxygen consumption decrease the time to desaturation (Fig. 16.8)[21] (also see Chapters 29 and 33).

Several techniques of preoxygenation exist with the goal of achieving an end-tidal oxygen level above 90%. Three minutes of tidal volume breathing of 100% $O_2$ is superior to four deep breaths in 30 seconds. Eight deep breaths in 60 seconds are equivalent to breathing 100% oxygen for 3 minutes.[22] Preoxygenation in a 25-degree head-up position in obese patients can increase the time to desaturation by decreasing atelectasis and improving ventilation/perfusion matching.[22,23] In addition, preoxygenation with noninvasive positive-pressure ventilation followed by a recruitment maneuver immediately after endotracheal intubation in obese patients can preserve lung volumes and oxygenation better than preoxygenation alone[24] (also see Chapter 29).

After induction of anesthesia, the face mask should be held to the patient's face with the fingers of the anesthesia provider's left hand lifting the mandible (chin lift, jaw thrust) to the face mask. Pressure on the submandibular soft tissue should be avoided because it can cause airway obstruction. The anesthesia provider's left thumb and index finger apply counterpressure on the face mask. Anterior pressure on the angle of the mandible (jaw thrust), atlanto-occipital joint extension, and chin lift combine to maximize the pharyngeal space. Differential application of pressure with individual fingers can improve the seal attained with the face mask. The anesthesia provider's right hand is used to generate positive pressure by squeezing the reservoir bag of the anesthesia breathing circuit. Ventilating pressure should be less than 20 cm $H_2O$ to avoid insufflation of the stomach.

### Managing Inadequate Ventilation Via a Mask

Signs of inadequate mask ventilation include absent or minimal chest rise, absent or inadequate breath sounds, cyanosis, gastric air entry, decreasing or inadequate oxygen saturation, absent or inadequate exhaled carbon dioxide, and hemodynamic changes associated with hypoxemia or hypercarbia, or both.[1]

Inadequate face mask ventilation is usually due to decreased compliance and increased resistance. An oral or nasal airway may help to generate sufficient positive pressure for adequate ventilation with the anesthesia breathing circuit. Oral and nasal airways are designed to create an air passage by displacing the tongue from the posterior pharyngeal wall. Aligning the airway device with the patient's profile and approximating the anatomic path that it will take can be used to estimate the appropriate size. The distal tip of the oral and nasal airway should be at the angle of the mandible when the proximal end is aligned with the mouth or the nose, respectively. An oral airway may generate a gag reflex or cause laryngospasm in an awake or lightly anesthetized patient. Nasal airways are better tolerated during lighter levels of anesthesia, but are relatively contraindicated in patients who have coagulation or platelet abnormalities, are pregnant, or have basilar skull fractures.

Presence of a beard or lack of teeth may result in inadequate seal between the patient's face and the mask making it difficult to deliver positive pressure. If the patient is amenable, shaving or trimming a beard can improve face mask seal. If a patient's dentures are well adhered, allowing them to be left in place or use of an oral airway can improve face mask seal in edentulous patients.

If oral and nasal airways do not optimize ventilation with a face mask, a two-handed face mask technique should be utilized. The anesthesia provider uses the right hand to mirror the hand position of the left to improve face mask seal and jaw thrust. A second person can assist by ventilating the patient with the reservoir bag. In spite of corrective measures, if difficult or impossible face mask ventilation continues, intubation or placement of a supraglottic airway should be attempted.[1]

## SUPRAGLOTTIC AIRWAY DEVICES

Supraglottic airway devices have become invaluable for routine and difficult airway management. For elective airway management, advantages over endotracheal intubation include the following: placement quickly and without the use of laryngoscope, less hemodynamic changes

with insertion and removal, less coughing and bucking with removal, no need for muscle relaxants, preserved laryngeal competence and mucociliary function, and less laryngeal trauma.[25] In the difficult airway scenario, they can be a lifesaving tool for oxygenation and ventilation as well as a conduit for intubation. Many of the factors that result in difficult mask ventilation and intubation do not overlap with those that influence supraglottic airway success. Therefore, when other oxygenation or ventilation techniques have failed, a supraglottic airway device may still succeed.[26] Difficult supraglottic airway placement or failure has been associated with small mouth opening, supra- or extraglottic disease, fixed cervical spine deformity, use of cricoid pressure, poor dentition or large incisors, male sex, surgical table rotation, and increased BMI.[18,27] The incidence of difficult supraglottic airway placement, indicated by inability of an anesthesiologist to provide adequate ventilation is 1.1%.[27]

Some contraindications for using supraglottic airway devices are as follows: patients at risk for regurgitation of gastric contents, nonsupine position, obesity, pregnant patients, long surgical time, and intraabdominal or airway procedures.[25] Although there have been numerous studies of patients in these categories in which supraglottic airways have been successfully used, one must consider the risk versus benefit of use in these situations. After placement of a supraglottic airway device, it is important to confirm correct positioning by observing end-tidal $CO_2$ and auscultation of breath sounds.

Reported complications of laryngeal mask airway (LMA) use in difficult airway patients include bronchospasm, postoperative swallowing difficulties, respiratory obstruction, laryngeal nerve injury, edema, and hypoglossal nerve paralysis.[1] Aspiration remains a concern with supraglottic airway placement and its risk increases with gastric inflation, high airway pressures, and poor supraglottic airway positioning over the glottis.[8] There are many different types of supraglottic airway devices in single-use and reusable forms, including intubating supraglottic airways and supraglottic airways allowing gastric decompression. Supraglottic airway devices are sized according to the patient's weight, and sizes vary by manufacturer. Selected devices are detailed next.

### Laryngeal Mask Airway

#### LMA Classic and Unique

The original LMA, the LMA Classic, is reusable, and the LMA Unique is the comparable single-use device. These LMAs consist of a flexible shaft connected to a silicone rubber mask (Classic) or polyvinylchloride (Unique) that seals with the airway in the hypopharynx (Fig. 16.9). The distal tip of the cuff should be against the upper esophageal sphincter (cricopharyngeus muscle), the lateral edges rest in the piriform sinuses, and the proximal end seats under the base of the tongue. Before placement, the cuff should be deflated, the device should be lubricated, and the head should be positioned in the sniffing position. These LMAs are designed to be inserted by holding the shaft between the index finger and thumb with the tip of the index finger at the junction of the mask and the tube. Upward pressure against the hard palate is applied as they are advanced toward the larynx until resistance is felt. Intubation through these devices can be facilitated by use of an intubation catheter and a fiberoptic bronchoscope (see later section regarding Aintree Intubation Catheter [AIC]). The LMA Classic and LMA Unique are available in sizes for infant, pediatric, and adult patients.

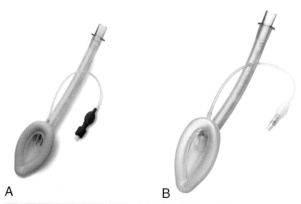

**Fig. 16.9** (A) The reusable laryngeal mask airway (LMA). (B) Classic and single-use LMA Unique. (Images courtesy of Teleflex, Morrisville, NC, modified with permission.)

### LMA Fastrach

The LMA Fastrach (intubating LMA, ILMA) was designed to obviate the problems encountered when attempting to blindly intubate the trachea through the LMA Classic. The ILMA is used with a specialized endotracheal tube that exits the laryngeal mask at a different angle than a standard endotracheal tube and results in better alignment with the airway. It is also available in a single-use version.

### LMA ProSeal/LMA Supreme

The reusable LMA ProSeal and single-use LMA Supreme are modifications of the LMA Classic (Fig. 16.10). Their cuffs are modified to extend onto the posterior surface of the mask, which results in an improved airway seal without increasing mucosal pressure. This allows for ventilation with higher airway pressures. They both contain a second lumen that opens at the distal tip of the mask to act as an esophageal vent to keep gases and fluid separate from the airway and facilitate placement of an orogastric tube. This is designed to decrease the risk of regurgitation and aspiration of gastric contents. In addition, placement of an orogastric tube can help confirm proper placement of these devices. The LMA ProSeal and Supreme also have built in bite blocks to decrease the chance of obstruction of the airway tube. The LMA Supreme may be more rapid and easier to insert, has lower cuff pressures, and has higher oropharyngeal leakage pressures when compared to the LMA Classic in patients undergoing surgery.[28] However, when there is difficulty with ventilation, the LMA Classic remains the "gold standard" supraglottic airway device.[26] Intubation through these devices can be achieved

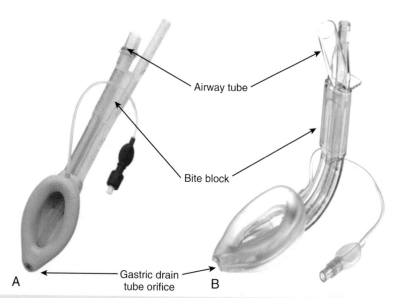

Airway tube

Bite block

Gastric drain tube orifice

**Fig. 16.10** (A) The reusable laryngeal mask airway (LMA) ProSeal. (B) The single-use LMA Supreme. These modifications of the LMA Classic have a gastric drain, built-in bite block, and modified cuffs for improved airway seals. (Images courtesy of Teleflex, Morrisville, NC, modified with permission.)

by using an intubation catheter and a fiberoptic broncho-scope. Both are available in pediatric and adult sizes.

### LMA Flexible

The LMA Flexible has a wire-reinforced, flexible airway tube that allows it to be positioned away from the surgical field while minimizing loss of seal. This can be useful for procedures involving the head and neck. Insertion of the LMA Flexible is more difficult than the LMA Classic.[25] Using a stylet or introducer may help with insertion of this device. It is available as a reusable or single-use device in adult and pediatric sizes.

## Air-Q Masked Laryngeal Airways

The Air-Q is a device that can be utilized either as a primary airway or as an intermediary channel for intubation of the trachea. It has an elliptical, inflatable, cuffed mask and a slightly curved airway tube with a detachable connector. Several features serve to aid intubation: a short shaft, no aperture bars within the mask, a detachable connector so that the wide lumen of the shaft can be used for intubation, and a distal airway tube shaped to direct an endotracheal tube toward the larynx.[25] When used as a conduit for intubation, each size of the Air-Q laryngeal mask has a corresponding maximum cuffed endotracheal tube size. After an endotracheal tube is placed, removal of the Air-Q device is aided by a removal stylet. The Air-Q is available in infant, pediatric, and adult sizes as a reusable or single-use airway device. The largest size can be used with up to an 8.5 mm standard endotracheal tube (Fig. 16.11).

## I-Gel

The I-Gel is a single-use supraglottic airway device composed of a soft, gel-like, noninflatable cuff. It has a widened, flattened stem with a rigid bite block that acts as a buccal stabilizer to reduce rotation and malpositioning, and a port for gastric tube insertion. It can be a primary airway, but also has a wide bore airway channel that can be used as a conduit for intubation with fiberoptic guidance.[29,30] This supraglottic airway device comes in infant, pediatric, and adult sizes. Adult sizes can accommodate endotracheal tube sizes 6.0 to 8.0 mm.

## Esophageal Tracheal Combitube and King Laryngeal Tube

The esophageal tracheal combitube (Combitube) and the King Laryngeal Tube (King LT) are primarily used for emergent airway control in prehospital settings when endotracheal intubation is not possible or feasible. The Combitube is an esophageal and tracheal double-lumen airway, whereas the King LT has a single lumen with a large proximal pharyngeal cuff and a distal esophageal cuff. The blind insertion techniques for these devices require minimal training and no movement of the head or neck. The Combitube is available in adult sizes, and the King LT is available in both pediatric and adult sizes.

A Combitube should be replaced after 8 hours of use owing to pressure the tube exerts on the pharyngeal mucosa. It can be replaced by deflating the oropharyngeal balloon and placing an endotracheal tube anterior or lateral to the Combitube.[31]

## ENDOTRACHEAL INTUBATION

Endotracheal intubation may be considered in every patient receiving general anesthesia (Box 16.1). Orotracheal intubation by direct laryngoscopy in anesthetized patients is routinely chosen unless specific circumstances or the patient's history and physical examination dictate a different approach. Equipment and drugs used for endotracheal intubation include a properly sized endotracheal tube, laryngoscope, functioning suction catheter, appropriate anesthetic drugs, and equipment for providing positive-pressure ventilation of the lungs with oxygen.

Proper positioning is crucial to successful direct laryngoscopy when alignment of the oral, pharyngeal, and laryngeal axes is necessary for creating a line of vision from the lips to the glottic opening. Elevation of the patient's head 8 to 10 cm with pads under the occiput (shoulders remaining on the table) and extension of the head at the atlanto-occipital joint serve to align these

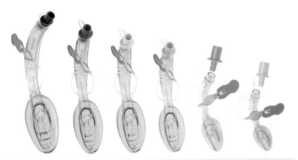

**Fig. 16.11** Air-Q disposable supraglottic airways in adult and pediatric sizes. The removable color-coded connector allows for intubation with a standard endotracheal tube. (Image courtesy of Cookgas, St. Louis, MO.)

> **Box 16.1** Indications for Endotracheal Intubation
>
> - Provide a patent airway
> - Prevent inhalation (aspiration) of gastric contents
> - Need for frequent suctioning
> - Facilitate positive-pressure ventilation of the lungs
> - Operative position other than supine
> - Operative site near or involving the upper airway
> - Airway maintenance by mask difficult

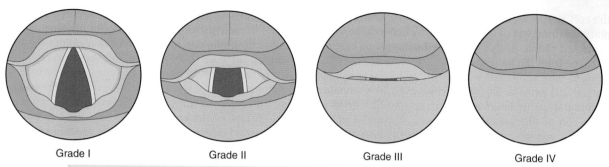

Grade I          Grade II          Grade III          Grade IV

**Fig. 16.12** Four grades of laryngoscopic view. Grade I is visualization of the entire laryngeal aperture, grade II is visualization of just the posterior portion of the laryngeal aperture, grade III is visualization of only the epiglottis, and grade IV is visualization of just the soft palate. (From Cormack RS, Lehane J. Difficult tracheal intubation in obstetrics. *Anaesthesia*. 1984;39(11):1105-1111.)

axes. The height of the operating table should be adjusted so that the patient's face is near the level of the standing anesthesia provider's xiphoid cartilage.

The laryngoscopic view obtained is classified according to the Cormack and Lehane score. Grade III or IV views are associated with difficult intubation (Fig. 16.12).[32]

Grade I: Most of the glottis is visible.

Grade II: Only the posterior portion of the glottis is visible.

Grade III: The epiglottis, but no part of the glottis, can be seen.

Grade IV: No airway structures are visualized.

## Difficult Airway Management

Difficult laryngoscopy is defined as the inability to visualize any portion of the vocal cords after multiple attempts at direct laryngoscopy. Difficult endotracheal intubation is defined as endotracheal intubation requiring multiple attempts. These occur in about 0.8% to 7.0% of patients in the operating room setting.[9,19] Failed intubation of the trachea occurs in about 1 in 2000 patients in an elective setting.[2,33]

The information obtained through a comprehensive airway assessment should allow development of a plan to manage the patient's airway. Airway devices have different advantages that make them beneficial in specific situations. Options include direct laryngoscopy, use of alternative airway devices such as video laryngoscopes and endotracheal tube guides, special techniques like awake or asleep fiberoptic endotracheal intubation, or rescue invasive techniques. In patients with anticipated or history of a difficult airway, the following management principles should be considered: (1) awake endotracheal intubation versus intubation after induction of general anesthesia, (2) initial intubation method via noninvasive versus invasive techniques, (3) video laryngoscopy as an initial approach to intubation, and (4) maintaining versus ablating spontaneous ventilation.[1] A patient's ability to

cooperate with airway management should be considered when making an initial plan and a difficult airway cart should be immediately available for management of back-up plans. Intubation attempts should be minimized, and repeat laryngoscopy should only occur when a different tactic is used.[19] The ASA difficult airway algorithm details approaches to alternative strategies of airway management once there is failure of a primary plan (see Fig. 16.1).[1]

## Direct Laryngoscopy

The laryngoscope is traditionally held in the anesthesia provider's left hand near the junction between the handle and blade of the laryngoscope. If not opened by extension of the head, the patient's mouth may be manually opened by counterpressure of the right thumb on the mandibular teeth and right index finger on the maxillary teeth ("scissoring"). Simultaneously with insertion of the laryngoscope blade, the patient's lower lip can be rolled away with the anesthesia provider's left index finger to prevent bruising by the laryngoscope blade. The blade is then inserted on the right side of the patient's mouth so that the incisor teeth are avoided and the tongue is deflected to the left. Pressure on the teeth or gums must be avoided as the blade is advanced forward and centrally toward the epiglottis. The anesthesia provider's wrist is held rigid as the laryngoscope is lifted along the axis of the handle to cause anterior displacement of the soft tissues and bring the laryngeal structures into view. The handle should not be rotated as it is lifted to prevent damaging the patient's upper teeth or gums. Manipulation of the patient's thyroid cartilage externally on the neck, commonly using backward upward rightward pressure (BURP), may facilitate exposure of the glottic opening.[19]

The endotracheal tube is held in the anesthesia provider's right hand like a pencil and introduced into the right side of the patient's mouth with the natural curve directed anteriorly. The endotracheal tube should be advanced toward the glottis from the right side of the mouth as midline insertion usually obscures visualization of the glottic opening. The tube is advanced until the proximal end of the cuff is 1 to 2 cm past the vocal cords, which should place the distal end of the tube midway between the vocal cords and carina. At this point, the laryngoscope blade is removed from the patient's mouth. The cuff of the endotracheal tube is inflated with air to create a seal against the tracheal mucosa. This seal facilitates positive-pressure ventilation of the lungs and decreases the likelihood of aspiration of pharyngeal or gastric contents. Use of the minimum volume of air in a low-pressure, high-volume cuff that prevents leaks during positive ventilation pressure (20 to 30 cm $H_2O$) minimizes the likelihood of mucosal ischemia resulting from prolonged pressure on the tracheal wall. After confirmation of correct placement (end-tidal $CO_2$, auscultation for bilateral breath sounds, ballottement of cuff in the suprasternal notch), the endotracheal tube is secured in position with tape. The success rate of endotracheal intubation using direct laryngoscopy in patients without a predicted difficult intubation is more frequent than 90%, and in patients with predicted difficult intubation is 84%.[34,35]

## Choice of Direct Laryngoscope Blade

The advantages of the curved blade, such as a Macintosh blade, include less trauma to teeth, more room for passage of the endotracheal tube, larger flange size that improves the ability to sweep the tongue, and less bruising of the epiglottis because the tip of the blade does not directly lift this structure. The advantages of the straight blade such as a Miller blade, are better exposure of the glottic opening and a smaller profile, which can be beneficial in patients with a smaller mouth opening.

The tip of the curved blade is advanced into the space between the base of the tongue and the pharyngeal surface of the epiglottis into the vallecula, which elevates the epiglottis and exposes the glottic opening (Fig. 16.13A). The tip of the straight blade is passed beneath the laryngeal surface of the epiglottis (see Fig. 16.13B). Forward and upward movement of the blade exerted along the axis of the laryngoscope handle directly elevates the epiglottis to expose the glottic opening.

Laryngoscope blades are numbered according to their length. A Macintosh 3 and Miller 2 are the standard intubating blades for adult patients. The Macintosh 4 and Miller 3 blades can be used for larger adult patients (Fig. 16.14).

## Video Laryngoscopes

Video laryngoscopes can help obtain a view of the larynx by providing indirect visualization of the glottic opening without alignment of the oral, pharyngeal, and tracheal axes and enable endotracheal intubation in patients who have conditions (limited mouth opening, inability to flex the neck) that can make traditional laryngoscopy difficult or impossible. Their ease of use is an advantage over fiberoptic bronchoscopy in these patients. They consist of a handle, light source, and a blade with a video camera at the distal end to enable the glottis to be visualized indirectly on a video monitor. Video laryngoscopes are classified as nonchanneled or channeled.

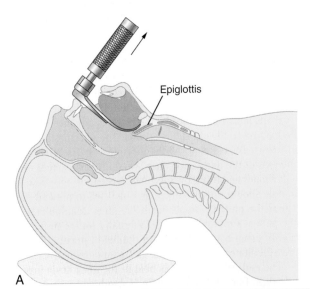
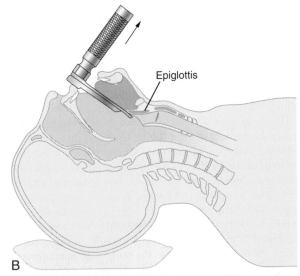

**Fig. 16.13** Schematic diagram depicting the proper position of the laryngoscope blade for exposure of the glottic opening. (A) The distal end of the curved blade is advanced into the space between the base of the tongue and the pharyngeal surface of the epiglottis. (B) The distal end of the straight blade is advanced beneath the laryngeal surface of the epiglottis. Regardless of blade design, forward and upward movement exerted along the axis of the laryngoscope handle, as denoted by the arrows, serves to elevate the epiglottis and expose the glottic opening.

Nonchanneled blades are Macintosh-style curved blades, Miller-style straight blades, and angulated blades.[18] Types of nonchanneled blades include Glide-Scope, C-MAC, and McGrath.

The Macintosh-style or Miller-style blades can be used for direct laryngoscopy or by viewing the monitor. These blades are inserted using the standard direct laryngoscopy techniques with or without a stylet in the endotracheal tube. The view obtained by looking at the monitor usually offers a slightly improved view compared to looking directly in the patient's mouth because the camera is more distally located and provides a wider visual field.[36] The advantage of these blades is user familiarity with the blade type and a display that can be used for instructional purposes.[36]

The angulated blades allow for a more anteriorly oriented view that can be obtained with minimal flexion or extension of the patient's head and neck.[37] The tip of the laryngoscope blade may be placed in the vallecula or be used to lift the epiglottis directly. These blades usually require a preshaped stylet that matches the curvature of the blade and are usually inserted midline in the mouth, unlike the Macintosh-style blades. An endotracheal tube with the preshaped stylet is advanced using direct visualization in the pharynx until it can be seen on the monitor, after which the tube is advanced into the trachea close to the blade, based on the image on the monitoring screen. Tonsillar and pharyngeal injuries can occur when using video laryngoscopy, especially with rigid stylets when the stylet is advanced through the oropharynx looking at the video screen and not under direct visualization.[38] A limitation of these devices is difficulty directing the endotracheal tube into the glottis despite good glottic visualization. This usually occurs when the laryngoscope is inserted too deeply.[36] Withdrawing the blade slightly, although often giving a poorer laryngoscopic

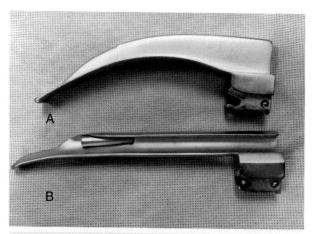

**Fig. 16.14** Examples of detachable laryngoscope blades that can be used interchangeably on the same handle. The Macintosh (A) is a curved blade, and the Miller (B) is a straight blade.

view, can improve the ability to direct the endotracheal tube through the glottic opening.

Channeled devices include the Airtraq and the King Vision Video Laryngoscope. These video laryngoscopes have a guide channel that directs an endotracheal tube toward the glottic opening via blades that are more angulated than traditional Macintosh blades.[36] The endotracheal tube is preloaded into the guide channel and the video laryngoscope is inserted midline in the mouth until the epiglottis is visualized. The blade is advanced into the vallecula or the epiglottis may be directly elevated by the tip of the blade until the cords are visualized. The glottis needs to optimally align on the screen for successful intubation via the channel. Channeled blades tend to have thicker blades than nonchanneled blades requiring a greater interincisor distance.

These techniques can be hindered if upper airway secretions obscure the optics. Video laryngoscopes can also be used on awake patients with topical application of local anesthetic to the airway and are as easy to perform with comparable patient discomfort as fiberoptic intubation.[39] Selected video laryngoscopes are detailed as follows.

### GlideScope

The GlideScope has two main blade types: an angulated style blade and a Macintosh-style blade. The reusable blades are made of either titanium or medical-grade plastic (AVL, GVL, and Ranger). The titanium blade offers the advantage of being thinner and hence a lower profile (allowing for insertion with a smaller interincisor distance). The angulated blade is anatomically shaped with a fixed (60-degree) angle and should be used with the GlideRite rigid stylet as this stylet matches the shape of the blade. The blades have a fog-resistant video camera embedded in the undersurface that transmits the digital image to a high-resolution color monitor that can be mounted on a pole. A portable (Ranger) device is also available. There are a variety of different pediatric and adult sizes in reusable and single-use blades (Fig. 16.15).

The GlideScope is associated with improved glottic visualization, especially in patients with potential difficult airways.[34] One study showed the overall success rate with the GlideScope to be 96% in patients with predicted difficult airways and 94% when used as a rescue device for failed direct laryngoscopy.[38] The high success rate of both direct laryngoscopy and video laryngoscopy in patients without a difficult airway emphasizes the advantage of the GlideScope for use in patients with clinical features suggestive of difficult intubation or as a rescue method after failed direct laryngoscopy.[34] Predictors that have been associated with difficult GlideScope use include abnormal neck anatomy, Cormack and Lehane grade 3 or 4 view on direct laryngoscopy, limited mandibular protrusion, and limited cervical spine mobility.[18,38]

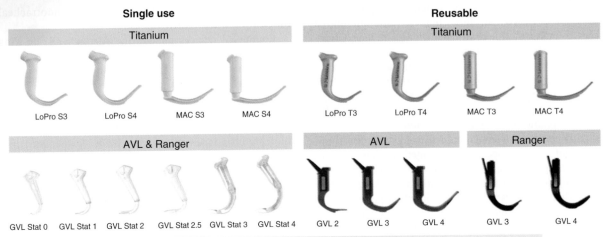

Single use — Titanium

LoPro S3    LoPro S4    MAC S3    MAC S4

Reusable — Titanium

LoPro T3    LoPro T4    MAC T3    MAC T4

AVL & Ranger

GVL Stat 0    GVL Stat 1    GVL Stat 2    GVL Stat 2.5    GVL Stat 3    GVL Stat 4

AVL

GVL 2    GVL 3    GVL 4

Ranger

GVL 3    GVL 4

Fig. 16.15 Comparison of the single-use and reusable GlideScope blades in different sizes and styles. (Image courtesy of Verathon, Bothell, WA.)

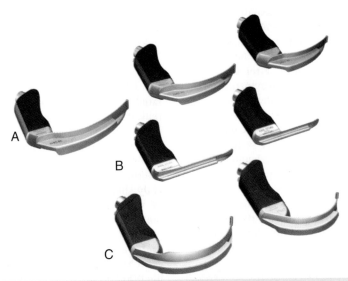

Fig. 16.16 Comparison of the different C-MAC blade types. (A) Macintosh style blade, (B) Miller style blade, and (C) D-blade. (Images courtesy of KARL STORZ Endoscopy, El Segundo, CA.)

## C-MAC

The C-MAC (KARL STORZ Endoscopy) has a stainless steel blade with a camera located on the distal end of the blade that displays on a high definition monitor. The interface between the laryngoscope blade and the monitor allows for easy interchange of different blades. The reusable blades come in several sizes and styles including Miller (sizes 0 and 1), Macintosh (sizes 2, 3, and 4), and an angulated D-blade (in pediatric and adult) for difficult airways (Fig.16.16). The D-blade and the Macintosh size 3 and 4 blades have a lateral guide for an oxygen or suction catheter. The C-MAC is also available in a single-use D-blade and Mac 3 or 4 blade. In difficult airway situations, using the D-Blade improves glottic view and has intubation success rates similar to the GlideScope when compared with direct laryngoscopy.[30,40]

## McGrath Scope

The McGrath video laryngoscope is a portable device that consists of an adjustable Macintosh style or angulated (McGrath series 5 or X-blade) single-use polycarbonate blade. The blades are attached to a battery-containing handle mounted with a color display monitor that can rotate and swivel to optimize the angle of visualization. The McGrath video laryngoscope comes in pediatric and adult sizes.

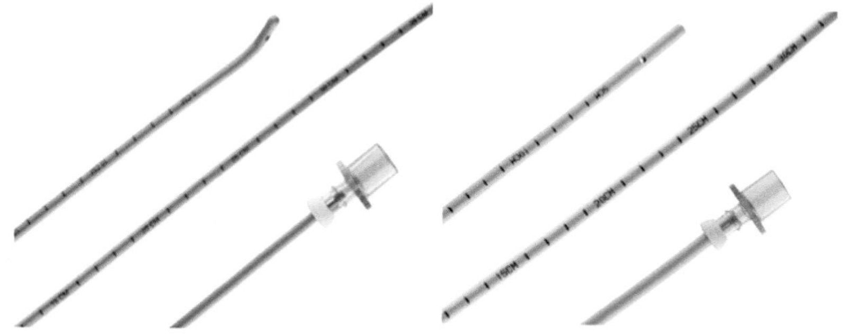

**Fig. 16.17** (A) Frova Intubating Introducer. (B) Aintree intubation catheter. (Images courtesy of Cook Medical, Bloomington, IN.)

### Channeled Scopes: Airtraq and King Vision Scope

The Airtraq is a single-use optical device that creates an image through prisms and mirrors to give a magnified angular view of the glottis. The device has two channels, one for viewing and the other for guiding, supporting, and directing the endotracheal tube toward the glottic opening.[30] Images are displayed on an adjusted screen by a camera. It comes in two models, the Avant with reusable optics and the entirely single-use SP model. The SP model comes in many sizes for infants, pediatric patients, nasotracheal intubations, and double-lumen tubes.

The King Vision Video Laryngoscope is fully portable with a reusable digital display and single-use channeled or nonchanneled blades.

## Endotracheal Tube Stylets, Introducers, and Airway Exchange Catheters

A variety of endotracheal tube stylets, introducers, and airway exchange catheters (AECs) may be used in selected patients to facilitate difficult endotracheal intubation, endotracheal tube exchange, and supraglottic airway exchange for an endotracheal tube. In addition, AECs can provide an airway conduit to assist with reintubation. Some of the devices have a hollow lumen and connectors to allow jet ventilation. Ventilation through the lumen should be used only in emergency situations because of the high risk of complications. When using intubating stylets in a patient with a difficult airway, intubation is successful in 78% to 100% of patients.[1] Complications of intubating stylets include bleeding, oropharyngeal trauma, tracheal trauma, and sore throat. Complications of endotracheal tube exchangers include tracheal/bronchial laceration and gastric perforation.[1]

### Stylet

Stylets are made from plastic coated, malleable metal that is used to stiffen and provide curvature to an endotracheal tube. After stylet placement through the lumen of an endotracheal tube, the tube can be bent into the desired shape, such as a curve matching a Macintosh blade or a "hockey stick" shape. Although stylets are not necessary with direct laryngoscopy, they can often help facilitate manipulation of the endotracheal tube in the airway. The tip of the stylet should not protrude past the end of the endotracheal tube. When an endotracheal tube is passed through the vocal cords, the stylet should be removed as the tube is advanced into the trachea to avoid trauma.

### Gum Elastic Bougie

A gum elastic bougie is a solid 60-cm long, 15-F stylet with a 40-degree curve approximately 3.5 cm from the distal tip. It is used to facilitate intubation in patients with a poor laryngoscopic view. It is passed under the epiglottis and into the airway. A characteristic bumping or clicking is felt in most tracheal placements as the bougie is advanced down the tracheal cartilages, but not felt in all esophageal placements. An endotracheal tube is then advanced over the bougie and into the airway.

### Frova Intubating Introducer

The Frova Intubating Introducer is available in a pediatric 35-cm long, 8-F, or an adult 65-cm long, 14-F stylet with a distal angulated tip and an internal channel to accommodate a stiffening rod or allow jet ventilation. The pediatric introducer can be used with endotracheal tubes 3.0 mm and wider and the adult introducer with endotracheal tubes 6.0 mm and wider. The Frova Intubating Introducer is inserted in a similar manner to the gum elastic bougie for patients with poor laryngoscopic views (Fig. 16.17A).

### Aintree Intubation Catheter

The AIC (Cook Medical) is 56-cm long, 19-F diameter and has a large, 4.7-mm lumen. It comes with two Rapi-Fit adapters. One is for jet ventilation, and the other for connection to an anesthesia circuit or Ambu bag. It can also be used to exchange supraglottic airways for endotracheal tubes size 7.0 mm or wider.[30]

For exchange of a supraglottic airway, the AIC is threaded onto a fiberoptic bronchoscope. The distal end of the fiberoptic bronchoscope is not covered by the AIC to allow for manipulation. The AIC and fiberoptic bronchoscope are then placed in the lumen of the supraglottic airway and advanced as a unit through the vocal cords into the trachea. The fiberoptic bronchoscope is then removed while the AIC remains in the trachea. The supraglottic airway is removed over the AIC and an endotracheal tube is then placed over the AIC into the trachea. Finally, the AIC is removed (Fig. 16.17B).

### Cook Airway Exchange Catheter

Cook AECs are available in pediatric and adult sizes (45- and 83-cm length and 8-, 11-, 14-, or 19-F) as well as an extra-firm soft tip version that is 100-cm long and 11- or 14 -F, for double-lumen tube exchange. They are designed for exchange of endotracheal tubes. They can also be used in the trachea after endotracheal tube removal to help with reintubation if necessary in patients with difficult airways. These catheters are hollow and can allow for jet ventilation or oxygenation through an anesthesia circuit or Ambu bag using Rapi-Fit adapters in emergency situations.[41] For orotracheal intubation, AEC insertion of 20 to 22 cm depth, and for nasotracheal intubation of 27 to 30 cm depth is sufficient for tube exchange and can help avoid complications. If placed deeper, there is risk of bronchial perforation or pneumothorax. To help with placement of an endotracheal tube over an AEC, laryngoscopy can displace tissues. Using a smaller endotracheal tube may also facilitate the use of AECs.

## Flexible Fiberoptic Endotracheal Intubation

Fiberoptic intubation was one of the first techniques introduced for difficult airway management and revolutionized the anesthesia provider's ability to safely care for these patients. Fiberoptic intubation can be performed through the nose and mouth in awake, sedated, or anesthetized patients. The decision to perform fiberoptic endotracheal intubation in an awake versus an anesthetized patient is dependent on the risk of a difficult airway and the cooperation of a patient. Fiberoptic endotracheal intubation may be advantageous in patients with unstable cervical spines. The technique does not require movement of the patient's neck and can be performed before induction of general anesthesia, thereby allowing for evaluation of the patient's neurologic function after endotracheal intubation and surgical positioning.

Patients who have sustained an injury to the upper airway from either blunt or penetrating trauma are at risk for the endotracheal tube creating a false passage by exiting the airway through the disrupted tissue during direct laryngoscopy. By performing a fiberoptic intubation, not only can the injury be assessed, but the endotracheal tube can also be placed beyond the level of the injury, thus minimizing the risk of subcutaneous emphysema.

A disadvantage of fiberoptic endotracheal intubation is that it requires time to set up and prepare the patient's airway. Another disadvantage is the fiberoptic bronchoscope needs space to pass through. Anything that impinges on upper airway size (edema of the pharynx or tongue, infection, hematoma, infiltrating masses) will make fiberoptic intubation more difficult. Inflating the cuff of the endotracheal tube to hold the pharyngeal walls open may be helpful. Blood and secretions can easily obscure the optics of a fiberoptic bronchoscope making it more challenging. Administering an antisialagogue before initiating fiberoptic intubation and suctioning can minimize view obstruction. A relative contraindication to fiberoptic intubation is the presence of a pharyngeal abscess, which could be disrupted as the endotracheal tube is advanced and result in aspiration of purulent material.

## Awake Fiberoptic Endotracheal Intubation

Awake fiberoptic intubation is commonly performed because of examination findings consistent with, or history of, a difficult airway, unstable cervical spine, or airway injury. Performing intubation before induction of anesthesia allows for continuation of spontaneous breathing, preservation of muscle tone, preservation of airway reflexes, and assessment of neurologic function after intubation. This is especially important in patients who are at risk for difficult mask ventilation or high aspiration risk. Patient cooperation is critical to this technique.

Awake fiberoptic intubation can be performed through the nose or mouth. In general, the nasal route is easier because the angle of curvature of the endotracheal tube naturally approximates that of the patient's upper airway. The risk of inducing bleeding is more frequent when the nasal route is used and therefore relatively contraindicated in patients at risk for bleeding, such as those with platelet abnormalities or coagulation disorders.

### Patient Preparation

The procedure should be fully explained to the patient. An antisialagogue (glycopyrrolate 0.2-0.4 mg intravenous [IV]) is recommended to inhibit the formation of secretions. The patient should be carefully sedated and monitored throughout the intubation of the trachea. There are many options for sedation, but the more difficult the airway, the less sedation should be used.

### Airway Anesthesia

Airway anesthesia is then completed by topical application of local anesthetic, or by specific nerve blocks. Topical application is effective and less invasive than nerve blocks and is usually the preferred method. It can be achieved by spraying (atomizing or nebulizing) or direct application (ointment, gels, or gargling solutions). Several commercial devices are available to assist with topical application of local anesthetic. The larger particle size of a spray tends to cause it to be deposited in the pharynx, with only a small proportion reaching the trachea. Conversely, the small particle size of a nebulized spray is carried more effectively into the trachea, but also into the smaller airways, where the anesthetic is not needed and undergoes more rapid systemic absorption. Lidocaine is the preferred topical local anesthetic because of its broad therapeutic window. Usually 1% and 2% solutions are used for nerve blocks and infiltration whereas 4% solutions are used topically.[42] Benzocaine is less preferred as it can cause methemoglobinemia even in therapeutic doses. Tetracaine has a very narrow therapeutic window, and the maximum allowable dose (1.2 mg/kg) can easily be exceeded. Cetacaine is a mixture of benzocaine and tetracaine and has the disadvantages of each local anesthetic.

### Nose and Nasopharynx

The nasal mucosa must be anesthetized and vasoconstriction with 0.05% oxymetazoline hydrochloride (HCL) spray is recommended. In addition to spraying, local anesthetic solutions can be applied directly in the nares on soaked cotton-tipped swabs or pledgets or by nasal airways covered in lidocaine ointment.

### Tongue and Oropharynx

Topical anesthesia may be achieved by spraying, direct application, or bilateral blocks of the glossopharyngeal nerve at the base of each anterior tonsillar pillar. Approximately 2 mL of 2% lidocaine injected at a depth of 0.5 cm is sufficient to block the glossopharyngeal nerves on each side. Aspiration with the syringe before injecting the local anesthetic solution is necessary to ensure that the needle is not intravascular or through the tonsillar pillar.

### Larynx and Trachea

Anesthesia of the larynx and trachea may be achieved by using the methods described earlier or by superior laryngeal nerve blocks and transtracheal block.

### Superior Laryngeal Nerve Block

Injecting local anesthetic solution bilaterally, in the vicinity of the superior laryngeal nerves where they lie between the greater cornu of the hyoid bone and the superior cornu of the thyroid cartilage as they traverse the thyrohyoid membrane to the submucosa of the piriform sinus, blocks the internal branch of the superior laryngeal nerve. The overlying skin is cleaned with antiseptic solution. The cornu of the hyoid bone or the thyroid cartilage may be used as a landmark. A 22- to 25-G needle is "walked" off the cephalad edge of the thyroid cartilage or the caudal edge of the hyoid bone, and approximately 2 to 3 mL of local anesthetic solution is injected on each side.

### Transtracheal Block

For a transtracheal block, the skin is prepared with antiseptic solution and a 20-G IV catheter is advanced through the cricothyroid membrane while simultaneously aspirating with an attached syringe filled with 4 mL of local anesthetic solution. When air is aspirated, the catheter is advanced into the trachea and the needle is withdrawn. The syringe is reattached to the catheter, aspiration of air is reconfirmed, and the local anesthetic solution is rapidly injected. This block is designed to block the sensory distribution of the recurrent laryngeal nerve and prevent coughing with placement of the endotracheal tube in the trachea.

### Technique

Nasal fiberoptic intubation of the trachea involves the use of a lubricated endotracheal tube that is at least 1.5 mm larger than the diameter of the fiberoptic bronchoscope. Softening the endotracheal tube in warm water before use makes it less likely to cause mucosal trauma or submucosal tunneling. The endotracheal tube is advanced through the nose into the pharynx by aiming perpendicular to the plane of the patient's face just above the inferior border of the nasal alar rim. If resistance is met at the back of the nasopharynx, 90 degrees of counterclockwise rotation allows the endotracheal tube to pass less traumatically because the bevel then faces the posterior pharyngeal wall. Secretions should be suctioned before inserting the fiberoptic bronchoscope through the endotracheal tube.

For oral fiberoptic intubation, using a channeled oral airway that fits an endotracheal tube can help keep the fiberoptic scope midline and create space in the oropharynx. Having an assistant gently extend the tongue out of the patient's mouth can help by elevating the epiglottis. The endotracheal tube can either be advanced in the mouth with the fiberoptic bronchoscope or can be secured at the top of the scope and advanced after the fiberoptic bronchoscope has entered the trachea. Inflation of the endotracheal tube cuff during advancement of the fiberoptic bronchoscope in the pharynx can create an enlarged pharyngeal space and help keep the optics of the fiberoptic bronchoscope from being obscured. The inflated cuff also further aims the tip of the endotracheal tube anteriorly. If the technique of cuff inflation is used to facilitate entry of the bronchoscope into the trachea, the provider should remember to deflate the cuff prior to advancement of the endotracheal tube into the trachea.

The fiberoptic bronchoscope is manipulated to bring the larynx into view, and the bronchoscope is advanced toward the glottic opening. The target should always be kept in the center of the anesthesia provider's field of vision by flexion/extension and rotation as the fiberoptic bronchoscope is slowly advanced. As the fiberoptic bronchoscope passes through the vocal cords, the tracheal rings will become visible. The scope should be placed just above the carina as the endotracheal tube is threaded over the scope. If resistance is encountered when advancing the endotracheal tube, force should not be exerted as the fiberoptic bronchoscope can become kinked and the endotracheal tube can pass into the esophagus and damage the fiberoptic bronchoscope. Resistance to advancement often means that the endotracheal tube is impacted on an arytenoid. Rotating the endotracheal tube as it is gently advanced can relieve this. The appropriate depth of endotracheal tube placement can be verified by observing the distance between the carina and the tip of the endotracheal tube as the fiberoptic bronchoscope is withdrawn. It is essential that the fiberoptic bronchoscope exit the tip of the endotracheal tube and not the Murphy eye. If there is any resistance when removing the fiberoptic bronchoscope, it is probably either through the Murphy eye or kinked in the pharynx. In both instances, the endotracheal tube and the scope must be withdrawn together to avoid damaging the fiberoptic bronchoscope.

### Fiberoptic Endotracheal Intubation After Induction of General Anesthesia

Alseep fiberoptic intubation is commonly performed because of examination findings consistent with or history of a difficult airway or unstable cervical spine when mask ventilation is not anticipated to be difficult. It is also an option when patients are not cooperative with awake fiberoptic intubation.

Fiberoptic intubation during general anesthesia can be done either through the nose or the mouth, with the patient breathing spontaneously or under controlled ventilation. To provide supplemental oxygenation during the procedure, a nasal airway can be placed and connected to the anesthesia breathing circuit with a 15-mm connector.

An important difference in performing fiberoptic laryngoscopy in an anesthetized patient is that the soft tissues of the pharynx, in contrast to the awake state, tend to relax and limit space for visualization with the fiberoptic bronchoscope. Using jaw thrust, specialized oral airways, inflating the endotracheal tube cuff in the pharynx, or applying traction on the tongue may overcome this problem. It is advisable to have a second person trained in anesthesia delivery assisting when a fiberoptic intubation is performed during general anesthesia because it is difficult to maintain the patient's airway, be attentive to the monitors, and perform the fiberoptic intubation alone.

When using the nasal approach, it is important to apply a vasoconstrictor to the nasal mucosa to decrease the risk of bleeding, which may obscure the optics of a fiberoptic bronchoscope.

The curvature of the endotracheal tube is not optimal for oral endotracheal intubation, and an appropriately sized channeled oral airway can help. Care must be taken to maintain the intubating airway in a midline position. Alternatively, a supraglottic airway provides an excellent channel for oral fiberoptic intubation.

### Endoscopy Mask

The single-use endoscopy mask is designed with a port that will accommodate an endotracheal tube and a fiberoptic bronchoscope through a diaphragm. This device allows for spontaneous or controlled ventilation while fiberoptic nasal or oral intubation is being performed. It is available in newborn, infant, pediatric, and adult sizes.

## Blind Nasotracheal Intubation

The use of blind nasotracheal intubation has decreased in frequency over the years with the introduction of other devices for difficult airway management. However, there are still clinical situations in which such a technique can be lifesaving.

A 6.0- to 7.0-mm internal diameter (ID) endotracheal tube is generally chosen for an adult. The endotracheal tube is advanced through the nose and into the pharynx while listening to breath sounds at the distal end of the endotracheal tube. Alternatively, the endotracheal tube can be attached to an anesthesia breathing circuit, and reservoir bag movement and carbon dioxide can be monitored to verify that the endotracheal tube is advancing into the trachea.

## Endotracheal Tube Sizes

Endotracheal tube sizes are specified according to their ID, which is marked on each tube. Endotracheal tubes are available in 0.5-mm ID increments. The endotracheal tube also has lengthwise centimeter markings starting at the distal tracheal end to permit accurate determination of the length inserted past the patient's lips. Endotracheal tubes are most often made of clear, inert polyvinyl chloride plastic that molds to the contour of the airway after softening on exposure to body temperature. Endotracheal tube material should also be radiopaque to ascertain the position of the distal tip relative to the carina and be transparent to permit visualization of secretions or airflow as evidenced by condensation of water vapor in the lumen of the tube ("breath fogging") during exhalation.

As noted previously, use the minimum volume of air in a low-pressure high-volume cuff that prevents leaks during positive-pressure ventilation (20 to 30 cm $H_2O$) to minimize risk of mucosal ischemia. Other serious complications attributable to endotracheal cuff pressures include tracheal stenosis, tracheal rupture, tracheoesophageal fistula, tracheocarotid fistula, and tracheoinnominate artery fistula.[43]

## Confirmation of Endotracheal Intubation

Confirmation of placement of the endotracheal tube in the trachea is verified by identification of carbon dioxide in the patient's exhaled tidal volume and clinical assessment. The presence of carbon dioxide in the exhaled gases from the endotracheal tube as detected by capnography (end-tidal $Pco_2 > 30$ mm Hg for three to five consecutive breaths) should be immediate and sustained. Carbon dioxide may initially be present in low concentrations, but will not persist in exhaled gases from a tube accidentally placed in the esophagus.

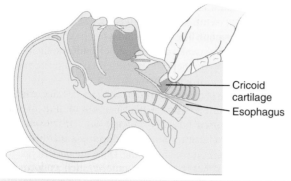

Cricoid cartilage

Esophagus

**Fig. 16.18** Cricoid pressure is provided by an assistant exerting downward pressure with the thumb and index finger on the cricoid cartilage (approximately 5-kg pressure) so that the cartilaginous cricothyroid ring is displaced posteriorly and the esophagus is thus compressed (occluded) against the underlying cervical vertebrae.

Symmetric chest rise with manual ventilation, bilateral breath sounds, and absence of breath sounds over the epigastrium is confirmed after endotracheal intubation. Palpation or balloting of the endotracheal tube cuff in the suprasternal notch can help determine endotracheal versus endobronchial intubation. Progressive decreases in oxygen saturation on a pulse oximeter may alert the anesthesia provider to a previously unrecognized esophageal intubation.

In adults, taping the endotracheal tube at the patient's lips corresponding to the 21- to 23-cm markings on the endotracheal tube usually places the distal end of the endotracheal tube in the midtrachea. Of note, flexion of the patient's head may advance and convert a tracheal placement into an endobronchial intubation, especially in children. Conversely, extension of the head can withdraw the tube and result in inadvertent extubation.

## Rapid Sequence Induction of Anesthesia With Cricoid Pressure

Cricoid pressure (Sellick maneuver) may prevent spillage of gastric contents into the pharynx during the period from induction of anesthesia (unconsciousness) to successful placement of a cuffed endotracheal tube. It can be applied by an assistant exerting downward external pressure with the thumb and index finger on the cricoid cartilage to displace the cartilaginous cricothyroid ring posteriorly and thus compress the underlying upper esophagus against the cervical vertebrae (Fig. 16.18). The magnitude of downward external pressure (30 newtons is recommended) that needs to be exerted on the cricoid cartilage to reliably occlude the esophagus is difficult to judge. The use of cricoid pressure has been questioned for several reasons including the following: (1) there is lack of validation in models other than cadavers, (2) there have been reports of aspiration despite its use, (3) it can cause relaxation of the lower esophageal sphincter, which can favor regurgitation, (4) it may cause complications such

as increasing the difficulty of mask ventilation or worsening laryngoscopic view or nausea, vomiting, and esophageal rupture, and (5) magnetic resonance imaging has shown that the esophagus may be lateral and not directly posterior to the cricoid cartilage in patients with or without application of cricoid pressure resulting in inadequate esophageal compression.[44,45] Other magnetic resonance imaging studies have suggested that although the esophagus is laterally displaced in some patients, the hypopharynx is the structure that is being compressed by cricoid pressure, and the cricoid and hypopharynx move together as a unit. Even if lateral movement occurs, there is compression of this structure.[46] The use of cricoid pressure remains controversial. It should probably be considered in selected patients with increased risk for regurgitation of gastric contents during induction of anesthesia, but can be released if it impedes oxygenation, ventilation, or view of glottic structures.

## TRANSTRACHEAL TECHNIQUES

In situations when ventilation and intubation are unsuccessful despite use of a supraglottic airway, emergency invasive access should be used.[1] Invasive emergency access consists of percutaneous or surgical airway, jet ventilation, and retrograde intubation. Predictors of difficult access through the cricothyroid membrane include increased neck circumference, overlying neck malformation, and a fixed cervical spine flexion deformity.[18,47]

### Cricothyrotomy

A cricothyrotomy can be a lifesaving procedure in a "cannot intubate, cannot ventilate" situation or can be used as a first-line technique to secure an airway when using a less invasive technique is not possible owing to factors such as facial trauma, upper airway bleeding, or upper airway obstruction. A cricothyrotomy is best performed with the patient in the sniffing position to optimize the ability to identify the cricothyroid membrane. A percutaneous cricothyrotomy uses the Seldinger technique. A needle is advanced at a 90-degree angle through the cricothyroid membrane while aspirating with an attached syringe. A change in resistance is felt as a pop when the needle enters the trachea and air is aspirated. The needle should be directed caudally at a 30- to 45-degree angle. A guidewire is then advanced through the needle, followed by removal of the needle, a small incision adjacent to the wire, and placement of a combined dilator and airway of adequate caliber (>4 mm). Finally, the wire and dilator are removed leaving the airway in place.[47]

The surgical technique involves a vertical or horizontal skin incision, followed by a horizontal incision through the cricothyroid membrane through which a standard endotracheal tube or tracheostomy tube is placed. A tracheal hook, dilator, AEC, or bougie can assist in placement of the airway.[48,49] A surgical cricothyrotomy can also be valuable as a rescue technique if a percutaneous cricothyrotomy is unsuccessful. There are commercial percutaneous and surgical cricothyrotomy kits available that require minimal assembly for use in emergency circumstances.

Both techniques can provide a cuffed endotracheal tube to bypass upper airway obstruction, provide ventilation, and protect against aspiration. There is no consensus on which technique is superior.[48,49] Success of either technique relies on knowledge, practice, proficiency, and performing the cricothyrotomy early when in a "cannot intubate, cannot ventilate" situation. Some relative contraindications to either technique are laryngeal or tracheal disruption and coagulopathy. Complications include bleeding, laryngeal, tracheal or esophageal injury, infection, and subglottic stenosis.[18,49]

## Transtracheal Jet Ventilation

Transtracheal jet ventilation is achieved by placement of an over-the-needle catheter in the trachea through the cricothyroid membrane. The cricothyroid membrane should be identified and a catheter over a needle connected to a syringe should puncture the membrane at a 90-degree angle until air is aspirated. The catheter should be advanced off the needle into the trachea at a 30- to 45-degree angle caudally. After reconfirming correct placement by aspiration of air, the catheter should be connected to a high-pressure oxygen source. Commercially available products contain kink-resistant catheters and specialized tubing for high-pressure (50 psi) ventilation. The risk for transtracheal jet ventilation includes pneumothorax, pneumomediastinum, bleeding, infection, and subcutaneous emphysema.[49] Contraindications to transtracheal jet ventilation are upper airway obstruction or any disruption of the airway.[50]

## Retrograde Endotracheal Intubation

Retrograde endotracheal intubation can be performed without identification of the glottic inlet. It has been used in cases of anticipated and unanticipated difficult airway management, particularly when there is bleeding, airway trauma, decreased mouth opening, or limited neck movement.

The cricothyroid membrane is punctured with a needle in the method previously described. Once in the trachea, the syringe is detached and a guide (usually a wire or catheter) is threaded through the needle in a *cephalad* direction. It is then retrieved from the mouth or nose. An endotracheal tube, with or without a fiberoptic bronchoscope, is threaded over the wire until it stops on impact with the anterior wall of the trachea. Tension on the guide can be relaxed to allow the endotracheal tube to pass further into the trachea before removing the wire. Commercially available kits have improved this technique by adding a guiding catheter that fits over the wire and inside the endotracheal tube. Contraindications include disease of the anterior aspect of the neck (tumors, infection, stenosis) or coagulopathy.[51]

## Endotracheal Extubation

Endotracheal extubation after general anesthesia requires skill and judgment. The patient must be either deeply anesthetized or fully awake at the time of endotracheal extubation. The risk and benefits of either technique should be taken into account when planning for extubation.

As with intubation, 100% $O_2$ should be administered prior to extubation. Any residual neuromuscular blockade should be reversed (also see Chapter 11). The oropharynx is suctioned and a bite block should be placed to prevent occlusion of the endotracheal tube. Once the patient has met routine endotracheal extubation criteria, such as spontaneous respirations with adequate minute ventilation, satisfactory oxygenation and acid base status, and hemodynamic stability, the endotracheal tube can be removed. Patients who are obese or have a history of obstructive sleep apnea may benefit from positioning with the head up for extubation.[52] For deep extubation, adequate anesthesia should be confirmed and for awake patients, they should be able to follow commands. Endotracheal extubation during a light level of anesthesia (disconjugate gaze, breath-holding or coughing, and not responsive to commands) increases the risk of laryngospasm. Laryngospasm is unlikely if the depth of anesthesia is sufficient so laryngeal reflexes are suppressed or the patient is allowed to awaken before endotracheal extubation so laryngeal reflexes are intact. A patient reaching for the endotracheal tube might indicate a localizing response to noxious stimulation despite not being awake enough from anesthesia to follow commands. The endotracheal tube cuff is then deflated and the endotracheal tube rapidly removed from the patient's trachea and upper airway while a positive-pressure breath is delivered to help expel any secretions. After endotracheal extubation, 100% $O_2$ is delivered by face mask and airway patency and adequate ventilation and oxygenation are confirmed.

Tracheal extubation before the return of protective airway reflexes (deep endotracheal extubation) is generally associated with less coughing and attenuated hemodynamic effects on emergence. This may be preferred in patients at risk from adverse effects of increased intracranial or intraocular pressure, bleeding into the surgical wound, or wound dehiscence. Previous difficult face mask ventilation or endotracheal intubation, high risk of aspiration, restricted access to the airway, obstructive sleep apnea or obesity, and a surgical procedure that may have resulted in airway edema, bleeding or increased irritability are relative contraindications to deep endotracheal extubation. Deep extubation may also predispose to airway obstruction owing to the remaining anesthetic drug present.

If a patient is at risk for failure of extubation and may be a difficult reintubation, a plan for reintubation must be made (Fig. 16.19). High-risk patients include those with airway edema, inadequate ventilation, and history of a difficult intubation.[18] Checking for a cuff leak can help determine if significant airway edema is present. This can be done easily in a spontaneously breathing patient by

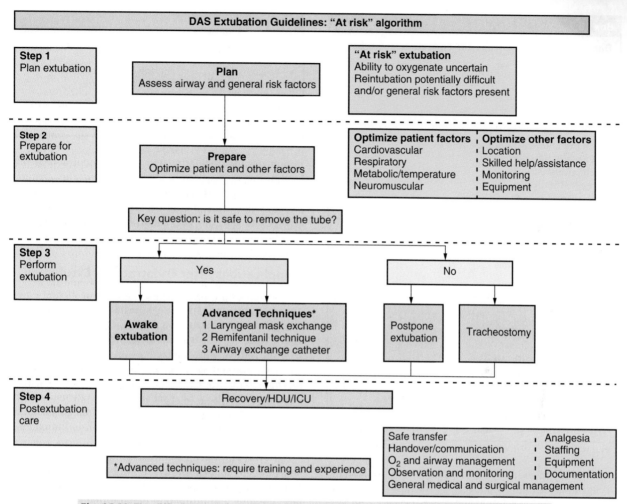

**Fig. 16.19** The difficult airway society (DAS) extubation guidelines for "at-risk" patients. *HDU,* high dependency unit; *ICU,* intensive care unit. (From Mitchell V, Dravid R, Patel A, et al. Difficult airway society guidelines for the management of tracheal extubation. *Anaesthesia.* 2012;67(3):318-340.)

removing him or her from the ventilation circuit, deflating the endotracheal tube cuff, and obstructing the end of the endotracheal tube. Breath sounds are evidence of air movement around the endotracheal tube. Extubation over an AEC or insertion of supraglottic airway prior to extubation provides a conduit to reintubation and allows for oxygenation and/or ventilation if necessary.[1,53] Extubation of the trachea is always elective, and postponing extubation may be appropriate in some cases when the patient has increased risk for requiring reintubation.

## COMPLICATIONS

Complications of endotracheal intubation are rare and should not influence the decision to place an endotracheal tube. Complications of endotracheal intubation may be categorized as those occurring (1) during direct laryngoscopy and endotracheal intubation, (2) while the endotracheal tube is in place, and (3) after endotracheal extubation (Box 16.2).

### Complications During Laryngoscopy and Endotracheal Intubation

Direct upper airway trauma is more likely to occur with difficult endotracheal intubation because often there is increased physical force applied to the patient's airway than normal, as well as the need for multiple attempts at intubation. One of the most common consequences of using increased physical force with a laryngoscope is dental damage (occurs in 1 in 4500 patients).[54] Other patients at risk for dental injury include those with preexisting poor dentition or fixed dental work. Use of a plastic shield placed over the upper teeth may help in selected patients but also decreases the interincisor distance, which may make laryngoscopy more difficult. Other risks include

---

**Box 16.2** Complications of Endotracheal Intubation

**During Direct Laryngoscopy and Endotracheal Intubation**
Dental and oral soft tissue trauma
Systemic hypertension and tachycardia
Cardiac dysrhythmias
Myocardial ischemia
Inhalation (aspiration) of gastric contents

**While the Endotracheal Tube Is in Place**
Endotracheal tube obstruction
Endobronchial intubation
Esophageal intubation
Endotracheal tube cuff leak
Pulmonary barotrauma
Nasogastric distention
Accidental disconnection from the anesthesia breathing circuit
Tracheal mucosa ischemia
Accidental extubation

**Complications After Endotracheal Extubation**
Laryngospasm
Inhalation (aspiration) of gastric contents
Pharyngitis (sore throat)
Laryngitis
Laryngeal or subglottic edema
Laryngeal ulceration with or without granuloma formation
Tracheitis
Tracheal stenosis
Vocal cord paralysis
Arytenoid cartilage dislocation

---

**Box 16.3** The Infant Airway Versus the Adult Airway

- Larynx positioned higher in the neck
- Tongue larger relative to mouth size
- Epiglottis larger, stiffer, and angled more posteriorly
- Head and occiput larger relative to body size
- Short neck
- Narrow nares
- Cricoid ring is the narrowest region

---

oral or pharyngeal injury, lip lacerations and bruises, and laryngeal, arytenoid, esophageal, or tracheal damage.

Laryngoscopy and intubation are associated with systemic hypertension, tachycardia, and increased intracranial pressure. These responses are generally short lived and of little consequence in most patients. In patients with preexisting hypertension, ischemic heart disease, or certain neurologic conditions, these responses can cause harm. Aspiration poses another potential risk, especially in patients who are not fasted, have symptomatic gastroesophageal reflux, have delayed gastric emptying, or are morbidly obese. Aspiration is the most common cause of death among major anesthesia airway complications.[8] If inadequate oxygenation or ventilation is prolonged after induction of anesthesia, patients may develop cardiac dysrhythmias and in rare cases cardiac arrest and brain damage.

## Complications While the Endotracheal Tube Is in Place

These complications include obstruction or accidental esophageal or endobronchial endotracheal tube placement. Obstruction of the endotracheal tube may occur as a result of secretions or kinking. The chance of endobronchial intubation or accidental extubation can be minimized by calculating the proper endotracheal tube length for the patient and then noting the centimeter marking on the tube at the point of fixation at the patient's lips. Care should be taken if the neck position changes to confirm the endotracheal tube is correctly positioned.

## Complications After Endotracheal Extubation

One third of adverse airway events occur during emergence or recovery from anesthesia.[8] Most of them are due to airway obstruction from factors such as laryngeal edema, laryngospasm, or bronchospasm. A patient who is lightly anesthetized at the time of endotracheal extubation is most at risk for laryngospasm. If laryngospasm occurs, oxygen delivered with positive pressure through a face mask and jaw thrust may be sufficient treatment. Administration of succinylcholine or an anesthetic drug, such as propofol, is indicated if laryngospasm persists.

Sore throat is present in about 40% of patients after laryngoscopy and endotracheal intubation and in 20% to 42% of patients after LMA placement.[55] Sore throat after laryngoscopy and intubation is more frequent in females and there is evidence of previous airway trauma in all genders. Use of larger endotracheal tubes and overinflating endotracheal tube cuffs may also increase the likelihood of sore throat. Sore throat is usually self-limiting and resolves in 24 to 72 hours.

The major complication of prolonged endotracheal intubation (>48 hours) is damage to the tracheal mucosa, which may progress to destruction of cartilaginous rings and subsequent fibrous scar formation and tracheal stenosis. Using high-volume, low-pressure cuffs and keeping cuff pressures less than 25 cm $H_2O$ can help prevent this complication.

## AIRWAY MANAGEMENT IN INFANTS AND CHILDREN

### Airway Management Differences Between Infants and Adults

Understanding the differences between the infant and adult airway is critical to proper airway management in pediatric anesthesia (Box 16.3; also see Chapter 34). The anatomic and physiologic differences between the infant airway and the adult airway decrease as the child grows; they resolve by about 10 to 12 years of age (also see Chapter 34).

The larynx in infants is located higher in the neck than in adults. In infants, the larynx is typically at the level of C3-C4 and in adults, the larynx is usually at the level of C4-C5. The higher larynx in infants causes the tongue to shift more superiorly, closer to the palate. As a result, the tongue more easily apposes the palate, which can cause airway obstruction in situations such as inhalation induction of anesthesia. An infant's tongue is also larger in proportion to the size of the mouth than in adults. The relatively large size of the tongue makes direct laryngoscopy more difficult and can contribute to obstruction of the upper airway during sedation, inhalation induction of anesthesia, and emergence from anesthesia. Anterior pressure on the angle of the mandible, commonly referred to as jaw thrust, will often shift the tongue to a more anterior position and resolve an upper airway obstruction. An oral or nasal airway can also be beneficial in these situations.

The epiglottis in an infant's airway is often described as relatively larger, stiffer, and more omega-shaped than an adult epiglottis. More importantly, an infant's epiglottis is typically angled in a more posterior position, thereby blocking the view of the vocal cords during direct laryngoscopy. In infants and small children, it is often necessary to lift the epiglottis with the tip of the blade of the laryngoscope to visualize the vocal cords and successfully intubate the trachea.

An infant's airway is often described as funnel-shaped, with a relatively large thyroid cartilage above and a relatively narrow cricoid cartilage below. The cricoid cartilage is the narrowest portion of an infant's airway; the vocal cords are the narrowest portion of an adult's airway. The cricoid cartilage is circular, allowing cuffed or uncuffed endotracheal tubes to successfully seal and protect the airway from aspiration.

An infant's head and occiput are relatively larger than an adult's. The proper position for direct laryngoscopy and endotracheal intubation in an adult is often described as the sniffing position with the head elevated and the neck flexed at C6-C7 and extended at C1-C2. An infant, on the other hand, requires a shoulder roll or neck roll to establish an optimal position for face mask ventilation and direct laryngoscopy. An infant's nares are relatively smaller than an adult's and can offer significant resistance to airflow and increase the work of breathing, especially when secretions, edema, or bleeding narrow them.

Oxygen consumption per kilogram is much higher in infants than in adults. This results in a much shorter allowable time for intubation before the infant desaturates, even after adequate preoxygenation (see Fig. 16.8). This can be a significant issue, especially in difficult intubations.

## Managing the Normal Airway in Infants and Children

A complete history and a focused physical examination are the first steps in managing the pediatric airway (also see Chapter 34).

### History

The history should include whether there were any problems with previous anesthetics; prior anesthetic records should be reviewed if they are available. A history of snoring should prompt additional questioning about whether the infant or child has obstructive sleep apnea. If present, respiratory obstruction may develop during the induction and emergence phases of anesthesia, as well as in the postoperative period, especially if opioids are used for pain management. There are numerous syndromes associated with difficult airway management, most of which involve mandibular hypoplasia or cervical spine abnormalities that limit flexion and extension (see Table 16.2).

### Physical Examination

It is often difficult to perform a complete physical examination on infants and children. Asking a child to look up at the sky and then down at the floor is one way of assessing neck extension and flexion, respectively. If there are any masses, tumors, or abscesses in the neck or upper airway that compromise neck flexion, extension, or breathing function, further evaluation is important and should include computed tomography to evaluate the location and degree of any airway compromise. Children will often voluntarily open their mouths to enable determination of a Mallampati classification. If an infant or child is uncooperative, external examination of the airway often reveals enough information to determine whether it is a normal or potentially difficult airway. Examining the profile of an infant or child can indicate whether the thyromental distance is short and whether the patient has micrognathia or a hypoplastic mandible.

The parent(s) and the child should be directly asked whether there are any loose teeth. If loose teeth are identified, care should be taken to avoid traumatizing these teeth during airway management. Very loose teeth should be removed before proceeding with airway management to prevent the possibility of dislodgement and aspiration.

## Preanesthetic Medication and Parental Presence During Induction of Anesthesia

Parental presence during induction of anesthesia is increasingly becoming the standard approach for pediatric patients. Parental presence can minimize the need for preanesthetic medication in infants and children (also see Chapter 34). Anxious parents can transfer their anxiety to their children. Therefore, it is important to spend adequate time preoperatively addressing any questions or concerns of both the child and the parents. Child-life services should be available preoperatively to use age-appropriate play therapy, preoperative instruction, and coping skills for both the child and the parents. The goal is to decrease anxiety and prepare them for the experience of the induction of anesthesia in the operating room. It is important to designate a member of the operating team to escort the parents from the operating room to the waiting area after the induction of anesthesia is completed and to address any worries parents may have after witnessing the procedure.

Preanesthetic medication can facilitate the induction of anesthesia in very anxious children. Preanesthetic medication is often not necessary in infants younger than 6 months because stranger anxiety does not usually develop until 6 to 9 months of age. If the child has an IV catheter in place, midazolam can be administered in small doses and titrated to effect. It is important to recognize that a higher per kilogram dose of IV midazolam is required in young children than in adults. Although the goal for premedication with midazolam in adults is often anxiolysis, the goal for premedication in young children is often sedation, thus, the higher per kilogram dosing.

If the child does not have an IV catheter in place, midazolam syrup can be given orally in a dose of about 0.5 mg/kg up to a maximum dose of about 20 mg. If the child is uncooperative with taking oral midazolam and preanesthetic medication is essential, midazolam can also be given intranasally, intramuscularly, or rectally. In rare cases in which older children are uncooperative, agitated, or violent, it may be necessary to administer intramuscular ketamine in a dose of about 3 mg/kg to facilitate IV placement and the induction of anesthesia.

## Induction of Anesthesia

If the infant or child has an IV catheter, induction of anesthesia with propofol is usually safer and quicker than an inhaled induction of anesthesia. After the infant or child loses consciousness and the ability to ventilate with a face mask is verified, either a supraglottic airway device can be inserted or a neuromuscular blocking drug can be given to facilitate direct laryngoscopy and endotracheal intubation. Although it is possible to perform laryngoscopy on infants and children without a neuromuscular blocking drug, using a neuromuscular blocking drug, such as rocuronium, facilitates laryngoscopy and intubation, decreases the incidence of laryngospasm, and decreases the amount of propofol required for the induction of anesthesia. For routine situations, a dose of 0.3 to 0.6 mg/kg of rocuronium is recommended (also see Chapter 11).

When the infant or child does not have an IV catheter in place, inhaled induction of anesthesia can be performed. Beginning the induction of anesthesia with the odorless mixture of nitrous oxide and oxygen through a face mask, then slowly increasing the concentration of sevoflurane is the best approach in a cooperative child. If the child is

uncooperative, it is better to induce with 8% sevoflurane. When the infant or child becomes unconscious, the nitrous oxide should be turned off to administer 100% oxygen to adequately preoxygenate prior to laryngoscopy. The increasing level of anesthesia will decrease skeletal muscle tone and can cause upper airway obstruction in infants and children. If upper airway obstruction occurs, it can usually be relieved by a jaw thrust, or by inserting an oral or nasal airway. An IV catheter should then be placed. Once the ability to ventilate the patient has been confirmed, either a supraglottic airway device can be inserted, or a neuromuscular blocking drug can be given to facilitate laryngoscopy and endotracheal intubation.

## Direct Laryngoscopy and Endotracheal Intubation

When performing direct laryngoscopy and endotracheal intubation in infants and children, it is important to appropriately position the infant or child with a roll under the neck or shoulders. The oropharynx should be visualized as divided into three compartments: (1) the tongue swept to the left by the laryngoscope blade, (2) the laryngoscope blade in the middle of the mouth, and (3) the endotracheal tube entering from the right side of the mouth. Gentle, external posterior pressure applied with the fingers of the anesthesia provider's right hand at the level of the thyroid or cricoid cartilage is sometimes necessary to bring the vocal cords into view.

Once the trachea is intubated, correct positioning of the endotracheal tube should be confirmed by end-tidal $CO_2$, by watching the chest rise and fall, and by auscultation of both right and left lungs. Because the trachea in infants and children is short, it is easy to accidentally intubate a main bronchus. The correct depth of a cuffed endotracheal tube can be estimated by palpating the endotracheal tube cuff in the suprasternal notch. The correct tracheal depth of an uncuffed endotracheal tube can be estimated by placing the double line at the distal end of the endotracheal tube at the vocal cords while performing direct laryngoscopy. In infants and children, it is important to reconfirm that the endotracheal tube is correctly positioned by listening for equal bilateral breath sounds after securing the endotracheal tube, and whenever there is a change in the patient's position.

### Airway Equipment
#### Nasal and Oral Airways
Nasal and oral airways can sometimes be useful in pediatric patients to relieve airway obstruction, especially during face mask ventilation at the beginning or end of anesthesia. The nasal airway should be carefully placed through one of the nares after lubricating its exterior. The nasal airway must be long enough to pass through the nasopharynx, but short enough that it still remains above the glottis.

Oral airways relieve airway obstruction by displacing the tongue anteriorly. Too large an oral airway will either obstruct the glottis or may cause coughing, gagging, or laryngospasm in a patient who is not deeply anesthetized. Too small an oral airway will push the tongue posteriorly and make the airway obstruction worse. Oral airways should be placed with care to prevent trauma to the teeth and oropharynx.

## Supraglottic Airway Devices

Supraglottic airway devices are placed in the patient's oropharynx to facilitate oxygenation and ventilation; they can also deliver inhalational anesthetics. They can be used for both routine airway management and difficult airway situations. Although supraglottic airway devices are ideally suited for situations in which the patient is breathing spontaneously, they can also be used to deliver positive-pressure ventilation. Care must be taken when using positive-pressure ventilation with a supraglottic airway device to minimize peak inspiratory pressure. Patients who have lung disease or whose peak inspiratory pressures are higher than normal are poor candidates for a supraglottic airway device. In these patients, air may leak into the esophagus resulting in distention of the stomach and increase the risk for emesis and aspiration. Supraglottic airway devices do not protect the airway from aspiration. They should not be routinely used in patients with full stomachs or those at increased risk for aspiration. Many supraglottic airway devices are available in both single-use and reusable versions.

## Laryngeal Mask Airways

LMAs are supraglottic airway devices that have proved to be very useful in managing the pediatric airway. The LMA Classic and the LMA Unique, which is the single-use version of the LMA Classic, are both available in seven sizes appropriate for a range of pediatric patients. The LMA ProSeal and the LMA Supreme, which is the single-use version of the LMA ProSeal, are also available in the same seven sizes. The LMA ProSeal and Supreme have an additional lumen that is designed to vent the esophagus. The LMA Flexible is essentially the LMA Classic with a wire-reinforced airway tube that resists kinking. It can minimize interference with surgical procedures involving the head and neck. The LMA Flexible is not available in sizes 1 and 1½. It is the most difficult LMA to insert; a stylet may be required to facilitate insertion.

The appropriate size LMA is most easily determined by using the weight of the infant or child (Table 16.5). An LMA that is too large will be more difficult to place. An LMA that is too small will not form a good seal, making positive-pressure ventilation more challenging.

After the LMA has been inserted and its cuff has been inflated, correct positioning should be confirmed by auscultation of breath sounds and by end-tidal $CO_2$. Ideally,

**Table 16.5** Appropriate-Size Laryngeal Mask Airway (LMA) Based on Patient Weight and Maximum Oral Endotracheal Tube Sizes

| LMA Size | Weight (kg) | Maximum Oral Endotracheal Tube Size (mm) |
|---|---|---|
| 1 | <5 | 3.0 uncuffed |
| 1.5 | 5-10 | 4.0 uncuffed, 3.5 cuffed |
| 2 | 10-20 | 4.5 uncuffed, 4.0 cuffed |
| 2.5 | 20-30 | 4.5 cuffed |
| 3 | 30-50 | 5.5 cuffed |
| 4 | 50-70 | 5.5 cuffed |
| 5 | 70-100 | 6.5 cuffed |
| 6 | >100 | 6.5 cuffed |

the cuff of the LMA should be inflated with just enough air to allow positive-pressure ventilation. Overinflation of the LMA cuff has been associated with mucosal damage and postoperative sore throat and may not decrease the leak pressure.[56,57] It is important to realize that the cuff pressure can be much higher than the leak pressure. Ideally, the pressure in the cuff of the LMA should be measured with a manometer (Fig. 16.20) and should be less than 30 to 40 cm $H_2O$.

## Air-Q Masked Laryngeal Airways

Air-Q intubating laryngeal airways (ILAs) are another type of supraglottic airway device used with infants and children. They are available in single-use and reusable versions. Their major advantage over LMAs is a design that facilitates endotracheal intubation with standard oral endotracheal tubes. The Air-Q's airway tube has a larger diameter than the LMA, allowing for intubation with a larger endotracheal tube than the correspondingly sized LMA. The Air-Q ILA can be used with a specially designed ILA removal stylet that stabilizes the endotracheal tube and allows controlled removal of the ILA, without dislodging the endotracheal tube from the trachea. The Air-Q ILA is available in seven sizes appropriate for a range of pediatric patients. As with the LMA, determining the appropriate size is most easily estimated by using the weight of the infant or child (Table 16.6). The 0.5 size Air-Q ILA is currently available only in the reusable version.

## Endotracheal Tubes

The appropriately sized endotracheal tube for infants and children can be estimated by using the following formula for uncuffed endotracheal tubes only:

$$(Age + 16)/4 = endotracheal\ tube\ (ID)\ size$$

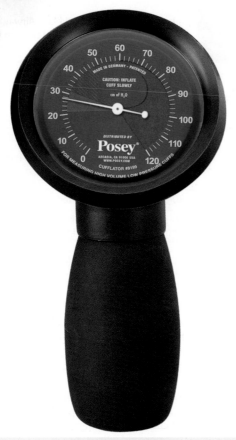

**Fig. 16.20** Posey 8199 Cufflator Endotracheal Tube Inflator and Manometer. (Image courtesy of Posey Company, Arcadia, CA.)

| Table 16.6 | Appropriate-Size Air-Q Masked Intubating Laryngeal Airway Size Recommendations and Maximum Cuffed Oral Endotracheal Tube Sizes | |
| --- | --- | --- |
| **Air-Q Size** | **Weight (kg)** | **Maximum Oral Endotracheal Tube Size** |
| 0.5 | <4 | 4.0 |
| 1 | 4-7 | 4.5 |
| 1.5 | 7-17 | 5.0 |
| 2.0 | 17-30 | 5.5 |
| 2.5 | 30-50 | 6.5 |
| 3.5 | 50-70 | 7.5 |
| 4.5 | 70-100 | 8.5 |

endotracheal tubes minimizes the need for repeated laryngoscopy, allows for lower fresh gas flows, decreases the amount of inhalational anesthetic used, and decreases the concentrations of anesthetic gases detectable in operating rooms.[58] Using cuffed endotracheal tubes does not increase the incidence of postextubation croup when compared to the use of uncuffed endotracheal tubes.[59,60]

When cuffed endotracheal tubes are used in infants and children, the cuff pressure should be measured and adjusted to maintain a cuff pressure of approximately 20 to 25 cm $H_2O$. A leak pressure may be used to approximate a cuff pressure, but ideally the cuff pressure should be measured directly with a manometer (see Fig. 16.20) as this will most closely correlate with the pressure of the cuff on the tracheal mucosa. If the cuff pressure is too low, it will be difficult to ventilate the patient with positive pressure. If the cuff pressure is too high, this can cause tracheal mucosal injury, postoperative sore throat, and postextubation croup.[61] In rare cases, often involving prolonged intubation, cuff pressures that are too high can result in tracheal stenosis. If nitrous oxide is used during the case, or in cases in which there is the potential for significant airway edema, the cuff pressure should be monitored periodically during the case. The cuff pressure should be measured and recorded in the anesthesia record.

When uncuffed endotracheal tubes are used in infants and children, the leak pressure should be checked. The correct size uncuffed endotracheal tube is one that results in a leak pressure of approximately 20 to 25 cm $H_2O$. If the uncuffed tube is too large, the leak pressure will be too high. In this situation, the endotracheal tube should be replaced with a smaller one to prevent tracheal mucosal injury, postextubation croup, and the possibility of subsequent tracheal stenosis. If the uncuffed tube is too small, the leak pressure will be too low. In this situation it will be difficult to ventilate the patient with positive pressure and the endotracheal tube should be replaced with a larger one. The leak pressure should be measured and documented in the anesthesia record.

To adapt this formula to cuffed endotracheal tubes it is necessary to subtract half a size from the calculated size, because the cuff is located on the outside of the endotracheal tube. Endotracheal tubes a half size larger and a half size smaller than calculated should always be available. Endotracheal tube size can also be based on patient age and body weight. An appropriately sized suction catheter should also always be available to suction secretions, blood, or fluid from the endotracheal tube (Table 16.7).

### Cuffed Versus Uncuffed Endotracheal Tubes

Historically, uncuffed endotracheal tubes were used in infants and smaller children, but more recently cuffed endotracheal tubes have been used increasingly in pediatric anesthesia. With cuffed endotracheal tubes, the cuff is on the outside of the endotracheal tube and adds to the external diameter. Using a cuffed tube often necessitates using a 0.5 mm ID smaller endotracheal tube than using an uncuffed tube. The smaller ID cuffed tube has more resistance to airflow and creates more work of breathing. The increased work of breathing in the slightly narrower cuffed tube is insignificant now that ventilators are available to decrease the work of breathing. Using cuffed

**Table 16.7** Endotracheal Tube, Suction Catheter, and Stylet Size Based on Age and Weight

| Age (yr) | Weight (kg) | Endotracheal Tube ID (mm) | Suction Catheter (F) | Stylet (F) |
|---|---|---|---|---|
| Premature | <1.5 | 2.5 | 6 | 6 |
| Premature | 1.5-2.5 | 3.0 | 6 | 6 |
| Newborn | 3.5 | 3.5 | 8 | 6 |
| 1 | 10 | 4.0 | 8 | 6 |
| 2-3 | 15 | 4.5 | 10 | 6 |
| 4-6 | 20 | 5.0 | 10 | 10 |
| 7-9 | 30 | 5.5 | 12 | 10 |
| 10-12 | 40 | 6.0 | 14 | 10 |
| 13-15 | 50 | 6.5 | 14 | 14 |
| >16 | >60 | 7.0 | 18 | 14 |

ID, Internal diameter.

## Microcuff Endotracheal Tubes

Microcuff pediatric endotracheal tubes offer several distinct advantages over conventional pediatric cuffed endotracheal tubes. Microcuff endotracheal tubes have a cuff made from a microthin polyurethane membrane that is 10 μm thick. The cuff is also cylindrical, rather than round or oval. These tubes seal the airway at lower cuff pressures than conventional endotracheal tubes, reducing the potential for tracheal mucosal edema and postextubation croup; however, using Microcuff endotracheal tubes does not eliminate the incidence of postextubation croup. The appropriately sized endotracheal tube must be used and the inflation pressure should be measured.[62] The cuff on the Microcuff endotracheal tube is also shorter and placed closer to the tip of the endotracheal tube, which increases the likelihood that the tube is correctly placed. In addition, the Microcuff endotracheal tube has an intubation depth mark indicating the correct depth for insertion, increasing the probability of correct placement. Microcuff endotracheal tubes are available in sizes ranging from 3.0 to 7.0 mm, in 0.5-mm increments, in both straight and curved versions.

## Stylet

Using a stylet stiffens the endotracheal tube and makes it easier to manipulate during direct laryngoscopy and endotracheal intubation. The appropriately sized stylet should always be immediately available (see Table 16.7).

## Laryngoscopes

In general, a straight-blade laryngoscope is easier to use in infants and small children than a curved blade. The smaller profile of the straight blade than the curved blade is easier to use in smaller mouths. The smaller tip of the straight blade more effectively lifts the epiglottis than the curved blade. However, curved blades have a larger flange that retracts the tongue to the left more effectively and may be useful in patients with larger than normal tongues (e.g., Beckwith-Wiedemann syndrome, trisomy 21).

In infants younger than 1 year, a Miller 1 straight laryngoscope blade is most useful. In children between 1 and 3 years of age, a 1½ straight laryngoscope blade, such as a Wis-Hipple, is recommended. A longer straight laryngoscope blade such as a Miller 2 is appropriate for most children between 3 and 10 years of age. The tracheas of children older than 11 years are often more easily intubated with a curved laryngoscope blade, such as a Macintosh 3. Both straight and curved laryngoscope blades of various sizes should always be immediately available.

## Video Laryngoscopes

Video laryngoscopes are very useful tools for managing both the unexpected and expected difficult pediatric intubation. Video laryngoscopes have a camera and a light source near the tip of the blade and a separate video display. Although direct laryngoscopy requires a direct line of sight to the glottic opening and vocal cords, video laryngoscopy allows the anesthesia provider to view the glottic opening indirectly, without the need for aligning the oral, pharyngeal, and laryngeal axes (see Fig. 16.7). Thus, the major advantage of video laryngoscopy over direct laryngoscopy is the ability to see "around the corner" to view the glottic opening and vocal cords, even in patients with limited neck extension, hypoplastic mandibles, or "anterior" airways.

Video laryngoscopy is easier to learn than fiberoptic bronchoscopy because it mimics the skills of direct laryngoscopy. Video laryngoscopy is a better tool than direct laryngoscopy for teaching both the routine and difficult airway because both the student and teacher can view the monitor at the same time.

Video laryngoscopy requires adequate mouth opening to allow space both for placing the video laryngoscope for an optimal view and for manipulating the endotracheal tube so that it is able to pass through the vocal cords. Video laryngoscopy has been shown in studies to improve the ability to see the glottic opening and vocal cords in pediatric patients with both normal and difficult airways. However, these studies have also demonstrated the need for increased time to intubate, as well as higher failed intubation rates compared to direct laryngoscopy.[34,63,64]

### GlideScope Video Laryngoscopes

The GlideScope video laryngoscope consists of different types of both single-use and reusable video laryngoscopes. Digital cameras are mounted at the tips of the blades or the video batons. The video image is viewed on a stand-alone, high-resolution monitor. The newest GlideScopes are the titanium models that are available in both single-use and reusable models (see Fig. 16.15). The T3 is a curved bladed style suitable for children weighing more than 10 kg and the T4 is suitable for children more than 40 kg. Titanium models are not currently available in sizes suitable for neonates, infants, and children less than 10 kg. The GlideScope AVL models consist of a video baton inserted into a single-use plastic blade. The GVL 0 is designed for infants weighing less than 1.5 kg, the GVL 1 for infants from 1.5 to 3.0 kg, the GVL 2 for infants from 1.8 to 10 kg, and the GVL 2.5 for children from 10 to 28 kg (Table 16.8).

### C-MAC Video Laryngoscopes

The C-MAC video laryngoscope consists of a camera with a wide-angle lens mounted at the tip of a reusable stainless steel blade, with a video display on a stand-alone, high-resolution monitor. The blades are available in curved Macintosh shape in sizes 2, 3, and 4, as well as straight Miller shape in sizes 0 and 1 for neonates and infants, respectively. There is also a D blade that is more curved than the Macintosh blade and is designed for difficult airways (see Fig. 16.6). The D blade is available in two sizes, pediatric and adult, but is too large for infants and small children (see Table 16.8).

### McGrath MAC Video Laryngoscopes

The McGrath MAC video laryngoscope consists of a reusable video laryngoscope that is inserted into a single-use plastic curved blade, with a video display mounted on the handle of the laryngoscope. It is available in sizes 2, 3, and 4 corresponding to regular Macintosh blade sizes 2, 3, and 4, respectively. The McGrath MAC video

laryngoscopes are most suitable for children 4 years of age or older (see Table 16.8).

### Fiberoptic Bronchoscopes

A flexible fiberoptic bronchoscope is another tool for managing a difficult pediatric airway. It is particularly valuable when the patient's mouth opening or neck mobility is limited. Disadvantages of a fiberoptic bronchoscope include a limited field of vision and interference from bleeding and secretions. The smallest fiberoptic bronchoscopes are 2.2 mm in diameter and can be used for endotracheal tubes as small as 3.0 mm ID. These small bronchoscopes, however, do not have a suction channel; they also have optics inferior to larger scopes. In general, the fiberoptic bronchoscope should be at least 1 mm smaller in outside diameter than the ID of the endotracheal tube.

Infants and children are unlikely to be able to cooperate with an awake fiberoptic intubation. Therefore, it is easier to perform an asleep fiberoptic intubation. Some anesthesia providers prefer to maintain spontaneous ventilation during fiberoptic laryngoscopy and endotracheal intubation, especially if there is concern about the ability to ventilate the patient's lungs with a face mask. Frequently, it is easier to administer neuromuscular blocking drugs to a pediatric patient to provide better viewing conditions, including less movement, less fogging of the bronchoscope, and less chance of laryngospasm. Using

| Table 16.8 | Video Laryngoscopes Suitable for Infants, Children, Teenagers, and Adults |
| --- | --- |

| Age Group | Weight | Model |
| --- | --- | --- |
| Premature infants | <2.5 kg | GlideScope GVL 0<br>C-MAC Miller 0 |
| Neonates | 2.5-5 kg | GlideScope GVL 1<br>C-MAC Miller 1 |
| Infants/toddlers | 5-15 kg | GlideScope GVL 2<br>C-MAC Miller 1 |
| Small children | 15-30 kg | GlideScope GVL 2.5<br>C-MAC Macintosh 2<br>McGrath MAC 2 |
| Children/teenagers | 30-70 kg | GlideScope GVL 3<br>GlideScope Titanium S3 or T3<br>C-MAC Macintosh 3 or C-MAC D Blade Pediatric<br>McGrath MAC 3 |
| Teenagers/adults | >70 kg | GlideScope GVL 4<br>GlideScope Titanium S4 or T4<br>C-MAC Macintosh 4.<br>C-MAC D Blade Adult<br>McGrath MAC 4 |

an elbow with a port that permits insertion of the fiberoptic bronchoscope allows for either continued spontaneous ventilation or assisted positive-pressure ventilation through the face mask.

For nasal fiberoptic laryngoscopy and endotracheal intubation, a vasoconstrictor, such as oxymetazoline hydrochloride 0.05% nasal spray, should be administered to the nasal mucosa to prevent or minimize nasal bleeding, which makes viewing the glottis and vocal cords more challenging. Phenylephrine should not be administered for vasoconstriction to the nasal mucosa of infants and small children because of the risk of phenylephrine toxicity.

For oral fiberoptic laryngoscopy and endotracheal intubation, a supraglottic airway device can provide an excellent channel directly to the vocal cords by shielding the bronchoscope from secretions and blood. It is recommended to select the largest endotracheal tube that will easily fit through the s upraglottic airway device and the largest bronchoscope that will fit through the endotracheal tube. If a supraglottic airway device is used as a conduit for oral fiberoptic laryngoscopy and endotracheal intubation, it is simplest to leave the supraglottic airway device in place until the end of the procedure, while partially deflating the cuff to prevent unnecessary pressure on the mucosa of the oropharynx.

## Managing the Difficult Airway in Infants and Children

The same general principles for managing a normal pediatric airway apply to managing both an unexpected and an expected difficult pediatric airway (also see Chapter 34). It is unlikely that infants and children will cooperate with procedures, such as an awake fiberoptic endotracheal intubation. Therefore, it is often necessary to induce anesthesia and manage the airway with the patient asleep. Infants and children desaturate much more rapidly than adults because their oxygen consumption per kilogram is much higher than adults. This time constraint presents an additional challenge when managing both an unexpected and expected difficult airway in infants and children.

### Unexpected Difficult Airway

When an unexpected difficult airway occurs in pediatric patients, the most important first step is to call for an additional anesthesia colleague to help (Fig. 16.21), as well as a surgeon adept in surgical airway management if an emergent surgical airway is necessary. A pediatric difficult airway cart should be obtained. The contents should include additional airway equipment including appropriately sized video laryngoscopes, fiberoptic bronchoscopes, and supraglottic, nasal, and oral airways. It is critical that the anesthesia provider not persist with repeated attempts at direct laryngoscopy. This can result in trauma to the upper airway,

edema, and bleeding. In most situations, a supraglottic airway device should be inserted to oxygenate and ventilate the patient, and allow time to obtain additional personnel and airway equipment. If blood or significant secretions are in the airway, a video laryngoscope is a better option than a pediatric fiberoptic bronchoscope for viewing the glottis and intubating the trachea. Using a supraglottic airway device as a conduit for fiberoptic intubation can provide a channel that minimizes blood and secretions and allows for successful fiberoptic intubation.

### Expected Difficult Airway

An expected difficult airway in pediatric patients should be approached with caution. Only preanesthetic medications that have minimal ventilatory depressant effects, such as midazolam, should be used. These preanesthetic medications should be administered in a location with appropriate airway equipment, including suction and a method of delivering oxygen with positive pressure. Pulse oximetry monitoring should be initiated.

An additional anesthesia colleague should be available for help during the induction of anesthesia, inserting an IV line, and securing the airway. A surgeon capable of establishing a surgical airway and emergency airway equipment should be in the operating room before beginning the induction of anesthesia. The most difficult decision in managing an expected difficult pediatric airway is whether to attempt direct laryngoscopy or to proceed directly to an alternative strategy for managing the airway (i.e., supraglottic airway device, fiberoptic intubation, video laryngoscopy, or surgical airway). The history and physical examination may indicate situations in which direct laryngoscopy will not

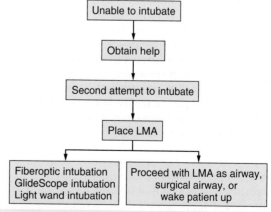

SIMPLIFIED DIFFICULT AIRWAY ALGORITHM
FOR INFANTS AND CHILDREN

Unable to intubate

Obtain help

Second attempt to intubate

Place LMA

Fiberoptic intubation
GlideScope intubation
Light wand intubation

Proceed with LMA as airway,
surgical airway, or
wake patient up

**Fig. 16.21** A suggested simplified algorithm for management of a difficult airway in infants and children. *LMA*, Laryngeal mask airway.

be successful, such as a patient in halo traction. In these cases, one should avoid direct laryngoscopy and proceed directly to an alternative strategy for managing the airway. As with the unexpected difficult airway, if direct laryngoscopy is not successful, one should not persist with direct laryngoscopy.

## Tracheal Extubation in Infants and Children

### Postextubation Croup
Infants and small children are at higher risk than adults for croup after endotracheal extubation (also see Chapter 34). Croup occurs most commonly when an uncuffed endotracheal tube that is too large or a cuffed endotracheal tube that is overinflated is used. The resulting pressure on the tracheal mucosa causes venous congestion and edema. In severe cases, the arterial blood supply can be compromised, causing mucosal ischemia. The resulting edema can narrow the tracheal lumen, especially in pediatric patients. Because resistance to flow through the airway is inversely proportional to the radius of the lumen to the fourth power, 1 mm of edema in a pediatric airway is much more significant than 1 mm of edema in an adult airway. Other risk factors for croup include multiple endotracheal intubation attempts, unusual positioning of the head during surgery, increased duration of surgery, and procedures involving the upper airway, such as rigid bronchoscopy.

### Manifestations
An infant or child with postextubation croup usually has respiratory distress in the postanesthesia care unit. Nasal flaring, retractions, an increased respiratory rate, audible stridor, and decreased oxygen saturation are common clinical findings.

### Treatment
Treatment of postextubation croup depends on the degree of respiratory distress. Mild symptoms can be managed with humidified oxygen and prolonged observation in the postanesthesia care unit. Severe cases may require aerosolized racemic epinephrine and postoperative observation in an intensive care unit. Patients whose respiratory distress is severe and not relieved with these measures may need to be reintubated with a smaller endotracheal tube. To prevent upper airway edema, steroids (e.g., dexamethasone) should be administered intravenously before the airway is instrumented in procedures such as rigid bronchoscopy.

### Obstructive Sleep Apnea
Infants and children with obstructive sleep apnea are at significant risk for airway obstruction, respiratory distress, and the potential for apnea in the postoperative period. At baseline, these infants and children hypoventilate, resulting in hypercapnia and often arterial hypoxemia when they sleep. Residual inhaled anesthetics or residual neuromuscular blockade can depress airway reflexes, decrease skeletal muscle tone and strength, and lower respiratory drive. This can result in significant airway compromise. Opioids must be very carefully titrated both intraoperatively and postoperatively, as they can depress the ventilatory drive and contribute to significant hypercapnia and arterial hypoxemia in these patients.

Tracheal extubation in patients with obstructive sleep apnea should occur only when they are fully awake. All infants and children with obstructive sleep apnea should be monitored postoperatively with pulse oximetry. High-risk patients should be monitored postoperatively in an intensive care unit setting.

### Laryngospasm
Infants and children are more prone to laryngospasm than older children and adults. Laryngospasm most commonly occurs during either inhalational induction of anesthesia or emergence from anesthesia, often after extubation or removal of a supraglottic airway device. Most of laryngospasm episodes in pediatric patients can be treated successfully with continuous positive-pressure ventilation via face mask with 100% $O_2$, while applying a chin lift and jaw thrust. The positive pressure may have to be as high as 50 cm $H_2O$ to successfully break the laryngospasm. If positive pressure is not successful and the infant or child is desaturating or bradycardic, further intervention is necessary. If there is IV access, laryngospasm should be treated with approximately 0.6 to 1.0 mg/kg of IV propofol and, if necessary, 0.2 to 0.3 mg/kg of IV rocuronium. If there is no IV access, laryngospasm should be treated with 0.6 to 1.0 mg/kg of intramuscular rocuronium or 1.5 to 2.0 mg/kg of intramuscular succinylcholine.[65]

### Extubation After a Difficult Intubation
Tracheal extubation of an infant or child after a difficult intubation should be considered carefully because reintubation can be more difficult than the initial intubation. The tracheas of infants and children with difficult airways should be extubated only when the patient is fully awake and there is no residual neuromuscular blockade. They should be extubated only when appropriate equipment and personnel are available for urgent reintubation.

Postoperative factors that can further compromise respiratory function must also be considered when extubating the trachea of an infant or child with a difficult intubation. For example, postoperative pain, especially if there is splinting from an abdominal or thoracic incision, may compromise respiratory function. Postoperative pain requiring significant opioid use will also compromise breathing by decreasing the respiratory drive. The use of regional anesthesia, such as a caudal or an epidural, may allow earlier extubation of these patients.

Edema of the airway from surgical trauma, positioning, or excessive fluid administration can significantly affect the ability to extubate the tracheas of infants and children with difficult intubations and can make emergency reintubation more difficult. Infants and children with postoperative airway edema and difficult airways should remain intubated until the edema has resolved. Fiberoptic bronchoscopy is an excellent tool for examining the supraglottic airway in the intubated infant or child for determining whether there is any significant residual airway edema.

## QUESTIONS OF THE DAY

1. What is the sensory and motor innervation of the larynx? What are the methods to provide topical anesthesia prior to awake fiberoptic intubation?
2. What physical examination findings predict difficult endotracheal intubation or difficult mask ventilation?
3. What are the risks and contraindications of using a supraglottic airway device instead of an endotracheal tube for airway management?
4. What are the advantages and disadvantages of video laryngoscopy versus conventional direct laryngoscopy or flexible fiberoptic laryngoscopy during routine airway management and difficult airway management?
5. What are the most important clinical differences in the following airway devices: plastic-coated metal endotracheal tube stylet, gum elastic bougie, and intubating stylet (e.g., Frova or Aintree)?
6. During a "cannot intubate, cannot ventilate" situation in which supraglottic airway placement has also failed, what are the relative advantages and disadvantages of cricothyrotomy versus transtracheal jet ventilation?
7. What are the most common complications after endotracheal extubation in adults and children? What is the expected time course of the complications?
8. What are the major differences between the airway anatomy of an infant compared to an adult?
9. When an uncuffed endotracheal tube is used in an infant, what steps should be taken to determine the appropriate size?

## REFERENCES

1. Apfelbaum JL, Hagberg CA, Caplan RA, et al. Practice guidelines for management of the difficult airway: an updated report by the American Society of Anesthesiologists Task Force on Management of the Difficult Airway. *Anesthesiology.* 2013;118(2):251–270.
2. Cook TM, MacDougall-Davis SR. Complications and failure of airway management. *Br J Anaesth.* 2012;109(suppl 1):i68–i85.
3. Sahin-Yilmaz A, Naclerio RM. Anatomy and physiology of the upper airway. *Proc Am Thorac Soc.* 2011;8(1):31–39.
4. Ovassapian A. *Fiberoptic Airway Endoscopy in Anesthesia and Critical Care.* New York: Raven Press; 1990.
5. Stackhouse RA. Fiberoptic airway management. *Anesthesiol Clin North Am.* 2002;20(4):933–951.
6. Patil VU, Stehling LC, Zauder HL. *Fiberoptic Endoscopy in Anesthesia.* St. Louis: Mosby; 1983.
7. Isaacs RS, Sykes JM. Anatomy and physiology of the upper airway. *Anesthesiol Clin North Am.* 2002;20(4):733–745.
8. Cook TM, Woodall N, Frerk C. Fourth National Audit Project. Major complications of airway management in the UK: results of the fourth national audit project of the royal college of anaesthetists and the difficult airway society. Part 1: anaesthesia. *Br J Anaesth.* 2011;106(5):617–631.
9. Shiga T, Wajima Z, Inoue T, Sakamoto A. Predicting difficult intubation in apparently normal patients: a meta-analysis of bedside screening test performance. *Anesthesiology.* 2005;103(2):429–437.
10. Baker P. Assessment before airway management. *Anesthesiol Clin.* 2015;33(2):257–278.
11. Khan ZH, Mohammadi M, Rasouli MR, et al. The diagnostic value of the upper lip bite test combined with sternomental distance, thyromental distance, and interincisor distance for prediction of easy laryngoscopy and intubation: a prospective study. *Anesth Analg.* 2009;109(3):822–824.
12. Mallampati SR, Gatt SP, Gugino LD, et al. A clinical sign to predict difficult tracheal intubation: a prospective study. *Can Anaesth Soc J.* 1985;32(4):429–434.
13. Samsoon G, Young J. Difficult tracheal intubation: a retrospective study. *Anaesthesia.* 1987;42(5):487–490.
14. Khan ZH, Kashfi A, Ebrahimkhani E. A comparison of the upper lip bite test (a simple new technique) with modified Mallampati classification in predicting difficulty in endotracheal intubation: a prospective blinded study. *Anesth Analg.* 2003;96(2):595–599.
15. El-Ganzouri AR, McCarthy RJ, Tuman KJ, et al. Preoperative airway assessment: predictive value of a multivariate risk index. *Anesth Analg.* 1996;82(6):1197–1204.
16. Bellhouse CP, Dore C. Criteria for estimating likelihood of difficulty of endotracheal intubation with the Macintosh laryngoscope. *Anaesth Intensive Care.* 1988;16(3):329–337.
17. Kheterpal S, Healy D, Aziz MF, et al. Incidence, predictors, and outcome of difficult mask ventilation combined with difficult laryngoscopy: a report from the multicenter perioperative outcomes group. *Anesthesiology.* 2013;119(6):1360–1369.
18. Law JA, Broemling N, Cooper RM, et al. The difficult airway with recommendations for management—part 2—the anticipated difficult airway. *Can J Anesth.* 2013;60(11):1119–1138.
19. Law JA, Broemling N, Cooper RM, et al. The difficult airway with recommendations for management—part 1—difficult tracheal intubation encountered in an unconscious/induced patient. *Can J Anesth.* 2013;60(11):1089–1118.
20. El-Orbany M, Woehlck HJ. Difficult mask ventilation. *Anesth Analg.* 2009;109(6):1870–1880.
21. Benumof JL, Dagg R, Benumof R. Critical hemoglobin desaturation will occur before return to an unparalyzed state following 1 mg/kg intravenous succinylcholine. *Anesthesiology.* 1997;87(4):979–982.
22. Bouroche G, Bourgain JL. Preoxygenation and general anesthesia: a review. *Minerva Anestesiol.* 2015;81(8):910–920.
23. Dixon BJ, Dixon JB, Carden JR, et al. Preoxygenation is more effective in the 25 degrees head-up position than in the supine position in severely obese patients: a randomized controlled study. *Anesthesiology.* 2005;(102):1110–1115.
24. Futier E, Constantin JM, Pelosi P, et al. Noninvasive ventilation and alveolar recruitment maneuver improve respiratory function during and after intubation of morbidly obese patients: a randomized controlled study. *Anesthesiology.* 2011;114(6):1354–1363.

25. Hernandez MR, Klock Jr PA, Ovassapian A. Evolution of the extraglottic airway: a review of its history, applications, and practical tips for success. *Anesth Analg.* 2012;114(2):349–368.

26. Timmermann A. Supraglottic airways in difficult airway management: successes, failures, use and misuse. *Anaesthesia.* 2011;66(suppl 2):45–56.

27. Ramachandran SK, Mathis MR, Tremper KK, et al. Predictors and clinical outcomes from failed laryngeal mask airway unique: a study of 15,795 patients. *Anesthesiology.* 2012;116(6):1217–1226.

28. Wong DT, Yang JJ, Jagannathan N. Brief review: the LMA supreme supraglottic airway. *Can J Anesth J.* 2012;59(5):483–493.

29. Cook T, Howes B. Supraglottic airway devices: recent advances. *Contin Educ Anaesth Crit Care Pain.* 2011;11(2):56–61.

30. Hagberg C. Current concepts in the management of difficult airway. *Anesthesiol News.* 2014;11(1):1–28.

31. Agro F, Frass M, Benumof JL, Krafft P. Current status of the Combitube: a review of the literature. *J Clin Anesth.* 2002;14(4):307–314.

32. Cormack R, Lehane J. Difficult tracheal intubation in obstetrics. *Anaesthesia.* 1984;39(11):1105–1111.

33. McKeen DM, George RB, O'Connell CM, et al. Difficult and failed intubation: incident rates and maternal, obstetrical, and anesthetic predictors. *Can J Anesth.* 2011;58(6):514–524.

34. Griesdale DE, Liu D, McKinney J, Choi PT. Glidescope® video-laryngoscopy versus direct laryngoscopy for endotracheal intubation: a systematic review and meta-analysis. *Can J Anesth.* 2012;59(1):41–52.

35. Aziz MF, Dillman D, Fu R, Brambrink AM. Comparative effectiveness of the C-MAC video laryngoscope versus direct laryngoscopy in the setting of the predicted difficult airway. *Anesthesiology.* 2012;116(3):629–636.

36. Cooper RM. Strengths and limitations of airway techniques. *Anesthesiol Clin.* 2015;33(2):241–255.

37. Paolini J, Donati F, Drolet P. Review article: video-laryngoscopy: another tool for difficult intubation or a new paradigm in airway management? *Can J Anesth.* 2013;60(2):184–191.

38. Aziz MF, Healy D, Kheterpal S, et al. Routine clinical practice effectiveness of the glidescope in difficult airway management: an analysis of 2,004 glidescope intubations, complications, and failures from two institutions. *Anesthesiology.* 2011;114(1):34–41.

39. Rosenstock CV, Thogersen B, Afshari A, et al. Awake fiberoptic or awake video laryngoscopic tracheal intubation in patients with anticipated difficult airway management: a randomized clinical trial. *Anesthesiology.* 2012;116(6):1210–1216.

40. Serocki G, Neumann T, Scharf E, et al. Indirect videolaryngoscopy with C-MAC D-blade and GlideScope: a randomized, controlled comparison in patients with suspected difficult airways. *Minerva Anestesiol.* 2013;79(2):121–129.

41. Duggan LV, Law JA, Murphy MF. Brief review: supplementing oxygen through an airway exchange catheter: efficacy, complications, and recommendations. *Can J Anesth.* 2011;58(6):560–568.

42. Simmons ST, Schleich AR. Airway regional anesthesia for awake fiberoptic intubation. *Reg Anesth Pain Med.* 2002;27(2):180–192.

43. Sengupta P, Sessler DI, Maglinger P, et al. Endotracheal tube cuff pressure in three hospitals, and the volume required to produce an appropriate cuff pressure. *BMC Anesthesiol.* 2004;4(1):8.

44. Smith KJ, Dobranowski J, Yip G, et al. Cricoid pressure displaces the esophagus: an observational study using magnetic resonance imaging. *Anesthesiology.* 2003;99(1):60–64.

45. Ovassapian A, Salem MR. Sellick's maneuver: to do or not do. *Anesth Analg.* 2009;109(5):1360–1362.

46. Rice MJ, Mancuso AA, Gibbs C, et al. Cricoid pressure results in compression of the postcricoid hypopharynx: the esophageal position is irrelevant. *Anesth Analg.* 2009;109(5):1546–1552.

47. Schaumann N, Lorenz V, Schellongowski P, et al. Evaluation of Seldinger technique emergency cricothyroidotomy versus standard surgical cricothyroidotomy in 200 cadavers. *J Am Soc Anesthesiol.* 2005;102(1):7–11.

48. Kristensen MS, Teoh WH, Baker PA. Percutaneous emergency airway access; prevention, preparation, technique and training. *Br J Anaesth.* 2015;114(3):357–361.

49. Hamaekers A, Henderson J. Equipment and strategies for emergency tracheal access in the adult patient. *Anaesthesia.* 2011;66(suppl 2):65–80.

50. Ross-Anderson DJ, Ferguson C, Patel A. Transtracheal jet ventilation in 50 patients with severe airway compromise and stridor. *Br J Anaesth.* 2011;106(1):140–144.

51. Dhara SS. Retrograde tracheal intubation. *Anaesthesia.* 2009;64(10):1094–1104.

52. Mitchell V, Dravid R, Patel A, et al. Difficult airway society guidelines for the management of tracheal extubation. *Anaesthesia.* 2012;67(3):318–340.

53. Cavallone LF, Vannucci A. Review article: extubation of the difficult airway and extubation failure. *Anesth Analg.* 2013;116(2):368–383.

54. Warner ME, Benenfeld SM, Warner MA, et al. Perianesthetic dental injuries: frequency, outcomes, and risk factors. *Anesthesiology.* 1999;90(5):1302–1305.

55. Hagberg C, Georgi R, Krier C. Complications of managing the airway. *Best Pract Res Clin Anaesthesiol.* 2005;19(4):641–659.

56. Schloss B, Rice J, Tobias JD. The laryngeal mask in infants and children: what is the cuff pressure? *Int J Pediatr Otorhinolaryngol.* 2012;76(2):284–286.

57. Jagannathan N, Sohn L, Sommers K, et al. A randomized comparison of the laryngeal mask airway supreme and laryngeal mask airway unique in infants and children: does cuff pressure influence leak pressure? *Pediatr Anesth.* 2013;23(10):927–933.

58. Tobias JD, Schwartz L, Rice J, et al. Cuffed endotracheal tubes in infants and children: should we routinely measure the cuff pressure? *Int J Pediatr Otorhinolaryngol.* 2012;76(1):61–63.

59. Weiss M, Dullenkopf A, Fischer JE, et al. European Paediatric Endotracheal Intubation Study Group. Prospective randomized controlled multi-centre trial of cuffed or uncuffed endotracheal tubes in small children. *Br J Anaesth.* 2009;103(6):867–873.

60. Litman RS, Maxwell LG. Cuffed versus uncuffed endotracheal tubes in pediatric anesthesia: the debate should finally end. *Anesthesiology.* 2013;118(3):500–501.

61. Liu J, Zhang X, Gong W, et al. Correlations between controlled endotracheal tube cuff pressure and postprocedural complications: a multicenter study. *Anesth Analg.* 2010;111(5):1133–1137.

62. Sathyamoorthy M, Lerman J, Lakshminrusimha S, Feldman D. Inspiratory stridor after tracheal intubation with a MicroCuff(R) tracheal tube in three young infants. *Anesthesiology.* 2013;118(3):748–750.

63. Sun Y, Lu Y, Huang Y, Jiang H. Pediatric video laryngoscope versus direct laryngoscope: a meta-analysis of randomized controlled trials. *Pediatr Anesth.* 2014;24(10):1056–1065.

64. Fiadjoe JE, Gurnaney H, Dalesio N, et al. A prospective randomized equivalence trial of the GlideScope cobalt® video laryngoscopy to traditional direct laryngoscopy in neonates and infants. *Anesthesiology.* 2012;116(3):622–628.

65. Orliaguet GA, Gall O, Savoldelli GL, Couloigner V. Case scenario: perianesthetic management of laryngospasm in children. *Anesthesiology.* 2012;116(2):458–471.

# 17 SPINAL, EPIDURAL, AND CAUDAL ANESTHESIA

## Alan J.R. Macfarlane, Richard Brull, and Vincent W.S. Chan

## PRINCIPLES

Spinal, epidural, and caudal blocks are collectively referred to as *central neuraxial blocks*. Significant technical, physiologic, and pharmacologic differences exist between the techniques, although all result in one or a combination of sympathetic, sensory, and motor blockade. Spinal anesthesia requires a small amount of drug to produce rapid, profound, reproducible, but finite sensory analgesia. In contrast, epidural anesthesia progresses more slowly, is commonly prolonged using a catheter, and requires a large amount of local anesthetic, which may be associated with

The editors and publisher would like to thank Drs. Kenneth Drasner and Merlin D. Larson for contributing to this chapter in the previous edition of this work. It has served as the foundation for the current chapter.

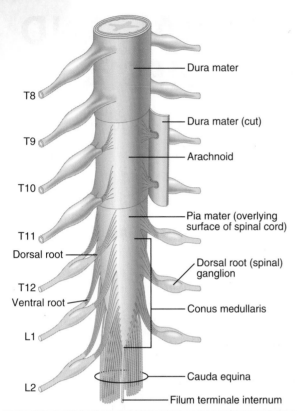

**Fig. 17.1** Terminal spinal cord and cauda equina. (From Bridenbaugh PO, Greene NM, Brull SJ. Spinal [subarachnoid] blockade. In Cousins MJ, Bridenbaugh PO, eds. *Neural Blockade in Clinical Anesthesia and Management of Pain.* Philadelphia: Lippincott-Raven; 1998:203-242.)

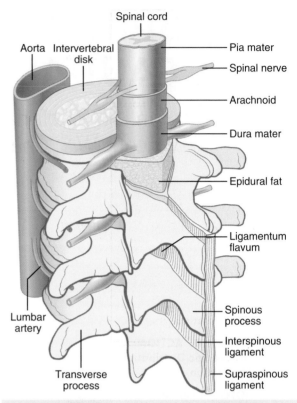

**Fig. 17.2** The spine in an oblique view. (From Afton-Bird G. Atlas of regional anesthesia. In Miller RD, ed. *Miller's Anesthesia.* Philadelphia: Elsevier; 2005.)

Chapter 44). Indwelling long-term spinal catheters may be inserted for chronic malignant and nonmalignant pain.

## ANATOMY

The spinal cord is continuous with the medulla oblongata proximally and terminates distally in the conus medullaris as the filum terminale (fibrous extension) and the cauda equina (neural extension) (Fig. 17.1). This distal termination varies from L3 in infants to the lower border of L1 in adults.

The spinal cord lies within the bony vertebral column, surrounded by three membranes: from innermost to outermost the pia mater, the arachnoid mater, and the dura mater (Fig. 17.2). Cerebrospinal fluid (CSF) resides in the *subarachnoid (or intrathecal) space* between the pia mater and the arachnoid mater. The pia mater is a highly vascular membrane that closely invests the spinal cord and brain. The arachnoid mater is a delicate, nonvascular membrane that functions as the principal barrier to drugs crossing into (and out of) the CSF.[4] The dura is a tough fibroelastic membrane.

Surrounding the dura is the epidural space, extending from the foramen magnum to the sacral hiatus. The epidural space is bounded anteriorly by the posterior longitudinal ligament, laterally by the pedicles and intervertebral foramina, and posteriorly by the ligamentum

## PRACTICE

Neuraxial blockade is widely utilized in surgery, obstetrics, acute postoperative pain management, and chronic pain relief. Single-injection spinal or epidural anesthesia is commonly used for surgery to the lower abdomen, pelvic organs (e.g., prostate), and lower limbs and for cesarean deliveries. Continuous catheter-based epidural infusions are used for obstetric labor analgesia and to provide postoperative pain relief for days after major surgery (e.g., thoracic, abdominal, lower limb). Neuraxial analgesia can reduce pulmonary and possibly cardiac morbidity, although the mortality benefits appear minimal.[1-3] More recently, the goals of epidural analgesia have shifted to facilitation of fast-track surgery recovery. Caudal blocks are mostly performed for surgical anesthesia and analgesia in children (also see Chapter 34) and for therapeutic analgesia in adults with chronic pain (also see

systemic side effects and complications unknown to spinal anesthesia. Combined spinal and epidural techniques blur some of these differences but add flexibility to clinical care.

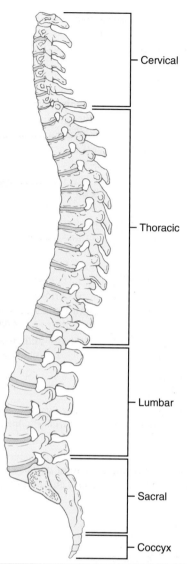

Fig. 17.3 The vertebral column from a lateral view exhibits four curvatures. (From Covino BG, Scott DB, Lambert DH. *Handbook of Spinal Anaesthesia and Analgesia*. Philadelphia: WB Saunders; 1994:12-24.)

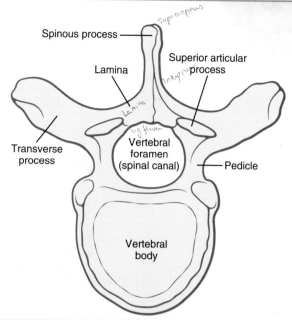

Fig. 17.4 Typical thoracic vertebra. (From Covino BG, Scott DB, Lambert DH. *Handbook of Spinal Anaesthesia and Analgesia*. Philadelphia: WB Saunders; 1994.)

flavum. Contents include nerve roots, fat, areolar tissue, lymphatics, and blood vessels.

The ligamentum flavum (the so-called "yellow ligament") also extends from the foramen magnum to the sacral hiatus. Although classically portrayed as a single ligament, it is actually composed of the right and left ligamenta flava, which join to form an acute midline angle with a ventral opening (see Fig. 17.2).[5] The ligamentum flavum thickness, distance to the dura, and skin-to-dura distance vary with the area of the vertebral canal. The vertebral canal is triangular and largest in area at the lumbar levels, and it is circular and smallest in area at the thoracic levels. Immediately posterior to the ligamentum flavum are either the lamina of vertebral bodies or the interspinous ligaments (that connect the spinous processes). Finally there is the supraspinous ligament, which extends from the external occipital protuberance to the coccyx and attaches to the vertebral spines (see Fig. 17.2).

There are 7 cervical, 12 thoracic, and 5 lumbar vertebrae and a sacrum (Fig. 17.3). The vertebral arch, spinous process, pedicles, and laminae form the posterior elements of the vertebra, and the vertebral body forms the anterior element (Fig. 17.4). The vertebrae are joined together anteriorly by the fibrocartilaginous joints with central disks containing the nucleus pulposus, and posteriorly by the zygapophyseal (facet) joints. Thoracic spinous processes are angulated more steeply caudad as opposed to the almost horizontal angulation of the lumbar spinous processes. The differences between the caudal and lumbar spinous processes are clinically important for needle insertion and advancement (Fig. 17.5).

The sacral canal contains the terminal portion of the dural sac, which typically ends at S2 in adults and lower in children. The sacral canal also contains a venous plexus.

## Spinal Nerves

Dorsal (afferent) and ventral (efferent) nerve roots merge distal to the dorsal root ganglion to form spinal nerves (Fig. 17.6). There are 31 pairs of spinal nerves (8 cervical, 12 thoracic, 5 lumbar, 5 sacral, and 1 coccygeal). The nerves pass through the intervertebral foramen, becoming ensheathed by the dura, arachnoid, and pia, which, respectively, become the epineurium, the perineurium, and the endoneurium. Preganglionic sympathetic fibers originate

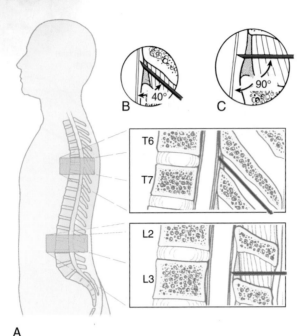

**A**

**Fig. 17.5** Lumbar and thoracic epidural technique. The increased angle of needle insertion during thoracic epidural cannulation may provide a slightly longer distance of "needle travel" before entering the epidural space (A). In contrast to lumbar epidural cannulation (B), the distance traveled is modified by a more perpendicular angle of needle insertion (C). (From Brull R, Macfarlane AJR, Chan VWS. Spinal, epidural, and caudal anesthesia. In Miller RD, Cohen NH, Eriksson LI, et al, eds. *Miller's Anesthesia*. 8th ed. Philadelphia: Saunders Elsevier; 2015:Fig. 56-9.)

in the intermediolateral gray columns between T1 and L2 and pass via the ventral nerve root to the paravertebral sympathetic ganglia and more distant plexuses (Fig. 17.7).

## Blood Supply

Two posterior spinal arteries supply the posterior one third of the spinal cord, whereas the anterior two thirds of the spinal cord are supplied by a single anterior spinal artery (Fig. 17.8). One of the largest anastomotic feeder arteries to the anterior system is the artery of Adamkiewicz, which arises from the aorta and enters an intervertebral foramen between T7 and L4 on the left. Ischemia within the anterior system leads to *anterior spinal artery syndrome,* manifested as anterior horn motor neuron injury along with disruption of pain and temperature sensation below the level affected. Ischemia may result from any one or a combination of profound hypotension, mechanical obstruction, vasculopathy, or hemorrhage.

Longitudinal anterior and posterior spinal veins communicate with segmental anterior and posterior radicular veins before draining into the internal vertebral venous plexus in the medial and lateral components of the epidural space. These drain into the azygous system.

## Anatomic Variations

Variations exist in size and structure of the spinal nerve roots as well as CSF volume, both of which may contribute to variability in spinal block quality, height, and regression time. Similarly, the epidural space is more segmented and less uniform than previously believed, which

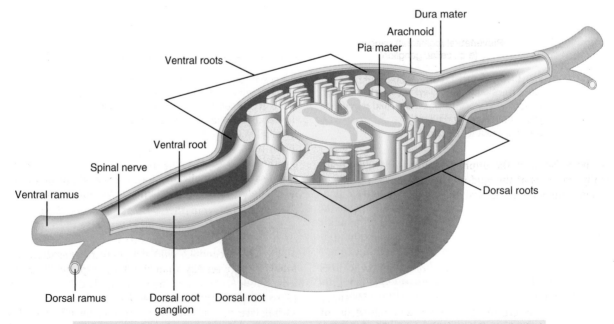

**Fig. 17.6** The spinal cord and nerve roots. (From Covino BG, Scott DB, Lambert DH. *Handbook of Spinal Anaesthesia and Analgesia*. Philadelphia: WB Saunders; 1994:19.)

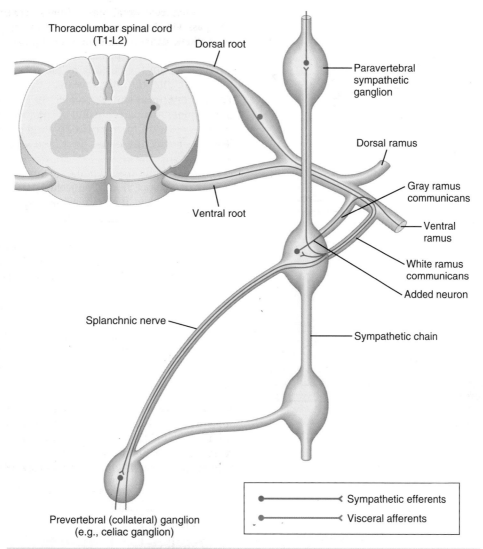

Thoracolumbar spinal cord
(T1-L2)

Dorsal root

Paravertebral
sympathetic
ganglion

Dorsal ramus

Gray ramus
communicans

Ventral
ramus

Ventral root

White ramus
communicans

Added neuron

Splanchnic nerve

Sympathetic chain

Prevertebral (collateral) ganglion
(e.g., celiac ganglion)

Sympathetic efferents

Visceral afferents

**Fig. 17.7** Cell bodies in the thoracolumbar portion of the spinal cord (T1-L2) give rise to the peripheral sympathetic nervous system. Preganglionic efferent fibers travel in the ventral root and then via the white ramus communicans to paravertebral sympathetic ganglia or more distant sites such as the celiac ganglion. Afferent fibers travel via the white ramus communicans to join somatic nerves, which pass through the dorsal root to the spinal cord.

may be a factor in the unpredictability of drug spread. Finally, contents of the epidural space also vary and can influence the volume of local anesthetic required.

## MECHANISM OF ACTION

Local anesthetics disrupt nerve transmission within the spinal cord, the spinal nerve roots, and the dorsal root ganglia. Nerves in the subarachnoid space are easily anesthetized, even with a small dose of local anesthetic, compared with the extradural nerves, which are often ensheathed by dura mater (the "dural

sleeve"). The speed of neural blockade depends on the size, surface area, and degree of myelination of the nerve fibers exposed to the local anesthetic. The small preganglionic sympathetic fibers (B fibers, 1 to 3 μm, minimally myelinated) are most sensitive to local anesthetic blockade. The C fibers (0.3 to 1 μm, unmyelinated), which conduct cold temperature sensation, are blocked more readily than the A-delta pinprick sensation fibers (1 to 4 μm, myelinated). The A-beta fibers (5 to 12 μm, myelinated), which conduct touch sensation, are the last sensory fibers to be affected. The larger A-alpha motor fibers (12 to 20 μm, myelinated) are the most resistant to local anesthetic blockade.

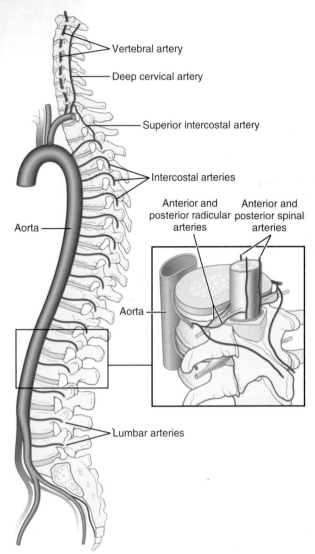

Vertebral artery

Deep cervical artery

Superior intercostal artery

Intercostal arteries

Anterior and posterior radicular arteries

Anterior and posterior spinal arteries

Aorta

Aorta

Lumbar arteries

**Fig. 17.8** Arterial blood supply to the spinal cord. (Modified from Covino BG, Scott DB, Lambert DH. *Handbook of Spinal Anaesthesia and Analgesia.* Philadelphia: WB Saunders; 1994:24.)

Regression of blockade ("recovery") follows in the reverse order.[6] Maximum block height varies according to each sensory modality, termed *differential sensory block.* Therefore, cold sensation (also an approximate level of sympathetic blockade) is most cephalad and is on average one to two spinal segments higher than the level of pinprick anesthesia, which in turn is one to two segments higher than anesthesia to touch.

## Drug Uptake and Distribution

Local anesthetic injected directly into the CSF diffuses from areas of high concentration toward other segments of the spinal cord.[7] Rostral spread, often evident within 10 to 20 minutes, is related to the CSF circulation time. Local anesthetic also diffuses through the pia mater and penetrates through the spaces of Virchow-Robin (extensions of the subarachnoid space accompanying the blood vessels that invaginate the spinal cord from the pia mater) to reach the deeper dorsal root ganglia. A portion of the subarachnoid drug diffuses outward to enter the epidural space, and some is taken up by the blood vessels of the pia and dura maters.

Drug penetration and uptake are directly proportionate to the drug mass, CSF drug concentration, contact surface area, lipid content (high in spinal cord and myelinated nerves), and local tissue vascular supply, but inversely related to nerve root size.

Epidural drug uptake and distribution are more complex. Some of the injected local anesthetic (<20%) moves from the epidural space into the CSF to exert its neural blocking effect, whereas some is lost through either vascular absorption, uptake into epidural fat, or exit via the intervertebral foramina. Other local anesthetic spreads by bulk flow longitudinally and circumferentially within the epidural space. Factors that may enhance the distribution of local anesthetic within the epidural space are small caliber (greater spread in the thoracic space), decreased epidural space compliance, decreased epidural fat content, decreased local anesthetic leakage through the intervertebral foramina (e.g., in the elderly and those with spinal stenosis), and increased epidural pressure (e.g., during pregnancy).[8] The direction of drug spread also varies with the vertebral level. Spread is mostly cephalad in the lumbar and low thoracic region, but caudad after a high thoracic injection.[8]

## Drug Elimination

No drug metabolism takes place in the CSF. Regression of neural blockade results from a decline in the CSF drug concentration caused by non-neural tissue uptake and, most importantly, vascular absorption. Increased spread exposes the drug to a larger area for vascular absorption and thus a shorter duration of action. Lipid-soluble local anesthetics (e.g., bupivacaine) bind to epidural fat to form a depot that can slow vascular absorption.

## PHYSIOLOGIC EFFECTS

Neuraxial anesthesia evokes blockade of the sympathetic and somatic (sensory and motor) nervous systems. The physiologic effects of epidural anesthesia are similar to those of spinal anesthesia, with the exception that local anesthetic blood levels reach concentrations sufficient enough to produce systemic effects on their own.

## Cardiovascular

Blockade of the peripheral (T1-L2) and cardiac (T1-T4) sympathetic fibers as well as adrenal medullary catecholamine secretion reduces systemic vascular resistance (SVR) and, to a much lesser extent, cardiac output. The degree to which arterial blood pressure decreases with either spinal or epidural technique depends on multiple factors.

### Systemic Vascular Resistance

The vasodilatory changes depend on both baseline sympathetic tone (i.e., higher sympathetic tone in the elderly equates to a greater hemodynamic change) and the extent of the sympathectomy (i.e., the height of the block). The sympathectomy typically extends for two to six dermatomes above the sensory block level with spinal anesthesia but the same level with epidural anesthesia.[9] If normal cardiac output is maintained, SVR should decrease only 15% to 18% after neuraxial blockade in healthy normovolemic patients, even with near total sympathectomy.

### Cardiac Output

Cardiac output is the product of heart rate and stroke volume and it is generally either maintained or slightly decreased during the onset of spinal anesthesia. Venous and arterial vasodilation reduces preload (venous return) and afterload (SVR), respectively. Because 75% of the total blood volume resides in the venous system, the venodilation effect predominates and stroke volume is reduced. Despite a compensatory baroreceptor-mediated sympathetic response (vasoconstriction and increased heart rate) above the level of blockade, the reduction in venous return and right atrial filling reduce signal output from intrinsic atrial and great vein chronotropic stretch receptors,[9] thereby increasing parasympathetic activity. The two opposing responses result in a minimal change in heart rate unless neuraxial anesthesia is extended to the T1 level when blockade of the cardioaccelerator fibers (in addition to a marked reduction in venous return) may result in severe bradycardia and even asystole. The Bezold-Jarisch reflex can also cause profound bradycardia and circulatory collapse after spinal anesthesia, especially in the presence of hypovolemia, when a small end-systolic left ventricular volume may trigger a mechanoreceptor-mediated bradycardia.[10]

### Coronary Blood Flow

A decrease in mean arterial pressure is paralleled by a decrease in coronary blood flow. However, a high thoracic block in patients with ischemic heart disease may be beneficial, with improvement in global and regional myocardial function and reversal of ischemic changes likely owing to reduced myocardial oxygen demand and left ventricular afterload.[11]

## Central Nervous System

Spinal anesthesia–induced hypotension may decrease regional cerebral blood flow (CBF) in elderly patients and those with preexisting hypertension. However, in studies that demonstrated a decrease in cerebral perfusion,[12] there was no postoperative change in cognitive function in any of the patients. Nevertheless avoiding hypotension would seem prudent.

## Respiratory

Alterations in pulmonary variables during neuraxial block are usually of little clinical importance. A decrease in vital capacity follows a reduction in expiratory reserve volume related to paralysis of the abdominal muscles necessary for forced exhalation rather than a decrease in phrenic or diaphragmatic function. These changes are more marked in obese patients and may affect patients with severe respiratory disease.[13] Respiratory arrest can rarely occur owing to hypoperfusion of the respiratory centers in the brainstem but this almost always disappears once cardiac output and arterial blood pressure are restored.

## Gastrointestinal

Neuraxial blockade from T6 to L1 disrupts splanchnic sympathetic innervation to the gastrointestinal tract, resulting in a contracted gut and hyperperistalsis because of unopposed parasympathetic (vagal) activity. Nausea and vomiting may occur in as many as 20% of patients. Atropine is effective in treating nausea associated with extensive (T5) subarachnoid anesthesia.

Thoracic epidural anesthesia (TEA) has a direct arterial blood pressure–dependent effect on intestinal perfusion.[14] Correction of systemic hypotension by vasopressor therapy (e.g., norepinephrine) reverses impaired colonic perfusion. Nevertheless, TEA may improve anastomotic mucosal blood flow in patients undergoing esophagectomy and may even reduce the rate of anastomotic leak after emergency laparotomy, esophageal surgery, and other gastrointestinal interventions.

## Renal

Despite a predictable decrease in renal blood flow accompanying neuraxial blockade, this decrease is of little physiologic importance. The belief that neuraxial blocks frequently cause urinary retention is questionable (see "Complications" later in the chapter).

## INDICATIONS

### Neuraxial Anesthesia

Single injection spinal anesthesia is useful for procedures of known duration that involve the lower extremities, perineum, pelvic girdle, or lower abdomen. It may also be indicated when patients wish to remain conscious or when some comorbid condition, such as severe respiratory disease or an airway that may be difficult to manage, increases the risks of using general anesthesia. Epidural anesthesia allows for more prolonged surgical anesthesia by catheter-based local anesthetic delivery. Indwelling catheter-based spinal anesthesia is less conventional, but may be useful when insertion of an epidural catheter is challenging or in the setting of severe cardiac disease when the reliability of a single-shot spinal anesthetic must be combined with more hemodynamically stable incremental dosing.

### Neuraxial Analgesia

Intrathecal or epidural local anesthetics along with other additives, such as opioids either alone or in combination, can provide excellent quality, long-lasting intra- and postoperative analgesia in labor and delivery[15] (also see Chapter 33), during and after hip[16] or knee replacement[17] (also see Chapter 32), in laparotomy,[18] in thoracotomy (also see Chapter 37),[19] and increasingly even in cardiac surgery (also see Chapter 25).[20] They may also be used in the management of chronic pain (also see Chapter 44).

## CONTRAINDICATIONS

### Absolute

The most important problems include patient refusal, localized sepsis, and an allergy to any of the drugs to be administered. A patient's inability to maintain stillness during needle puncture (which could expose the neural structures to traumatic injury),[21] as well as increased intracranial pressure (which may theoretically predispose to brainstem herniation)[22] may be absolute contraindications to a neuraxial technique.

### Relative

Relative contraindications can be approached by system and must be weighed against the potential benefits of neuraxial blockade.

#### Neurologic
##### Myelopathy or Peripheral Neuropathy
Although preexisting central or peripheral neurologic deficit has never been definitively demonstrated to increase susceptibility of injury following neuraxial anesthesia or analgesia (the double-crush phenomenon), the risk-benefit ratio of performing neuraxial techniques should be considered especially in patients with preexisting central or peripheral neurologic diseases such as multiple sclerosis (MS) or diabetic polyneuropathy. Chronic low back pain without neurologic deficit is not a contraindication to neuraxial blockade.

#### Spinal Stenosis
There is an association between the presence of spinal stenosis and nerve injury following neuraxial techniques,[23] but the relative contribution of surgical factors and natural history of the spinal disease itself is unknown.

#### Spine Surgery
Previous spine surgery does not predispose patients to an increased risk of neurologic complications.[23] However, in the presence of scar tissue, adhesions, hardware, or bone grafts, needle access to the CSF or epidural space and epidural catheter insertion may be challenging or impossible. In addition, the resultant spread of local anesthetic in the CSF or epidural space in particular can be unpredictable and incomplete.

#### Multiple Sclerosis
Patients with MS may be more sensitive to neuraxial local anesthetics and exhibit a prolonged motor and sensory blockade. Any association between neuraxial anesthesia and exacerbation of MS symptoms is not based in evidence.[24]

#### Spina Bifida
Depending on the severity of the neural tube defect the potential for traumatic needle injury to the spinal cord may be increased. The spread of local anesthetic in the CSF and epidural space (if present) can be markedly variable. In any of these circumstances, a careful evaluation of neurologic status must first be undertaken and noted along with documentation of the discussion of the risks and benefits.

#### Cardiac (Also See Chapter 25)
##### Aortic Stenosis or Fixed Cardiac Output
The potential rapid and significant reduction in SVR after spinal anesthesia is in theory a risk in preload-dependent patients and may dangerously decrease coronary perfusion.[25] In the presence of aortic stenosis, neuraxial anesthesia must be considered on an individual patient basis in the context of disease severity, left ventricular function, and case urgency. A catheter-based neuraxial anesthetic with repeated small doses of local anesthetic may allow better hemodynamic control.

## Hypovolemia

An exaggerated hypotensive response because of vasodilatory effects may occur.

## Hematologic

### Thromboprophylaxis and Anticoagulants

Catastrophic cases of spinal hematoma causing paralysis associated with low-molecular-weight heparin (LMWH) have occurred. A summary of the American Society of Regional Anesthesia and Pain Medicine (ASRA) and other professional society guidelines regarding neuraxial techniques (including catheter removal) in patients receiving antithrombotic or thrombolytic therapy is reproduced in Table 17.1.

### Inherited Coagulopathy

Hemorrhagic complications after neuraxial techniques in patients with known hemophilia, von Willebrand disease, or idiopathic thrombocytopenic purpura appear infrequently when factor levels are more than 0.5 IU/mL for factor VIII, von Willebrand factor, and ristocetin cofactor activity, or when the platelet count is more than $50 \times 10^9$/L before block performance. The minimum safe factor levels and platelet count for neuraxial blockade remain undefined in both the obstetric and general populations.[26]

## Infection

Theoretical concerns exist regarding iatrogenic seeding of the neuraxis in the setting of a systemic infection, particularly if a catheter is left in situ. This, along with profound vasodilation, may be sufficient reason to avoid neuraxial techniques in patients with significant bacteremia or septic shock. Some providers avoid neuraxial techniques in febrile patients yet a lumbar puncture is a critical component of the investigation of fever of unknown origin. Patients with evidence of systemic infection may safely undergo neuraxial anesthesia once antibiotic therapy has demonstrated a response.[27]

## SPINAL ANESTHESIA

## Factors Affecting Block Height

The dermatomal levels required for various surgical procedures are outlined in Fig. 17.9. Intra-abdominal structures such as the peritoneum (T4), bladder (T10), and uterus (T10) have a spinal segment innervation that may be much more cephalad than the corresponding skin incision used to operate on these structures. Drug, patient, and procedural factors can all affect the distribution of local anesthetic spread within the intrathecal space,[28] but not all are controllable by the anesthesia provider, leading to significant interpatient variability (Table 17.2). Ultimately dose, baricity, and patient positioning are most important.

## Drug Factors

### Baricity

Baricity is the ratio of the density of a local anesthetic solution to the density of CSF. It is conventionally defined at 37° C because density varies inversely with temperature. Plain bupivacaine 0.5%, for example, may be isobaric at 24° C but is slightly hypobaric at 37° C. The density of CSF is 1.00059 g/L. Local anesthetic solutions that have the same density as CSF are termed *isobaric*, those that have a higher density than CSF are termed *hyperbaric*, and those with a lower density are termed *hypobaric*. Dextrose and sterile water are commonly added to render local anesthetic solutions either hyperbaric or hypobaric respectively. Hyperbaric solutions have a more predictable spread,[29] preferentially moving to the dependent regions of the spinal canal. Hypobaric solutions spread to nondependent regions whereas isobaric solutions tend not to be influenced by gravitational forces. The administration of hyperbaric local anesthetic to patients in the lateral decubitus position will therefore preferentially affect the dependent side. The natural curvatures of the vertebral column influence local anesthetic spread in patients placed in the horizontal supine position immediately after intrathecal administration. Hyperbaric local anesthetics injected at the L3-L4 or L4-L5 interspace will spread from the height of the lumbar lordosis down toward the trough of the thoracic kyphosis, resulting in a higher level of anesthetic effect than isobaric or hypobaric solutions.[28]

### Dose, Volume, and Concentration

Dose, volume, and concentration are inextricably linked (volume × concentration = dose), but dose is the most reliable determinant of local anesthetic spread (and thus block height) of isobaric and hypobaric solutions.[30] Hyperbaric local anesthetic injections are primarily influenced by baricity.

The choice of local anesthetic or additive drugs (other than opioids) does not influence spread if all other factors are controlled. Opioids may increase mean spread,[28] possibly as a result of pharmacologic enhancement at the extremes of the spread where the local anesthetic block alone would have been subclinical.[31]

### Patient Factors

Many patient factors can influence the number of spinal levels which are anesthetized (blocked) from a spinal anesthetic. These factors include extremes of height (short or tall), weight (thin or obese), age (children or the elderly), and gender. Within the range of "normal-sized" adults, a patient's height does not affect the spread of spinal anesthesia. However, the vertebral column length, which is related to the local anesthetic spread, should influence the dosage.

Although lumbosacral CSF pressure is fairly constant, the CSF volume varies between patients, which influences peak block height and regression.[32] Although block height

III

**Table 17.1**  Neuraxial[a] Anesthesia in the Patient Receiving Thromboprophylaxis

| Resource | Antiplatelet Medications | Subcutaneous UFH | Intravenous UFH | LMWH |
|---|---|---|---|---|
| German Society for Anaesthesiology and Intensive Care Medicine[b] | NSAIDs: no contraindication; hold LMWH, fondaparinux 36-42 h Thienopyridines and GPIIb/IIIa are contraindicated | Needle placement 4 h after heparin; heparin 1 h after needle placement or catheter removal | Needle placement and/or catheter removal 4 h after discontinuing heparin, heparinize 1 h after neuraxial technique; delay bypass surgery 12 h if traumatic | Neuraxial technique 10-12 h after LMWH; next dose 4 h after needle or catheter placement Delay block for 24 h after therapeutic dose |
| Belgian Association for Regional Anesthesia[c] | NSAIDs: no contraindication Discontinue ticlopidine 14 d, clopidogrel 7 d, GPIIb/IIIa inhibitors 8-48 h in advance | Not discussed | Heparinize 1 h after neuraxial technique Remove catheter during normal aPTT; reheparinize 1 h later | Neuraxial technique 10-12 h after LMWH; next dose 4 h after needle or catheter placement Delay block for 24 h after therapeutic dose |
| American Society of Regional Anesthesia and Pain Medicine | NSAIDs: no contraindication. Discontinue ticlopidine 14 d, clopidogrel 7 d, GPIIb/IIIa inhibitors 8-48 h in advance | No contraindication with twice-daily dosing and total daily dose <10,000 U; consider delay heparin until after block if technical difficulty anticipated. The safety of neuraxial blockade in patients receiving doses greater than 10,000 units of UFH daily, or more than twice daily dosing of UFH has not been established. | Heparinize 1 h after neuraxial technique, remove catheter 2-4 h after last heparin dose; no mandatory delay if traumatic | Twice-daily dosing: LMWH 24 h after surgery, regardless of technique; remove neuraxial catheter 2 h before first LMWH dose Single-daily dosing: according to European statements BUT with no additional hemostasis-altering drugs Therapeutic dose: delay block for 24 h |
| American College of Chest Physicians[d] | NSAIDs: no contraindication Discontinue clopidogrel 7 d before neuraxial block | Needle placement 8-12 h after dose; subsequent dose 2 h after block or catheter withdrawal | Needle placement delayed until anticoagulant effect is minimal | Needle placement 8-12 h after dose; subsequent dose 2 h after block or catheter withdrawal Indwelling catheter safe with twice-daily dosing Therapeutic dose: delay block for 18+ h |

[a]For patients undergoing deep plexus or peripheral block, follow American Society of Regional Anesthesia (ASRA) recommendations for neuraxial techniques.
[b]Modified from the German Society of Anesthesiology and Intensive Care Medicine Consensus guidelines.
[c]Modified from the Belgian Association for Regional Anesthesia. Working party on anticoagulants and central nerve blocks.
[d]Modified from the American College of Chest Physicians.

aPTT, Activated partial thromboplastin time; GPIIb/IIIa, glycoprotein IIb/IIIa; LMWH, low-molecular-weight heparin; NSAIDs, nonsteroidal antiinflammatory drugs; UFH, unfractionated heparin.
From Horlocker TT, Wedel DJ, Rowlingson JC, et al. Regional Anesthesia in the Patient Receiving Antithrombotic or Thrombolytic Therapy American Society of Regional Anesthesia and Pain Medicine Evidence-Based Guidelines (Third Edition). Reg Anesth Pain Med. 2010;35(1):64-101.

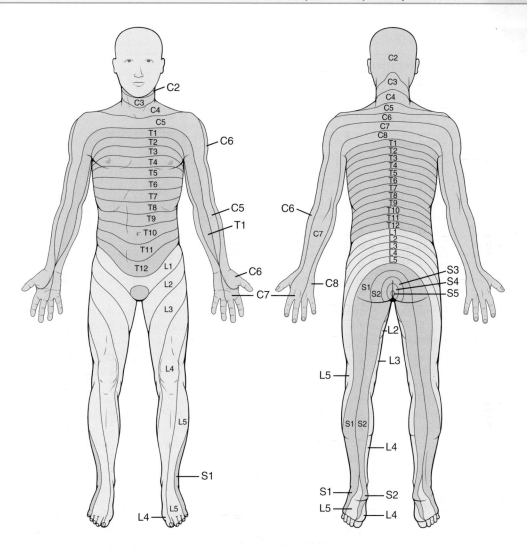

**Sensory level anesthesia necessary for surgical procedures**

| Sensory level | Type of surgery |
| --- | --- |
| S2-S5 | Hemorrhoidectomy |
| L2-L3 (knee) | Foot surgery |
| L1-L3 (inguinal ligament) | Lower extremity surgery |
| T10 (umbilicus) | Hip surgery<br>Transurethral resection<br>of the prostate<br>Vaginal delivery |
| T6-T7 (xiphoid process) | Lower abdominal surgery<br>Appendectomy |
| T4 (nipple) | Upper abdominal surgery<br>Cesarean section |

**Fig. 17.9** Areas of sensory innervation by spinal nerves and the sensory level required for various surgical procedures. Note that the thoracic nerves supply the thorax and abdomen and the lumbar and sacral nerves supply the lower limb. (Modified from Veering BT, Cousins MJ. Epidural neural blockade. In Cousins MJ, Bridenbaugh PO, Carr DB, Horlocker TT, eds. *Neural Blockade in Clinical Anesthesia and Management of Pain*. Philiadelphia: Lippincott-Raven; 2009:241-295.)

**Table 17.2** Factors Affecting Spinal Local Anesthetic Distribution and Block Height

| Factors | More Important | Less Important | Not Important |
|---|---|---|---|
| Drug factors | Dose<br>Baricity | Volume<br>Concentration<br>Temperature of injection<br>Viscosity | Additives other than opioids |
| Patient factors | CSF volume<br>Advanced age<br>Pregnancy | Weight<br>Height<br>Spinal anatomy<br>Intra-abdominal pressure | Menopause<br>Gender |
| Procedure factors | Patient position<br>Epidural injection postspinal | Level of injection (hypobaric more than hyperbaric)<br>Fluid currents<br>Needle orifice direction<br>Needle type | |

CSF, Cerebrospinal fluid.
Modified from Greene NM. Distribution of local anesthetic solutions within the subarachnoid space. *Anesth Analg*. 1985;64(7):715-730.

varies indirectly with CSF volume, CSF volume itself does not correlate well with simple anthropomorphic measurements other than body weight.[32] The increased abdominal mass in obese patients, and possible increased epidural fat, may in theory decrease CSF volume and therefore increase the spread of local anesthetic and block height.[33]

CSF density varies depending on gender, menopausal status, and pregnancy (also see Chapter 33), but the clinical relevance of these factors is probably unimportant.

Advanced age is associated with increased block height (also see Chapter 35). In older patients, CSF volume decreases, whereas its specific gravity increases. Further, the nerve roots are likely more sensitive to local anesthetics in the aged population.

In the lateral position, the broader shoulders of males relative to their hips make this position slightly more head-up whereas the reverse is true in females. Despite this, whether males actually have reduced cephalad spread as compared to females in the lateral position is not clear.

Variations of the spine such as scoliosis can make needle insertion more difficult but have little effect on local anesthetic spread if the patient is turned supine. Kyphosis, however, in a supine patient may affect the spread of a hyperbaric solution.

Spread of local anesthetic is enhanced by changes in the lumbar lordosis during pregnancy, as well as by the volume and density of CSF, by twin pregnancies compared with singletons, by intra-abdominal pressure increases (possibly), and by a progesterone-mediated increase in neuronal sensitivity (also see Chapter 33).

### Procedure Factors

The spread of local anesthetic within the subarachnoid space appears to stop 20 to 25 minutes after injection; thus, positioning of the patient is most important during this period, particularly in the initial few minutes. Although a 10-degree head-up tilt can reduce the spread of hyperbaric solutions without hemodynamic compromise, a head-down tilt does not always increase the spread of hyperbaric bupivacaine. Flexion of the hips in combination with the Trendelenburg position flattens the lumbar lordosis and increases cephalad spread of hyperbaric solutions.[34] A "saddle block" in which only the sacral nerve roots are anesthetized can be achieved with a small dose of hyperbaric local anesthetic while the patient remains sitting for up to 30 minutes. Block height is more extensive with hypobaric solutions if they are administered to patients who are in the sitting position.

The specific needle type and orientation of the orifice may affect block quality. With hypobaric solutions, cephalad alignment of the orifice of Whitacre, but not Sprotte, needles produces greater spread.[35] The orientation of the needle orifice does not appear to affect the spread of hyperbaric solutions. When directing the needle orifice to one side (and using hyperbaric anesthetic), a more marked unilateral block is achieved again when using a Whitacre rather than a Quincke needle.[36]

The level of injection does not affect block height with hyperbaric solutions. With isobaric solutions, the block height is generally higher the more cephalad the injection.[37] Injection rate and barbotage (repeated aspiration and reinjection of CSF) of isobaric and hyperbaric solutions have not consistently been shown to affect block height. The injection of local anesthetic or even saline into the epidural space after a spinal anesthetic increases the block height and is discussed later.

### Duration of the Block

Duration is affected primarily by the dose,[38] the intrinsic properties of the local anesthetic (which affect elimination from the subarachnoid space), and the use of additives (if applicable). Hyperbaric solutions have a shorter duration of action than isobaric solutions.[38]

**Table 17.3**   Dose, Block Height, Onset Times, and Duration of Commonly[a] Used Spinal Anesthetics

| Local Anesthetic Mixture | Dose (Mg) | | Duration (Min) | | |
|---|---|---|---|---|---|
| | To T10 | To T4 | Plain | Epinephrine (0.2 mg) | Onset (Min) |
| Lidocaine 5% (with/without dextrose) | 40-75 | 75-100 | 60-150[b] | 20-50% | 3-5 |
| Mepivacaine 1.5% (no dextrose) | 30-45[c] | 60-80[d] | 120-180[e] | - | 2-4 |
| Chloroprocaine 3% (with/without dextrose) | 30-40 | 40-60 | 40-90[f] | N/R | 2-4 |
| Bupivacaine 0.5-0.75% (no dextrose) | 10-15 | 12-20 | 130-230[g] | 20-50% | 4-8 |
| Levobupivacaine 0.5% (no dextrose) | 10-15 | 12-20 | 140-230[g] | - | 4-8 |
| Ropivacaine 0.5-1% (with/without dextrose) | 12-18 | 18-25 | 80-210[h] | - | 3-8 |

Note that duration depends on how the regression of the block is measured, which varies widely between studies.
[a]Lidocaine is not commonly used now.
[b]Regression to T12.
[c]Note peak with these doses was T12, and not in all cases.
[d]Median peak block height in this study with 60 mg was T5, not T4.
[e]Regression to S1 for block duration.
[f]Regression to L1.
[g]Regression to L2.
[h]Regression to S2.
*N/R,* Not recommended.
From Brull R, Macfarlane AJR, Chan VWS. Spinal, epidural, and caudal anesthesia. In Miller RD, Cohen NH, Eriksson LI, et al, eds. *Miller's Anesthesia.* 8th ed. Philadelphia: Saunders Elsevier; 2015:1696, Table 56-4.

## Pharmacology

The clinical effects of intrathecal local anesthetics are mediated by drug uptake and distribution within the CSF, and elimination. These variables in turn are dictated in part by the pKa (dissociation ionization constant), lipid solubility, and protein binding of the local anesthetic solution. Rather than their pharmacologic structure (i.e. amide or ester), local anesthetics are usually classified by their duration of action. The choice and dose of local anesthetic depend on both the expected duration and the nature (location, ambulatory) of surgery. Table 17.3 shows a range of local anesthetics commonly used for spinal anesthesia with corresponding doses, onset times, and durations of action.

### Short- and Intermediate-Acting Local Anesthetics

*Procaine* is an ester local anesthetic and one of the oldest spinal anesthetics. It is not commonly used because of a more frequent failure rate than lidocaine, significantly more nausea, and a slower time to recovery.

*Chloroprocaine* is an ultra–short-acting ester that is rapidly metabolized by pseudocholinesterase with minimal systemic or fetal effects. Preservative-free chloroprocaine is of interest in ambulatory surgery owing to reliable, short-duration spinal anesthesia,[39] with a faster recovery time than procaine, lidocaine, and bupivacaine. Transient neurologic symptoms (TNS) can occur, albeit at a considerably lesser rate (0.6%) than lidocaine (14%).[40]

*Articaine* is an ester metabolized by nonspecific cholinesterases and has been widely used for dental nerve blocks. It has not been used in spinal anesthesia.

*Lidocaine* is a hydrophilic, relatively poorly protein-bound amide local anesthetic with a rapid onset and intermediate duration. Because of an association with both permanent nerve injury and TNS (discussed later, under "Complications") the use of intrathecal lidocaine has declined.

*Prilocaine* is an amide local anesthetic with an intermediate duration of action. It is rarely associated with TNS and may be used in the ambulatory surgery setting (also see Chapter 37). In large doses (>600 mg; not used in spinal anesthesia), prilocaine can result in methemoglobinemia.

*Mepivacaine* is an amide local anesthetic but the incidence of TNS after hyperbaric mepivacaine was similar to that of lidocaine.[40] TNS occur less frequently with the isobaric preparation.

## Long-Acting Local Anesthetics

*Tetracaine* is an ester packaged either as niphanoid crystals or as an isobaric 1% solution. A 0.5% hyperbaric preparation can be created for perineal and abdominal surgery. Tetracaine is usually combined with a vasoconstrictor additive because the duration of tetracaine alone can be unreliable. Although such combinations can provide up to 5 hours of anesthesia, the addition of phenylephrine in particular has been associated with TNS.

*Bupivacaine* is a highly protein-bound amide with a slow onset because of its relatively high pKa, and a duration of action of 2.5 to 3 hours.[41] Doses as low as 4 to 5 mg of bupivacaine are used in ambulatory procedures.[42] Bupivacaine is rarely associated with TNS.

*Levobupivacaine* is the pure S(–) enantiomer of racemic bupivacaine. Although levobupivacaine potency appears to be slightly less than bupivacaine, the majority of clinical studies using identical doses of levobupivacaine and bupivacaine have found no significant difference in clinical efficacy for spinal anesthesia. Levobupivacaine is less cardiotoxic than bupivacaine, but this is only a theoretical risk in spinal anesthesia.

*Ropivacaine* is another highly protein-bound amide local anesthetic. With the same pKa (8.1) as bupivacaine, it also has a slow onset and a long duration of action, but it is less potent. The proposed advantages of spinal ropivacaine were less cardiotoxicity and greater motor-sensory block differentiation, resulting in less motor block. When given in an equivalent dose to bupivacaine, there is slightly less motor block and earlier recovery with ropivacaine.[43]

## Spinal Additives

A variety of medications may exert a direct analgesic effect on the spinal cord and nerve roots, or prolong the duration of sensory and motor blockade. The coadministration of such drugs often allows a reduction in the dose of local anesthetic, with the advantage of motor block sparing and faster recovery while still producing the same degree of analgesia.

Opioids added to the CSF are complex because of a combination of direct spinal cord dorsal horn opioid receptor activation, cerebral opioid receptor activation after CSF transport, and peripheral and central systemic effects after vascular uptake. The effect at each site depends on both the dose administered and the physicochemical properties of the opioid, particularly lipid solubility. Highly lipid-soluble drugs such as fentanyl and sufentanil have a more rapid onset and shorter duration of action than more hydrophilic opioids. Greater lipid solubility also results in rapid uptake into both blood vessels (with a resultant systemic effect) and fatty tissue. The spread of lipophilic opioids within the CSF is therefore more limited than hydrophilic opioids such as (preservative-free) morphine, which demonstrate greater spread as a result of slower uptake and elimination from the CSF.

As a result, hydrophilic opioids have a more frequent risk of late respiratory depression. The extent of neural tissue and vascular uptake also affects the potency of intrathecal opioids. For example, the relative intrathecal to intravenous potency of morphine is 200:1 to 300:1, whereas for fentanyl and sufentanil it is only 10:1 to 20:1.[44] Other side effects of intrathecal opioids are discussed under "Complications."

### Hydrophilic Opioids

Preservative-free morphine is widely used, providing analgesia for up to 24 hours.[45] Adequate analgesia with minimal side effects is achieved with 100 µg for cesarean deliveries (also see Chapter 33). The most efficacious dose for major orthopedic surgery is less clear,[46] but side effects increase without improvement in analgesia with doses of 300 µg or more. Spinal opioids alone are commonly given as a simple alternative to epidural local anesthetic–based analgesia. For major abdominal surgery or thoracotomies, 500 µg or more may be used. However, the optimal dose remains unclear.

Diamorphine is a lipid-soluble prodrug that crosses the dura faster than morphine and is cleared from the CSF more quickly than morphine. It is converted to morphine and 6-monoacetyl morphine, both of which are µ-agonists with a relatively long duration of action.

Hydromorphone is not commonly used for spinal analgesia and does not provide any advantage compared with morphine. Also, few data are available.

Meperidine is an opioid of intermediate lipid solubility, but it also has some local anesthetic properties. Although it has been administered as the sole intrathecal anesthetic in both obstetric and general surgery, it is rarely used. The neurotoxicity profile is unclear.

### Lipophilic Opioids

Fentanyl and sufentanil are used frequently in obstetrics for labor analgesia and cesarean delivery as discussed elsewhere (also see Chapter 33). Fentanyl is useful in ambulatory surgery because of its rapid onset time of 10 to 20 minutes and relatively short duration of 4 to 6 hours.

### Vasoconstrictors

Epinephrine and phenylephrine prolong sensory and motor blockade when added to local anesthetics. The $\alpha_1$-adrenergic-mediated vasoconstriction reduces systemic local anesthetic uptake and epinephrine may also enhance analgesia via a direct $\alpha_2$-adrenergic-mediated effect. Tetracaine, lidocaine, and bupivacaine spinal anesthesia can all be prolonged by epinephrine. Although there are no human data to support the theory, there is a concern that potent vasoconstrictive action places the blood supply of the spinal cord at risk. Phenylephrine prolongs both lidocaine and tetracaine spinal anesthesia but is associated with TNS.

### α₂-Agonists

Intrathecal clonidine, dexmedetomidine, and epinephrine all act on prejunctional and postjunctional α₂–adrenergic receptors in the dorsal horn of the spinal cord. Clonidine prolongs sensory and motor blockade by approximately 1 hour and improves analgesia. It likely causes less urinary retention than morphine but can cause (non–dose-related) hypotension and sedation lasting up to 8 hours. Dexmedetomidine is approximately 10-fold more α₂-receptor selective than clonidine and can prolong motor and sensory block without hemodynamic compromise.

### Other Drugs

Intrathecal neostigmine prolongs motor and sensory blockade and reduces postoperative analgesic requirements, but its benefits are limited by nausea, vomiting, bradycardia, and, in higher doses, lower extremity weakness. Midazolam also increases sensory and motor block without adverse effects and appears to be safe. Intrathecal ketamine, adenosine, tramadol, magnesium, and nonsteroidal antiinflammatory drugs are unlikely to have any clinical value.

## Technique

Technique can be classified into a series of steps: preparation, position, projection, and puncture (i.e., the four Ps).

### Preparation

Informed consent must be obtained, and risks documented. Resuscitation equipment must be available, intravenous access should be secured, and standard monitoring is necessary.

The most important characteristics of a spinal needle are the shape of the tip and the needle diameter. Needle tip shapes either cut (Pitkin and the Quincke-Babcock) or spread (Whitacre and Sprotte) the dura (Fig 17.10). In the latter group, needles have a conical, pencil-point tip that provides better tactile sensation but, more importantly, reduces the incidence of post–dural puncture headache. Using smaller needles reduces the incidence of post–dural puncture headache from 40% with a 22-G needle to less than 2% with a 29-G needle. The failure rate is increased however, with 29-G needles,[47] so pencil-point needles of 25 G, 26 G, and 27 G probably represent the optimal needle choice.

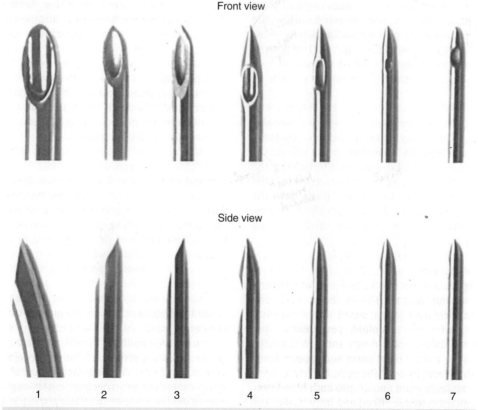

Front view

Side view

1 2 3 4 5 6 7

**Fig. 17.10** Comparative needle configuration for (1) 18-gauge Tuohy, (2) 20-gauge Quincke, (3) 22-gauge Quincke, (4) 24-gauge Sprotte, (5) 25-gauge Polymedic, (6) 25-gauge Whitacre, and (7) 26-gauge Gertie Marx. (From Schneider MC, Schmid M. Postdural puncture headache. In Birnbach DJ, Gatt SP, Datta S, eds. *Textbook of Obstetric Anesthesia*. Philadelphia: Churchill Livingstone; 2000:487-503.)

Strict aseptic technique is of utmost importance. One of the most common organisms responsible for postspinal bacterial meningitis is the oral commensal *Streptococcus viridans,* emphasizing the purpose of wearing a mask. A combination of chlorhexidine and alcohol together is the most effective solution to clean the back.[48] Chlorhexidine must be allowed to dry completely before skin puncture because chlorhexidine is neurotoxic.

Current consensus guidelines state that neuraxial blocks should be performed with the patient awake,[21] except when the physician and patient conclude that benefit outweighs the risk. General anesthesia or heavy sedation can prevent a patient from recognizing warning signs of pain or paresthesia if the needle is in close proximity to nerve tissue.

## Position (Also See Chapter 19)

The two primary patient positions are lateral decubitus and sitting. The prone position is rarely used. The superiority of any one particular position is unclear. The lateral decubitus position facilitates administration of sedative medication if required and is likely more comfortable. Patients are placed with their back parallel to the edge of the operating table, thighs flexed onto the abdomen, with the neck flexed to allow the forehead to be as close as possible to the knees in an attempt to "open up" the vertebral spaces. The patient should be positioned so that spread of hypobaric, isobaric, or hyperbaric solution to the operative site is optimized.

Identification of the midline may be easier when the patient is placed in the sitting position, especially when obesity or scoliosis renders midline anatomy difficult to examine. An assistant helps to maintain the patient in a vertical plane while flexing the patient's neck and arms over a pillow, relaxing the shoulders, and asking the patient to "push out" the lower back to open up the lumbar vertebral spaces. Hypotension may be more common in the sitting position.

## Projection and Puncture

The spinal cord ends at the level of L1-L2, and so needle insertion above this level should be avoided. The intercristal line is the line drawn between the two iliac crests. This, albeit with incomplete reliability, corresponds to the level of the L4 vertebral body or the L4-L5 interspace.[49] Once the appropriate space (usually L3-L4, L2-L3, or L4-L5) has been selected, local anesthesia is infiltrated and an introducer is inserted at a slight cephalad angle of 10 to 15 degrees through skin, subcutaneous tissue, and supraspinous ligament to reach the interspinous ligament. The needle, with its bevel parallel to the midline, is advanced slowly until the characteristic change in resistance is noted as the needle passes through the ligamentum flavum and dura. On passing through the dura, a slight "click" or "pop" sensation often occurs. The stylet is then removed, and clear CSF should appear at the needle hub. If the CSF does not flow, the needle might be obstructed and rotation in 90-degree increments can be undertaken until CSF appears. If CSF does not appear in any quadrant, the needle should be advanced a few millimeters and rechecked. If CSF still has not appeared the needle should be withdrawn and the insertion steps repeated. A common reason for failure is insertion of the needle off the midline. After CSF is freely obtained the anesthetic dose is injected at a rate of approximately 0.2 mL/sec. After completion of the injection, CSF can be aspirated into the syringe and reinjected into the subarachnoid space to reconfirm location.

The paramedian approach may be especially useful in the setting of diffuse calcification of the interspinous ligament. A skin wheal is raised 1 cm lateral and 1 cm caudad to the corresponding spinous process. The spinal introducer and needle are inserted 10 to 15 degrees off the sagittal plane in a cephalomedial plane (Fig. 17.11). If the needle contacts bone, it is redirected slightly in a cephalad direction and the needle "walked up" the lamina. The characteristic feel of the ligamentam flavum and dura is possible, but with this approach the needle is not passing through the supraspinous and interspinous ligaments.

## Special Spinal Techniques

*Continuous spinal anesthesia* allows incremental dosing of local anesthetic and therefore predictable titration of the block to an appropriate level, with better hemodynamic stability than a single-shot spinal injection.[50] This approach is useful in controlling arterial blood pressure in patients with severe aortic stenosis or pregnant women with complex cardiac disease. It may also be used in prolonged cases rather than the combined spinal-epidural (CSE) technique, or when previous spinal surgery may hinder epidural spread. Spinal microcatheters exist, but small-gauge catheters (less than 24 G in particular) have been associated with cauda equina syndrome,[51] probably because of lumbosacral pooling of local anesthetic. Catheter-over-the-needle devices are also available for use with continuous spinal anesthesia, with the advantage of minimizing leakage of CSF around the catheter, but they may be more difficult to insert.

The terms *unilateral spinal anesthesia* and *selective spinal anesthesia* overlap slightly, but both refer to small-dose techniques that capitalize on baricity and patient positioning to hasten recovery. For example, 4 to 5 mg of hyperbaric bupivacaine with unilateral positioning can be adequate for knee arthroscopy. In selective spinal anesthesia, minimal local anesthetic doses are used with the goal of anesthetizing only the sensory fibers to a specific area.[52]

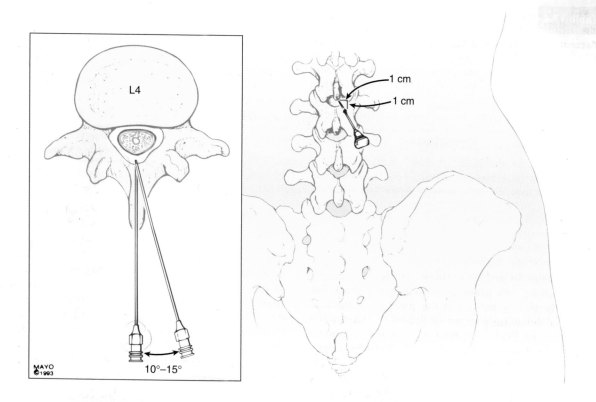

**Fig. 17.11** Vertebral anatomy of the midline and paramedian approaches to central neuraxis blocks. The midline approach highlighted in the inset requires anatomic projection in only two planes: sagittal and horizontal. The paramedian approach shown in the inset and in the posterior view requires an additional oblique plane to be considered, although the technique may be easier in patients who are unable to cooperate in minimizing their lumbar lordosis. The paramedian needle is inserted 1 cm lateral and 1 cm caudad to the caudad edge of the more superior vertebral spinous process. The paramedian needle is inserted approximately 15 degrees off the sagittal plane, as shown in the inset. (Courtesy of the Mayo Foundation, Rochester, Minn.)

## Monitoring of the Block

Once the spinal anesthetic has been administered, the onset, extent, and quality of the sensory and motor blocks must be assessed while heart rate and arterial blood pressure should be monitored for any resultant sympathetic blockade. Cold sensation and pinprick representing C fibers and A-delta fibers respectively are used most often to assess sensory block. Loss of sensation to cold usually occurs first, verified using an ethyl chloride spray, ice, or alcohol, followed by the loss of sensation to pinprick, verified using a needle that does not pierce the skin.[6] Finally, loss of sensation to touch occurs. The modified Bromage scale (Box 17.1) is most commonly used to measure motor block, although this represents only lumbosacral motor fibers.[53] Ensuring that the level of block using cold or pinprick is two to three segments above the expected level of surgical stimulus, and the presence of a motor block is commonly considered adequate.

**Box 17.1** Modified Bromage Scale

0 No motor block
1 Inability to raise extended leg; able to move knees and feet
2 Inability to raise extended leg and move knee; able to move feet
3 Complete block of motor limb

From Brull R, Macfarlane AJR, Chan VWS. Spinal, epidural, and caudal anesthesia. In Miller RD, Cohen NH, Eriksson LI, et al, eds. *Miller's Anesthesia*. 8th ed. Philadelphia: Saunders Elsevier; 2015, Box 56-1.

## EPIDURAL ANESTHESIA

### Factors Affecting Epidural Block Height

Drug Factors
The volume and total mass of injectate are the most important drug-related factors. As a general principle, 1 to 2 mL of solution should be injected per segment to be

**Table 17.4**    Factors Affecting Epidural Local Anesthetic Distribution and Block Height

| Factors | More Important | Less Important | Not Important |
|---|---|---|---|
| Drug factors | Volume<br>Dose | Concentration | Additives |
| Patient factors | Elderly age<br>Pregnancy | Weight<br>Height<br>Pressure in adjacent body cavities | |
| Procedure factors | Level of injection | Patient position | Speed of injection<br>Needle orifice direction |

Visser WA, Lee RA, Gielen MJM. Factors affecting the distribution of neural blockade by local anesthetics in epidural anesthesia and a comparison of lumbar versus thoracic epidural anesthesia. *Anesth Analg.* 2008;107(2):708-721.

blocked. Bicarbonate, epinephrine, and opioids influence onset, quality, and duration of analgesia and anesthesia, and these do not affect spread (Table 17.4).

### Patient Factors

Age can influence epidural block height. Up to 40% less volume may be required in thoracic epidurals in the elderly, possibly because of decreased leakage of local anesthetic through intervertebral foramina, decreased compliance of the epidural space, or an increased sensitivity of the nerves (also see Chapter 35). Only the extremes of patient height influence local anesthetic spread in the epidural space. Weight is not well correlated with block height. Less local anesthetic is required to produce the same epidural spread of anesthesia in pregnant patients, in part because of engorgement of epidural veins secondary to increased abdominal pressure (also see Chapter 33). Continuous positive airway pressure increases the height of a thoracic epidural block.

### Procedure Factors

The level of injection is the most important procedural-related factor that affects epidural block height. In the upper cervical region, spread of injectate is mostly caudal, in the midthoracic region spread is equally cephalad and caudal, and in the low thoracic region spread is primarily cephalad.[54] After a lumbar epidural, spread is more cephalad than caudal. Some studies suggest that the total number of segments blocked is less in the lumbar region compared with thoracic levels for a given volume of injectate. Patient position affects lumbar epidural injections, with preferential spread and faster onset to the dependent side in the lateral decubitus position. The sitting and supine positions do not affect epidural block height. However, the head-down tilt position does increase spread in obstetric patients. Needle bevel direction and speed of injection do not appear to influence the spread of a bolus injection.

## Pharmacology

Local anesthetics for epidural use may be classified into short-, intermediate-, and long-acting drugs. A single bolus dose of local anesthetic can provide surgical anesthesia ranging from 45 minutes up to 4 hours depending on the type administered and the use of any additives (Table 17.5). Most commonly, however, an epidural catheter is left in situ so that anesthesia or analgesia can be extended indefinitely.

### Short-Acting and Intermediate-Acting Local Anesthetics

*Procaine* is not commonly used because the resultant block can be unreliable and of poor quality.

*Chloroprocaine* is available in 2% and 3% preservative-free solutions. Prior to preservative-free preparations, large volumes of chloroprocaine had been associated with deep, burning lumbar back pain.[55] This was thought to be secondary to the ethylenediaminetetraacetic acid that chelated calcium and caused a localized hypocalcemia.

*Articaine* is not widely used for epidural anesthesia and has not been studied extensively.

*Lidocaine* is available in 1% and 2% solutions. Unlike spinal anesthesia, TNS is not commonly associated with epidural lidocaine.

*Prilocaine* is available in 2% and 3% solutions. The 2% solution produces a sensory block with minimal motor block. In large doses, prilocaine is associated with methemoglobinemia.

*Mepivacaine* is available as 1%, 1.5%, and 2% preservative-free solutions. The 2% preparation has an onset time similar to that for lidocaine of approximately 15 minutes, but a slightly longer duration (up to 200 minutes with epinephrine).

### Long-Acting Local Anesthetics

*Tetracaine* is not widely used because of unreliable block height and, in larger doses, systemic toxicity.

*Bupivacaine* is available in 0.25%, 0.5%, and 0.75% preservative-free solutions. More dilute concentrations such

| Table 17.5 | Comparative Onset Times and Analgesic Durations of Local Anesthetics Administered Epidurally in 20- to 30-mL Volumes | | | |
|---|---|---|---|---|
| | | | **Duration (min)** | |
| **Drug** | **Conc. (%)** | **Onset (min)** | **Plain** | **1 : 200,000 Epinephrine** |
| 2-Chloroprocaine | 3 | 10-15 | 45-60 | 60-90 |
| Lidocaine | 2 | 15 | 80-120 | 120-180 |
| Mepivacaine | 2 | 15 | 90-140 | 140-200 |
| Bupivacaine | 0.5-0.75 | 20 | 165-225 | 180-240 |
| Etidocaine | 1 | 15 | 120-200 | 150-225 |
| Ropivacaine | 0.75-1.0 | 15-20 | 140-180 | 150-200 |
| Levobupivacaine | 0.5-0.75 | 15-20 | 150-225 | 150-240 |

Data from Cousins MJ, Bromage PR. Epidural neural blockade. In Cousins MJ, Bridenbaugh PO, eds. *Neural Blockade in Clinical Anesthesia and Management of Pain.* Philadelphia: JB Lippincott; 1988:255; Brown DL. Spinal, epidural, and caudal anesthesia. In Miller RD, Cohen NH, Eriksson LI, et al, eds. *Miller's Anesthesia.* 7th ed. Philadelphia: Saunders Elsevier; 2010:1611-1638.

as 0.125% to 0.25% can be used for analgesia. However, disadvantages include cardiac and central nervous system toxicity and potential motor block from larger doses.

*Levobupivacaine* administered epidurally has the same clinical characteristics as bupivacaine and is less cardiotoxic. Liposomal bupivacaine is not licensed for epidural use.

*Ropivacaine* is available in 0.2%, 0.5%, 0.75%, and 1.0% preservative-free preparations. It is associated with a superior safety profile compared with bupivacaine, with a higher seizure threshold and less cardiotoxicity.

### Epidural Additives
#### Vasoconstrictors

Epinephrine reduces vascular absorption of local anesthetics in the epidural space. The effect is greatest with lidocaine,[56] mepivacaine, and chloroprocaine (up to 50% prolongation); less with bupivacaine and levobupivacaine; and limited with ropivacaine, which already has intrinsic vasoconstrictive properties (see Table 17.5). Epinephrine itself may also have some analgesic benefits owing to absorption into CSF, and dorsal horn $\alpha_2$-receptor activation. Phenylephrine is used less widely and is less effective than epinephrine.

#### Opioids

Opioids synergistically enhance the analgesic effects of epidural local anesthetics, without prolonging motor block. A combination of local anesthetic and opioid reduces the dose-related adverse effects of each drug independently. Opioid-related side effects are dose-dependent and there appears to be a therapeutic ceiling effect above which only side effects increase. Opioids may also be used alone. Epidural opioids cross the dura and arachnoid membrane to reach the CSF and spinal cord dorsal horn. Lipophilic opioids, such as fentanyl and sufentanil, partition into epidural fat and therefore are found in lower concentrations in CSF than hydrophilic opioids, such as morphine and hydromorphone. Fentanyl and sufentanil are also readily absorbed into the systemic circulation, which may be the principal analgesic mechanism.

Epidural morphine can be administered as a bolus (duration of up to 24 hours) or continuously. The optimal bolus analgesic dose that minimizes side effects is 2.5 to 3.75 mg.[57] Hydromorphone is more hydrophilic than fentanyl but more lipophilic than morphine, and has a duration of 18 hours. Epidural fentanyl and sufentanil have a faster onset but a shorter duration (only 2 to 3 hours). Diamorphine is available in the United Kingdom. Depodur is an extended-release liposomal formulation of morphine used as a single-shot lumbar epidural dose, potentially avoiding issues of continuous local anesthetic infusions and indwelling catheters.

#### $\alpha_2$-Agonists

Epidural clonidine can prolong sensory block to a longer extent than motor block and reduces both epidural local anesthetic and opioid requirements. Clonidine may also reduce immune stress and cytokine response, but side effects include hypotension, bradycardia, dry mouth, and sedation. Dexmedetomidine can reduce intraoperative anesthetic requirements, improve postoperative analgesia, and prolong both sensory and motor block.

#### Other Drugs

Ketamine, neostigmine, midazolam, tramadol, dexamethasone, and droperidol have all been studied but are not commonly used.

**Table 17.6** Suggested Epidural Insertion Sites for Common Surgical Procedures

| Nature of Surgery | Suggested Level of Insertion | Remarks |
|---|---|---|
| Hip surgery<br>Lower extremity<br>Obstetric analgesia | Lumbar L2-L5 | |
| Colectomy, anterior resection<br>Upper abdominal surgery | Lower thoracic<br>T6-T8 | Spread more cranial than caudal |
| Thoracic | T2-T6 | Midpoint of surgical incision |

Modified from Visser WA, Lee RA, Gielen MJM. Factors affecting the distribution of neural blockade by local anesthetics in epidural anesthesia and a comparison of lumbar versus thoracic epidural anesthesia. *Anesth Analg.* 2008;107(2):708-721.

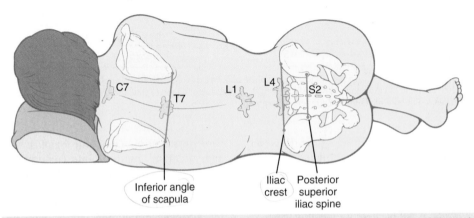

**Fig. 17.12** Surface landmarks are a guide to the vertebral level. (From Brown DL, ed. *Atlas of Regional Anesthesia.* Philadelphia: WB Saunders; 1992.)

### Carbonation and Bicarbonate

Both carbonation of the solution and adding bicarbonate increase the solution pH, and therefore the nonionized free-base proportion of local anesthetic. Although this may theoretically increase the speed of onset and quality of the block by producing more rapid intraneural diffusion and more rapid penetration of connective tissue surrounding the nerve trunk, data suggest that there are no clinical advantages for carbonated solutions.[58,59]

## Technique

### Preparation

Patient preparation as previously described for spinal anesthesia must equally be applied to epidural anesthesia, namely consent, monitoring, resuscitation equipment, and intravenous access. Sterility is arguably even more important than spinal anesthesia because a catheter is often left in situ. The nature and the duration of surgery must be understood so that the epidural may be inserted at the appropriate level (Table 17.6) and the appropriate drugs chosen.[8] The risks and benefits will vary depending on the severity of patient comorbid conditions. Tuohy needles are most commonly used

(see Fig. 17.10). They are usually 16 to 18 G and have a shaft marked in 1-cm intervals with a 15- to 30-degree curved, blunt Huber needle tip designed to both reduce the risk of accidental dural puncture and guide the catheter cephalad. The catheter is made of a flexible, calibrated, radiopaque plastic with either a single end hole or multiple side orifices near the tip. Multiple orifices can improve analgesia but may increase epidural vein cannulation in parturients.

### Position

The sitting and lateral decubitus positions necessary for epidural puncture are the same as those for spinal anesthesia, and success rates are comparable. As with spinal anesthesia, epidurals are ideally performed with the patient awake.[21]

### Projection and Puncture

Important surface landmarks include the intercristal line (corresponding to the L4-L5 interspace), the inferior angle of the scapula (corresponding to the T7 vertebral body), the root of the scapular spine (T3), and the vertebra prominens (C7) (Fig. 17.12). Ultrasonography may be useful to identify the correct thoracic space.

A variety of different needle approaches exist: midline, paramedian, modified paramedian (Taylor approach), and caudal. A midline approach, in which the angle of approach is only slightly cephalad, is commonly chosen for lumbar and low thoracic approaches. In the midthoracic region, the approach should be more cephalad because of the significant downward angulation of the spinous processes (see Fig. 17.5). The needle should be advanced in a controlled fashion with the stylet in place through the supraspinous ligament and into the interspinous ligament, at which point the stylet can be removed and the syringe attached. This method may increase the chance of a false loss-of-resistance, possibly because of defects in the interspinous ligament.

Air or saline (or a combination) is commonly used to detect a loss-of-resistance when identifying the epidural space (Fig. 17.13). Each involves intermittent (for air) or constant (for saline) gentle pressure applied to the bulb of the syringe with the dominant thumb while the needle is advanced with the nondominant hand. Usually the ligamentum flavum is identified as a tougher structure with increased resistance, and when the epidural space is subsequently entered, the pressure applied to the syringe plunger allows the solution to flow without resistance into the epidural space. Air is likely less reliable in identifying the epidural space, results in a possible chance of incomplete block, and may cause both pneumocephalus (which can result in headaches) and even venous air embolism in rare cases. Nevertheless, adverse outcomes in obstetric patients do not vary when air versus saline was studied.[60] Fluid inserted through the epidural needle before catheter insertion can also reduce the risk of epidural vein cannulation by the catheter.[61] However, saline may make it more difficult to detect an accidental dural puncture.

With the hanging-drop technique, a drop of solution such as saline is placed within the hub of the needle after the needle is placed in the ligamentum flavum. When the needle tip reaches the epidural space, the solution is "sucked in" as a result of subatmospheric pressure inside the epidural space.

When a lumbar midline approach is used, the depth from skin to the ligamentum flavum in most (80%) patients is between 3.5 and 6 cm. Ultrasonography can predict this depth before needle insertion. When the epidural space is identified, the depth should be noted, the syringe removed, and a catheter gently threaded to leave 4 to 6 cm in the space. Less than 4 cm in length in the epidural space may increase the risk of catheter dislodgement and inadequate analgesia. Threading more catheter increases the likelihood of catheter malposition or complications.[62] The Tsui test can be used to confirm catheter tip location using a special electrically conducting catheter.[63] This stimulates the spinal nerve roots with a low electrical current resulting in twitches of the corresponding muscles.

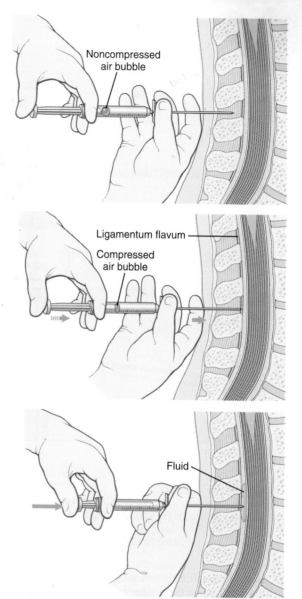

**Fig. 17.13** Loss-of-resistance technique. The needle is inserted into the ligamentum flavum, and a syringe containing saline and an air bubble is attached to the hub. After compression of the air bubble is obtained by applying pressure on the syringe plunger, the needle is carefully advanced until its entry into the epidural space is confirmed by the characteristic loss of resistance to syringe plunger pressure, and the fluid enters the space easily. (From Afton-Bird G. Atlas of regional anesthesia. In Miller RD, ed. *Miller's Anesthesia*. Philadelphia: Elsevier; 2005.)

### Paramedian Approach

The paramedian approach is particularly useful in the mid- to high-thoracic region, where the angulation of the spine is steeper and the spaces narrower. The needle should be inserted 1 to 2 cm lateral to the inferior tip of the spinous process corresponding to the vertebra above the desired

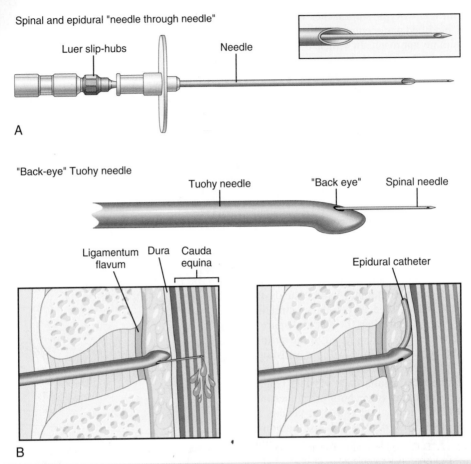

Spinal and epidural "needle through needle"

Luer slip-hubs

Needle

A

"Back-eye" Tuohy needle

Tuohy needle     "Back eye"     Spinal needle

Ligamentum flavum   Dura   Cauda equina

Epidural catheter

B

**Fig. 17.14** (A) A spinal needle and epidural needle are used for the combined spinal-epidural technique. (B) Tuohy needle with a "back eye" that permits placement of the spinal needle directly into the subarachnoid space *(left panel)* and subsequent threading of the epidural catheter into the epidural space after removal of the spinal needle. (Modified from Veering BT, Cousins MJ. Epidural neural blockade. In Cousins MJ, Bridenbaugh PO, Carr DB, Horlocker TT, eds. *Neural Blockade in Clinical Anesthesia and Management of Pain.* Philadelphia: Lippincott-Raven; 2009:241-295.)

interspace. The needle is then advanced horizontally until the lamina is reached and then redirected medially and cephalad to enter the epidural space. The Taylor approach is a modified paramedian approach via the L5-S1 interspace, which may be useful in trauma patients who cannot tolerate or are not able to maintain a sitting position. The needle is inserted 1 cm medial and 1 cm inferior to the posterior superior iliac spine and is angled medially and cephalad at a 45- to 55-degree angle. Before initiating an epidural local anesthetic infusion, a test dose may be administered. The purpose of this is to exclude intrathecal or intravascular catheter placement.

## COMBINED SPINAL-EPIDURAL ANESTHESIA

CSE anesthesia allows the flexibility of a rapid-onset spinal block while the epidural catheter allows anesthesia or analgesia to be extended as the spinal resolves. This is particularly useful in obstetrics (also see Chapter 33). Another advantage is the ability to administer a low dose of intrathecal local anesthetic, and, if necessary, use the epidural catheter to extend the block. Adding either local anesthetic or saline alone to the epidural space via the catheter compresses the dural sac and increases the block height. This latter technique of epidural volume extension (EVE) allows smaller doses of intrathecal local anesthetic to be used while significantly hastening motor recovery.[64] This sequential technique also provides greater hemodynamic stability for high-risk patients.

### Technique

Most commonly the epidural needle is placed first, followed by either a "needle through needle" technique using specially available kits (Fig. 17.14) or an altogether separate spinal needle insertion at either the same or

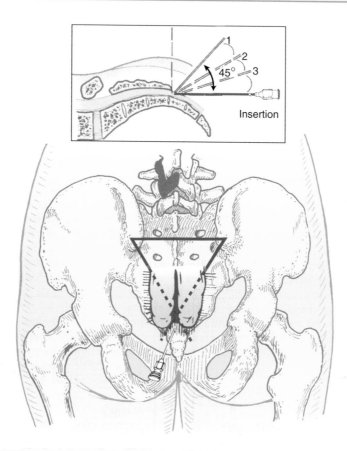

**Fig. 17.15** Caudal technique. Palpating fingers locate the sacral cornua by using the equilateral triangle. Needle insertion is completed by insertion and withdrawal in a stepwise fashion (inset, so-called "1-2-3 insertion") until the needle can be advanced into the caudal canal and the solution can be injected easily (without creation of a subcutaneous "lump" of fluid). (From Brull R Macfarlane AJR, Chan VWS. Spinal, epidural, and caudal anesthesia. In Miller RD, Cohen NH, Eriksson LI, et al, eds. *Miller's Anesthesia*. 8th ed. Philadelphia: Saunders Elsevier; 2015:Fig. 56-10.)

different interspace. The separate needle insertion technique[65] has the advantage of being able to confirm that the epidural catheter is functional before spinal anesthesia is administered but does theoretically risk shearing the in situ epidural catheter.

## CAUDAL ANESTHESIA

Caudal anesthesia is popular in pediatric anesthesia (also see Chapter 34). In adults, caudal anesthesia is unpredictable when upper abdominal or thoracic spread is required. Therefore its indications in adults are the same as those for lumbar epidural anesthesia. It is most useful when sacral anesthetic spread is desired (e.g., perineal, anal, rectal procedures), where a spinal surgery scar may prevent a lumbar anesthetic technique, or more commonly, in chronic pain and cancer pain management (also see Chapter 44). Both fluoroscopy and ultrasonography can help guide correct needle placement.

## Pharmacology

The local anesthetics used are similar to those described for epidural anesthesia and analgesia. In adults, approximately twice the lumbar epidural dose is required to achieve a similar block with the caudal approach.

## Technique

Patient preparation as described before applies equally to caudal anesthesia. The prone position, lateral decubitus position, and the knee-chest position may be used. Caudal anesthesia requires identification of the sacral hiatus. The sacrococcygeal ligament (i.e., extension of ligamentum flavum) overlies the sacral hiatus, between the two sacral cornua. The posterior superior iliac spines should be located, and by using the line between them as one side of an equilateral triangle, the location of the sacral hiatus can be approximated (Fig. 17.15).

After the sacral hiatus is identified, local anesthetic is infiltrated and the caudal needle (or Tuohy needle if a catheter is to be placed) is inserted at an angle of approximately 45 degrees to the sacrum. A decrease in resistance to needle insertion should be appreciated as the needle enters the caudal canal. The needle is advanced until bone (i.e., the dorsal aspect of the ventral plate of the sacrum) is contacted and then slightly withdrawn, and then redirected so that the angle of insertion relative to the skin surface is decreased. In male patients, this angle is almost parallel to the coronal plane; in female patients, a slightly steeper angle (15 degrees) is necessary. During redirection of the needle, loss-of-resistance is sought to confirm entry into the epidural space, and the needle advanced no more than approximately 1 to 2 cm into the caudal canal. In adults, the tip should never be advanced beyond the S2 level (approximately 1 cm inferior to the posterior superior iliac spine), which is the level to which the dural sac extends. Additional advancement increases the risk of dural puncture and unintentional intravascular cannulation. Before injection of any drugs, aspiration to see if CSF can be withdrawn should be performed and a test dose administered to exclude intravascular or intrathecal placement.

## COMPLICATIONS

Clear distinction should be made between the physiologic effects of the neuraxial technique and complications, which imply some harm to the patient.[66] The material risks associated with neuraxial anesthesia must be intimately understood and respected because catastrophic injury is not unknown.

### Neurologic

Serious neurologic complications associated with neuraxial anesthesia are rare.

#### Paraplegia

The frequency is reported to be approximately 0.1 per 10,000.[67] The mechanism of such a severe injury is likely multifactorial. Direct needle trauma to the spinal cord is possible, but the intrathecal injectate can be neurotoxic. In the early 1980s, several patients developed adhesive arachnoiditis, cauda equina syndrome, or permanent paresis possibly related to a combination of low pH and the antioxidant sodium bisulfite preservative used in early (and discontinued) preparations of the short-acting ester local anesthetic chloroprocaine.[68]

Profound hypotension or ischemia of the spinal cord can also be an important contributing factor. Anterior spinal artery syndrome, characterized by potentially irreversible, painless loss of motor and sensory function with sparing of proprioception was described earlier.

#### Cauda Equina Syndrome

The rate of cauda equina syndrome is approximately 0.1 per 10,000 and invariably results in permanent neurologic deficit.[69] The lumbosacral roots of the spinal cord may be particularly vulnerable to direct exposure of large doses of local anesthetic, whether it is administered as a single injection of relatively highly concentrated local anesthetic (e.g., 5% lidocaine) or prolonged exposure to a local anesthetic through a (small gauge in particular as described earlier) continuous catheter.

#### Epidural Hematoma

Bleeding within the vertebral canal can cause ischemic compression of the spinal cord and lead to permanent neurologic deficit if not recognized and evacuated expeditiously. Many risk factors have been associated with the development of an epidural hematoma, including difficult or traumatic needle or catheter insertion, coagulopathy, elderly age, and female gender.[70] Radicular back pain, prolonged blockade longer than the expected duration of the neuraxial technique, and bladder or bowel dysfunction are features commonly associated with a space-occupying lesion within the vertebral canal and should prompt magnetic resonance imaging on an urgent basis. The rate is about 0.07 per 10,000.[67]

#### Nerve Injury

The current conclusion is that epidural (including CSE) anesthesia is associated with a more frequent rate of radiculopathy or peripheral neuropathy compared with spinal anesthesia,[69] and that neuraxial anesthesia performed in adults for the purposes of perioperative anesthesia or analgesia is associated with an increased likelihood of neurologic complications compared with that performed in the obstetric, pediatric, and chronic pain settings.[67] The rate of permanent nerve injury is around 0.1 per 10,000.[67] Radicular pain or paresthesia occurring during the procedure is a risk factor.

#### Post-Dural Puncture Headache

This headache is relatively common and results from unintentional or intentional puncture of the dura membrane. The incidence is approximately 1% in spinal anesthesia and is minimized by using smaller gauge, noncutting tip spinal needles and orientating the needle bevel parallel with the axis of the spine. In obstetrics, accidental dural puncture may occur in around 1.5% of patients with between 52% and 80% of these patients subsequently developing a post–dural puncture headache.[71] Additional risk factors for post-spinal puncture headache are listed in Box 17.2.

The loss of CSF through the dura may cause traction on pain-sensitive intracranial structures as the brain loses support and sags (Fig. 17.16). Perhaps the loss of CSF initiates compensatory yet painful intracerebral vasodilation to offset the decreased intracranial pressure.[72] The characteristic feature of a post–dural puncture headache is a frontal or occipital headache that worsens with the upright or seated posture and is relieved by lying supine. Associated symptoms can include nausea, vomiting, neck pain, dizziness, tinnitus, diplopia, hearing loss, cortical blindness, cranial nerve palsies, and even seizures. Symptoms usually begin within 3 days of the procedure, and 66% start within the first 48 hours. Spontaneous resolution usually occurs within 7 days in the majority (72%) of cases, whereas 87% of cases resolve by 6 months.

---

**Box 17.2** Relationships Among Variables and Post Dural Puncture Headache

**Factors That Can Increase the Incidence of Headache After Spinal Puncture**
- Age: Younger, more frequent
- Sex: Females > males
- Needle size: larger > smaller
- Needle bevel: less when the needle bevel is placed in the long axis of the neuraxis
- Pregnancy: more when pregnant
- Dural punctures: more with multiple punctures

**Factors That Do Not Increase the Incidence of Headache After Spinal Puncture**
- Continuous spinal infusion
- Timing of ambulation

From Brull R, Macfarlane AJR, Chan VWS. Spinal, epidural, and caudal anesthesia. In Miller RD, Cohen NH, Eriksson LI, et al, eds. *Miller's Anesthesia*. 8th ed. Philadelphia: Saunders Elsevier; 2015:Box 56-2.

---

Conservative management for post–dural puncture headache includes supine positioning, hydration, caffeine, and oral analgesics. The use of sumatriptan has varying effects. Epidural blood patch is the definitive therapy for post–dural puncture headache[73] with a single patch resulting in a 90% initial improvement rate and persistent resolution of symptoms in 61% to 75% of cases. A blood patch is ideally performed 24 hours after dural puncture and after the development of classic post–dural puncture headache symptoms. Prophylactic epidural blood patching is not efficacious. It is recommended inserting the blood patch needle at or caudad to the level of the dural puncture, with 20 mL of blood being a reasonable starting target volume.[74] A second epidural blood patch may be performed 24 to 48 hours if the first is ineffective.

### Transient Neurologic Symptoms

TNS are characterized by bilateral or unilateral pain in the buttocks radiating to the legs or, less commonly, isolated buttock or leg pain. Symptoms occur within 24 hours of the resolution of an otherwise uneventful spinal anesthetic and are not associated with any neurologic deficits or laboratory abnormalities. Pain can be mild or severe but typically resolves spontaneously in less than 1 week. TNS are more likely after intrathecal lidocaine and mepivacaine and are far less frequent with bupivacaine.[75] The phenomenon is related to the concentration of lidocaine, the addition of dextrose or epinephrine, and solution osmolarity. TNS are less commonly associated with

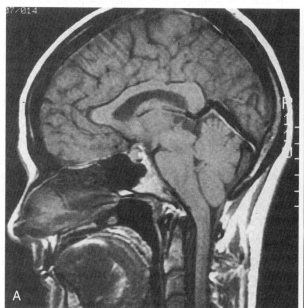
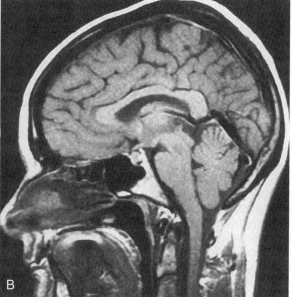

**Fig. 17.16** Anatomy of a "low-pressure" headache. (A) A T1-weighted sagittal magnetic resonance image demonstrates a "ptotic brain" manifested as tonsillar herniation below the foramen magnum, forward displacement of the pons, absence of the suprasellar cistern, kinking of the chiasm, and fullness of the pituitary gland. (B) A comparable image of the same patient after an epidural blood patch and resolution of the symptoms demonstrates normal anatomy. (From Drasner K, Swisher JL. In Brown DL, ed. *Regional Anesthesia and Analgesia*. Philadelphia: WB Saunders; 1996.)

epidural procedures. The risk is also more likely in the lithotomy position for surgery. Nonsteroidal antiinflammatory drugs are the first line of treatment, but opioids may be required.

## Cardiovascular

### Hypotension

Hypotension is more likely with peak block height higher than or equal to T5, at an age of 40 years or older, baseline systolic blood pressure less than 120 mm Hg, combined spinal and general anesthesia, spinal puncture at or above the L2-L3 interspace, and the addition of phenylephrine to the local anesthetic. Hypotension is also independently associated with chronic alcohol consumption, history of hypertension, body mass index (BMI), and the urgency of surgery.[76] Nausea is a common symptom of hypotension in the setting of neuraxial anesthesia; other symptoms include vomiting, dizziness, and dyspnea.

### Bradycardia

The mechanism has been described earlier but factors that may increase the likelihood of exaggerated bradycardia include baseline heart rate less than 60 beats/min, age younger than 37 years, male gender, nonemergency status, β-adrenergic blockade, and prolonged duration of surgery.

### Cardiac Arrest

This event is rare, and the cause of sudden cardiac arrest after spinal anesthesia is not understood. Hypoxemia and oversedation may be a factor in the severe bradycardia and asystole that can occur suddenly during well-conducted spinal anesthesia. Curiously, these rare events are associated with spinal anesthesia rather than epidural techniques.

## Respiratory

The risk of respiratory depression associated with neuraxial opioids is dose-dependent, with a reported frequency that approaches 3% after the administration of 0.8 mg of intrathecal morphine.[77] Respiratory depression may stem from rostral spread of opioids within the CSF to the chemosensitive respiratory centers in the brainstem. With lipophilic anesthetics, respiratory depression is generally an early phenomenon occurring within the first 30 minutes (and has not been reported after 2 hours), whereas with intrathecal morphine late respiratory depression may occur up to 24 hours after injection. Respiratory monitoring for the first 24 hours after the administration of intrathecal morphine is recommended. Patients with sleep apnea can be especially sensitive and considerable caution must be exercised in this group.[78] Older patients also have a more frequent risk of respiratory depression, and therefore, the dose of neuraxial opioids should be

reduced (also see Chapter 35). Coadministration of systemic sedatives also increases this risk.

## Infection

Bacterial meningitis and epidural abscess are rare but potentially catastrophic complications. Staphylococcal infections arising from organisms on the patient's skin are one of the most common epidural-related infections, whereas oral bacteria such as *S. viridans* are a common cause of infection after spinal anesthesia. The presence of a concomitant systemic infection, diabetes, immunocompromised states, and prolonged maintenance of an epidural (or spinal) catheter are risk factors. The rate of serious neuraxial infection is less than 0.3 per 10,000[79] for spinal anesthesia, whereas infectious complications after epidural techniques may be at least twice as common.[67] Obstetric patients are less likely to develop deep infections related to epidural analgesia. Chlorhexidine in an alcohol base is the most effective antiseptic for the purposes of neuraxial techniques.

## Backache

There is no association between epidural analgesia and new-onset back pain up to 6 months postpartum.

## Nausea and Vomiting

Nausea and vomiting may be secondary to either direct exposure of the chemoreceptor trigger zone in the brain to emetogenic drugs (e.g., opioids), hypotension, or gastrointestinal hyperperistalsis secondary to unopposed parasympathetic activity. Nausea or vomiting after spinal anesthesia is more likely with the addition of phenylephrine or epinephrine to the local anesthetic, peak block height more than or equal to T5, baseline heart rate more rapid than 60 beats/min, use of procaine, history of motion sickness, and the development of hypotension during spinal anesthesia. Intrathecal morphine has the highest risk of opioid-induced nausea or vomiting, whereas fentanyl and sufentanil carry the lowest risk.[80] Again these side effects are dose-dependent. Using less than 0.1 mg morphine reduces the risk, without compromising the analgesic effect.

## Urinary Retention

Urinary retention can occur in as many as one third of patients after neuraxial anesthesia. Local anesthetic blockade of the S2, S3, and S4 nerve roots inhibits urinary function as the detrusor muscle is weakened. Neuraxial opioids can further complicate urinary function by suppressing detrusor contractility and reducing the sensation of urge.[81] Spontaneous return of normal bladder function is expected once the sensory level decreases to less than S2-S3. Along with male gender and age, intra-thecal morphine has also been linked to urinary retention after neuraxial anesthesia.[81]

## Pruritus

Pruritus can be distressing and is the most common side effect related to the intrathecal administration of opioids with rates between 30% and 100%.[82] It is not dependent on the type or dose of opioid administered, although reducing the dose can reduce the likelihood of pruritus. Naloxone, naltrexone, or the partial agonist nalbuphine can be used for treatment. Ondansetron and propofol are also useful therapies.

## Shivering

The rate of shivering is as frequent as 55%[83] and is more related to epidural than spinal anesthesia. One postulated cause is the relatively cold temperature of the epidural injectate, which can affect the thermosensitive basal sinuses. The addition of neuraxial opioids, specifically fentanyl and meperidine, reduces the likelihood of shiv-ering.[83] Prewarming the patient with a forced air warmer and avoiding the administration of cold epidural and intravenous fluids can reduce the incidence of shivering.

## Complications Unique to Epidural Anesthesia

### Intravascular Injection

Epidural anesthesia can produce local anesthetic–induced systemic toxicity, primarily through the unintentional administration of drug into an epidural vein. The frequency of vascular puncture by needle or catheter can reach 10%, with rates highest in the obstetric population, in whom these vessels are relatively dilated.[84] Seizures related to epidural anesthesia may be as frequent as 1%.[79] In obstet-rics (also see Chapter 33), the likelihood of intravascular injection is decreased by placing the patient in the lateral position during needle and catheter insertion, administer-ing fluid through the epidural needle before catheter inser-tion, using a single-orifice rather than multiorifice catheter or a wire-embedded polyurethane compared with polyam-ide epidural catheter, and advancing the catheter less than 6 cm into the epidural space. The paramedian approach, and the use of a smaller-gauge epidural needle or catheter, does not reduce the risk of epidural vein cannulation.

Using epinephrine mixed with local anesthetic as a test dose can be unreliable and so prevention of systemic tox-icity should always involve aspiration of the catheter and incremental administration of the local anesthetic.

### Subdural Injection

The subdural extra-arachnoid space is easily entered in autopsy attempts in humans. It is an infrequent clinical problem with epidural anesthesia (<1%). Yet, when an epidural block is performed and a higher-than-expected block develops 15 to 30 minutes after injection, subdu-ral placement of local anesthetic must be considered. With a subdural block, the motor block will be modest compared to the extent of the sensory block, and the sympathetic block may be exaggerated. The treatment is symptomatic.

## RECENT ADVANCES IN ULTRASONOGRAPHY

Preprocedural ultrasound imaging can accurately iden-tify the intervertebral levels, the midline spinous process, the midline interspinous window, and the paramedian interlaminar window.[49] Imaging of the lumbar spine is significantly easier than that of the thoracic spine, which has narrower interspinous and interlaminar windows. Through these windows the hyperechoic dura (a bright line), the subarachnoid space, and the posterior aspect of the vertebral body may be visualized. Visualization of the ligamentum flavum and epidural space is often more difficult. Ultrasound facilitates identification of the opti-mal location for needle insertion and an estimation of the skin-to-dura distance. This can be useful in patients with difficult surface anatomic landmarks (e.g., obesity), spine disorders (e.g., scoliosis), or previous spine surgery. Real-time guidance is a highly challenging technique. Ultrasonography in the pediatric population is impres-sive because of limited ossification of the vertebral col-umn. The epidural catheter tip, dural displacement, and the extent of cranial spread of a fluid bolus can all be visualized.

## QUESTIONS OF THE DAY

1. What is the distal termination of the spinal cord in adults and infants? Why is this landmark important to know when performing spinal anesthesia?
2. How does the shape of the spinous processes change from the thoracic to lumbar region? What is the implication for epidural block technique?
3. What is the mechanism of differential sensory block during spinal anesthesia? What is the clinical impli-cation when assessing block height?
4. What are the cardiovascular, respiratory, and gastro-intestinal effects of neuraxial anesthesia?
5. What are the absolute and relative contraindications to neuraxial anesthesia?
6. How does local anesthetic baricity impact local anes-thetic spread during spinal anesthesia? What patient positions can alter the spread of hyperbaric spinal anesthesia?

III

7. What local anesthetics are available for spinal use in your institution? How do they differ in terms of duration of action or side effect profile?

8. What is the effect of the following spinal anesthesia additives on quality and/or duration of anesthesia: opioids, vasoconstrictors, alpha agonists?

9. What factors affect epidural anesthesia block height?

10. What are the possible neurologic complications of neuraxial anesthesia? What are the risk factors for each?

## REFERENCES

1. Guay J, Choi PT, Suresh S, et al. Neuraxial anesthesia for the prevention of postoperative mortality and major morbidity: an overview of Cochrane Systematic Reviews. *Anesth Analg.* 2014;119:716–725.
2. Leslie K, McIlroy D, Kasza J, et al. Neuraxial block and postoperative epidural analgesia: effects on outcomes in the POISE-2 trial. *Br J Anaesth.* 2016;116:100–112.
3. Beattie WS, Badner NH, Choi P. Epidural analgesia reduces postoperative myocardial infarction: a meta-analysis. *Anesth Analg.* 2001;93:853–858.
4. Bernards CM, Hill HF. Morphine and alfentanil permeability through the spinal dura, arachnoid, and pia mater of dogs and monkeys. *Anesthesiology.* 1990;73:1214–1219.
5. Zarzur E. Anatomic studies of the human ligamentum flavum. *Anesth Analg.* 1984;63:499–502.
6. Liu S, Kopacz DJ, Carpenter RL. Quantitative assessment of differential sensory nerve block after lidocaine spinal anesthesia. *Anesthesiology.* 1995;82:60–63.
7. Greene NM. Distribution of local anesthetic solutions within the subarachnoid space. *Anesth Analg.* 1985;64:715–730.
8. Visser WA, Lee RA, Gielen MJM. Factors affecting the distribution of neural blockade by local anesthetics in epidural anesthesia and a comparison of lumbar versus thoracic epidural anesthesia. *Anesth Analg.* 2008;107:708–721.
9. Greene NM. *Physiology of Spinal Anesthesia.* 3rd ed. Baltimore: Williams & Wilkins; 1981.
10. Crystal GJ, Salem MR. The Bainbridge and the "reverse" Bainbridge reflexes: history, physiology, and clinical relevance. *Anesth Analg.* 2012;114:520–532.
11. Olausson K, Magnusdottir H, Lurje L, et al. Anti-ischemic and anti-anginal effects of thoracic epidural anesthesia versus those of conventional medical therapy in the treatment of severe refractory unstable angina pectoris. *Circulation.* 1997;96:2178–2182.
12. Minville V, Asehnoune K, Salau S, et al. The effects of spinal anesthesia on cerebral blood flow in the very elderly. *Anesth Analg.* 2009;108:1291–1294.
13. Groeben H. Epidural anesthesia and pulmonary function. *J Anesth.* 2006;20:290–299.
14. Freise H, Fischer LG. Intestinal effects of thoracic epidural anesthesia. *Curr Opin Anaesthesiol.* 2009;22:644–648.
15. Hawkins JL. Epidural analgesia for labor and delivery. *N Engl J Med.* 2010;362:1503–1510.
16. Macfarlane AJR, Prasad GA, Chan VWS, Brull R. Does regional anaesthesia improve outcome after total hip arthroplasty? A systematic review. *Br J Anaesth.* 2009;103:335–345.
17. Macfarlane AJR, Prasad GA, Chan VWS, Brull R. Does regional anesthesia improve outcome after total knee arthroplasty? *Clin Orthop Relat Res.* 2009;467:2379–2402.
18. Nishimori M, Low JHS, Zheng H, Ballantyne JC. Epidural pain relief versus systemic opioid-based pain relief for abdominal aortic surgery. *Cochrane Database Syst Rev.* 2012;(7):CD005059.
19. Joshi GP, Bonnet F, Shah R, et al. The comparative effects of postoperative analgesic therapies on pulmonary outcome: cumulative meta-analyses of randomized, controlled trials. *Anesth Analg.* 2008;107:1026–1040.
20. Svircevic V, van Dijk D, Nierich AP, et al. Meta-analysis of thoracic epidural anesthesia versus general anesthesia for cardiac surgery. *Anesthesiology.* 2011;114:271–282.
21. Neal JM, Barrington MJ, Brull R, et al. The Second ASRA Practice Advisory on Neurologic Complications Associated With Regional Anesthesia and Pain Medicine: executive Summary 2015. *Reg Anesth Pain Med.* 2015;40(5):401–430.
22. Hilt H, Gramm HJ, Link J. Changes in intracranial pressure associated with extradural anaesthesia. *Br J Anaesth.* 1986;58:676–680.
23. Hebl JR, Horlocker TT, Kopp SL, Schroeder DR. Neuraxial blockade in patients with preexisting spinal stenosis, lumbar disk disease, or prior spine surgery: efficacy and neurologic complications. *Anesth Analg.* 2010;111:1511–1519.
24. Perlas A, Chan VWS. Neuraxial anesthesia and multiple sclerosis. *Can J Anaesth.* 2005;52:454–458.
25. McDonald SB. Is neuraxial blockade contraindicated in the patient with aortic stenosis? *Reg Anesth Pain Med.* 2004;29:496–502.
26. Choi S, Brull R. Neuraxial techniques in obstetric and non-obstetric patients with common bleeding diatheses. *Anesth Analg.* 2009;109:648–660.
27. Wedel DJ, Horlocker TT. Regional anesthesia in the febrile or infected patient. *Reg Anesth Pain Med.* 2006;31:324–333.
28. Hocking G, Wildsmith JAW. Intrathecal drug spread. *Br J Anaesth.* 2004;93:568–578.
29. Tetzlaff JE, O'Hara J, Bell G, et al. Influence of baricity on the outcome of spinal anesthesia with bupivacaine for lumbar spine surgery. *Reg Anesth.* 1995;20:533–537.
30. Van Zundert AA, Grouls RJ, Korsten HH, Lambert DH. Spinal anesthesia: volume or concentration—what matters? *Reg Anesth.* 1996;21:112–118.
31. Sarantopoulos C, Fassoulaki A. Systemic opioids enhance the spread of sensory analgesia produced by intrathecal lidocaine. *Anesth Analg.* 1994;79:94–97.
32. Carpenter RL, Hogan QH, Liu SS, et al. Lumbosacral cerebrospinal fluid volume is the primary determinant of sensory block extent and duration during spinal anesthesia. *Anesthesiology.* 1998;89:24–29.
33. Taivainen T, Tuominen M, Rosenberg PH. Influence of obesity on the spread of spinal analgesia after injection of plain 0.5% bupivacaine at the L3-4 or L4-5 interspace. *Br J Anaesth.* 1990;64:542–546.
34. Kim JT, Shim JK, Kim SH, et al. Trendelenburg position with hip flexion as a rescue strategy to increase spinal anaesthetic level after spinal block. *Br J Anaesth.* 2007;98:396–400.
35. Urmey WF, Stanton J, Bassin P, Sharrock NE. The direction of the Whitacre needle aperture affects the extent and duration of isobaric spinal anesthesia. *Anesth Analg.* 1997;84:337–341.
36. Casati A, Fanelli G, Cappelleri G, et al. Effects of spinal needle type on lateral distribution of 0.5% hyperbaric bupivacaine. *Anesth Analg.* 1998;87:355–359.

37. Sanderson P, Read J, Littlewood DG, et al. Interaction between baricity (glucose concentration) and other factors influencing intrathecal drug spread. *Br J Anaesth.* 1994;73:744–746.

38. Malinovsky JM, Renaud G, Le Corre P, et al. Intrathecal bupivacaine in humans: influence of volume and baricity of solutions. *Anesthesiology.* 1999;91:1260–1266.

39. Goldblum E, Atchabahian A. The use of 2-chloroprocaine for spinal anaesthesia. *Acta Anaesthesiol Scand.* 2013;57:545–552.

40. Zaric D, Pace NL. Transient neurologic symptoms (TNS) following spinal anaesthesia with lidocaine versus other local anaesthetics. *Cochrane Database Syst Rev.* 2009;(2):CD003006.

41. Casati A, Vinciguerra F. Intrathecal anaesthesia. *Curr Opin Anaesthesiol.* 2002;15:543–551.

42. Nair GS, Abrishami A, Lermitte J, Chung F. Systematic review of spinal anaesthesia using bupivacaine for ambulatory knee arthroscopy. *Br J Anaesth.* 2009;102:307–315.

43. Whiteside JB, Burke D. Comparison of ropivacaine 0.5% (in glucose 5%) with bupivacaine 0.5% (in glucose 8%) for spinal anaesthesia for elective surgery. *Br J Anaesth.* 2003;90:304–308.

44. Hamber EA, Viscomi CM. Intrathecal lipophilic opioids as adjuncts to surgical spinal anesthesia. *Reg Anesth Pain Med.* 1999;24:255–263.

45. Meylan N, Elia N, Lysakowski C, Tramèr MR. Benefit and risk of intrathecal morphine without local anaesthetic in patients undergoing major surgery: meta-analysis of randomized trials. *Br J Anaesth.* 2009;102:156–167.

46. Murphy PM, Stack D, Kinirons B, Laffey JG. Optimizing the dose of intrathecal morphine in older patients undergoing hip arthroplasty. *Anesth Analg.* 2003;97:1709–1715.

47. Flaatten H, Rodt SA, Vamnes J, et al. Postdural puncture headache. A comparison between 26- and 29-gauge needles in young patients. *Anaesthesia.* 1989;44:147–149.

48. Hebl JR. The importance and implications of aseptic techniques during regional anesthesia. *Reg Anesth Pain Med.* 2006;31:311–323.

49. Chin KJ, Karmakar MK, Peng P. Ultrasonography of the adult thoracic and lumbar spine for central neuraxial blockade. *Anesthesiology.* 2011;114:1459–1485.

50. Moore JM. Continuous spinal anesthesia. *Am J Ther.* 2009;16:289–294.

51. Rigler ML, Drasner K, Krejcie TC, et al. Cauda equina syndrome after continuous spinal anesthesia. *Anesth Analg.* 1991;72:275–281.

52. Vaghadia H, Viskari D, Mitchell GW, Berrill A. Selective spinal anesthesia for outpatient laparoscopy. I: characteristics of three hypobaric solutions. *Can J Anaesth.* 2001;48:256–260.

53. Bromage PR. A comparison of the hydrochloride and carbon dioxide salts of lidocaine and prilocaine in epidural analgesia. *Acta Anaesthesiol Scand Suppl.* 1965;16:55–69.

54. Visser WA, Liem TH, van Egmond J, Gielen MJ. Extension of sensory blockade after thoracic epidural administration of a test dose of lidocaine at three different levels. *Anesth Analg.* 1998;86:332–335.

55. Stevens RA, Urmey WF, Urquhart BL, Kao TC. Back pain after epidural anesthesia with chloroprocaine. *Anesthesiology.* 1993;78:492–497.

56. Marinacci AA. Neurological aspects of complications of spinal anesthesia, with medicolegal implications. *Bull Los Angeles Neurol Soc.* 1960;25:170–192.

57. Sultan P, Gutierrez MC, Carvalho B. Neuraxial morphine and respiratory depression: finding the right balance. *Drugs.* 2011;71:1807–1819.

58. Covino BG, Scott DB, McClure JH. *Handbook of Epidural Anaesthesia and Analgesia.* Fribourg, Switzerland: Mediglobe; 1999.

59. Morison DH. Alkalinization of local anaesthetics. *Can J Anaesth.* 1995;42:1076–1079.

60. Schier R, Guerra D, Aguilar J, et al. Epidural space identification: a meta-analysis of complications after air versus liquid as the medium for loss of resistance. *Anesth Analg.* 2009;109:2012–2021.

61. Mhyre JM, Lou VH, Greenfield M, et al. A systematic review of randomized controlled trials that evaluate strategies to avoid epidural vein cannulation during obstetric epidural catheter placement. *Anesth Analg.* 2009;108:1232–1242.

62. Afshan G, Chohan U, Khan FA, et al. Appropriate length of epidural catheter in the epidural space for postoperative analgesia: evaluation by epidurography. *Anaesthesia.* 2011;66:913–918.

63. Tsui BC, Gupta S, Finucane B. Confirmation of epidural catheter placement using nerve stimulation. *Can J Anaesth.* 1998;45:640–644.

64. Lew E, Yeo SW, Thomas E. Combined spinal-epidural anesthesia using epidural volume extension leads to faster motor recovery after elective cesarean delivery: a prospective, randomized, double-blind study. *Anesth Analg.* 2004;98:810–814.

65. Rawal N. Combined spinal-epidural anaesthesia. *Curr Opin Anaesthesiol.* 2005;18:518–521.

66. Mackey D. Physiologic effects of regional block. In: Brown DL, ed. *Regional Anesthesia and Analgesia.* Philadelphia: WB Saunders; 1996.

67. Cook TM, Counsell D, Wildsmith JAW. Royal College of Anaesthetists Third National Audit Project. Major complications of central neuraxial block: report on the Third National Audit Project of the Royal College of Anaesthetists. *Br J Anaesth.* 2009;102:179–190.

68. Moore DC, Spierdijk J, vanKleef JD, et al. Chloroprocaine neurotoxicity: four additional cases. *Anesth Analg.* 1982;61:155–159.

69. Brull R, McCartney CJL, Chan VWS, El-Beheiry H. Neurological complications after regional anesthesia: contemporary estimates of risk. *Anesth Analg.* 2007;104:965–974.

70. Horlocker TT. What's a nice patient like you doing with a complication like this? Diagnosis, prognosis and prevention of spinal hematoma. *Can J Anaesth.* 2004;51:527–534.

71. Choi PT, Galinski SE, Takeuchi L, et al. PDPH is a common complication of neuraxial blockade in parturients: a meta-analysis of obstetrical studies. *Can J Anaesth.* 2003;50:460–469.

72. Turnbull DK, Shepherd DB. Post-dural puncture headache: pathogenesis, prevention and treatment. *Br J Anaesth.* 2003;91:718–729.

73. Harrington BE. Postdural puncture headache and the development of the epidural blood patch. *Reg Anesth Pain Med.* 2004;29:136–163.

74. Paech MJ, Doherty DA, Christmas T, Wong CA. Epidural Blood Patch Trial Group. The volume of blood for epidural blood patch in obstetrics: a randomized, blinded clinical trial. *Anesth Analg.* 2011;113:126–133.

75. Gozdemir M, Muslu B, Sert H, et al. Transient neurological symptoms after spinal anaesthesia with levobupivacaine 5 mg/ml or lidocaine 20 mg/ml. *Acta Anaesthesiol Scand.* 2010;54:59–64.

76. Hartmann B, Junger A, Klasen J, et al. The incidence and risk factors for hypotension after spinal anesthesia induction: an analysis with automated data collection. *Anesth Analg.* 2002;94:1521–1529.

77. Gwirtz KH, Young JV, Byers RS, et al. The safety and efficacy of intrathecal opioid analgesia for acute postoperative pain: seven years' experience with 5969 surgical patients at Indiana University Hospital. *Anesth Analg.* 1999;88:599–604.

78. American Society of Anesthesiologists Task Force on Neuraxial Opioids, Horlocker TT, Burton AW, Connis RT, et al. Practice guidelines for the prevention, detection, and management of respiratory depression associated with neuraxial opioid administration. *Anesthesiology.* 2009;110:218–230.

79. Auroy Y, Benhamou D, Bargues L, et al. Major complications of regional anesthesia in France: the SOS Regional Anesthesia Hotline Service. *Anesthesiology*. 2002;97:1274–1280.

80. Borgeat A, Ekatodramis G, Schenker CA. Postoperative nausea and vomiting in regional anesthesia: a review. *Anesthesiology*. 2003;98:530–547.

81. Kuipers PW, Kamphuis ET, van Venrooij GE, et al. Intrathecal opioids and lower urinary tract function: a urodynamic evaluation. *Anesthesiology*. 2004;100:1497–1503.

82. Rathmell JP, Lair TR, Nauman B. The role of intrathecal drugs in the treatment of acute pain. *Anesth Analg*. 2005;101(5 suppl):S30–S43.

83. Crowley LJ, Buggy DJ. Shivering and neuraxial anesthesia. *Reg Anesth Pain Med*. 2008;33:241–252.

84. Bell DN, Leslie K. Detection of intravascular epidural catheter placement: a review. *Anaesth Intensive Care*. 2007;35:335–341.

# 18 PERIPHERAL NERVE BLOCKS

## Edward N. Yap and Andrew T. Gray

## INTRODUCTION

### The Role of Regional Anesthesia

Peripheral nerve blocks can provide surgical anesthesia and postoperative pain relief (Table 18.1). Paresthetic techniques and peripheral nerve blocks have been used for decades. However, the main emphasis of this chapter will be on ultrasound guidance for peripheral nerve blocks. In addition, ultrasound guidance and nerve stimulation technologies can be combined for some regional blocks.

### Preparation to Perform a Regional Nerve Block

#### Foundation of Knowledge
To perform safe and effective peripheral nerve blocks, an understanding of peripheral neuroanatomy, ultrasound technology, local anesthetic pharmacology, and risks associated with peripheral nerve blocks is needed.

#### Patient and Surgeon Factors
The willingness of the patient and the surgeon, as well as the anatomic location of the surgery, must be taken into consideration when incorporating peripheral nerve blocks into an anesthetic plan. A thorough preoperative review of the patient's medical history, including any comorbid diseases, allergies, prior neuropathy, and concurrent anticoagulation medications, must be performed to rule out any contraindications in providing a peripheral nerve block.

#### Monitors and Equipment
Peripheral nerve blocks may be performed preoperatively in a dedicated block area or in the operating room. The patient must have a functional peripheral intravenous line, and monitoring equipment including pulse oximetry,

The editors and publisher would like to thank Dr. Adam B. Collins for contributing a chapter on this topic to the prior edition of this work. It has served as the foundation for the current chapter.

electrocardiogram (ECG), and noninvasive blood pressure machine. Supplemental oxygen as well as emergency medications and airway equipment must be readily accessible. Sedation may be indicated, depending on the patient's anxiety and magnitude of pain.

The patient, ultrasound machine, and anesthesia provider must be positioned in a way to optimize the nerve block being performed. For most blocks, the provider is positioned on the ipsilateral side and the ultrasound on the contralateral side of the block region. The choice of the ultrasound probe (Fig. 18.1) and needle is dependent on the location of the peripheral nerve block as well, and the addition of placing a catheter will depend on the type of surgery being performed, the duration of hospital stay, and patient and surgeon preference.

## Choice of Local Anesthetic

The choice of local anesthetic for peripheral nerve blockade depends on a number of factors, including the desired onset, duration, and degree of conduction block (see Chapter 10). Lidocaine and mepivacaine, 1% to 1.5%, produce surgical anesthesia in 10 to 20 minutes that lasts 2 to 3 hours. Ropivacaine, 0.5%, and bupivacaine, 0.375% to 0.5%, have a slower onset and produce less motor blockade, but the effect lasts for at least 6 to 8 hours. The

addition of epinephrine, 1:200,000 (5 µg/mL), can serve as a marker for intravascular injection and can increase the duration of a conduction block. In addition, through a decrease in the rate of systemic absorption, epinephrine can reduce peak plasma levels of local anesthetic. Considerations for the choice of local anesthetic solution for intravenous regional anesthesia are different from those for peripheral nerve blocks (see the later discussion under "Intravenous Regional Anesthesia [Bier Block]").

## Regional Block Checklist

A standardized regional block checklist should be reviewed prior to performing a peripheral nerve block to improve safety.[1] The checklist should include surgical consent and site marking, allergies and anticoagulation status, proposed peripheral nerve block and local anesthetic dose, side of the block, monitors implemented, emergency equipment available, and sedation plan.

## Risks and Prevention

### Infection

Infectious risk associated with a peripheral nerve block or placement of a peripheral nerve catheter is rare.[2] However, an infection can cause significant morbidity and may lead to permanent neurologic injury. By performing proper hand hygiene, using maximal barriers during nerve block and catheter placement, and providing antiseptic solution at the site of insertion, the rate of infection can be reduced.

### Hematoma

The risk of developing a hematoma depends on location of the peripheral nerve block being performed, the proximity to vascular structures, and vascular compressibility. With the use of ultrasound and proper aspiration technique, vascular puncture can be reduced.[3] A review of the patient's medical history with an emphasis on any anticoagulation medications is important. The American Society of Regional Anesthesia and Pain Medicine provides guidelines on anticoagulation management.[4]

### Local Anesthetic Systemic Toxicity (Also See Chapter 10)

Local anesthetic systemic toxicity (LAST) secondary to local anesthetic absorption can range from mild symptoms to major neurologic and cardiovascular toxicity. A variety of

| **Table 18.1** | Examples of Peripheral Nerve Blocks |
| --- | --- |

| Origin | Specific Block |
| --- | --- |
| Cervical plexus | Superficial |
| Brachial plexus | Interscalene |
| | Supraclavicular |
| | Infraclavicular |
| | Axillary |
| Lumbar plexus | Lateral femoral cutaneous[a] |
| | Femoral |
| | Adductor canal |
| | Saphenous |
| | Obturator[a] |
| Sacral plexus | Proximal sciatic |
| | Popliteal sciatic |

[a]Not covered.

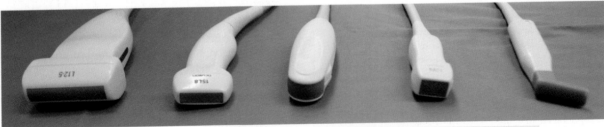

**Fig. 18.1** Ultrasound transducers for regional blocks. (From Gray AT. *Atlas of Ultrasound-Guided Regional Anesthesia.* 2nd ed. Philadelphia: Elsevier; 2013:22.

factors including patient risk factors, concurrent medications, total local anesthetic dose, and anatomic location of the peripheral nerve block play a role in the risk of LAST. There is no single measure to prevent LAST; however, using the smallest effective dose, an incremental injection, aspiration prior to injection, an intravascular marker (i.e., epinephrine), and ultrasound guidance may decrease the risk of LAST. Lipid emulsion resuscitation remains the cornerstone of therapy to treat patients with LAST.[5]

### Nerve Injury

Nerve injury may result from direct needle trauma, inadvertent intraneural injection, or drug neurotoxicity. Serious neurologic injury from a peripheral nerve block is rare; however, the rate of transient paresthesia that resolves within days to weeks postoperatively is substantially higher.[6,7] The use of ultrasound to identify nerves, limiting the injection pressure, and patient feedback may help decrease the rate of nerve injury, although clinical outcome data are limited.

### Wrong-Sided Block

Wrong site, wrong procedure, and wrong patient peripheral nerve blocks are potentially serious medical errors that are inherent risks in performing any medical procedure.[8] Although rare, this complication can be reduced by having a universal protocol that includes a checklist to ensure the correct patient, the proper surgery site, and correct laterality (Table 18.2).

## ULTRASOUND BASICS

An understanding of ultrasound imaging and transducer manipulation is important in providing safe and effective peripheral nerve blocks.

### Basic Ultrasound Physics

Ultrasound imaging uses sound waves with frequency greater than 20 kHz. The use of ultrasound for medical purposes was first recognized in the 1930s. Since then, improvements in technology have paved the way to produce real-time images to help in diagnostics and interventions. Medical ultrasound machines use piezoelectric crystals in the transducer that convert electrical currents into mechanical pressure waves and vice versa, sending and receiving ultrasound echoes to thereby generate images.

As ultrasound waves pass through different body tissues the resistance to the propagation of ultrasound waves, or acoustic impedance, changes depending on the density of the tissue. Solid tissues have denser particles that effectively reflect waves that will be received by the transducer, displayed as brighter or hyperechoic structures. Less dense tissue does not reflect ultrasound waves as effectively, displayed as darker or hypoechoic structures. Tissues that do not reflect any ultrasound waves are considered anechoic.

Improving image resolution, or the ability to distinguish one structure from another, will optimize performance of peripheral nerve blocks. Increasing the frequency of the ultrasound wave will improve resolution of the image but will decrease the penetration of the ultrasound waves. Decreasing the frequency will lower the resolution but will improve the penetration to deeper tissue because there is less attenuation. Increasing the receiver gain (i.e., amplification of the returning echo signal) can to some extent compensate for attenuation.

## Echogenic Properties of Nerves and Tissue

Peripheral nerves can be recognized on ultrasound scans by their fascicular echotexture. Central nerves (such as the cervical ventral rami) and very small nerves (such as the phrenic nerve) have a monofascicular or oligofascicular appearance (Fig. 18.2). Most peripheral nerves have a polyfascicular appearance, which consists of a collection

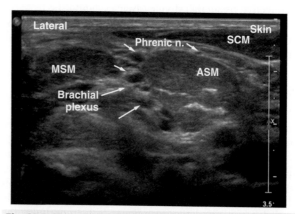

**Fig. 18.2** This sonogram of the right side of the neck shows the roots of the brachial plexus as they pass between the anterior and middle scalene muscles. The core of these large peripheral nerves is less echogenic than the surrounding muscle. The phrenic nerve is a small hypoechoic structure seen on the anterior surface of the anterior scalene muscle. *ASM*, Anterior scalene muscle; *MSM*, middle scalene muscle; *SCM*, sternocleidomastoid muscle.

| Table 18.2 | Approximate Incidence of Adverse Events During Peripheral Nerve Blocks | |
|---|---|---|
| **Adverse Event** | **Approximate Incidence** | |
| Anesthetic systemic toxicity | 1 in 1000 | |
| Peripheral nerve injury | 1 in 1000 | |
| Wrong side/site block | 1 in 10,000 | |

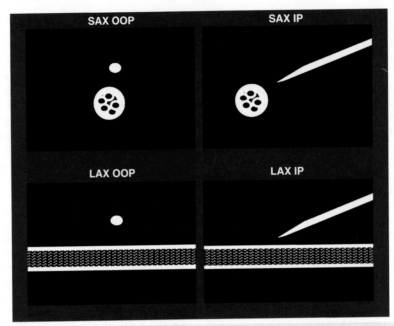

**Fig. 18.3** Approaches to regional block with ultrasound. *LAX IP*, Long-axis imaging, in-plane needle approach; *LAX OOP*, long-axis imaging, out-of-plane needle approach; *SAX IP*, short-axis imaging, in-plane needle approach; *SAX OOP*, short-axis imaging, out-of-plane needle approach. (From Gray AT. *Atlas of Ultrasound-Guided Regional Anesthesia*. 2nd ed. Philadelphia: Elsevier; 2013:32, Fig. 12-1.)

of small round hypoechoic dots (from the nerve fascicles or nerve fiber content) surrounded by hyperechoic stroma (from the nerve connective tissue). This pattern can be referred to as "honeycomb" or "bunch of grapes." Although we use the term *nerve fascicles*, it is understood that only a subset of the total number of fascicles will be evident on an ultrasound scan because thin layers of connective tissue that divide fascicles cannot be resolved on the image.[9] Nerves have a relatively constant cross-sectional area along their course, which helps distinguish these anatomic structures from tendons.

### Ergonomics and Transducer Manipulation

Proper ergonomics are essential for ultrasound-guided interventions. It is important to maintain proper posture and position to reduce anesthesia provider fatigue (e.g., optimize patient position, bed height, and position of the display). A comfortable grip on the ultrasound transducer and resting the ulnar aspect of the transducer hand on the patient will promote stability. There are five basic transducer manipulation techniques to help optimize the ultrasound image: sliding, tilting, rocking, rotation, and compression. Peripheral nerves exhibit anisotropy, which means that the reflected echoes depend on the angle of insonation.[10] The transducer can be tilted to maximize the returning echoes for the peripheral nerve. Slide and rotate the transducer to find the needle tip while maintaining nerve visibility. For some regional blocks the soft

tissue will allow the transducer to rock back and reduce the angle of insonation, thereby improving needle tip visibility. Visual inspection is a good technique before using ultrasound guidance or if needle lineups are difficult.[11] Most practitioners compress adjacent veins while introducing the needle to reduce the chance of venous puncture.

### Regional Block Technique

There are multiple approaches to peripheral nerve blocks. Most blocks can be performed with a short-axis view of the nerve to be blocked. This view is stable for nerves with a relatively straight path. The in-plane technique, with the entire needle shaft and tip within the plane of imaging, is often used to guide needle placement (Fig. 18.3). Alternatively, the out-of-plane approach can be used so that the needle tip crosses the plane of imaging as an echogenic dot. The quality of imaging and identification of structures is more important than approach. Differences in outcomes have been difficult to show when comparing various approaches to blocks in clinical studies.

### Peripheral Nerve Catheters

Catheters can be placed adjacent to peripheral nerves for postoperative analgesia by infusion of dilute local anesthetic solutions. Continuous peripheral nerve blocks can be used in the hospital setting to facilitate vigorous

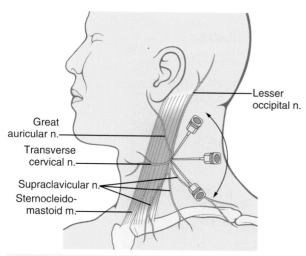

**Fig. 18.4** Anatomic landmarks and method of needle placement for a superficial cervical plexus block. With the patient's head turned to the side, local anesthetic is infiltrated along the posterolateral border of the sternocleidomastoid muscle. (Modified from Brown DL, Factor DA, eds. *Regional Anesthesia and Analgesia*. Philadelphia: WB Saunders; 1996:245.)

early joint mobilization following orthopedic surgery. They can also be used to provide potent analgesia for outpatient surgery (also see Chapter 37). For placement of these catheters, the peripheral nerve should be first located in a fashion similar to that for single-injection blocks (typically ultrasound guidance with a large-bore needle), and then the catheter is threaded. Injection of a local anesthetic or dextrose solution immediately prior to catheter placement can be useful by creating more space adjacent to the nerve. Peripheral nerve catheters are more prone to dislodgment than epidural catheters because movement of skin near the catheter entry point is more likely.

## CERVICAL PLEXUS BLOCK

The cervical plexus is formed by the second, third, and fourth cervical nerves. With the patient's head turned to the opposite side, the superficial cervical plexus can be blocked by infiltration of local anesthetic solution just deep to the platysma and investing fascia of the neck along the posterior lateral border of the sternocleidomastoid muscle (Fig. 18.4). The anesthesia produced by a cervical plexus block includes the area from the inferior surface of the mandible to the level of the clavicle. A cervical plexus block is used most often to provide anesthesia in conscious patients undergoing carotid endarterectomy (see Chapter 25). Although combined superficial and deep cervical plexus blocks have traditionally been used for this surgical procedure, a superficial block alone is often sufficient.

## UPPER EXTREMITY BLOCKS

### Brachial Plexus

The brachial plexus is a network of nerves that is composed of five nerve roots (C5, C6, C7, C8, and T1) that provide both motor control and sensory input for almost the entire upper extremity (Fig. 18.5). The skin over the shoulder is supplied by the supraclavicular nerves of the cervical plexus, and the medial aspect of the arm is supplied by the intercostobrachial branch of the second intercostal nerve (Fig. 18.6). The C5 to T1 nerve roots form ventral rami and trunks in the space between the anterior and middle scalene muscles in the cervical region and then pass over the first rib and under the clavicle. The trunks form three anterior and three posterior divisions, which recombine to create three cords in the infraclavicular region. These cords divide into terminal branches in the axillary region. The location of the surgery, experience of the anesthesia provider, and patient factors, such as body habitus, help determine where along the brachial plexus a peripheral nerve block should be performed (Table 18.3).

### Interscalene Block

An interscalene block targets the ventral rami of the brachial plexus (derived from C5, C6, C7, C8, and T1 nerve roots) and is therefore suited for surgeries that involve the distal clavicle, shoulder, and upper arm.[12] The interscalene block can spare the inferior trunk (from C8 and T1, partly the ulnar distribution of the brachial plexus), and thus is not always suitable for distal forearm and hand surgeries.

An interscalene block is traditionally performed near the C6 vertebral level, where the brachial plexus emerges in between the anterior and middle scalene muscles. The patient's head is turned toward the contralateral side of the block to help expose the interscalene groove. A linear ultrasound probe is placed in a transverse plane at the C6 vertebral level, providing a short-axis view of the brachial plexus. Anatomic structures that are identified should be the middle scalene muscle, anterior scalene muscle, sternocleidomastoid muscle, and brachial plexus (Fig. 18.7). The obtained view has a "stop-light" appearance of the brachial plexus that refers to the C5, C6, and C7 ventral rami as aligned in a parallel fashion from cephalad to caudad.

In the in-plane technique the needle is inserted in the lateral to medial direction through the middle scalene muscle toward the brachial plexus. Once the needle passes into the brachial plexus fascia sheath, local anesthetic is injected. To ensure an adequate block, spread of the local anesthetic should be seen along the cervical ventral rami.

Interscalene block has the potential risk of Horner syndrome, recurrent laryngeal nerve block, epidural or subarachnoid injection, vertebral artery injection, and

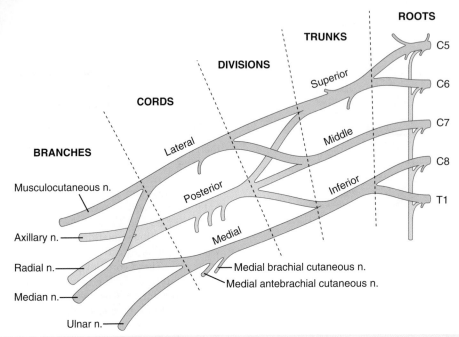

**Fig. 18.5** Roots, trunks, divisions, cords, and branches of the right brachial plexus. (Modified from Horlocker TT, Kopp SL, Wedel DJ. Nerve blocks. In Miller RD, ed. *Miller's Anesthesia*. 8th ed. Philadelphia: Elsevier; 2015:1724, Fig. 57-3.)

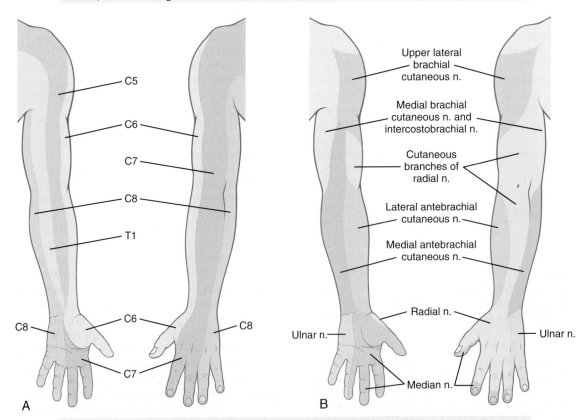

**Fig. 18.6** (A) Cutaneous distribution of the cervical and thoracic roots of the upper extremity. (B) Cutaneous distribution of the peripheral nerves of the upper extremity. (Modified from Horlocker TT , Kopp SL, Wedel DJ. Nerve blocks. In Miller RD, ed. *Miller's Anesthesia*. 8th ed. Philadelphia: Elsevier; 2015:1725, Fig. 57-4.)

**Table 18.3**   Techniques for Brachial Plexus Block

| Technique | Level | Advantage | Potential Drawback(s) |
|---|---|---|---|
| Interscalene | Roots/trunks | Shoulder coverage | Hemidiaphragmatic paresis Inferior trunk sparing |
| Supraclavicular | Trunks/divisions | Overall completeness | Pneumothorax risk |
| Infraclavicular | Cords | Catheter placement | Deep to pectoral muscles |
| Axillary | Branches | Shallow block | Musculocutaneous nerve sparing |

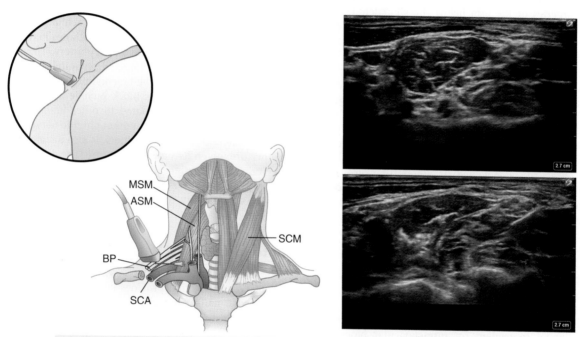

**Fig. 18.7** The brachial plexus passes between the anterior and middle scalene muscles and joins the subclavian artery as it passes over the first rib *(left, lower drawing)*. Interscalene block of the brachial plexus is performed with the patient supine and the head turned to the contralateral side *(left, upper drawing)*. The interscalene groove is imaged with high-frequency ultrasound *(right, upper sonogram)*. The needle advances from lateral to medial within the plane of imaging. Interscalene block is performed by infiltrating local anesthetic around the roots of the brachial plexus as they pass between the anterior and middle scalene muscles *(right, lower sonogram)*. *ASM,* Anterior scalene muscle; *BP,* brachial plexus; *MSM,* middle scalene muscle; *SCA,* subclavian artery; *SCM,* sternocleidomastoid muscle.

pneumothorax. The risk of transient phrenic nerve block and resultant hemidiaphragmatic paresis can be reduced with interscalene injections lower in the neck with a smaller volume and lower concentration of local anesthetic.[13,14]

### Supraclavicular Block

Supraclavicular block of the brachial plexus is achieved by injecting 20 to 30 mL of local anesthetic solution around the brachial plexus where it is usually tightly bundled and adjacent to the subclavian artery, just cephalad to the clavicle. Pneumothorax is the most common serious complication of a supraclavicular block (about a 1% incidence) and can be manifested initially as cough, dyspnea, or pleuritic chest pain. Block of the phrenic nerve occurs frequently (50% of procedures) but generally causes no clinically significant symptoms. Bilateral supraclavicular blocks are not recommended for fear of bilateral pneumothorax or phrenic nerve paralysis. Likewise, patients with chronic obstructive pulmonary disease may not be ideal candidates for a supraclavicular block. Advantages of a supraclavicular block are rapid onset and ability to perform the block with the arm in any position. The increased risk for pneumothorax may limit the use of supraclavicular block for outpatients. Because of these risks, many practitioners have advocated the use of ultrasound imaging to guide supraclavicular blocks.

The supraclavicular block can be performed with a similar technique to interscalene blocks described previously. The ultrasound probe is moved closer to the clavicle and faces caudally to facilitate imaging of the brachial plexus adjacent to the subclavian artery and over the first rib. In this location, almost all practitioners utilize in-plane technique because of the proximity of the pleura.

## Infraclavicular Block

The infraclavicular block targets the medial, lateral, and posterior cords of the brachial plexus and is suitable for surgeries of the arm below the shoulder. The cords of the brachial plexus are named in relation to the axillary artery as the plexus travels underneath the clavicle toward the axilla.

The infraclavicular block is performed with the short-axis in-plane approach (Fig. 18.8). A linear or curvilinear ultrasound transducer with a small footprint may be used. The choice of needle is dependent on the patient's body habitus and whether a continuous catheter will be placed. The patient is positioned supine with the arm abducted, elbow flexed, and arm externally rotated if possible. This will retract the clavicle and straighten the neurovascular bundle. The ultrasound transducer is placed medial to the coracoid process in a parasagittal plane (about halfway between supraclavicular and axillary regions). Key structures to identify on the ultrasound image are the pectoral major and minor muscles, axillary artery and vein, and cords of the brachial plexus. Although the cords of the brachial plexus may be visualized around the axillary artery, they can be difficult to delineate on the ultrasound image.

The needle approaches in plane from cephalad to caudad (lateral to medial) for infraclavicular block. After a skin wheal of local anesthetic is placed, the needle is directed toward the space between the lateral cord and the axillary artery. The goal of the infraclavicular block is to spread the local anesthetic around the axillary artery in a U-shaped manner, as this will assure blockade of all three cords of the brachial plexus.

The advantages of the infraclavicular block are the close proximity of the brachial plexus to the artery, relatively consistent anatomy, and a stable site for placement of a continuous peripheral nerve catheter. Because of the close proximity to the clavicle and the depth of the block, performing this block can be challenging in some patients.

## Axillary Block

The axillary block targets the terminal branches of the brachial plexus in the axilla: the median, ulnar, radial, and musculocutaneous nerves. The axillary block is suitable for surgeries of the elbow, forearm, wrist, and hand.

Axillary block is typically performed with a linear transducer using a short-axis view of the nerves and vessels in the axilla and in-plane approach (Fig. 18.9). The patient is positioned supine with the arm to be blocked abducted and externally rotated. The ultrasound image should display the axillary artery and vein(s), terminal branches of the brachial plexus, conjoint tendon, and the biceps, triceps, and coracobrachialis muscles.[15] The relation of the terminal branches to the axillary artery are usually as follows: median (superficial), ulnar (medial), radial (posterior), and musculocutaneous (lateral, traversing through the coracobrachialis muscle). The block is performed with a 5- to 7-cm needle, approaching in plane from cephalad to caudad (lateral to medial) toward the branches of the brachial plexus. The goal is to surround each terminal branch of the brachial plexus with local anesthetic, often leading to local anesthetic spread circumferentially around the axillary artery. The musculocutaneous nerve can be targeted separately after block of the other branches of the brachial plexus.[16]

The advantages of this block include a lower risk of complications when compared to other brachial plexus blocks (e.g., no risk of concomitant phrenic nerve block or pneumothorax). The axillary block is also a simpler block to perform given its superficial nature. The disadvantages include the potential risk of intravascular injection and hematoma given the proximity of the axillary artery and veins, unsuitability for a peripheral nerve catheter, and lack of coverage for the upper arm and shoulder.

## Intercostobrachial Nerve Block

The intercostobrachial nerve is a thoracic nerve (derived from T2 and T3) that provides cutaneous innervation to the medial half of the arm. This block may be used as a supplement to brachial plexus blocks to improve tolerance of an arm tourniquet or to improve surgical conditions for proximal arm surgery. The intercostobrachial nerve can be blocked by subcutaneous infiltration in the medial half of the arm with 2 to 3 mL of local anesthetic.

## LOWER EXTREMITY BLOCKS

The lower extremity nerves originate from the lumbar and sacral plexuses (Fig. 18.10). The lumbar plexus is composed of the first four lumbar nerves (L1-L4). Lower extremity nerves that arise from the lumbar plexus include the lateral femoral cutaneous, femoral, and obturator nerves. The sacral plexus is composed of the first four sacral nerves (S1-S4) and also receives contributions from L4 and L5. This plexus gives rise to the sciatic nerve.

## Femoral Nerve

### Femoral Nerve Block

The femoral nerve is the largest branch of the lumbar plexus and derives from the ventral rami of L2 to L4. This nerve provides motor innervation to the quadriceps

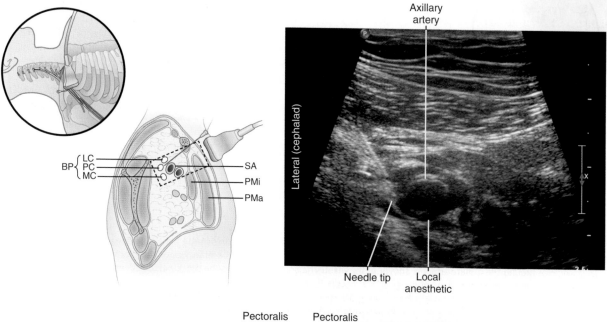

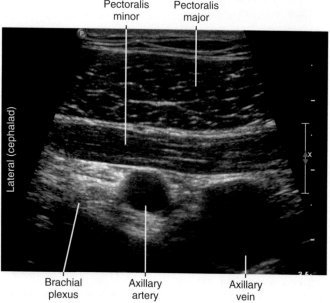

**Fig. 18.8** Technique of infraclavicular block. *(Left)* With the patient supine and the arm abducted and externally rotated, an ultrasound transducer is placed inferior to the clavicle to visualize the subclavian artery and adjacent cords of the brachial plexus. A needle is advanced caudally within the plane of imaging until its tip lies within the fascial sheath that surrounds the brachial plexus deep to the axillary artery. In the sonograms *(right)* the needle tip passes between the lateral and medial cords of the brachial plexus and injects local anesthetic that surrounds the three cords. *BP*, Brachial plexus; *LC*, lateral cord; *MC*, medial cord; *PC*, posterior cord; *PMa*, pectoralis major muscle; *PMi*, pectoralis minor muscle; *SA*, subclavian artery. (Sonograms from Gray AT. *Atlas of Ultrasound-Guided Regional Anesthesia.* 2nd ed. Philadelphia: Elsevier; 2013:93, Figs. 31-2 and 31-3.)

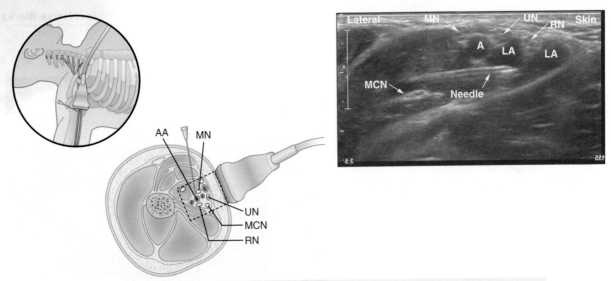

**Fig. 18.9** Axillary block. The arm is abducted 90 degrees. Key structures in the right axilla are visualized with a high-frequency ultrasound transducer. The arrangement of the branches of the brachial plexus around the axillary artery is shown in the inset. The sonogram shows the block needle advancing from lateral within the plane of imaging. The needle tip passes deep to the artery and injects local anesthetic that surrounds the radial nerve. Additional injections ensure local anesthetic spread around the ulnar and median nerves. *A* and *AA*, Axillary artery; *LA*, local anesthetic; *MCN*, musculocutaneous nerve; *MN*, median nerve; *RN*, radial nerve; *UN*, ulnar nerve.

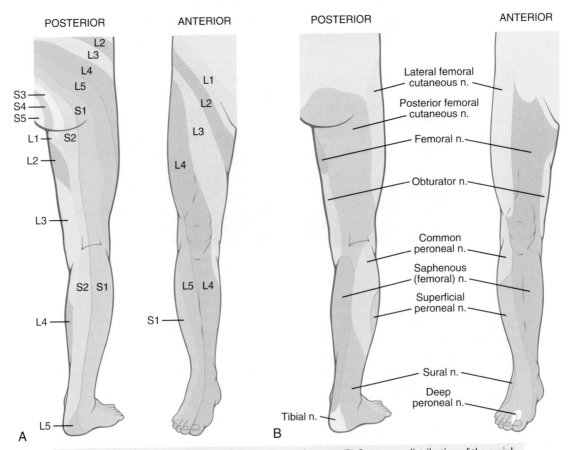

**Fig. 18.10** (A) Cutaneous distribution of the lumbosacral nerves. (B) Cutaneous distribution of the peripheral nerves of the lower extremity. Note that the cutaneous distribution of the obturator nerve is highly variable, but shown here on the medial aspect of the thigh. (Modified from Horlocker TT , Kopp SL, Wedel DJ. Nerve blocks. In Miller RD, ed. *Miller's Anesthesia*. 8th ed. Philadelphia: Elsevier; 2015)

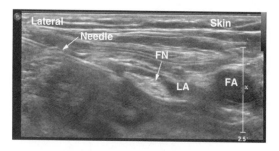

**Fig. 18.11** Femoral nerve block. The femoral nerve runs over the surface of the iliopsoas muscle as it passes under the inguinal ligament. The iliac fascia invests the femoral nerve and iliopsoas muscle, which is anatomically separate from the femoral sheath. Femoral nerve block is performed with short-axis imaging of femoral nerve and artery. In the sonogram, the block needle passes from lateral to medial, deep to the fascia iliaca and injects local anesthetic that surrounds the femoral nerve. *FA*, Femoral artery; *FN*, femoral nerve; *LA*, local anesthetic.

and sensation from the anterior thigh and medial leg. The femoral nerve descends through the psoas muscle and then travels between the psoas and iliacus muscles, exiting the pelvis under the inguinal ligament. Femoral nerve block is suitable for surgeries of the anterior thigh (e.g., quadriceps tendon surgery) and provides analgesia for hip, femur, and knee surgeries.

The femoral nerve block is typically performed distal to the point at which the femoral nerve passes under the inguinal ligament (Fig. 18.11). The nerve block is performed with a 5- to 7-cm echogenic needle with a linear transducer and short-axis in-plane approach. The patient is positioned supine, and the transducer is placed in a transverse plane 1 to 2 cm distal to the inguinal ligament. Important structures to identify in the ultrasound image are the femoral artery and vein, femoral nerve, sartorius and iliopsoas muscles, and the fascia lata and fascia iliaca (which can be difficult to delineate). The femoral nerve is lateral to the femoral artery and can be seen as a flat oval or triangular polyfascicular structure under both fascia lata and fascia iliaca. The needle is advanced from lateral to medial toward the lateral corner of the femoral nerve, and typically two "pops" can be felt as the needle is advanced through the fascia lata and fascia iliaca. Once the needle tip is under the fascia iliaca and adjacent to the femoral nerve, local anesthetic is injected to surround the nerve.

The advantage of femoral nerve block is its reliability in providing analgesia to the anterior thigh and medial leg. It is a good location for a peripheral nerve catheter because it is away from the thigh tourniquet and surgical site. Its predictable and shallow anatomy makes it a relatively easy block to master. However, femoral nerve block does cause quadriceps muscle weakness, which may not be favorable for early mobilization and may increase the risk of falls postoperatively.[17]

### Adductor Canal and Saphenous Nerve Blocks

The adductor canal block targets distal branches of the femoral nerve as they travel deep to the sartorius muscle in the thigh. Sensory nerves from the femoral nerve are still present near the adductor canal (e.g., the saphenous nerve and infrapatellar nerve). However, many motor nerves have already branched off and innervated their corresponding muscles (all except the nerves to the vastus medialis muscle). Therefore, the advantage of the adductor canal block includes analgesia for knee surgery, with minimal quadriceps muscle weakness.[18,19]

The patient is positioned supine with the leg to be blocked slightly externally rotated and bent at the knee (Fig. 18.12). A short-axis in-plane approach with a linear transducer is used. A 5- to 7-cm echogenic needle is appropriate for this block. The adductor canal block is performed midthigh where the superficial femoral artery is near the middle of the undersurface of the sartorius muscle belly. The subsartorial nerves may be visible just lateral to the superficial femoral artery; however, in many

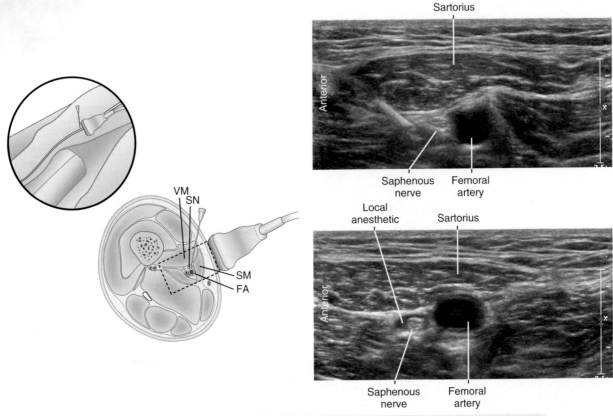

**Fig. 18.12** Saphenous nerve block near the adductor canal. With the patient supine and leg externally rotated, the medial thigh is scanned in axial section with high-frequency ultrasound. The needle advances from anterior to posterior within the plane of imaging. The saphenous nerve is not always visible, but it courses with the superficial femoral artery, deep to the sartorius muscle. Local anesthetic surrounds the saphenous nerve. *FA*, Femoral artery; *SM*, sartorius muscle; *SN*, saphenous nerve; *VM*, vastus medialis muscle. (Sonograms from Gray AT. *Atlas of Ultrasound-Guided Regional Anesthesia.* 2nd ed. Philadelphia: Elsevier; 2013:165, Fig. 41-2C and D.)

cases these nerves are difficult to discern. The goal is to direct the needle from lateral to medial and anterior to posterior and achieve local anesthetic spread under the thick fascia that covers the posterior surface of the sartorius muscle, lateral to the superficial femoral artery.

The saphenous nerve is a terminal branch of the femoral nerve that carries sensory nerve fibers from the medial aspect of the leg, ankle, and foot. Depending on the desired location of blockade, the saphenous nerve can be blocked at the thigh, leg, or ankle. Many practitioners use the adductor canal approach described earlier to block the saphenous nerve in the thigh.

## Sciatic Nerve

### Proximal Sciatic Nerve Block

The sciatic nerve is the largest branch of the sacral plexus and consists of the L4, L5, and S1 to S4 spinal nerves. It provides motor innervation and sensation of the posterior thigh and most of the leg. As the sciatic nerve exits the pelvis via the greater sciatic foramen, it travels along the posterior thigh anterior to the gluteus maximus and biceps femoris and posterior to the adductor magnus muscles. The sciatic nerve block is suitable for surgeries involving the posterior thigh, lower leg, foot and ankle and can also improve analgesia following knee surgery.

There are three main approaches to the sciatic nerve block: the anterior, the transgluteal, and the subgluteal approaches. Only the transgluteal approach will be described here. For the transgluteal approach, the patient is placed in the lateral position with the block leg up and the leg slightly flexed at the hip (Fig. 18.13). A transverse short-axis in-plane approach with a low-frequency linear or curvilinear transducer and a 10-cm echogenic needle is used for the block. The sciatic nerve can reliably be located traveling halfway between the greater trochanter of the femur and the ischial tuberosity, deep to the gluteus maximus muscle. The nerve at this level appears as a hyperechoic polyfascicular triangular structure. The needle is directed lateral to medial and posterior to anterior

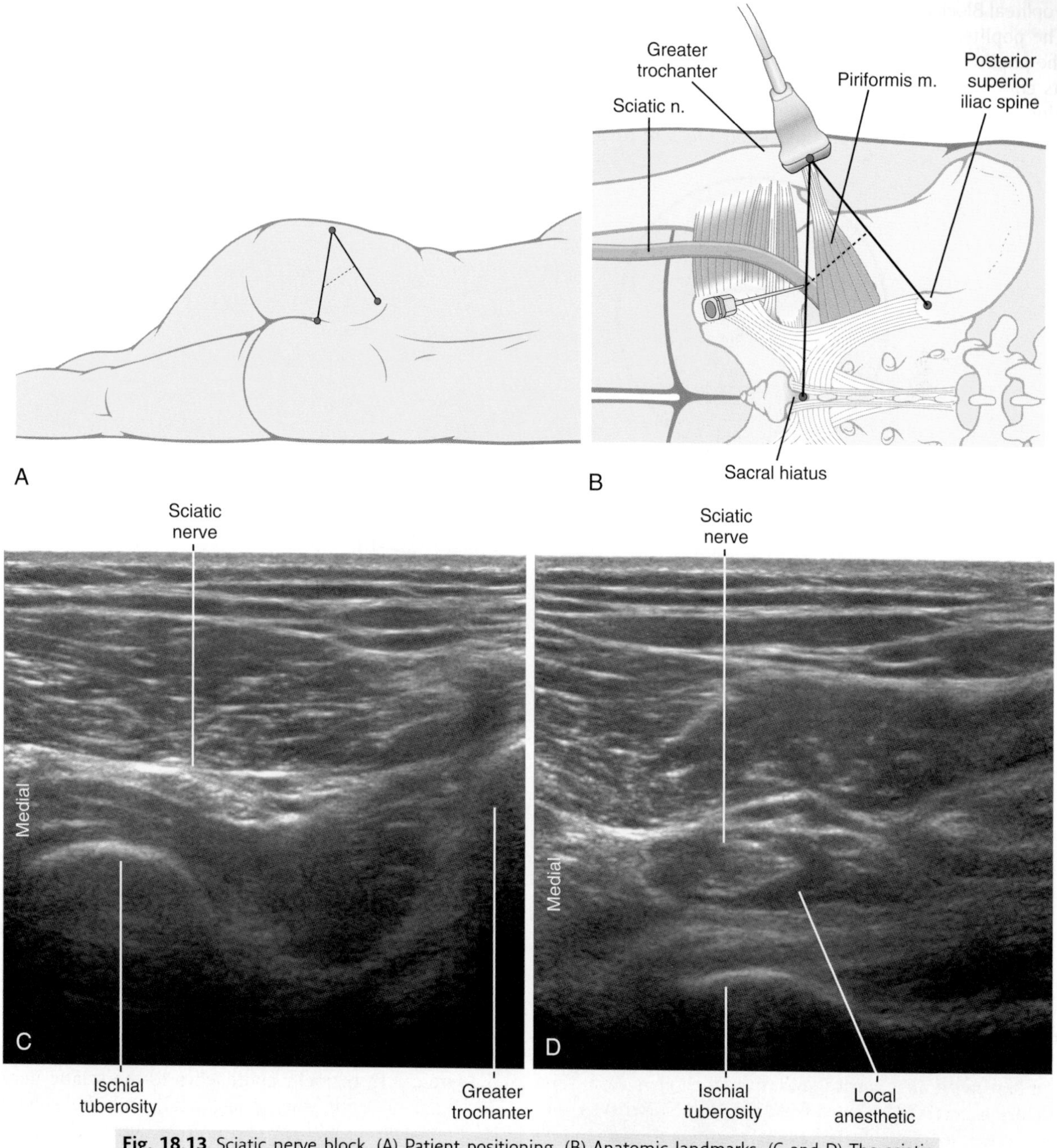

**Fig. 18.13** Sciatic nerve block. (A) Patient positioning. (B) Anatomic landmarks. (C and D) The sciatic nerve lies beneath a point 5 cm caudad along a perpendicular line that bisects a line joining the posterior iliac spine and the greater trochanter of the femur. This point is also usually the intersection of that perpendicular line with a line joining the greater trochanter and the sacral hiatus. (C and D from Gray AT. *Atlas of Ultrasound-Guided Regional Anesthesia*. 2nd ed. Philadelphia: Elsevier; 2013:182, Fig. 43-8A and B.)

toward the lateral border of the sciatic nerve. The goal is to place the needle below the fascial plane of the gluteus maximus muscle and have the local anesthetic spread around the nerve.

The advantages of the sciatic nerve block are the reliable posterior thigh and leg analgesia for the surgeries mentioned previously. This location is away from the thigh tourniquet or surgical site for placement of a continuous peripheral nerve catheter. Disadvantages of the sciatic nerve block are the hamstring weakness, as well as potential procedural discomfort and difficulty due to the increased depth of the block.

## Popliteal Block of the Sciatic Nerve

The popliteal block targets the sciatic nerve as it enters the popliteal fossa, at which point the nerve divides into its common peroneal and tibial nerve components. This block is commonly used for foot and ankle surgery, usually combined with a saphenous nerve block to cover the medial aspect of the leg. The patient is placed in lateral position with the block leg elevated and knee extended.[20] A transverse short-axis in-plane approach is used with a linear transducer and a 5- to 7-cm echogenic needle (Fig. 18.14). The ultrasound transducer is placed in the popliteal fossa, locating the sciatic nerve posterior to

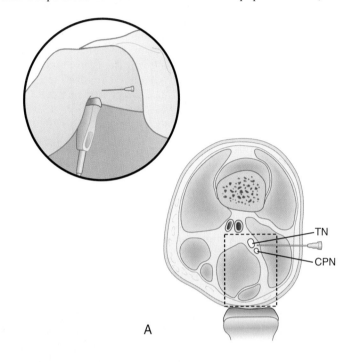

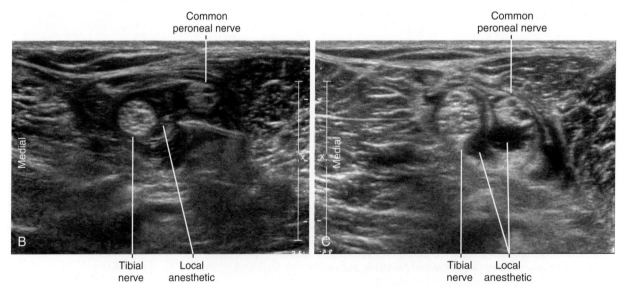

**Fig. 18.14** Popliteal block of the sciatic nerve: (A) The patient is positioned supine with the leg elevated to allow the popliteal fossa to be scanned from below with high-frequency ultrasound. (B and C) The block needle passes from the lateral thigh through the biceps femoris muscle and injects local anesthetic around the tibial and common peroneal nerves. *CPN,* Common peroneal nerve; *TN,* tibial nerve. (B and C from Gray AT. *Atlas of Ultrasound-Guided Regional Anesthesia.* 2nd ed. Philadelphia: Elsevier; 2013:192, Fig. 45-6A and B.)

the popliteal vein and artery. The nerve is blocked at the bifurcation of the sciatic nerve into the tibial and common peroneal nerves, which can be located by sliding the ultrasound transducer cephalad and caudad. The needle is advanced from lateral to medial, with the goal of local anesthetic distribution around both components of the sciatic nerve, creating a "donut" of local anesthetic around each nerve. After injection the tranducer can be slid distally to verify tracking of the local anesthetic with the common peroneal and tibial nerves as they separate in the distal popliteal fossa.

## Ankle Block

All five peripheral nerves that supply the foot can be blocked (ankle block) at the level of the malleoli (Fig. 18.15). The tibial nerve is the major nerve to the sole of

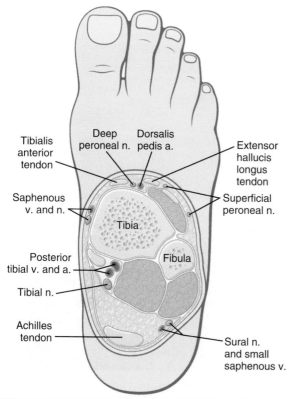

**Fig. 18.15** Cross-sectional anatomy for an ankle block. An ankle block is performed by injecting local anesthetic solution at five separate nerve locations. The superficial peroneal nerve, sural nerve, and saphenous nerve are usually blocked by subcutaneous infiltration because they may have already branched as they cross the ankle joint. The tibial and deep peroneal nerves require deeper injection adjacent to the accompanying blood vessels (the posterior tibial and anterior tibial arteries, respectively). Because the block needle approaches the ankle from many angles, it is convenient to elevate the foot by supporting the calf. (Modified from Brown DL, Factor DA, eds. *Regional Anesthesia and Analgesia.* Philadelphia: WB Saunders; 1996.)

the foot. This nerve lies on the heel side of the posterior tibial artery and can be blocked by infiltrating 3 to 5 mL of local anesthetic solution in a fanning pattern around this artery. The sural nerve innervates the lateral side of the foot and can be blocked by injecting 5 mL of local anesthetic solution in the groove between the lateral malleolus and the calcaneus near the small saphenous vein. The saphenous nerve innervates the medial aspect of the foot. Infiltration of 5 mL of local anesthetic solution anterior to the medial malleolus near the great saphenous vein blocks this nerve. The deep peroneal nerve innervates the webbing between the first and second toes and is blocked by injecting 5 mL of local anesthetic solution adjacent to the anterior tibial artery. Alternatively, if arterial pulsation is absent, the deep peroneal nerve can also be blocked deep to the extensor hallucis longus tendon and extensor retinaculum. The dorsum of the foot is innervated by the superficial peroneal nerve. The superficial branches of this nerve are blocked by injecting a subcutaneous ridge of local anesthetic between the medial and lateral malleoli over the anterior surface of the foot. Because the foot does not have a generous blood supply, systemic toxicity after an ankle block is rare.

## CHEST AND ABDOMEN BLOCKS

Peripheral nerve blocks for the chest and abdomen can provide intraoperative and postoperative analgesia, reduce systemic pain medications, improve patient satisfaction, and improve patient discharge times from the postanesthesia care unit.

### Intercostal Nerve Block

Intercostal nerve blocks target the ventral rami of the thoracic spinal nerves. The intercostal nerves travel inferior to the associated rib within the subcostal groove and inferior to the accompanying intercostal vein and artery. At the angle of the ribs these nerves travel in the space between the internal intercostal and innermost intercostal muscles. These blocks are beneficial for thoracic and upper abdominal surgery, as well as following chest wall trauma. However, because of the proximity of the pleura there is a potential risk of a pneumothorax. LAST is possible due to the high-peak plasma levels after injection, as well as the need for multiple nerve blocks for adequate dermatomal coverage of the surgical incision.

For this block, the patient is positioned prone, and a linear transducer placed in a short-axis parasagittal plane is used at the midscapular line. A 5-cm echogenic needle is used to inject 3 to 5 mL of local anesthetic at each level, proceeding in a caudad to cephalad direction. The ultrasound image should demonstrate the intercostal muscles, pleura, and adjacent ribs and their acoustic shadows. The goal of the block is to have spread of local anesthetic in between the innermost and internal intercostal muscles along the inferior border of the rib.

### Transversus Abdominis Plane Block

The transversus abdominis plane (TAP) block is an abdominal wall field block targeting the ventral rami of the thoracic and lumbar spinal nerves (T7 to L1) as they travel in the plane between the transversus abdominis and internal oblique muscles. The block provides analgesia for lower abdominal surgery and may help with laparoscopic surgery. Because the block relies on a large volume of local anesthetic for appropriate spread, there is some risk of local anesthetic toxicity. There also is a small potential for intraperitoneal injection and intrahepatic injection.

For this block, the patient is positioned supine, and a linear transducer is placed in a transverse plane at the midaxillary line (Fig. 18.16). The ultrasound image should demonstrate the external oblique, internal oblique, and transversus abdominis muscles. A 7- to 10-cm echogenic needle is used to inject at least 20 mL of local anesthetic per side. The needle is directed in the anterior to posterior direction, with the goal of local anesthetic distribution between the transversus abdominis and internal oblique muscles.

## INTRAVENOUS REGIONAL ANESTHESIA (BIER BLOCK)

Intravenous regional anesthesia (or Bier block, named after August Bier) is a method of producing anesthesia of the arm or leg. This anesthetic technique is used for surgical procedures with minimal postoperative pain and duration of 2 hours or less. The technique involves intravenous injection of large volumes of dilute local anesthetic into an extremity after exsanguination and isolation of the circulation by a tourniquet. Contraindications to Bier block include contraindications to a tourniquet (e.g., sickle cell disease, ischemic vascular disease, or infection in the extremity). Lacerations to the blocked arm may cause escape of local anesthetic, and patients with fractures may experience pain during exsanguination of the extremity. Tourniquet pain and the maximum allowable tourniquet time limit the duration of the block. Intravenous regional sympathetic blocks with guanethidine, reserpine, or bretylium are sometimes used for chronic pain management.

To perform the Bier block, a small peripheral intravenous catheter (e.g., 22 G) is placed in the distal portion of the extremity being blocked (Fig. 18.17). The extremity is then exsanguinated by wrapping with an Esmarch bandage from distal to proximal, and then a tourniquet is inflated to 250 to 275 mm Hg (at least 100 mm Hg above the patient's systolic blood pressure). Plain local anesthetic solution (40 to 50 mL for an arm tourniquet in

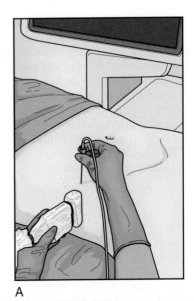

A

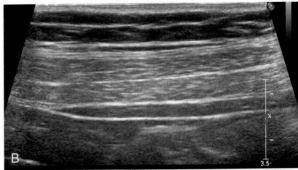

B

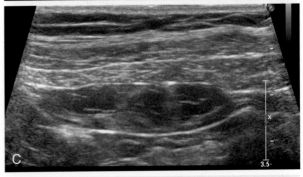

C

**Fig. 18.16** Transversus abdominis plane (TAP) block. (A) For the classic posterior TAP block the patient is in the supine position with the transducer placed near the midaxillary line between the costal margin and pelvic brim. (B and C) The needle travels through the external oblique and internal oblique muscles to enter the fascial plane between the internal oblique and underlying transversus abdominis muscles. The injection should be performed near the posterior border of the transversus abdominis muscle so that the injection distributes with well-defined margins where the nerves enter the plane. (Redrawn from Gray AT. *Atlas of Ultrasound-Guided Regional Anesthesia.* 2nd ed. Philadelphia: Elsevier; 2013:245, Fig. 54-2A.)

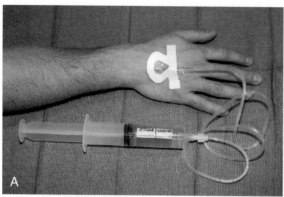
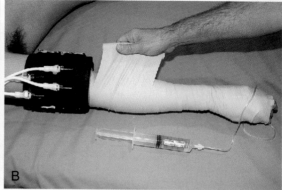

**Fig. 18.17** (A) Placement and securing of a small intravenous catheter. (B) Exsanguination of the arm with an Esmarch bandage before inflation of the tourniquet and injection of the local anesthetic solution through the catheter.

adults) is injected through the intravenous catheter and then the catheter is removed. Patients may begin experiencing pain at the tourniquet site after 45 minutes; a double-tourniquet technique may be employed to help mitigate this. With a double tourniquet, the proximal cuff is initially inflated, and once the patient experiences pain, the distal cuff is inflated over the anesthetized arm and the proximal cuff deflated.

## Selection of Local Anesthetic

Commonly used local anesthetic solutions for intravenous regional anesthesia are 0.5% lidocaine or chloroprocaine (plain solutions without epinephrine). Racemic bupivacaine is avoided because of potential systemic toxicity, which can include malignant ventricular cardiac dysrhythmias leading to refractory cardiac arrest. Preservative-free solutions of local anesthetic are recommended because preservatives have been associated with thrombophlebitis.

## Characteristics of the Block

The onset of anesthesia rapidly follows the intravenous administration of local anesthetic solution into the isolated extremity. The duration of surgical anesthesia depends on the time that the tourniquet is inflated and not on the local anesthetic drug selected. Technically, a regional intravenous anesthesia block is easier and faster to perform than a brachial plexus block or lower extremity block and is readily applicable to all age groups, including pediatric patients.

## Risks

The principal risk associated with intravenous regional anesthesia is the potential systemic toxicity that may occur when the tourniquet is deflated and large amounts of local anesthetic solution from the previously isolated

part of the extremity enter the systemic circulation. Local anesthetic levels peak approximately 2 to 5 minutes after tourniquet deflation. One approach to reduce the risk of toxicity is to keep the tourniquet inflated for at least 20 minutes, even if the surgical procedure is completed in less time. If 40 minutes has elapsed, the tourniquet can be deflated in a single maneuver. If surgical duration is between 20 and 40 minutes, the tourniquet can be deflated, reinflated immediately, and finally deflated after 1 minute. This method will reduce the peak plasma level of local anesthetic. Limitation of extremity movement (including avoidance of extremity elevation) after release of the tourniquet is also useful for minimizing local anesthetic blood levels.

If the extremity is not adequately exsanguinated, the skin will have a blotchy appearance after injection of the local anesthetic. In this situation, the quality of the block and surgical field will be poor.

## QUESTIONS OF THE DAY

1. Can a supraclavicular block be performed successfully without the use of ultrasound? Does the use of ultrasound improve the rate of success? How would you position the patient, anesthesia providers, monitors, and ultrasound machine in order to optimize performance of the block? How can proper ergonomics facilitate block placement?
2. How can peripheral nerves be recognized on ultrasound scans? What features set them apart from other structures such as tendons, veins, and arteries? What transducer manipulation techniques can improve nerve visualization?
3. A patient is scheduled for open reduction of a distal radius fracture. What are the advantages and disadvantages of axillary versus interscalene block for this procedure?

4. What are the potential benefits of femoral nerve block for a patient undergoing knee surgery?

5. A transversus abdominis plane (TAP) block would provide suitable analgesia for what types of surgeries?

6. What type of surgery is most appropriate for an intravenous regional (Bier) block? What precautions can be taken to minimize the risk of systemic toxicity with this block?

## REFERENCES

1. Mulroy MF, Weller RS, Liguori GA. A checklist for performing regional nerve blocks. *Reg Anesth Pain Med.* 2014;39:195–199.

2. Alakkad H, Naeeni A, Chan VW, et al. Infection related to ultrasound-guided single-injection peripheral nerve blockade: a decade of experience at Toronto Western hospital. *Reg Anesth Pain Med.* 2015;40:82–84.

3. Barrington MJ, Kluger R. Ultrasound guidance reduces the risk of local anesthetic systemic toxicity following peripheral nerve blockade. *Reg Anesth Pain Med.* 2013;38:289–297.

4. Horlocker TT, Wedel DJ, Rowlingson JC, et al. Regional anesthesia in the patient receiving antithrombotic or thrombolytic therapy: American Society of Regional Anesthesia and Pain Medicine Evidence-Based Guidelines (Third Edition). *Reg Anesth Pain Med.* 2010;35(1):64–101.

5. Weinberg GL. Lipid emulsion infusion: resuscitation for local anesthetic and other drug overdose. *Anesthesiology.* 2012;117:180–187.

6. Sites BD, Taenzer AH, Herrick MD, et al. Incidence of local anesthetic systemic toxicity and postoperative neurologic symptoms associated with 12,668 ultrasound-guided nerve blocks: an analysis from a prospective clinical registry. *Reg Anesth Pain Med.* 2012;37:478–482.

7. Neal JM, Barrington MJ, Brull R, et al. The Second ASRA Practice Advisory on Neurologic Complications Associated With Regional Anesthesia and Pain Medicine: executive Summary 2015. *Reg Anesth Pain Med.* 2015;40(5):401–430.

8. Hudson ME, Chelly JE, Lichter JR. Wrong-site nerve blocks: 10 yr experience in a large multihospital healthcare system. *Br J Anaesth.* 2015;114:818–824.

9. Silvestri E, Martinoli C, Derchi LE, et al. Echotexture of peripheral nerves: correlation between US and histologic findings and criteria to differentiate tendons. *Radiology.* 1995;197:291–296.

10. Soong J, Schafhalter-Zoppoth I, Gray AT. The importance of transducer angle to ultrasound visibility of the femoral nerve. *Reg Anesth Pain Med.* 2005;30:505.

11. Lam NC, Fishburn SJ, Hammer AR, et al. A randomized controlled trial evaluating the see, tilt, align, and rotate (STAR) maneuver on skill acquisition for simulated ultrasound-guided interventional procedures. *J Ultrasound Med.* 2015;34(6):1019–1026.

12. Kapral S, Greher M, Huber G, et al. Ultrasonographic guidance improves the success rate of interscalene brachial plexus blockade. *Reg Anesth Pain Med.* 2008;33:253–258.

13. Kessler J, Schafhalter-Zoppoth I, Gray AT. An ultrasound study of the phrenic nerve in the posterior cervical triangle: implications for the interscalene brachial plexus block. *Reg Anesth Pain Med.* 2008;33:545–550.

14. Gautier P, Vandepitte C, Ramquet C, et al. The minimum effective anesthesia volume of 0.75% ropivacaine in ultrasound-guided interscalene brachial plexus block. *Anesth Analg.* 2011;113:951–955.

15. Gray AT. The conjoint tendon of the latissimus dorsi and teres major: an important landmark for ultrasound-guided axillary block. *Reg Anesth Pain Med.* 2009;34:179–180.

16. Schafhalter-Zoppoth I, Gray AT. The musculocutaneous nerve: ultrasound appearance for peripheral nerve block. *Reg Anesth Pain Med.* 2005;30:385–390.

17. Ilfeld BM. Single-injection and continuous femoral nerve blocks are associated with different risks of falling. *Anesthesiology.* 2014;121:668–669.

18. Andersen HL, Gyrn J, Møller L, et al. Continuous saphenous nerve block as supplement to single-dose local infiltration analgesia for postoperative pain management after total knee arthroplasty. *Reg Anesth Pain Med.* 2013;38:106–111.

19. Machi AT, Sztain JF, Kormylo NJ, et al. Discharge readiness after tricompartment knee arthroplasty: adductor canal versus femoral continuous nerve blocks—a dual-center, randomized trial. *Anesthesiology.* 2015;123(2):444–456.

20. Gray AT, Huczko EL, Schafhalter-Zoppoth I. Lateral popliteal nerve block with ultrasound guidance. *Reg Anesth Pain Med.* 2004;29:507–509.

# 19 PATIENT POSITIONING AND ASSOCIATED RISKS

Kristine E. W. Breyer

Patient positioning in the operating room facilitates surgical procedures; however, positioning can be a source of patient injury and can alter intraoperative physiology. Positioning injuries during surgery remain a significant source of perioperative morbidity. Anesthesia providers share a critical responsibility for the proper positioning of patients in the operating room.[1] This chapter will review general physiologic changes during positioning, general intraoperative positions, some specific positioning concerns, and intraoperative positioning related injuries.

## PHYSIOLOGIC ASPECTS OF POSITIONING

Physiologic responses play an essential role in blunting hemodynamic changes that would otherwise occur from positional changes in our day-to-day lives. Central, regional, and local mechanisms are involved. When a person reclines from an upright to a supine position, venous return to the heart increases and this increases preload, stroke volume, and cardiac output. These changes cause a brief increase in arterial blood pressure, which in turn activates afferent baroreceptors from the aorta (via the vagus nerve) and within the walls of the carotid sinuses (via the glossopharyngeal nerve) to decrease sympathetic outflow and to increase parasympathetic impulses to the sinoatrial node and myocardium. This parasympathetic outflow counters the increase in arterial blood pressure from increased preload and as a result systemic arterial blood pressure is maintained within a narrow range during postural changes in the nonanesthetized setting.

Central, regional, and local physiologic responses are important in maintaining hemodynamics when changing positions during a normal day-to-day life. During various types of anesthesia some of these responses can

The editors and publisher would like to thank Drs. Jae-Woo Lee and Lydia Cassorla for contributing to this chapter in the previous edition of this work. It has served as the foundation for the current chapter.

be blunted, which can change a patient's hemodynamic responses to positional changes.

Pulmonary physiology is also altered by positional changes, which are further exaggerated during anesthesia. For example, when nonanesthetized people lie down, their functional residual capacity (FRC) decreases as a result of the diaphragm shifting upward. In anesthetized patients, the decrease in FRC is more dramatic, and often closing capacity exceeds FRC, leading to increases in ventilation-perfusion ($\dot{V}/\dot{Q}$) mismatching and hypoxemia. Furthermore, positioning that limits diaphragmatic movement pushes on the chest wall or abdomen, causing intrapulmonary shunting from atelectasis.

## GENERAL POSITIONING

Proper positioning requires the cooperation of anesthesia providers, surgeons, and nurses to ensure patient well-being and safety while permitting surgical exposure. Positioning also involves maintaining spine and extremity neutrality, proper padding, and securing the patient in order to prevent inadvertent changes in position. Patients often remain in the same position for long periods; therefore, prevention of positioning-related complications often requires compromise and judgment. During normal sleep we change positions, which prevents prolonged compression and excessive stretch. During anesthesia patients lose the ability to both sense injury and change position, increasing their risk for injury.[2] Ideally, patients are placed in a surgical position that they can tolerate when awake. The duration of more extreme positions, when necessary, should be limited as much as possible. Tissues overlying all bony prominences, such as the heels and sacrum, must be padded to prevent soft tissue ischemia due to pressure. Maintaining neutrality of the patient's spine and extremities prevents undue stretch.

### Supine

The supine position, also called the dorsal decubitus position, is the most common position for surgery (Fig. 19.1A). In the classic supine position the head, neck, and spine all retain neutrality. One or both arms can be abducted or adducted alongside the patient. Arm abduction should be limited to less than 90 degrees in order to prevent brachial plexus injury from the head of the humerus pushing into the axilla.

Hands and forearms are either supinated or kept in a neutral position with the palm toward the body to reduce external pressure on the ulnar nerve (Fig. 19.1B). When the arms are adducted, they are usually held alongside the body with a "draw sheet" that passes under the body and over the arm and is then tucked directly under the torso (not the mattress) to ensure that the arm remains properly placed next to the body. The anesthesia provider should pad all bony prominences as well as stopcocks or intravenous lines that may exert pressure on the skin during the operation (Fig. 19.1C).[3]

### Variations of the Supine Position

Variations of the supine position are also frequently used such as the lawn-chair position, frog-leg position, and Trendelenburg positions. The lawn-chair position (Fig. 19.1D) flexes the hips and knees slightly, which reduces stress on the back, hips, and knees. This modified supine position is often better tolerated by patients who are awake or undergoing monitored anesthesia care. The legs are placed slightly above the level of the heart, which facilitates venous drainage from the lower extremities. Furthermore, the xiphoid to pubic distance is decreased, reducing tension on the abdominal musculature. Typically the back of the bed is raised, the legs below the knees are lowered to an equivalent angle, and a slight Trendelenburg tilt is used to level the hips with the shoulders.

The frog-leg position, in which the hips and knees are flexed and the hips are externally rotated with the soles of the feet facing each other, facilitates procedures to the perineum, medial thighs, genitalia, and rectum. The knees must be supported in order to minimize stress or dislocation of the hips.

Tilting a supine patient head-down with the pubic symphysis as the highest part of the trunk is called the Trendelenburg position (Fig. 19.1E). It is named after a 19th century German surgeon who first described its use for abdominal surgery. Walter Cannon, a Harvard physiologist, is credited with popularizing the use of Trendelenburg positioning to improve hemodynamics for patients in hypovolemic shock during World War I. Trendelenburg positioning is commonly used today to increase venous return during hypotension, improve exposure during abdominal and laparoscopic surgery, and prevent air emboli during central line placement.

The Trendelenburg position does produce hemodynamic and respiratory changes. Initially, placement of the patient head-down causes an autotransfusion from the legs with about a 9% from baseline increase in cardiac output in 1 minute. However, these changes are not sustained and within 10 minutes many hemodynamic variables, including cardiac output, return to baseline values. Nevertheless, Trendelenburg positioning is still part of the initial resuscitative efforts to treat hypovolemia. The abdominal contents are displaced toward the diaphragm, which decreases FRC and can also decrease pulmonary compliance necessitating higher airway pressures during mechanical ventilation. Intraocular pressure and intracranial pressure (ICP) can also increase. In patients with increased ICP and impaired cerebral autoregulation, Trendelenburg positioning should be avoided. For patients receiving general anesthesia who will be placed in the Trendelenburg position, endotracheal intubation is strongly recommended over supraglottic airways because of the risk of pulmonary aspiration of gastric contents.

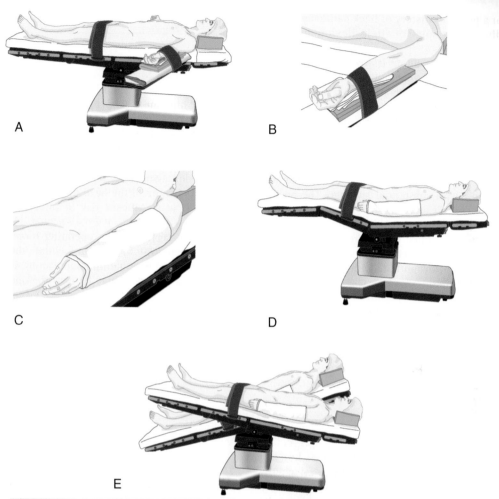

**Fig. 19.1** (A) Supine positioning. Note the asymmetry of the base of the table, placing the patient's center of gravity over the base if positioned in the usual direction. (B) Arm position on the arm board. Abduction of the arm should be limited to less than 90 degrees whenever possible. The arm is supinated, and the elbow is padded. (C) Arm tucked at patient's side. Arm in neutral position with palm to hip. The elbow is padded, and one needs to ensure that the arm is supported. (D) Lawn-chair position. Flexion of the hips and knees decreases tension on the back. (E) Trendelenburg position (head tilted down) and reverse Trendelenburg position (head tilted up). Shoulder braces should be avoided to prevent brachial plexus compression injuries.

Prolonged head-down position can lead to swelling of the face, conjunctivae, larynx, and tongue with an increased potential for postoperative upper airway obstruction. An air leak should be verified around the endotracheal tube or the larynx visualized prior to extubation.[4]

When placing a patient in the Trendelenburg position, measures should be taken to ensure the patient does not slide or shift. Nonsliding mattresses are recommended to prevent the patient from sliding cephalad. Caution should be exerted when shoulder braces are used because of considerable risk of compression or stretch injury to the brachial plexus.

Conversely, the reverse Trendelenburg position (Fig. 19.1E) tilts the supine patient upward so that the head is higher than any other part of the body. This position is most often used to facilitate upper abdominal surgery. Again, patients must be prevented from slipping on the table. Patients in reverse Trendelenburg, particularly those patients who are hypovolemic, are at risk for hypotension due to decreased venous return. Invasive arterial blood pressure monitoring should be calibrated (i.e., zeroed) at the level of the external auditory meatus in order to optimize cerebral perfusion.

Complications

Backache may occur in the supine position as the normal lumbar lordotic curvature is lost during general anesthesia with muscle relaxation or a neuraxial blockade. Consequently, patients with extensive kyphosis, scoliosis, or a previous history of back pain may require extra padding of the spine or slight flexion at the hip and knee.

With obese patients, caution is advised when placing them in reverse axis on the operating room table (also see Chapter 29). The base of the operating room table is asymmetric, with the torso usually over the foot of the table. However, patients are often positioned with the torso over the open side of the table to improve surgical access or to permit use of equipment such as C-arm x-ray devices. This places the heaviest portion of the body, and therefore the patient's center of gravity, opposite the weighted foot of the table, with substantial leverage. The operating room table can tilt and tip over if sufficient weight is placed away from the base, particularly if extensions are used or the bed is tilted in the Trendelenburg position. Operating room table weight limits should be strictly observed; they differ substantially with regard to normal and reverse positioning.

## Lithotomy

Lithotomy position (Fig. 19.2A to C) is frequently used during gynecologic, rectal, and urologic surgeries. The legs are abducted 30 to 45 degrees from the midline, the knees are flexed, and legs are held by supports. The patient's hips are flexed to varying degrees depending upon the type of lithotomy required for the procedure; standard, low, or high lithotomy. Legs should be raised and lowered simultaneously in order to prevent spine torsion. The lower extremities should be padded to prevent compression against the leg rests. The common peroneal nerve wraps around the head of the fibula on the lateral leg and is at significant risk of injury if insufficiently padded.

The foot section of the operating room table is lowered or taken away in order to facilitate the procedure. If the arms are on the operating table alongside the patient, the hands and fingers may lie near the open edge of the

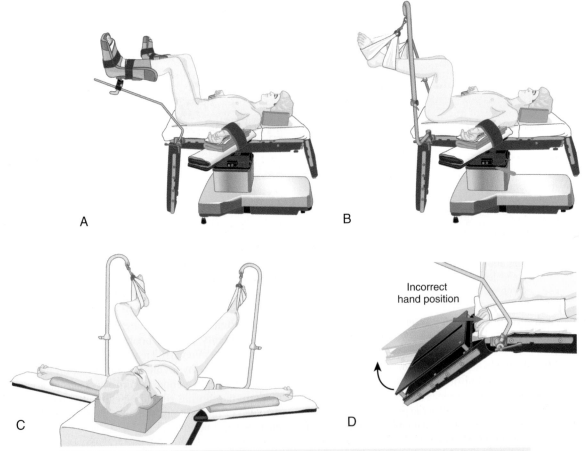

**Fig. 19.2** (A) Lithotomy position. Hips are flexed 80 to 100 degrees with the lower leg parallel to the body. Arms are on armrests away from the hinge point of the foot section. (B) Lithotomy position with "candy cane" supports. (C) Lithotomy position with correct position of "candy cane" stirrups away from lateral fibular head. (D) Improper position of arms in lithotomy position with fingers at risk for compression when the lower section of the bed is raised.

lowered section of the table. When the foot of the bed is raised again at the end of the procedure strict attention to the position of the hand must be paid to avoid a potentially disastrous crush injury to the fingers (Fig. 19.2D). For this reason, positioning the arms on armrests far from the table hinge point is recommended at all times when patients are in the lithotomy position.

The lithotomy position causes some physiologic changes. When the legs are elevated, preload increases, causing a transient increase in cardiac output. In addition, the lithotomy position causes the abdominal viscera to displace the diaphragm cephalad, reducing lung compliance and potentially resulting in a decreased tidal volume. Again, the normal lordotic curvature of the lumbar spine is lost in this position, potentially aggravating any previous lower back pain.

Lower extremity compartment syndrome is a rare but devastating complication associated with the lithotomy position. It occurs when perfusion to an extremity is inadequate because of either restricted arterial flow (from leg elevation) or obstructed venous outflow (direct limb compression or excessive hip flexion). This results in ischemia, edema, and rhabdomyolysis from increased tissue pressure within a fascial compartment. In a large retrospective review of 572,498 surgeries, the incidence of compartment syndromes was higher in the lithotomy (1 in 8720) and lateral decubitus (1 in 9711) positions as compared to the supine (1 in 92,441) position. Long surgical procedure time was the only distinguishing characteristic of the surgeries in which patients developed lower extremity compartment syndromes.[5] In a retrospective multicenter review of 185 urologic patients who were placed in high lithotomy position, the overall complication rate due to positioning was 10%. Neurapraxia was the most common positioning-related complication (12 of 18 patients). Two patients from this cohort had compartment syndrome, and for both of these patients the time in high lithotomy exceeded 5 hours.[6] Therefore, it is recommended to periodically lower the legs to the level of the body if surgery extends beyond several hours.

## Lateral Decubitus

In the lateral decubitus position the patient lies on the non-operative side in order to facilitate surgery in the thorax, retroperitoneum, or hip (Fig. 19.3A). The patient must be well secured to avoid falling or tilting forward to backward. Often a beanbag or bedding rolls are used. A kidney rest is sometimes also used to help secure the patient.

The extremities must be carefully positioned in order to prevent injury. The dependent leg should be somewhat flexed. A pillow or other padding is generally placed between the knees with the dependent leg flexed to minimize excessive pressure on bony prominences and stretch of lower extremity nerves. The dependent arm is placed in front of the patient on a padded arm board. The non-dependent arm is often supported over folded bedding or

suspended with an armrest or foam cradle (Fig. 19.3B). Neither arm should be abducted more than 90 degrees in order to prevent injury to the brachial plexus from the humeral head. Additionally, an axillary roll should be placed underneath the patient just caudal to the axilla, *not* placed in the axilla itself. The axillary roll prevents compression injury to the dependent brachial plexus and dependent axillary vascular structures (Fig. 19.3C). Sometimes an axillary roll is not used if an inflatable beanbag is being used for positioning; however, the team must ensure that there is no compression in the axilla. With invasive arterial monitoring consider placing the catheter in the dependent arm in order to detect positioning compression of the axillary neurovascular structures.

The patient's head must be kept in a neutral position to prevent excessive lateral rotation of the neck and stretch injuries to the brachial plexus. This positioning may require additional head support (Fig. 19.3B). The dependent ear should be checked to avoid folding and undue pressure. The eyes should be securely taped before repositioning if the patient is asleep. The dependent eye must be checked frequently for external compression.

Lastly, the lateral decubitus position changes pulmonary function. In a patient who is mechanically ventilated, the combination of the lateral weight of the mediastinum and disproportionate cephalad pressure of abdominal contents on the dependent diaphragm decreases compliance of the dependent lung and favors ventilation of the nondependent lung. Simultaneously pulmonary blood flow to the dependent lung increases because of the effect of gravity. This causes ventilation-perfusion mismatching and can affect alveolar ventilation and gas exchange.

## Prone

The prone or ventral decubitus position (Fig. 19.4A) is used primarily for surgical access to the posterior fossa of the skull, the posterior spine, the buttocks and perirectal area, and the lower extremities. When general anesthesia is required in the prone position, endotracheal intubation, intravenous access, Foley catheter, and invasive hemodynamic access should all be obtained in the supine position first while the patient is still on a gurney. Make sure all lines and tubes are very well secured to prevent dislodgement during turning and to prevent tube migration during the case.

Turning the patient from supine to prone requires coordination of all operating room providers. The anesthesia provider is primarily responsible for coordinating the move and for the repositioning of the head. An exception is in cases in which the head is placed in rigid pin fixation and the surgeon holds the pin frame. During the turn to prone, the head, neck, and spine are maintained in a neutral position. Some patients requiring prone positioning have unstable spines necessitating surgical operation. Also, strokes apparently can occur from presumed carotid

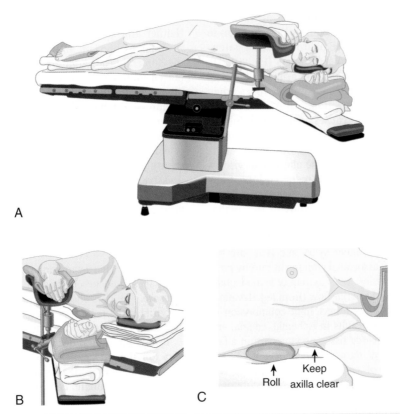

**Fig. 19.3** (A) Lateral decubitus position. Note flexion of the lower leg, padding between the legs, and proper support of both arms. (B) Lateral decubitus position showing placement of arms and head. Note additional padding under headrest to ensure alignment of head with spine. Headrest should be kept away from the dependent eye. (C) Use of axillary roll in lateral decubitus position. The roll, in this case a bag of intravenous fluid, is placed well away from the axilla to prevent compression of the axillary artery and brachial plexus.

and vertebral artery injury during turning. For some cases when neuromonitoring will be used for the surgical procedure "pre-flip," baseline recordings are obtained prior to turning the patient prone for safety documentation.

In order to minimize risk of dislodgement, disconnect as many monitors and lines as is safe and possible before turning the patient from supine to the prone position. This is particularly helpful for lines and monitors on the side that rotates the furthest (the outside arm). Our practice is to disconnect the endotracheal tube during movement and to reconnect immediately upon prone positioning.

The position of the head is very important. In most cases, the head is maintained in a neutral position using a surgical pillow, horseshoe headrest, or Mayfield rigid head pins. Several commercially available pillows are specially designed for the prone position. Most, including disposable foam versions, support the forehead, malar regions, and the chin with a cutout for the eyes, nose, and mouth. The prone position is a risk factor for perioperative visual loss, which is discussed in a separate section later in this chapter. Mirror systems are available to facilitate checking face positioning

(Fig. 19.4B). The anesthesia provider must ensure that the eyes and nose are free from pressure and document these findings at regular intervals throughout the case. Facial pressure wounds are a complication of prone positioning. The horseshoe headrest supports only the forehead and malar regions and allows excellent access to the airway (Fig. 19.4C and D). Rigid fixation pins support the head without any direct pressure on the face, allow access to the airway, and hold the head firmly in one position that can be finely adjusted for optimal neurosurgical exposure (Fig. 19.5A). Patient movement must be prevented when the head is held in rigid pins; slipping out of pins can result in scalp lacerations, skull fractures, and even cervical spine injury.

The legs should be padded and flexed slightly at the knees and hips. Both arms may be positioned to the patient's sides, tucked in the neutral position as described for the supine patient, or placed next to the patient's head on arm boards. Again, the arms should not be abducted greater than 90 degrees to prevent excessive stretching of the brachial plexus. Extra padding under the elbow will be needed to prevent compression of the ulnar nerve.

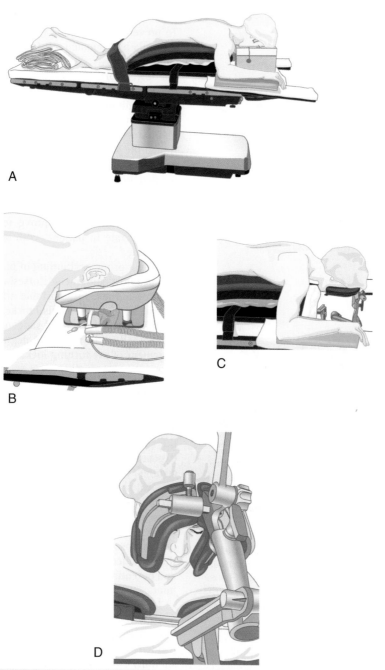

**Fig. 19.4** (A) Prone position with Wilson frame. Arms are abducted less than 90 degrees whenever possible. Pressure points are padded, and chest and abdomen are supported away from the bed to minimize abdominal pressure and preserve pulmonary compliance. Foam head pillow has cutouts for eyes and nose and a slot to permit the endotracheal tube to exit. Eyes must be checked frequently. (B) Mirror system for prone position. Bony structures of the head and face are supported, and monitoring of eyes and airway is facilitated with a plastic mirror. (C) Prone position with horseshoe adapter. Head height is adjusted to position neck in a neutral position. (D) Prone position, face seen from below. Horseshoe adapter permits superior access to airway and visualization of eyes. Width may be adjusted to ensure proper support by facial bones.

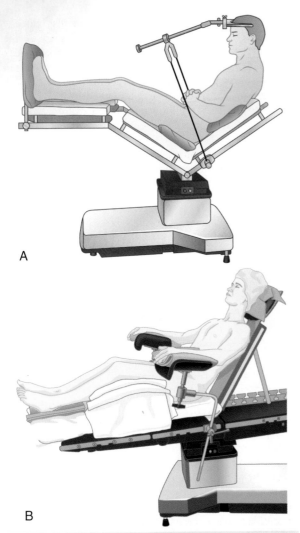

A

B

**Fig. 19.5** (A) Sitting position with Mayfield head pins. The patient is typically semirecumbent rather than sitting as the legs are kept as high as possible to promote venous return. Arms must be supported to prevent shoulder traction. Note that the head holder support is preferably attached to the back section rather than the thigh section of the table so that the patient's back may be adjusted or lowered emergently without first detaching the head holder. (B) Sitting position adapted for shoulder surgery. Note the absence of pressure over the ulnar area of the elbow.

The abdomen should hang relatively freely for patients in the prone position. This alleviates external pressure on the abdomen, which can otherwise cause problems with ventilation and hypotension by compressing the inferior vena cava and reducing venous return. The thorax should be supported by firm rolls or bolsters placed along each side from the clavicle to the iliac crest. Multiple commercial rolls and bolsters are available including the Wilson frame (Fig. 19.4A), Jackson table, Relton frame, and the Mouradian/Simmons modification of the Relton frame. All devices and special operating room tables for the

prone position serve to minimize abdominal compression. To prevent tissue injury, pendulous structures (e.g., male genitalia and female breasts) should be clear of compression; the breasts should be placed medial to the bolsters. The lower portion of each roll or bolster must be placed under its respective iliac crest to prevent pressure injury to the genitalia and the femoral vasculature.

Similar to the supine position, hemodynamics are well maintained, and pulmonary function is actually superior to the supine position. The FRC is actually improved compared to the supine positioning, leading to improved oxygenation. For obese patients, pulmonary compliance is improved in the prone position with the abdomen hanging freely (also see Chapter 29). The prone position has been utilized to improve respiratory function and mortality rate in patients with adult respiratory distress syndrome.[7]

Proper prone positioning of patients relies on the table and headrest equipment. Horseshoe and rigid fixation pin headrests attach to adjustable articulating supports; any slippage or failure of this bracketing device may lead to complications if the head suddenly drops. Jackson tables can actually tilt or flip 180 degrees as a result of disengagement of the turning locking mechanisms.

## Sitting

In the sitting position (Fig. 19.5B) the patient's head and also the operative field are located above the level of the heart. Sitting position can provide excellent surgical exposure for some cervical spine and neurosurgical procedures, particularly of the posterior fossa and superior cervical spine. Blood loss may also be reduced owing to decreased venous pressure in the operative field.[8] A variation of the sitting position, the "beach chair" position, has been increasingly used for shoulder surgeries including arthroscopic procedures. This position offers access to the shoulder from both the anterior and posterior aspect, and potential for great mobility of the arm at the shoulder joint.

In the sitting position, the patient's head must be adequately fixed. This can be done either with a head strap, tape, or rigid fixation. The arms should be supported and padded. The anesthesia provider should ensure that the shoulders are even or very mildly elevated in order to avoid stretch injury between the neck and shoulders. The knees are usually slightly flexed for balance and to reduce stretching of the sciatic nerve, and the feet are also supported and padded.

The most significant complication from the sitting position is risk of venous air embolism (VAE). During intracranial procedures, a significant amount of air can be entrained through the open dural venous sinuses. Low venous pressure in the operative field creates a gradient for air entry into the venous system, similar to the risk of venous air entry during central line placement.

The important fear is the occurrence of a paradoxical air embolism. Patients undergoing planned surgery in the sitting position should be first evaluated to rule-out anatomic intracardiac shunts. If an intracardiac shunt is present, even small amounts of entrained venous air may result in a stroke or myocardial infarction. Transesophageal echocardiography (TEE) has shown some degree of venous air in most patients undergoing neurosurgery in the sitting position even as high as 100%. Clinically significant VAE has a much smaller incidence of 0.5% to 3%.[8,9] Currently TEE is the gold standard for detection of intracardiac shunts. Even with screening, contrast echocardiography septal patency may not always be detected. A recent meta-analysis assessing accuracy of TEE for detection of intracardiac shunts compared to autopsy, cardiac catheterization, or surgery found a sensitivity of 89% and specificity of 91% for TEE. Other means of evaluating for intracardiac shunts include transthoracic echocardiography (TTE) and transcranial Doppler (TCD). Recent studies comparing TTE or TCD to TEE reveal sensitivities and specificities of 46% and 99% for TTE and 97% and 93% for TCD, respectively.[9-12] Other complications of VAE include arrhythmias, acute pulmonary hypertension, and circulatory collapse. Preoperative diagnosis of an intracardiac shunt is a contraindication to surgery in the sitting position. With adequate intravascular volume, the use of intraoperative TEE or precordial Doppler ultrasound may aid in early detection of entrained air.[13]

Patients are at risk for hypotension from pooling of blood in the lower body. The lower extremities are often wrapped in Ace bandages or compression stockings. Intravenous fluids and vasopressors are usually required in order to raise mean arterial pressure. Invasive arterial blood pressure monitoring is recommended for these cases and should be measured at the level of the external auditory meatus in order to optimize cerebral perfusion pressure. Central venous catheter (CVC) access is also recommended for these cases. Long-arm CVCs provide intravenous access without being near the surgical field. Multiorifice CVCs offer an advantage over conventional CVCs for improved aspiration of air should a VAE occur.

Pneumocephalus occurs in almost all patients undergoing cervical spine or posterior fossa surgery in the sitting position if diagnosed on postoperative imaging. Clinically significant pneumocephalus is more rare and occurs because of the lower pressure of cerebrospinal fluid in the sitting position. Symptomatic patients may experience headache, confusion, seizures, or even temporary hemiparesis. Patients experiencing any of these symptoms need to also be evaluated to rule out other postoperative complications, such as intravascular bleeding or stroke. Complications from head and neck positioning are also a risk of the sitting position. Excessive flexion of the cervical spine can impede cerebral venous outflow contributing to swelling and can also impede cerebral arterial inflow causing hypoperfusion of the brain. Macroglossia can also occur with excessive neck flexion. TEE monitoring combined with neck flexion can cause compression of laryngeal structures and the tongue. A minimum distance of two fingerbreadths between the mandible and the sternum is recommended for a normal-sized adult in order to prevent these complications. If preoperative examination reveals that the patient has a further decreased range of motion, then intraoperative positioning should not extend beyond the patient's normal limitations.[14]

## POSITIONING FOR ROBOTIC SURGERY

Robotic surgery came into use around 1999 and has quickly become the norm for many urologic operations as well as in gynecologic surgery where it is also dramatically increasing.[12,13,15,16] For surgeons, robotic surgery offers advantages regarding range of motion and accuracy of laparoscopic instrumentation. However, robotic surgery does introduce some new positioning challenges. Robotic surgery is generally performed with the patient in steep Trendelenburg (30 to 45 degrees) and lithotomy with arms tucked in neutral position bilaterally to the sides. The patient must be very well secured in order to avoid slipping in steep Trendelenburg position.

Many medical institutions use a nonslip mattress (such as a bean bag and foam) on the bed. In order to better secure the patient, the chest straps are placed in an X configuration over the chest. Use of shoulder braces can also help, although there are case reports of brachial plexus injuries because of stretch between the shoulder and neck. If shoulder braces are employed, monitor for excessive stretch at the patient's neck. The endotracheal tube should be well secured to avoid migration. Often a metal tray or table is placed above the patient's face in order to provide protection from laparoscopic equipment.[14-19]

Once the robot is docked, direct access to the patient is limited. The anesthesia provider should place all monitors, intravenous lines, and invasive lines that might be required during the case prior to docking the robot. It is prudent to perform a test by placing the patient in steep Trendelenburg position prior to docking the robot to ensure that the patient is properly positioned and does not slip, and to ensure that the patient can tolerate steep Trendelenburg positioning from a physiologic standpoint.

Physiologic changes during robotic surgery are due to both laparoscopic insufflation as well as the steep Trendelenburg positioning. Hemodynamic changes are largely due to laparoscopic insufflation, whereas changes in respiratory mechanics are also affected by positioning. FRC decreases with laparoscopy and the addition of steep Trendelenburg, which further decreases it. This is due to the combination of pressures of abdominal contents from laparoscopy and Trendelenburg pushing up on the diaphragm. It can also be worsened by chest fixation that is applied to prevent the patient from slipping off the table. Peak and plateau airway pressures have been shown to rise as much as 50%. Between changes in pulmonary compliance, decreased FRC, and the need for increased minute ventilation with carbon dioxide insufflation, intraoperative mechanical ventilation can be quite challenging during these cases.[14-20]

Other complications from robotic laparoscopic surgeries include laryngeal edema and optic neuropathy. Consider checking for airway leak at the start and at the end of the surgical procedure prior to extubation.

## PRESSURE INJURIES

Pressure injuries are due to prolonged pressure that inhibits capillary blood flow over a bony prominence. In animal models, damage has been shown to start within 2 hours with 70 mm Hg force. Classification of pressure ulcers is according to the consensus panel from the National Pressure Sore Advisory Panel. Stages range from intact, nonblanchable erythema (stage 1) to full-thickness tissue loss (stage 4). Muscle damage occurs before skin and subcutaneous tissue damage and is likely due to increased oxygen requirements of muscle. In the supine position, areas most at risk include the sacrum, heels, and occiput. In the prone position, the chest and knees are at the most frequent risk for pressure injury and in the sitting position, the ischial tuberosities are at the most frequent risk.[18,21]

Most intraoperative pressure injuries (>80%) are discovered within 72 hours of surgery and occur most often in operations lasting more than 3 hours. The longer the surgery the higher the incidence of pressure injury. Cardiac, thoracic, orthopedic, and vascular patients had the highest incidences.

Aside from pressure injuries over bony prominences, pressure injuries in the lips, tongue, and nasal alae can occur from endotracheal tubes, nasogastric tubes, and other medical devices. One should ensure that pressure from medical devices is minimized. This is particularly important during hypotension or hypothermia when the tissue is more vulnerable to pressure-induced injuries.

## BITE INJURIES

Transcranial motor-evoked potentials (Tc-MEPs) are becoming more commonly used for both spine surgical procedures and neurosurgical procedures. Tc-MEPs involve contraction of the temporalis and masseter muscle, which has been implicated in tongue, lip, and even tooth injuries because of biting motion. A retrospective review of over 17,000 cases employing Tc-MEPs found an overall incidence of 0.14% and the tongue was most frequently injured (~80% of all associated injuries).[19,22] Severity of injury ranged from minor bruising to the necessity of laceration repair by suture in 25 of 111 patients. Some medical institutions use bite blocks between the right and left molars ("double-bite blocks") for these cases in order to prevent these injuries. Even so, approximately 50% of injured patients did have double-bite blocks in place. There are commercial devices available, but they often are of questionable additional benefit.

## PERIPHERAL NERVE INJURIES

Peripheral nerve injury remains a serious perioperative complication and a significant source of professional liability despite its low incidence. The incidence of peripheral nerve injury is between 0.03% to 0.11%, according to the American Society of Anesthesiologists (ASA) Closed Claims Project database. Peripheral nerve injuries represented 22% of all claims. Injuries occur when peripheral nerves are subjected to compression, stretch, ischemia, metabolic derangement, and direct trauma/laceration during surgery.[23] Because sensation is blocked by unconsciousness or regional anesthesia, early warning symptoms of pain with normal spontaneous repositioning are absent.[1,20,24]

Peripheral nerve injury is a complex phenomenon with a multifactorial cause. The ASA released an updated practice advisory in 2010 to help prevent perioperative neuropathies (Box 19.1). Ulnar neuropathy is the most common lesion representing 28% of all peripheral nerve injury claims, followed by injury to the brachial plexus (20%), lumbosacral nerve root (16%), and spinal cord (13%) (Table 19.1). Interestingly the distribution of nerve injury claims has changed over time. Ulnar neuropathy decreased from 37% in 1980 to 1984 to 17% in the 1990s, and spinal cord injury increased from 8% in 1980 to 1984 to 27% in the 1990s. Spinal cord injury and lumbosacral nerve root neuropathy were predominantly associated with regional anesthesia. Epidural hematoma and chemical injury represented 29% of the known mechanisms of injury among the claims filed. The injuries were probably related to the use of neuraxial block in patients who are receiving anticoagulation drugs and the increased usage of blocks for chronic pain management (Table 19.2).[1,21,25,26]

There is no direct evidence that positioning or padding alone can prevent perioperative neuropathies. Most injuries, particularly injuries to nerves of the upper extremity such as the ulnar nerve and brachial plexus, occurred in the presence of adequate positioning and

**Box 19.1** An Updated Report by the American Society of Anesthesiologists Task Force on Prevention of Perioperative Peripheral Neuropathies

### I. Preoperative History and Physical Assessment

- When judged appropriate, it is helpful to ascertain that patients can comfortably tolerate the anticipated operative position.
- Body habitus, preexisting neurologic symptoms, diabetes mellitus, peripheral vascular disease, alcohol dependency, arthritis, and gender (e.g., male gender and its association with ulnar neuropathy) are important elements of a preoperative history.

### II. Positioning Strategies for the Upper Extremities

- Arm abduction in supine patients should be limited to 90 degrees. Patients who are positioned prone may comfortably tolerate arm abduction greater than 90 degrees.
  - *Supine Patient With Arm on an Arm Board:* The upper extremity should be positioned to decrease pressure on the postcondylar groove of the humerus (ulnar groove). Either supination or the neutral forearm positions facilitates this action.
  - *Supine Patient With Arms Tucked at Side:* The forearm should be in a neutral position. Flexion of the elbow may increase the risk of ulnar neuropathy, but there is no consensus on an acceptable degree of flexion during the perioperative period. Prolonged pressure on the radial nerve in the spiral groove of the humerus should be avoided. Extension of the elbow beyond the range that is comfortable during the preoperative assessment may stretch the median nerve. Periodic perioperative assessments may ensure maintenance of the desired position.

### III. Specific Positioning Strategies for the Lower Extremities

- *Stretching of the Hamstring Muscle Group:* Positions that stretch the hamstring muscle group beyond the range that is comfortable during the preoperative assessment may stretch the sciatic nerve.
- *Limiting Hip Flexion:* Because the sciatic nerve or its branches cross both the hip and the knee joints, extension and flexion of these joints, respectively, should be considered when determining the degree of hip flexion. Neither extension nor flexion of the hip increases the risk of femoral neuropathy. Prolonged pressure on the peroneal nerve at the fibular head should be avoided.

### IV. Protective Padding

- *Padded Arm Boards:* Padded arm boards may decrease the risk of upper extremity neuropathy
- *Chest Rolls:* The use of chest rolls in the laterally positioned patient may decrease the risk of upper extremity neuropathy.
- *Padding at the Elbow:* Padding at the elbow may decrease the risk of upper extremity neuropathy.
- *Padding to Protect the Peroneal (Fibular) Nerve:* The use of specific padding to prevent pressure of a hard surface against the peroneal nerve at the fibular head may decrease the risk of peroneal neuropathy.
- *Complications From the Use of Padding:* The inappropriate use of padding (e.g., padding too tight) may increase the risk of perioperative neuropathy.

### V. Equipment

The use of properly functioning automated blood pressure cuffs on the arm (i.e., placed above the antecubital fossa) does not change the risk of upper extremity neuropathy. The use of shoulder braces in a steep head-down position may *increase* the risk of perioperative neuropathies.

### VI. Postoperative Assessment

A simple postoperative assessment of extremity nerve function may lead to early recognition of peripheral neuropathies.

### VII. Documentation

Documentation of specific perioperative positioning actions may be useful for continuous improvement processes and may result in improvements by helping practitioners focus attention on relevant aspects of patient positioning and providing information on positioning strategies that eventually leads to improvements in patient care.

From American Society of Anesthesiologists Task Force on Prevention of Perioperative Peripheral Neuropathies. Practice advisory for the prevention of perioperative peripheral neuropathies: an updated report by the American Society of Anesthesiologists Task Force on Prevention of Perioperative Peripheral Neuropathies. *Anesthesiology.* 2011;114(4):741-754.

padding. Stretch injuries in peripheral nerves are due to compromise of the vascular plexus (vasa nervorum) that runs alongside supplying these nerves. This can be due to either an obstruction in venous outflow or an obstruction to arterial inflow. Compression injuries can manifest in several different ways. Neurapraxia is caused by a relatively short ischemia time and usually causes only a transient dysfunction. Axonotmesis is a demyelinating injury. Neurotmesis is due to a severed or disrupted nerve and usually deficits are permanent.[2]

Because the cause of peripheral nerve injuries is often not clear, identification of modifiable factors for prevention is difficult to ascertain. Generally, maintaining neutral positioning as much as possible is advised. Stretch, overflexion, and overextension should all be avoided. Superficial nerves, especially near bony prominences, should be padded (common peroneal at fibular head, ulnar nerve at elbow). Padding and support should distribute weight as evenly as possible. Ensure that equipment (such as laparoscopic equipment, C-arms, and other x-ray equipment) is never resting directly on the patient.

In a retrospective study of 1000 consecutive spine surgeries that used somatosensory evoked potential (SSEP) monitoring, five arm positions were compared with regard to SSEP changes in the upper extremities. A modification of arm position reversed 92% of upper extremity SSEP changes. The incidence of position-related upper

**Table 19.1** Nerve Injury Claims in the American Society of Anesthesiologists Closed Claims Project Database

| | Distribution of Claims for Nerve Injury | | | |
|---|---|---|---|---|
| Nerve | Number of Claims in Current Database (*N* = 4183) | Percentage of Total (*N* = 670) | Number of Claims Since 1990 Report | Percentage of Total Since 1990 (*N* = 445) |
| Ulnar | 190 | 28 | 113 | 25 |
| Brachial plexus | 137 | 20 | 83 | 19 |
| Lumbosacral nerve root | 105 | 16 | 67 | 15 |
| Spinal cord | 84 | 13 | 73 | 16 |
| Sciatic[a] | 34 | 5 | 23 | 5 |
| Median | 28 | 4 | 19 | 4 |
| Radial | 18 | 3 | 13 | 3 |
| Femoral | 15 | 2 | 9 | 2 |
| Other single nerves | 43 | 6 | 35 | 8 |
| Multiple nerves | 16 | 2 | 10 | 2 |
| Total | 670 | 100 | 445 | 100 |

[a]Includes peroneal nerve.
From Cheney FW, Domino KB, Caplan RA, Posner KL. Nerve injury associated with anesthesia: a closed claims analysis. *Anesthesiology*. 1999;90(4):1062-1069.

**Table 19.2** Most Common Nerve Injuries in American Society of Anesthesiologists Closed Claims Project Database After 1990

| Nerve Injury | Recommendations for Prevention |
|---|---|
| Ulnar nerve (25%) | Avoid excessive pressure on the postcondylar groove of the humerus. Keep the hand and forearm either supinated or in a neutral position. |
| Brachial plexus (19%) | Avoid the use of shoulder braces in patients in the Trendelenburg position (use nonsliding mattresses). Avoid excessive lateral rotation of the head either in the supine or prone position. Limit abduction of the arm to less than 90 degrees in the supine position. Avoid the placement of high "axillary" roll in the decubitus position—keep the roll out of the axilla. Use ultrasound imaging to find the internal jugular vein for central line placement. |
| Spinal cord (16%) and lumbosacral nerve root (15%) | Be aware that the fraction of spinal cord injuries is increasing, probably in relation to use of epidural catheters for pain management. Follow current guidelines for regional anesthesia in anticoagulated patients. |
| Sciatic and peroneal (5%) nerves | Minimize time of surgery in the lithotomy position. Use two assistants to coordinate the simultaneous movement of both legs to and from the lithotomy position. Avoid excessive flexion of the hips, extension of the knees, or torsion of the lumbar spine. Avoid excessive pressure on peroneal nerve at the fibular head. |
| Median (4%) and radial (3%) nerves | Be aware that 25% of injuries to the median and radial nerves were associated with axillary block, and 25% of injuries were associated with traumatic insertion or infiltration of an intravenous line. |

From Cheney FW, Domino KB, Caplan RA, Posner KL. Nerve injury associated with anesthesia: a closed claims analysis. *Anesthesiology*. 1999;90(4):1062-1069; Cheney FW. The American Society of Anesthesiologists Closed Claims Project: what have we learned, how has it affected practice, and how will it affect practice in the future? *Anesthesiology*. 1999;91(2):552-556.

extremity SSEP changes was significantly more frequent in the prone "superman" (7%) and lateral decubitus (7.5%) positions compared with the supine arms out, supine arms tucked, and prone arms tucked positions (1.8% to 3.2%). Reversible SSEP changes were not associated with postoperative deficits.[22,27]

### Ulnar Nerve

The incidence of ulnar neuropathy from intraoperative positioning is low, but the degree of morbidity can be severe. Ulnar deficits result in the inability to abduct the fifth finger and cause decreased sensation to the fourth and fifth fingers giving the appearance of a "claw" hand. Multiple studies have attempted to elucidate causes and risk factors for ulnar neuropathy. In a large retrospective review of perioperative ulnar neuropathy lasting longer than 3 months, risk factors were patients who were either very thin or obese and those with prolonged postoperative bed rest. In this study there was no association with intraoperative patient position or anesthetic technique. In the ASA Closed Claims Project database, diabetes, alcoholism, cigarette smoking, and cancer were found to be risk factors. In this study 9% of ulnar injury claims had an explicit mechanism of injury, and in 27% of claims, the padding of the elbows was explicitly stated.[1,23,28]

### Brachial Plexus

The brachial plexus is susceptible to injury from stretching and compression because of its superficial course in the axilla and proximity to the humeral head. Motor and sensory deficits are wide ranging, although sensory deficits in the ulnar nerve distribution are most commonly associated with arm abduction more than 90 degrees, lateral rotation of the head, asymmetric retraction of the sternum for internal mammary artery dissection during cardiac surgery, and direct trauma. In cardiac surgery patients requiring median sternotomy, brachial plexus injury has been specifically associated with the C8-T1 nerve roots. Patients should be positioned with the head midline, arms kept at the sides, the elbows mildly flexed, and the forearms supinated.

### Other Upper Extremity Nerves

Isolated injuries to the radial and median nerves are rare. Injury to the radial nerve can cause wrist drop, the inability to abduct the thumb, and the inability to extend the fingers from the metacarpophalangeal joints. The most superficial portion of the radial nerve is in the lower one third of the upper arm where the nerve goes across the spiral groove of the humerus. The median nerve is relatively protected with its most vulnerable location being in the antecubital fossa adjacent to veins used for intravenous access.

### Lower Extremity Nerves

Injuries to the sciatic and common peroneal nerves occur most often in the lithotomy position. The sciatic nerve can be injured with stretch from external rotation of the leg and also from hyperflexion at the hip. As previously mentioned, the common peroneal nerve is most at risk for injury as it wraps around the head of the fibula. Injury to the common peroneal nerve can cause footdrop, inversion of the foot, and sensory deficit. A femoral neuropathy will present with decreased flexion of the hip, decreased extension of the knee, or a loss of sensation over the superior aspect of the thigh and medial/anteromedial side of the leg. The obturator nerve can be injured during a difficult forceps delivery, in the lithotomy position, or by excessive flexion of the thigh to the groin. An obturator neuropathy will present with inability to adduct the leg and decreased sensation over the medial thigh. A cadaveric study revealed that abduction of the hips of greater than 30 degrees puts significant strain on the obturator nerve. This strain was significantly reduced or eliminated by adding at least 45 degrees of hip flexion.[24,29]

According to a prospective study of close to 1000 patients the overall incidence of nerve injury in the lithotomy position is 1.5%. The obturator nerve was most frequently injured, followed closely by the lateral femoral cutaneous nerve, as well as sciatic and peroneal nerves. Neuropathy was evident within 4 hours of the surgical end time. Symptoms were paresthesias and pain, and interestingly no motor weakness was found in this study. Length of surgery greater than 2 hours was the only risk factor found in this study.[25,30] For 14 of 15 patients with nerve injury the symptoms resolved within 4 months of surgery. In a previous retrospective study, the same authors found the incidence of severe motor disability in patients undergoing surgery in the lithotomy position to be 1 in 3608, and in this study the lateral femoral cutaneous nerve was the most common motor neuropathy from lithotomy.[27,31]

## EVALUATION AND TREATMENT OF PERIOPERATIVE NEUROPATHIES

When a nerve injury becomes apparent postoperatively, it is essential that a directed physical examination be performed to correlate and document the extent of sensory or motor deficits with the preoperative examination as well as any intraoperative events. A neurologic consultation can help define the neurogenic basis, localize the site of the lesion, and determine the severity of injury for guiding prognostication. With proper diagnosis and management, most injuries resolve, but months to years may be required.

Most sensory neuropathies are generally transient and require only reassurance to the patient with follow-up, whereas most motor neuropathies include demyelination of peripheral fibers of a nerve trunk (neurapraxia) and generally take 4 to 6 weeks for recovery to the axon within an intact nerve sheath (axonotmesis) or complete nerve disruption (neurotmesis) can cause severe pain and disability. When reversible, recovery often takes 3 to 12 months. Interim physical therapy is recommended to prevent contractures and muscle atrophy.

If a new sensory or motor deficit is found postoperatively, electrophysiologic evaluation by a neurologist within the first week may provide useful information concerning the characteristic and temporal pattern of the injury. However, another examination after 4 weeks when enough time has elapsed for the electrophysiologic changes to evolve will provide more definitive information about the site, nature, and severity of the nerve injury. Regardless, electrophysiologic testing must be interpreted within the clinical content for which it was obtained. No single test can define the cause of injury.

## PERIOPERATIVE EYE INJURY AND VISUAL LOSS

The incidence of perioperative eye injuries is approximately 0.05%, and they account for 3% of claims in the ASA Closed Claims Project database (also see Chapter 31). Greater monetary settlements were associated with ocular injuries as compared to nonocular injuries. Perioperative eye injuries include corneal abrasions and postoperative vision loss (POVL).[1,28,32]

Corneal abrasions are by far the most common type of perioperative ocular injury with an incidence of 0.11% in a recent study.[33] During general anesthesia the natural lid reflex is abolished and tear production is decreased, which place the cornea at risk. Symptoms most commonly manifest as sensation of a foreign body in the eye upon awakening from anesthesia, photophobia, blurry vision, and erythema. Risk factors include increased age, length of surgery, prone position, Trendelenburg position, and supplemental oxygen delivery in the postanesthesia care unit.[33] Precautionary measures to reduce the incidence of corneal abrasion include early and careful taping of the eyelids following induction of anesthesia, care regarding dangling objects when leaning over patients, and close observation as patients awaken. Ophthalmic ointments may add an additional layer of protection and combat dry eye. Patients often try to rub their eyes or nose with pulse oximeter probes, arm boards, and intravenous lines attached before they are fully awake.

POVL is a devastating complication that has been associated with specific surgeries and patient risk factors. The incidence varies and is the lowest for non-cardiac surgery and ranges up to 0.09% for patients undergoing spine surgery in the prone position.[28,32] Ischemic optic neuropathy (ION) and to a lesser extent central retinal arterial occlusion from direct retinal pressure are the conditions most cited as potential causes. Perioperative factors associated with an increased risk of ION include prolonged hypotension, long duration of surgery, large blood loss, large crystalloid use, anemia or hemodilution, and increased intraocular or venous pressure from the prone position. Patient risk factors associated with ION include hypertension, diabetes, atherosclerosis, morbid obesity, and tobacco use. However, with the exception of obvious external compression of the eyes, the cause of POVL appears to be multifactorial in nature with no consistent underlying mechanism.[30,34]

In 1999, the ASA Committee on Professional Liability established the ASA Postoperative Visual Loss Registry to better understand the complication. By 2005, 131 cases were reported to the registry; 73% of these reported cases involved patients undergoing spine surgeries and 9% involved cardiac surgery. Of 93 patients with POVL following prone spine surgery, Lee and associates reported that 89% were diagnosed with ION, predominantly posterior, and 11% with central retinal artery occlusion (CRAO). In patients who were diagnosed with ION, 66% had documented bilateral involvement, of which 42% had eventual improvement in vision although often clinically insignificant. Compared to CRAO, patients with ION had significantly higher anesthetic duration (9.8 ± 3.1 vs. 6.5 ± 2.2 hours), estimated blood loss (median 2 vs. 0.75 L), and crystalloid infusion (9.7 ± 4.7 vs. 4.6 ± 1.7 L). Patients with ION were also relatively healthy (64% ASA I and II), and 72% were male. In 2006, the ASA issued a practice advisory for perioperative visual loss associated with spine surgery (also see Chapter 32). Unfortunately, no definite recommendations were made concerning the issue of induced hypotension, use of vasopressors, or transfusion threshold owing to the multifactorial nature and the low incidence of the injury. Despite a lack of direct evidence, several suggestions were made for high-risk patients undergoing complex spine surgery.[31,32,35,36]

Until the causative factors of this devastating type of injury are better defined, patient management strategies will continue to be debated. With regard to patient positioning, the anesthesia provider should be aware that intraocular pressures are increased in the dependent eye in the lateral position and both eyes in the prone position in the absence of any external pressure. Eye checks should be frequently performed and documented. Time in the prone position should be limited whenever possible. Fortunately, in a retrospective review of 5.6 million patients in the National (Nationwide) Inpatient Sample, the largest United States all-payer hospital inpatient care database, the rate of POVL decreased from 1996 to 2005, perhaps because of an increase in awareness of this complication.[33,37]

## ANESTHESIA OUTSIDE THE OPERATING ROOM

Anesthesia care providers are increasingly involved with procedures performed in remote locations such as for gastrointestinal endoscopy, cardiac catheterization, interventional radiology, neuroradiology, magnetic resonance imaging/computed tomography, and office-based procedures (also see Chapter 38). Vigilance is particularly important outside the operating room to maintain patient safety because of the less familiar environment, relative lack of positioning equipment, and variability in staff and nursing training with regard to patient positioning. For example, many locations do not routinely have safety straps or arm supports available. In some settings, such as magnetic resonance imaging, radiation therapy, and computed tomography, the anesthesia provider is not continuously in direct proximity to the patient. In such an environment, where practice patterns have often evolved in the context of nonanesthetized patients, the anesthesia provider will be primarily responsible for verifying the safety of each patient's position and for implementing guidelines for patients receiving anesthesia.

## CONCLUSION

The positioning of patients under anesthesia is an essential aspect of intraoperative care. Each position has different physiologic effects on ventilation and circulation. Despite provider awareness, position-related complications including peripheral nerve injuries continue to remain a significant source of patient morbidity. The entire operative team, including anesthesia providers, must work together when positioning each patient to ensure the patient's comfort and safety in addition to the desired surgical exposure. Ideally, the final position should appear natural: a position that the patient would comfortably tolerate if awake and not sedated for the anticipated duration of the procedure.

## QUESTIONS OF THE DAY

1. What are the physiologic effects of the Trendelenburg position after 1 minute? After 10 minutes? What are the long-term complications of prolonged Trendelenburg position (>2 hours)?

2. What are the risks of the lithotomy position? What steps can be taken to reduce the risks?

3. A patient is placed in the lateral decubitus position. How can the risk of axillary neurovascular compression be reduced?

4. What factors contribute to the risk of postoperative visual loss during spine surgery in the prone position?

5. What are the clinical manifestations of venous air embolism (VAE) in the sitting position? Which monitors are the most sensitive for detection of VAE?

6. What positioning strategies should be used for the upper extremities in order to reduce the risk of perioperative peripheral neuropathy? What positioning strategies should be used for the lower extremities to reduce the risk of neuropathy?

## REFERENCES

1. Cheney FW, Domino KB, Caplan RA, Posner KL. Nerve injury associated with anesthesia: a closed claims analysis. Anesthesiology. 1999;90(4):1062-1069.

2. Johnson RL, Warner ME, Staff NP, Warner MA. Neuropathies after surgery: anatomical considerations of pathologic mechanisms. Clin Anat. 2015;28(5):678-682.

3. American Society of Anesthesiologists Task Force on Prevention of Perioperative Peripheral Neuropathies. Practice advisory for the prevention of perioperative peripheral neuropathies: an updated report by the American Society of Anesthesiologists Task Force on Prevention of Perioperative Peripheral Neuropathies. Anesthesiology. 2011;114(4):741-754.

4. Geerts BF, van den Bergh L, Stijnen T, et al. Comprehensive review: is it better to use the Trendelenburg position or passive leg raising for the initial treatment of hypovolemia? J Clin Anesth. 2012;24(8):668-674.

5. Warner ME, LaMaster LM, Thoeming AK, et al. Compartment syndrome in surgical patients. Anesthesiology. 2001;94(4):705-708.

6. Anema JG, Morey AF, McAninch JW, et al. Complications related to the high lithotomy position during urethral reconstruction. J Urol. 2000;164(2):360-363.

7. Guérin C, Reignier J, Richard JC, PROSEVA Study Group, et al. Prone positioning in severe acute respiratory distress syndrome. N Engl J Med. 2013;368(23):2159-2168.

8. Black S, Ockert DB, Oliver WC Jr, et al. Outcome following posterior fossa craniectomy in patients in the sitting or horizontal positions. Anesthesiology. 1988;69:49-56.

9. Ganslandt O, Merkel A, Schmitt H, et al. The sitting position in neurosurgery: indications, complications and results, a single institution experience of 600 cases. Acta Neurochir (Wien). 2013;155(10):1887-1893.

10. Mojadidi MK, Bogush N, Caceres JD, et al. Diagnostic accuracy of transesophageal echocardiogram for the detection of patent foramen ovale: a meta-analysis. Echocardiography. 2014;31(6):752-758.

11. Mojadidi MK, Roberts SC, Winoker JS, et al. Accuracy of transcranial Doppler for the diagnosis of intracardiac right-to-left shunt: a bivariate meta-analysis of prospective studies. JACC Cardiovasc Imaging. 2014;7(3):236-250.

12. Mojadidi MK, Winoker JS, Roberts SC, et al. Accuracy of conventional transthoracic echocardiography for the diagnosis of intracardiac right-to-left shunt: a meta-analysis of prospective studies. *Echocardiography.* 2014;31(9):1036-1048.

13. Mammoto T, Hayashi Y, Ohnishi Y, et al. Incidence of venous and paradoxical air embolism in neurosurgical patients in the sitting position: detection by transesophageal echocardiography. *Acta Anaesthesiol Scand.* 1998;42:643-647.

14. Warner M. Positioning the head and neck. In: Martin JT, Warner MA, eds. *Positioning in Anesthesia and Surgery.* 3rd ed. Philadelphia: WB Saunders; 1997.

15. Hu JC, Gu X, Lipsitz SR, et al. Comparative effectiveness of minimally invasive vs open radical prostatectomy. *JAMA.* 2009;302(14):1557-1564.

16. Wright JD, Ananth CV, Lewin SN, et al. Robotically assisted vs laparoscopic hysterectomy among women with benign gynecologic disease. *JAMA.* 2013;309(7):689-698.

17. Gainsburg DM. Anesthetic concerns for robotic-assisted laparoscopic radical prostatectomy. *Minerva Anestesiol.* 2012;78(5):596-604.

18. Hsu RL, Kaye AD, Urman RD. Anesthetic challenges in robotic-assisted urologic surgery. *Rev Urol.* 2013;15(4):178-184.

19. Kalmar AF, De Wolf AM, Hendrickx JFA. Anesthetic considerations for robotic surgery in the steep Trendelenburg position. *Adv Anesth.* 2012;30:75-96.

20. Lestar M, Gunnarsson L, Lagerstrand L, et al. Hemodynamic perturbations during robot-assisted laparoscopic radical prostatectomy in 45 degrees Trendelenburg position. *Anesth Analg.* 2011;113(5):1069-1075.

21. Cushing CA, Phillips LG. Evidence-based medicine: pressure sores. *Plast Reconstr Surg.* 2013;132(6):1720-1732.

22. Tamkus A, Rice K. The incidence of bite injuries associated with transcranial motor-evoked potential monitoring. *Anesth Analg.* 2012;115(3):663-667.

23. Winfree CJ, Kline DG. Intraoperative positioning nerve injuries. *Anesthesiology.* 2009;111:490-497.

24. Welch MB, Brummett CM, Welch TD, et al. Perioperative peripheral nerve injuries: a retrospective study of 380,680 cases during a 10-year period at a single institution. *Anesthesiology.* 2009;111(3):490-497.

25. Fitzgibbon DR, Posner KL, Domino KB, et al. Chronic pain management: American Society of Anesthesiologists Closed Claims Project. *Anesthesiology.* 2004;100(1):98-105.

26. Cheney FW. The American Society of Anesthesiologists Closed Claims Project: what have we learned, how has it affected practice, and how will it affect practice in the future? *Anesthesiology.* 1999;91(2):552-556.

27. Kamel IR, Drum ET, Koch SA, et al. The use of somatosensory evoked potentials to determine the relationship between patient positioning and impending upper extremity nerve injury during spine surgery: a retrospective analysis. *Anesth Analg.* 2006;102(5):1538-1542.

28. Warner MA, Warner ME, Martin JT. Ulnar neuropathy. Incidence, outcome, and risk factors in sedated or anesthetized patients. *Anesthesiology.* 1994;81(6):1332-1340.

29. Litwiller JP, Wells RE Jr, Halliwill JR, et al. Effect of lithotomy positions on strain of the obturator and lateral femoral cutaneous nerves. *Clin Anat.* 2004;17(1):45-49.

30. Warner MA, Warner DO, Harper CM, et al. Lower extremity neuropathies associated with lithotomy positions. *Anesthesiology.* 2000;93(4):938-942.

31. Warner MA, Martin JT, Schroeder DR. Lower-extremity motor neuropathy associated with surgery performed on patients in a lithotomy position. *Anesthesiology.* 1994;81(1):6-12.

32. Roth S, Thisted RA, Erickson JP, et al. Eye injuries after nonocular surgery. A study of 60,965 anesthetics from 1988 to 1992. *Anesthesiology.* 1996;85(5):1020-1027.

33. Segal KL, Fleischut PM, Kim C, et al. Evaluation and treatment of perioperative corneal abrasions. *J Ophthalmol.* 2014;2014:901901.

34. Cheng MA, Todorov A, Tempelhoff R, et al. The effect of prone positioning on intraocular pressure in anesthetized patients. *Anesthesiology.* 2001;95(6):1351-1355.

35. American Society of Anesthesiologists Task Force on Perioperative Visual Loss. Practice advisory for perioperative visual loss associated with spine surgery: an updated report by the American Society of Anesthesiologists Task Force on Perioperative Visual Loss. *Anesthesiology.* 2012;116(2):274-285.

36. Lee LA, Roth S, Posner KL, et al. The American Society of Anesthesiologists Postoperative Visual Loss Registry: analysis of 93 spine surgery cases with postoperative visual loss. *Anesthesiology.* 2006;105(4):652-659; quiz 867-868.

37. Shen Y, Drum M, Roth S. The prevalence of perioperative visual loss in the United States: a 10-year study from 1996 to 2005 of spinal, orthopedic, cardiac, and general surgery. *Anesth Analg.* 2009;109(5):1534-1545.

# 20

# ANESTHETIC MONITORING

James Szocik, Magnus Teig, and Kevin K. Tremper

INTRODUCTION
Overview

RESPIRATORY SYSTEM
Oxygenation
Ventilation

CIRCULATORY SYSTEM
Measurement of the Electrocardiogram
Blood Pressure and Flow
Measures of Intravascular Volume
Responsiveness
Central Venous Monitoring

CENTRAL NERVOUS SYSTEM
Processed Electroencephalograph Monitoring
Minimum Alveolar Concentration Alert
Intracranial Pressure Monitoring
Cerebral Oximetry

PERIPHERAL NERVOUS SYSTEM
Neuromuscular Monitoring

TEMPERATURE

MAGNETIC RESONANCE IMAGING AND
ADVERSE CONDITIONS

MONITORS AND ALARMS

QUESTIONS OF THE DAY

## INTRODUCTION

Anesthesiologists have long been at the forefront of patient monitoring. This has been of necessity, because we are responsible for continuously assessing the patient's physiologic status and the effects of surgery and anesthetic drugs. The following is an introduction to the basic function and utility of the wide array of monitors employed in modern anesthesia care. Monitoring devices will be organized by the organ or organ system that they are monitoring, not the physical property or technique on which that monitor derives its information. Because the monitors for each organ system may employ the same physical properties, such as light absorption or pressure transduction, each monitor will be described as it is used for a specific organ, but the description of the principle may refer to another section within the chapter. For an in-depth review of these principles the reader is referred to a more comprehensive text.[1]

### Overview

In 1986 the American Society of Anesthesiologists (ASA) established a set of basic monitoring standards, stating that the patient's oxygenation, ventilation, circulation, and temperature shall be continually evaluated.[2] These standards, the first of their kind (last affirmed in 2015), should be viewed as a minimum requirement and many situations will require additional monitoring. All of the organ systems monitored are perfused by the circulatory system (Fig. 20.1). Monitoring the patient permits the anesthesia provider to continuously assess if the patient's state is "normal" or "abnormal," and to correct the cause of the abnormality, or at least treat the abnormal number generated by the monitor. However, the limitations of monitors and how to use

The editors and publisher would like to thank Dr. Anil de Silva for contributing to this chapter in the previous edition of this work. It has served as the foundation for the current chapter.

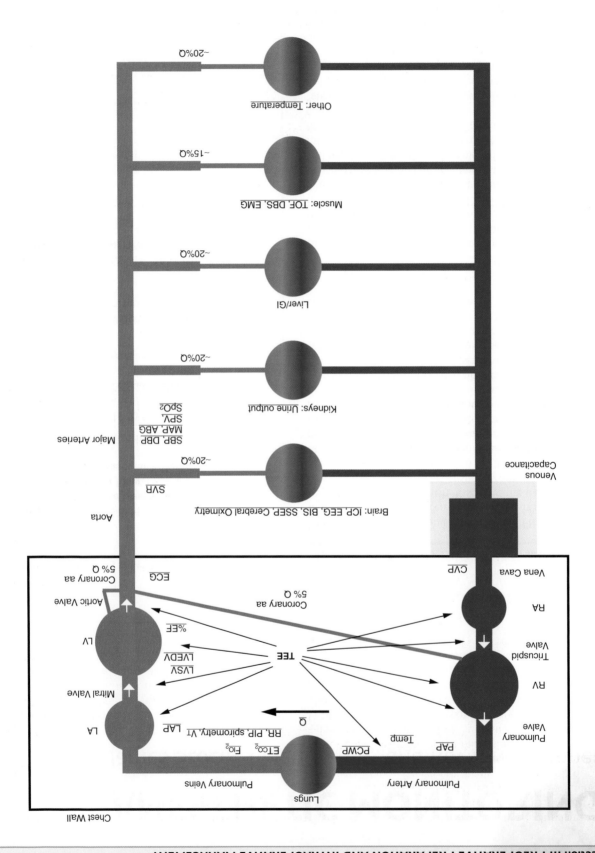

data from multiple devices must be understood in order to confirm the diagnosis and follow the prescribed treatment.

## RESPIRATORY SYSTEM

Oxygen ($O_2$) is a colorless, odorless gas critical for cellular respiration. Lack of delivery of oxygen to tissues will result in cellular death. Carbon dioxide is a consequence of cellular metabolism and must be removed from the tissues to maintain acid-based homeostasis. This section will review monitors of patient oxygenation and patient ventilation.

### Oxygenation

Inspired Oxygen content (or fraction of inspired $O_2$, $Fio_2$) can be measured by a variety of methods. Anesthesia machines most commonly use an amperometric sensor to measure $O_2$ in the fresh gas flow. Calibration is recommended, as the sensor, which is basically a fuel cell that consumes oxygen and generates current, has "drift"; that is, the readings in a constant concentration of oxygen will not be constant. It is a slow responding device, meaning that it cannot be used to measure inspired/expired oxygen, which rapidly changes. An alternative method of measuring inspired oxygen uses the fact that oxygen is paramagnetic. A paramagnetic oxygen sensor can be autocalibrating, using room air as a source of 21% $O_2$. The gradient between the sample and the room air can be measured by a pressure transducer or a torsion wire. The fast response time allows the measurement of both inspired and expired oxygen content. Measuring expired $O_2$ ($Feo_2$) concentration during preoxygenation (just prior to induction of anesthesia) also allows the determination of complete preoxygenation/denitrogenation.

### Pulse Oximetry

The pulse oximeter provides a continuous noninvasive estimate of arterial hemoglobin saturation ($Sao_2$) by analyzing red and infrared light transmitted through living tissue, such as a fingertip or earlobe (Fig. 20.2).[3] It uses the physical principle known as *Beer's law*, which relates the concentration of a dissolved substance to the log of the ratio of the incident and transmitted light intensity through a known distance. Because of the differing amounts of red and infrared light absorbed by oxyhemoglobin and reduced hemoglobin the device makes this estimate using only two wavelengths of light emitted by light-emitting diodes, or LEDs (red at 660 nm and infrared at 940 nm) detected by a photodiode. The device determines the signal related to arterial hemoglobin saturation by analyzing the pulsatile component of the absorbents, hence the name pulse oximeter (Fig. 20.3). The device continuously determines the ratio of pulse-added red to pulse-added infrared light absorbance:

$$R = \frac{AC_{red}/DC_{red}}{AC_{IR}/DC_{IR}}$$

Eq. 1

This ratio (R) of absorbance is empirically calibrated to estimate $Sao_2$. That is, the device uses $Sao_2$ data derived from human volunteers to determine the relationship between the pulse oximeter saturation ($Spo_2$) and the ratio of light absorbance (Fig. 20.4).

#### Dyes and Dyshemoglobins

Standard pulse oximeters using two wavelengths of light can determine functional saturation, that is, the percent of oxyhemoglobin ($HbO_2$) over $HbO_2$ plus reduced hemoglobin (Hb). Two equations are used to solve for two unknowns:

$$Sao_2 = \frac{HbO_2}{HbO_2 + Hb}$$

Eq. 2

Functional saturation

$$So_2 = \frac{HbO_2}{COHb + MetHb + HbO_2 + Hb}$$

Eq. 3

Fractional saturation

**Fig. 20.1** A summary of monitors and the circulation. Anatomic features are listed around the periphery, with monitored variables central and underlined (see Table 20.1 for normal values of monitored variables). The blood flows in a circuit with a cardiac output of roughly 20% each to the brain, kidneys, liver, GI tract, muscle mass, and other organs (skin, etc.). The systemic vascular resistance (SVR) is a calculated variable, reflecting the totality of blood flow and pressure. Roughly 70% of the blood is on the venous side. The venous capacitance is highly variable and acts as a buffer for changes in volume. Some variables may be measured or derived, depending on methodology. *aa,* Arteries; *ABG,* arterial blood gas; *BIS,* bispectral index; *CVP,* central venous pressure; *DBP,* diastolic blood pressure; *DBS,* double burst stimulation; *ECG,* electrocardiogram; *EEG,* electroencephalography; *EF,* ejection fraction; *EMG,* electromyography; *ETco$_2$,* end-tidal CO$_2$; *Fio$_2$,* fraction of inspired oxygen; *GI,* gastrointestinal; *ICP,* intracranial pressure; *LA,* left atrium; *LAP,* left atrial pressure; *LV,* left ventricle; *LVEDV,* left ventricular end-diastolic volume; *LVSV,* left ventricular systolic volume; *MAP,* mean arterial pressure; *PAP,* pulmonary artery pressure; *PCWP,* pulmonary capillary wedge pressure; *PIP,* peak inspiratory pressure; *Q,* cardiac output; *RA,* right atrium; *RR,* respiratory rate; *RV,* right ventricle; *SBP,* systolic blood pressure; *Spo$_2$,* arterial O$_2$ saturation; *SPV,* systolic pressure variation; *SSEP,* somatosensory evoked potential; *TEE,* transesophageal echocardiography; *TOF,* train-of-four; *VT,* tidal volume.

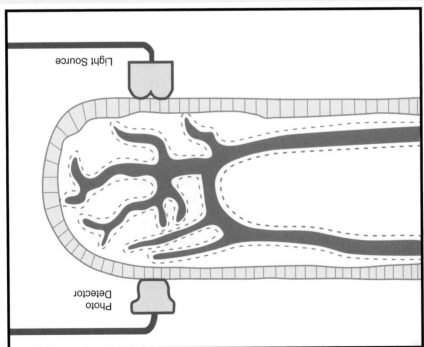

**Fig. 20.2** Pulse oximeter. Pulse oximeters (Spo₂) provide an estimate of arterial hemoglobin saturation (Sao₂) by analyzing the pulsatile absorbance of two frequencies of light (660nm and 940 nm) emitted by light-emitting diodes (LEDs), the light source, and detected by a photodiode on the opposite side of the tissue bed of the finger. The photodiode generates a current when it detects any light: red or infrared, or room light. For that reason, the photodiode alternates a pulse of red light and room light with a pulse of infrared light and the room light. Then, when both LEDs are off, it measures room light alone, then subtracts the room light signal from the previous two signals, continuously correcting for changes in room light. It thereby derives a signal associated with the pulsing LED signals. The signal may be improved by decreasing ambient light by covering the probe with an opaque material.

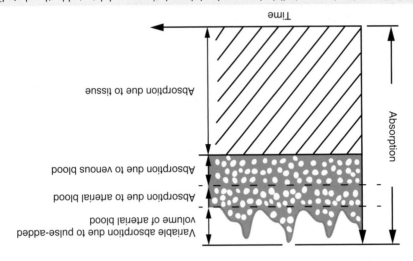

**Fig. 20.3** Tissue absorbances. As light is transmitted through tissues and detected by the photodiode it is absorbed by all the tissues between the light source and the detector, that is, the muscle, bone, and blood. Because the pulse oximeter wants to determine a signal related only to arterial blood, it analyzes only the pulsatile absorbance noted at the top of the figure. The pulse oximeter, therefore, makes the assumption that whatever is pulsing must be arterial blood. In most cases this is true, but in some situations (e.g., patient motion) there can be large venous pulsations that can produce erroneously low saturation values.

Pulse oximeters are calibrated using human volunteers who have little carboxyhemoglobin (COHb) or methemoglobin (MetHb). Therefore, if either carboxyhemoglobin (carbon monoxide poisoning) or methemoglobin (methemoglobin toxicity from benzocaine, for example) is present the devices will produce an erroneous saturation value. In the case of carboxyhemoglobin, because it is red and absorbs red light similarly to that of oxyhemoglobin, the pulse oximeter will give a reading approximately equal to the sum of carboxyhemoglobin and oxyhemoglobin, giving the impression the patient is adequately saturated with oxyhemoglobin even when he has severe carboxyhemoglobin toxicity. In the case of methemoglobin, which is dark and absorbs both red and infrared light to a high degree, it causes the ratio of absorbance to tend toward one. From the calibration curve it can be seen that a ratio of 1 will produce an Spo2 of 85% (see Fig. 20.4 [calibration curve]). Therefore, if there is a significant (>20%) amount of methemoglobin present, the pulse oximeter value will tend toward 85%. Thus, it will produce falsely low values when the patient has high Sao2, and falsely "high" values of 85% when the patient is severely hypoxemic. Dyes produce similar errors, as does methemoglobin; that is, they force the saturation toward 85%, although because they are cleared from the circulation quickly this error is only transient. Newer eight-wavelength pulse oximeters are available that can detect all saturations: oxyhemoglobin, carboxyhemoglobin, and methemoglobin.[4] Motion artifact will also cause the Spo2 value to tend toward 85% because the motion artifact produces noise in the numerator and denominator, the ratio R is forced toward 1.0, as occurs with methemoglobin. In fact, any situation that results in a small signal-to-noise ratio may cause the Spo2 to trend toward 85%.[3]

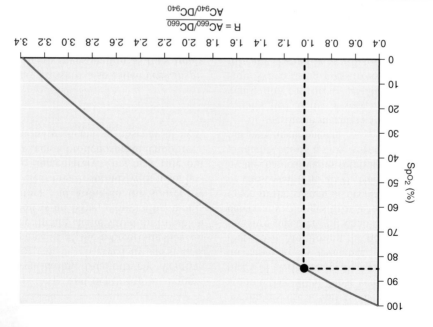

$$R = \frac{AC_{660}/DC_{660}}{AC_{940}/DC_{940}}$$

**Fig. 20.4** Pulse oximeter calibration curve. Because of all the absorbances between the light source and the photo detector, the concentrations of oxyhemoglobin and reduced hemoglobin cannot be measured specifically; that is, the exact path length of the light is unknown. Using the pulse-added absorbance from both the infrared and red light source, a ratio of these pulse-added absorbance (see Eq. 1) can be empirically related to Spo2. That is, volunteer subjects breathe low inspired oxygen concentrations to produce desaturation while blood samples are obtained for Sao2 measurement. These Sao2 measurements are calibrated to the ratio of red to infrared pulsatile absorbance to develop the calibration curve, which is incorporated into the device. Note the ratio ranges from approximately 0.4 to 3.4 as the saturation decreases from 100% to 0%. The volunteer data are only available from 100% saturation down to 75% and all values below that are extrapolated from the data. Note that at approximately Spo2 85% the ratio of the two absorbances is 1.0. Therefore, any situation that causes the ratio of pulse-added red to pulse-added infrared light to tend toward a ratio of 1.0 produces a saturation of approximately 85%. This occurs with motion artifact, dyes, and methemoglobin toxicity. AC, Alternating current; DC, direct current.

## Ventilation

The respiratory rate, pattern, and depth are all important descriptors of ventilation. Qualitatively, ventilation depth and pattern can be observed by chest rise, auscultation, or reexpansion of the rebreathing bag on the anesthesia machine. In any acute situation in which adequacy of ventilation is an issue, eliminating monitoring devices altogether and going to the source by listening for bilateral clear breath sounds with a stethoscope should be done immediately. This may rule out tension pneumothorax, acute bronchospasm, endobronchial intubation, pulmonary edema, or absence of ventilation altogether.

### Airway Pressures

Increases in peak airway pressure, also called *peak inspiratory pressure (PIP)*, merit investigation as they imply an acute increase in airflow resistance or reduction in lung/chest wall compliance. Setting the ventilator to produce an end-inspiratory pause will allow measurement of a plateau pressure, which will be a reflection of lung/chest wall compliance only. The difference between peak and plateau pressure will be a reflection of airway resistance only. If peak airway pressure is increased and plateau pressure is increased a similar amount, this signifies reduced lung/chest wall compliance, which can be caused by conditions such as tension pneumothorax or pulmonary edema. Other clinical findings can help to determine the specific cause, such as accompanying arterial hypotension with tension pneumothorax or visible frothy fluid in the endotracheal tube (ETT) with pulmonary edema. External obstruction of an ETT (from a patient biting on the tube or tube kinking) can cause an increase in PIP with a lesser increase in the plateau pressure. This can be easily ruled out by passing a suction catheter down the ETT. A loss or abrupt decrease in airway pressure is not specific but can indicate a variety of major problems, including circuit disconnections, leaks, extubation of the trachea, failure to deliver fresh gases, failure to set the ventilator properly, excess scavenging, and other anesthesia machine issues.[5] Airway pressure can be measured with analog gauges or electronic pressure transducers.

### Tidal Volume

One large study demonstrated improved pulmonary outcomes after major abdominal surgery by using tidal volume of 6 to 8 mL/kg of ideal body weight (based on height and gender) as well as recruitment maneuvers and positive end-expiratory pressure (PEEP).[6] These settings are similar to those associated with improved outcomes in patients with acute respiratory distress syndrome (also see Chapter 41). Once these tidal volumes are set, the respiratory rate should be adjusted to maintain an end-tidal $CO_2$ ($ETCO_2$) in the normal range of 35 to 40 mm Hg. Modern ventilators use a variety of modes to achieve this tidal volume (Fig. 20.5). Most ventilators have pressure limits that will alert when peak pressures are exceeded owing to increased airway resistance in the circuit or in the patient (Fig. 20.6). Monitoring the tidal volume and peak airway pressure together will enable the practitioner to quickly detect any changes in resistance to airflow due to resistance in the system or decreased compliance in the lung or chest wall (Fig. 20.7). Tidal volumes can be measured by mechanical vanes rotating in the gas stream, pressure gradients across a flow restriction (fixed or variable), and hot wire anemometers.

All anesthesia machines require a "disconnect" alarm, usually tied to the airway pressure reading. Inadequate ventilation can occur despite a nominally normal pressure. When using pressure-controlled ventilation, a significant change in ventilator volume can occur without an alarm condition occurring. Mechanical alarms and indicators of ventilation do not ensure tracheal intubation. An esophageal intubation can return "adequate" pressures and volumes and, with transmission of sounds, appear to have bilateral breath sounds. With an intact circulation, measurement of expired $CO_2$ is the best monitor of ventilation as discussed in detail in the next section.

### Capnography/End-Tidal $CO_2$

Capnography is the analysis of the continuous waveform of expired $CO_2$. Gas is continuously sampled from the ventilator circuit just on the patient side of the Y connector. The gas sample is drawn through a small tube into an infrared analyzer and the $CO_2$ waveform is displayed on the physiologic monitor (Figs. 20.8 and 20.9). Carbon dioxide generated in the tissues is delivered to the right side of the heart through the venous system into the lungs via the pulmonary arteries. Exchange of the carbon dioxide into the alveolar space is fairly efficient because $CO_2$ has 20 times the solubility in water as does oxygen. Therefore, well-perfused alveoli achieve equilibrium with carbon dioxide in the blood. During expiration alveolar gas leaves the lungs, exiting the trachea through the ETT where the aspirated gas is sampled by the capnometer, producing a peak expired $CO_2$ close to the arterial carbon dioxide tension ($PaCO_2$) in healthy patients ($ETCO_2$ is usually 3 to 5 mm Hg less than $PaCO_2$ during general anesthesia).

The respiratory tidal volume is composed of alveolar gas volume and dead space. Approximately one third of the tidal volume in healthy patients is dead space (see Fig. 20.8 for details). Because the inspired gas contains no carbon dioxide (unless the $CO_2$ absorber is malfunctioning and allowing rebreathing of $CO_2$ to occur), dead space gases will not contain carbon dioxide. When expiration begins in the respiratory cycle, the first gas detected is apparatus dead space, followed by the anatomic dead space. Neither of these spaces contains carbon dioxide.

Alveolar dead space may be increased in chronic obstructive lung disease (also see Chapter 41) in which large emphysematous areas of the lung increase the alveolar dead space and produce a large gradient between the $ET_{CO_2}$ and $Pa_{CO_2}$. In other situations, acute changes in alveolar dead space occur. The classic case involves pulmonary emboli that completely obstruct blood flow to some capillaries, causing an acute increase in alveolar dead space and resulting in an acute decrease in the $ET_{CO_2}$ value (Fig. 20.10D). Increased dead space can also occur when there is a ventilation-perfusion mismatch causing decreased perfusion to well-ventilated areas of the lung. For example, when a patient is placed in the lateral position (see Chapter 19) the dependent lung is well perfused and ventilated but the elevated lung is less well perfused and therefore has more alveolar dead

so the capnogram will remain at zero during the initial phase I of the capnogram (see Fig. 20.9). As the gas from the alveolar space (well perfused) and the alveolar dead space mix and are detected at the sampling tube, the carbon dioxide waveform will increase from zero up to a plateau value producing a rough square wave until inspiration begins and the $CO_2$ waveform immediately returns to zero. The final plateau value of the capnogram ($ET_{CO_2}$) will approximately equal the arterial $CO_2$ value if there is no alveolar dead space. The $ET_{CO_2}$ value will always be less than the $Pa_{CO_2}$ value: the degree of this gradient will be in direct proportion to the amount of alveolar dead space in the expired volume, relative to the alveolar gas. The larger the proportion of dead space, the smaller the $ET_{CO_2}$ value. Common abnormalities of the capnogram are depicted in Fig. 20.10.

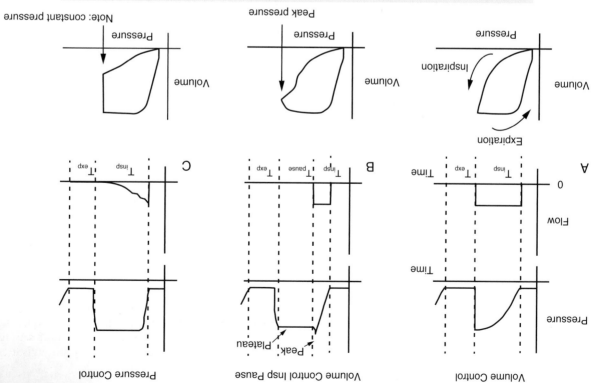

**Fig. 20.5** Ventilator pressure time curves. Three commonly employed modes of ventilation generate characteristic curves. (A) In volume-controlled ventilation, the pressure and volume smoothly increase until expiration (which is passive). (B) With the addition of an inspiratory pause, the pressure drops with minimal change in volume. (C) In pressure-controlled ventilation, the pressure is constant as volume increases, until expiration. Only four variables determine volume-based mechanical ventilation: (1) inspiratory time ($T_{insp}$), (2) inspiratory pause time ($T_{pause}$), (3) expiratory time ($T_{exp}$), and (4) inspiratory flow rate. In ventilators that have control loops, faulty monitoring can lead to inadequate or hazardous ventilation. The compliance of the lung can be measured by dividing the tidal volume by the distending pressure (peak or plateau pressure minus PEEP). Dynamic compliance reflects the compliance during airflow, so it includes the resistance of the endotracheal tube as well as the compliance of the lungs. With an inspiratory pause (B), both the dynamic compliance and the static compliance (of the lungs and chest wall) can be measured by using either the peak pressure or the plateau pressure, respectively. The pressure-volume loops are different for the various ventilation modes as well. *PEEP,* Positive end-expiratory pressure.

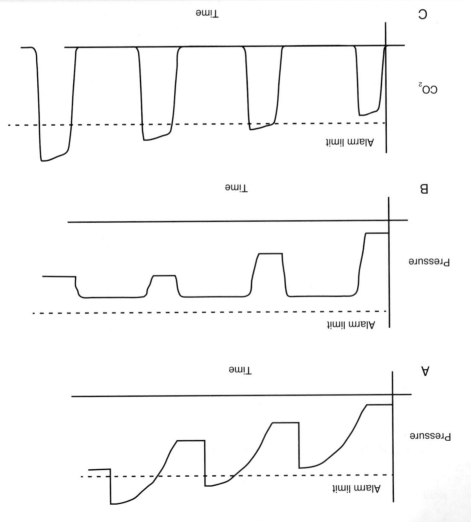

**Fig. 20.6** Stacking breaths. In both volume control (A) and pressure ventilation (B), insufficient expiratory time leads to "stacking" of breaths and changes in the pressure waveform. In the case of volume control ventilation, the pressure can increase, triggering an alarm. With pressure control ventilation, tidal volumes decrease and pressure remains constant (this may trigger a high PEEP alarm). (C) The capnogram also demonstrates decreased ventilation (increasing $CO_2$) and a change in the shape of the $CO_2$ curve. *PEEP*, Positive end-expiratory pressure.

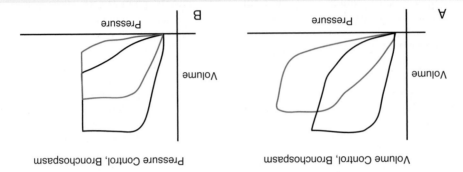

**Fig. 20.7** Bronchospasm. With volume control ventilation (A), the set tidal volume is attempted to be delivered, with an increase in pressure. This results in the pressure volume loop being shifted to the right and flattened. In pressure control ventilation (B), the stiffness of the lung results in a decreased tidal volume, without a change in the pressure (because that is the ventilator setpoint).

space, again producing a decrease in the $ET_{CO_2}$ value compared to the $Pa_{CO_2}$. Finally, a progressive increase in alveolar dead space may occur because of a global lack of perfusion when the cardiac output decreases (see Fig. 20.10D). For example, if cardiac output suddenly decreases from 5 L/min to 2.5 L/min with alveolar ventilation remaining constant, less blood flow will flow per unit time to perfuse the same number of ventilated alveoli. The result is an increase in alveolar dead space and a decrease in $ET_{CO_2}$. For this reason the $ET_{CO_2}$ capnogram is often referred to as the "poor man's measure of cardiac output." Any significant decrease in cardiac output is associated with a decrease in $ET_{CO_2}$ (see Fig. 20.10D). In the most acute situation of cardiac arrest when cardiopulmonary resuscitation (CPR) is initiated (also see Chapter 45), the most important monitor to follow to assure the adequacy of chest compressions during CPR is the capnogram. A capnogram showing $ET_{CO_2}$ greater than 20 mm Hg with every ventilated breath during CPR ensures both ventilation and perfusion of the lung. If

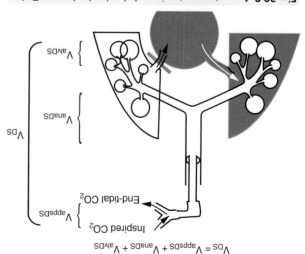

$$V_{Ds} = V_{appsDS} + V_{anaDS} + V_{alvDS}$$

**Fig. 20.8** Apparatus, anatomic, and alveolar dead space. To interpret the capnogram one must first understand alveolar dead space and its components. This schematic shows the heart, lung, and ventilator circuit up to the Y connector. Dead space volume ($V_{Ds}$) is defined as any portion of the tidal volume that does not participate in gas exchange. $V_{Ds}$ is further divided into three components: apparatus dead space ($V_{appsDS}$), anatomic dead space ($V_{anaDS}$), and alveolar dead space ($V_{alvDS}$). Apparatus dead space is the volume of gas between the Y connector and the end of the endotracheal tube. Anatomic dead space is the dead space of the trachea and all connecting airways down to the alveoli. In this figure the lung on the right has no blood flow so all those alveoli are not perfused and at the end of expiration will have zero carbon dioxide. The lung on the left is well perfused and those alveoli can be assumed at end of expiration to equilibrate to the arterial carbon dioxide ($Pa_{CO_2}$) value. The expired mixture of the alveolar gas ($Pa_{CO_2}$) and alveolar dead space gas (no $CO_2$) produces the end-tidal $CO_2$ ($ET_{CO_2}$).

the capnogram shows $ET_{CO_2}$ less than 20 mm Hg during chest compressions, it is likely that cardiac output is inadequate. In this situation, the CPR should be adjusted until $ET_{CO_2}$ is more than 20 mm Hg. The other advantage of monitoring the capnogram during CPR is that there is no motion artifact associated with a capnogram unlike nearly every other monitor during CPR or chest compressions, such as electrocardiogram (ECG) and the pulse oximeter. Because of the utility of the continuous capnogram waveform assuring that there is intact ventilation and perfusion (i.e., cardiac output), some consider the capnogram to be the most important monitor used during general anesthesia.

Although the sampling tube can be placed on nasal cannula or around the mouth in patients whose tracheas are not intubated, a reliable capnographic waveform is achieved only in a patient whose trachea is intubated. In nonclosed systems (where the sampling tube is placed by the airway under a mask or a nasal cannula), there may be aspiration of room air (with no carbon dioxide), which will dilute the capnographic sample.

## CIRCULATORY SYSTEM

Multiple characteristics of the circulation can be measured, including the heart rate, ECG, blood pressure, urine output, central venous pressures (CVPs), pulmonary artery pressures (PAPs), cardiac output, and systolic pressure variation (SPV) (Table 20.1). Some of these are difficult to measure and all require interpretation. Many important variables cannot be measured, such as venous capacitance, organ blood flow/perfusion, and circulating blood volume. Other values are derived from combinations of measured values (e.g., stroke volume, vascular resistance). No single characteristic determines adequacy of perfusion, and a solid understanding of the underlying physiology is necessary to interpret even the simplest monitor.

## Measurement of the Electrocardiogram

Continuous monitoring of the ECG is one of the standards of the ASA, yielding information on heart rate and rhythm. Simply, the ECG is the electrical activity of the heart, measured at the body surface. Technically, it is the net dipole moment of the heart displayed on the vertical axis in millivolts versus time on the horizontal axis. The operating room is an electrically noisy environment and subtle ECG changes can be obscured by the filtering, and artifacts (false positives) can be introduced. ECG monitors in the operating room have a filtering mode that reduces the electrical interference, but they may produce artifacts that look like concerning ECG changes, such as T-wave changes. These monitors also have a "diagnostic mode" that removes all filtering and the artifacts it may induce.

Therefore, if the ECG on the monitor looks different from the preoperative ECG, it is best to switch the filters off and place the monitor in the diagnostic mode to see if those changes are real. A three-lead system, which uses electrodes placed on both shoulders and left abdomen below the rib cage, provides leads I, II, and III. The preferred method is a five-lead system, using a single precordial lead placed in the $V_5$ position (Fig. 20.11). A majority of the dysrhythmias and ischemia seen during anesthesia can be detected by a combination of monitoring leads II and $V_5$.[7] Monitoring the ECG allows dysrhythmias, such as heart block, atrial fibrillation, ventricular fibrillation, bradycardia, asystole, and tachycardia to be diagnosed (and treatment evaluated). The ECG can also aid in diagnosing myocardial ischemia and electrolyte disturbances (Table 20.2).

## Blood Pressure and Flow

The primary utility of the circulatory system is to maintain a constant supply of blood flow to all organs to allow them to function and maintain aerobic metabolism. This system is composed of a basic pump, the heart; conduits, the blood vessels; and resistance as blood flows through the microcirculation. This is an Ohm's law system, $V = IR$, where V (blood pressure) equals blood flow (cardiac output) multiplied by resistance (systemic vascular resistance). The pressure difference across the circulation of any organ is defined as the perfusion pressure, that is, the pressure on the upstream side of that system minus the pressure on the downstream side. For the systemic circulation, the pressure difference is the mean arterial pressure (MAP) minus the CVP; and for the pulmonary circulation it is the mean pulmonary artery pressure (MPAP) minus the left atrial pressure, usually estimated by a pulmonary artery wedge pressure (PAWP). Mean pressure is approximated by the formula:

$$\text{Mean BP} = \text{Diastolic BP} + \frac{(\text{Systolic BP} - \text{Diastolic BP})}{3} \qquad \text{Eq. 4}$$

For the most vital of organs, the brain and heart, these perfusion pressures are slightly different. For the brain it is the MAP minus the intracranial pressure (ICP) (see "Intracranial Pressure Monitoring") and for the heart

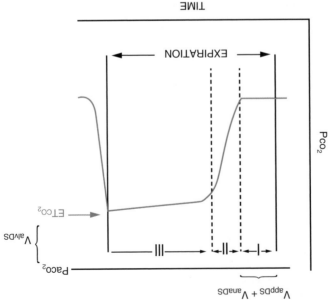

**Fig. 20.9** Normal capnogram. A capnogram is a continuous tracing of the carbon dioxide concentration sampled at the Y connector on an intubated, ventilated patient and plotted versus time during the inspiratory and expiratory cycle. It can be divided into three phases. Phase I is the beginning of expiration when the apparatus dead space ($V_{appDS}$) and anatomic dead space ($V_{anaDS}$) are being sampled, both of which have zero carbon dioxide. Phase II starts when the mixed alveolar gases are detected and the capnogram rises and reaches a plateau value. Phase III has only a slight rise as the mixed alveolar gases are sampled during the end of the expiratory cycle. With the initiation of inspiration the $CO_2$ value drops to zero and stays at zero until the next expiration. Note the end peak value is the end-tidal $CO_2$ ($ETCO_2$). The $ETCO_2$ is always lower than the $PaCO_2$; the magnitude of this gap is directly proportional to the ratio of alveolar dead space to alveolar gas.

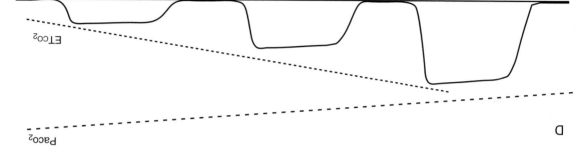

**Fig. 20.10** Capnogram abnormalities. (A) The normal Paco₂ to ETco₂ gradient is 2 to 5 mm Hg. (B) This rightward slant of the initiation of the alveolar gas detection is seen when there is the presence of asthma or chronic obstructive pulmonary disease. The greater the slant to the right, the worse the expiratory airway resistance. The gradient of Paco₂ to ETco₂ has increased. (C) This waveform shows a progressive rise in the baseline CO₂ value; that is, there is a progressive increase in inspiratory carbon dioxide, noting a CO₂ rebreathing most commonly due to an exhausted CO₂ absorber. (D) This waveform signifies a progressive drop in the ETco₂, that is, a decrease in the height of the waveform. This form is noted whenever there is abrupt reduction in pulmonary blood flow (cardiac output), as occurs with a pulmonary embolism or a cardiac arrest. *ETco₂,* End-tidal carbon dioxide.

it is the systemic diastolic pressure minus the right side of the heart, or coronary sinus pressure. Because the heart perfuses itself during diastole, the diastolic pressure is used as the upstream pressure head. In all these systems, blood pressure correlates directly to blood flow assuming the resistance is constant. Unfortunately, in some situations the pressure may be normal but the flow may be reduced because of a high resistance. The reverse is certainly true: as the arterial blood pressure decreases, the blood flow to that organ, or the body in general, will eventually be insufficient to perfuse organs adequately. Therefore, the purpose of

constant and repeated measurements of arterial blood pressure is to ensure that hypotension is not occurring. Fig. 20.12 presents a decision tree for the diagnosis of hypotension.

**Blood Pressure: Hypotension**

Documentation of pulse rate and arterial blood pressure at least every 5 minutes is one of the ASA standards. Yet, despite this long history of measuring arterial blood pressure at frequent intervals, the definition of hypotension based on clinical outcomes was determined relatively recently. In 2009, an association between a MAP

### Table 20.1   Normal Values

| Measured Variable (Abbreviation) | Normal Value |
| --- | --- |
| Systolic blood pressure (SBP) | 90–140 mm Hg |
| Diastolic blood pressure (DBP) | 60–90 mm Hg |
| Mean arterial pressure (MAP) | 70–105 mm Hg |
| Systolic pressure variation (SPV) | 5 mm Hg |
| Pulse pressure variation (PPV) | 10%–13% |
| Central venous pressure (CVP) | 2–6 mm Hg |
| Right ventricular pressure | 15–30/2–8 mm Hg |
| Pulmonary artery pressure (PAP) | 15–30/5–15 mm Hg |
| Mean pulmonary artery pressure | 9–20 mm Hg |
| Pulmonary capillary wedge pressure (PCWP) | 6–12 mm Hg |
| Left atrial pressure (LAP) | 4–12 mm Hg |
| Heart rate (HR) | 60–90 beats/min |
| Arterial $O_2$ saturation (SpO$_2$) | 95%–100% |
| Cardiac output (Q or CO) | 4–8 L/m |
| Cardiac index (CI) | 2.4–4.0 L/min/m² |
| Ejection fraction (EF) | 55%–70% |
| End-diastolic volume | 65–240 mL |
| **Calculated Values** | |
| Stroke volume (SV), stroke volume index (SVI) | 50–100 mL/beat, 33–47 mL/m²/beat |
| Systemic vascular resistance (SVR) | 800–1300 dynes · sec/cm⁵ |
| Pulmonary vascular resistance (PVR) | <250 dynes · sec/cm⁵ |
| **Respiratory Parameters** | |
| Respiratory rate (RR) | 12–20 breaths/min |
| Peak inspiratory pressure (PIP) | 15–20 cm $H_2O$ |
| Tidal volume (Vt) | 6–8 mL/kg ideal body weight |
| End-tidal $CO_2$ (ETco$_2$) | 35–40 mm Hg |
| **Cerebral Parameters** | |
| Intracranial pressure (ICP) | 5–15 mm Hg |
| Electroencephalography (EEG) | Waveform varies by state of consciousness |
| Somatosensory evoked potential (SSEP) | Normal amplitude and latency |
| Bispectral index (BIS) | 80–100 awake |
| **Muscle Parameters** | |
| Train-of-four (TOF) | 4 twitches present |
| TOF ratio | >0.9 |
| Double burst stimulation (DBS) | No fade |
| Tetany | No fade |
| Electromyography (EMG) | Depends on stimulus |

The range of normal values for monitored and measured variables in clinical practice are shown in this table. Indices are commonly obtained by dividing the value by the body surface area (BSA).

of less than 50 mm Hg or a 40% decrease in MAP from the preoperative arterial blood pressure for more than 10 minutes was associated with an increased incidence of postoperative cardiac events (i.e., troponin increases).[8] In 2013, the cumulative time with a mean MAP less than 55 mm Hg was noted to be associated with progressively increasing incidences of postoperative renal and cardiac injury (increased creatinine and troponin in the postoperative period).[9] In 2015, it was noted that mean MAPs less than approximately 50 mm Hg and less than 60 mm Hg for as short a duration as 5 and 10 minutes, respectively, were associated with an increased 30-day postoperative mortality rate.[10] Therefore, intraoperative hypotension for adults can be defined as mean MAP between 55 to 60 mm Hg.

### Noninvasive Blood Pressure

The use of an automatic noninvasive cuff, which measures blood pressure by the oscillometric method, is the routine in anesthetic care. The cuff inflates beyond systolic pressure and slowly deflates until it detects a pulse, continues deflating until it reaches maximal pulsations (the MAP), and further deflates until a pulse is not detected. Although it presents systolic and diastolic blood pressures, the most accurate pressure of an oscillometric cuff is the MAP

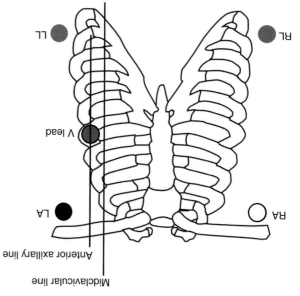

**Fig. 20.11** Electrocardiograph lead placement. The limb leads (RA, LA, RL, LL) are placed peripherally on the chest (or on the limbs if available). The V lead is placed in the fifth intercostal space in the anterior axillary line (between the middle of the clavicle and the middle of the axilla).

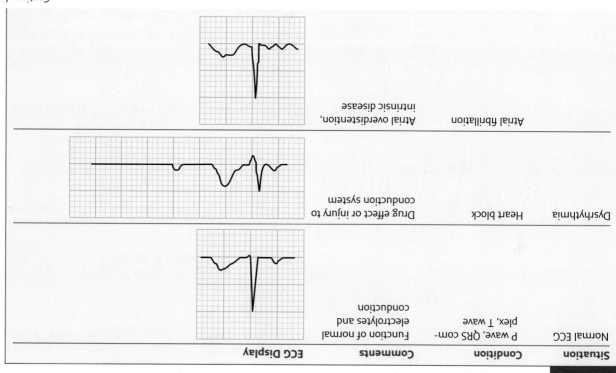

**Table 20.2** Electrocardiographic Monitoring

| Situation | Condition | Comments | ECG Display |
|---|---|---|---|
| Normal ECG | P wave, QRS complex, T wave | Function of normal electrolytes and conduction | |
| Dysrhythmia | Heart block | Drug effect or injury to conduction system | |
| Atrial fibrillation | Atrial overdistention, intrinsic disease | | |

**Table 20.2** Electrocardiographic Monitoring—cont'd

| Situation | Condition | Comments | ECG Display |
|---|---|---|---|
| Sinus tachycardia | | Hypovolemia, light anesthesia, hypoxia, hypercarbia | 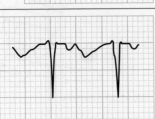 |
| Sinus bradycardia | | Excess vagal tone, drug effects, hypoxia | |
| Asystole | | Extreme vagal tone, extreme hypoxia | |
| Torsades | | Genetic ion channel differences, long QT syndrome, drugs | 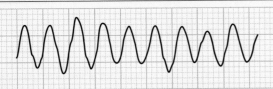 |
| Ventricular tachy-cardia | | Coronary artery disease, mechanical irritation from central line | 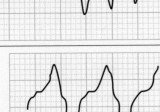 |
| Ventricular fibrillation | | Intrinsic myocardial disease | 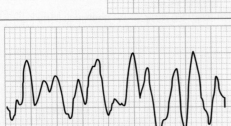 |
| Active ischemia | ST-segment changes | Ischemia, demand or supply | |

**Table 20.2** Electrocardiographic Monitoring—cont'd

| Situation | Condition | Comments | ECG Display |
|---|---|---|---|
| Completed old infarction | Q waves | Localized to area of injury | |
| Electrolyte | Hypokalemia | Depressed T wave, U wave | |
| | Hyperkalemia | Peaked T waves, sinusoidal ECG in the extreme | |
| | Hypercalcemia | Shortened QT interval, possible J wave | |
| Temperature | Hypothermia | Osborne J wave | |

The electrocardiogram (ECG) changes induced in many physiologic conditions are neither sensitive nor specific but may be confirmatory. The ECG changes for heart rhythm are diagnostic.

the intravascular status volume by measuring SPV or other measures of volume responsiveness (see following section, "Measures of Intravascular Volume Responsiveness").

The radial artery is most commonly used because it has the least associated risk and is most easily palpable. Other sites such as the brachial, femoral, or dorsalis pedis arteries may be used. Table 20.3 provides a comparison of different techniques of blood pressure measurement and sites of arterial cannulation. The arterial line is connected to a pressure transducer, which converts the mechanical energy of the arterial pulse into an electrical signal. This fluid-filled tube/transducer setup is an underdamped system that can cause amplification artifact of the systolic blood pressure. This artifact is worsened by an increasing pulse rate and increasing amount of fluid (length of tubing) in the system; however, the MAP should remain accurate.[1] Placement of an arterial line is a sterile procedure, with many technical variations on placement. Some institutions have created protocols to be followed for any line placement.

## Measures of Intravascular Volume Responsiveness

### Systolic Pressure Variation

The gold standard for determining the adequacy of intravascular volume and cardiac function is transesophageal echocardiography (TEE). Although TEE is extremely useful for diagnosing and in some cases monitoring cardiac performance, it is not necessary or practical during use of most anesthetics. Yet, there are many procedures that cause intravascular volume shifts and lead to questions about cardiac performance, resulting in a need for more information than is available with standard monitors. In situations in which CVP monitoring is not necessary or feasible, substantial information can be derived from analyzing the variations of a continuous arterial pressure waveform associated with positive-pressure ventilation. Measuring the degree to which a positive-pressure breath can result in a decrease in the systolic pressure can predict the responsiveness of a patient to an intravascular fluid challenge[12] (Table 20.4). Responsiveness is typically defined as an improvement in stroke volume, blood pressure, or cardiac output.[12] SPV is defined as the difference between maximum and minimum systolic blood pressure during a positive-pressure respiratory cycle. SPV may be manually calculated by freezing the arterial waveform on the physiologic monitor and scrolling up and down, subtracting the average value of arterial peak pressures between positive-pressure breaths from the lower peak arterial pressure values during the breaths (Fig. 20.14). The decrease in arterial pressure associated with positive-pressure ventilation is due in part to the positive intrathoracic pressure transiently impeding venous return to the right side of the heart (see Fig. 20.1). This in turn reduces right-sided heart stroke volume, which in turn reduces left-sided heart stroke volume and arterial blood pressure.

glucose and other blood constituents, and assessment of sampling of hematocrit, analysis of arterial blood gases, beat-to-beat blood pressure measurement, allows for blood great value (also see Chapter 41). An arterial line provides from an invasive catheter (usually in the radial artery) is of a continuous arterial blood pressure measurement shifts, disease or the procedure is expected to have large fluid In cases in which a patient has significant cardiovascular

### Invasive Arterial Blood Pressure Monitoring

(Fig. 20.13).[11] The size of the blood pressure cuff will influence the resultant blood pressure measurement. If the cuff is properly sized its width will be approximately 40% of the circumference of the arm. If the cuff is too small the blood pressure measurement will be too high, if it is too large the measurement will be too low. The oldest noninvasive method of determining blood pressure is the Riva-Rocci technique, which uses a cuff to occlude the arterial flow, slowly deflating the cuff, and noting the pressure when the flow returns (as determined by palpation, Doppler, or any other method). By using a Doppler probe, this method can be successful in patients with hypotension or nonpulsatile flow, including patients with a left ventricular assist device (LVAD).

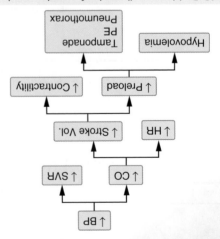

**Fig. 20.12** Decision tree diagnosis of acute hypotension. Given that the cardiovascular system is a pressure = flow × resistance "circuit," the diagnosis and acute management of hypotension should follow the principles outlined in the text. This schematic does not account for increasing venous compliance. Decreases in blood pressure (BP) must be due to a drop in either resistance or cardiac output (CO). If there is no obvious reason for an acute drop in resistance (e.g., a sympathectomy from spinal anesthesia), then the CO drop must be due to a decrease in either heart rate (HR) or stroke volume. If the HR has not decreased, then the decrease in stroke volume must be due to a decrease in either preload or contractility. If there must be due to a decrease in either preload or contractility. If there is no reason for a drop in contractility and the preload is decreased, it is most commonly due to a lack of relative volume, frequently due to the increase in venous capacitance with anesthetics. One should always keep in mind the three acute mechanical obstructions to blood flow: cardiac tamponade, pulmonary embolism (PE), and tension pneumothorax. *SVR,* Systemic vascular resistance.

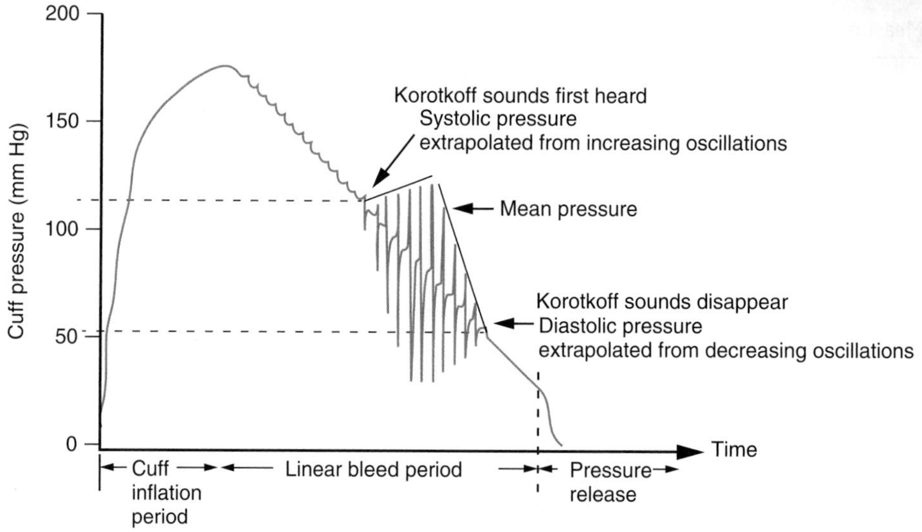

**Fig. 20.13** Oscillometric cuff and Korotkoff sounds. Initial Korotkoff sounds correlate with the increasing cuff oscillations. The magnitude of the oscillations increase progressively to a peak, and then decrease. The peak in oscillations is a measure of the mean arterial pressure, which is the most accurate measurement in an oscillometric cuff. The oscillometric systolic and diastolic pressures are inferred from the slope of the envelope around the oscillations. The decreasing oscillations correlate with the diastolic pressure and disappearance of Korotkoff sounds. (Adapted from Ehrenwerth J, Eisenkraft J, Berry J. *Anesthesia Equipment: Principles and Applications.* 2nd ed. Philadelphia: Elsevier Saunders; 2013.)

**Table 20.3**  Arterial Blood Pressure Measurement

| Method | How Obtained | Advantage/Benefit/Indication | Disadvantage/Risk |
|---|---|---|---|
| Riva-Rocci | Palpate pulse, inflate cuff, slowly deflate until pulse returns | Can be used without a stethoscope, by palpation of pulse or Doppler flow detection | Only gives a systolic pressure, can work with nonpulsatile flow |
| Korotkoff | Auscultate over antecubital fossa, inflate cuff, slowly deflate, noting first auscultation sounds and last sounds | Gives diastolic as well as systolic pressure | Needs stethoscope, quiet environment |
| Noninvasive blood pressure (NIBP) | Choose correct cuff size, initiate cuff inflation | Can be automated, for routine monitoring, measures mean pressure, interpolates systolic and diastolic pressure | Does not work with severe hypotension, motion artifact, or patient with left ventricular assist device |
| Invasive | Connect intra-arterial catheter to transducer | Wide range of pressure, measures a mean pressure, systolic and diastolic pressure, useful when there is hemodynamic instability, vasopressor administration. Can serve as access route for blood draws | Invasive, potential for amplification artifact, dampening, hemorrhage, hematoma, infection, injury to artery or distal areas |
| Radial |  | Most commonly used as generally accessible; hand typically has dual blood supply | Can produce artificially low values with severe systemic vasoconstriction |
| Brachial |  | Sometimes available when radial site is not | No redundant blood supply, uncomfortable, cannot flex arm |
| Femoral |  | Large vessel, can give accurate values with profound vasoconstriction | Prone to infection, affected by prone positioning |
| Dorsalis pedis |  | May be an accessible site when others are not | Some amplification of waveform |

| Table 20.4 | Measures of Volume Responsiveness to Intravenous Fluid Bolus^a | |
| --- | --- | --- |
| | **Fluid Responsive** | **Not Fluid Responsive** |
| SPV | >10 mm Hg | <5 mm Hg |
| PPV | >15% | <7% |
| SVV | <15% | <5% |

The three measures of volume responsiveness are systolic pressure variation (SPV), pulse pressure variation (PPV), and stroke volume variation (SVV). As the table indicates, there is a "gray zone" between levels of responsiveness where it is unclear if the patient would benefit from the treatment.[13]

^aDefined as improved stroke volume or end-diastolic area as assessed by transesophageal echocardiography.

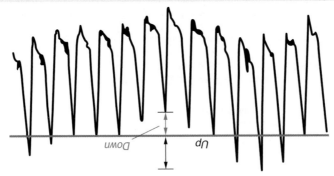

**Fig. 20.14** Systolic pressure variation. A positive-pressure breath can result in a transient decrease in the systolic blood pressure. The mechanism is predominantly related to the positive intrathoracic pressure causing a decrease in venous return and subsequent decrease in right-sided heart stroke volume, and ultimately left-sided heart stroke volume, which causes the systolic pressure to decrease. The magnitude of the drop in systolic blood pressure can predict the responsiveness of a patient to an intravascular fluid challenge

The SPV is an indirect assessment of the venous capacitance, which when abnormal, indicates a potential of the blood pressure to improve with fluid administration. One of the major limitations of SPV is that the patient must have a regular heartbeat, that is, it cannot be used in atrial fibrillation, which itself causes irregular variations in systolic blood pressure. The values may also be affected by increased lung or chest wall compliance, prone positioning, and high PEEP and will not be usable when there is an open thoracic cavity. The newer generation of physiologic monitors automatically calculates SPV.

Pulse Pressure Variation

Another method of deriving similar information is measuring the relative changes in pulse pressure during the respiratory cycle, known as *pulse pressure variation (PPV)*. In this situation, the pulse pressure between breaths minus the pulse pressure during the positive-pressure breath is subtracted and then divided by the mean pulse pressure times 100%.

Eq. 5

$$PPV\% = \frac{PP_{max} - PP_{min} \times 100}{\dfrac{PP_{max} + PP_{min}}{2}}$$

PPV can be used to predict a response to an intravenous fluid bolus, similar to the SPV.[13]

Stroke Volume Variation

Stroke volume variation is another technique using the arterial waveform to assess volume responsiveness. In this situation, a pulse contour algorithm is employed to estimate the stroke volume from the arterial pulse wave.[14] These estimates of arterial pulse volume are compared during the respiratory cycle in an analogous fashion to SPV and PPV described previously. The percent reduction in estimated stroke volume associated with positive-pressure ventilation is used to assess whether the patient would benefit from additional fluid. All of these measures of volume responsiveness require positive-pressure ventilation in a closed chest with a regular cardiac rhythm without excessively high levels of PEEP (see Table 20.4).

Central Venous Monitoring

As described in the preceding theoretical analysis, blood pressure alone is not a sufficient variable to evaluate perfusion (also see Chapter 25). Knowledge of CVP, PAP, and cardiac output (CO) may be helpful in guiding patient therapy. Additionally, central venous access may be necessary for administration of certain drugs and may act as secure access for administration of large volumes of resuscitation fluids. Table 20.5 lists a comparison of different sites for central line placement.

Central Venous Pressure

Information obtained from a CVP line includes the CVP pressure and waveforms (Fig. 20.15). The CVP waveform has several elements, each reflecting the underlying cardiovascular physiology. The *a wave* reflects atrial contraction against the closed tricuspid valve, the *c wave* reflects tricuspid bulging as the ventricle contracts, the *x descent* corresponds to atrial relaxation, the *v wave* occurs during atrial filling, and the *y descent* reflects atrial emptying. Despite the physiologic basis for the waveform, CVP is a minimally helpful guide for intravascular fluid therapy because of the complexity of the relationships between intravascular volume, venous capacitance, venous return, cardiac performance, and arterial blood pressure.[15] Although CVP values are not considered to be very predictive of intravascular volume status, they may be useful in the extremes. That is, a CVP under 2 mm Hg may suggest a beneficial cardiovascular effect from intravenous fluid administration, whereas a value of more than 15 mm Hg suggests that more fluid may not be needed. This approach to assessing the utility of a physiologic variable has been described as a "gray zone analysis." That is, in the extremes the variable provides useful information, but in the range between those extremes, or the normal range, is an area where the utility of the variable is less valuable in assessing clinical status. However, even at extreme values, the decision whether to administer

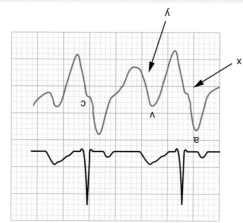

**Fig. 20.15** Central venous pressure waveform. The mean central venous pressure (CVP) value can be used to assess right-sided heart filling pressure. The waveform can also be instructive.

**Table 20.5** Central Venous Access and Pressure Measurement

| Route | Indications | Risk | Benefit |
|---|---|---|---|
| Any central venous pressure (CVP) catheter | Unable to obtain peripheral access, route for potent vasoactive medications | Bleeding, infection | Stable IV access |
| RIJ (right internal jugular) | Unable to obtain peripheral access, route for potent vasoactive medications | Carotid artery injury | Straight path to heart for pulmonary artery (PA) catheter |
| LIJ (left internal jugular) | Unable to use RIJ | Carotid artery injury, thoracic duct injury, short distance to innominate vein | Can use if RIJ not available |
| Subclavian | Unable to use RIJ or LIJ | Pneumothorax risk, injury to brachial plexus, subclavian artery/vein | More comfortable for patient after surgery, can insert with cervical collar in place; lower infection risk |
| Femoral | Disease of head and neck precluding use of neck access | Increased infection risk | Can apply pressure if bleeding |
| PA catheter | Unstable patient | In addition to CVP risks: PA rupture, dysrhythmias | Can obtain cardiac output information |

Practice guidelines for pulmonary artery catheterization have been published: American Society of Anesthesiologists Task Force on Pulmonary Artery Catheterization. Practice guidelines for pulmonary artery catheterization: an updated report by the American Society of Anesthesiologists Task Force on Pulmonary Artery Catheterization. *Anesthesiology.* 2003;99(4):988–1014. These guidelines highlight three areas: (1) patient disease (Does the patient have serious cardiac disease for which knowledge of the cardiac output and filling pressures may alter treatment?), (2) surgery (Is the surgery a major procedure in which there will be fluid shifts or changes that will be reflected in the monitor?), and (3) setting (Do the practitioners have the expertise to perform the procedure with minimum potential risk and maximum potential benefit?).

fluid or remove fluid (with diuretics) should be based on the individual patient's clinical circumstances.

### Central Venous Catheter Placement

Before placing a central venous catheter, informed consent must be obtained because of such risks as bleeding, infection, and potential damage to surrounding structures (nerves, lymph, vessels, lung, pneumothorax, and more); and to apprise the patient of the risks and benefits. The ASA has an excellent practice guideline for central venous access.[16]

### Pulmonary Artery Pressure and Cardiac Output

A pulmonary artery catheter (PAC) is an access catheter advanced from the right atrium to the right ventricle into a wedge position in the pulmonary artery by following the pressure waveforms as noted in Fig. 20.16. Data from a PAC can be used to diagnose a variety of conditions owing to its ability to measure right- and left-sided heart filling pressures as well as cardiac output. Under normal conditions, because the pulmonary vascular system is a very low resistance system, the PA diastolic pressure

and the PA wedge pressure are very similar. Table 20.6 describes a variety of acute causes of severe hypotension and the results of specific monitored parameters.

### Methods of Measuring Cardiac Output

Thermodilution is a common method of measuring cardiac output. A measured amount of "cold" fluid is injected into the central circulation via the proximal port of a PAC, and a thermister measures the temperature at the distal port. These temperature readings are recorded as a curve over time. The area under the curve is proportional to the cardiac output. Typically, several measurements are averaged at different points of the respiratory cycle. Special PACs can measure and display cardiac output on a continuous basis. In spite of all the hemodynamic data provided by the PAC, there have been no studies documenting improved outcomes in surgical patients.[17] The risks are substantial, including line sepsis, thrombosis, and pulmonary artery rupture. If a PAC is utilized for the management of severe hemodynamic compromise, it should be removed as soon as

**Table 20.6** Differential Diagnosis of Severe Hypotension

| Diagnosis | CVP | PAP | PCWP | CO | Airway Pressure |
| --- | --- | --- | --- | --- | --- |
| Pneumothorax | ↑ | ↑ | ↓ | ↓ | ↑ |
| Tamponade | ↑ | ↑ | ↑ | ↓ | ↔ |
| Pulmonary embolism | ↑ | ↑ | ↓ | ↓ | ↔ |
| Hypovolemic shock | ↓ | ↓ | ↓ | ↓ | ↔ |
| Cardiogenic shock | ↑ | ↑ | ↑ | ↓ | ↔ |
| Septic shock | ↓ | ↓ | ↓ | ↑ | ↔ |

The changes in invasive hemodynamic and airway pressures are associated with specific causes of hypotension.
*CO*, Cardiac output; *CVP*, central venous pressure; *PAP*, pulmonary artery pressure; *PCWP*, pulmonary capillary wedge pressure.

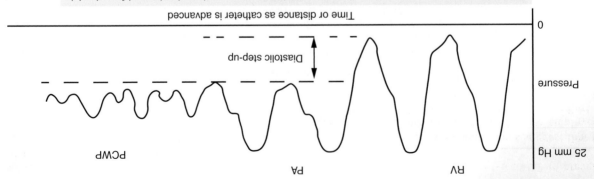

**Fig. 20.16** A trace of pressure versus distance as a pulmonary artery catheter is advanced from the right atrium through the right ventricle (RV) into the pulmonary artery and ultimately resting in a wedge position in the pulmonary artery. Note as the catheter is advanced from the right ventricle into the pulmonary artery, the diastolic pressure is cut off and rises to the PA diastolic, which is only slightly higher than the pulmonary artery wedge pressure. *PA*, Pulmonary artery; *PCWP*, pulmonary artery capillary wedge pressure.

possible. Although the use of PACs in surgery and critical care has dramatically decreased, there has been an increase in echocardiography for immediate diagnosis of cardiac disease.

Transesophageal Echocardiogram Monitoring

One way to quickly determine the cardiac status is to perform a TEE (also see Chapter 25). An ultrasound probe is inserted into the esophagus and various views of the heart are obtained in real time. Information on cardiac structure (heart valves, chamber size), contractile activity (ejection fraction), systolic and diastolic dysfunction, and pericardial disease (effusion, tamponade) can all be diagnosed with a TEE. It has therefore become the gold standard in cardiac evaluation. Limitations of TEE include the need for expertise on the part of the provider, access to the head of the patient, and the risk of esophageal injury.

## CENTRAL NERVOUS SYSTEM

### Processed Electroencephalograph Monitoring

Although the electrical activity of the brain can be monitored with the multichannel electroencephalograph (EEG), processed EEG monitors focused on the frontal area have been developed for the sake of convenience. These devices are derived through an empirical comparison of the awake and anesthetized EEG and provide output as an index generated through a multistep process. EEG features are extracted, artifact is minimized, and an algorithm converts the EEG features to a numerical index, often ranging from 100 (awake) to 0 (isoelectric EEG). These monitors are intended to assess anesthetic depth and reduce the incidence of awareness with postoperative recall (also see Chapter 47) (avoiding subtherapeutic dosing) and minimize unnecessary anesthetic administration (avoiding supratherapeutic dosing). The incidence of recall is between 1:500 to 1:1000.[18,19] The most definitive work on these devices—in particular, the bispectral index (BIS) monitor—has demonstrated a reduction in the incidence of postoperative recall of intraoperative events, compared to no monitoring of anesthetic depth, but not to a greater degree than alerts based on the expired anesthetic concentrations.[18,19] (also see Chapter 47).

### Minimum Alveolar Concentration Alert Monitoring

The minimum alveolar concentration (MAC) was developed as a method to assess and compare the relative potency of inhaled anesthetics. MAC is the end-expired concentration of an anesthetic at equilibrium at which 50% of the subjects would move in response to a noxious stimulus. In clinical anesthesia it has been used to assess depth of anesthesia and randomized controlled clinical trials suggest keeping MAC above 0.5 to 0.7 to prevent recall of intraoperative events.

The results in large randomized trials suggest that in cases in which inhalational anesthetics are employed, alerts related to the expired anesthetic age-adjusted MAC (0.5 to 0.7) are equivalent to the BIS monitor in preventing awareness with postoperative recall.[20] These studies also noted that patients monitored by either method had lower incidence of recall than patients without any anesthetic depth monitoring. When total intravenous anesthesia (TIVA) is used without any inhaled anesthetic, no calculated MAC alert can be produced and use of a neurologic monitor is recommended, especially if a nondepolarizing muscle relaxant is employed[20] (also see Chapter 11).

A 2012 study demonstrated an association between the simultaneous occurrence of a low BIS (<45), a low MAC (<0.8), and a low MAP (<75)—a so-called "triple-low" state—and increased 30-day mortality rate. One of two subsequent studies of the triple-low state has demonstrated the same weak independent association, though it is unclear whether changing one of the three parameters (BIS, MAC, MAP) would alter mortality rate.[21,22]

### Intracranial Pressure Monitoring

Because the brain is enclosed in a fixed cranial vault, the perfusion pressure of the brain (cerebral perfusion pressure, CPP) is defined as the MAP minus the ICP. For that reason, under conditions when cerebral edema or increased cerebrospinal fluid may dramatically increase the ICP, continuous monitoring of ICP may be useful to ensure brain perfusion. Two methods are commonly employed to monitor ICP (also see Chapter 30). The first is a ventriculostomy catheter, inserted percutaneously into a lateral ventricle of the brain. ICP is transduced with a traditional disposable transducer zeroed at the tragus of the ear. An advantage of ICP monitoring with a ventriculostomy is that cerebrospinal fluid may be removed to reduce intracranial volume and thus ICP. A second technique of measuring ICP employs a device with a fiberoptic pressure transducer on the tip of a catheter, which can be inserted into the brain parenchyma or the subdural space. These devices do not require zeroing.

### Cerebral Oximetry

The oxygenation of a portion of the brain (i.e., portion of the cerebral cortex) can be monitored with a reflectance oximeter. This device uses near infrared light in a fashion similar to a pulse oximeter. However, instead of using the pulsatile absorbance of light transmitted through tissue to estimate arterial saturation, it uses the reflected infrared light through the scalp and skull from a portion of the cerebral cortex beneath it. This parameter is called *regional oxygen saturation (rSo2).* The light is reflected predominantly from the hemoglobin in the red blood cells within the vasculature of the cerebral cortex. The device presents a number between 1% and 100% saturation, again similar to a pulse oximeter. The algorithms for determining this saturation are proprietary to the manufacturers. These devices have been used in cardiac and vascular surgical procedures when there is a concern of decreased cerebral oxygenation because of poor perfusion of the brain. One study of shoulder surgery in the beach chair position demonstrated that rSo2 may be helpful in determining when changes in Fio2 or ventilation may be needed.[23] rSo2 values are usually about 70% (like mixed venous blood). Those values less than 50% or with a 20% decrease from the baseline values may be associated with decreased cerebral oxygenation.

## PERIPHERAL NERVOUS SYSTEM

### Neuromuscular Monitoring

The use of neuromuscular blocking drugs is an important part of many anesthetics (also see Chapter 11). Monitoring the effects of drugs that block neuromuscular transmission at the synaptic junction is vital to prevent patient motion at inopportune times during the surgery and to prevent partial paralysis with risks of awareness, aspiration of gastric contents, and hypoventilation at the end of surgery. In the past few years, residual neuromuscular blockade postoperatively has been a major concern. Whether the neuromuscular blockade has been reversed by neostigmine or sugammadex can only be confidently determined by the results of monitoring with a peripheral nerve stimulator.

#### Basic Physiology and Pharmacology

Normal neuromuscular transmission starts with a motor nerve impulse arriving at the end plate. Quanta of acetylcholine are released in response to the depolarization, diffuse across the neuromuscular synaptic cleft, bind to the postsynaptic nicotinic cholinergic receptor, and trigger depolarization of the nerve, opening calcium channels with subsequent activation of actin–myosin chains and muscle contraction. Most of the acetylcholine is hydrolyzed enzymatically by acetylcholinesterase. The resulting choline is recycled into the nerve terminal. Nondepolarizing neuromuscular blocking drugs act by competitively inhibiting the binding of acetylcholine with the receptor. Although the blockade is competitive, it can be overcome with additional quanta of acetylcholine. The nondepolarizing blockers demonstrate fade with repeated stimulation, thought to be due to a presynaptic α3β2 acetylcholine receptor exhaustion.[24-26] Succinylcholine acts differently by binding to the receptor and activating it, resulting in prolonged depolarization and blockade of transmission.

#### Neuromuscular Blockade Monitor

The most common method to follow the effects of a nondepolarizing neuromuscular blocking drug is to use a "twitch monitor" and follow a train-of-four (TOF) count. The TOF monitor generates four supramaximal stimuli at 0.5-second intervals (2 Hz). As the degree of blockade deepens, the twitches first fade, then are progressively lost (Table 20.7). Assessment of very deep or profound levels of blockade can be done by using a posttetanic count. A tetanic stimulus for 5 seconds primes the nerve terminal with more acetylcholine allowing a posttetanic count to be done. Even low levels of blockade may be associated with adverse results. To test for lower levels of blockade a double-burst stimulation can be performed. Despite being quantitative there is a great degree of subjectivity in the monitor. Newer monitors are more quantitative, allowing the measurement of TOF ratio and detection of lighter levels of blockade, which may still be clinically significant. Succinylcholine induces a noncompetitive blockade, which can be followed by a single twitch.[25,26]

#### Evoked Potential

Evoked potential (EP) monitoring is indicated for procedures in which there may be neurologic injury because of either mechanical trauma or ischemia such as spinal surgery, thoracic abdominal aneurysm, or surgery of the face or neck. Monitoring of EPs requires constant attention of trained personnel. It is important for anesthesia providers to understand their use and limitations, for they will affect the choice of anesthetic. The most commonly employed EPs are somatosensory evoked potentials (SSEPs) and motor evoked potentials (MEPs). Both involve a stimulating electrode and a sensing electrode continuously assessing the function of the sensory or motor nerve track.

SSEPs involve delivering a small current to a sensory nerve and measuring the response on the sensory cortex with a scalp electrode. The response is viewed as voltage versus time plot. To reduce background noise, multiple responses are averaged to produce an SSEP waveform. Nerve injury or ischemia is associated with a decrease in amplitude and an increase in latency of the peaks in the waveform compared to the baseline waveform. Inhaled anesthetics (halogenated ethers and nitrous oxide) also produce marked decreases in amplitude and increases in latency at larger doses. Patients with preexisting compromise of brain or spinal cord integrity are especially susceptible to the effects of inhaled anesthetics. Propofol is considered the best drug choice for maintenance of unconsciousness during EP monitoring. Dexmedetomidine has also been used as an anesthetic adjunct with minimal depression of neurophysiologic signals in adults. A limitation of SSEPs for spine surgery is that they monitor sensory tracts but not motor tracts (the ventral spinal cord). Therefore, there can be false negatives; that is, procedures can have intact SSEPs when there is in fact damage to the motor tracts.

### Table 20.7 Assessment of Neuromuscular Blockade by Monitor

| % Blockade | PTC | TOF | DBS | TOF Ratio | Tetany | Clinical Response |
|---|---|---|---|---|---|---|
| >100% | 0 | 0/4 | 0 | N/A | | Flaccid |
| >100% | 0<PTC<10 | 0 | 0 | N/A | | |
| 90% | PTC < 10 | 1 of 4 | N/A | N/A | | |
| 80% | | 2 of 4 | N/A | | | May breathe, maintain ET$CO_2$, but lack airway patency |
| 75% | | 3 of 4 | N/A | | | |
| 0–75% | N/A | 4 of 4 | Significant fade | 0.2 | | |
| | N/A | | Fade detectable | | | Risk of aspiration still present |
| | N/A | | Some fade | 0.4 | | Head lift > 5 sec |
| | N/A | | | 0.7 | | Fade at 50 Hz |
| | N/A | | | 0.9 | Fade at 50 Hz | |
| 60% | N/A | | | | No fade at 50 Hz, fade at 100 Hz | |
| 30% | N/A | | | | Fade at 200 Hz | |
| 0% | N/A | | | 1.0 | | |

The table provides the responses of a neuromuscular blockade monitor as a function of block versus the stimulus. Posttetanic count (PTC), train-of-four (TOF), double-burst suppression (DBS), train-of-four ratio (TOF ratio), tetany, and the clinical response are given as a function of the percentage of neuromuscular blockade.

MEPs involve stimulating the motor cortex and detecting a response in muscle. MEPs therefore have the advantage of ensuring an intact ventral spinal cord and are more sensitive to both neural injury and anesthetic drugs. The disadvantage is that they require an intact neuromuscular junction, that is, the avoidance of neuromuscular nondepolarizing muscle relaxants during anesthetic care. MEPs are more profoundly affected by volatile anesthetics and nitrous oxide than SSEPs; therefore, intravenous anesthetics are commonly used. It is common to combine SSEP and MEP monitoring as well as electromyography (EMG) in a patient undergoing major spinal surgery. There should be close communication among the anesthesia provider, monitoring technician, and surgeon at all times during surgery.

## TEMPERATURE

Anesthetics interfere with normal temperature autoregulation and can cause abrupt increases in temperature associated with malignant hyperthermia (MH).[27] Therefore, the patient's temperature is monitored to manage intraoperative hypothermia (inadvertent or desired), prevent hyperthermia, and to confirm and detect MH (although rising temperature is often a later finding in MH). Historically, core body temperature was measured orally or rectally with liquid thermometers. Although accurate, these were slow to respond, fragile, and cumbersome in an operating room environment. Infrared scanners directed at the tympanic membrane are used extensively pre- and postoperatively. The infrared response time is faster, but readings are subject to errors caused by cerumen and other obstructions to the optical path. Intraoperative, low mass, small thermisters are often used. These work by converting changes in temperature to a change in electrical resistance, which is converted and displayed. The acceptable accuracy is +/- 0.5° C.

True core temperature is measured by probes in the pulmonary artery, distal esophagus, tympanic membrane, or nasopharyngeal zones. Other sites that can approximate core temperature include oral, axillary, and bladder. Bladder temperature is highly affected by urine output, approaching true core temperature at high urine flows. Rectal and skin temperatures are highly variable relative to true core temperature (Table 20.8).

For short-duration anesthetics (under 30 minutes), the primary mechanism for the drop in core temperature is redistribution of heat from the core to the periphery.

## MAGNETIC RESONANCE IMAGING AND ADVERSE CONDITIONS

Magnetic resonance imaging (MRI) uses radiofrequency pulses to change the rotation of nuclei in atoms aligned in a very strong magnetic field (also see Chapter 38). As the pulse is removed, the energy is released and can be imaged in multiple dimensions. Because different body tissues have different relaxation rates, better tissue differentiation (e.g., white vs. gray matter in the central nervous system) can be obtained.

The magnetic field strength decreases with distance from the coil. The actual rate of decrease is nonlinear and depends on multiple factors, including the shape and orientation of the magnet. A safe distance in one direction may not be a safe distance in another direction. MRI suites have demarcation lines indicating the field strength at various distances. Better designed suites have a series of rooms, so that direct access to the high magnetic environment is not possible without being screened. Equipment that functions at a certain distance may not work closer to the magnet (and may become a projectile).

All monitors are affected by the MRI environment.[28] Noise levels in an MRI suite are up to 95 dB, making auscultation

| **Table 20.8** | Temperature Monitoring Sites | |
|---|---|---|
| **Site** | **Advantages** | **Disadvantages** |
| Pulmonary arterial | Gives true blood temperature | Extremely invasive |
| Tympanic | Gives "brain" temperature | May cause injury to tympanic membrane |
| Esophageal | Tends to reflect core temperature | Subject to cooling by respiratory gases |
| Nasopharyngeal | Gives "brain" temperature | Nosebleeds, ambient cooling/heating |
| Oral | Comfortable in awake patient | Not easily done in sleeping patient |
| Bladder | Easily done if a Foley catheter is in place | Depends on urine output to reflect core temperature |
| Skin | Easy, noninvasive | Doesn't reflect core temperature, ambient temperature |
| Rectal | | May not reflect true core, invasive, nonsterile area |

All temperature readings are dependent upon blood flow to the area. Alterations in blood flow may result in erroneous temperature readings. Surgical site can compromise monitoring; for example, an open thorax can change esophageal temperature readings.

of any sounds difficult (breath sounds, heart tones, Korotkoff sounds). The magnetic field will interfere with ECG monitoring as well. The rapidly changing magnetic field orientation can induce a current in any loop, causing heating and burns (also applies to pulse oximetry equipment). Extended ventilation and sampling tubing helps keep sensitive equipment away from the magnet. The converse is true as well, in that monitors may affect the quality of the MRI.

## MONITORS AND ALARMS

False positives are the bane of alarm settings. Too sensitive a setting and alarm fatigue ensues. A setting not sensitive enough can lead to critical states occurring without notification. For this reason, the pulse tone of the pulse oximeter (decreasing with decreasing saturation) is the only continuous audible "alarm" used in the operating room. The ventilator disconnect (a low circuit pressure) is the most commonly employed true audible alarm active in the operating room. In an attempt to try to address the alarm overdose/alarm fatigue issues associated with multiple monitoring systems, a newer generation of integrated alerting systems have been developed, such as AlertWatch.[29]

## QUESTIONS OF THE DAY

1. How is the accuracy of pulse oximetry affected by abnormal hemoglobins such as carboxyhemoglobin or methemoglobin?
2. During mechanical ventilation, how should an increase in peak airway pressure be investigated to determine the clinical cause?
3. What are the advantages and disadvantages of noninvasive arterial blood pressure measurement compared to invasive arterial blood pressure measurement with an arterial line?
4. What is the rationale for using systolic blood pressure variation, pulse pressure variation, or stroke volume variation as a measure of intravascular volume responsiveness? In what clinical circumstances would the systolic pressure variation be inaccurate as a measure of intravascular volume responsiveness?
5. A patient requires a central venous line because of poor peripheral intravenous access. What factors should be used to determine the site of cannulation?
6. Which monitoring sites most closely reflect core body temperature?

III

## REFERENCES

1. Szocik J, Barker SJ, Tremper KK. Fundamental principles of monitoring instrumentation. In: Miller RD, Cohen NH, Eriksson LI, et al., eds. *Miller's Anesthesia*. 8th ed. Philadelphia: Elsevier Saunders; 2014:1315–1344.
2. American Society of Anesthesiologists. Standards for Basic Anesthetic Monitoring, Approved on October 21, 1986, and last amended on October 20, 2010, and last affirmed on October 28, 2015. http://www.asahq.org/~/media/Sites/ASAHQ/Files/Public/Resources/standards-guidelines/standards-for-basic-anesthetic-monitoring.pdf. TG. Accessed on September 2, 2015.
3. Tremper KK, Barker SJ. Pulse oximetry. *Anesthesiology*. 1989;70:98–108.
4. Barker SJ, Curry J, Redford D, Morgan S. Measurement of carboxyhemoglobin and methemoglobin by pulse oximetry. *Anesthesiology*. 2006;105:892–897.
5. Raphael DT. The low-pressure alarm condition: safety considerations and the anesthesiologist's response. *Anesthesia Patient Safety Foundation Newsletter*. 1998-1999;13(4). Winter.
6. Futier E, Constantin JM, Paugam-Burtz C, et al. A trial of intraoperative low-tidal-volume ventilation in abdominal surgery. *N Engl J Med*. 2013;369:428–437.
7. Landesberg G, Mosseri M, Wolf Y, et al. Perioperative myocardial ischemia and infarction: identification by continuous 12-lead electrocardiogram with online ST-segment monitoring. *Anesthesiology*. 2002;96:264–270.
8. Kheterpal S, O'Reilly M, Englesbe MJ, et al. Preoperative and intraoperative predictors of cardiac adverse events after general, vascular, and urological surgery. *Anesthesiology*. 2009;110:58–66.
9. Walsh M, Devereaux PJ, Garg AX, et al. Relationship between intraoperative mean arterial pressure and clinical outcomes after noncardiac surgery. *Anesthesiology*. 2013;119:507–515.
10. Monk TG, Bronsert MR, Henderson WG, et al. Association between intraoperative hypotension and hypertension and 30-day postoperative mortality in noncardiac surgery. *Anesthesiology*. 2015;123:307–319.
11. Ehrenwerth J, Eisenkraft JB, Berry JM. *Anesthesia Equipment: Principles and Applications*. 2nd ed. Philadelphia: Elsevier Saunders; 2013.
12. Perel A, Minkovich L, Preisman S, et al. Assessing fluid-responsiveness by a standardized ventilatory maneuver (the respiratory systolic variation test). *Anesth Analg*. 2005;100:942–945.
13. Cannesson M, Slieker J, Desebbe O, et al. The ability of a novel algorithm for automatic estimation of the respiratory variations in arterial pulse pressure to monitor fluid responsiveness in the operating room. *Anesth Analg*. 2008;106:1195–1200.
14. Lahner D, Kabon B, Marscalek C, et al. Evaluation of stroke volume variation obtained by arterial pulse contour analysis to predict fluid responsiveness intraoperatively. *Br J Anaesth*. 2009;103(3):346–351.
15. Marik PE, Cavallazzi R. Does the central venous pressure predict fluid responsiveness? An updated meta-analysis and a plea for some common sense. *Crit Care Med*. 2013;41:1774–1781.
16. American Society of Anesthesiologists Task Force on Central Venous Access, Rupp SM, Apfelbaum JL, Blitt C, et al. Practice guidelines for central venous access: a report by American Society of Anesthesiologists Task Force on Central Venous Access. *Anesthesiology*. 2012;116(3):539–573.
17. Sandham JD, Hull RD, Brant RF, et al. A randomized, controlled trial of the use of pulmonary-artery catheters in high risk surgical patients. *N Engl J Med*. 2003;348:5–14.
18. Avidan MS, Jacobsohn E, Glick D, et al. Prevention of intraoperative awareness in a high-risk surgical population. *N Engl J Med*. 2011;365:591–600.
19. Mashour GA, Shanks A, Tremper KT, et al. Prevention of intraoperative awareness with explicit recall in an unselected surgical population. A randomized comparative effectiveness trial. *Anesthesiology*. 2012;117:717–725.
20. Mashour GA, Orser BA, Avidan M. Intraoperative awareness from neurobiology to clinical practice. *Anesthesiology*. 2011;114:1218.
21. Sessler DI, Sigl JC, Kelley SD, et al. Hospital stay and mortality are increased in patients having a "triple low" of low blood pressure, low bispectral index, and low minimum alveolar concentration of volatile anesthesia. *Anesthesiology*. 2012;116:1195–1203.
22. Willingham MD, Karren E, Shanks AM, et al. Concurrence of intraoperative hypotension, low minimum alveolar concentration, and low bispectral index is associated with postoperative death. *Anesthesiology*. 2015;123:775–785.
23. Picton P, Dering A, Alexander A, et al. Influence of ventilation strategies and anesthetic techniques on regional cerebral oximetry in the beach chair position: a prospective interventional study with a randomized comparison of two anesthetics. *Anesthesiology*. 2015;123(4):765–774.
24. Fagerlund MJ, Eriksson LI. Current concepts in neuromuscular transmission. *Br J Anaesth*. 2009;103(1):108–114.
25. Murphy GS, Brull SJ. Residual neuromuscular block: lessons unlearned. Part I: definitions, incidence, and adverse physiologic effects of residual neuromuscular block. *Anesth Analg*. 2010;111:120–128.
26. Brull SJ, Murphy GS. Residual neuromuscular block: lessons unlearned. Part II: methods to reduce the risk of residual weakness. *Anesth Analg*. 2010;111:129–140.
27. Sessler D. Temperature monitoring and perioperative thermoregulation. *Anesthesiology*. 2008;109:318–338.
28. Patteson SK, Chesney JT. Anesthetic management for magnetic resonance imaging: problems and solutions. *Anesth Analg*. 1992;74:121–128.
29. Sathishkumar S, Lai M, Picton P, et al. Behavioral modification of intraoperative hyperglycemia management with a novel real-time audiovisual monitor. *Anesthesiology*. 2015;123:29–37.

# 21

# ACID-BASE BALANCE AND BLOOD GAS ANALYSIS

Linda L. Liu

The concentrations of hydrogen and bicarbonate ions in plasma must be precisely regulated to optimize enzyme activity, oxygen transport, and rates of chemical reactions within cells. Each day approximately 15,000 mmol of carbon dioxide (which can generate carbonic acid as it combines with water) and 50 to 100 mEq of nonvolatile acid (mostly sulfuric acid) are produced and must be eliminated safely. The body is able to maintain this intricate acid-base balance by utilizing buffers, pulmonary excretion of carbon dioxide, and renal elimination of acid. This chapter will define concepts important for understanding acids and bases, discuss clinical measurements of blood gases and their interpretation, and present a diagnostic approach to common acid-base disturbances.

## DEFINITIONS

### Acids and Bases

Bronsted and Lowry defined an acid as a molecule that can act as a proton ($H^+$) donor and a base as a molecule that can act as a proton acceptor. In physiologic solutions, a strong acid is a substance that readily and irreversibly gives up an $H^+$, and a strong base avidly binds $H^+$. In contrast, biologic molecules are either weak acids or bases, which reversibly donate $H^+$ or reversibly bind $H^+$.

### Acidemia and Acidosis

A blood pH less than 7.35 is called *acidemia* and a pH greater than 7.45 is called *alkalemia*, regardless of the mechanism. The underlying process that lowers the pH is called an *acidosis*, and the process that raises the pH is known as an *alkalosis*. A patient can have a mixed disorder with both an acidosis and an alkalosis concurrently, but can only be either acidemic or alkalemic. The last two terms are mutually exclusive.

## Base Excess

Base excess (BE) is usually defined as the amount of strong acid (hydrochloric acid for BE greater than zero) or strong base (sodium hydroxide for BE less than zero) required to return 1 L of whole blood exposed in vitro to a $P_{CO_2}$ of 40 mm Hg to a pH of 7.4.[1] Instead of an actual titration, the blood gas machine calculates the BE with algorithms utilizing plasma pH, blood $P_{CO_2}$, and hemoglobin concentration. The number is supposed to refer to the nonrespiratory or metabolic component of an acid-base disturbance. A BE less than zero (also called a *base deficit*) suggests the presence of a metabolic acidosis, and a value greater than zero suggests the presence of a metabolic alkalosis. In vitro, the number has been accurate, but in the living organism, because ions do cross beyond vascular and cellular boundaries, a primary acute change in $Pa_{CO_2}$ sometimes can cause the BE to move in the opposite direction, despite an unchanged metabolic acid-base status.[2] In clinical practice, the BE is often used as a surrogate measure for lactic acidosis, which is one measurement to help determine adequacy of intravascular volume resuscitation.

# REGULATION OF THE HYDROGEN ION CONCENTRATION

At 37° C, the normal hydrogen ion concentration in arterial blood and extracellular fluid is 35 to 45 nmol/L, which is equivalent to an arterial pH of 7.45 to 7.35, respectively. The normal plasma bicarbonate ion concentration is 24 ± 2 mEq/L. The intracellular hydrogen ion concentration is approximately 160 nmol/L, which is equivalent to a pH of 6.8.

Physiologic changes to acid-base disturbances are corrected by three systems—buffers, ventilation, and renal response. The buffer systems provide an immediate chemical response. The ventilatory response occurs in minutes whenever possible, and, lastly, the renal response can slowly provide nearly complete restoration of the pH, but it can take days.

## Buffer Systems

A buffer is defined as a substance within a solution that can prevent extreme changes in pH. A buffer system is composed of a base molecule and its weak conjugate acid. The base molecules of the buffer system bind excess hydrogen ions, and the weak acid protonates excess base molecules. The *dissociation ionization constant* (pKa) indicates the strength of an acid and is derived from the classic Henderson-Hasselbalch equation (Fig. 21.1). The pKa is the pH at which an acid is 50% protonated and 50% deprotonated. Hydrochloric acid, a strong acid, has a pKa of −7, whereas carbonic acid, a weak acid, has a pKa of 6. The most important buffer systems in blood, in

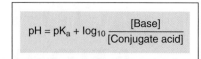

Fig. 21.1 Henderson-Hasselbalch equation. *[Base]*, Concentration of base; *[Conjugate acid]*, concentration of conjugate acid.

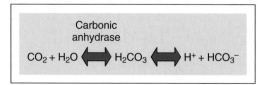

Fig. 21.2 Hydration of carbon dioxide results in carbonic acid, which dissociates into bicarbonate and hydrogen ions.

order of importance, are the (1) bicarbonate buffer system ($H_2CO_3/HCO_3^-$), (2) hemoglobin buffer system (HbH/Hb), (3) other protein buffer systems (PrH/Pr⁻), (4) phosphate buffer system ($H_2PO_4^-/HPO_4^{2-}$), and (5) ammonia buffer system ($NH_3/NH_4^+$).

### Bicarbonate Buffer System

Carbon dioxide, generated through aerobic metabolism, slowly combines with water to form carbonic acid, which spontaneously and rapidly deprotonates to form bicarbonate (Fig. 21.2). In this system, the base molecule is bicarbonate, and its weak conjugate acid is carbonic acid. Less than 1% of the dissolved carbon dioxide undergoes this reaction because it is so slow. However, the enzyme carbonic anhydrase, present in the endothelium, erythrocytes, and kidneys, catalyzes this reaction to accelerate the formation of carbonic acid and make this the most important buffering system in the human body when combined with renal control of bicarbonate and pulmonary control of carbon dioxide.

### Hemoglobin Buffer System

The hemoglobin protein is the second most important buffering system because of multiple histidine residues. Histidine is an effective buffer from pH 5.7 to 7.7 (pKa 6.8) because it contains multiple protonatable sites on the imidazole side chains. Buffering by hemoglobin depends on the bicarbonate system to facilitate the movement of carbon dioxide intracellularly. Carbon dioxide freely diffuses into erythrocytes, where carbonic anhydrase resides. There, carbon dioxide combines with water to form carbonic acid, which rapidly deprotonates. The generated protons are bound by hemoglobin. The bicarbonate anions are exchanged electroneutrally back into plasma with extracellular chloride (chloride or Hamburger shift) (Fig. 21.3). At the lungs, the reverse process occurs. Chloride ions move out of the red blood cells as bicarbonate enters for conversion back to carbon dioxide. The carbon

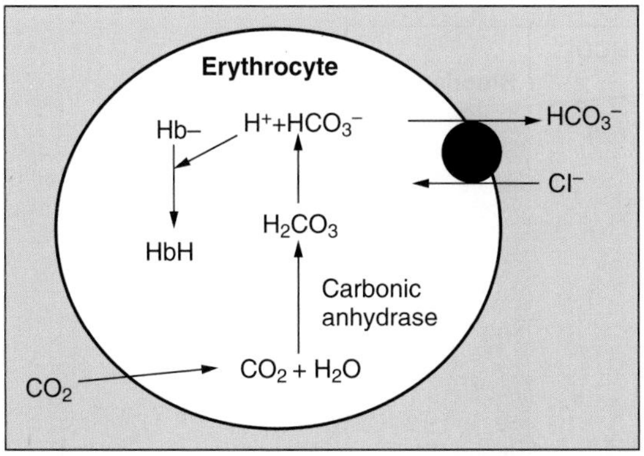

**Fig. 21.3** Hemoglobin buffering system: Carbon dioxide freely diffuses into erythrocytes, where it combines with water to form carbonic acid, which rapidly deprotonates. The protons generated are bound up by hemoglobin. The bicarbonate anions are exchanged back into plasma with chloride.

dioxide is released back into plasma and is eliminated by the lungs. This process allows a large fraction of extrapulmonary carbon dioxide to be transported back to the lungs as plasma bicarbonate.

Oxygenated and deoxygenated hemoglobin have different affinities for hydrogen ions and carbon dioxide. Deoxyhemoglobin takes up more hydrogen ions, which shifts the carbon dioxide/bicarbonate equilibrium to produce more bicarbonate and facilitates removal of carbon dioxide from peripheral tissues for release into the lungs. Oxyhemoglobin favors the release of hydrogen ions and shifts the equilibrium to more carbon dioxide formation. At physiologic pH, a small amount of carbon dioxide is also carried as carbaminohemoglobin. Deoxyhemoglobin has a greater affinity (3.5 times) for carbon dioxide, so venous blood carries more carbon dioxide than arterial blood. These two mechanisms combine to account for the difference in carbon dioxide content of arterial versus venous plasma (25.6 mmol/L vs. 27.7 mmol/L, respectively) (Haldane effect).

## Ventilatory Response

Central chemoreceptors lie on the anterolateral surface of the medulla and respond to changes in cerebrospinal fluid pH. Carbon dioxide diffuses across the blood-brain barrier to elevate cerebrospinal fluid (CSF) hydrogen ion concentration, which activates the chemoreceptors and increases alveolar ventilation. The relationship between $Pa_{CO_2}$ and minute ventilation is almost linear except at very high arterial $Pa_{CO_2}$, when carbon dioxide narcosis develops, and at very low arterial $Pa_{CO_2}$, when the apneic threshold is reached. There is a very wide variation in individual $Pa_{CO_2}$/ventilation response curves, but minute ventilation generally increases 1 to 4 L/min for every 1 mm Hg increase in $Pa_{CO_2}$. During general anesthesia, spontaneous

ventilation will cease when the $Pa_{CO_2}$ decreases to less than the apneic threshold, whereas in the awake patient, cortical influences prevent apnea, so the apneic threshold is not ordinarily observed.

Peripheral chemoreceptors are located at the bifurcation of the common carotid arteries and surrounding the aortic arch. The carotid bodies are the principal peripheral chemoreceptors and are sensitive to changes in $Pa_{O_2}$, $Pa_{CO_2}$, pH, and arterial perfusion pressure. They communicate with the central respiratory centers via the glossopharyngeal nerves. Unlike the central chemoreceptors, which are more sensitive to hydrogen ions, the carotid bodies are most sensitive to $Pa_{O_2}$. Bilateral carotid endarterectomies abolish the peripheral chemoreceptor response, and these patients have almost no hypoxic ventilatory drive (also see Chapter 25).

The stimulus from central and peripheral chemoreceptors to either increase or decrease alveolar ventilation diminishes as the pH approaches 7.4 such that complete correction or overcorrection is not possible. The pulmonary response to metabolic alkalosis is usually less than the response to metabolic acidosis. The reason is because progressive hypoventilation results in hypoxemia when breathing room air. Hypoxemia activates oxygen-sensitive chemoreceptors and limits the compensatory decrease in minute ventilation. Because of this, the $Pa_{CO_2}$ usually does not rise above 55 mm Hg in response to metabolic alkalosis for patients not receiving oxygen supplementation.

## Renal Response

Renal effects are slower in onset and may not be maximal for up to 5 days. The response occurs via three mechanisms: (1) reabsorption of the filtered $HCO_3^-$, (2) excretion of titratable acids, and (3) ammonia (Fig. 21.4).[3] Carbon dioxide combines with water in the renal tubular cell. With the help of carbonic anhydrase, the bicarbonate produced enters the bloodstream while the hydrogen ion is exchanged with sodium and is released into the renal tubule. There, H⁺ combines with filtered bicarbonate and dissociates into carbon dioxide and water with help from carbonic anhydrase located in the luminal brush border, and the carbon dioxide diffuses back into the renal tubular cell. The proximal tubule reabsorbs 80% to 90% of the bicarbonate this way, while the distal tubule takes care of the remaining 10% to 20%. Once the bicarbonate is reclaimed, further hydrogen ions can combine with $HPO_4^{2-}$ to form $H_2PO_4^-$, which is eliminated in the urine. The last important urinary buffer is ammonia. Ammonia is formed from deamination of glutamine, an amino acid. The ammonia passively crosses the cell membrane to enter the tubular fluid. In the tubular fluid, it combines with hydrogen ion to form $NH_4^+$, which is trapped within the tubule and excreted in the urine. All of these

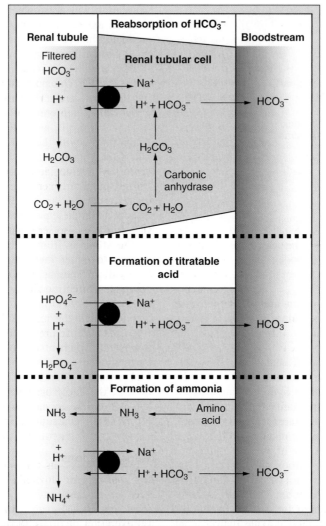

**Fig. 21.4** Three mechanisms of renal compensation during acidosis to sequester hydrogen ions and reabsorb bicarbonate: (1) reabsorption of the filtered $HCO_3^-$, (2) excretion of titratable acids, and (3) production of ammonia.

steps allow for generation and return of bicarbonate into the bloodstream. The large amount of bicarbonate filtered by the kidneys allows for rapid excretion if necessary for compensation during alkalosis. The kidneys are highly effective in protecting the body against alkalosis except in association with sodium deficiency or mineralocorticoid excess.

## ANALYSIS OF ARTERIAL BLOOD GASES

The ability to measure arterial blood gas (ABG) and venous blood gas has revolutionized patient care during anesthesia and in the intensive care unit. Although pulse oximetry and capnography can be monitored continuously, analysis of ABGs has increased our diagnostic ability and the accuracy of our measurements.

### Blood Gas and pH Electrodes

#### pH Electrode
The pH electrode is a silver/silver chloride electrode encased in a special pH-sensitive glass that contains a buffer solution with a known pH. The electrode is placed in a blood sample and measures changes in voltage. The potential difference generated across the glass and a reference electrode is proportional to the difference in hydrogen ion concentration. Both electrodes must be kept at 37° C and calibrated with buffer solutions of known pH.

### Oxygen Electrode

The $O_2$ electrode is known as the Clark or polarographic electrode.[4] It has a silver/silver chloride reference electrode that is immersed in a potassium chloride solution. Electrons are formed by the oxidation reaction of the silver with the chloride ions of the potassium chloride electrolyte solution. The electrons are then free to combine with $O_2$ molecules at the platinum cathode. The platinum surface is covered with an oxygen-permeable membrane (polyethylene), on the other side of which is placed the unknown sample. Current flow is increased if oxygen concentration is higher and more electrons are taken up. The current is directly proportional to the $Po_2$.

### Carbon Dioxide Electrode

The carbon dioxide sensor was first described by Stow in 1957 and then modified by Bradley and Severinghaus.[5] The carbon dioxide electrode is a pH electrode immersed in a sodium bicarbonate solution and is separated from the blood specimen by a Teflon semipermeable membrane. The carbon dioxide in the sample diffuses into the sodium bicarbonate solution producing hydrogen ions and bicarbonate. The measured pH in the bathing solution is altered in direct proportion to the logarithm of the $Pco_2$.

## Sampling

Arterial blood is most often obtained percutaneously from the radial, brachial, or femoral artery. In certain clinically stable situations, peripheral venous blood may serve as an approximation and save an arterial puncture. Venous pH is only 0.03 to 0.04 less than arterial values. Venous blood cannot be used for estimation of oxygenation because venous $Po_2$ ($Pvo_2$) is significantly less than $Pao_2$. Also, depending on the site of the venous blood draw, differences in tissue metabolic activity may alter $Pvo_2$. The correlation between arterial and venous blood gas measurements varies with the hemodynamic stability of the patient. Periodic correlations of arterial and venous measurements should be performed especially when venous measurements are used for serial monitoring in critically ill patients.[6]

A heparinized, bubble-free, fresh blood sample is required for blood gas analysis. In the past, liquid heparin was aspirated into a syringe and then expelled. This small amount of heparin remaining in the syringe was enough to anticoagulate the sample. Excessive amounts of anticoagulant in the sampling syringe could falsely dilute the measured $Po_2$, $Pco_2$, and ionized calcium. Commercially prepared syringes with preweighed lyophilized electrolyte-balanced heparin are used in most hospitals now. Air bubbles should be removed because equilibration of oxygen and carbon dioxide in the blood with the corresponding partial pressures in the air bubble could influence the measured results. A delay in analysis can lead to oxygen consumption and carbon dioxide generation by the metabolically active white blood cells. Usually this error is small and can be reduced by placing the sample on ice. In some leukemia patients with a markedly increased white blood cell count, this error can be large and lead to a falsely low $Po_2$ even though the patient's oxygenation is acceptable. This phenomenon is often referred to as *leukocyte larceny* and has also been described with extreme thrombocytosis (platelet larceny).[7]

## Temperature Correction

Decreases in temperature decrease the partial pressure of a gas in solution, even though the total gas content does not change. Both $Pco_2$ and $Po_2$ decrease during hypothermia, but serum bicarbonate is unchanged. This leads to an increase in pH if the blood could be measured at the patient's temperature. A blood gas with a pH of 7.4 and $Pco_2$ of 40 mm Hg at 37° C will have a pH of 7.58 and a $Pco_2$ of 23 mm Hg at 25° C.[8] Unfortunately, all blood gas samples are measured at 37° C, which raises the issue of how to best manage the ABG measurement in hypothermic patients. This has led to two schools of thought: alpha stat and pH stat.

### Alpha Stat

Alpha refers to the protonation state of the imidazole side chain of histidine. The pKa of histidine changes with temperature so that its protonation state is relatively constant regardless of temperature. The term *alpha stat* developed because as the patient's pH was allowed to drift with temperature, the protonation state of the histidine residues remained *static*. This concept arose from the observation that *cold-blooded* poikilothermic animals functioned well over a wide range of body temperatures, yet they relied on a similar complement of enzymes as *warm-blooded* homeothermic animals. During cardiopulmonary bypass, an anesthesia provider using alpha stat would manage the patient based on an ABG measured at 37° C and strive to keep that pH at 7.4, but the patient's true pH would be higher. No extra adjustments would be made for the patient's hypothermia.

### pH Stat

pH stat is different from alpha stat in that it requires keeping a patient's pH static at 7.4 based on the core temperature (similar to that of a hibernating, homeothermic animal). During cardiopulmonary bypass, an anesthesia provider using pH stat would manage the patient based on an ABG that is corrected for the patient's temperature. With hypothermia, this usually means adding carbon dioxide so that the patient's temperature-correct (hypothermic) blood gas has a pH of 7.4. The lower pH and higher $Pco_2$ maintained during pH stat may improve cerebrovascular perfusion during hypothermia; however, there is still debate about which method provides better outcomes.[9]

## Oxygenation

The same physical properties exist for oxygen and hypothermia as for carbon dioxide. Decreases in temperature decrease the partial pressure of a gas in solution, so temperature correction of $Po_2$ remains relatively important for assessing oxygenation at the extremes of temperature. To be exact, the change in $Po_2$ with respect to temperature depends on the degree that hemoglobin is saturated with oxygen, but as a guideline, the $Po_2$ is decreased approximately 6% for every 1° C that the patient's body temperature is below 37° C. $Po_2$ is increased approximately 6% for every 1° C that the body temperature exceeds 37° C.

## DIFFERENTIAL DIAGNOSIS OF ACID-BASE DISTURBANCES

Acid-base disturbances are categorized as respiratory or metabolic acidosis (pH less than 7.35) or alkalosis (pH more than 7.45). These disorders are further stratified into acute versus chronic based on their duration, which is gauged clinically by the patient's compensatory responses.[10] It must be kept in mind that a patient may have a mixed acid-base disorder. The approach to managing acid-base disorders should first involve searching for the causes, rather than an immediate attempt to normalize the pH. Sometimes the treatment may be more detrimental than the original acid-base problem.

### Adverse Responses to Acidemia and Alkalemia

Adverse responses can be associated with severe acidemia or alkalemia. Consequences of severe acidosis can occur regardless of whether the acidosis is of respiratory, metabolic, or mixed origin. Acidemia usually leads to decreased myocardial contractility and release of catecholamines. With mild acidosis, the release of catecholamines mitigates the myocardial depression. Permissive hypercapnia, which is used as a protective lung ventilation strategy for acute respiratory distress syndrome (ARDS) patients, has been quite well tolerated. No significant impact on systemic vascular resistance, pulmonary vascular resistance, cardiac output, or systemic oxygen delivery has been seen.[11] With severe acidemia (pH < 7.2), myocardial responsiveness to catecholamines decreases, so myocardial depression and hypotension predominates (Fig. 21.5). Respiratory acidosis may produce more rapid and profound myocardial dysfunction than metabolic acidosis because of the rapid entry of carbon dioxide into the cardiac cell. In the brain, this rapid increase in carbon dioxide can lead to confusion, loss of consciousness, and seizures. This is probably due to an abrupt decrease of intracellular pH, because chronic increases in carbon dioxide as high as 150 mm Hg are typically well tolerated.

Severe alkalemia (pH > 7.6) can lead to decreased cerebral and coronary blood flow as a result of arteriolar

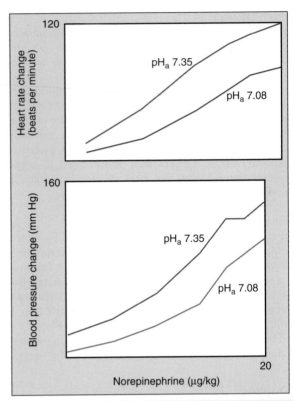

**Fig. 21.5** Diminished hemodynamic response to intravenously administered norepinephrine in a canine model of lactic acidosis. pHa = arterial pH. (From Ford GD, Cline WH, Fleming WW. Influence of lactic acidosis on cardiovascular response to sympathomimetic amines. *Am J Physiol.* 1968;215(5):1123-1129, used with permission.)

vasoconstriction. The consequences of severe alkalosis are also more prominent with respiratory than with metabolic causes because of the rapid movement of carbon dioxide across cell membranes.[12] Acute hyperventilation can produce confusion, myoclonus, depressed consciousness, and seizures.

### Respiratory Acidosis

Respiratory acidosis occurs when alveolar minute ventilation is inadequate relative to carbon dioxide production (Box 21.1). It can occur with a normal or increased minute ventilation if carbon dioxide production is increased from sepsis or overfeeding or if there is decreased carbon dioxide elimination from ARDS or obstructive lung disease. Decreased carbon dioxide elimination from a decreased minute ventilation can occur with volatile or intravenous anesthetics (see Chapter 8), neuromuscular blocking drugs (see Chapter 11), or neuromuscular disease. Increased rebreathing or absorption, found with exhausted soda lime, an incompetent one-way valve, or laparoscopic surgery can cause respiratory acidosis.

**Box 21.1** Causes of Respiratory Acidosis

Increased $CO_2$ production
    Malignant hyperthermia
    Hyperthyroidism
    Sepsis
    Overfeeding
Decreased $CO_2$ elimination
    Intrinsic pulmonary disease (pneumonia, ARDS, fibrosis, edema)
    Upper airway obstruction (laryngospasm, foreign body, OSA)
    Lower airway obstruction (asthma, COPD)
    Chest wall restriction (obesity, scoliosis, burns)
    CNS depression (anesthetics, opioids, CNS lesions)
    Decreased skeletal muscle strength (residual effects of neuromuscular blocking drugs, myopathy, neuropathy)
Increased $CO_2$ rebreathing or absorption
    Exhausted soda lime
    Incompetent one-way valve in breathing circuit
    Laparoscopic surgery

*ARDS*, Acute respiratory distress syndrome; *CNS*, central nervous system; *$CO_2$*, carbon dioxide; *COPD*, chronic obstructive pulmonary disease; *OSA*, obstructive sleep apnea.

## Compensatory Responses and Treatment

Over the course of hours to days, the kidneys compensate for the respiratory acidosis by increased hydrogen ion secretion and bicarbonate reabsorption. After a few days, the $P_{CO_2}$ will remain increased, but the pH will be near normal, which is the hallmark of a chronic respiratory acidosis. Respiratory acidosis with a pH less than 7.2 indicates the need for tracheal intubation or increased ventilatory support. In patients with chronic respiratory acidosis, the key is to avoid hyperventilation. The alkalosis from excessive ventilation and relative hypocapnia can result in central nervous system (CNS) irritability and cardiac ischemia. Also, the kidneys will now start to lose bicarbonate. The increased bicarbonate has allowed the patient to maintain a normal pH with a relatively smaller alveolar minute ventilation. Losing the bicarbonate will increase the work of breathing when ventilatory support is decreased, making it difficult to wean from the ventilator.

## Respiratory Alkalosis

Respiratory alkalosis occurs when alveolar minute ventilation is increased relative to carbon dioxide production. The increased alveolar minute ventilation can be related to a variety of causes (Box 21.2). $Paco_2$ is diminished relative to bicarbonate levels, resulting in a pH more than 7.45. The decreased $Paco_2$ and increased pH trigger the peripheral and central chemoreceptors to decrease the stimulus to breathe. During prolonged respiratory alkalosis, active transport of bicarbonate ions out of CSF causes the central chemoreceptors to reset to a lower $Paco_2$ level.

**Box 21.2** Causes of Respiratory Alkalosis

Increased minute ventilation
    Hypoxia (high altitude, low $F_{IO_2}$, severe anemia)
    Iatrogenic (mechanical ventilation)
    Anxiety and pain
    CNS disease (tumor, infection, trauma)
    Fever, sepsis
    Drugs (salicylates, progesterone, doxapram)
    Liver disease
    Pregnancy
    Restrictive lung disease
    Pulmonary embolism

*CNS*, Central nervous system; *$F_{IO_2}$*, fractional concentration of inspired oxygen.

**Box 21.3** Causes of Metabolic Acidosis

**Anion Gap Acidosis**
Methanol, ethylene glycol
Uremia
Lactic acidosis = CHF, sepsis, cyanide toxicity
Ethanol
Paraldehyde
Aspirin, INH
Ketones = starvation, diabetic ketoacidosis

**Nongap Acidosis**
Excessive chloride administration
GI losses—diarrhea, ileostomy, neobladder, pancreatic fistula
Renal losses—RTA
Drugs—acetazolamide

*CHF*, Congestive heart failure; *GI*, gastrointestinal; *INH*, isoniazid; *RTA*, renal tubular acidosis.

## Compensatory Responses and Treatment

Respiratory alkalosis is compensated for by decreased reabsorption of bicarbonate ions from the renal tubules and increased urinary excretion of bicarbonate. Treatment of respiratory alkalosis is directed at correcting the underlying disorder. Mild alkalemia usually does not require treatment. In rare cases, severe acute respiratory alkalosis (pH > 7.6) may require sedation. During general anesthesia, acute respiratory alkalosis is easily remedied by decreasing total minute ventilation.

## Metabolic Acidosis

Metabolic acidosis is present when accumulation of any acid in the body other than carbon dioxide results in a pH lower than 7.35 (Box 21.3). A compensatory increase in ventilatory elimination of carbon dioxide starts within minutes after the development of metabolic acidosis to provide a near normal pH. Some patients, however, may not be able to sustain the increased minute ventilation and require tracheal intubation and mechanical ventilation.

$$Anion\ gap = [Na^+] - ([Cl^-] + [HCO_3^-])$$

**Fig. 21.6** Calculation of the anion gap: the difference between the cations and the anions equals the concentration of unmeasured anions in serum.

## Anion Gap

The best way to categorize the differential diagnosis for a metabolic acidosis is to divide these causes into those that cause or do not cause an anion gap. The anion gap is the difference between measured cations (sodium) and measured anions (chloride and bicarbonate) and represents the concentration of anions in serum that are unaccounted for in this equation (Fig. 21.6). A normal anion gap value is 8 to 12 mEq/L and is mostly composed of anionic serum albumin.[13] A patient with a low serum albumin concentration will likely have a narrower anion gap value (each 1.0 g/dL decrease or increase in serum albumin less or more than 4.4 g/dL decreases or increases the actual concentration of unmeasured anions by approximately 2.5 mEq/L). An increase in the anion gap occurs when the anion replacing bicarbonate is not one that is routinely measured. The most common unmeasured anions are lactic acid and keto acids. Metabolic acidosis with a normal anion gap occurs when chloride replaces the lost bicarbonate such as with a bicarbonate-wasting process in the kidneys (renal tubular acidosis) or gastrointestinal tract (diarrhea). Aggressive fluid resuscitation with normal saline (>30 mL/kg/h) will induce a nongap metabolic acidosis secondary to excessive chloride administration, which impairs bicarbonate reabsorption in the kidneys.[14]

## Strong Ion Difference

A second way to categorize metabolic acidoses is the strong ion difference (SID) introduced by Peter Stewart in the 1980s.[15] His major tenet is that although serum bicarbonate and BE can be used to determine the extent of a clinical acid-base disorder, they do not help determine the mechanism of the abnormality. Instead, he proposed that the independent variables responsible for changes in acid-base balance are the SID (the difference between the completely dissociated cations and anions in plasma) (Fig. 21.7), the plasma concentration of nonvolatile weak acids ($A_{TOT}$), and the arterial carbon dioxide tension ($Paco_2$). The strong ion approach distinguishes six primary acid-base disturbances (acidosis due to decreased SID, alkalosis due to increased SID, acidosis due to increased $A_{TOT}$, alkalosis due to decreased $A_{TOT}$, respiratory acidosis, or respiratory alkalosis) instead of the four primary acid-base disturbances (respiratory acidosis or alkalosis, or metabolic acidosis or alkalosis) differentiated by the traditional Henderson-Hasselbalch equation. Under normal conditions, the SID is approximately 40 mEq/L. Processes that increase the SID increase blood pH, whereas processes that reduce it decrease pH. For instance, in the case of massive volume resuscitation with normal saline, the major ions are $Na^+$ and $Cl^-$, which gives the fluid an SID of 0. Because infusions of saline would lower the normal SID of 40, this leads to a strong ion acidosis. With the Stewart approach, administering a solution with a high SID, such as sodium bicarbonate, should treat the resultant strong ion acidosis.

The major practical difference between the two theories (Stewart vs. Henderson-Hasselbalch) is the inclusion of the serum albumin concentration in the Stewart approach, which provides some increase in accuracy in certain clinical settings. If changes in serum albumin concentration are accounted for in measurement of the anion gap, the more complex Stewart approach does not appear to offer a clinically significant advantage over the traditional approach to acid-base disturbances.[16]

## Compensatory Responses and Treatment

The compensatory responses for a metabolic acidosis include increased alveolar ventilation from carotid body stimulation and renal tubule secretion of hydrogen ions into urine. Chronic metabolic acidosis, as seen with chronic renal failure, is commonly associated with loss of bone mass because buffers present in bone are used to neutralize the nonvolatile acids.

Treatment of metabolic acidosis is based on whether an anion gap is present or not. Intravenous administration of sodium bicarbonate is often given for a nongap metabolic acidosis because the problem is bicarbonate loss. Management of an anion gap metabolic acidosis is guided by diagnosis and treatment of the underlying cause in order to remove the nonvolatile acids from the circulation. Tissue hypoxia leading to lactic acidosis should be corrected if possible with oxygen, fluid resuscitation, and circulatory support. Diabetic ketoacidosis requires intravenous fluid and insulin therapy. Minute ventilation can be increased in a patient who is mechanically ventilated to compensate until more definitive treatment takes effect.

Bicarbonate therapy is more controversial, but may be considered in the setting of extreme metabolic acidosis as a temporizing measure, particularly when a patient is hemodynamically unstable. Sodium bicarbonate administration generates carbon dioxide, which, unless eliminated by ventilation, can worsen any intracellular and extracellular acidosis. A common approach is to administer a small dose of sodium bicarbonate, and then repeat the pH measurement and monitor hemodynamics to determine the impact of treatment. Alkalinizing drugs, because of their osmotic properties, introduce the risk of causing hypervolemia and hypertonicity.

$$SID = [\text{strong cations}] - [\text{strong anions}]$$
$$= [Na^+] + [K^+] + [Ca^{2+}] + [Mg^{2+}] - ([Cl^-] + [SO_4^{2-}] + [\text{organic acids}^-])$$
$$\approx [Na^+] + [K^+] - [Cl^-]$$

**Fig. 21.7** Calculation of the strong ion difference (SID): the difference between the completely dissociated cations and anions in plasma.

## Metabolic Alkalosis

Metabolic alkalosis is present when the pH is higher than 7.45 due to gain of bicarbonate ions or loss of hydrogen ions. The loss of hydrogen ions is usually from the gastrointestinal tract or the kidney. The stimulus for bicarbonate reabsorption or gain is usually from hypovolemia, hypokalemia, or hyperaldosteronism (Box 21.4). In hypovolemia, because of insufficient chloride ions, bicarbonate is reabsorbed with sodium. With the adoption of low tidal volumes (4 to 6 mL/kg) and permissive hypercapnia for ventilatory management of ARDS patients, a compensatory metabolic alkalosis is often a common finding for the critically ill patient.

### Compensatory Responses and Treatment

Compensatory responses for metabolic alkalosis include increased reabsorption of hydrogen ions by renal tubule cells, decreased secretion of hydrogen ions by renal tubule cells, and alveolar hypoventilation. The efficiency of the renal compensatory mechanism is dependent on the presence of cations (sodium, potassium) and chloride. Lack of these ions impairs the ability of the kidneys to excrete excess bicarbonate and results in incomplete renal compensation. Respiratory compensation for pure metabolic alkalosis, in contrast to metabolic acidosis, is never more than 75% complete. As a result, the pH remains increased in patients with primary metabolic alkalosis. Treatment of metabolic alkalosis should be aimed at reducing the acid loss (e.g., by stopping gastric drainage) or fluid repletion with saline and potassium chloride, which allows the kidneys to excrete excess bicarbonate ions. Occasionally, a trial of acetazolamide may be useful in causing a bicarbonaturia. Life-threatening metabolic alkalosis is rarely encountered.

## Diagnosis

The diagnosis of an acid-base disorder should occur in a structured fashion. Fig. 21.8 shows a stepwise algorithm for blood gas interpretation. Step 1, which determines oxygenation, will be discussed later in this chapter. Step 2 involves determining whether the patient is acidemic (pH < 7.35) or alkalemic (pH > 7.45). Step 3 looks at whether the cause is from a primary metabolic or respiratory process. Metabolic processes involve a change in bicarbonate concentration from 24 mEq/L, and respiratory processes involve a change in $P_{CO_2}$ from 40 mm Hg. If the primary process

---

**Box 21.4** Causes of Metabolic Alkalosis

**Chloride Responsive**
Renal loss—diuretic therapy
GI loss—vomiting, NG suction
Alkali administration—citrate in blood products, acetate in
   TPN, bicarbonate

**Chloride Resistant**
Hyperaldosteronism
Refeeding syndrome
Profound hypokalemia

*GI*, Gastrointestinal; *NG*, nasogastric; *TPN*, total parenteral nutrition.

---

is respiratory in origin, then step 4 assesses whether the abnormality is chronic or acute (Box 21.5). If a metabolic alkalosis is present, then the next step is to skip to step 7 and determine whether appropriate respiratory compensation is present (Box 21.6). If the measured $P_{CO_2}$ is more than expected, a concurrent respiratory acidosis is present. If the measured $P_{CO_2}$ is less than expected, then a concurrent respiratory alkalosis is present. If a metabolic acidosis is present, then an anion gap should be calculated (step 5). If there is a gap, then a $\Delta$gap should be determined. The $\Delta$gap is the excess anion gap (anion gap minus 12) added back to the serum bicarbonate level. If the number is less than 22 mEq/L, then a concurrent nongap metabolic acidosis is present. If the number is more than 26 mEq/L, then a concurrent metabolic alkalosis is present. The last step, step 7, determines whether an appropriate respiratory compensation is present for the metabolic acidosis. If the measured $P_{CO_2}$ is more than expected [as calculated by the formula $P_{CO_2} = (0.7 \times HCO_3^-) + 21$], then a concurrent respiratory acidosis is present. If the measured $P_{CO_2}$ is less than calculated, then a concurrent respiratory alkalosis is present. See sample calculations in Fig. 21.9.

## OTHER INFORMATION PROVIDED BY ANALYSIS OF ARTERIAL BLOOD GASES AND pH

Aside from acid-base problems, additional measurements and information available from a blood gas analysis include the patient's ability to ventilate and oxygenate and cardiac output estimates.

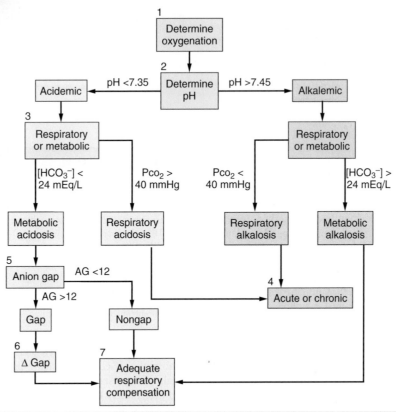

**Fig. 21.8** Seven steps for acid-base diagnosis. Δgap = anion gap − 12 + [HCO₃⁻]. If Δgap is less than 22 mEq/L, then concurrent nongap metabolic acidosis exists. If Δgap is greater than 26 mEq/L, then concurrent metabolic alkalosis exists. *AG,* Anion gap.

---

**Box 21.5** Determining Whether Respiratory Process Is Acute or Chronic

**Acute Process**
pH Δ 0.08 for every 10 mm Hg Δ in Pco₂ from 40 mm Hg

**Chronic Process**
pH Δ 0.03 for every 10 mm Hg Δ in Pco₂ from 40 mm Hg

---

**Box 21.6** Determining Appropriate Compensation in Acid-Base Disorders

**Metabolic Alkalosis**
$Pco_2 = (0.7 \times HCO_3^-) + 21$
 If measured $Pco_2$ > calculated $Pco_2$, then concurrent respiratory acidosis is present.
 If measured $Pco_2$ < calculated $Pco_2$, then concurrent respiratory alkalosis is present.

**Metabolic Acidosis**
Winter's formula:
 $Pco_2 = (1.5 \times HCO_3^-) + 8$
 If measured $Pco_2$ > calculated $Pco_2$, then concurrent respiratory acidosis is present.
 If measured $Pco_2$ < calculated $Pco_2$, then concurrent respiratory alkalosis is present.

## Ventilation

$Paco_2$ reflects the adequacy of ventilation for removing carbon dioxide from blood. A measured $Paco_2$ above 45 mm Hg suggests that a patient is hypoventilating relative to carbon dioxide production, whereas a $Paco_2$ below 35 mm Hg suggests that a patient is hyperventilating. Increased dead space ventilation markedly decreases the efficiency of ventilation. The Vᴅ/Vᴛ ratio is the fraction of each tidal volume that is involved in dead space ventilation. This value is usually around 0.25 to 0.3 because of anatomic dead space. When minute ventilation is held constant during anesthesia, the gradient between $Paco_2$ and end-tidal $CO_2$ (ETCO₂) will increase if dead space is increased (e.g., pulmonary embolus or reduced cardiac output).

## Oxygenation

Oxygenation is assessed by measurement of $Pao_2$. Arterial hypoxemia may be caused by (1) a low $Po_2$ in the inhaled gases (altitude, accidental occurrence during anesthesia), (2) hypoventilation, or (3) venous admixture with or

A 23-year-old man with insulin-dependent diabetes presents to the emergency room with somnolence, influenza-like symptoms, nausea, vomiting, and anorexia.

Laboratory values: Na 130 mEq/L, Cl 80 mEq/L, $HCO_3^-$ 10 mEq/L
ABG: pH 7.20, $P_{CO_2}$ 35 mm Hg, $P_{O_2}$ 68 mm Hg on room air

**Step 1**: Determine oxygenation:

$$\text{A-a gradient} = [(P_B - P_{H_2O})F_{IO_2} - Pa_{CO_2}/RQ] - Pa_{O_2}$$
$$= (150 - Pa_{CO_2}/0.8) - Pa_{O_2}$$
$$= (150 - 35/0.8) - 68$$
$$= 38$$

There is an A-a gradient, possibly from pneumonia or aspiration.

**Step 2**: Determine pH: pH <7.4, so there is an acidosis.

**Step 3**: $[HCO_3^-]$ <24 mEq/L and $P_{CO_2}$ <40 mm Hg
Primary abnormality is from metabolic acidosis.

**Step 4**: Not applicable here since we are going down metabolic acidosis pathway.

**Step 5**: Determine anion gap

$$\text{Anion gap} = [Na] - ([Cl] + [HCO_3^-]) \text{ should be } <12$$
$$= 130 - (80 + 10)$$
$$= 40 \text{ mEq/L}$$

There is an anion gap, probably from starvation or diabetic ketoacidosis.

**Step 6**: Determine $\Delta$ gap

$$\Delta \text{ gap} = \text{anion gap} - 12 + [HCO_3^-]$$
$$= 40 - 12 + 10$$
$$= 38 \text{ mEq/L}$$

There is a concurrent metabolic alkalosis probably from vomiting.

**Step 7**: Is there appropriate respiratory compensation?

$$\text{Winter's formula} = 1.5 [HCO_3^-] + 8 = \text{expected } P_{CO_2}$$
$$= 1.5 (10) + 8$$
$$= 23 \text{ mm Hg}$$

There is also a respiratory acidosis probably from somnolence.

**Fig. 21.9** Example for calculating acid-base abnormalities. *ABG,* Arterial blood gas.

without decreased mixed venous oxygen content. Acute hypoxemia causes activation of the sympathetic nervous system with endogenous catecholamine release, which augments blood pressure and cardiac output despite the vasodilating effects of hypoxemia. The increased cardiac output will increase oxygen delivery from the lungs to peripheral tissues.

### Alveolar Gas Equation

The alveolar gas equation estimates the partial pressure of alveolar oxygen by accounting for barometric pressure, water vapor pressure, and the inspired oxygen concentration (Fig. 21.10). Atmospheric oxygen is a constant 21% of barometric pressure; however, barometric pressure diminishes with altitude such that the decrease in inspired oxygen can become significant. Hypoventilation leads to increased $P_{CO_2}$, which encroaches on the space available in the alveolus for oxygen and dilutes the oxygen concentration. The alveolar gas equation estimates this decrease in alveolar oxygen concentration by subtracting an amount equal to the carbon dioxide divided by the respiratory quotient.

### Alveolar-Arterial Gradient

Calculation of the alveolar-arterial (A-a) gradient provides an estimate of venous admixture as the cause of hypoxemia (see Fig. 21.10). Venous admixture refers to deoxygenated venous blood mixing with oxygenated arterial blood through shunting. The A-a gradient formula calculates the difference in oxygen partial pressure between alveolar ($PA_{O_2}$) and arterial ($Pa_{O_2}$) blood. Normally, the A-a gradient is less than 15 mm Hg while breathing room air as a result of shunting via the thebesian and bronchial veins. Age increases the A-a gradient because of progressive increase in closing capacity relative to functional residual capacity (FRC). Increased fractional concentration of inspired oxygen ($FI_{O_2}$) can lead to a larger gradient (up to 60 mm Hg

---

Alveolar gas equation: $P_{AO_2} = (P_b - P_{H_2O})F_{IO_2} - P_{aCO_2}/RQ$

$P_{AO_2}$ = alveolar partial pressure oxygen (mm Hg)
$P_B$ = barometric pressure (760 mm Hg at sea level)
$P_{H_2O}$ = partial pressure of water vapor (47 mm Hg at 37° C)
$F_{IO_2}$ = fraction inspired oxygen concentration
$R\bar{Q}$ = respiratory quotient (0.8 for normal diet)

A-a gradient  = $P_{AO_2} - P_{aO_2}$

For patient with $P_{aO_2}$ of 363 mm Hg and $P_{aCO_2}$ of 40 mm Hg breathing $F_{IO_2}$ 1.0

$$P_{AO_2} = (760 - 47)(1.0) - 40/0.8$$
$$= (713) - 50$$
$$= 663 \text{ mm Hg}$$

A-a gradient = 663 – 363
         = 300 mm Hg

% shunt  = 1% for every 20 mm Hg of A-a gradient
       = 300/20
       = 15%

**Fig. 21.10** The alveolar gas equation, calculation of alveolar-arterial (A-a) gradient, and estimation of percentage of shunt.

while breathing $F_{IO_2}$ 1.0). Vasodilating drugs (nitroglycerin, nitroprusside, inhaled anesthetics), which inhibit hypoxic pulmonary vasoconstriction and increase ventilation/perfusion ($\dot{V}/\dot{Q}$ mismatch), can also increase the A-a gradient.

Larger A-a gradients suggest the presence of pathologic shunting, such as right-to-left intrapulmonary shunts (atelectasis, pneumonia, endobronchial intubation) or intracardiac shunts (congenital heart disease). The A-a gradient provides an assessment of the patient's shunt fraction and is more sensitive than pulse oximetry. A patient may have an $S_{aO_2}$ of 100% but have a $P_{aO_2}$ of only 90 mm Hg while breathing 100% oxygen. Significant shunting secondary to a pulmonary or cardiac process has occurred despite the reassuring pulse oximeter reading. In patients with large shunts (>50%), administration of 100% oxygen will be unable to raise $P_{aO_2}$.

To estimate the amount of shunt present, when $P_{aO_2}$ is higher than 150 mm Hg, the shunt fraction is approximately 1% of cardiac output for every 20 mm Hg difference in the A-a gradient. When $P_{aO_2}$ is less than 150 mm Hg or when cardiac output is increased relative to metabolism, this guideline will underestimate the actual amount of venous admixture.

### $P_{aO_2}/F_{IO_2}$ Ratio

The $P_{aO_2}/F_{IO_2}$ (P/F) ratio is a simple alternative to the A-a gradient to communicate the degree of hypoxemia. Standards have been created to define the P/F ratio for acute lung injury (ALI) versus ARDS in order to recruit more homogeneous research subjects. Patients with mild ARDS have a P/F ratio below 300, whereas patients with moderate ARDS have a P/F ratio below 200.[17] A ratio under 200 suggests a shunt fraction greater than 20%.

### Cardiac Output Estimates

Normal mixed venous $P_{O_2}$ ($P\bar{v}_{O_2}$) is 40 mm Hg and is a balance between oxygen delivery and tissue oxygen consumption. A true $P\bar{v}_{O_2}$ should reflect blood from the superior and inferior vena cava and the heart. It is usually obtained from the distal port of an unwedged pulmonary artery (PA) catheter. Owing to the complexity and risks of placing a PA catheter, many clinicians simply follow the trend from a central line placed in the superior vena cava.[18] If tissue oxygen consumption is unchanged, changes in $P\bar{v}_{O_2}$ reflect direct changes in cardiac output. The $P\bar{v}_{O_2}$ will decrease when there is inadequate cardiac output because the peripheral tissues have to increase oxygen extraction for aerobic metabolism. The $P\bar{v}_{O_2}$ will increase when there is high cardiac output (sepsis), peripheral shunting (arteriovenous [AV] fistulas), or impaired oxygen extraction (cyanide toxicity).

### Fick Equation

If $P_{aO_2}$, $P\bar{v}_{O_2}$, and hemoglobin are measured, the cardiac output can then be calculated by using the Fick equation (Fig. 21.11), which states that the delivery of oxygen in the veins must equal the delivery of oxygen in the arteries minus what is consumed ($V_{O_2}$). The delivery of oxygen is cardiac output multiplied by the amount of

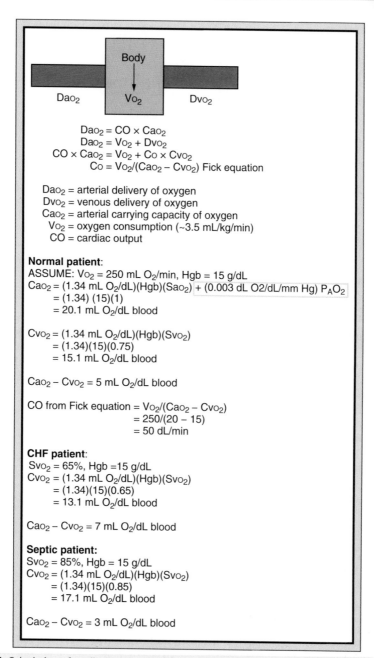

$$Da_{O_2} = CO \times Ca_{O_2}$$
$$Da_{O_2} = V_{O_2} + Dv_{O_2}$$
$$CO \times Ca_{O_2} = V_{O_2} + CO \times Cv_{O_2}$$
$$CO = V_{O_2}/(Ca_{O_2} - Cv_{O_2}) \text{ Fick equation}$$

$Da_{O_2}$ = arterial delivery of oxygen
$Dv_{O_2}$ = venous delivery of oxygen
$Ca_{O_2}$ = arterial carrying capacity of oxygen
$V_{O_2}$ = oxygen consumption (~3.5 mL/kg/min)
$CO$ = cardiac output

**Normal patient:**
ASSUME: $V_{O_2}$ = 250 mL $O_2$/min, Hgb = 15 g/dL
$Ca_{O_2}$ = (1.34 mL $O_2$/dL)(Hgb)($Sa_{O_2}$) + (0.003 dL O2/dL/mm Hg) $P_A{O_2}$
    = (1.34) (15)(1)
    = 20.1 mL $O_2$/dL blood

$Cv_{O_2}$ = (1.34 mL $O_2$/dL)(Hgb)($Sv_{O_2}$)
    = (1.34)(15)(0.75)
    = 15.1 mL $O_2$/dL blood

$Ca_{O_2} - Cv_{O_2}$ = 5 mL $O_2$/dL blood

CO from Fick equation = $V_{O_2}/(Ca_{O_2} - Cv_{O_2})$
                        = 250/(20 − 15)
                        = 50 dL/min

**CHF patient:**
$Sv_{O_2}$ = 65%, Hgb =15 g/dL
$Cv_{O_2}$ = (1.34 mL $O_2$/dL)(Hgb)($Sv_{O_2}$)
    = (1.34)(15)(0.65)
    = 13.1 mL $O_2$/dL blood

$Ca_{O_2} - Cv_{O_2}$ = 7 mL $O_2$/dL blood

**Septic patient:**
$Sv_{O_2}$ = 85%, Hgb = 15 g/dL
$Cv_{O_2}$ = (1.34 mL $O_2$/dL)(Hgb)($Sv_{O_2}$)
    = (1.34)(15)(0.85)
    = 17.1 mL $O_2$/dL blood

$Ca_{O_2} - Cv_{O_2}$ = 3 mL $O_2$/dL blood

**Fig. 21.11** Calculation of cardiac output via Fick equation, arterial and mixed venous oxygen content, and arteriovenous difference in normal, septic, and heart failure patients. *CHF,* Congestive heart failure.

oxygen carried in the blood. The total amount of oxygen in the blood is the amount bound to hemoglobin and the amount dissolved in solution. Because the vast majority of the oxygen content in blood is bound to hemoglobin, the amount dissolved can often be left out of the equation in order to simplify calculations. The amount dissolved becomes important in situations such as severe anemia, when the amount carried by hemoglobin is low.

### Arteriovenous Difference

The difference between the arterial and mixed venous oxygen content (AV difference) is a good estimate of the adequacy of oxygen delivery (see Fig. 21.11). The normal AV difference is 4 to 6 mL/dL of blood. When tissue oxygen consumption is constant, a decreased cardiac output (congestive heart failure) leads to higher oxygen extraction, which increases the AV difference.

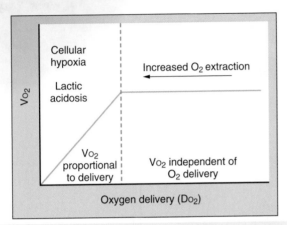

**Fig. 21.12** Relationship of oxygen consumption ($V_{O_2}$) to oxygen delivery ($D_{O_2}$): When oxygen consumption becomes supply dependent, cellular hypoxia occurs, which leads to progressive lactic acidosis and eventually death.

An increased cardiac output (sepsis) or lower extraction (cyanide poisoning) leads to a lower AV difference.

When the delivery of oxygen is first reduced, oxygen consumption remains normal because of the body's ability to increase extraction. With further reductions in oxygen delivery, a critical point is reached when oxygen consumption becomes proportional to delivery. When oxygen consumption becomes supply dependent, cellular hypoxia occurs, which leads to progressive lactic acidosis and eventual death if uncorrected (Fig. 21.12).

## QUESTIONS OF THE DAY

1. What is the expected increase in minute ventilation for every 1 mm Hg increase in $PaCO_2$? What does the term *apneic threshold* mean in the context of a spontaneously breathing patient receiving general anesthesia?

2. A patient with lung disease develops chronic respiratory acidosis. What is the expected renal compensation and the time course of the compensatory response?

3. A hypothermic patient has an arterial blood gas drawn for analysis. Assuming unchanged ventilation and oxygenation, how do the serum bicarbonate, $PaCO_2$, and $PaO_2$ change with hypothermia?

4. What are the physiologic mechanisms for development of acute respiratory acidosis? If a patient receiving laparoscopic surgery developed increased end-tidal $PCO_2$, how would you determine the cause?

5. A patient presents to the emergency department with metabolic acidosis. How would you determine whether the process was acute or chronic? How would measurement of the anion gap help to determine the cause of the acidosis?

6. What is the alveolar gas equation? How is it used to calculate the alveolar-arterial (A-a) gradient in a patient? What are the causes of large A-a gradients?

## REFERENCES

1. Adrogue HJ, Gennari FJ, Galla JH, et al. Assessing acid-base disorders. *Kidney Int.* 2009;76:1239–1247.
2. Morgan TJ. The Stewart approach—one clinician's perspective. *Clin Biochem Rev.* 2009;30:41–54.
3. McNamara J, Worthley LIG. Acid-base balance: part 1, physiology. *Crit Care Resusc.* 2001;3(3):181–187.
4. Clark LC. Monitor and control of blood and tissue $O_2$ tensions. *Trans Am Soc Artif Intern Organs.* 1956;2:41–48.
5. Severinghaus JW, Bradley AF. Electrodes for blood $pO_2$ and $pCO_2$ determination. *J Appl Physiol.* 1958;13:515–520.
6. Malinoski DJ, Todd SR, Slone S, et al. Correlation of central venous and arterial blood gas measurements in mechanically ventilated trauma patients. *Arch Surg.* 2005;140:1122–1125.
7. Mehta A, Lichtin AE, Vigg A, et al. Platelet larceny: spurious hypoxaemia due to extreme thrombocytosis. *Eur Respir J.* 2008;31:469–472.
8. Ashwood ER, Kost G, Kenny M. Temperature correction of blood-gas and pH measurements. *Clin Chem.* 1983;29:1877–1885.
9. Piccioni MA, Leirner AA, Auler JO. Comparison of pH-stat versus alpha-stat during hypothermic cardiopulmonary bypass in the prevention and control of acidosis in cardiac surgery. *Artif Organs.* 2004;28:347–352.
10. Adrogue HJ, Madias NE. Secondary responses to altered acid-base status: the rules of engagement. *J Am Soc Nephrol.* 2010;21:920–923.
11. McIntyre RC, Haenel JB, Moore FA, et al. Cardiopulmonary effects of permissive hypercapnia in the management of adult respiratory distress syndrome. *J Trauma.* 1994;37:433–438.
12. Adrogue HJ, Madias NE. Management of life-threatening acid-base disorders. *N Engl J Med.* 1998;338(1):26–34. 1998;338(2):107–111.
13. Fidkowski C, Helstrom J. Diagnosing metabolic acidosis in the critically ill: bridging the anion gap, Stewart, and base excess methods. *Can J Anaesth.* 2009;56:247–256.
14. Lira A, Pinsky MR. Choices in fluid type and volume during resuscitation: impact on patient outcomes. *Ann Intensive Care.* 2014;4:1–13.
15. Stewart PA. Modern quantitative acid-base chemistry. *Can J Physiol Pharmacol.* 1983;61:1444–1461.
16. Dubin A, Menises MM, Masvicius FD, et al. Comparison of three different methods of evaluation of metabolic acid-base disorders. *Crit Care Med.* 2007;35:1254–1270.
17. The ARDS Definition Task Force; Ranieri VM, Rubenfeld GD, Thompson BT, et al. Acute respiratory distress syndrome: the Berlin definition. *JAMA.* 2012;307(23):2526–2533.
18. Dueck MH, Klimek M, Appenrodt S, et al. Trends but not individual values of central venous oxygen saturation agree with mixed venous oxygen saturation during varying hemodynamic conditions. *Anesthesiology.* 2005;103:249–257.

# HEMOSTASIS

## Lindsey L. Huddleston and Linda L. Liu

Hemostasis is the formation of blood clot at the site of vessel injury. Physiologic hemostasis involves a complex interplay of four components: vascular endothelium, platelets, coagulation factors, and the fibrinolytic system. This intricate system of checks and balances allows blood to maintain its fluidity within a vessel, promotes clot at the site of vessel injury, dismantles clot, and prevents thrombus formation at other sites. If dysfunction of one component or imbalance between components occurs, abnormal bleeding or pathologic thrombosis may occur. Both congenital and acquired disease states, as well as medications, can disrupt the equilibrium of this complex system and lead to bleeding or thrombosis.

## PRIMARY HEMOSTASIS

Primary hemostasis refers to initial vascular endothelial injury leading to platelet deposition at the site of injury (or platelet plug). Under normal conditions and blood flow, platelets do not adhere to the endothelial surface or aggregate with each other, but with vascular injury, the endothelial matrix is exposed. This initial trigger leads to platelet adhesion to collagen or von Willebrand factor (vWF) via multiple surface receptors.

Platelet activation then plays a critical role in the aggregation of platelets. Integrins that are normally present on the platelet surface in inactive forms are activated and bind multiple ligands, including vWF, collagen, fibrinogen, fibronectin, and vitronectin. The activated platelets degranulate and release agonists that act on G protein–coupled receptors to further propagate aggregation and formation of the platelet plug. These agonists include adenosine diphosphate (ADP), thromboxane $A_2$ ($TxA_2$), serotonin, epinephrine, and vasopressin. Along

The editors and publisher would like to thank Dr. Greg Stratmann for contributing to this chapter in the previous edition of this work. It has served as the foundation for the current chapter.

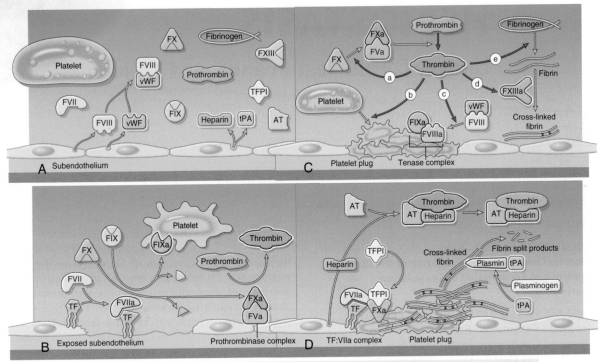

**Fig. 22.1** (A) Normal endothelium. Procoagulants (factors [F] VII, VIII, IX, X, XIII, prothrombin), fibrinogen, and platelets circulate in their inactive forms. Anticoagulants (tissue factor pathway inhibitor [TFPI], heparin, and tissue plasminogen activator [tPA]) actively prevent endothelial spontaneous thrombus formation. (B) Vascular injury, initial phase. Subendothelial tissue factor (TF) exposed to circulating FVII forms a TF:VII complex. TF:VII activates FIX and FX. FIXa binds to platelets. FXa activates FV (FVa) to form prothrombinase complex, which converts localized, small amounts of prothrombin to thrombin. (C) Vascular injury, role of thrombin. Thrombin (a) activates FX and FV to form prothrombinase complexes that generate the secondary thrombin burst, (b) activates platelets, (c) separates FVIII from von Willebrand factor (vWF) and activates FVIII, (d) converts fibrinogen to fibrin, (e) activates factor XI, and (f) activates FXIII, the stabilizer of cross-linked fibrin. Stable clot is formed. (D) Control of coagulation and fibrin clot dissolution. Antithrombin (AT) binds heparin and potently inhibits thrombin activity. TFPI binds to FXa to inhibit the TF:VIIa complex. Plasminogen is activated to plasmin by tPA and cleaves fibrin into soluble fibrin split products. (From Stratmann G. Hemostasis. In Miller RD, Pardo MC, eds. *Basics of Anesthesia.* 6th ed. Philadelphia: Elsevier; 2011.)

with the activated integrins on platelet surfaces, each of these agonists target and activate phospholipase C (PLC). PLC activation leads to the release of large amounts of calcium, which catalyzes degranulation and induces a change in the platelet shape, making them extremely adhesive.

Following platelet activation, the most abundant receptor on the platelet surface, glycoprotein IIb/IIIa (GPIIb/IIIa), undergoes a conformational change and gains high affinity for fibrinogen, thus promoting platelet aggregation and stablization of the platelet plug. In addition, the cytosolic portion of GPIIb/IIIa binds to the platelet cytoskeleton to mediate platelet spreading and clot retraction. By integrating receptor-ligand interactions with cytosolic events, GPIIb/IIIa is the final common pathway for platelet aggregation.[1]

## SECONDARY HEMOSTASIS

### Clotting Cascade and Propagation of the Clot

Proteases cleave inactive precursor proteins (zymogens) to active enzymes that assemble into complexes that subsequently activate thrombin and propagate clot formation. Traditionally, the clotting cascade has been described as consisting of intrinsic, extrinsic, and common pathways. Although this view is useful for providing a structural framework to understand coagulation and to interpret in vivo coagulation tests (e.g., prothrombin time [PT], partial thromboplastin time [PTT]), the current view is that after formation of the platelet plug, coagulation proceeds via an interplay of mechanisms, which include tissue factor (TF) activation of clotting factors, amplification of clotting factors, and propagation of clot formation by thrombin[2] (Fig. 22.1).

The primary physiologic event thought to initiate clotting is the interaction of TF at the site of vascular injury with activated factor VII (factor VIIa). The TF-VIIa complex then activates factors X and IX. Factor Xa then complexes with and activates factor V (which is released from platelet granules during platelet activation) forming the prothrombinase complex. This complex converts a small amount of prothrombin (factor II) to thrombin. This small amount of thrombin amplifies the cascade by activating additional factors V, VIII, XI, and platelets. Factor IXa and factor VIIIa form a complex (the tenase complex) on the surface of activated platelets. The tenase complex activates additional factor X, leading to increased production of the prothrombinase complex and increased thrombin formation. Once sufficient levels of thrombin are available, fibrin is generated from fibrinogen. Finally, to form a strong blood clot, fibrin activates factor XIII to cross-link the fibrin monomers.

## Control and Termination of Coagulation

Three main regulatory molecules control coagulation and facilitate the termination of the coagulation cascade: (1) antithrombin (AT) (formerly antithrombin III), (2) TF pathway inhibitor (TFPI), and (3) activated protein C (aPC). AT inhibits thrombin (factor IIa) and factors Xa, IXa, XIa, and VIIa. When heparin binds to AT, a conformational change occurs and the inactivating process is accelerated by over 100-fold. Endogenous heparin is found on normal endothelial cell surface and prevents spontaneous clot formation, thus limiting the coagulation process to only damaged endothelium. TFPI directly inhibits factor Xa and also complexes with factor Xa to inhibit the TF–factor VIIa complex. Protein C becomes activated when thrombin binds to thrombomodulin on the endothelial cell surface as clot progresses. The thrombin-thrombomodulin complex no longer promotes platelet activation or the formation of fibrin, but instead activates protein C. aPC inactivates factors Va and VIIIa, thus inactivating the prothrombinase and intrinsic tenase complexes. This process is greatly enhanced by the presence of protein S.

## Fibrinolysis

Under normal physiologic conditions, plasmin circulates in its inactive plasminogen form. Plasminogen activator inhibitor type 1 (PAI-1) is synthesized by endothelial cells and secreted to prevent the activation of plasminogen. Injured endothelium secretes tissue plasminogen activator (tPA), which cleaves plasminogen to its active form, plasmin. Because tPA also binds fibrin, the generation of plasmin takes place on the fibrin clot surface, localizing the action of plasmin to the area of clot. Fibrin is cleaved by plasmin into soluble products (D-dimer, fibrin degradation products), which also inhibit thrombin activity.

Like the formation of clot, clot resolution is a highly regulated process. Plasmin that is unbound to the fibrin clot and circulating is inhibited by $\alpha_2$-antiplasmin. If plasmin activation goes unchecked, systemic fibrinolysis and massive hemorrhage may develop.[3]

## DISEASES ASSOCIATED WITH BLEEDING

Certain hereditary or acquired disorders, systemic diseases, and environmental conditions can predispose a patient to excessive bleeding after tissue injury, including surgery. This is the result of a disruption of the hemostatic process and involves a complex interaction between coagulation factors, platelets, fibrinolysis, and vascular integrity. Patients with less than 20% to 30% normal coagulation factor values or platelet counts of less than 50,000 cells/$\mu$L are more likely than patients with normal values to have uncontrolled intraoperative bleeding. Bleeding diatheses vary in clinical presentation depending on what component of the hemostatic system is affected.

Diseases involving coagulation factor deficiencies may present in early childhood with subcutaneous, intramuscular, or intra-articular hemorrhage after only minor trauma. Diseases involving decreased or dysfunctional platelets are typically associated with mucosal bleeding, epistaxis, prolonged bleeding after dental procedures, and menorrhagia. A careful history and physical examination, laboratory evaluation, and consultation with a hematologist when appropriate are necessary to evaluate any patient with suspected bleeding disorders.

## Inherited Coagulation Factor Deficiencies

### Hemophilia A and B

Hemophilia A and hemophilia B are X-linked recessive disorders that are the most common inherited deficiencies of specific coagulation factors. Hemophilia A is a deficiency of factor VIII and occurs in approximately 1 in 5000 live male births. Hemophilia B is a deficiency of factor IX and occurs in approximately 1 in 30,000 live male births. Severe disease, defined by less than 1% of coagulation factor activity, occurs in approximately two thirds of patients with hemophilia A and one half of patients with hemophilia B. Laboratory evaluation shows a prolonged activated PTT (aPTT) that corrects in mixing studies, with a normal platelet count and PT. Plasma von Willebrand factor antigen (vWF:Ag) is normal in hemophilia, distinguishing factor VIII deficiency from von Willebrand disease (vWD). Many patients with hemophilia A (up to 25%) and some with hemophilia B (approximately 3% to 5%) will develop inhibitory antibodies as a response to exogenous factor. In these cases, the aPTT does not correct in mixing studies and alternative treatment is necessary.

Acquired factor deficiencies are caused by autoantibodies, most commonly to factor VIII. Acquired factor inhibitors can develop in patients who have received infusions of factor concentrates, are pregnant (also see Chapter 33), or have underlying systemic disease such as lupus erythematosus or rheumatoid arthritis, or as a drug reaction. In contrast to hemophilia, these acquired factor inhibitors typically occur in adulthood. In addition, mixing studies fail to show correction of the aPTT that is characteristic of hemophilia.

Other Factor Deficiencies

Less common inherited factor deficiencies include deficiencies of factors XI, XII, and XIII. Factor XI deficiency, also known as hemophilia C or Rosenthal disease, is an autosomal recessive disorder that can be associated with bleeding and is characterized by a prolonged aPTT. Factor XII deficiency can result in a prolonged aPTT but is associated with clotting rather than bleeding. Factor XIII is involved in stabilizing the fibrin clot. Patients with factor XIII deficiency present with delayed bleeding after hemostasis, impaired wound healing, and, occasionally, pregnancy loss. Laboratory evaluation shows a normal aPTT and PT with low factor XIII levels.

von Willebrand Disease

vWD is the most common inherited bleeding disorder. The estimated prevalence is 1% of the general population; however, the true prevalence is likely more frequent because of the highly polymorphic von Willebrand gene and variable phenotypes of the disorder. vWF is synthesized by megakaryocytes and endothelial cells. Once released from these cells, it circulates as a series of multimers formed from a basic dimer subunit. The most active forms of vWF are high-molecular-weight multimers that have multiple binding sites for both platelet receptors and subendothelial structures. In normal hemostasis, vWF binds to both platelets and the extracellular matrix at the site of endothelial injury, thus contributing to primary hemostasis by facilitating platelet adhesion. vWF also plays a role in the coagulation cascade and fibrin clot formation by acting as a carrier protein for factor VIII, increasing its concentration and prolonging its half-life. vWD is classified into three types according to vWF levels and protein function (Table 22.1).

In addition to the inherited forms for vWD, several disease states are associated with acquired vWD. These consist of autoimmune, lymphoproliferative, myeloproliferative, neoplastic, and cardiovascular disorders. The underlying pathophysiology of acquired vWD includes autoantibodies to vWF, increased clearance of vWF from plasma, enhanced proteolysis after shear stress, and decreased synthesis.

## Acquired Coagulation Factor Disorders

Vitamin K Deficiency

Vitamin K is an essential fat-soluble vitamin that is required for the carboxylation of factors II, VII, IX, and X and proteins C and S. Without carboxylation, these factors

| Table 22.1 | Classification of von Willebrand Disease | | | | |
|---|---|---|---|---|---|
| **Type** | **Characteristic** | **Frequency** | **Inheritance** | **Diagnosis** | **Treatment** |
| 1 | Not enough vWF | 70-80% | AD | vWF:Ag, vWF:RCo, FVIII | 1. DDAVP<br>2. FVIII/vWF concentrate |
| 2 | Qualitative defect of vWF | 15-20% | AD | | |
| A | ↓ binding of vWF to platelets, ↓ large multimers | Common | | vWF:RCo << vWF:Ag (↓ large multimers) | |
| B | ↑ binding of vWF to platelets, ↓ large multimers | | | RIPA (much less ristocetin required for aggregation) | FVIII/vWF concentrate (DDAVP contraindicated) |
| M | ↓ vWF function despite normal large multimers | Rare | | ↓ vWF:RCo compared with vWF:Ag | 1. FVIII/vWF concentrate<br>2. DDAVP |
| N | ↓ binding of VWF to FVIII | Rare | | | 1. FVIII/vWF concentrate?<br>2. DDAVP? |
| 3 | Absent vWF | Very rare | AR | vWF:Ag | 1. FVIII/vWF concentrate/rFVIII<br>2. Platelet concentrate |

*AD*, Autosomal dominant; *AR*, autosomal recessive; *DDAVP*, desmopressin acetate; *FVIII*, coagulation factor VIII; *rFVIIa*, recombinant factor VIIa; *RIPA*, ristocetin-induced platelet aggregation; *vWF*, von Willebrand factor; *vWF:Ag*, von Willebrand factor antigen; *vWF:RCo*, von Willebrand factor ristocetin cofactor activity; ↓, decreased; ↑, increased; <<, much lower than; *?*, uncertain.
From Stratmann G. Hemostasis. In Miller RD, Pardo MC, eds. *Basics of Anesthesia*. 6th ed. Philadelphia: Elsevier; 2011.

cannot bind to the phospholipid membrane of platelets during secondary hemostasis. Vitamin K is in dietary sources (leafy greens) and is also synthesized by bacteria in the gastrointestinal tract. Patients who are fasting, who have poor dietary intake or are receiving total parenteral nutrition, and those with impaired intestinal absorption (obstructive jaundice, intestinal ileus or obstruction, or total parenteral nutrition) are susceptible to vitamin K deficiency. Newborns, who have not yet developed normal intestinal flora, and patients undergoing oral antibiotic therapy that alters gut flora are also prone to vitamin K deficiency.

### Liver Disease

Multiple causes for bleeding diatheses occur in patients with severe liver disease. Primary hemostasis may be impaired because of thrombocytopenia secondary to platelet sequestration by the spleen in patients with portal hypertension and decreased production of thrombopoietic factors. In addition, comorbid conditions such as renal failure and infection can lead to dysfunctional platelets. Secondary hemostasis can be compromised because plasma clotting factors, with the exception of factor VIII, are synthesized in the liver. Laboratory values of platelets, PT, and aPTT may overestimate the bleeding risk in these patients, because the liver is also responsible for the synthesis of anticoagulant factors: protein C, protein S, and AT. Often, this deficiency of both procoagulant and anticoagulant factors leads to a tenuous hemostatic balance, which can be altered by any small disturbance.

## Treatment of Clotting Factor Deficiencies

### Hemophilia A and Hemophilia B

Patients with known hemophilia should have a thorough preoperative evaluation, including bleeding history, and laboratory evaluation for levels of factor and presence of inhibitors. Given the significant variability of individual response to factor replacement, consultation with a hematologist is necessary to manage perioperative care. Factor concentrates are the treatment of choice for patients with hemophilia A (factor VIII concentrate) and hemophilia B (factor IX concentrate). Dose calculations are targeted to achieve at lease 50% of normal factor activity levels for minor surgery and 80% to 100% of normal factor activity levels for major surgery. Treatment with factor concentrates should continue postoperatively until wound healing is complete. Patient response and the type of surgery determine the necessary duration of treatment.

In resource-limited areas, treatment with cryoprecipitate and fresh frozen plasma (FFP) may be necessary, although not optimal. Cryoprecipitate contains large quantities of factor VIII, vWF, fibrinogen, and factor XIII, but it does not contain factor IX and should not be used for replacement therapy in hemophilia B. Sufficient levels of factor VIII or factor IX levels are difficult to achieve with FFP alone because of inadequate levels of factor and the need for a large volume administration. Prothrombin complex concentrates (PCCs) contain factor IX and can be used for bleeding control in hemophilia B when factor IX concentrates are unavailable. However, PCCs induce a higher thrombotic risk than pure factor IX concentrate and extreme caution should be used when administering concomitant antifibrinolytics. Other adjuvant therapies include desmopressin acetate (DDAVP), which increases plasma levels of factor VIII and vWF and can be useful for hemophilia A, and antifibrinolytics (tranexamic acid [TXA], ε-aminocaproic acid [EACA]), which may decrease the bleeding risk.

### von Willebrand Disease

DDAVP is the treatment of choice in type 1 vWD. One dose of DDAVP (0.3 μg/kg) will produce a complete or near complete response in the majority of patients.[4] In addition, cryoprecipitate and intermediate-purity factor VIII concentrates, which both contain high levels of vWF, can be used to attenuate surgical bleeding. DDAVP is contraindicated in type 2b vWD because it causes a transient thrombocytopenia. In addition, patients with severe vWD (type 3) do not respond to DDAVP and should be treated with a combination of factor VIII and vWF concentrates. Antifibrinolytics may also be useful adjuvants in the management of perioperative bleeding in this patient population.

### Acquired Coagulation Disorders

Vitamin K deficiency can be treated with vitamin K replacement via oral, intravenous, intramuscular, or subcutaneous administration. In cases of serious bleeding, intravenous vitamin K is the recommended therapy, beginning with a dose of 5 mg. In isolated vitamin K deficiency, correction of the PT will occur within 3 to 4 hours of intravenous vitamin K administration.

Treatment of severe bleeding in the setting of liver failure is most often guided by laboratory abnormalities (also see Chapter 28). Platelets are administered for thrombocytopenia, FFP for prolonged PT, and cryoprecipitate may be necessary to treat bleeding in the setting of hypofibrinogenemia (also see Chapter 24). Because of the complex balance between deficiencies of procoagulant and anticoagulant factors, routine administration of blood products to correct laboratory values in the absence of bleeding or major surgery is not recommended in these patients. Whether blood product replacement in nonbleeding patients with liver failure should be used for minimal risk procedures, such as central line placement, is not well established.

Treatment of patients with acquired factor inhibitors is complex, as these patients may not respond to standard therapy with factor concentrates. "Bypassing agents" treat bleeding by producing thrombin through pathways that do not require factor VIII or factor IX. "Bypassing agents" are the mainstay of therapy for bleeding patients with high levels of inhibitor in whom administration of factor concentrate is ineffective.[5] Currently available "bypassing agents" include recombinant factor VIIa (rFVIIa) and PCCs. Another treatment strategy in the nonurgent clinical setting is "immune tolerance induction" when patients are exposed to prolonged, high concentrations of factor in an effort to eliminate a coagulation inhibitor.

## Platelet Disorders

Both decreased platelet numbers (thrombocytopenia) and qualitative platelet disorders can result in severe bleeding. Inherited platelet disorders are rare congenital diseases that typically affect qualitative function of platelets. In addition to inherited disorders, a multitude of acquired disorders can affect platelet number, platelet function, or both. Both inherited and acquired disorders of platelet function are characterized by prolonged bleeding time and abnormal platelet function tests.

### Thrombocytopenia

Low platelet counts can be the result of decreased platelet production, increased destruction, or sequestration. Decreased platelet production in the bone marrow occurs in myelodysplastic syndromes, infections (especially in the setting of sepsis), and nutrient deficiencies. Patients with these disorders typically present with pancytopenia because production of all cell lines in the bone marrow is impaired. Other causes of impaired production of platelets include immune thrombocytopenia (idiopathic thrombocytopenic purpura [ITP]) and drug-induced bone marrow suppression. Peripheral platelet destruction by antiplatelet antibodies can be induced by certain medications or ingested substances, as well as in the setting of specific autoimmune diseases. Heparin-induced thrombocytopenia (HIT) occurs in less than 5% of patients exposed to heparin. Antibodies to platelet factor 4 can cause thrombocytopenia and platelet activation, potentially leading to life-threatening arterial and venous thrombosis. Increased platelet consumption within thrombi is seen in disseminated intravascular coagulation (DIC) and thrombotic thrombocytopenic purpura/hemolytic uremic syndromes (TTP-HUS). Diseases that cause splenomegaly or splenic congestion through portal hypertension (e.g., cirrhosis) lead to sequestration of platelets in the spleen, inhibiting their release into circulation.

Multiple disorders of pregnancy result in thrombocytopenia including gestational thrombocytopenia, preeclampsia, and pregnancy-associated hypertensive disorders (also see Chapter 33). The most severe of these disorders is the HELLP syndrome (hemolysis, elevated liver function test results, low platelet counts), which necessitates emergent delivery before life-threatening maternal complications occur.

### Qualitative Platelet Disorders

Even with adequate platelet numbers, poor function can increase bleeding risk and affect measures of platelet aggregation. Several common drugs impair platelet function including aspirin, nonsteroidal antiinflammatory drugs (NSAIDs), alcohol, dipyridamole, and clopidogrel. Uremia, when severe, is associated with increased clinical bleeding. Proposed pathophysiologic mechanisms include intrinsic platelet metabolic defects, impaired platelet granule release, and impaired platelet–endothelial cell interactions. Normal platelet function is also impaired in conditions with high levels of abnormal circulating proteins (multiple myeloma, dysproteinemia, transfused dextran solutions). Many rare conditions involve inherited disorders of platelet function. Glanzmann thrombasthenia is an autosomal recessive disorder characterized by defective GPIIb/IIIa receptors on platelets leading to impaired platelet aggregation. Giant platelet disorders include platelet glycoprotein abnormalities, as in Bernard-Soulier syndrome. Wiskott-Aldrich syndrome is an X-liked recessive disorder in which patients have immunodeficiency, severely dysfunctional platelets, and thrombocytopenia. This syndrome is an example of a storage pool disorder, in which granule deficiencies lead to impaired platelet aggregation.

### Treatment of Platelet Disorders (Also See Chapter 24)

In the nonbleeding patient, treatment of thrombocytopenia in the form of platelet transfusion is usually withheld until the platelet count is less than 10,000 cells/μL. In the patient who is actively bleeding or requires surgical intervention, platelet transfusion is recommended to a goal of 50,000 cells/μL, or in some cases, such as intracranial hemorrhage or neurosurgery, 100,000 cells/μL. A major concern with the transfusion of platelets is the potential for human leukocyte antigen (HLA) or human platelet antigen antibodies to form. If multiple platelet transfusions are expected, platelets should be HLA-matched whenever possible. For patients with normal platelet counts but suspected dysfunctional platelets, administration of platelets is often ineffective because the patient's underlying condition causes transfused platelets to function abnormally. In these cases, DDAVP may be effective.

## DISEASES ASSOCIATED WITH THROMBOSIS

Development of venous thrombosis (most commonly deep venous thrombosis [DVT] or pulmonary embolus) is a common occurrence in the surgical population and leads to increased morbidity and mortality rates. The classic teaching for the pathogenesis of venous thromboembolism (VTE), often referred to as Virchow triad, proposes that VTE occurs as a result of (1) stasis of blood flow, (2) endothelial injury, and (3) a hypercoagulable state (inherited or acquired).

Patients with inherited thrombophilia (deficiencies of protein C, protein S, and AT; factor V Leiden and prothrombin gene mutations) have an increased tendency for VTE. Numerous other conditions such as malignancy, pregnancy, immobilization, trauma, DIC, antiphosholipid syndrome, infection, drugs (e.g., oral contraceptives), and recent surgery also predispose patients to VTE.

## Hereditary Hypercoagulable States

### Factor V Leiden and Prothrombin Gene Mutation

The most common inherited thrombophilias are the factor V Leiden mutation and the prothrombin gene mutation, accounting for 50% to 60% of cases. Individuals with factor V Leiden have an abnormal mutation of factor V that is resistant to the action of aPC. aPC regulates the coagulation process by inhibiting factor V from forming excessive fibrin in normal individuals. The prothrombin gene mutation (prothrombin 20210) leads to overproduction of prothrombin (factor II) and makes the blood more likely to clot. Individuals with factor V Leiden or the prothrombin gene mutation are at increased risk of developing DVTs, with homozygotes having the highest risk. Despite the increased relative risk, the absolute risk of blood clots in these patients remains low in the absence of other risk factors for hypercoagulability.

### Protein C and Protein S Deficiencies

Under normal physiologic conditions, aPC inactivates factors Va and VIIIa (enhanced by protein S). In addition, aPC acts directly on cells to protect the endothelial barrier function and also has antiinflammatory activities. Protein C deficiency is an autosomal dominant trait affecting approximately 1 in 500 individuals in the general population. Clinical manifestations of the deficiency include VTE, neonatal purpura (in homozygous neonates), fetal loss, and warfarin-induced skin necrosis. Protein S is a cofactor for aPC and is synthesized by hepatocytes, endothelial cells, and megakaryocytes. Forty to 50% of protein S circulates as the free form, the only form with aPC cofactor activity. In the presence of protein S, aPC inactivates factors Va and VIIIa at an accelerated rate. Protein S also serves as a cofactor for protein C enhancement of fibrinolysis and can directly inhibit prothrombin activation. Individuals with protein S deficiency present similarly to those with other inherited thrombophilias and are at increased risk of VTE, superficial thrombophlebitis, and pulmonary embolism (PE).

Both protein C and protein S deficiencies can be acquired secondary to underlying disease. Acquired protein C deficiency can be seen in liver disease, severe infection (especially meningococcemia), septic shock, and DIC. Acquired protein S deficiency has been associated with pregnancy, use of oral contraceptives, DIC, human immunodeficiency virus (HIV) infection, nephrotic syndrome, and liver disease.

## Acquired Hypercoagulable States

### Antiphospholipid Syndrome

The antiphospholipid (antibody) syndrome (APS) is a condition characterized by both venous and arterial thromboses or recurrent pregnancy complications (also see Chapter 33). Patients with this syndrome have persistent circulating antiphospholipid antibodies (aPLs), which include lupus anticoagulant, anticardiolipin antibody, or anti-β2GPI antibodies. It is one of the few prothrombotic states in which arterial and venous thromboses occur. Most cases of APS are sporadic or acquired. Rarely, the condition runs in families; yet it does not exhibit a clear pattern of inheritance.

DVT is the most common venous thrombosis and stroke is the most common arterial thrombosis. Diagnosis is made by clinical criteria (arterial/venous thromboses, recurrent pregnancy complications) and by the presence of one or more of the three aPLs detected on two or more occasions at least 12 weeks apart. Patients who have persistently positive aPLs (especially those with multiple differing aPLs), who present with arterial thromboses, or who have recurrent thromboses in the setting of anticoagulation are most likely at risk for thrombosis. The lupus anticoagulant, although often found in patients with systemic lupus erythematosus, can also be associated with medications (phenothiazines, phenytoin, hydralazine, quinine, and antibiotics), inflammatory bowel disease (Crohn disease and ulcerative colitis), infections, and certain kinds of tumors. Catastrophic APS (CAPS) is a rare accelerated form of APS in which patients present with coagulopathy, ischemic necrosis of the extremities, and multiorgan failure in the setting of positive circulating aPLs and histopathologic evidence of small vessel occlusion. Although CAPS occurs in less than 1% of patients with APS, mortality rate is approximately 30%.[6] Early recognition and treatment with anticoagulation and immunosuppressant therapy are paramount to survival.

### Disseminated Intravascular Coagulation

DIC is an acquired disorder caused by an underlying condition (most commonly, sepsis) that is characterized by widespread systemic activation of coagulation (also see Chapter 24). This results in uncontrolled intravascular thrombin generation and fibrin deposition in small blood vessels. The formation of microvascular thrombi ultimately leads to end-organ dysfunction and multiorgan failure. Excessive consumption of circulating coagulation factors, platelets, and fibrinogen occurs simultaneously with microvascular thrombi formation, which can result in life-threatening bleeding. A patient with DIC may present with both thrombotic and hemorrhagic complications.

No single laboratory test identifies DIC; however, a combination of laboratory tests in the setting of a condition known to cause DIC can be sufficient for diagnosis (Table 22.2). The most common laboratory abnormalities

| Table 22.2 | Conditions Associated With Disseminated Intravascular Coagulation |
|---|---|

| Category | Conditions |
|---|---|
| Infections | Bacterial (gram-negative bacilli, gram-positive cocci)<br>Viral (CMV, EBV, HIV, VZV, hepatitis)<br>Fungal (histoplasma)<br>Parasites (malaria) |
| Malignancy | Hematologic (AML)<br>Solid tumors (prostate cancer, pancreatic cancer)<br>Malignant tumors (mucin-secreting adenocarcinoma) |
| Obstetric causes | Amniotic fluid embolism<br>Preeclampsia/eclampsia<br>Placental abruption<br>Acute fatty liver of pregnancy<br>Intrauterine fetal demise |
| Massive inflammation | Severe trauma<br>Burns<br>Traumatic brain injury<br>Crush injury<br>Severe pancreatitis |
| Toxic/immunologic | Snake envenomation<br>Massive transfusion<br>ABO blood type incompatibility<br>Graft versus host disease |
| Other | Liver disease/fulminant hepatic failure<br>Vascular disease (aortic aneurysms, giant hemangiomas)<br>Ventricular assist devices |

*AML,* Acute myelogenous leukemia; *CMV,* cytomegalovirus; *EBV,* Epstein-Barr virus; *HIV,* human immunodeficiency virus; *VZV,* varicella zoster virus.

associated with DIC are thrombocytopenia, elevated fibrin degradation products (D-dimers), prolonged PT and aPTT, and low fibrinogen. Because laboratory abnormalities in DIC can be seen in other conditions such as massive blood loss, liver failure, HIT, and thrombotic microangiopathy, a scoring system has been developed by the International Society on Thrombosis and Hemostasis (ISTH). The ISTH scoring system uses simple laboratory tests (platelet count, PT, aPTT, fibrinogen, D-dimer) plus the presence of a triggering underlying condition to diagnose DIC. It has a high sensitivity and specificity (91% and 97%, respectively) and is an independent predictor of mortality risk.[7]

## Treatment of Hypercoagulable States

Inherited thrombophilias are relatively rare in the general population, and screening for the presence of these diseases in the absence of VTE is not recommended. In patients with a known thrombophilia but no history of VTE (or pregnancy complications), primary prophylaxis with anticoagulation is not recommended. Patients who present with VTE and test positive for an inherited thrombophilia are anticoagulated for their acute presentation. Continuation of anticoagulation after resolution of acute VTE is determined by severity of presentation, presence of more than one thrombophilia, and homozygosity or heterozygosity for thrombophilia.[8] In the case of pregnant patients with known thrombophilia, anticoagulation is often recommended in the antepartum and postpartum setting (also see Chapter 33). The necessary duration and type of anticoagulation therapy are not clear because of the rarity of these diseases; a hematologist should manage all patients. Patients with antiphospholipid syndrome (APS) have an increased risk of recurrent thrombosis and are most often treated with long-term anticoagulation. The specific treatment and targets for optimal anticoagulation therapy remain controversial.

For DIC, the mainstay of therapy is to treat the underlying cause. Supportive care for actively bleeding patients is guided by laboratory tests to ensure appropriate transfusion therapy (also see Chapter 24). In patients with active bleeding and suspected fibrinolysis, antifibrinolytics, such as TXA, may be used. Transfusions for non-bleeding patients are typically withheld unless platelets, fibrinogen, or coagulation factors are severely low, or if patients undergo an invasive procedure. Anticoagulation in patients with DIC remains controversial, and therapy with heparin is rarely initiated unless severe thrombosis is present.

## LABORATORY EVALUATION OF HEMOSTASIS

Currently, the coagulation tests that are commonly performed in the laboratory have limited clinical value and are poor at predicting surgical bleeding (Table 22.3; also see Chapter 24). Although routine coagulation tests have been standardized to guide heparin and warfarin therapy and certainly play a role in the diagnosis and management of factor deficiencies (e.g., hemophilia), they were not developed with the intent to manage the actively bleeding patient. Newer global coagulation assays (thromboelastography, rotational thromboelastometry) may provide a more detailed picture of complex hemostasis and help guide therapy toward specific abnormalities of coagulation or fibrinolysis.

### Tests of Coagulation

#### Prothrombin Time
PT can be used to assess what was traditionally thought of as the extrinsic pathway of clotting. Prolonged PT will occur with low levels of TF, factor VII, factor II, factor

**Table 22.3**  Common Laboratory Tests of Hemostasis and Normal Ranges

| Platelet Tests | Coagulation Tests | Fibrinolysis Tests |
|---|---|---|
| Platelet count: 140,000-450,000 cells/µL | Prothrombin time: 11.5-14.5 sec[a] | Thrombin time: 22.1-31.2 sec |
| Bleeding time: <11 min | Partial thromboplastin time: 24.5-35.2 sec[a] | Fibrinogen-fibrin degradation products: >5 µg/dL |
| Platelet function analysis | Thrombin time: 22.1-31.2 sec[a] | Fibrin D-dimer assay: <250 µg/mL |
| Collagen/epinephrine: 94-193 sec | Fibrinogen: 175-433 mg/dL | |
| Collagen/adenosine diphosphate: 71-118 sec | Activated coagulation time: 70-180 sec | |
| Platelet aggregation (response to aggregating agents: collagen, adenosine diphosphate, epinephrine, and ristocetin) | | |

[a]The normal range varies with reagent lots.

From Stratmann G. Hemostasis. In Miller RD, Pardo MC, eds. *Basics of Anesthesia*. 6th ed. Philadelphia: Elsevier; 2011.

V, factor X, and fibrinogen. For the test, citrated patient plasma is recalcified in the presence of thromboplastin (which activates factor X in the presence of factor VII). The end point of the test is the time to formation of fibrin clot, as measured by visual, optical, or electromechanical means. Because the PT can measure reduced activity of the vitamin K–dependent factors, it is used to monitor warfarin therapy. Heparin, low-molecular-weight heparin (LMWH), and fondaparinux inhibit thrombin and therefore should prolong the PT. However, most PT reagents contain heparin-binding chemicals that block this effect and thus PT remains normal in the setting of these therapies. Because PT reagents can vary widely between laboratories and lead to differing values, the international normalized ratio (INR) was developed by the World Health Organization to standardize PT and allow the values to be directly compared between laboratories.

### Activated Partial Thromboplastin Time

The aPTT is used to assess the integrity of the intrinsic and common coagulation pathways. It can detect low levels of prekallikrein; high-molecular-weight kininogen; factors XII, XI, IX, and VIII (intrinsic pathway); as well as low levels of factors II, V, and X and fibrinogen (final common pathway). Citrated plasma is recalcified in the presence of a thromboplastic material that does not have TF activity. A negatively charged substance such as kaolin, celite, ellagic acid, or silica provides a surface for contact activation of factor and speeds up the reaction. As with the PT, the end point of the aPTT is formation of fibrin clot. Both hemophilias A and B as well as vWD (because of potentially low levels of factor VIII) will prolong aPTT. Unfractionated heparin (UFH) therapy and therapy with parenteral direct thrombin inhibitors (DTIs) (argatroban) are monitored with aPTT levels.

### Thrombin Time

The thrombin time measures the conversion of fibrinogen to fibrin, which is the final step in the clotting pathway. The test is performed by recalcifying citrated plasma and adding thrombin. Time to clot formation is measured in seconds. Conditions that prolong the thrombin time include therapy with anticoagulants (including heparin and DTIs), hypofibrinogenemia (<100 mg/dL), the presence of abnormal fibrinogen or fibrinogen degradation products, high concentrations of serum proteins (multiple myeloma, amyloidosis), and circulating bovine thrombus antibodies (after exposure during surgery).

### Fibrinogen Level

A number of methods are available for measuring fibrinogen. The most common method uses the Clauss assay, in which diluted plasma is exposed to a high concentration of thrombin. The time to clot formation is compared to a standard calibration curve, and the fibrinogen concentration is deduced. Immunologic fibrinogen assays are used when clotting-based fibrinogen assays suggest reduced fibrinogen for no obvious clinical reason, or when dysfibrinogenemia is suspected.

### Activated Clotting Time

The activated clotting time (ACT) measures the time in seconds for formation of a clot after an activating agent (e.g., celite, kaolin) is added to a sample of freshly drawn whole blood. The aPTT has replaced this test in many clinical situations, except in the operating room. In the setting of high heparin concentrations (>1 unit/mL), the aPTT becomes infinitely prolonged; therefore, for procedures that require high heparin doses such as coronary artery bypass surgery or percutaneous coronary interventions (PCIs), the ACT is still used for heparin monitoring.

## Tests of Fibrinolysis

Laboratory analysis of fibrinolysis is difficult because of the complexity of the fibrinolytic system and the interchange between hemostasis and fibrinolysis proteins. Current assays in clinical studies are poor predictors of thrombosis or bleeding. Furthermore, other inflammatory states can increase the concentrations of fibrin degradation products in the absence of fibrinolysis. Global tests of fibrinolysis, including clot lysis time and thromboelastography, have shown promise in the perioperative setting in predicting bleeding and allowing for targeted treatment of fibrinolysis with antifibrinolytics and cryoprecipitate. These global assays allow for fast, real-time analysis of hemostasis, and are especially useful in cases with increased risk of hemorrhage such as trauma (also see Chapter 42), liver transplant (also see Chapter 36), postpartum hemorrhage (also see Chapter 33), cardiac surgery (also see Chapter 25), or multiple blood transfusions (also see Chapter 24).

### Fibrin Degradation Products

Elevated levels of different fibrin degradation products result from the action of plasmin on fibrin and fibrinogen during fibrinolysis. D-dimer is formed when plasmin cleaves cross-linked fibrin polymers at the D fragment site and has been used as a marker of fibrinolytic states. Increased D-dimer concentrations have predictive and prognostic value in states of fibrinolysis, such as DIC, and in thrombotic disorders such as pulmonary embolus or DVT. Although an increased D-dimer level is nearly 90% sensitive (in the case of DIC), it is not very specific and therefore is not often used to detect fibrinolysis.

### Global Coagulation Assays

There are currently two available semiautomated devices that use viscoelastic measures to analyze time to blood clot formation, maximal clot stability, and resolution of clot due to fibrinolysis (Fig. 22.2). Thromboelastography (TEG) uses fresh whole blood placed in a cup that continuously rotates around a pin. As clot forms, there is increased resistance to rotation of the cup, which is transmitted to the sensor pin and displayed graphically. In rotational thromboelastometry (ROTEM), a similar rotational method and graphic display are used; however, in this case, the cup with fresh whole blood is fixed while the pin rotates. Since the advent of viscoelastic measurements of coagulation in 1948, improvements in technique have led to easier use and the ability to perform point-of-care testing with rapid results. The addition of various trigger reagents provides further information on the extrinsic pathway, levels of fibrinogen, effects or presence of heparin, and resistance to lysis.[9] Although viscoelastic measurements can assess platelet aggregation, these tests do not measure platelet

dysfunction (either inherited or drug induced). In addition, they are unable to detect the effects of vWF. Other concerns include difficulty with quality control and the ability to standardize these measurements across different centers. Despite these limitations, TEG and ROTEM clearly can help detect coagulopathy, guide transfusion therapy, and even decrease the need for some blood transfusions (Fig. 22.3) (also see Chapter 24).

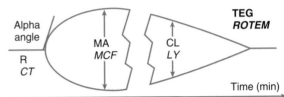

| Variable | TEG | ROTEM |
|---|---|---|
| From start to 2-mm amplitude (clot initiation) | R (reaction time) | CT (clotting time) |
| From 2-mm to 20-mm amplitude (clot kinetics) | K (kinetics) | CFT (clot formation time) |
| Alpha angle | Slope between R and K | Angle of tangent at 2-mm amplitude |
| Maximum strength (clot strength) | MA (maximum amplitude) | MCF (maximum clotting time) |
| Clot lysis (at minutes) | CL 30, CL 60 | LY 30, LY 60 |

**Fig. 22.2** Comparison of common variables for the global coagulation assays TEG (thromboelastography) and ROTEM (rotational thromboelastometry). *CL,* Clot lysis; *LY,* lysis.

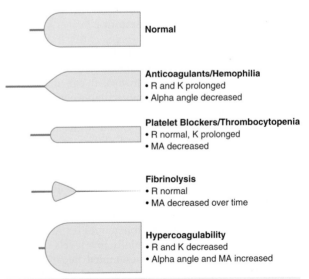

**Fig. 22.3** Common thromboelastography examples with analysis. *K,* Kinetics; *MA,* maximum amplitude; *R,* reaction time.

## Tests of Platelet Function

### Platelet Count

Platelet count is determined as part of the complete blood count and is performed by automated machines that use optical, impedance, or flow cytometry methods. Platelet clumping (that results from minimal platelet activation) and the presence of giant platelets can lead to artificially decreased platelet counts. Conversely, if samples contain cellular debris (thalassemias, leukemias, TTP), the platelet count may be overestimated by some methods.

### Bleeding Time

The bleeding time has been used as a screening test for platelet function in the past, however, because of the difficulty in performing an accurate test, it is rarely used in clinical practice today. To perform the test, a blood pressure cuff is inflated on the upper part of the arm to 40 mm Hg and a standardized 9-mm long and 1-mm deep incision is made on the volar surface of the forearm. Blood is blotted away every 30 seconds with filter paper and a prolonged bleeding time (>11 minutes) can signify either platelet dysfunction or platelet count of less than 100,000 cells/μL.

### Platelet Aggregation Studies

Platelet aggregation studies are not commonly used in the perioperative setting, but they may be useful in the preoperative evaluation of patients with potential platelet disorders. A platelet agonist (e.g., collagen, ADP, epinephrine, or ristocetin) is added to platelet rich plasma, and then platelet aggregration is measured by decreased light scatter. These studies can help differentiate between inherited disorders of platelet dysfunction (e.g., Glanzmann thrombasthenia, Bernard-Soulier syndrome, vWD) as well as monitor antiplatelet therapy with aspirin or clopidogrel.

### Platelet Function Analysis

Platelets within citrated blood are exposed to a membrane coated with collagen and either ADP or epinephrine to initiate adhesion. The test measures the time to instrument aperture occlusion as a result of platelet thrombus. Abnormal closure times indicate platelet dysfunction; however, the result is not specific for any disorder. Because the test is simple, rapid, and does not require special training, it may be useful as a screening tool to assess for platelet dysfunction.

## ANTITHROMBOTICS AND PROCOAGULANTS

Antithrombotic drugs are usually used to treat cardiovascular disease, stroke, and DVT or PE. They can be further subdivided into antiplatelet agents, anticoagulants (Table 22.4), and thrombolytics.

### Antiplatelet Drugs

Platelets are involved in the formation of pathologic thrombus leading to coronary artery disease. Antiplatelet drugs can be divided into three classes: (1) cyclooxygenase (COX) inhibitors, (2) P2Y12 receptor antagonists, and (3) platelet GPIIb/IIIa antagonists.

#### Cyclooxygenase Inhibitors

There are two primary COX isozymes: COX-1 and COX-2. COX-1 maintains the integrity of the gastric lining and renal blood flow and initiates the formation of $TxA_2$, which is important for platelet aggregation. COX-2 is responsible for synthesizing the prostaglandin mediators in pain and inflammation.

**Table 22.4**  Common Anticoagulants with the Required Monitoring and Possible Reversal Drugs for Emergencies

| Anticoagulants | Drug Name | Monitoring | Reversal Agents |
|---|---|---|---|
| Vitamin K antagonists | Warfarin | PT, INR | PCC, FFP, vitamin K |
| Heparins | Unfractionated heparin (UFH) | aPTT | Protamine |
| | Low-molecular-weight heparin (LMWH) | None required, but anti–factor Xa assay can monitor levels | Partially reversed by protamine |
| Pentasaccharide | Fondaparinux | None required, but anti–factor Xa assay can monitor levels | None |
| Direct thrombin inhibitors | Hirudin, argatroban, bivalirudin | aPTT or ACT | None |
| | Dabigatran | None required | Idarucizumab, dialysis may remove drug |
| Factor Xa inhibitors | Rivaroxaban, apixaban | None required | None |

*ACT,* Activated clotting time; *aPTT,* activated partial thromboplastin time; *FFP,* fresh frozen plasma; *INR,* international normalized ratio; *PCC,* prothrombin complex concentrate; *PT,* prothrombin time.

Small doses of aspirin irreversibly inhibit COX-1. Large doses of aspirin irreversibly inhibit both COX-1 and COX-2, which leads to antiinflammatory and analgesic effects. Because platelets have no deoxyribonucleic acid (DNA), they are unable to synthesize new COX-1 once aspirin has irreversibly inhibited the enzyme, which means despite its short half-life (15 to 20 minutes), aspirin works for 7 to 10 days, the expected lifetime of anucleated platelets. The recovery of platelet function after aspirin depends on platelet turnover. Generally, megakaryocytes generate 10% to 12% of platelets daily, so near normal hemostasis is expected in 2 to 3 days after the last dose of aspirin, assuming platelet turnover is normal. Otherwise, immediate reversal can only be achieved with platelet transfusions.

Most NSAIDs are nonselective reversible COX inhibitors (also see Chapters 40 and 44). Platelet function returns to normal 3 days after discontinuing the use of NSAIDs. Selective COX-2 antagonists such as celecoxib were developed to provide pain relief without the gastrointestinal bleeding complications, but recent clinical trials with selective COX-2 antagonists have reported increased risks for cardiovascular complications.[10] COX-2 specific inhibitors do not affect platelet function because platelets do not express COX-2. The increased cardiovascular risk is likely due to inhibition of prostacyclin ($PGI_2$) without inhibition of $TxA_2$, thus tipping the balance toward thrombosis. Current recommendations are to use COX-2 inhibitors only when necessary and then with the smallest effective dose possible along with low-dose aspirin.

### P2Y12 Receptor Antagonists

These drugs (ticlopidine, clopidogrel, prasugrel, ticagrelor) interfere with platelet function by inhibiting the P2Y12 receptor, which prevents the expression of GPIIb/IIIa on the surface of activated platelets and inhibits platelet adhesion and aggregation. Clopidogrel (Plavix) is the most commonly prescribed drug in this class. Platelet functions normalize 7 days after discontinuing clopidogrel and 14 to 21 days after discontinuing ticlopidine.

Clopidogrel, a noncompetitive and irreversible antagonist, is a prodrug that requires CYP2C19 for activation. It has wide interindividual variability in inhibiting ADP-induced platelet function. Although many factors may be involved, genetic factors deserve consideration. Patients treated with clopidogrel who have decreased CYP2C19 activity were shown to have significantly increased risk of major cardiovascular events. The Food and Drug Administration (FDA) put a black box warning on clopidogrel to make patients and health care providers aware that patients who are CYP2C19-poor metabolizers, which represents up to 14% of patients, are at high risk of treatment failure and that genotype testing may be helpful.

Ticagrelor has much lower interindividual variability because it binds to a separate site on the P2Y12 receptor to inhibit G-protein activation and signaling, and ticagrelor is not a prodrug. Because it is much shorter acting than clopidogrel, ticagrelor must be dosed twice daily.

### Glycoprotein IIb/IIIa Antagonists

The GPIIb/IIIa receptor mediates platelet aggregation by binding fibrinogen and vWF. Available drugs that block the receptor are abciximab (ReoPro), eptifibatide (Integrilin), and tirofiban (Aggrastat). They are given intravenously in order to (1) stop ongoing arterial thrombosis and (2) eliminate excessive platelet reactivity in diseased vessels so that occlusive thrombi and restenosis do not occur. Abciximab is a noncompetitive irreversible inhibitor of GPIIb/IIIa, whereas eptifibatide and tirofiban are competitive, reversible GPIIb/IIIa antagonists. The inhibition provided by abciximab continues at various levels for several days after the infusion has stopped. Platelet aggregation normalizes 24 to 48 hours after discontinuing abciximab and 8 hours after discontinuing eptifibatide and tirofiban. All of these drugs cause thrombocytopenia, but the effect is strongest with abciximab (incidence of about 2.5%).

## Anticoagulants

### Vitamin K Antagonists

Warfarin, the most frequently used oral vitamin K antagonist (VKA), disrupts the formation of factors II, VII, IX, and X and proteins C and S. Without vitamin K, these proteins do not undergo carboxylation and therefore cannot actively bind to the phospholipid membrane of platelets during hemostasis (Fig. 22.4).

Warfarin has a long half-life (40 hours), and the complete anticoagulant effects take 48 to 72 hours to develop after administration because of the half-lives of the preexisting coagulation factors. Prothrombin (factor II) has the longest half-life (~60 hours). Factor VII and protein C have the shortest half-lives (3 to 6

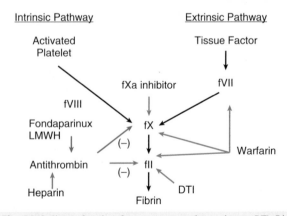

**Fig. 22.4** Sites of action for common anticoagulants. *DTI,* Direct thrombin inhibitor; *f,* factor; *LMWH,* low-molecular-weight heparin.

hours). Early reductions in the anticoagulant protein C can cause an imbalance toward a hypercoagulable state during the initiation of warfarin therapy, resulting in thrombosis or warfarin-induced skin necrosis. Patients at high risk for thromboembolism must be bridged with another anticoagulant (usually heparin) until the target INR is achieved.

The therapeutic range for warfarin anticoagulation is generally an INR of 2.0 to 3.0, except for patients with mechanical heart valves, in whom higher values are necessary (INR 2.5 to 3.5). The INR is not calibrated to evaluate coagulation deficiencies in liver disease and should not be used to evaluate therapeutic effects of other anticoagulants. Warfarin is difficult to manage because of a very narrow therapeutic window. Drugs, foods, and alcohol can profoundly alter the pharmacokinetic profile of warfarin, making frequent laboratory monitoring a necessity. Warfarin is contraindicated in pregnancy because fetal exposure can lead to embryopathy.

Warfarin's pharmacology is also affected by genetic variations in the metabolism of the drug (cytochrome P450, CYP2C9). Pharmacogenetic testing for polymorphisms that affect the metabolism of warfarin may be considered when there is difficulty achieving a target INR.

### Unfractionated Heparin
UFH indirectly inhibits thrombin and factor Xa by binding to AT (see Fig. 22.1). Heparin therapy is monitored with the aPTT or ACT. Benefits of heparin are its short half-life and ability to be fully reversed with protamine, a positively charged protein isolated from salmon. Patients may be resistant to UFH if they have hereditary insufficiency of AT or an acquired deficiency of AT from prolonged heparin administration. Treatment should be with FFP transfusions, which will replenish AT levels.

Full-dose heparin for cardiac surgery is administered as an intravenous bolus of 300 to 400 U/kg. An ACT greater than 400 seconds is usually considered safe for initiation of cardiopulmonary bypass. One mg protamine to 100 units of heparin is the reversal dose used at the conclusion of cardiopulmonary bypass.

The main complication of heparin, aside from bleeding risk, is HIT. UFH and to a lesser degree LMWH can stimulate the production of antibodies against the heparin–platelet factor 4 (PF4) complex. HIT is the most feared nonhemorrhagic complication of heparin and has a mortality rate of 20% to 30%. These antibodies can activate platelets to induce thrombosis and cause HIT. HIT should be suspected if the platelet count decreases to less than 100,000 cells/μL or less than 50% of baseline 5 to 10 days after the initiation of heparin therapy. If thrombocytopenia or thrombosis develops in a patient on heparin, HIT antibodies testing should be undertaken to confirm the diagnosis. The enzyme-linked immunosorbent assay

(ELISA) is sensitive but not as specific as the serotonin release assay, which is currently the gold standard. Patients with suspected HIT must be started on an alternate anticoagulant (not UFH or LMWH) immediately, while test results are pending. The most commonly used agents are the parenteral DTIs such as bivalirudin, argatroban, and lepirudin. Warfarin is contraindicated for HIT treatment because the initial decreased synthesis of proteins C and S enhances the patient's prothrombotic state. Platelet transfusions should also be held unless the patient is severely thrombocytopenic (<20,000 cells/μL) with signs of bleeding.

A difficult decision about anticoagulation arises when patients with a history of HIT require cardiopulmonary bypass. If time allows, antibody titers to heparin–PF4 complex should be measured. If titers are low, then a single dose of heparin can be considered for cardiac bypass. Otherwise, bivalirudin, the shortest acting DTI, is the alternative agent for anticoagulation while on bypass. Presurgical treatment with plasmapheresis for rapid antibody clearance is an alternative plan, but risks and benefits should be discussed with a hematologist.

### Low-Molecular-Weight Heparin and Fondaparinux
LMWH, produced by cleaving heparin into shorter fragments, and fondaparinux, a synthetic pentasaccharide, act more specifically to inhibit factor Xa via AT. LMWH and fondaparinux do not affect the aPTT assay, and coagulation testing is usually not needed. However, if necessary, the drugs' plasma activity levels can be assessed with factor Xa levels. This may be helpful in patients with renal failure, which affects drug excretion, or in pregnant women, obese patients, and neonates for whom drug levels are less certain after subcutaneous injection. LMWH and fondaparinux have longer half-lives than heparin and can be administered subcutaneously either once or twice daily. Protamine is only partially effective in reversing LMWH and not effective for fondaparinux. LMWH is contraindicated in HIT. Although the incidence of HIT is relatively rare for fondaparinux, cases have been reported, and it is not approved for use in HIT.

### Direct Thrombin Inhibitors
All DTIs inhibit thrombin in its free and fibrin-bound states, unlike heparin, which only has an effect on free thrombin. Clinical effects can be monitored with aPTT or ACT in the operating room. Hirudin is a naturally occurring anticoagulant found in leeches. Lepirudin is recombinant hirudin derived from yeast cells, whereas argatroban and bivalirudin are synthetic agents. Argatroban, which has a half-life of 45 minutes, is the preferred DTI in patients with renal insufficiency because it is hepatically eliminated. Bivalirudin is a reversible DTI and is metabolized by plasma proteases and renally excreted.

It has the shortest half-life and is the drug of choice for patients with both renal and hepatic dysfunction. There are no antidotes for any of the DTIs, so reversal depends upon their clearance. All DTIs will interfere with the INR, but argatroban will prolong the INR the most, which can complicate transition to warfarin therapy for long-term anticoagulation.

### New Oral Anticoagulants

During the past few years, several direct oral anticoagulants (DOACs) have been introduced into the market. These new drugs have more predictable pharmacokinetics and pharmacodynamics and fewer interactions with foods and other drugs. The predictability allows for fixed daily dosing without the need for monitoring, but the drawback is the lack of specific antidotes for anticoagulation reversal and a paucity of evidence to guide placement of neuraxial/peripheral blocks (also see Chapter 40).

The DOACs have a shorter half-life than warfarin and have demonstrated noninferior efficacy to warfarin. A meta-analysis of phase II and phase III randomized clinical trials comparing DOACs with VKAs in patients with atrial fibrillation showed that use of DOACs was associated with a significant reduction in major bleeding (relative risk [RR] 0.86, 95% confidence interval [CI] 0.72-1.02) and significantly decreased the risk of intracranial hemorrhage (RR 0.46, 95% CI 0.39 to 0.56).[11] Comparison of apixaban, a factor Xa inhibitor, versus warfarin in patients with atrial fibrillation showed a reduction of stroke along with a significant reduction in major bleeding.[12]

Dabigatran (Pradaxa), an oral DTI, is approved for the prevention of ischemic stroke in patients with nonvalvular atrial fibrillation and the treatment of VTE. Direct factor Xa inhibitors, rivaroxaban (Xarelto) and apixaban (Eliquis), are new drugs whose activity is directed against the active site of factor Xa. These drugs are approved for use in DVT/PE prophylaxis, stroke prophylaxis in patients with atrial fibrillation, and VTE treatment.

Although monitoring is not routine, it would be useful in patients presenting with relatively high or low body weight, renal insufficiency (dabigatran), patients taking other medications that alter P-glycoprotein and cytochrome P450 metabolism, overdoses, life-threatening bleeding, or need for emergent surgery. The perfect laboratory test would be the dilute thrombin time or ecarin clotting time for DTI and an anti–factor Xa assay calibrated for the specific direct factor Xa inhibitor; however, these tests are currently not widely available.

There are limited data regarding the use of these new anticoagulants with regional anesthesia, which includes neuraxial techniques. Most recommendations are based exclusively on the pharmacokinetics and pharmacodynamics of these drugs.[13]

In the event of an emergency, antidotes are becoming available. Idarucizumab, a specific antidote for dabigatran, is a humanized antibody fragment that binds to dabigatran with an affinity 350 times greater than thrombin. Andexanet alfa, a recombinant factor Xa, was developed to reverse the factor Xa inhibitors. Lastly, ciraparantag (PER977), a small, synthetic, water-soluble, cationic molecule, binds and neutralizes UFH, LMWH, fondaparinux, dabigatran, and the new factor Xa inhibitors through hydrogen bonding and charge-charge interactions. Idarucizumab has been approved by the FDA whereas andexanet alfa and ciraparantag are still undergoing clinical trials.

Because dabigatran and rivaroxiban/apixaban are competitive inhibitors of thrombin and factor Xa, respectively, in theory, it would make physiologic sense to attempt reversal with a PCC, but randomized controlled in vivo studies are lacking. There are some case reports that hemodialysis can eliminate dabigatran. Further research is needed to document the best method for reversing the clinical effects of these NOACs. Fortunately, their half-lives are relatively short, so time and supportive medical care are often enough to manage the acute clinical situation.

### Thrombolytics

Thrombolytic therapy is used to break up or dissolve blood clots during acute myocardial infarctions (within 12 hours), strokes (within 3 hours), or massive pulmonary embolus. Thrombolysis may be given through an intravenous line systemically or directly to the site of the blockage. Most thrombolytic agents are serine proteases that work by converting plasminogen to plasmin, which then lyses the clot by breaking down fibrinogen and fibrin.

Fibrinolytic drugs are divided into two categories: (1) fibrin-specific drugs and (2) non–fibrin-specific drugs. Recombinant tPAs (e.g., alteplase, reteplase, and tenecteplase) are fibrin-specific drugs that theoretically produce less plasminogen conversion in the absence of fibrin. Non–fibrin-specific drugs (e.g., streptokinase) catalyze systemic fibrinolysis. Streptokinase, produced by β-hemolytic streptococci, is highly antigenic and can cause immunologic sensitization and allergic reactions, particularly with repeat administration. Streptokinase is not widely used in the United States but is still used elsewhere because of its lower cost.

tPAs are both thrombolytics and anticoagulants because fibrinolysis generates increased amounts of circulating fibrin degradation products, which inhibit platelet aggregation by binding to platelet surfaces. Surgery or puncture of noncompressible vessels is contraindicated within a 10-day period after the use of thrombolytic drugs.

## Procoagulants

There are really only two main causes of perioperative bleeding. The first and most common is surgical bleeding, which will not be discussed here (see Chapter 24). The second is nonsurgical bleeding, or failure of the hemostatic pathways. Causes for this failure include massive blood transfusion (leading to thrombocytopenia, low fibrinogen, and coagulopathy) (also see Chapter 24), fibrinolysis (induced by the surgical procedure such as prostatectomy, orthotopic liver transplant [also see Chapter 36], or exposure to a foreign graft material), DIC (from sepsis, cardiopulmonary bypass [also see Chapter 25]), or transfusion reactions [also see Chapter 24]), an undetected preexisting bleeding disorder, or a combination of the foregoing possibilities.

The mainstays of massive blood loss management include replacement of red blood cells, platelets, clotting factors, and fibrinogen. The patient needs to be kept warm and frequent laboratory reports are necessary to help guide transfusions and electrolyte replacements. A basic laboratory profile in the operating room should include hematocrit, platelet count, PT, aPTT, and fibrinogen level. Although blood products and transfusion thresholds are discussed separately in Chapter 24, some other procoagulants exist that could be helpful to the anesthesia provider when the patient is bleeding at a rapid rate.

### Antifibrinolytics

There are two types of antifibrinolytics: (1) the lysine analogs, EACA and TXA, and (2) a serine protease inhibitor, aprotinin. Aprotinin was removed from the U.S. market and is now only available in Europe and Canada. The lysine analogs work by competitively inhibiting the binding site on plasminogen and preventing its cleavage to plasmin. TXA and EACA likely have equivalent efficacy and decrease perioperative blood loss in cardiac surgery, liver transplantation, and orthopedic surgery.

In trauma patients (also see Chapter 42), TXA administration may reduce mortality rate (14.5% vs. 16%, $p$ = 0.0035), including the risk of death due to bleeding (4.9% vs. 5.8%, $p$ = 0.0077), without an increase in fatal or nonfatal vascular occlusive events.[14] Early treatment (≤1 hour) after traumatic injury significantly reduced the risk of death due to bleeding events in the tranexamic acid group (5.3%) versus placebo group (7.7%). Overall, the lysine analogs (TXA and EACA) likely should be considered for use in major surgery or critical bleeding.

### Recombinant Factor VIIa

rFVIIa increases the generation of thrombin (factor II), which enhances hemostasis. The drug was originally FDA approved for use in hemophiliac patients. It works by having an effect on both pathways of the coagulation system. In the TF dependent or extrinsic system, rFVIIa binds to TF at the site of vessel injury, causing activation of factor X. In the TF independent or intrinsic system, rFVIIa binds to the surface of the activated platelet, activating factor X. Both mechanisms result in a "burst" of thrombin and fibrin generation, which leads to clot formation. The half-life of rFVIIa is only 2 to 2.5 hours, so the initial dose may require repeating until the bleeding is controlled.

rFVIIa has generated a great deal of interest because of its ability to enhance hemostasis in patients with severe bleeding. The off-label uses of rFVIIa have been quite varied and include intracranial hemorrhage, cardiac surgery, trauma, traumatic brain injury, and liver transplantation. If all trials are analyzed together, there is a slight reduction in the number of patients who need packed red blood cell transfusions, but there is no evidence that the use of rFVIIa changed overall survival rate.

Because of concern for arterial and venous thrombosis, prophylactic use of rFVIIa is questionable. Considering that no randomized controlled trial has been able to demonstrate a significant benefit in terms of intensive care unit (ICU) stay, hospital stay, or mortality rate, each clinician will have to weigh the risk of thromboembolic events against the benefit of clotting for the individual patient.

### Prothrombin Complex Concentrate

PCCs are commercially available formulations containing varying amounts of coagulation factors (factors II, VII, IX, and X) as well as one or more types of anticoagulants (protein C or S). Three-factor PCCs differ from four-factor PCCs in that they do not contain significant amounts of factor VII. Most of the factors are administered in the inactive state, which is supposed to decrease the thrombogenic risks. PCCs are now the drug of choice for emergent reversal of VKAs in place of rFVIIa or FFP. Although PCCs are derived from human plasma, they are treated with at least one viral reduction process, which reduces the risk for infectious and noninfectious transfusion reactions.

## PERIOPERATIVE MANAGEMENT OF ANTICOAGULATION

The perioperative management of patients who require chronic anticoagulation or antiplatelet therapy involves two major risk determinations: (1) the risk of a thrombotic complication for that patient and (2) the risk of a major bleeding complication from the procedure being performed. A multidisciplinary team should evaluate patients a few weeks prior to elective surgery to perform these necessary risk assessments and make management decisions regarding continuation, stoppage, and reinstitution of anticoagulation or antiplatelet therapy.

For those patients taking VKAs, the current recommendation is to stop VKAs 5 days prior to surgery for

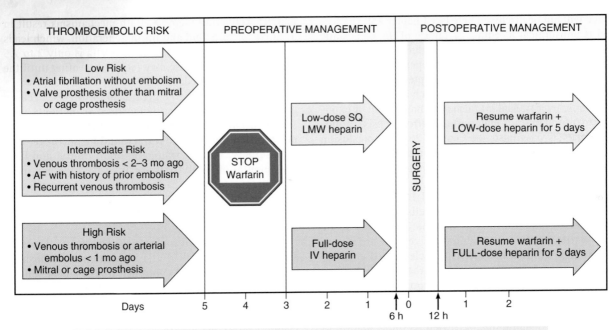

**Fig. 22.5** Perioperative management of an anticoagulated patient. *AF*, Atrial fibrillation; *IV*, intravenous; *LMW*, low-molecular-weight; *SQ*, subcutaneous. (From Stratmann G. Hemostasis. In Miller RD, Pardo MC, eds. *Basics of Anesthesia.* 6th ed. Philadelphia: Elsevier; 2011.)

those patients who are at low risk for perioperative VTE. VKAs should be restarted 12 to 24 hours postoperatively. For patients at high risk of VTE, the current recommendation is bridging with heparin or LMWH after discontinuation of VKAs prior to surgery. No clear evidence exists for patients who are at moderate risk for VTE with regard to discontinuation of VKAs and bridging, so the approach chosen is based on the individual patient and surgical risk factors. For those patients receiving bridging therapy with UFH, the infusion should be stopped 4 to 6 hours prior to surgery and resumed without a bolus dose no sooner than 12 hours postoperatively. In surgeries with increased postoperative bleeding risk, resumption of UFH should be delayed 48 to 72 hours. In patients receiving bridging therapy with LMWH, the last dose of LMWH should be administered 24 hours prior to surgery and dosing should be resumed 24 hours postoperatively (or delayed until 48 to 72 hours postoperatively for surgeries with high bleeding risk)[15] (Fig. 22.5).

For patients receiving antiplatelet therapy, risk assessment is based on the patient's risk of a perioperative cardiovascular event, whether the surgery is a minor procedure, noncardiac major procedure, or cardiac procedure, and the timing and type of stent placement for those patients who have undergone recent PCI. Many studies have examined management

of aspirin therapy perioperatively, but there are fewer data for management of clopidogrel in the perioperative setting. For patients undergoing minor procedures who are receiving acetylsalicylic acid (ASA) or aspirin for the secondary prevention of cardiovascular events, ASA should be continued throughout the perioperative period. In addition, patients who are at high or moderate risk for cardiovascular events, as well as those undergoing cardiac or vascular surgery, should continue ASA throughout the perioperative period. Patients who are at low risk for cardiovascular events and who are undergoing noncardiac surgery should discontinue ASA therapy 7 to 10 days prior to surgery. Patients on dual antiplatelet therapy (ASA and clopidogrel) should discontinue clopidogrel 5 days prior to cardiac or noncardiac surgery.

Lastly, for patients who have undergone recent PCI with coronary stent placement, surgery should be delayed for at least 6 weeks after placement of a bare-metal stent (BMS) and for at least 6 months after placement of a drug-eluting stent (DES). If surgery is required before this time has passed, dual antiplatelet therapy should be continued unless the risk of bleeding outweighs the risk of stent thrombosis.

In addition to surgical bleeding risk assessment, many patients who are receiving anticoagulant or antiplatelet therapy can potentially benefit from neuraxial

| Table 22.5 | University of California San Francisco Guidelines for the Use of Antithrombotic Drugs in the Setting of Neuraxial Procedures | | | |
|---|---|---|---|---|
| Anticoagulant | Minimum Time Between the Last Dose and When Neuraxial Catheter Can Occur | Minimum Time After Catheter Placement to Drug Start | Minimum Time Between Last Dose and Catheter Removal | Minimum Time Between Neuraxial Catheter Removal and When Next Dose Can Be Given |
| NSAIDs/ASA | No restrictions for catheter placement or removal | | | |
| Heparin SQ bid | No restrictions for catheter placement or removal | | | |
| Heparin SQ tid | 4 hours | 2 hours | 4 hours | 2 hours |
| Lovenox qd | 12 hours | 6 hours | 12 hours | 4 hours |
| Clopidogrel | 7 days | Contraindicated while catheter in place | | 2 hours |
| Ticlodipine | 14 days | Contraindicated while catheter in place | | 2 hours |
| Dabigatran | 5 days | Contraindicated while catheter in place | | 6 hours |
| Rivaroxaban | 3 days | Contraindicated while catheter in place | | 6 hours |
| Apixaban | 3 days | Contraindicated while catheter in place | | 6 hours |
| Abciximab | 48 hours | Contraindicated while catheter in place | | 2 hours |
| Eptifibatide | 8 hours | Contraindicated while catheter in place | | 2 hours |
| Alteplase | 10 days | Contraindicated while catheter in place | | 10 days |

ASA, Acetylsalicylic acid; bid, twice a day; NSAIDs, nonsteroidal antiinflammatory drugs; qd, every day; SQ, subcutaneous; tid, three times a day.

anesthesia procedures. Given the abundance of different antithrombotic medications being used in the perioperative setting to treat thrombosis and prevent postoperative thrombotic events, anesthesia providers must be aware of the risks of bleeding and neurologic injury associated with each therapy. These guidelines and recommendations will continue to be updated as evidence emerges on the bleeding risk and pharmacologic profiles of the newer anticoagulants. In the absence of concrete data, many hospital committees are setting local practice guidelines (Table 22.5).

Management of perioperative anticoagulation is becoming increasingly more complex with the advent of the DOACs and the number of patients who are now receiving chronic anticoagulation. Continued research on thromboembolic events and bleeding risk in the setting of these novel therapies is needed before official recommendations can be made regarding management. Early preoperative assessment of patients receiving anticoagulation and a multidisciplinary team approach between the patient, primary care physician, surgeon, anesthesia provider, and hematologist is essential to ensure the perioperative safety of these patients.

## QUESTIONS OF THE DAY

1. What are the steps in the coagulation cascade after the initial formation of a platelet plug at the site of vascular endothelial injury?
2. Which regulatory molecules facilitate termination of the coagulation cascade?
3. A patient presents with a history of von Willebrand disease (vWD). What are the different types of vWD?
4. What are the two most common hereditary hypercoagulable states? What is the mechanism of the prothrombotic state in each?
5. What are the clinical manifestations of heparin-induced thrombocytopenia (HIT)? What diagnostic tests can be used to confirm the diagnosis? If a patient with HIT requires ongoing anticoagulation, what medications can be used as an alternative?
6. A patient develops diffuse bleeding during surgery. How can thromboelastography be used to assess coagulation status?
7. What coagulation factors are present in prothrombin complex concentrate (PCC)? What are the indications for administration of this concentrate?

## REFERENCES

1. Stalker TJ, Welsh JD, Brass LF. Shaping the platelet response to vascular injury. *Curr Opin Hematol.* 2014;21(5):410–417.
2. Berndt MC, Metharom P, Andrews RK. Primary haemostasis: newer insights. *Haemophilia.* 2014;20(suppl 4):15–22.
3. Chapin JC, Hajjar KA. Fibrinolysis and the control of blood coagulation. *Blood Rev.* 2015;29(1):17–24.
4. Mensah PK, Gooding R. Surgery in patients with inherited bleeding disorders. *Anaesthesia.* 2015;70(suppl 1):112–120. e39–e40.
5. Kempton CL, Meeks SL. Toward optimal therapy for inhibitors in hemophilia. *Blood.* 2014;124(23):3365–3372.
6. Lim W. Antiphospholipid syndrome. *Hematology Am Soc Hematol Educ Program.* 2013;2013:675–680.
7. Venugopal A. Disseminated intravascular coagulation. *Indian J Anaesth.* 2014;58(5):603–608.
8. De Stefano V, Rossi E. Testing for inherited thrombophilia and consequences for antithrombotic prophylaxis in patients with venous thrombo-embolism and their relatives. A review of the Guidelines from Scientific Societies and Working Groups. *Thromb Haemost.* 2013;110(4):697–705.
9. Lancé MD. A general review of major global coagulation assays: thromb-elastography, thrombin generation test and clot waveform analysis. *Thromb J.* 2015;13:1–6.
10. Coxib and traditional NSAID Trialists' (CNT) Collaboration. Vascular and upper gastrointestinal effects of non-steroidal anti-inflammatory drugs: meta-analyses of individual participant data from randomised trials. *Lancet.* 2013;382:769–779.
11. Dentali F, Riva N, Crowther M, et al. Efficacy and safety of the novel oral anticoagulants in atrial fibrillation: a systematic review and meta-analysis of the literature. *Circulation.* 2012;126:2381–2391.
12. Granger CB, Alexander JH, McMurray JJ, et al. Apixaban versus warfarin in patients with atrial fibrillation. *N Engl J Med.* 2011;365:981–992.
13. Horlocker T, Wedel D, Rowlingson J, et al. Regional anesthesia in the patient receiving antithrombotic or thrombolytic therapy: American Society of Regional Anesthesia and Pain Medicine Evidence-Based Guidelines (third edition). *Reg Anesth Pain Med.* 2010;35:64–101.
14. Shakur H, Roberts I, Bautista R, et al. Effects of tranexamic acid on death, vascular occlusive events, and blood transfusion in trauma patients with significant hemorrhage (CRASH2): a randomized, placebo controlled trial. *Lancet.* 2010;376(9734):23–32.
15. Douketis JD, Spyropoulos AC, Spencer FA, et al. American College of Chest Physicians. Perioperative management of antithrombotic therapy and Prevention of Thrombosis, 9th ed: American College of Chest Physicians Evidence-Based Clinical Practice Guidelines. *Chest.* 2012;141(suppl 2): e326S–e350S.

# FLUID MANAGEMENT

## Elizabeth A.M. Frost

The goals of perioperative fluid management are purported to provide appropriate amounts of parenteral fluid to maintain intravascular volume and cardiac preload, oxygen-carrying capacity, optimal coagulation status, acid-base homeostasis, and electrolyte balance. Just how these goals may be achieved remains controversial and often elusive. Over the past few years there has been a paradigm shift in perioperative fluid management not only in quantity but also in quality owing in part to changes in surgical and anesthetic techniques and also to the status of the patient population.

## BACKGROUND

Prior to the explanation of the heart and vascular system by Harvey in 1628, little was understood about the circulation.[1] The need for intravenous fluid replacement probably started during the cholera epidemic that broke out in India in 1827, spreading to Russia in 1829 and to England in 1831, finally reaching the United States in 1832.[2]

O'Shaughnessy, a recent Edinburgh graduate, performed an analysis on the blood and excreta of several victims and concluded that the blood . . .

> "has lost a large proportion of its water . . . it has lost also a great proportion of its neutral saline ingredients."[2] . . . the indications of cure . . . are two in number-viz. 1st to restore the blood to its natural specific gravity; 2nd to restore its deficient saline matters . . . the first of these can only besic, (sic) effected by absorption, by imbibition, or by the injection of aqueous fluid into the veins. . . . When absorption is entirely suspended . . . in those desperate cases . . . the author recommends the injection into the veins of tepid water holding a solution of the normal salts of the blood."[3]

Although intravenously administered anesthetics used to induce anesthesia became a standard approach during the second half of the 20th century, intravenous fluid

The editors and publisher would like to thank Dr. Alan David Kaye for contributing to this chapter in the previous edition of this work. It has served as the foundation for the current chapter.

infusions were restricted to extreme and complicated cases. Rather, through the 1950s it was standard practice to secure a vein with a right-angle steel needle. A moveable arm with a rubber patch on the outside of the skin was then moved to cover the hole of the needle within the vein. Should fluid or blood be required, small amounts could be injected via syringe or by presterilized and packaged infusion sets. These sets did not have filters when blood was given.

## OVERVIEW OF FLUID AND ELECTROLYTE PHYSIOLOGY

Water, the major component of fluid compartments in the body, makes up about 60% of body weight or 600 mL/kg. In a 70-kg individual that would represent about 40 L. Age, gender, adiposity, and physical activity are major factors that alter these percentages. Body water is divided between intracellular (66%) and extracellular (34%) spaces, separated by water-permeable cell membranes. The extracellular compartment comprises blood volume (60 to 65 mL/kg) and the interstitial fluid volume (120 to 165 mL/kg). The percentage of plasma, the noncellular component of blood, is a fraction of the blood, as measured by the hematocrit, and averages about 30 to 35 mL/kg. About 15% of blood is in the arterial side and 85% in the venous (and capillary) side. The higher oncotic pressure of plasma due to the protein content (20 mm Hg greater than interstitial pressure) helps to maintain intravascular volume. Daily maintenance requirements for adults approximate 1.5 to 2.5 L of water, 50 to 100 mEq sodium, 50 to 100 g glucose, and 40 to 80 mEq potassium.[4] The normal electrolyte composition in body compartments is shown in Table 23.1.

## PERIOPERATIVE FLUID BALANCE

Traditionally, preoperative fasting produces a fluid deficit, which is calculated as the maintenance fluid requirement

| Table 23.1 | Normal Electrolyte Composition in Body Compartments | | |
|---|---|---|---|
| Electrolyte | Plasma Fluid (mEq/L) | Intracellular Fluid (mEq/L) | Extracelluar Fluid (mEq/L) |
| Sodium | 142 | 10 | 140 |
| Potassium | 4 | 150 | 4.5 |
| Magnesium | 2 | 40 | 2 |
| Calcium | 5 | 1 | 5 |
| Chloride | 103 | 103 | 117 |
| Bicarbonate | 25 | 7 | 28 |

Modified from Rhoades RA, Tanner GA. *Medical Physiology*. Boston: Little Brown; 1995.

multiplied by the duration of fasting since fluid intake. After fasting for 8 to 10 hours, the normal state after sleep, requirements in the noncomatose individual may be little more than 250 mL. Very few patients are likely to require 1500 to 2000 mL fluid within the first 1 to 2 hours of surgery. Preoperative fasting causes a slight decrease in extracellular fluid while maintaining intravascular volume.[5] Current fasting requirements encourage clear fluids for up to 2 hours before anesthesia. The use of evanescent anesthetics ensures a rapid return to consciousness. Also, insensible losses are decreased with laparoscopic incisions and by constant irrigation of the wound. The preoperative use of bowel preps has also decreased significantly. Finally, antidiuretic hormone release during anesthesia severely curtails the ability of the kidneys to remove excess fluid.

The concept of the "third space" grew out of a study in the 1960s with two groups of patients: group 1 consisted of 5 patients undergoing minor surgery with general anesthesia (cyclopropane and ether); group 2 (13 patients) had elective major surgical procedures (cholecystectomy, gastrectomy, and colectomy). Plasma volume, red blood cell mass, and extracellular fluid volumes were measured in all patients on two occasions during the operative period by using [131]I-tagged serum albumin, [51]Cr-labeled red blood cells, and [35]S-tagged sodium sulfate. The authors determined that the loss of functional extracellular fluid in group 2 was due to an internal redistribution because of surgery; in other words, there is a "third space" that must be replaced.[6] This conclusion was argued by Moore who wrote that the redistribution was due to antidiuretic hormone release and that intravenous fluid administration should follow a more restricted approach.[7] Although both groups later recommended moderation, the concept of the "third space" became firmly established. Although inadequate fluid administration can be harmful, excessive fluid replacement is also associated with poorer outcome. Although the concept of the "third space" may have some validity, its overall validity has been questioned.[8]

Currently, patients undergoing major surgical procedures do require fluid replacement based mainly on losses from the surgical site as well as hourly needs, which will be defined later.

## FLUID REPLACEMENT SOLUTIONS

Many crystalloid and colloid solutions are available and appropriate for adults (Table 23.2). Blood and blood products are discussed in Chapter 24. The British Consensus Guidelines on Intravenous Fluid Therapy for Adult Surgical Patients contains many evidence-scored recommendations to assist in intravenous fluid management.[4] However, controversy in fluid replacement is still common, and many recommendations are seriously challenged.[9]

## Crystalloids

Crystalloids are grouped as balanced, isotonic, hypertonic, and hypotonic salt solutions in water, depending on the amount of electrolytes they contain. They cross rapidly from the vascular to the interstitial spaces (e.g., gut, lungs, dependent parts) with only about one third remaining intravascular.

### Balanced Salt Solutions

The electrolyte composition of balanced salt solutions is similar to that of extracellular fluid. Examples include lactated Ringer solution (similar to Hartmann solution), Plasma-Lyte, and Normosol. These solutions are hypotonic with respect to sodium. The added buffer (e.g., lactate) is metabolized in vivo to generate bicarbonate. They each contain small amounts of other electrolytes such as potassium, magnesium, and calcium. A Cochrane database review concluded that the administration of buffered fluids is equally safe as nonbuffered saline-based fluids and is associated with less metabolic derangements, especially hyperchloremia and metabolic acidosis.[10]

### Normal Saline

Normal saline (0.9% NaCl) is hypertonic with equal concentrations of $Na^+$ and $Cl^-$ even though the plasma concentration of $Na^+$ normally is 40 mEq/L higher than that of $Cl^-$. Concerns have been raised that normal saline, which is probably the most widely used of all solutions for resuscitation, is associated with significant hyperchloremic metabolic acidosis and the need for renal replacement therapy, as compared to resuscitation with balanced crystalloid solutions.[4,11] These effects may well be dose dependent and in otherwise healthy individuals may be of no clinical significance.[9] Avoiding an increased $Cl^-$ concentration or using fluids that lessen the increase in $Cl^-$ reduces the risk of renal dysfunction, infections, and possibly even death.[12] Either normal saline or Plasma-Lyte may be used for diluting packed red blood cells, but lactated Ringer solution should be avoided as it contains calcium.

### Hypertonic Saline

Use of hypertonic solutions generally is restricted to specific situations such as control of intracranial hypertension or the need for rapid intravascular resuscitation. The sodium concentrations range from 250 to 1200 mEq/L; the inverse relation between the concentration of sodium and the amount of fluid required is due to the osmotic gradient from the intracellular to the extracellular spaces. Patients predisposed to tissue edema might benefit from use of a hypertonic solution. However, the half-life of hypertonic solutions is similar to that of isotonic solutions. Sustained expansion of plasma volume is not achieved unless colloids are present. Also, the osmolarity may cause hemolysis at the point of injection.

### Five Percent Dextrose

Five percent dextrose is similar to free water as the dextrose is metabolized. It is iso-osmotic and does not cause hemolysis. With the realization that hyperglycemia is associated with poor outcome and the stress of the operative period causes blood sugar levels to increase, 5% dextrose solutions are seldom used currently except for the treatment and/or prevention of hypoglycemia or hypernatremia.

| Table 23.2 | Composition of Replacement Fluids | | | | | |
| --- | --- | --- | --- | --- | --- | --- |
| **Fluid** | **Na (mEq/L)** | **K (mEq/L) (g/L)** | **Glucose (g/L)** | **Osm** | **pH** | **Other** |
| 5% Albumin | 145 ± 15 | <2.5 | 0 | 330 | 7.4 | COP 32-35 mm Hg |
| Plasmanate | 145 ± 15 | <2.0 | | | 7.4 | COP 20 mm Hg |
| 10% Dextran 40 | 0 | 0 | 0 | 255 | 4.0 | |
| HES 450/0.7 | 154 | 0 | 0 | 310 | 5.9 | |
| 0.9% NaCl | 154 | 0 | 0 | 308 | 6.0 | |
| Lactated Ringer | 130 | 4 | 0 | 273 | 6.5 | Lactate 28 mEq/L |
| 5% Dextrose | 0 | 0 | 50 | 252 | 4.5 | |
| D5LR | 130 | 4 | 50 | 525 | 5.0 | |
| D50.45% NaCl | 77 | 0 | 50 | 406 | 4.0 | |
| Normosol-R | 140 | 5 | 0 | 294 | 6.6 | Mg 3 mEq/L, acetate 27 mEq/L, gluconate 23 mEq/L |
| Plasma-Lyte A | 140 | 5 | 0 | 295 | 7.4 | |

*COP*, Colloid oncotic pressure; *D5LR*, 5% dextrose in lactated Ringer's solution; *D50.45% NaCl*, 5% dextrose in 0.45% NaCl; *HES*, hydroxyethyl starches; *Osm*, osmolarity.

From Kaye AD. Fluid management. In Miller RD, Pardo MC Jr, eds. *Basics of Anesthesia*. 6th ed. Philadelphia: Elsevier; 2011:364.

## Colloids

Colloid solutions, albumin, and starches contain large-molecular-weight substances that remain in the intravascular space for significantly longer periods than crystalloids. The synthetic starches have little to no risk of infection, but allergic reactions can occur. They are more expensive than crystalloids but less expensive with fewer risks than with blood replacement.

### Albumin

Albumin is supplied as a 5% or 25% solution. Albumin comprises about 50% of plasma proteins. The initial volume of distribution is equivalent to the plasma volume, and it remains in the intravascular space for a longer duration than crystalloids. Preparation removes viruses and bacteria. There is little effect on coagulation.

### Dextran

First discovered by Pasteur as a microbial product in wine, dextrans are complex branched polysaccharides composed of chains of lengths varying from 3 to 2000 kilodaltons (kDa). The two used medically are dextran 40 (40 kDa) and dextran 70 (70 kDa). Dextrans are used as antithrombotics to reduce blood viscosity, and as intravascular volume expanders in hypovolemia. Dextrans are synthesized from sucrose by lactic acid bacteria, such as *Leuconostoc mesenteroides* and *Streptococcus mutans*. The antithrombotic effect is due to binding of erythrocytes, platelets, and vascular endothelium, increasing the electronegativity and reducing erythrocyte aggregation and platelet adhesiveness. Dextrans also reduce factor VIII-Ag von Willebrand factor and, hence, platelet function. By inhibiting $\alpha_2$-antiplasmin, dextran serves as a plasminogen activator, and so possesses thrombolytic features. Dextrans remain intravascular, are potent osmotic agents, and have been used to treat hypovolemia, although less so nowadays. The hemodilution caused by intravascular volume expansion also improves blood flow, which provides a theoretical advantage in promoting patency of microanastomoses and reducing thrombosis. However, a recent study did not find antithrombotics, including dextrans, of value in improving free flap survival.[13]

Both solutions are degraded to glucose. Side effects include anaphylactic or anaphylactoid reactions in about 1:3300 administrations, increased bleeding times, and rarely, noncardiogenic pulmonary edema.

### Hydroxyethyl Starch

Hydroxyethyl starches (HES) are nonionic starch derivatives and were one of the most frequently used intravascular volume expanders. These synthetic colloids are modifications of natural polysaccharides. They are characterized by concentration and molecular weight. Six percent solutions are isotonic. Molecular weights vary from under 70 kDa to over 450 kDa. The molar

substitution and C2/C6 ratios are also factors. The molar substitutions refer to the number of hydroxyethyl residues per 10 glucose subunits. Preparations with 7 hydroxyethyl residues per 10 glucose units (a ratio of 0.7) are hetastarches. The larger the molecular weight and molar substitution, the longer the duration of the increase in intravascular volume effect but at the expense of more side effects. The C2/C6 ratio describes the pattern of hydroxyethyl substitution on specific carbon atoms of the HES glucose subunits. HES preparations with higher C2/C6 ratios are more resistant to breakdown by amylase, and have a prolonged duration of effect without an increase in side effects. Several preparations are available: Hespan (B. Braun Medical Inc.) is 6% HES 450/0.7; Hextend (Biotime Inc.) is 6% HES 670/0.7; Voluven (Fresenius Kabi) is 6% HES 130/0.4 in 0.9% NaCl, or Volvulyte (Fresenius Kabi) is 6% HES 130/0.4 in a balanced electrolyte solution. Pentastarch is a subgroup of HES with 5 hydroxyethyl groups out of each 11 hydroxyls, giving it approximately 50% hydroxyethylation, which compares with tetrastarch at 40% and HES at 70% hydroxyethylation, respectively.

HES interferes with von Willebrand, factor VIII, and platelet function. The dose-dependent risk of dilutional coagulopathy differs between colloids (dextran > hetastarch > pentastarch > tetrastarch, gelatins > albumin). Monitoring for early signs of side effects can include use of rotational thromboelastometry/thromboelastography to assess the deterioration not only in clot strength but also in clot formation and in platelet interaction.[14]

Higher molecular weight preparations may have side effects related to the solvent, as Hespan is dissolved in saline and Hextend in a balanced salt solution. The most common complication associated with HES administration is pruritus, which occurs in up to 22% of patients.

A systematic review of HES administration in intensive care unit (ICU) patients requiring intravascular volume resuscitation revealed an association of HES use and risk of mortality and acute kidney injury.[15] The FDA (Food and Drug Administration) accordingly issued a black box warning in 2013, advising that HES solutions not be used in adult critically ill patients, including those with sepsis.[16]

The choice of fluid for intravenous administration should be guided by the cause of the hypovolemia, the cardiovascular state of the patient, and the renal function, as well as the serum osmolarity, comorbid conditions, and any coexisting acid-base and electrolyte disorders.[17]

## Crystalloids Versus Colloids

The debate over crystalloid versus colloid persists and has stimulated many clinical studies—primarily in the adult critical care patient population. The fundamental principles are described in this section (also see Chapter 41).

Crystalloids dilute plasma proteins and decrease plasma oncotic pressure. Fluid is extravasated to interstitial compartments causing edema of the gastrointestinal tract and all dependent parts and extra lung fluid. Colloids given after blood loss in a ratio of 1:1 restores intravascular blood volume more rapidly. Colloids, although remaining in the vascular space longer, have more complications and are expensive. A Cochrane review of 78 randomized controlled trials of intravascular fluid resuscitation in critically ill patients concluded that resuscitation with colloid (albumin mainly) did not reduce the risk of death and HES might increase mortality rate.[18] Another Cochrane study of kidney function in patients receiving HES versus other fluid therapies for volume depletion reviewed over 40 randomized controlled trials. HES use was associated with increased risk of acute kidney injury and need for renal replacement therapy.[19] A safe volume of HES was not determined. The Surviving Sepsis Campaign (SSC) has issued international guidelines regarding management of patients with severe sepsis and septic shock, including the management of fluid therapy.[20] Recommendations include use of crystalloids as the initial fluid choice, avoidance of HES fluids, and use of albumin when patients require substantial amounts of crystalloid. The Saline versus Albumin Fluid Evaluation (SAFE) study of albumin versus saline for intravascular fluid resuscitation in the ICU evaluated almost 7000 patients in a randomized controlled trial. At 28 days, there was no difference in outcomes (including death, ICU length of stay, or organ failure), but a small subgroup of patients with traumatic brain injury had increased mortality rate after resuscitation with albumin.[21]

Although the aforementioned studies are primarily in the adult critical care population, they may be relevant in the perioperative setting as well, especially for complex or prolonged surgical procedures.

## PERIOPERATIVE FLUID STRATEGIES

Although it might seem simple to arrive at a fluid management formula that could be applied universally in the perioperative setting, many difficulties have arisen. First, there has been little consensus as to what represents liberal (20 mL/kg/h), standard (5 to 10 mL/kg/h), or restrictive fluid replacement (2 to 5 mL/kg/h). Most studies have not been standardized, so reasonable comparisons cannot be performed. The specific clinical targets are also open to speculation (Box 23.1). Many clinicians are unwilling to change established protocols in their practice. There is no clear differentiation between major and minor surgery. Perhaps the target that has been most closely associated with adverse outcome is that of weight gain. A small study of primarily postcardiac surgery ICU patients demonstrated increased mortality rate in the patients with the greatest postoperative weight

| Box 23.1 | Study Targets |
| --- | --- |
| Weight gain | Need for revision surgery |
| Postoperative nausea and vomiting | Speed of wound healing |
| | Infection |
| Pain | Cardiovascular complications |
| Tissue oxygenation | Length of hospital stay |
| Postoperative ileus | Development of coagulopathies |
| Pneumonia | |

increase during their ICU stay.[22] Although this does not demonstrate a cause-effect relationship, it does raise the question of "how much is too much fluid?" By way of contrast, for healthy patients having minor elective surgery (e.g., young women undergoing short gynecologic procedures), liberal fluid administration (20 to 30 mL/kg) was associated with less nausea and vomiting and improved pain control.[8]

How did perioperative fluid management evolve? Following the discovery of the "third space" by Shires and associates[6] in the 1960s, protocols were developed to compensate for it and for other supposed intraoperative requirements. The 4:2:1 or 100-50-20 rule was developed and has remained in general use despite its lack of relevance to current anesthetic practice.[23] Fluids are infused depending on weight: 4 mL/kg/h for the first 10 kg, 2 mL/kg/h for the next 10 kg, and finally 1 mL/kg/h thereafter; or looking at daily replacement, 100 mL/kg for the first 10 kg, 50 mL/kg for the next 10 kg, and 20 mL/kg for weight over that. Holliday's article[23] of almost 60 years ago was intended as a general guide to daily needs of children and was not meant specifically for intraoperative application. It was based on three theories from even earlier work:

1. Surface area can estimate water expenditure.[24]
2. Caloric needs depend on age, weight, activity, and food.[25]
3. Urinary output and insensible losses correspond to age.[26]

"Rules" for fluid replacement, therefore, were developed without scientific evidence, and much information was based on unpublished data. Apart from the fact that the formulas were not meant for adults, anesthetic and surgical techniques have changed drastically. The relevance in today's practice should be questioned.

A recent meta-analysis shows that larger fluid volumes are required to meet the same targets if a goal-directed approach is used with crystalloids than with colloids, with an estimated ratio of 1.5 (1.36-1.65).[27] Again, there is little consistency among studies and the reasons behind such heterogeneity are unclear. The suggested crystalloid-colloid ratio has decreased over the years as less crystalloid is infused. Differences in ratios correlate mainly with the concentration of albumin solutions.

**Table 23.3** Assumptions Underlying "Classic" Approaches to Perioperative Fluid Management

| Assumption | Problems With Assumption |
| --- | --- |
| The patient is fasted preoperatively and is thus hypovolemic. | BUT current fasting guidelines allow water ingestion up to 2 hours prior to surgery. The so-called fluid deficit in elective surgery is negligible. |
| Insensible losses continue during surgery and must be accounted for. | BUT with laparoscopic and other minimally invasive surgery there is little insensible loss. |
| Fluid shifts to the "third space" must be replaced. | BUT it is unlikely that the "third space" exists. |
| Blood loss must be replaced with three to four times the amount of crystalloid. | BUT there should be an assessment of fluid responsiveness to guide administration of fluid after blood loss. |
| Hypotension following induction of anesthesia is due to vasodilation, and the vascular space must be filled. | BUT anesthetic-induced vasodilation is better managed with vasopressors and/or lighter anesthesia to maintain peripheral vascular resistance. |
| Urine output must be taken into consideration and replaced. | BUT antidiuretic hormone excretion (ADH) during surgery makes urine output as a guide very unreliable. |
| Even if the patient has an excessive intravascular volume, the kidneys will regulate. | BUT the kidneys are already stressed by ADH, and it may take days or weeks to excrete a large fluid load. |

## Intraoperative Fluids

Several previous assumptions regarding preoperative fluid therapy need to be modified. Some of these assumptions are listed in Table 23.3.

Based on current findings, appropriate fluid replacement strategies for elective surgical procedures should consider the following principles:

1. No excessive administration of intravenous fluids at the start of a case or prior to epidural analgesia
2. No fluid replacement of "third space" or urine output
3. Replacement of surgical blood loss on a 1:1 basis with colloid
4. Use of colloid on a restricted basis for hypovolemia
5. Limit volume of crystalloids administered intraoperatively (e.g., limit to 100 to 200 mL/hr in the adult)
6. Preference for balanced salt solutions rather than normal saline
7. Postoperative restriction of fluids and use of diuretics if weight gain exceeds 1 kg

## Monitoring Adequacy of Fluid Replacement

Assessment of the adequacy of intravascular volume is essential in assuring appropriate vascular volume, cardiac function, and tissue oxygenation. Traditional measurements such as arterial blood pressure and heart rate react slowly to changes in intravascular volume, depending also on contractility and compensation.[28,29] Unfortunately, these measurements may not change with an intravascular fluid challenge, especially in elderly patients or those receiving cardiovascular medications (also see Chapters 25 and 35). Surgical stimulation and anesthetic drugs can also impact these basic vital signs without changing intravascular volume status. Central venous pressure (CVP) records pressure from the right atrium and does not reliably indicate circulating blood volume or intravascular volume responsiveness. CVP may remain "normal" long after both blood pressure and heart rate have declined. The use of pulmonary artery catheters has decreased in frequency of use. Serial hemoglobin levels are also notoriously subject to intraoperative variability.

Arterial pulse pressure variation induced by mechanical ventilation has been appreciated for decades as an indicator of "fluid responsiveness." Computerized analyses that incorporate information from the pulse oximeter arterial waveform provide an estimate of stroke volume variability and a prediction of response to intravascular fluid challenge. Several commercial monitors are available including Edwards Vigileo, System-Flo Trac, and Lidco, among others.[30,31] Also, transesophageal echocardiography (TEE) can be used to assess cardiac output and preload in order to guide fluid therapy (also see Chapter 20). A combination monitor of TEE and pulse pressure variation (PPV) is available as the Cardio–EDM.[32] Other monitors incorporate sensors on endotracheal tubes, and on finger probes again measuring PPV. Thus, intravascular fluid versus vasopressor therapy can be tailored to a patient's needs rather than general application of formulas.

Although controversy still exists as to how much and which fluids to use, the current recommendations are becoming clearer. Older formulas have little or no place in currently practiced perioperative care. Our standard monitors do not give accurate information and should be supplemented with newer techniques such as pulse pressure or stroke volume variation measurements. Above all, patients must be treated as individuals and their complete history and physical examination taken into account to allow sound clinical judgment to prevail.

## QUESTIONS OF THE DAY

1. What is the rationale for intravenous fluid replacement of the so-called preoperative fasting deficit? Do clinical studies support this practice?
2. What metabolic abnormalities are associated with normal saline administration, as compared to balanced salt solutions?
3. What are the potential adverse affects of hydroxyethyl starch (HES) administration? Which patient populations should not receive HES solutions?
4. What common assumptions about perioperative fluid management should be challenged?

## REFERENCES

1. Harvey W. Exercitatio Anatomica de Motu Cordis et Sanguinis in Animalibus. Frankfurt am Main, Germany: Sumptibus Guilielmi Fitzeri; 1628. Retrieved June 30, 2015. http://special.lib.gla.ac.uk/exhibns/month/june2007.html

2. O'Shaughnessy WB. The cholera in the North of England. *Lancet*. 1831;1:401–404.

3. O'Shaughnessy WB. Chemical pathology of cholera. *Lancet*. 1832;2:225–232.

4. National Institute for Health and Care Excellence. CG174 Intravenous Fluid Therapy in Adults in Hospital: guidelines, issued December 2013. http://www.nice.org.uk (under "search" CG 175). Accessed August 10, 2015.

5. Jacob M, Chappell D, Conzen P, et al. Blood volume is normal after pre-operative overnight fasting. *Acta Anaesthesiol Scand*. 2008;52(4):522–529.

6. Shires T, Williams J, Brown F. Acute changes in extracellular fluids associated with major surgical procedures. *Ann Surg*. 1961;154:803–810.

7. Moore FD. Common patterns of water and electrolyte changes in injury, surgery and disease. *N Engl J Med*. 1958;258(7):325–333.

8. Doherty M, Buggy DJ. Intraoperative fluids: how much is too much? *Br J Anaesth*. 2012;109(1):69–79.

9. Woodcock T. GIFTAHo; an improvement on GIFTASuP? New NICE guidelines on intravenous fluids. *Anaesthesia*. 2014;69(5):410–415.

10. Burdett E, Dushianthan A, Bennett-Guerrero E, et al. Perioperative buffered versus non-buffered fluid administration for surgery in adults. *Cochrane Database Syst Rev*. 2012;12:CD004089.

11. McCluskey SA, Karkouti K, Wijeysundera D, et al. Hyperchloremia after noncardiac surgery is independently associated with increased morbidity and mortality: a propensity-matched cohort study. *Anesth Analg*. 2013;117(2):412–421.

12. Magder S. Balanced versus unbalanced salt solutions: what difference does it make? *Best Pract Res Clin Anaesthesiol*. 2014;28(3):235–247.

13. Lee KT, Mun GH. The efficacy of postoperative antithrombotics in free flap surgery: a systematic review and meta-analysis. *Plast Reconstr Surg*. 2015;135(4):1124–1139.

14. Kozek-Langenecker SA. Fluids and coagulation. *Curr Opin Crit Care*. 2015;21(4):285–291.

15. Zarychanski R, Abou-Setta AM, Turgeon AF. Association of hydroxyethyl starch administration with mortality and acute kidney injury in critically ill patients requiring volume resuscitation: a systematic review and meta-analysis. *JAMA*. 2013;309(7):678–688.

16. Food and Drug Administration. FDA Safety Communication: Boxed warning on increased mortality and severe renal injury, and additional warning on risk of bleeding, for use of hydroxylethyl starch solutions in some settings. November 25, 2013. http://www.fda.gov/BiologicsBloodVaccines/SafetyAvailability/ucm358271.htm. Accessed April 26, 2016.

17. Liamis G, Filippatos TD, Elisaf MS. Correction of hypovolemia with crystalloid fluids: individualizing infusion therapy. *Postgrad Med*. 2015;127(4):405–412.

18. Perel P, Roberts I, Ker K. Colloids versus crystalloids for fluid resuscitation in critically ill patients. *Cochrane Database Syst Rev*. 2013;2:CD000567.

19. Mutter TC, Ruth CA, Dart AB. Hydroxyethyl starch (HES) versus other fluid therapies: effects on kidney function. *Cochrane Database Syst Rev*. 2013;7:CD007594.

20. Dellinger RP, Levy MM, Rhodes A, et al. Surviving sepsis campaign: international guidelines for management of severe sepsis and septic shock: 2012. *Crit Care Med*. 2013;41(2):580–637.

21. SAFE Study Investigators, Infer S, Bellomo R, Boyce N, et al. A comparison of albumin and saline for fluid resuscitation in the intensive care unit. *N Eng/ J Med*. 2004;350:2247–2256.

22. Lowell JA, Schifferdecker C, Driscoll DF, et al. Postoperative fluid overload: not a benign problem. *Crit Care Med*. 1990;18(7):728–733.

23. Holliday MA, Segar WE. The maintenance need for water in parenteral fluid therapy. *Pediatrics*. 1957;19:823–832.

24. Crawford JD, Terry ME, Rourke GM. Simplification of drug dosage calculation by application of the surface area principle. *Pediatrics*. 1950;5:783–790.

25. Darrow DC, Pratt EL. Fluid therapy; relation to tissue composition and the expenditure of water and electrolyte. *JAMA*. 1950;143(4):365–373.

26. Wallace WM. Quantitative requirements of the infant and child for water and electrolyte under varying conditions. *Am J Clin Pathol*. 1953;23(11):1133–1141.

27. Orbegozo Cortés D, Gamarano Barros T, Njimi H, Vincent JL. Crystalloids versus colloids: exploring differences in fluid requirements by systematic review and meta-regression. *Anesth Analg*. 2015;120(2):389–402.

28. Arulkumaran N, Corredor C, Hamilton MA, et al. Cardiac complications associated with goal directed therapy in high-risk surgical patients: a meta-analysis. *Br J Anaesth*. 2014;112(4):648–659.

29. Zheng H, Guo H, Ye J, et al. Goal directed fluid therapy in gastrointestinal surgery in older coronary heart disease patients; a randomized trial. *World J Surg*. 2013;37:2820–2829.

30. Auler Jr JO, Galas F, Hajjar L, et al. Online monitoring of pulse pressure variation to guide fluid therapy after cardiac surgery. *Anesth Analg*. 2008;106(4):1201–1206.

31. Peng K, Li J, Cheng H, Ji FH. Goal-directed fluid therapy based on stroke volume variations improves fluid management and gastrointestinal perfusion in patients undergoing major orthopedic surgery. *Med Princ Pract*. 2014;23(5):413–420.

32. Chytra I, Pradi R, Bosman R, et al. Esophageal Doppler-guided fluid management decreases blood lactate levels in multiple-trauma patients: a randomized controlled trial. *Crit Care*. 2007;11(1):R24.

# 24 BLOOD THERAPY

## Ronald D. Miller

Allogeneic blood transfusions are given for inadequate oxygen-carrying capacity/delivery and correction of coagulation deficits. Also, blood transfusions provide additional intravascular fluid volume. The American Society of Anesthesiologists (ASA) Committee on Standards and Parameters and a Task Force on Perioperative Blood Management analyzed the literature and solicited many opinions that were published in 2015.[1] The "Practice Guidelines for Perioperative Blood Management" had a major impact on the writing of this chapter, as did the earlier 2006 version of this report, which served as the foundation for this chapter in the 6th edition.[2]

In the past 5 to 10 years, many new conceptual terms have been added to the blood transfusion literature. These terms include *transfusion trigger, patient blood management (PBM), transfusion ratios*, and *preoperative anemia*. These terms and concepts have tended to clarify how safety can be enhanced in transfusion medicine. Conversely, a few terms emphasize the severe complications that can occur when multiple transfusions are given to a patient. For example, the term *lethal triad* describes hypothermia, acidosis, and coagulopathy and is an important negative indicator of transfusion medicine.[3] The *50/50 rule* has recently been introduced and has received considerable attention.[4] Basically, a 10% increase in mortality rate was observed with every 10 units of blood given. So, when 50 units of blood are given, there is a 50% mortality rate. While an individual clinician rarely gives 50 units of blood to a patient, the 50/50 rule simply confirms the logical conclusion that patients who require increasing numbers of transfusions have medical or surgical conditions that are very serious with increasing mortality rates. Yet, red blood cell transfusions given for specific clinical situations can decrease mortality rates.[5,6] Clearly, indications for blood transfusion should be well defined and, if utilized, are often clinically beneficial and even lifesaving.

Refining the preciseness of the indications for blood transfusions is complex. For example, older adult patients are more likely to receive a blood transfusion as compared to younger patients.[7] A recommendation was even made to develop an evidence-based decision aid for blood transfusions.[8]

## BLOOD THERAPY PROCEDURES

Determination of the blood types of the recipient and donor is the first step in selecting blood for transfusion therapy. Routine typing of blood is performed to identify the antigens (A, B, Rh) on the membranes of erythrocytes (Table 24.1). Naturally occurring antibodies (anti-B, anti-A) are formed whenever erythrocyte membranes lack A or B antigens (or both). These antibodies are capable of causing rapid intravascular destruction of erythrocytes that contain the corresponding antigens.

### Crossmatch

The major crossmatch occurs when the donor's erythrocytes are incubated with the recipient's plasma. Incubation of the donor's plasma with the recipient's erythrocytes constitutes a minor crossmatch. Agglutination occurs if either the major or minor crossmatch is incompatible. The major crossmatch also checks for immunoglobulin G antibodies (Kell, Kidd). Type-specific blood means that only the ABO-Rh type has been determined. The chance of a significant hemolytic reaction related to the transfusion of type-specific blood is about 1 in 1000.

### Emergency Transfusion

In an emergency situation that requires transfusion before compatibility testing is completed, the most desirable approach is to transfuse type-specific, partially crossmatched blood. The donor erythrocytes are mixed with recipient plasma, centrifuged, and observed for macroscopic agglutination. If the time required to complete this examination (typically < 10 minutes) is not acceptable, the second option is to administer type-specific, non-crossmatched blood if available or else O-negative packed red blood cells. O-negative whole blood is not selected because it may contain high titers of anti-A and anti-B hemolytic antibodies. For adult patients, except female patients of childbearing age, emergency administration of O-positive blood is considered acceptable practice until the patient's blood type is determined. If the patient's blood type becomes known and available after 2 units of type O-negative packed red blood cells have been transfused, classic teaching was that subsequent transfusions should probably continue with O-negative blood. However, it is not clear if this practice is necessary and the generally recommended approach is to switch to type-specific blood when it is available.

Soon after blood is typed, crossmatched, and stored, the functional platelets begin to disappear. Fresh whole blood is extremely effective in restoring normal coagulation after severe injury. The effectiveness of fresh whole blood depends on how long it has been stored and its temperature. In the military in Vietnam in the late 1960s,[9] type-specific blood that was maintained at room temperature and stored for no longer than 24 hours was extremely effective in preventing and treating trauma and fluid-induced (e.g., crystalloids) coagulopathies. In the past 50 years, this deduction has been confirmed many times including by retrospective analysis.[10] Not surprisingly, the use of fresh whole blood by forward surgical teams in Afghanistan is associated with improved survival compared to component therapy without platelets.[10]

In an urgent clinical situation, blood needs to be released from the blood bank on an urgent basis. Even a nontrauma hospital should be able to release blood rapidly. At the author's institution (UCSF Medical Center), a massive transfusion and emergency release protocol ensure that blood products are available at all times. A call activating the massive transfusion protocol will automatically release 4 units of uncrossmatched red blood cells (type O-negative), 4 units of fresh frozen plasma, and 1 unit of platelets. The red blood cells will be released

**Table 24.1** Blood Groups: Typing and Crossmatching

| Blood Group | Antigen on Erythrocyte | Plasma Antibodies | Incidence (%) | |
| --- | --- | --- | --- | --- |
| | | | White | African American |
| A | A | Anti-B | 40 | 27 |
| B | B | Anti-A | 11 | 20 |
| AB | AB | None | 4 | 4 |
| O | None | Anti-A, anti-B | 45 | 40 |
| Rh | Rh | | 42 | 17 |

in 5 minutes, with the other products available in 10 minutes. Most acute care hospitals have some type of emergency release or massive transfusion policy.

## Type and Screen

Blood that has been typed and screened has been typed for A, B, and Rh antigens and screened for common antibodies. This approach is used when the scheduled surgical procedure is unlikely to require transfusion of blood (hysterectomy, cholecystectomy) but is one in which blood should be available. Blood typing and screening permit more cost-efficient use of stored blood because the blood is available to more than one patient. The chance of a significant hemolytic reaction related to the use of typed and screened blood is approximately 1 in 10,000 units transfused.

## Blood Storage

Blood can be stored in a variety of solutions that contain phosphate, dextrose, and possibly adenine at temperatures of 1° C to 6° C. Storage time (70% viability of transfused erythrocytes 24 hours after transfusion) is 21 to 35 days, depending on the storage medium. Adenine increases erythrocyte survival by allowing the cells to resynthesize the adenosine triphosphate needed to fuel metabolic reactions. Changes that occur in blood during storage reflect the length of storage and the type of preservative used. For many years, fresher blood (<5 days of storage) has been recommended for critically ill patients in an effort to improve the delivery of oxygen (2,3-diphosphoglycerate [2,3-DPG] concentrations better maintained). Administration of younger blood (i.e., stored < 14 days) has been associated with better outcomes (e.g., decreased mortality rate and fewer postoperative complications), especially with major surgery.[11] Yet, some authors occasionally conclude that red blood cell quality cannot be determined by duration of storage.[12] More recently, Heddle and associates concluded that the death rate among a general hospital population was not related to the duration of blood storage.[13] Yet, each specialty publishes guidelines for giving blood transfusions, which often includes storage time. These differences even vary within a specialty.[13] Nevertheless, the transfusion-related evidence supported by specialty committees and clinical experience increasingly concludes that the clinician must consider the duration of storage as one of the criteria for selection of a blood product for transfusion.

## DECISION TO TRANSFUSE

The decision to transfuse should be based on a combination of factors: (1) PBM and preoperative anemia; (2) monitoring of blood loss; (3) assessment of how much additional blood loss may occur; (4) monitoring for inadequate perfusion and oxygenation of vital organs; (5) quantitation of intravenous fluids given overall; and (6) monitoring for transfusion indicators, especially the hemoglobin concentration.

## Patient Blood Management

PBM has been a major part of our transfusion terminology for the past 5 to 10 years. One of the major components of PBM has been the presence of preoperative anemia.[14] For example, preoperative anemia is a risk factor for a poorer clinical outcome and a predisposing factor for intraoperative blood transfusions. Also, the increasingly common term *precision medicine* is a broad call for practicing more precise medicine including specifying the indications for a blood transfusion.[15] A major limitation of these conclusions concerns placing attention on one or two variables when many others exist. For example, we cannot forget that hypothermia frequently occurs in patients with severe injury.[16]

## Monitoring for Blood Loss

Visual estimation is the simplest technique for quantifying intraoperative blood loss. The estimate is based on a combination of visualization and gravimetric measurements of blood on sponges and drapes and in suction devices. Specifically, differences in weight between dry and blood-soaked gauze pads can routinely be determined. However, these methods for measuring blood loss are only modestly accurate.

## Monitoring for Inadequate Perfusion and Oxygenation of Vital Organs

Standard monitors, such as the electrocardiogram and those measuring arterial blood pressure, heart rate, urine output, and oxygen saturation, are commonly used. Analysis of arterial blood gases, mixed venous oxygen saturation, and echocardiography may be useful in selected patients. Tachycardia is an insensitive and nonspecific indicator of hypovolemia, especially in patients receiving a volatile anesthetic. Maintenance of adequate arterial blood pressure and central venous pressure (6 to 12 mm Hg) suggests adequate intravascular blood volume. Urinary output usually decreases during moderate to severe hypovolemia and the resulting tissue hypoperfusion. Arterial pH may decrease only when tissue hypoperfusion becomes severe.

## Monitoring for Transfusion Indicators (Especially Hemoglobin Concentration)

The decision to transfuse is based on the risk anemia poses to a patient and the patient's ability to compensate for decreased oxygen-carrying capacity, as well as the inherent risks associated with transfusion (also see Chapter 20). As a member of the UCSF Transfusion Committee for over 20 years, this author can affirm that many of the variables used to guide transfusion therapy are based on clinical judgment rather than peer review studies.

In the past 20 years, new terminology on blood transfusion policy has appeared. A clinician may be using a *restrictive* blood policy, meaning "give blood only when absolutely necessary." This restrictive approach evolved many years ago when fear of transmitting hepatitis and human immunodeficiency virus (HIV) was widespread. However, transmission of such diseases is now rare. Blood transfusions given in response to proper indications should decrease patient mortality rates with various conditions.[17,18] Proper preoperative preparation can reduce the number of blood transfusions used intraoperatively. For example, preoperative anemia should be treated (e.g., with recombinant human erythropoietin and iron). This action decreases not only the need for intraoperative blood transfusions but the overall morbidity and mortality rates.[19]

In parallel with the new terminology, a general standard of care has evolved that healthy patients with hemoglobin values more than 10 g/dL rarely required transfusion, whereas those with hemoglobin values less than 6 g/dL almost always required transfusion, especially when anemia or surgical bleeding (or both) were acute and continuing. Determination of whether intermediate hemoglobin concentrations (6 to 10 g/dL) justify or require transfusion should be based on the patient's risk for complications of inadequate oxygen delivery. For example, certain clinical situations (e.g., coronary artery disease, chronic lung disease, surgery associated with large blood loss) may warrant transfusion of blood at a higher hemoglobin value than that in otherwise healthy patients. A hemoglobin concentration of 8 g/dL may be an appropriate threshold for transfusion in surgical patients with no risk factors for ischemia, whereas a transfusion threshold of 10 g/dL may be justified in patients who are considered to be at risk for ischemia (emphysema, coronary artery disease). Controlled studies to determine the hemoglobin concentration at which blood transfusion improves outcome in a surgical patient with acute blood loss are few. Yet, to center on hemoglobin values in a complex clinical situation must be done with caution.

More recently, the PBM policy has focused on the words *restrictive* and *liberal* for blood transfusions. This policy was dominated by using a hemoglobin value as the indicator. A liberal policy would allow giving blood when hemoglobin levels were more than 9 g/dL. A restrictive policy allowed giving blood only when the hemoglobin levels were preferably 8 g/dL or lower. Analysis of the literature clearly favors the restrictive approach. However, some groups have recommended a liberal approach to sicker patients. One such group is Fominskiy

and associates, who wrote, "According to randomized published evidence, perioperative adult patients have an improved survival when receiving a liberal blood transfusion policy."[20]

Another problem is that the proponents of the restrictive approach do not state what the policy should be for the repetitive or additional administration of blood. Should the indications for the initial administration of blood be the same for each subsequent administration of blood? Clearly the clinician should also estimate whether additional blood will be lost in the actively bleeding patient.

Transfusion of packed red blood cells in patients with hemoglobin concentrations higher than 10 to 12 g/dL does not substantially increase oxygen delivery. Further decreases in the hemoglobin concentration can sometimes be offset by increases in cardiac output. The exact hemoglobin value at which cardiac output increases varies among individuals and is influenced by age, whether the anemia is acute or chronic, and sometimes by anesthesia. For example, the cardiovascular response to anemia in the elderly is decreased, as it is with general anesthesia. Yet, the focus on hemoglobin as a *transfusion indicator* has existed for many years and still continues.[21] Furthermore, a relatively new noninvasive spectrophotometric monitor (Masimo SpHb) attached to a finger allows the continuous monitoring of hemoglobin levels. Whether this monitor currently can be used for transfusion decisions without a laboratory co-oximeter determination is not clear.[22] For sure, this monitor will provide more opportunity for defining the relationship between hemoglobin levels and transfusion requirements.

The aforementioned considerations indicate that the decision to give a blood transfusion requires a careful thought process that is based on objective clinical indications and a knowledge of transfusion medicine overall.

## BLOOD COMPONENTS

### Packed Red Blood Cells

Packed red blood cells (250- to 300-mL volume with a hematocrit of 70% to 80%) are used for treatment of anemia usually associated with surgical blood loss. The major goal is to increase the oxygen-carrying capacity of blood. Although packed red blood cells can increase intravascular fluid volume, nonblood products, such as crystalloids and colloids, can also achieve that end point. A single unit of packed red blood cells will increase adult hemoglobin concentrations approximately 1.0 to 1.5 g/dL. Administration of packed red blood cells can be facilitated by reconstituting them in crystalloid solutions, such as 50 to 100 mL of saline. The use of hypotonic glucose solutions may theoretically cause hemolysis, whereas the calcium present in lactated Ringer solution may cause clotting if mixed with packed red blood cells.

## Complications

Complications associated with packed red blood cells are similar to those of whole blood. An exception would be the chance for development of citrate intoxication, which would be less with packed red blood cells than with whole blood because less citrate is infused. Removal of plasma decreases the concentration of factors I (fibrinogen), V, and VIII as compared with whole blood.

### Decision to Administer Packed Red Blood Cells

The decision to administer packed red blood cells should be based on measured blood loss and inadequate oxygen-carrying capacity.

### Acute Blood Loss

Acute blood loss in the range of 1500 to 2000 mL (approximately 30% of an adult patient's blood volume) may exceed the ability of crystalloids to replace blood volume without jeopardizing the oxygen-carrying capacity of the blood. Hypotension and tachycardia are likely, but these compensatory responses may be blunted by anesthesia or other drugs (e.g., β-adrenergic blocking drugs). Compensatory vasoconstriction may conceal the signs of acute blood loss until at least 10% of the blood volume is lost, and healthy patients may lose up to 20% of their blood volume before signs of hypovolemia occur. To ensure an adequate oxygen content in blood, packed red blood cells should be administered when blood loss is sufficiently large. Administration of whole blood, when available, decreases the incidence of hypofibrinogenemia and perhaps coagulopathies associated with administration of packed red blood cells.[2] In the Vietnam conflict, fresh whole blood (typed and crossmatched, but not cooled) was quite effective, especially with massive transfusion-associated coagulopathies.[9] Forty years later in Iraq, military physicians administered fresh whole blood from prescreened "walking donors," which also can treat or prevent thrombocytopenia. In fact, warm fresh whole blood may be more efficacious than stored component therapy when treating critically ill patients requiring massive blood transfusions.[23] Also, whole blood may be preferable to packed red blood cells when replacing blood losses that exceed 30% of the blood volume. Alternatively, specific ratios of red blood cell transfusions with fresh frozen plasma (FFP) and platelets are being recommended.[24] For example, a ratio of 1.5 units red blood cells with 1 unit of FFP has been proposed. Then 1 unit platelets for 6 units of red blood cells has been recommended in patients with large blood losses and trauma.[24]

With acute blood loss, interstitial fluid and extravascular protein are transferred to the intravascular space, which tends to maintain plasma volume. For this reason, when crystalloid solutions are used to replace blood loss, they should be given in amounts equal to about three times the amount of blood loss, not only to replenish intravascular fluid volume but also to replenish the fluid lost from interstitial spaces. Albumin and hetastarch are examples of solutions that are useful for acute expansion of the intravascular fluid volume. In contrast to crystalloid solutions, albumin and hetastarch are more likely to remain in the intravascular space for prolonged periods (about 12 hours). These solutions avoid complications associated with blood-containing products but do not improve the oxygen-carrying capacity of the blood and, in large volumes (>20 mL/kg), may cause coagulation defects.

## Platelets

Administration of platelets allows specific treatment of thrombocytopenia without the infusion of unnecessary blood components. Platelets are derived from volunteer donors (cytapheresis and plateletpheresis). Pooled platelet concentrates are derived from whole blood donation and can be called *random-donor platelets*. During surgery, platelet transfusions are probably not required unless the platelet count is less than 50,000 cells/mm$^3$ as determined by laboratory analysis or in predetermined ratios with red blood cells as described previously.

### Complications

The risks associated with platelet concentrate infusions are (1) sensitization reactions because of human leukocyte antigens on the cell membranes of platelets and (2) transmission of infectious diseases, which is rare. One of the leading causes of transfusion-related fatalities in the United States is bacterial contamination, which is most likely to occur in platelet concentrates (Table 24.2). Platelet-related sepsis can be fatal and occurs as frequently as 1 in 5000 transfusions; it is probably underrecognized because of the many other confounding variables present in critically ill patients. When donor platelets are cultured before infusion (and not released until the culture is negative after a minimum of 24 hours' incubation), the incidence of sepsis may be significantly reduced, but sepsis is still possible. The fact that platelets are stored at 20° C

| Table 24.2 | Estimated Risk of Infection Transmitted by Blood Transfusion |
|---|---|
| **Infection** | **Risk** |
| Hepatitis B | 1 in 220,000 |
| Hepatitis C | 1 in 1.6 million |
| HIV | 1 in 1.8 million |
| HTLV-I | 1 in 640,000 |
| West Nile virus | 1 in >1 million |

*HIV*, Human immunodeficiency virus; *HTLV-I*, human T-cell lymphotropic virus type I.

to 24° C instead of 4° C probably accounts for the greater risk of bacterial growth than with other blood products. As a result, any patient in whom a fever develops within 6 hours of receiving platelet concentrates should be considered to possibly be manifesting platelet-induced sepsis, and empirical antibiotic therapy should be instituted.

## Fresh Frozen Plasma

FFP is the fluid portion obtained from a single unit of whole blood that is frozen within 6 hours of collection. All coagulation factors, except platelets, are present in FFP, which explains the use of this component for the treatment of hemorrhage from presumed coagulation factor deficiencies. FFP transfusions during surgery are probably not necessary unless the prothrombin time (PT) or partial thromboplastin time (PTT), or both, are at least 1.5 times longer than normal. More recently, FFP is given in specific ratios with red blood cells in trauma patients (see Chapter 42). Other indications for FFP are urgent reversal of warfarin and management of heparin resistance. The role of FFP as a cause of transfusion-related acute lung injury (TRALI) will be discussed later.

## Cryoprecipitate

Cryoprecipitate is the fraction of plasma that precipitates when FFP is thawed. This component is useful for treating hemophilia A (contains high concentrations of factor VIII in a small volume) that is unresponsive to desmopressin. Cryoprecipitate can also be used to treat hypofibrinogenemia (as induced by packed red blood cells) because it contains more fibrinogen than FFP.

## COMPLICATIONS OF BLOOD THERAPY

Blood transfusions are extremely valuable in clinical medicine and have become increasingly safer, mainly because of more effective donor screening and pretransfusion blood testing (see Table 24.3). Complications of blood therapy, like an adverse effect of any therapy, must be considered when evaluating the risk-to-benefit ratio for treatment of individual patients with blood products.

The Food and Drug Administration (FDA) analyzes and publishes fatality and related outcomes from blood transfusions. Table 24.3 lists types of fatal reactions associated with blood transfusions from 2010 to 2015 on a cumulative basis and in 2015 alone. For several years, the conclusion has been that fatal reactions are rare and have been similar in occurrence for the last 5 years and that the risk of having a fatal outcome from blood transfusion is remote but possible. The leading causes of a fatal outcome from blood transfusion are TRALI, transfusion-associated circulatory overload (TACO), and hemolytic transfusion reactions (see Table 24.3). For the last 5 years,

the FDA has reported that blood transfusions are safer than at any time in history, but still should be given only when absolutely necessary. Historically, transmission of infectious diseases, hepatitis, and HIV and hemolytic transfusion reactions have probably been the most feared complications of transfusion therapy.

Yet, the previous optimistic description must be cautious. Another cause of transfusion-related infections is health care–associated infections.[25] The concept is that transfusions make a patient increasingly susceptible to infections. Patients who are older or sicker require more transfusions and therefore are exposed to more infectivity.[25] All specialties should have indications for blood transfusion that closely match the 2016 general guidelines from the United Kingdom's National Clinical Guideline Centre (NCGC) as published in *JAMA*.[26] These indications are compatible with the values given in this chapter. Of prime importance is the use of restrictive red blood cell transfusion thresholds (7 to 9 g/dL) for patients who do not have major hemorrhage or acute coronary syndrome (ACS).

## Transmission of Infectious Diseases

Historically, the incidence of infection from blood transfusions has markedly decreased. For example, in 1980, the incidence of hepatitis was as high as 10%. Improved donor blood testing and screening have dramatically decreased the risk of transmission of hepatitis C and HIV to less than 1 in 1 million transfusions. Although many factors account for the marked decrease in the incidence of transmission of infectious agents by blood transfusion, the most important one is improved testing of donor blood. Currently, hepatitis C, HIV, and West Nile virus are

| **Table 24.3** | Comparison of Transfusion-Related Fatalities in the United States Between 2011 and 2015 | | |
|---|---|---|---|
| **Cause** | **No. 2011 Through 2015** | | **No. 2015 Alone** |
| TRALI | 66 | 38% | 12 |
| TACO | 41 | 24% | 11 |
| HTR (Non-ABO) | 24 | 14% | 4 |
| HTR (ABO) | 13 | 7.5% | 2 |
| Microbial infection | 18 | 10% | 5 |
| Anaphylaxis | 8 | 5% | 2 |
| Hypotensive | 2 | 1% | 1 |
| Other | 1 | 0.5% | - |

*HTR,* Hemolytic transfusion reaction; *TACO,* transfusion-associated circulatory overload; *TRALI,* transfusion-related acute lung injury.
From Fatalities Reported to FDA Following Blood Collection and Transfusion. Annual Summary for Fiscal Year 2015. Accessed online November 28, 2016. http://www.fda.gov/BiologicsBloodVaccines/SafetyAvailability/ReportaProblem/TransfusionDonationFatalities/.

tested by nucleic acid technology. In 2002, more than 30 cases of transfusion-transmitted West Nile virus occurred. By 2003, nearly universal screening of donor blood by nucleic acid technology reduced the incidence to that of HIV.

The most recent infectious concern is the possible transmission of the Zika virus. As of November 2016, there were no confirmed transmissions via blood transfusions of the Zika virus in the United States. Yet, the Zika virus has been transmitted via platelet transfusions in Brazil. The FDA has recommended use of a blood screening test.

Other less commonly transmitted infectious agents include Chagas disease, hepatitis B, human T-cell lymphotropic virus, cytomegalovirus, malaria, and possibly variant Creutzfeldt-Jakob disease.

## Noninfectious Hazards of Transfusion

The causes of noninfectious serious hazards of transfusion (NISHOT) are numerous and dominated by TRALI and transfusion-related immunomodulation.

### Transfusion-Related Acute Lung Injury
TRALI is the leading cause of transfusion-related deaths (see Table 24.3). TRALI is acute lung injury that occurs within 6 hours after transfusion of a blood product, especially packed red blood cells or FFP. Exclusion of female blood donors and fresher blood (i.e., storage <14 days) may decrease the risk of TRALI.[27] It is characterized by dyspnea and arterial hypoxemia secondary to noncardiogenic pulmonary edema. The diagnosis of TRALI is confirmed when pulmonary edema occurs in the absence of left atrial hypertension and the pulmonary edema fluid has a high protein content. Immediate actions to take when TRALI is suspected include (1) stopping the transfusion, (2) supporting the patient's vital signs, (3) determining the protein concentration of the pulmonary edema fluid via the endotracheal tube, (4) obtaining a complete blood count and chest radiograph, and (5) notifying the blood bank of possible TRALI so that other associated units can be quarantined.

Because the diagnosis is sometimes difficult to make, follow-up paperwork is especially important, including sending a blood specimen and bags of units of blood given to the blood bank. All copies of transfusion forms and anesthetic records will be required by the blood bank.

### Transfusion-Related Immunomodulation
Blood transfusion suppresses cell-mediated immunity, which when combined with similar effects produced by surgical trauma, may place patients at risk for postoperative infection. The association with long-term prognosis in cancer surgery is unclear, but there is a suggestion of a correlation between tumor recurrence and blood transfusions.[28,29] Conversely, patients who receive blood transfusions may have more extensive disease and a poorer prognosis independent of the administration of blood. As such, the role of blood transfusions in postoperative infections and cancer is difficult to ascertain. Packed red blood cells, which contain less plasma than whole blood does, may produce less immunosuppression, thus suggesting that plasma contains an undefined immunosuppressive factor.

Removing most of the white blood cells from blood and platelets (leukoreduction) is becoming increasingly common. This practice reduces the incidence of nonhemolytic febrile transfusion reactions and the transmission of leukocyte-associated viruses. Other possible benefits (reduction of cancer recurrence and postoperative infections) are more speculative.

## Metabolic Abnormalities

Metabolic abnormalities that accompany the storage of whole blood include accumulation of hydrogen ions and potassium and decreased 2,3-DPG concentrations. The citrate present in the blood preservative may produce changes in the recipient.

### Hydrogen Ions
The addition of most preservatives promptly increases the hydrogen ion content of stored whole blood. Continued metabolic function of erythrocytes results in additional production of hydrogen ions with the pH of stored blood being as low as 7.0. Despite these changes, metabolic acidosis is not a consistent occurrence in recipients of blood products, even with rapid infusion of large volumes of stored blood. Therefore, intravenous administration of sodium bicarbonate to patients receiving transfusions of whole blood should be determined by measurement of pH and not be based on arbitrary regimens.

### Potassium
The potassium content of stored blood increases progressively with the duration of storage, but even massive transfusions rarely increase plasma potassium concentrations. Failure of plasma potassium concentrations to increase most likely reflects the small amount of potassium actually present in 1 unit of stored blood. For example, because 1 unit of whole blood contains only 300 mL of plasma, a measured potassium concentration of 21 mEq/L would represent the administration of less than 7 mEq of potassium to the patient.

### Decreased 2,3-Diphosphoglycerate
Storage of blood is associated with a progressive decrease in concentrations of 2,3-DPG in erythrocytes, which results in increased affinity of hemoglobin for oxygen (decreased $P_{50}$ values). Conceivably, this increased affinity could make less oxygen available for

tissues and jeopardize tissue oxygen delivery. There is speculation that fresh blood (with more oxygen available for tissues) should be used for critically ill patients. Despite these observations, the clinical significance of the 2,3-DPG oxygen affinity changes remains unconfirmed.

### Citrate

Citrate metabolism to bicarbonate may contribute to metabolic alkalosis, whereas binding of calcium by citrate could result in hypocalcemia. Indeed, metabolic alkalosis rather than metabolic acidosis can follow massive blood transfusions. Hypocalcemia as a result of citrate binding of calcium is rare because of mobilization of calcium stores from bone and the ability of the liver to rapidly metabolize citrate to bicarbonate. Therefore, arbitrary administration of calcium in the absence of objective evidence of hypocalcemia (prolonged QT intervals on the electrocardiogram, measured decrease in plasma ionized calcium concentrations) is not indicated. Supplemental calcium may be needed when (1) the rate of blood infusion is more rapid than 50 mL/min, (2) hypothermia or liver disease interferes with the metabolism of citrate, or (3) the patient is a neonate. Patients undergoing liver transplantation are the most likely to experience citrate intoxication, and these patients may require calcium administration during a massive transfusion of stored blood.

## Hypothermia

Administration of blood stored at less than 6° C can result in a decrease in the patient's body temperature. Passage of blood through specially designed warmers greatly decreases the likelihood of transfusion-related hypothermia. Unrecognized malfunction of these warmers, causing them to overheat, may result in hemolysis of the blood being transfused.

## Coagulation

The conclusion that excessive microvascular bleeding is occurring should be the combined judgment of both the surgical and anesthesia teams. Laboratory tests are only a supplement to clinically determined excessive microvascular bleeding. Blood loss should be determined by checking suction canisters, surgical sponges, and drains. A decision needs to be made regarding whether the blood loss is from inadequate surgical control of vascular bleeding or a coagulopathy. A platelet count, PT or international normalized ratio (INR), PTT, and fibrinogen level can confirm both the presence and type of coagulopathy. Platelet concentrates may be administered if the platelet count is less than 50,000 cells/mm[3].[9,17] A qualitative platelet defect (antiplatelet drugs, cardiopulmonary bypass) may require platelet concentrates to be given, even with a normal platelet count. Administration of FFP should be considered when the PT is longer than 1.5 times normal or the INR is more than 2.0 and if laboratory tests are unavailable, more than one blood volume (about 70 mL/kg) has been transfused, and excessive microvascular bleeding is present. The dose of FFP (10 to 15 mL/kg) should achieve at least 30% of most plasma factor concentrations. As indicated previously, specific ratios of FFP and platelets with administration of red blood cells seem to decrease coagulation problems in patients with trauma and massive blood loss. The previous description is based on laboratory-derived coagulation values (e.g., platelet count), which takes some time. Use of point-of-care viscoelastic testing with rotational thromboelastography (ROTEM) has been successfully used in several clinical situations. However, most of the published studies on transfusion medicine and bleeding are based on standard laboratory tests.

Cryoprecipitate should be considered if fibrinogen levels are less than 100 mg/dL. Also, a highly purified, lyophilized virus-inactivated fibrinogen concentrate from human plasma (Riastap, CSL Behring, Kankakee, IL) can be used to treat hypofibrinogenemia and is effective in some broader based coagulopathies.[30] Low blood fibrinogen levels are increasingly associated with coagulopathies and massive blood transfusions. Accordingly, fibrinogen administration via Riastap or cryoprecipitate is increasingly recognized as being important in treating patients with significant blood loss.[31] In addition, desmopressin or a topical hemostatic (fibrin glue) may be used for excessive bleeding. Recombinant activated factor VII may be considered as a "rescue" drug when standard therapy has failed to successfully treat a coagulopathy (microvascular bleeding).[32] It apparently enhances thrombin generation on already activated platelets. It also has the risk of inducing thromboembolic complications.[32]

## Transfusion Reactions

Although transfusion reactions are traditionally categorized as febrile, allergic, and hemolytic, anesthesia, especially general anesthesia, may mask the signs and symptoms of all types of transfusion reactions.[33] The possibility of a transfusion reaction during anesthesia should be suspected in the presence of hyperthermia, increased peak airway pressure, or an acute change in urine output or color.

In considering the occurrence of transfusion reactions, it is important to periodically check for signs and symptoms of bacterial contamination, TRALI, and hemolytic transfusion reactions, including urticaria, hypotension, tachycardia, increased peak airway pressure, hyperthermia, decreased urine output, hemoglobinuria, and microvascular bleeding.[2] Before instituting therapy for transfusion reactions, stop the blood transfusion and order appropriate diagnostic testing.[2]

### Febrile Reactions

Febrile reactions are the most common adverse nonhemolytic response to the transfusion of blood, and they accompany 0.5% to 1% of transfusions. The most likely explanation for febrile reactions is an interaction between recipient antibodies and antigens present on the leukocytes or platelets of the donor. The patient's temperature rarely increases above 38° C, and the condition is treated by slowing the infusion and administering antipyretics. Severe febrile reactions accompanied by chills and shivering may require discontinuation of the blood transfusion.

### Allergic Reactions

Allergic reactions to properly typed and crossmatched blood are manifested as increases in body temperature, pruritus, and urticaria. Treatment often includes intravenous administration of antihistamines and, in severe cases, discontinuation of the blood transfusion. Examination of plasma and urine for free hemoglobin is useful to rule out hemolytic reactions.

### Hemolytic Reactions

Hemolytic reactions occur when the wrong blood type is administered to a patient. The common factor in the production of intravascular hemolysis and the development of spontaneous hemorrhage is activation of the complement system. With the exception of hypotension, the immediate signs (lumbar and substernal pain, fever, chills, dyspnea, skin flushing) of hemolytic reactions are masked by general anesthesia. Even hypotension may be attributed to other causes in an anesthetized patient. The appearance of free hemoglobin in plasma or urine is presumptive evidence of a hemolytic reaction. Acute renal failure reflects precipitation of stromal and lipid contents (not free hemoglobin) of hemolyzed erythrocytes in distal renal tubules. Disseminated intravascular coagulation causing a coagulopathy is initiated by material released from hemolyzed erythrocytes.

### Treatment

Treatment of acute hemolytic reactions is immediate discontinuation of the incompatible blood transfusion and maintenance of urine output by infusion of crystalloid solutions and administration of mannitol or furosemide. The use of sodium bicarbonate to alkalinize the urine and improve the solubility of hemoglobin degradation products in the renal tubules is of unproven value, as is the administration of corticosteroids.

## AUTOLOGOUS BLOOD TRANSFUSIONS

Types of autologous blood transfusion are (1) predeposited (preoperative) autologous donation (PAD), (2) intraoperative and postoperative blood salvage, and (3) normovolemic hemodilution. Two primary reasons for the use of autologous blood are to decrease or eliminate complications from allogeneic blood transfusions and to conserve blood resources. In the 1980s, both patient and physician fear escalated because of a legitimate concern regarding infectious diseases, especially hepatitis C and HIV. Although there is still an inherent belief that PAD blood is safer, the markedly reduced rate of infectious disease transmission from allogeneic blood makes that view difficult to prove. Furthermore, PAD blood is more expensive and not very effective in reducing allogeneic blood transfusion. Therefore, PAD is not generally a cost-effective alternative to allogeneic blood.

### Predeposited Autologous Donation

Patients scheduled for elective surgery who may require transfusion of blood may choose to predonate (predeposit) blood for possible transfusion in the perioperative period. Patient-donors must have a hemoglobin concentration of at least 11 g/dL. Most patients can donate 10.5 mL/kg of blood approximately every 5 to 7 days (maximum, 2 to 3 units), with the last unit collected 72 hours or more before surgery to permit restoration of plasma volume. Oral iron supplementation is recommended when blood is withdrawn within a few days preceding surgery. Treatment with recombinant erythropoietin is very expensive, but it increases the amount of blood that patients can predeposit by as much as 25%.

### Intraoperative and Postoperative Blood Salvage

Intraoperative blood salvage for reinfusion into the patient decreases the amount of allogeneic blood needed. Typically, semiautomated systems are used in which the red blood cells are collected and washed and then delivered to a reservoir for future administration either intraoperatively or postoperatively. The presence of infection or malignant disease at the operative site is considered a contraindication to blood salvage. Complications of intraoperative salvage include dilutional coagulopathy, reinfusion of excessive anticoagulant (heparin), hemolysis, air embolism, and disseminated intravascular coagulation. A documented quality assurance program, as recommended by the American Association of Blood Banks, is required for those who use intraoperative salvage techniques.

### Normovolemic Hemodilution

Normovolemic hemodilution consists of withdrawing a portion of the patient's blood volume early in the intraoperative period and concurrent infusion of crystalloids or colloids to maintain intravascular volume. The end point is a hematocrit of 27% to 33%, depending on the patient's cardiovascular and respiratory status. By initially hemodiluting the patient, fewer red blood cells will be lost per millimeter of blood loss during surgery. At the conclusion of surgery, the patient's blood, with its enhanced oxygen-carrying capacity by virtue of a higher hematocrit and its greater clotting ability by virtue of platelets and other coagulation factors, is reinfused. Whether the use of this technique actually decreases allogeneic blood administration is questionable. The survival of recovered red blood cells appears to be similar to that of transfused allogeneic cells.

## CONCLUSIONS AND FUTURE DIRECTIONS

Transfusion of blood products has become increasingly safer, especially because of the dramatically decreased incidence of infectious disease transmission (see Table 24.2). If given in accordance with proper indications, patient mortality rate is not increased because of receiving blood transfusions per se.[17,18] As indicated previously, increasingly, emphasis is being placed on defining ratios of blood products that should be given (e.g., 1:1 packed red blood cells with fresh frozen plasma or platelets).[34,35] Alternatively, perhaps in the future whole blood will be given more often. Other possibilities include hemoglobin-based oxygen carriers (HBOCs) (synthetic blood). For over 20 years with all of their advantages (e.g., no typing and crossmatching), we hoped that one or more of these products would partially replace human blood transfusions. However, an FDA and National Institutes of Health conference in 2008 indicated that HBOC products will not be available soon.[36] Also, the ultimate impact that the length of time blood has been stored will have on transfusion practice overall is not clear.[11] Lastly, consistent with the practice of medicine overall, well-designed protocols will increasingly be the basis upon which transfusion practice is based.[37]

## QUESTIONS OF THE DAY

1. A patient requires emergency packed red blood cell transfusion. How is a crossmatch performed? What are the risks of hemolytic transfusion reaction if type-specific, non-crossmatched red blood cells are administered instead?
2. What factors are used to determine whether a red blood cell transfusion is indicated during surgery?
3. What are the most common causes of fatality related to blood transfusions in the United States?
4. What are the possible metabolic abnormalities associated with blood product transfusion?
5. What are the manifestations of hemolytic transfusion reaction in a patient receiving general anesthesia? What is the appropriate initial management?
6. What are the complications of intraoperative blood salvage?

## REFERENCES

1. American Society of Anesthesiologists Task Force on Perioperative Blood Management. Practice guidelines for perioperative blood management: an updated report by the American Society of Anesthesiologists Task Force on Perioperative Blood Management. *Anesthesiology*. 2015;122: 241–275.
2. American Society of Anesthesiologists Task Force on Perioperative Blood Transfusion and Adjuvant Therapies. Practice guidelines for perioperative blood transfusion and adjuvant therapies: an updated report by the American Society of Anesthesiologists Task Force on Perioperative Blood Transfusion and Adjuvant Therapies. *Anesthesiology*. 2006;105:198–208.
3. Holcomb JB, Hoyt DB. Comprehensive injury research. *JAMA*. 2015;313: 1463–1435.
4. Frank SM. 50/50 rule ties blood transfused to increasing mortality. *Anesthesiol News*. 2015;41:10–15.
5. Park DW, Chun BC, Kwon SS, et al. Red blood cell transfusions are associated with lower mortality in patients with severe sepsis and septic shock: a propensity-matched analysis. *Crit Care Med*. 2012;40:3140–3145.
6. Goudie R, Sterne JA, Verheyden V, et al. Risk scores to facilitate preoperative prediction of transfusion and large volume blood transfusion associated with adult cardiac surgery. *Br J Anaesth*. 2015;114:757–766.
7. Brown CH 4th, Savage WJ, Masear CG, et al. Odds of transfusion for older adults compared to younger adults undergoing surgery. *Anesth Analg*. 2014;118:1168–1178.
8. Toledo P. Shared decision-making and blood transfusions: is it time to share more? *Anesth Analg*. 2014;118:1151–1153.
9. Miller RD. Massive blood transfusions: the impact of Vietnam military data on modern civilian transfusion medicine. *Anesthesiology*. 2009;110:1412–1416.
10. Nessen SC, Eastridge BJ, Cronk D, et al. Fresh whole blood use by forward surgical teams in Afghanistan is associated with improved survival compared to component therapy without platelets. *Transfusion*. 2013;53(suppl 1): 107S–113S.
11. Adamson JW. New blood, old blood, or no blood? *N Engl J Med*. 2008;358: 1295–1296.
12. Spinella PC, Acker J. Storage duration and other measures of quality of red blood cells for transfusions. *JAMA*. 2015;314:2509–2510.
13. Heddle NM, Cook RJ, Arnold DM, et al. Effect of short-term vs. long-term blood storage on mortality after transfusion. *N Engl J Med*. 2016;375(20):1937–1945.
14. Muñoz M, Gómez-Ramírez S, Kozek-Langeneker SK, et al. "Fit to fly": overcoming barriers to preoperative haemoglobin optimization in surgical patients. *Br J Anaesth*. 2015;115(1): 15–24.

15. Klein HG, Flegel WA, Natanson C. Red blood cell transfusion: precision vs imprecision medicine. *JAMA.* 2015;314:1557–1558.

16. Perlman R, Callum J, Laflamme C, et al. A recommended early goal-directed management guideline for prevention of hypothermia-related transfusion, morbidity and mortality in severely injured trauma patients. *Crit Care.* 2016;20:107.

17. Vincent JL, Sakr Y, Sprung C, et al. Are blood transfusions associated with greater mortality rates? *Anesthesiology.* 2008;108:31–39.

18. Weightman WM, Gibbs NM, Sheminant MR, et al. Moderate exposure to allogeneic blood products is not associated with reduced long-term survival after surgery for coronary artery disease. *Anesthesiology.* 2009;111:327–333.

19. Beattie WS, Karkouti K, Wijeysundera DN, et al. Risk associated with preoperative anemia in noncardiac surgery. *Anesthesiology.* 2009;110:574–581.

20. Fominskiy E, Putzu A, Monaco F, et al. Liberal transfusion strategy improves survival in perioperative but not in critically ill patients. A meta-analysis of randomized trials. *Br J Anaesth.* 2015;115(4):511–519.

21. Weiskopf RB. Emergency transfusion for acute severe anemia: a calculated risk. *Anesth Analg.* 2010;111:1088–1092.

22. Miller RD, Ward TA, Shiboski S, et al. A comparison of three methods of hemoglobin monitoring in patients undergoing spine surgery. *Anesth Analg.* 2011;112:858–863.

23. Spinella PC. Warm fresh whole blood transfusion for severe hemorrhage: U.S. military and potential civilian applications. *Crit Care Med.* 2008;36:S340–S345.

24. Inaba K, Lustenberger T, Talving P, et al. The impact of platelet transfusions in massively transfused trauma patients. *J Am Coll Surg.* 2010;211:573–579.

25. Rohde JM, Dimcheff DE, Blumberg N, et al. Health care-associated infection after red blood cell transfusion: a systematic review and meta-analysis. *JAMA.* 2014;311:1317–1326.

26. Alexander J, Cifu AS. Transfusion of red blood cells. *JAMA.* 2016;316:2038–2039.

27. Benson AB, Moss M. Trauma and acute respiratory distress syndrome. *Anesthesiology.* 2009;110:216–217.

28. Spahn DR, Moch H, Hofmann H, et al. Patient blood management. *Anesthesiology.* 2008;109:951–953.

29. Arad S, Glasner A, Abiri N, et al. Blood transfusion promotes cancer progression: a critical role for aged erythrocytes. *Anesthesiology.* 2008;109:989–997.

30. Rahe-Meyer N, Pichlmaier M, Haverich A, et al. Bleeding management with fibrinogen concentrate targeting a high-normal plasma fibringogen level: a pilot study. *Br J Anaesth.* 2009;102:785–792.

31. Stinger HK, Spinella PC, Perkins JG, et al. The ratio of fibrinogen to red cells transfused affects survival in casualties receiving massive transfusions at an army combat support hospital. *J Trauma.* 2008;64:S79–S85.

32. Aledort LM. Off-label use of recombinant activated factor VII—safe or not safe? *N Engl J Med.* 2010;363:1853–1854.

33. Kopko PM, Holland PV. Mechanisms of severe transfusion reaction. *Transfus Clin Biol.* 2001;8:278–281.

34. Holcomb JB, Wade CE, Michalek JE, et al. Increased plasma and platelet to red blood cell ratios improves outcome in 466 massively transfused civilian trauma patients. *Ann Surg.* 2008;248:447–458.

35. Perkins JG, Andrew PC, Blackbourne LH, et al. An evaluation of the impact of apheresis platelets used in the setting of massively transfused trauma patients. *J Trauma.* 2009;66:S77–S84.

36. Silverman TA, Weiskoph RB. Planning committee: hemoglobin-based oxygen carriers. *Anesthesiology.* 2009;111:946–963.

37. Cotton BA, Dossett LA, Au BK, et al. Room for (performance) improvement: provider-related factors associated with poor outcomes in massive transfusions. *J Trauma.* 2009;67:1004–1012.

# SPECIAL ANESTHETIC CONSIDERATIONS

# 25 CARDIOVASCULAR DISEASE

## Arthur Wallace

Cardiovascular disease is the leading cause of global death with an estimated 17 million deaths per year, and by 2030 this number could be more than 23 million. It is the leading cause of death in the United States.[1,2] Many of the risk factors identified to predict perioperative fatality are cardiovascular in origin. Coronary artery disease (CAD), peripheral vascular disease (PVD), and risk for CAD increase operative risk.[3,4] Recent myocardial infarction, the presence of congestive heart failure (CHF), and aortic stenosis are among the most important risk factors. Management of anesthesia for patients with cardiovascular disease requires an understanding of the pathophysiology of the disease process, appropriate preoperative testing, application of perioperative risk reduction strategies, and careful selection of anesthetic, analgesic, neuromuscular, and autonomic blocking drugs. The use of appropriate monitors to match the needs created by cardiovascular disease is very important.

## CORONARY ARTERY DISEASE

CAD (ischemic heart disease), often asymptomatic, is a common accompaniment of aging in the American population (also see Chapter 35). Of the adult patients who undergo surgery annually in the United States, about 40% will either have or be at risk for CAD.[1] The presence of CAD in patients who undergo anesthesia for noncardiac surgery may be associated with increased morbidity and mortality rates. History, physical examination with specific attention to cardiac and respiratory disease, and cardiac risk factors are very important. In addition, determination of the presence of the patient's exercise tolerance, cardiac symptoms, and electrocardiogram (ECG) are important components of the routine preoperative cardiac evaluation (also see Chapter 13).[5] The presence of symptoms of cardiac disease include shortness of breath with exercise in men and fatigue in women. People with severe CAD frequently state that they have no chest pain or shortness of breath with walking or activity. When asked about walking up stairs, they readily admit to shortness of breath. The presence of angina, angina at rest, orthopnea, paroxysmal nocturnal dyspnea, and dizziness or fainting can also be signals of cardiovascular disease.

More specialized procedures, such as ambulatory ECG monitoring (Holter monitoring), exercise stress testing, transthoracic or transesophageal echocardiography (TEE), radionuclide ventriculography (determination of ejection fraction), dipyridamole-thallium scintigraphy (mimics the coronary vasodilator response but not the heart rate response associated with exercise), cardiac catheterization, and angiography, are performed on selected patients. There is no evidence that invasive preoperative testing adds appreciably to the information provided by routine history and physical examination and electrocardiographic data for predicting adverse outcomes.[1] For example, echocardiographic determination of ejection fraction may not provide information that improves upon the ability to predict the presence of a preoperative myocardial infarction beyond that provided by a careful preoperative clinical evaluation.[6] Thallium scintigraphy, which evaluates adequacy of coronary blood flow, does not predict patients at risk for perioperative cardiac events.[7,8] Ultimately, the history and physical examination with specific attention to signs and symptoms of new onset of angina, change in anginal pattern, unstable angina, recent myocardial infarction, CHF, or aortic stenosis, and presence of appropriate medical therapy should determine whether patients are in the best medical condition possible before elective cardiac or noncardiac surgery.[6]

## Patient History

Important aspects of the history taken from patients with CAD before noncardiac surgery include cardiac reserve, characteristics of angina pectoris, the presence of a prior myocardial infarction, and the medical, interventional cardiology, prior percutaneous coronary intervention (PCI), and cardiac surgical therapy for those conditions. Potential interactions of medications used in the treatment of CAD with drugs used to produce anesthesia must also be considered. Coexisting noncardiac diseases that are often present in these patients include hypertension, PVD, chronic obstructive pulmonary disease (COPD) from cigarette smoking, renal dysfunction associated with chronic hypertension, and diabetes mellitus. As stated previously, a thorough evaluation is especially important because patients can remain asymptomatic despite 50% to 70% stenosis of a major coronary artery.

### Cardiac Reserve

Limited exercise tolerance in the absence of significant pulmonary disease is the most striking evidence of decreased cardiac reserve. Inability to lie flat, awakening from sleep with angina or shortness of breath, or angina at rest or with minimal exertion are evidence of significant cardiac disease. If a patient can climb two to three flights of stairs without symptoms, cardiac reserve is probably adequate. It is very common for patients with severe CAD requiring revascularization to state that they are able to walk as much as they would like but then admit to not being able to climb a single flight of stairs without shortness of breath. The ability to walk slowly on level ground requires only minimal exertion.

### Angina Pectoris

Angina pectoris is considered to be stable when no change has occurred for at least 60 days in precipitating factors, frequency, and duration. Chest pain or shortness of breath produced with less than normal activity or at rest, or increasing in frequency, or lasting for increasingly longer periods is considered characteristic of unstable angina pectoris and may signal an impending myocardial infarction. Dyspnea following the onset of angina pectoris may be indicative of acute left ventricular dysfunction due to myocardial ischemia. Angina pectoris due to spasm of the coronary arteries (variant or Prinzmetal angina) differs from classic angina pectoris in that it may occur at rest and then be absent during vigorous exertion. Silent myocardial ischemia does not evoke angina pectoris (asymptomatic) and usually occurs at a heart rate and systemic arterial blood pressure less than those present during exercise-induced myocardial ischemia. About 70% of ischemic episodes are not associated with angina pectoris and as many as 15% of acute myocardial infarctions are silent. Women and diabetics are more likely to have painless myocardial ischemia and infarctions. The most common angina symptom in men is shortness of breath with exertion (e.g., stair climbing), and the most common symptom in women is fatigue.

The heart rate and systolic blood pressure at which angina pectoris or evidence of myocardial ischemia is indicated on the ECG are useful preoperative information. An increased heart rate is more likely than hypertension to produce signs of myocardial ischemia (Fig. 25.1). Tachycardia increases myocardial oxygen requirements while at the same time decreases the duration of diastole, thereby decreasing left ventricular coronary blood flow, which occurs in diastole, and the delivery of oxygen to the left ventricle. Conversely, increased systolic and diastolic blood pressure, while increasing oxygen consumption, simultaneously increases coronary perfusion despite the presence of atherosclerotic coronary arteries.

## Prior Myocardial Infarction

The incidence of myocardial reinfarction in the perioperative period is related to the time elapsed since the previous myocardial infarction (Table 25.1).[9-12] The incidence of perioperative myocardial reinfarction generally does not stabilize at 5% to 6% until 6 months after the prior myocardial infarction. Thus, a common recommendation is to delay elective surgery, especially thoracic, upper abdominal, or other major procedures, for a period of 2 to 6 months after a myocardial infarction.[6] The exact duration

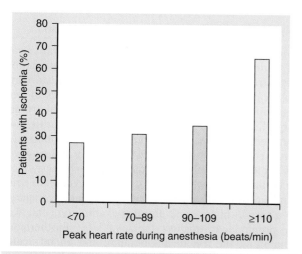

**Fig. 25.1** The incidence of myocardial ischemia increases with heart rates with the greatest effect at heart rates above 110 beats/min. (From Slogoff S, Keats AS. Does chronic treatment with calcium entry blocking drugs reduce perioperative myocardial ischemia? *Anesthesiology.* 1988;68:676-680, used with permission.)

of suggested delay is not clear. Even after 6 months, the 5% to 6% incidence of myocardial reinfarction is about 50 times higher than the 0.13% incidence of perioperative myocardial infarction in patients undergoing similar operations but in the absence of a prior myocardial infarction.[13] Most perioperative myocardial reinfarctions occur in the first 48 to 72 hours postoperatively. However, if ischemia is initiated by the stress of surgery, there can be an increased risk of myocardial infarction for several months after surgery.[3,14]

Several factors influence the incidence of myocardial infarction in the perioperative period. For example, the incidence of myocardial reinfarction is increased in patients undergoing intrathoracic or intraabdominal operations lasting longer than 3 hours. Factors that do not predispose to a myocardial reinfarction include the (1) site of the previous myocardial infarction, (2) history of prior aortocoronary bypass graft surgery, (3) site of the operative procedure if the duration of the surgery is shorter than 3 hours, and (4) techniques used to produce anesthesia. In patients with CAD or PVD, appropriate use of β-adrenergic blocking drugs reduces the risk of cardiac morbidity (myocardial infarction or cardiac death) (also see Chapter 6).[6] Statin therapy with fluvastatin for 30 days before and after surgery, in addition to β-adrenergic blockade, reduces risk of myocardial infarction and death by an additional 50%.[15] Intensive hemodynamic monitoring using an intra-arterial catheter and prompt pharmacologic intervention or fluid infusion to treat physiologic hemodynamic alterations from the normal range may decrease the risk of perioperative cardiac morbidity in high-risk patients (see Table 25.1).[11]

## Current Medications

Drugs most likely to be taken by patients with CAD are β-adrenergic antagonists, nitrates, calcium channel blockers, angiotensin-converting enzyme inhibitors, drugs that decrease blood lipids, diuretics, antihypertensives, and platelet inhibitors. Knowledge of the pharmacology of these drugs and potential adverse interactions with anesthetics is an important preoperative consideration (see Chapters 6 and 8). Accordingly, patients with known CAD, known PVD, or those receiving β-adrenergic blocking drugs should be monitored throughout the perioperative

**IV**

| Table 25.1 | Incidence of Perioperative Myocardial Infarction | | | |
|---|---|---|---|---|
| **Time Elapsed Since Previous Myocardial Infarction** | **Reported Incidence** | | | |
| | Tarhan et al[9] | Steen et al[10] | Rao et al[11] | Shah et al[12] |
| 0-3 months | 37% | 27% | 5.7% | 4.3% |
| 4-6 months | 16% | 11% | 2.3% | 0 |
| >6 months | 5% | 6% | | 5.7% |

**Table 25.2**    Area of Myocardial Ischemia as Reflected by the Electrocardiogram

| Electrocardiogram Leads | Coronary Artery Responsible for Myocardial Ischemia | Area of Myocardium That May Be Involved |
| --- | --- | --- |
| II, III, aVF | Right coronary artery | Right atrium<br>Sinus node<br>Atrioventricular node<br>Right ventricle |
| $V_3$-$V_5$ | Left anterior descending coronary artery | Anterolateral aspects of the left ventricle |
| I, aVL | Circumflex coronary artery | Lateral aspects of the left ventricle |

period.[6] Although COPD is not a contraindication to perioperative β-adrenergic blockade,[16,17] reactive asthma is. Patients with CAD or vascular disease should receive a statin type of drug unless there is a specific contraindication.[15] Despite the potential for adverse drug interactions, cardiac medications being taken preoperatively should be continued without interruption through the perioperative period. Discontinuation of β-adrenergic blockers,[18] calcium channel blockers, nitrates, statins, angiotensin-converting enzyme inhibitors,[19,20] or angiotensin receptor blockers[21] in the perioperative period can increase risk of perioperative morbidity and mortality and should not be discontinued.

## Electrocardiogram

Preoperative evaluation of a resting 12-lead ECG is reasonable for patients with known coronary heart disease, significant arrhythmia(s), peripheral arterial disease, cerebrovascular disease, or other significant structural heart disease and may be indicated for some asymptomatic patients without known coronary heart disease (also see Chapter 20). Preoperative resting 12-lead ECG is not indicated in patients undergoing low-risk surgery.[6] The preoperative ECG should be examined for evidence of (1) myocardial ischemia, (2) prior myocardial infarction, (3) cardiac hypertrophy, (4) abnormal cardiac rhythm and conduction disturbances, and (5) electrolyte abnormalities. The exercise ECG simulates sympathetic nervous system stimulation as may accompany perioperative events such as direct laryngoscopy, tracheal intubation, surgical incision, postoperative pain, and recovery. The resting ECG in the absence of angina pectoris may be normal despite extensive CAD. Nevertheless, an ECG demonstrating ST-segment depression more than 1 mm, particularly during angina pectoris, confirms the presence of myocardial ischemia. Furthermore, the ECG lead demonstrating changes of myocardial ischemia can help determine the specific diseased coronary artery (Table 25.2). It is of particular importance that a prior myocardial infarction, especially if subendocardial, may not be accompanied by persistent changes on the ECG. The preoperative presence of ventricular premature beats may signal their likely occurrence intraoperatively. A prolonged PR interval on the ECG (longer than 200 ms) may be related to medication therapy such as amiodarone, digoxin, pregabalin, or dolasetron. Conversely, the block of conduction of cardiac impulses below the atrioventricular node (right bundle branch block, left bundle branch block, or intraventricular conduction delay) most likely reflects pathologic changes rather than drug effect.

## Risk Stratification Versus Risk Reduction

One of the standard approaches to the perioperative care of patients with cardiac disease is risk stratification. Risk stratification consists of a preoperative history and physical examination followed by some series of tests thought to predict perioperative cardiac morbidity and mortality risks. These tests may include persantine thallium, echocardiography, Holter monitoring, dobutamine stress echocardiography, and angiography and may lead to angioplasty with or without an intracoronary stent or coronary artery bypass surgery. Yet, preoperative risk stratification with invasive testing may not be superior to a careful history and physical examination followed by prophylactic medical therapy.[6-8,17,22] Furthermore, combining the risk of angiography and an intracoronary stent or coronary artery bypass graft (CABG) to a surgical procedure may not reduce total risk.[6,23,24] The combined risk of two procedures may exceed that of the original operation.[23,25,26] Despite the lack of proven benefit of prophylactic invasive testing combined with either CABG or coronary angioplasty with stenting over medical therapy, the American College of Cardiology (ACC) and American Heart Association (AHA) have developed a protocol entitled ACC/AHA Guideline Perioperative Cardiovascular Evaluation for Noncardiac Surgery.[6,27-30] Fig. 25.2 provides a suggested protocol for preoperative evaluation. Unfortunately, the ACC/AHA protocol has been studied and found to be difficult to apply in practice with conflicting guidance on indications for testing with physicians ordering more tests than suggested by the guidelines.[31] Perioperative risk reduction therapy with β-adrenergic blockers and

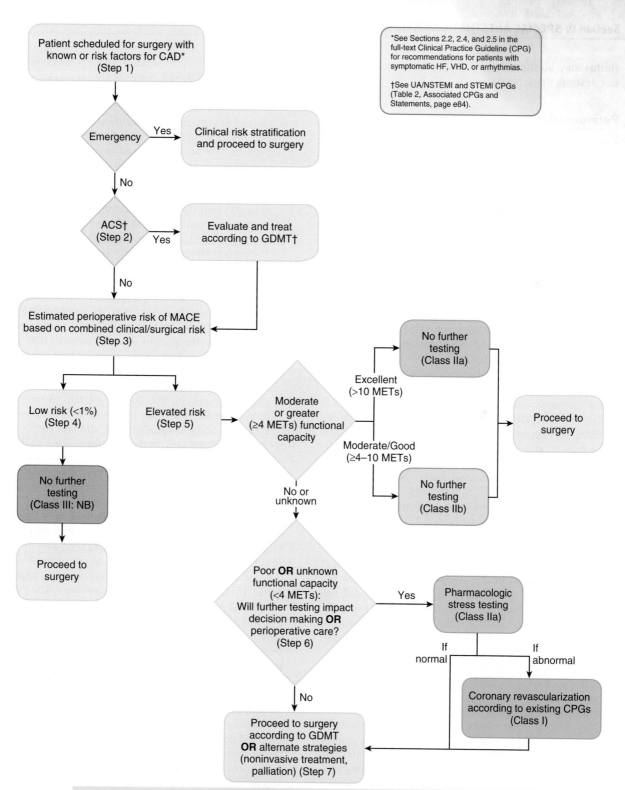

**Fig. 25.2** Stepwise approach to perioperative cardiac assessment for coronary artery disease (CAD). *ACS,* Acute coronary syndrome; *CPG,* clinical practice guideline; *GDMT,* guideline-directed medical therapy; *HF,* heart failure; *MACE,* major adverse cardiac event; *MET,* metabolic equivalent; *NB,* no benefit; *STEMI,* ST-segment elevation myocardial infarction; *UA/NSTEMI,* unstable angina/non–ST-segment elevation myocardial infarction; *VHD,* valvular heart disease. (From Fleisher L, Fleischmann K, Auerbach AD, et al. 2014 ACC/AHA Guideline on Perioperative Cardiovascular Evaluation and Management of Patients Undergoing Noncardiac Surgery. A report of the American College of Cardiology/American Heart Association Task Force on Practice Guidelines. *J Am Coll Cardiol.* 2014;64(22):e77-e137.)

statins may be superior to risk stratification with invasive testing, angioplasty, and CABG.[6,15-17,23,32-35]

## Perioperative Cardiac Risk Reduction Therapy

There is some controversy after the publication of the POISE study on the use of prophylactic perioperative β-adrenergic blockade.[36,37] Continuation of anti-ischemic drugs in the perioperative period is recommended.[6,32,33] Perioperative use of β-adrenergic blockers in patients with known CAD or PVD is recommended.[6] Prophylactic addition of β-adrenergic blockers to patients at risk for CAD is recommended in patients with significant cardiac risk (revised cardiac risk index [RCRI] ≥ 3) and in those patients with intermediate- or high-risk preoperative tests.[6] If initiation of β-adrenergic blocker administration is planned, it should begin long enough in advance of surgery to assess safety and tolerability, preferably more than 1 day.[6] Large-dose β-adrenergic blocker[36,37] therapy should not be started on the day of surgery.[6,16,17] The following β-adrenergic blocker protocol[14,17] has been tested in 40,000 patients and has been shown to reduce risk.[32,33]

1. All patients who have either CAD, PVD, or two risk factors for CAD (age ≥ 60 years, cigarette smoking, diabetes, hypertension, cholesterol ≥ 240 mg/dL) should receive perioperative β-adrenergic blockade unless they have a specific intolerance to β-adrenergic blockers. Patients with renal failure or renal insufficiency may also benefit from therapy.

2. β-Adrenergic blockade should be started as soon as the patient is identified as having CAD, PVD, or risk factors. If the surgeon identifies the patient as having risk, the surgeon should start the medication. If the anesthesia preoperative clinic identifies the patient, it should be started in the preoperative clinic (also see Chapter 13). If the patient is not identified until the morning of surgery, intravenous atenolol or metoprolol should be used. If the drug is started prior to the day of surgery, atenolol 25 mg by mouth (PO) per day (qd) is an appropriate starting dose.

3. β-Adrenergic blockade should be continued until at least 30 days postoperatively, if not indefinitely, in patients with CAD or PVD. In patients with only risk factors, 7 days may be sufficient.

4. The optimal time to start β-adrenergic blockade is at the time of identification of the risk. This process should be multitiered to avoid missing patients. The following approach should be used to provide the maximum benefit at the minimum cost.
   a. The surgeon should give a β-adrenergic blocker if the patient has CAD, PVD, or two risk factors. Atenolol 25 mg PO daily is an appropriate starting dose.
   b. If a medical or cardiology consult is requested by surgery, the most common advice is: start a β-adrenergic blocker.
   c. The anesthesia preoperative clinic checks to see if the patients at risk are receiving a β-adrenergic blocker. If the patient is not getting adequate β-adrenergic blockade, the dose is increased.
   d. On the day of surgery, treatment with or increasing the dose of intravenously (IV) administered β-adrenergic blockers should be considered. Intravenous metoprolol in 5-mg boluses is used. Standard dose is 10 mg IV (withhold for heart rate less than 50 beats/min or systolic blood pressure less than 100 mm Hg). Intraoperative doses are used as needed. The patient should receive additional doses in the postanesthesia care unit as needed.
   e. The patient should receive the drug postoperatively for 30 days. If the patient is nil per os (NPO, or nothing by mouth), the patient receives intravenous metoprolol (10 mg IV q12h) unless systolic blood pressure is less than 100 mm Hg or heart rate is less than 50 beats/min. If the patient is taking oral medications, the patient receives atenolol 100 mg PO daily if the heart rate is more rapid than 65 beats/min and the systolic blood pressure is more than 100 mm Hg. If the heart rate is between 55 and 65 beats/min, the dose is 50 mg. There is a hold order for heart rate less than 50 beats/min or systolic blood pressure less than 100 mm Hg.
   f. The patient remains on the drug for at least 30 days postoperatively.
   g. Many patients should remain on the drug for life (patients with known CAD, known PVD, and hypertension).

5. Preoperative testing and revascularization[26] should only be used as needed for specific indications not prophylaxis.[38] If a patient is identified with new-onset angina, unstable angina, a change in the anginal pattern, or CHF, then further risk stratification is appropriate. If the patient is stable with known CAD, PVD, or two risk factors for CAD, the patient should receive a β-adrenergic blocker.[16,17,32,33]

6. Care should be taken with patients who have CHF, aortic stenosis, intracoronary stents on platelet inhibitors, or renal failure. All patients who have CHF should be evaluated by a cardiologist for the initiation of β-adrenergic blocker therapy. β-Adrenergic blocker therapy reduces the risk of death from CHF. Many patients with CHF are profoundly improved by β-adrenergic blockade; however, the dose must be titrated slowly and usually under the supervision of a cardiologist. Patients with aortic stenosis should be evaluated by cardiology and β-adrenergic blockade initiated with a cardiologist's supervision.

7. Patients with intracoronary stents on platelet inhibitors should be seen by a cardiologist. WARNING: Discontinuation of platelet inhibitors in patients with intracoronary stents can be lethal.[24,39,40] Patients with renal failure should be treated with appropriate drugs, but special attention is needed.

8. Patients with an indication for statin therapy and especially those with known CAD or PVD should be considered for statin therapy.[15] Therapy should be started 30 days prior to surgery and continued for at least 30 days after surgery,[15] possibly indefinitely.

## Management of Anesthesia

Anesthesia care for patients with known CAD, known PVD, or two risk factors for CAD (age ≥ 60 years, hypertension, diabetes, significant smoking history, or hyperlipidemia) should begin as soon as the patient is identified as needing surgery.[16,17,32,33] All patients with new-onset angina, a change in anginal pattern, unstable angina, angina without medical therapy, aortic stenosis, CHF, or an intracoronary stent receiving a platelet inhibitor should be referred to cardiology. Patients with recently placed intracoronary stents receiving platelet inhibitors have a high risk of intracoronary thrombosis and death when the platelet inhibitors are discontinued for perioperative care.[24,39,40] Patients with bare metal stents may require 3 or more months of antiplatelet therapy.[40] Patients with drug-eluting intracoronary stents may require platelet inhibitors for a year or more.[39] Patients with stable coronary disease on medical therapy with no evidence of CHF or aortic stenosis should receive an oral β-adrenergic blocker (atenolol or metoprolol 25 mg/day PO) and a statin drug.[15] Patients with CHF should have β-adrenergic blockers initiated by cardiology over a prolonged period. The dose of β-adrenergic blockers should be increased as tolerated. β-Adrenergic blockers should be avoided in patients with a history of high-grade atrioventricular (AV) block without a pacemaker, reactive asthma, or an intolerance for β-adrenergic blockers. Diabetes is an indication for perioperative β-adrenergic blockade. For maximal effect, β-adrenergic blockers should be started as soon as the patient is identified as needing surgery.[14,17] Starting high-dose β-adrenergic blockers on the day of surgery is not indicated.[6,36,37] If a patient is identified on the day of surgery, intravenous atenolol or metoprolol can be started in the preoperative area (atenolol or metoprolol 10 mg IV if the heart rate is more rapid than 55 beats/min or systolic blood pressure is higher than 100 mm Hg) and continued postoperatively.[16] Perioperative β-adrenergic blockers should be continued for at least 7 days postoperatively.[16] In patients with higher risks (those with known CAD or PVD), β-adrenergic blockers should be continued at least 30 days if not indefinitely.[14,17] Esmolol boluses during surgery do not constitute perioperative β-adrenergic blockade and are not adequate to reduce perioperative cardiac risk.[41] Appropriate dosing of β-adrenergic blockers is prudent to avoid sequelae related to hypotension and bradycardia.[37]

The intraoperative anesthetic management as well as postoperative pain management (also see Chapter 40) of patients with CAD should permit the modulation of sympathetic nervous system responses and provide for the rigorous control of hemodynamic variables.[1] Management of anesthesia in these patients is based on a preoperative evaluation of left ventricular function and the maintenance of a favorable balance between myocardial oxygen requirements and myocardial oxygen delivery so as to prevent myocardial ischemia (Table 25.3 and Box 25.1). Any event associated with persistent tachycardia, systolic hypertension, arterial hypoxemia, or diastolic hypotension can adversely influence this delicate balance. Heart rate higher than 100 beats/min increases the risk of postoperative death in patients with risk for CAD; heart rates higher than 120 beats/min significantly increase risk.

Persistent and excessive changes in heart rate and systemic arterial blood pressure should be minimized (see Fig. 25.1).[42] Maintaining heart rate and systemic arterial blood pressure within 20% of the awake values is commonly recommended. Monitoring with an intra-arterial catheter greatly improves the ability to maintain stable systemic arterial blood pressures. Nevertheless, an estimated one half of all new perioperative ischemic episodes are not preceded by or associated with significant changes in heart rate or systemic arterial blood pressure.[43]

| Table 25.3 | Evaluation of Left Ventricular Function | |
|---|---|---|
| **Assessment Feature** | **Good Function** | **Impaired Function** |
| Previous myocardial infarction | No | Yes |
| Evidence of congestive heart failure | No | Yes |
| Ejection fraction | >0.55 | <0.4 |
| Left ventricular end-diastolic pressure | <12 mm Hg | >18 mm Hg |
| Cardiac index | >2.5 L/min/m² | <2 L/min/m² |
| Areas of ventricular dyskinesia | No | Yes |

**Box 25.1** Determinants of Myocardial Oxygen Requirements and Delivery

**Myocardial Oxygen Requirements**
- Heart rate
- Systolic blood pressure
- Myocardial contractility
- Ventricular volume

**Myocardial Oxygen Delivery**
- Coronary blood flow
- Oxygen content of arterial blood

A single 1-minute episode of myocardial ischemia detected by a 1-mm ST-segment elevation or depression increases the risk of cardiac events 10-fold and the risk for death 2-fold.[3,4] Tachycardia for 5 minutes above 120 beats/min in the postoperative period can increase the risk of death 10-fold. The only clinically proven method to reduce the risk of perioperative myocardial ischemia and associated death is perioperative β-adrenergic blockade (atenolol or metoprolol).[16,17,32,33]

## Monitoring (Also See Chapter 20)

Anticipation of problems and avoidance of potential disasters are key components for successful anesthetic management of patients with cardiovascular disease. Prophylactic therapy and more extensive monitoring reduce risk. Continuous intra-arterial pressure monitoring can reduce the risk of hemodynamic events by early identification of problems. Continuous ECG monitoring rapidly identifies arrhythmias, tachycardia, and myocardial ischemia. Monitoring should be continuous if possible. Rapid changes in hemodynamics can quickly lead to cardiac arrest; monitoring can quickly identify those changes and permits prompt therapy before further complications develop. When operations are completed, monitoring should be continued into the recovery room or intensive care unit (ICU). When patients are transferred from the operating room table to the gurney or ICU bed, or are turned from supine to prone or back to supine, monitoring should be as continuous as possible. Unconscious patients with cardiac disease may have rapid hemodynamic collapse with transfers from the operating room table to the gurney or ICU bed or when turned over and should be monitored during transfers. If arterial blood pressure, ECG, and saturation are monitored, the problem can be quickly identified and corrected prior to serious sequelae. Intravascular volume, vasoconstrictors, β-agonists, β-adrenergic blockers, anticholinergics, and vasodilator drugs should be immediately available. Loss of a pulse oximeter signal or desaturation can imply hypoxia or inadequate arterial blood pressure or cardiac output and should signal an immediate search for a cause and initiation of corrective action. The pulse oximeter is a monitor of both oxygen saturation and perfusion. If the pulse oximeter loses a signal, adequacy of perfusion should be assessed. Loss of the pulse oximeter signal may occur simply from the finger becoming cold, or much more importantly, may be the first warning of hemodynamic collapse. Continuous monitoring and prophylactic therapy can reduce the risk in patients with cardiovascular disease.

The intensity of monitoring in the perioperative period is influenced by the complexity of the operative procedure and the severity of the cardiovascular disease. The five-lead ECG serves as a noninvasive monitor of the balance between myocardial oxygen requirements and myocardial oxygen delivery in unconscious patients (also see

Chapter 20). When this balance is unfavorably altered, myocardial ischemia occurs, as evidenced on the ECG by at least a 1-mm downsloping of the ST segment from the baseline. A precordial $V_5$ lead is a useful selection for detecting ST-segment changes characteristic of ischemia of the left ventricle during anesthesia. Intra-arterial pressure monitoring can speed the identification and treatment of hemodynamic changes. Monitoring should be continuous if possible. Ventricular wall motion abnormalities observed by TEE may be the most sensitive indicator of myocardial ischemia, but this monitor is expensive, is invasive, and requires additional training before its use as a routine method for detecting an imbalance between myocardial oxygen delivery and myocardial oxygen requirements. Intraoperative monitoring of pulmonary artery pressures or use of TEE should be reserved for selected high-risk patients (cardiac surgery, recent myocardial infarction, current CHF, unstable angina).[1] Continuous cardiac output monitoring with stroke volume variation (SVV) measurement of fluid responsiveness may improve intravascular fluid management.[44]

## Induction of Anesthesia

Preoperative anxiety can lead to preoperative myocardial ischemia.[41] Myocardial ischemia predisposes to subsequent myocardial ischemia. Preoperative β-adrenergic blocker therapy reduces the incidence of myocardial ischemia.[17,41] Patients should receive their routine medications except for oral hypoglycemic drugs. Preoperative sedative medication is intended to produce sedation and reduce anxiety, which, if unopposed, could lead to secretion of catecholamines and an increase in myocardial oxygen requirements because of an increase in heart rate and systemic arterial blood pressure. Oral administration of benzodiazepines (diazepam or lorazepam PO) is an effective pharmacologic approach to allay severe anxiety. Supplemental oxygen may be needed if narcotics are combined with benzodiazepines for sedation.

Induction of anesthesia is acceptably accomplished with the intravenous administration of rapidly acting drugs. Preinduction placement of an intra-arterial catheter to monitor arterial blood pressure allows rapid pharmacologic manipulations and a very stable induction of anesthesia. An infusion of phenylephrine (0.2 to 0.4 µg/kg/min) started prophylactically stabilizes arterial blood pressure and can eliminate most hemodynamic changes with induction. Etomidate is a popular anesthetic to induce anesthesia because of its limited inhibition of the sympathetic nervous system and limited hemodynamic effects[45] (also see Chapter 8). The lack of inhibition of autonomic reflexes by etomidate may lead to hypertension with laryngoscopy and endotracheal intubation. Propofol is popular secondary to its antiemetic effects and rapid recovery, but the dose should be reduced to avoid hypotension with induction. Fentanyl and midazolam in combination with an infusion of phenylephrine and a nondepolarizing muscle relaxant cause minimal associated changes in arterial blood pressure or heart rate.

Ketamine is not often used to induce anesthesia for patients with coronary disease because of the associated increase in heart rate and systemic arterial blood pressure, which may increase myocardial oxygen requirements. When giving desflurane, the inspired concentration should be slowly increased to avoid sympathetic stimulation and associated tachycardia, pulmonary hypertension, myocardial ischemia, and bronchospasm.[46] Tracheal intubation is facilitated by the administration of succinylcholine or a nondepolarizing neuromuscular blocking drug (also see Chapter 11).

Myocardial ischemia may accompany the tachycardia and hypertension that result from the stimulation of direct laryngoscopy as necessary for tracheal intubation. Adequate anesthesia and a brief duration of direct laryngoscopy are important in minimizing the magnitude of these circulatory changes. When the duration of direct laryngoscopy is not likely to be brief, or when hypertension coexists, the addition of other drugs to minimize the pressor response produced by tracheal intubation should be considered. For example, laryngotracheal lidocaine (2 mg/kg) administered just before placing the tube in the trachea produces rapid topical anesthesia of the tracheal mucosa and minimizes the magnitude and duration of the systemic arterial blood pressure increase. Alternatively, lidocaine (1.5 mg/kg IV), administered just before initiating direct laryngoscopy, is efficacious (also see Chapter 16).

Administration of opioids (fentanyl, sufentanil, alfentanil, or remifentanil) before initiating direct laryngoscopy reduces the stimulation produced by tracheal intubation. β-Adrenergic blockers are effective in attenuating heart rate increases associated with tracheal intubation. Tachycardia should be avoided in all patients with coronary disease, vascular disease, or risk factors for coronary disease.

### Maintenance of Anesthesia

The choice of anesthesia is often based on the patient's left ventricular function (see Table 25.3). For example, patients with CAD but normal left ventricular function may develop tachycardia and hypertension in response to intense stimulation. Controlled myocardial depression produced by a volatile anesthetic with or without nitrous oxide may be appropriate if the primary goal is to prevent increased myocardial oxygen requirements. Equally acceptable for maintenance of anesthesia is the use of a nitrous oxide–opioid technique with the addition of a volatile anesthetic as necessary to treat acute increases in systemic arterial blood pressure as produced by a change in the level of surgical stimulation. When hypertension is treated with a volatile anesthetic (isoflurane, desflurane, sevoflurane), the drug-induced decrease in systemic vascular resistance (SVR) is more responsible for decreases

in systemic arterial blood pressure than is drug-induced myocardial depression. The ability to rapidly increase the alveolar concentration of sevoflurane makes this drug uniquely efficacious for treating sudden increases in systemic arterial blood pressure. Abrupt and large increases in the delivered concentrations of desflurane may be accompanied by stimulation of the sympathetic nervous system and transient increases in systemic arterial blood pressure, heart rate, pulmonary hypertension, and myocardial ischemia[51] (also see Chapter 7).

Volatile anesthetics are vasodilators. Under unusual clinical circumstances, potent coronary vasodilators can divert blood flow from ischemic areas of myocardium (blood vessels already fully dilated) to nonischemic areas of myocardium supplied by vessels capable of vasodilation. Regional myocardial ischemia associated with drug-induced vasodilation is known as coronary artery steal. There are reports that the incidence of myocardial ischemia is either unchanged or increased in patients with CAD and anesthetized with isoflurane compared with those receiving a different volatile anesthetic or an opioid-based anesthetic.[47-49] Volatile anesthetics to varying degrees (halothane, isoflurane, sevoflurane, and desflurane) induce ischemic preconditioning and may protect the myocardium from subsequent ischemia.[50,51] All facts considered, volatile anesthetics may be either beneficial in patients with CAD because they decrease myocardial oxygen requirements and induce ischemic preconditioning, or detrimental because they decrease systemic arterial blood pressure and coronary perfusion pressure or produce coronary artery steal (isoflurane) or tachycardia (desflurane).[46] A large clinical trial in patients undergoing cardiac surgery failed to demonstrate a difference between halothane, enflurane, isoflurane, and narcotic-based anesthetics.[52] Avoiding tachycardia with the use of long-acting β-adrenergic blockers (metoprolol or atenolol) is more important than anesthetic choice.[16,17,32,33] Intraoperative bolus doses of short-acting β-adrenergic blockers (esmolol) have not been shown to be effective in reducing perioperative cardiac risk. Prophylactic perioperative administration of long-acting β-adrenergic blockers (metoprolol or atenolol) is needed to reduce perioperative risk.[41]

Patients with impaired left ventricular function, as associated with a prior myocardial infarction, may not tolerate direct myocardial depression produced by volatile anesthetics. In these patients, the use of short-acting opioids with nitrous oxide may be a more acceptable selection. Nitrous oxide, when administered to patients who have received opioids for anesthesia, may produce undesirable decreases in systemic arterial blood pressure and cardiac output. High-dose fentanyl (50 to 100 µg/kg IV) or equivalent doses of sufentanil or alfentanil as the primary anesthetic with benzodiazepines added to ensure amnesia may be useful for patients who cannot tolerate the myocardial depression from even low concentrations

**IV**

of anesthesia. Yet, this technique is not clearly better than moderate dose narcotics with an inhaled or intravenous anesthetic.[52] Infusions of dexmedetomidine combined with smaller-dose fentanyl (1-10 µg/kg) and inhaled anesthetics work well and apparently reduce postoperative delirium in patients undergoing CABG.[53]

A regional anesthetic is an excellent technique in patients with CAD (also see Chapters 17 and 18). Regional anesthesia for peripheral surgery (orthopedic, podiatric, peripheral vascular) and lower abdominal surgery (gynecologic and urologic) is a very safe technique for patients with cardiac risk. However, flow through critically narrowed coronary arteries is pressure-dependent. Therefore, decreases in systemic arterial blood pressure associated with a regional anesthetic that are more than 20% of the preblock value probably should be treated with an intravenous infusion of crystalloid solutions or a vasoconstrictor such as phenylephrine. Phenylephrine improves coronary perfusion pressure but at the expense of increasing afterload and myocardial oxygen requirements. Nevertheless, the increase in coronary perfusion pressure is likely to more than offset any increase in myocardial oxygen requirements. Perioperative β-adrenergic blockers should be used in patients with cardiac risk undergoing surgery using regional anesthesia.

### Neuromuscular Blocking Drugs (Also See Chapter 11)

The choice of nondepolarizing neuromuscular blocking drugs during maintenance of anesthesia for patients with CAD may be influenced by the circulatory effects of these drugs. Vecuronium, rocuronium, and cisatracurium do not evoke histamine release and associated decreases in systemic arterial blood pressure, even with the rapid intravenous administration of large doses. Likewise, the systemic arterial blood pressure lowering effects of atracurium and mivacurium are usually modest, especially if the drug is injected over 30 to 45 seconds to minimize the likelihood of drug-induced histamine release. None of these neuromuscular blocking drugs will adversely alter myocardial oxygen requirements. Pancuronium increases heart rate and systemic arterial blood pressure, but these changes are usually less than 15% above predrug values, making this drug a possible choice for administration to patients with CAD. Furthermore, circulatory changes produced by pancuronium can be used to offset negative inotropic or chronotropic effects of drugs being used for anesthesia. In contrast to pancuronium, the other nondepolarizing neuromuscular blocking drugs would not be expected to offset decreases in systemic arterial blood pressure or heart rate as associated with the administration of large doses of opioids. With the increased use of more selective neuromuscular blocking drugs (vecuronium, rocuronium, and cisatracurium), use of pancuronium has markedly decreased and in some cases has been eliminated.

Nondepolarizing neuromuscular blockade in patients with CAD can be safely antagonized with anticholinesterase drugs (i.e., neostigmine) combined with an anticholinergic drug. Glycopyrrolate has more titratable chronotropic effects than atropine. Tachycardia after reversal of nondepolarizing muscle relaxants can still occur. One of the common causes of postoperative myocardial ischemia and infarction is tachycardia after emergence, which may be the result of the combination of emergence, surgical pain, and reversal of nondepolarizing muscle relaxants. The addition of long-acting intravenous β-adrenergic blockers should be used to avoid tachycardia, which may lead to myocardial ischemia in this period.

Sugammadex has been used in many countries and now the United States (also see Chapter 11 for details). Sugammadex does not have significant cardiovascular effects. Readers are advised to read the Food and Drug Administration (FDA) prescribing information, which provides an excellent description of its pharmacology.

### Treatment of Myocardial Ischemia

The appearance of signs of myocardial ischemia on the ECG supports the aggressive treatment of adverse changes in heart rate or systemic arterial blood pressure. Only 5% of perioperative myocardial ischemia found on Holter ECG is identified by clinicians. Prophylactic therapy with long-acting β-adrenergic blockers is essential to reduce perioperative risk.[16,17,32,33] Tachycardia is treated with the administration of atenolol, metoprolol, propranolol, or esmolol. Excessive increases in systemic arterial blood pressure respond to narcotics, increases in inhaled anesthetics, β-adrenergic blockers, or continuous intravenous infusion of nitroprusside. Nitroglycerin is a more appropriate choice than nitroprusside when myocardial ischemia is associated with a normal systemic arterial blood pressure. Hypotension should be treated with a phenylephrine infusion to rapidly restore pressure-dependent perfusion through atherosclerotic coronary arteries. In addition to drugs, the intravenous infusion of fluids to restore systemic arterial blood pressure can improve myocardial oxygen supply. A disadvantage of this approach is the time necessary for intravenous fluid treatment to be effective.

Although few or no data support the use of pulmonary artery catheters,[54,55] in selected patients a pulmonary artery catheter in combination with a TEE probe may be helpful for monitoring responses to intravenous fluid replacement and the therapeutic effects of drugs on left ventricular function and cardiac output. Continuous measurement of SVV or pulse pressure variation (PPV) can predict fluid responsiveness and be used to optimize fluid administration as part of goal-directed therapy. Right atrial (central venous) pressure does not predict left-sided heart volume status.[56] In healthy patients who have a reduced need for monitoring and in patients with CAD when the ejection fraction is higher than 0.5 and when there is no evidence of left ventricular dysfunction, right atrial pressure is more likely to correlate with pulmonary artery occlusion pressure.[57,58] Pressures measured with pulmonary artery catheters correlate poorly with volume status in patients with diastolic dysfunction, myocardial ischemia, mitral regurgitation or stenosis, pulmonary hypertension, positive end-expiratory pressure (PEEP), pulmonary stenosis, or tricuspid regurgitation. Abrupt increases in the pulmonary artery pressure may also reflect acute myocardial ischemia or acute mitral regurgitation. When compared with TEE, monitoring with a pulmonary artery catheter is not a highly sensitive approach for detecting myocardial ischemia. TEE also provides an assessment of regional wall motion, global ventricular function, valvular function, intravascular fluid volume, and associated ventricular filling. TEE is more expensive than pulmonary artery catheterization, but the information is more accurate and useful than pulmonary artery catheter data.

Decreases in body temperature that occur intraoperatively may predispose to shivering on awakening, leading to abrupt increases in myocardial oxygen requirements. Attempts to minimize decreases in body temperature and provision of supplemental oxygen are of obvious importance. Postoperative pain relief is important as pain-induced activation of the sympathetic nervous system can increase myocardial oxygen requirements.

## Postoperative Care

Postoperative care of the patient with CAD is based on provision of perioperative anti-ischemic drugs (β-adrenergic blockers, or statins), analgesia, and, if needed, sedation to blunt excessive sympathetic nervous system activity and facilitate rigorous control of hemodynamic variables (also see Chapter 39). Intensive and continuous postoperative monitoring is useful for detecting myocardial ischemia, which is often asymptomatic. Episodes of myocardial ischemia lead to increased risk and increasingly frequent occurrences.[3,17,59] Reducing the incidence of myocardial ischemia with β-adrenergic blockers reduces 30-day and 2-year mortality rates.[17,41] Patients with known CAD, known PVD, or two risk factors for CAD (≥60 years of age, hypertension, vascular disease, diabetes, significant smoking history, or hyperlipidemia) should be placed on a perioperative β-adrenergic blocker unless there is a specific contraindication.[16,17,32,33] They should receive β-adrenergic blockers as soon as they are identified as being at risk for cardiac complications.[6,16,17,32,33] Patients with a lower risk should take the drug for at least 7 days postoperatively.[16,17] Patients with known coronary disease or vascular disease should remain on the drug for at least 30 days if not permanently. COPD is not a contraindication to perioperative β-adrenergic blockade, but reactive asthma is. Diabetes is not a contraindication for perioperative β-adrenergic blockade; it is an indication. All medications have a therapeutic index and β-adrenergic blockers are no exception. The dose of perioperative β-adrenergic blockers should follow standard manufacturer guidelines to avoid hypotension, bradycardia, morbidity, and death.[37]

The major determinant of pulmonary complications (atelectasis, pneumonia) after cardiac surgery is poor cardiac function. Early mobilization and pain control are likely to minimize the incidence of clinically significant pulmonary complications.

## VALVULAR HEART DISEASE

The most frequently encountered forms of valvular heart disease produce pressure overload (mitral stenosis, aortic stenosis) or volume overload (mitral regurgitation, aortic regurgitation).[60] The net effect of valvular heart disease is interference with forward flow of blood from the heart into the systemic circulation. TEE has revolutionized the evaluation and intraoperative management of valvular heart disease (Box 25.2). Selection of anesthetic drugs for patients with valvular heart disease is often based on the likely effects of drug-induced changes in cardiac rhythm, heart rate, systemic arterial blood pressure, SVR, and pulmonary vascular resistance (PVR) relative to maintenance of cardiac output in these patients. Although no specific general anesthetic is superior, when cardiac reserve is minimal, an anesthetic combination of opioids, an amnestic benzodiazepine, and an inhaled anesthetic is common. Dexmedetomidine infusions may be extremely useful in combination with other drugs. Patients with valvular heart disease should receive appropriate antibiotics in the perioperative period for protection against infective endocarditis. Monitoring intra-arterial pressure is helpful in patients with clinically significant valvular heart disease.

### Mitral Stenosis

Mitral stenosis is characterized by mechanical obstruction of left ventricular diastolic filling secondary to a progressive decrease in the orifice of the mitral valve. The obstruction produces an increase in left atrial and pulmonary venous pressure. Increased PVR is likely when the left atrial pressure is chronically higher than 25 mm Hg. Distention of the left atrium predisposes to atrial fibrillation, which can result in stasis of blood, the formation

---

**Box 25.2** Diagnosis: Echocardiography and Valvular Heart Disease

- Determine significance of cardiac murmurs (most often aortic stenosis).
- Identify hemodynamic abnormalities associated with physical findings (most often mitral regurgitation).
- Determine transvalvular pressure gradient.
- Determine cardiac valve regurgitation.
- Evaluate prosthetic valve function.

of thrombi, and systemic emboli. Chronic anticoagulation or antiplatelet therapy (or both) of patients with atrial fibrillation can reduce the risk of systemic embolic events. Mitral stenosis is commonly due to the fusion of the mitral valve leaflets during the healing process of acute rheumatic carditis. Symptoms of mitral stenosis do not usually develop until about 20 years after the initial episode of rheumatic fever. A sudden increase in the demand for cardiac output as produced by pregnancy or sepsis, however, may unmask previously asymptomatic mitral stenosis.

Patients with mitral stenosis who are being chronically treated with digitalis for the control of heart rate should continue to take this drug throughout the perioperative period. Adequate digitalis effect for heart rate control is generally reflected by a ventricular rate less than 80 beats/min. Because diuretic therapy is common in these patients, the serum potassium concentration should be measured preoperatively. Other common antiarrhythmic drugs such as β-adrenergic blockers should also be continued. The discontinuation of anticoagulant or antiplatelet therapy should be discussed with the surgeon and cardiologist. Patients should be switched from warfarin (Coumadin) therapy to heparin therapy prior to surgery depending on the type of case. Also, patients with mitral stenosis can be more susceptible than normal individuals to the ventilatory depressant effects of sedative drugs used for preoperative medication. If patients are given sedative drugs, supplemental oxygen may increase the margin of safety. Most medications that patients are taking, except anticoagulants, antiplatelet drugs, and oral hypoglycemic agents, should be continued throughout the preoperative period.

### Management of Anesthesia

Preinduction of anesthesia placement of an intra-arterial pressure monitoring line can speed the identification and treatment of hemodynamic changes in patients with clinically significant valvular disease. Induction of anesthesia in the presence of mitral stenosis can be achieved with intravenous drugs, with the possible exception of ketamine, which may be avoided because of its propensity to increase the heart rate. Tracheal intubation is facilitated by the administration of a neuromuscular blocking drug. Drugs used for maintenance of anesthesia should cause minimal changes in heart rate and in SVR and PVR. Furthermore, these drugs should not greatly decrease myocardial contractility. No one anesthetic has been proved to be superior. These goals can be achieved with combinations of an opioid and low concentrations of a volatile anesthetic or intravenous anesthetics such as propofol or dexmedetomidine. Although nitrous oxide can increase PVR, this increase is not sufficient to justify avoiding this drug in all patients with mitral stenosis.[61] The effect of nitrous oxide on PVR, however, seems to be accentuated when coexisting pulmonary hypertension is severe. Avoiding the use of nitrous oxide allows higher inspired oxygen concentrations and may reduce pulmonary vasoconstriction. Rapid increases in the concentration of desflurane may cause tachycardia, bronchospasm, and pulmonary hypertension and should be avoided.[46] Control of arterial blood pressure with a prophylactic intravenous infusion of the vasoconstrictor phenylephrine can reduce hemodynamic changes with induction of anesthesia.

Nondepolarizing neuromuscular blocking drugs with minimal circulatory effects are useful in patients with mitral stenosis. The adverse effects of drug-induced tachycardia in response to drug-assisted antagonism of nondepolarizing neuromuscular blocking drugs should be avoided (Box 25.3). Sugammadex, which can replace neostigmine, does not cause cardiovascular changes. If cases are prolonged and neuromuscular blockade is not required for the conduct of the case, allowing the nondepolarizing neuromuscular blockade to be eliminated through metabolism may reduce the risk of tachycardia with drug-assisted antagonism. Intraoperative intravenous fluid therapy must be carefully titrated because these patients are susceptible to intravascular volume overload and to the development of left ventricular failure and pulmonary edema. Likewise, the head-down position may not be well tolerated because the pulmonary blood volume is already increased.

Monitoring intra-arterial pressure and SVV or PPV is a helpful guide to the adequacy of intravascular fluid replacement. If central pressures are measured, an increase in right atrial pressure could also reflect pulmonary vasoconstriction, suggesting the need to check for causes, which may include nitrous oxide, desflurane, acidosis, hypoxia, increased mitral regurgitation, or light anesthesia.

Postoperatively, patients with mitral stenosis are at high risk for developing pulmonary edema and right-sided heart failure. Mechanical ventilation may be necessary, particularly after major thoracic or abdominal surgery. The shift from positive-pressure ventilation to spontaneous ventilation with weaning and extubation may lead to increased venous return and increased central venous pressures with worsening of heart failure.

---

**Box 25.3** Anesthetic Considerations in Patients With Mitral Stenosis

- Avoid sinus tachycardia or rapid ventricular response rate during atrial fibrillation.
- Avoid marked increases in central blood volume associated with overtransfusion or head-down position.
- Avoid drug-induced decreases in systemic vascular resistance.
- Avoid events such as arterial hypoxemia or hypoventilation that may exacerbate pulmonary hypertension and evoke right ventricular failure.

## Mitral Regurgitation

Mitral regurgitation is characterized by left atrial volume overload and decreased left ventricular forward stroke volume due to the backflow of part of each stroke volume through the incompetent mitral valve back into the left atrium. This regurgitant flow is responsible for the characteristic V waves seen on the recording of the pulmonary artery occlusion pressure.[62] Mitral regurgitation secondary to rheumatic fever usually has a component of mitral stenosis. Dilated cardiomyopathy, which may be from ischemia, multiple myocardial infarctions, viral or parasitic infections, or other causes, may cause mitral regurgitation. Isolated mitral regurgitation may be acute, reflecting papillary muscle dysfunction after a myocardial infarction or rupture of chordae tendineae secondary to infective endocarditis.

### Management of Anesthesia

Management of anesthesia in patients with mitral regurgitation should avoid decreases in the forward left ventricular stroke volume. Conversely, cardiac output can be improved by mild increases in heart rate and mild decreases in SVR (Box 25.4). Preinduction placement of intra-arterial pressure monitoring can speed the identification and treatment of hemodynamic changes in patients with clinically significant valvular disease.

A general anesthetic is the usual choice for patients with significant mitral regurgitation. Although decreases in SVR are theoretically beneficial, the rapid onset and uncontrolled nature of this response with a spinal anesthetic may detract from the use of this technique. Local or regional anesthesia may be used safely for surgery on peripheral body sites. Continuous spinal anesthetics may allow a slow titration of the regional block and can be a good choice of anesthetic. Maintenance of general anesthesia can be provided with volatile anesthetic, with or without nitrous oxide, or a continuous infusion of intravenous anesthetic. The concentration of volatile anesthetic can be adjusted to attenuate undesirable increases in systemic arterial blood pressure and SVR that can accompany surgical stimulation. Avoiding the use of nitrous oxide allows higher inspired oxygen concentrations and may reduce pulmonary vasoconstriction. Rapid increases in the concentration of desflurane may cause tachycardia, bronchospasm, and

---

> **Box 25.4** Anesthetic Considerations in Patients With Mitral or Aortic Regurgitation
>
> - Avoid sudden decreases in heart rate.
> - Avoid sudden decreases in systemic vascular resistance.
> - Minimize drug-induced myocardial depression.
> - Monitor the magnitude of the V wave as a reflection of mitral regurgitant flow.
> - Maintain sinus rhythm.
> - Maintain diastolic pressure if possible.

---

pulmonary hypertension and should be avoided.[46] Control of arterial blood pressure with a prophylactic intravenous infusion of the vasoconstrictor phenylephrine can reduce hemodynamic changes with induction. Intravascular fluid volume must be maintained by prompt replacement of blood loss to ensure adequate venous return and ejection of an optimal forward left ventricular stroke volume.

## Aortic Stenosis

Aortic stenosis is characterized by increased left ventricular systolic pressure to maintain the forward stroke volume through a narrowed aortic valve. The magnitude of the pressure gradient across the valve serves as an estimate of the severity of valvular stenosis. Hemodynamically significant aortic stenosis is associated with pressure gradients more than 50 mm Hg or valve areas less than 1.2 cm². A peak systolic gradient exceeding 50 mm Hg in the presence of a normal cardiac output or an effective aortic orifice less than about 0.75 cm² in an average-sized adult (i.e., 0.4 cm²/m² of body surface area or less than approximately one fourth of the normal orifice) is generally considered to represent critical aortic stenosis. The combination of symptoms (angina, congestive failure, or fainting), signs (serious left ventricular dysfunction and progressive cardiomegaly), and a reduced valve area also indicate the diagnosis of critical aortic stenosis requiring surgical replacement. Increased intraventricular pressures are accompanied by compensatory increases in the thickness of the left ventricular wall. Angina pectoris occurs often in these patients in the absence of CAD, reflecting an increased myocardial oxygen demand because of the increased amounts of ventricular muscle associated with myocardial hypertrophy in combination with higher intraventricular pressures. There is a decrease in oxygen delivery secondary to the aortic valve pressure gradient in combination with an increase in oxygen requirements from the increase in left ventricular pressure and stroke work. Thus, aortic stenosis results in an increase in left ventricular stroke work and oxygen requirements (increased demand) while reducing coronary blood flow (reduced supply). The factors determining coronary blood flow are described by the following equation:

$$\text{Coronary blood flow} = (\text{aortic diastolic pressure} - \text{left ventricular end diastolic pressure})/\text{coronary vascular resistance}.$$

Isolated nonrheumatic aortic stenosis usually results from progressive calcification and stenosis of a congenitally abnormal (usually bicuspid) valve. Aortic stenosis due to rheumatic fever almost always occurs in association with mitral valve disease. Likewise, aortic stenosis is usually accompanied by some degree of aortic regurgitation. Regardless of the cause of aortic stenosis, the natural

IV

history of the disease includes a long latent period, often 30 years or more, before symptoms occur. Because aortic stenosis may be asymptomatic, it is important to listen for this cardiac murmur (systolic murmur in the second right intercostal space that may radiate to the right carotid) in patients scheduled for surgery. The incidence of sudden death is increased in patients with aortic stenosis.

### Management of Anesthesia

With the advent of transcatheter aortic valve replacement (TAVR) the indications for aortic valve replacement (AVR) have changed, and many patients previously thought too high risk for surgical AVR (SAVR) are now considered candidates for TAVR. Patients with critical aortic stenosis or aortic stenosis with reduced left ventricular function or symptoms of angina or CHF should be evaluated for AVR prior to elective surgery.

Goals during management of anesthesia in patients with aortic stenosis are avoidance of arterial hypotension, maintenance of normal sinus rhythm, and avoidance of extreme and prolonged alterations in heart rate, SVR, and intravascular fluid volume (Box 25.5). Hypotension on induction can rapidly lead to myocardial ischemia from high myocardial oxygen requirements secondary to a constant load on the left ventricle from the stenotic valve combined with a decrease in coronary perfusion pressure secondary to an increase in left ventricular end-diastolic pressure and a relative diastolic hypotension. The most critical issue on induction of anesthesia is the avoidance of hypotension. Preservation of normal sinus rhythm is critical because the left ventricle is dependent on properly timed atrial contractions to ensure optimal left ventricular filling and stroke volume. Marked increases in heart rate (more than 100 beats/min) decrease the time for left ventricular filling and ejection and decrease coronary blood flow while increasing myocardial oxygen consumption. Coronary blood flow to the left ventricle occurs during diastole, and changes in heart rate primarily affect diastolic time. Bradycardia (less than 50 beats/min) can lead to acute overdistention of the left ventricle. Tachycardia may lead to myocardial ischemia and ventricular dysfunction. In view of the obstruction to left ventricular ejection, decreases in SVR may be associated with large decreases in systemic arterial blood pressure and coronary

blood flow and result in myocardial ischemia. Intra-arterial pressure monitoring is essential prior to induction of anesthesia and throughout the anesthetic period and can speed identification and treatment of hemodynamic changes. Prophylactic infusions of vasoconstrictors such as phenylephrine started prior to induction, may reduce hemodynamic changes.

A general anesthetic may be preferred to a regional anesthetic because sympathetic nervous system blockade can lead to undesirable decreases in SVR. If surgery is peripheral, a regional anesthetic with careful intra-arterial pressure monitoring can be equally successful. Maintenance of general anesthesia can be achieved with both intravenous and volatile anesthetics. A potential disadvantage of volatile inhaled anesthetics is depression of sinus node automaticity, which may lead to junctional rhythm and decreased left ventricular filling due to loss of properly timed atrial contractions. Techniques with peripheral vasodilation should be used carefully. The most important aspect of management for patients with aortic stenosis is intra-arterial pressure monitoring with careful avoidance of hypotension.

Intravascular fluid volume must be maintained by prompt replacement of blood loss and liberal administration of intravenous fluids. If a pulmonary artery catheter is placed, it should be remembered that the occlusion pressure may overestimate the left ventricular end-diastolic volume because of the decreased compliance of the left ventricle that accompanies chronic aortic stenosis. It is difficult to demonstrate any benefit in patient outcomes with pulmonary artery catheter monitoring. A cardiac defibrillator should be promptly available when anesthesia is administered to patients with aortic stenosis because external cardiac compressions are unlikely to generate an adequate stroke volume across a stenosed aortic valve. Cardiopulmonary resuscitation (CPR) has a lower success rate in patients with aortic stenosis secondary to low coronary perfusion pressures as a result of the stenotic aortic valve.

## Aortic Regurgitation

Aortic regurgitation is characterized by decreased forward left ventricular stroke volume due to regurgitation of part of the ejected stroke volume from the aorta back into the left ventricle through an incompetent aortic valve. A gradual onset of aortic regurgitation results in marked left ventricular hypertrophy and eventually dilation. Increased myocardial oxygen requirements secondary to left ventricular hypertrophy, plus a characteristic decrease in aortic diastolic pressure that decreases coronary blood flow, can manifest as angina pectoris in the absence of CAD. Coronary blood flow to the left ventricle occurs during diastole. In severe or acute aortic regurgitation with low diastolic pressures and elevated end-diastolic ventricular pressures, coronary blood flow can be

---

**Box 25.5** Anesthetic Considerations in Patients With Aortic Stenosis

- Intra-arterial pressure monitoring
- Rapid availability or prophylactic administration of intravenous vasoconstrictors (phenylephrine)
- Maintenance of normal sinus rhythm
- Avoidance of extreme bradycardia or tachycardia
- Avoidance of sudden decreases in systemic vascular resistance
- Optimization of intravascular fluid volume

severely compromised. The combination of a low diastolic pressure from aortic regurgitation with the increase in left ventricular diastolic pressure substantially decreases the coronary perfusion pressure gradient. Acute aortic regurgitation is most often due to infective endocarditis, trauma, or dissection of a thoracic aortic aneurysm. Chronic aortic regurgitation is usually due to prior rheumatic fever. In contrast to aortic stenosis, the occurrence of sudden death in patients with aortic regurgitation is rare.

### Management of Anesthesia

Management of anesthesia for noncardiac surgery in patients with aortic regurgitation is similar to the approach described for patients with mitral regurgitation (see Box 25.4). Preinduction intra-arterial pressure monitoring can speed the identification and treatment of hemodynamic changes and should be used for patients with significant aortic regurgitation. Anesthetics with minimal effects on SVR or cardiac function should be selected.

## Mitral Valve Prolapse

Mitral valve prolapse (click-murmur syndrome, Barlow syndrome) is characterized by an abnormality of the mitral valve support structure that permits prolapse of the valve into the left atrium during contraction of the left ventricle.[63] Previous estimates that mitral valve prolapse was present in 5% to 15% of individuals are most likely erroneously high.[64] Transesophageal or transthoracic echocardiography can confirm the diagnosis of mitral valve prolapse, particularly in the absence of the characteristic systolic murmur. The incidence of mitral valve prolapse in patients probably increases with musculoskeletal abnormalities, including Marfan syndrome, pectus excavatum, and kyphoscoliosis.

Despite the prevalence of mitral valve prolapse, most patients are asymptomatic, emphasizing the usually benign course of this abnormality. Nevertheless, serious complications may accompany mitral valve prolapse (Box 25.6). For example, mitral valve prolapse is probably the most common cause of pure mitral regurgitation, which may progress to the need for surgical intervention. Infective endocarditis is a potential complication, and transient ischemic attacks in patients

---

**Box 25.6 Complications Associated With Mitral Valve Prolapse**

- Mitral regurgitation
- Infective endocarditis
- Transient ischemic events
- Cardiac dysrhythmias
- Sudden death (extremely rare)

---

younger than 45 years of age are often associated with mitral valve prolapse. Sudden death is an extremely rare complication of mitral valve prolapse and, when it occurs, is presumed to be due to a ventricular cardiac dysrhythmia.

### Management of Anesthesia

The important principle in the management of anesthesia in patients with mitral valve prolapse is the avoidance of events that can increase cardiac emptying and subsequently accentuate prolapse of the mitral valve into the left atrium.[65] Perioperative events that can increase cardiac emptying include (1) sympathetic nervous system stimulation, (2) decreased SVR, and (3) performance of surgery with patients in the head-up or sitting position. It is important to optimize intravascular fluid volume in the preoperative period. Although intravenous anesthetics can be used to induce anesthesia, a sudden prolonged decrease in SVR must be avoided. Also, preinduction placement of intra-arterial pressure monitoring can speed the identification and treatment of hemodynamic changes and should be used with patients who have clinically significant mitral valve prolapse. Prophylactic infusions of phenylephrine can reduce systemic vasodilation during anesthesia induction.

Maintenance of anesthesia is most often achieved with a volatile anesthetic with or without nitrous oxide, and a narcotic to minimize sympathetic nervous system activation because of noxious intraoperative stimulation. The dose of volatile anesthetic is titrated to avoid excessive decreases in SVR. A regional anesthetic could also produce undesirable decreases in SVR but can be used with careful monitoring and rapid hemodynamic therapy if needed. Prompt replacement of blood loss and generous administration of intravenous fluids will contribute to maintenance of an optimal intravascular fluid volume and decrease the potential adverse effects of positive-pressure ventilation of the patient's lungs. Lidocaine, amiodarone, metoprolol, and esmolol should be available to treat cardiac dysrhythmias. If a vasoconstrictor is needed to treat hypotension, an α-agonist, such as phenylephrine, should probably be used.

## DISTURBANCES OF CARDIAC CONDUCTION AND RHYTHM

The ECG is a valuable tool for diagnosing disturbances of cardiac conduction and rhythm (also see Chapter 20). Ambulatory ECG monitoring (Holter monitoring) is useful in documenting the occurrence of life-threatening cardiac dysrhythmias and assessing the efficacy of antidysrhythmic drug therapy. The incidence of intraoperative cardiac dysrhythmias depends on the definition (benign versus life threatening), patient characteristics, and the type of surgery (frequent incidence during cardiothoracic

IV

surgery).[65] The following questions should be asked when interpreting the ECG:

1. What is the heart rate?
2. Are P waves present, and what is their relationship to the QRS complexes?
3. What is the duration of the PR interval (normal 120 to 200 ms)?
4. What is the duration of the QRS complex (normal 50 to 120 ms)?
5. Is the ventricular rhythm regular?
6. Are there early cardiac beats or abnormal pauses after a preceding QRS complex?
7. Is there evidence of prior myocardial infarction or ventricular hypertrophy?
8. Is there evidence of myocardial ischemia?
9. Is there a conduction disturbance such as left bundle branch block, right bundle branch block, or intraventricular conduction delay?

## Heart Block

Disturbances of conduction of cardiac impulses can be classified according to the site of the conduction block relative to the atrioventricular node (Box 25.7). Heart block occurring above the atrioventricular node is usually benign and transient. Heart block occurring below the atrioventricular node tends to be progressive and permanent.

A theoretical concern in patients with bifascicular heart block is that perioperative events, such as alterations in systemic arterial blood pressure, arterial oxygenation, or electrolyte concentrations, might compromise conduction in the one remaining intact fascicle, leading to the acute onset intraoperatively of third-degree atrioventricular heart block. However, surgery performed during general or regional anesthesia does not predispose to the development of third-degree atrioventricular

---

**Box 25.7** Classification of Heart Block

- First-degree atrioventricular heart block
- Second-degree atrioventricular heart block
- Mobitz type I (Wenckebach)
- Mobitz type II
- Unifascicular heart block
- Left anterior hemiblock
- Left posterior hemiblock
- Right bundle branch block
- Left bundle branch block
- Bifascicular heart block
- Right bundle branch block plus anterior hemiblock
- Right bundle branch block plus posterior hemiblock
- Third-degree (trifascicular, complete) atrioventricular heart block

---

heart block in patients with coexisting bifascicular block. Therefore, placement of a prophylactic artificial cardiac pacemaker is not required before anesthesia and surgery, but it should be available.

Third-degree atrioventricular heart block is treated by placement of an artificial cardiac pacemaker. An artificial cardiac pacemaker can be inserted intravenously (endocardial lead) or by the subcostal approach (epicardial or myocardial lead). An alternative to emergency transvenous artificial cardiac pacemaker placement is noninvasive transcutaneous or temporary esophageal cardiac pacing. A continuous intravenous infusion of isoproterenol acting as a pharmacologic cardiac pacemaker may be necessary to maintain an adequate heart rate until artificial electrical cardiac pacing can be established.

## Sick Sinus Syndrome

Sick sinus syndrome is characterized by inappropriate sinus bradycardia associated with degenerative changes in the sinoatrial node. Frequently, bradycardia due to this syndrome is complicated by episodes of supraventricular tachycardia. Artificial cardiac pacemakers may be indicated when therapeutic plasma concentrations of drugs necessary to control tachycardia result in bradycardia. The increased incidence of pulmonary embolism in these patients may be a reason to initiate anticoagulation.

## Ventricular Premature Beats

Ventricular premature beats, also known as premature ventricular complexes (PVCs), are recognized on the ECG by (1) premature occurrence, (2) the absence of a P wave preceding the QRS complex, (3) a wide and often bizarre QRS complex, (4) an inverted T wave, and (5) a compensatory pause that follows the premature beat. The primary goal with PVCs should be to identify any underlying cause (myocardial ischemia, arterial hypoxemia, hypercarbia, hypertension, hypokalemia, mechanical irritation of the ventricles) if possible and correct it. PVCs can be treated with lidocaine (1 to 2 mg/kg IV) when they (1) are frequent (more than 6 premature beats/min), (2) are multifocal, (3) occur in salvos of three or more, or (4) take place during the ascending limb of the T wave (R on T phenomenon) that corresponds to the relative refractory period of the ventricle.

## Ventricular Tachycardia

Ventricular tachycardia is defined as the appearance of at least three consecutive wide QRS complexes (longer than 120 ms) on the ECG occurring at an effective heart rate more rapid than 120 beats/min. Ventricular tachycardia not associated with hypotension is initially treated with the intravenous administration of amiodarone, lidocaine, or procainamide. Torsades de pointes responds to magnesium. Symptomatic ventricular tachycardia is best treated with external electrical cardioversion. The presence of ventricular tachycardia should elicit an immediate search for a cause such as myocardial ischemia, hypoxia, electrolyte abnormalities, or myocardial stimulation by the surgeons.

## Preexcitation Syndromes

Preexcitation syndromes are characterized by activation of a portion of the ventricles by cardiac impulses that travel from the atria via accessory (anomalous) conduction pathways. These pathways bypass the atrioventricular node such that activation of the ventricles occurs earlier than it would if impulses reached the ventricles by normal pathways.

### Wolff-Parkinson-White Syndrome

The Wolff-Parkinson-White syndrome is the most common of the preexcitation syndromes, with an incidence that may approach 0.3% of the general population. The lack of physiologic delay in transmission of cardiac impulses along the Kent fibers results in the characteristic short PR interval (less than 120 ms) on the ECG. The wide QRS complex and delta wave on the ECG reflect the composite of cardiac impulses conducted by normal and accessory pathways. Paroxysmal atrial tachycardia is the most frequent cardiac dysrhythmia associated with this syndrome. An increasing number of patients with Wolff-Parkinson-White syndrome are being treated by catheter ablation of accessory pathways as identified by electrophysiologic mapping. Supraventricular tachycardias such as atrial fibrillation or atrial flutter with one-to-one conduction may lead to hemodynamic collapse in patients with Wolff-Parkinson-White syndrome.

### Management of Anesthesia

The goal during management of anesthesia in the presence of a preexcitation syndrome is to avoid events (anxiety) or drugs (anticholinergics, ketamine, pancuronium) that might increase sympathetic nervous system activity and predispose to tachydysrhythmias.[65] All cardiac antidysrhythmic drugs should be continued throughout the perioperative period. Anesthesia can be induced with intravenous drugs, with the possible exception of ketamine. Tracheal intubation should be performed only after a sufficient concentration or dose of anesthetic has been given to reliably blunt sympathetic nervous system stimulation evoked by instrumentation of the upper airway. Intravenous β-adrenergic blockers (atenolol, metoprolol, propranolol, or esmolol) can be used to avoid tachycardia during induction of anesthesia. Neuromuscular blocking drugs with minimal effects on heart rate should be used.

The onset of paroxysmal atrial tachycardia or fibrillation in the perioperative period can be treated with the intravenous administration of drugs that abruptly prolong the refractory period of the atrioventricular node (adenosine) or lengthen the refractory period of accessory pathways (procainamide). β-Adrenergic blockers may be used for heart rate control. Digitalis and verapamil may decrease the refractory period of accessory pathways responsible for atrial fibrillation, resulting in an increase in ventricular response rate during this dysrhythmia and should be avoided. Electrical cardioversion is indicated when tachydysrhythmias are life threatening.

## Prolonged QT Interval Syndrome

A prolonged QT interval (longer than 440 ms on the ECG) syndrome is associated with ventricular dysrhythmias, syncope, and sudden death. Treatment should include β-adrenergic antagonists or left stellate ganglion block. The effectiveness of a left stellate ganglion block supports the hypothesis that this syndrome results from a congenital imbalance of autonomic innervation to the heart produced by decreases in right cardiac sympathetic nerve activity. Management of anesthesia includes avoidance of events or drugs that are likely to activate the sympathetic nervous system and availability of β-antagonists (metoprolol, atenolol, propranolol, or esmolol) or electrical cardioversion to treat life-threatening ventricular dysrhythmias.[65] The effect of inhaled and intravenous anesthetics can prolong the QT interval on the ECG in normal patients. Fortunately, these anesthetics do not produce additional prolonged QT interval in those patients with this syndrome in a predictable manner.[66] Many medications have the potential to prolong the QT interval (e.g., droperidol)[67,68] and should be avoided, if possible, in patients with prolonged QT syndrome.

## ARTIFICIAL CARDIAC PACEMAKERS

Preoperative evaluation of the patient with an artificial cardiac pacemaker in place includes determination of the reason for placing the pacemaker, assessment of its present function, as well as the brand, model, magnet mode, and availability of a programmer for this specific device and a person who knows how to operate the programmer.[69] Many implanted electrical devices can be used. A device under the skin may not be a pacemaker. Implanted devices include deep brain stimulators, automatic implantable cardiac defibrillators, intravenous pumps, spinal stimulators for chronic pain, bladder stimulators for neurogenic bladder, gastric stimulators for the treatment of obesity, intravenous ports, and vagal stimulators for sleep.

Special considerations are necessary for devices when the patient's life depends on the device. If a device is a cardiac pacemaker placed for third-degree heart block, special considerations for the continuous operation of that device and monitoring of its operation should be taken.

IV

If a pacemaker implanted for third-degree heart block is to be disconnected to change the stimulator, transvenous pacing may be needed. If the device is an automatic defibrillator, it will need to be inactivated during electrical-surgical cautery to avoid the device erroneously detecting ventricular dysrhythmias and defibrillating, which would waste battery life and possibly cause R-on-T phenomenon and ventricular fibrillation. The device should be reactivated after the surgical procedure and interrogated for proper function. The magnet mode of many implanted devices is now programmable. The magnet mode cannot automatically be assumed to be "safe." The specific magnet mode for a patient's device should be identified as some magnet modes change with device state or are programmable. Magnet mode for many pacemakers is asynchronous at 99 beats/min. If the patient has a spontaneous heart rate of 60 to 80 beats/min, the asynchronous mode at 99 beats/min would be safe. However, in some devices, the magnet mode shifts to asynchronous at 50 beats/min at the end of battery life. Asynchronous pacing at 50 beats/min may lead to R-on-T phenomenon if the patient has a spontaneous heart rate above 50 beats/min. The specific magnet mode should be identified and used only when needed given the circumstances of the case.

Intraoperative monitoring of patients with artificial cardiac pacemakers includes the ECG and possible intra-arterial pressure monitoring so as to detect the appearance of asystole promptly. Atropine, isoproterenol, and an external pacemaker should be available if the artificial cardiac pacemaker ceases to function. If electrocautery interferes with the ECG, monitoring the intra-arterial pressure, or arterial oxygenation, auscultation through an esophageal stethoscope or a palpable pulse confirms continued cardiac activity. Monitoring systemic arterial blood pressure with an intra-arterial catheter provides immediate evidence of loss of pacemaker function and should be considered in patients with third-degree heart block. Inhibition of pulse generator activity by electromagnetic interference most commonly from electrosurgical cautery, which is interpreted as spontaneous cardiac activity by the artificial cardiac pacemaker, is most likely when the ground plate for electrocautery is placed too near the pulse generator or unipolar cautery is used. For this reason, the ground plate should be placed as far as possible from the pulse generator. Bipolar electrocautery may also reduce interference between electrosurgical cautery and the pacemaker. If surface pads are placed for external pacing or defibrillation, they should be placed away from the implanted device to reduce current passing down the pacing lead and hyperpolarizing a small segment of myocardium, which could interfere with pacemaker capture after defibrillation. Automatic implantable cardioversion devices sense ventricular fibrillation or ventricular tachycardia. They provide a cardioversion shock through implanted cardiac leads. Electrocautery signals can be misinterpreted as ventricular dysrhythmias, thus triggering unnecessary shocks and decreasing battery life. These devices should be reprogrammed to the standby mode prior to elective surgery and returned postoperatively to full function with interrogation of proper operation (also see Chapter 13).

Selection of drugs or techniques for anesthesia is not influenced by the presence of artificial cardiac pacemakers as there is no evidence that the threshold and subsequent response of these devices is altered by drugs administered in the perioperative period. However, patients with artificial cardiac pacemakers or implanted cardioversion devices have a frequent incidence of coexisting cardiac disease and should be monitored carefully and anesthetized with care. Patients with defibrillators frequently have poor ventricular function. Insertion of a pulmonary artery catheter will not disturb epicardial electrodes but might dislodge recently placed (less than 2 weeks) transvenous endocardial electrodes.[70]

## ESSENTIAL HYPERTENSION

Essential hypertension is arbitrarily defined as sustained increases in systemic arterial blood pressure (systolic blood pressure higher than 160 mm Hg or a diastolic blood pressure higher than 90 mm Hg) independent of any known cause. Treatment of essential hypertension with appropriate drug therapy decreases the incidence of stroke and CHF. Hypertension is a risk factor for CAD, and the longer the patient has hypertension the higher the risk of end organ damage.

### Management of Anesthesia

Management of anesthesia for patients with essential hypertension includes preoperative evaluation of drug therapy and the extent of the disease plus a consideration of the implications of exaggerated systemic arterial blood pressure responses elicited by preoperative anxiety and painful intraoperative stimulation.[71]

### Preoperative Evaluation

Preoperative evaluation of patients with essential hypertension begins with a determination of the adequacy of systemic arterial blood pressure control and a review of the pharmacology of the antihypertensive drugs being used for therapy (see Chapters 6 and 13). Antihypertensive drugs should be continued throughout the perioperative period. Evidence of major organ dysfunction (CHF, CAD, cerebral ischemia, renal dysfunction) must be sought. Patients with essential hypertension have an elevated risk of CAD. Evidence of PVD should be recognized, as all patients with PVD have some degree of CAD. It can be assumed that nearly one half of patients with evidence of PVD will have more than 50% stenosis of one or more coronary arteries even in the absence of angina pectoris and the presence of a normal resting ECG. Additional monitoring, including intra-arterial catheter monitoring, is justified for significant operations. Patients with increased pulse pressure have increased perioperative and long-term complications.[72] Essential hypertension is associated with a shift to the right of the curve for the autoregulation of cerebral blood flow, emphasizing that these patients are more vulnerable to cerebral ischemia should perfusion pressures decrease. Detection of renal dysfunction due to chronic hypertension may influence the selection of drugs, particularly if elimination from the plasma depends on renal clearance or metabolites of the drugs are known potential nephrotoxins (e.g., fluoride from metabolism of sevoflurane).

Hypertension should be treated preoperatively because the incidence of hypotension and evidence of myocardial ischemia on the ECG during the maintenance of anesthesia is increased in patients who remain hypertensive before the induction of anesthesia.[57] Patients who are treated with antihypertensives prior to surgery should be continued on those medications in the perioperative period. Discontinuation of antihypertensive and antianginal medications in the perioperative period increases operative risk.[6,19,21,32,33] Prophylactic cardiac risk reduction therapy with β-adrenergic blockers of patients with CAD, PVD, or two risk factors (age ≥ 60, hypertension, cholesterol > 240 mg/dL, diabetes, or smoking) reduces risk of perioperative death.[14,32,33,41] Appropriate dosing of β-adrenergic blockers is important to avoid sequelae.[6,37]

Despite therapy, systemic arterial blood pressure increases during the intraoperative period are more likely to occur in patients with a history of essential hypertension regardless of the degree of pharmacologic control of systemic arterial blood pressure established preoperatively. Furthermore, the incidence of postoperative cardiac complications is not increased when hypertensive patients undergo elective operations as long as the preoperative diastolic blood pressure is not more than 110 mm Hg and heart rate is controlled. Pretreatment with a β-adrenergic blocker may be useful in blunting exaggerated sympathetic nervous system responses and reduces perioperative mortality risk.[16,17,41]

## Induction of Anesthesia

Induction of anesthesia with intravenous drugs is acceptable, remembering that an exaggerated decrease in systemic arterial blood pressure may occur, particularly if hypertension is present preoperatively. Thiopental, propofol, midazolam, synthetic opioids (fentanyl, sufentanil, alfentanil, remifentanil), and etomidate all have been used to induce anesthesia. Any anesthetic is acceptable if used with appropriate dosing and careful monitoring. Etomidate or combinations of midazolam and fentanyl are frequently used for induction because of their limited hemodynamic effects. Ketamine is rarely selected for induction of anesthesia in patients with essential hypertension because it can increase systemic arterial blood pressure and cause tachycardia, which may lead to myocardial ischemia. Placement of an intra-arterial pressure monitor prior to induction of anesthesia and prophylactic infusions of the vasoconstrictor phenylephrine can reduce hemodynamic perturbations with induction of anesthesia. Hemodynamic changes with induction most likely reflect unmasking of decreased intravascular fluid volume due to chronic hypertension combined with a stiffening of the arterial vasculature.

Hypertension can occur during direct laryngoscopy for tracheal intubation in patients with essential hypertension but may be attenuated with administration of opioids and β-adrenergic blockers. Tachycardia may lead to episodes of myocardial ischemia. A single 1-minute episode of myocardial ischemia increases the risk of perioperative cardiac morbidity 10-fold and death 2-fold. The risk of myocardial ischemia can be reduced by prophylactic therapy with β-adrenergic blockers.[16,17,41]

Maximal attenuation of sympathetic nervous system responses should be attempted during direct laryngoscopy by administering anesthetics, intravenous opioids, and β-adrenergic blockers before attempting tracheal intubation. Careful attention to the airway is critical in all anesthetics, and the risks are greater in patients with cardiac disease. If the patient has a recognized difficult airway precluding direct laryngoscopy, hemodynamic control with specific attention to heart rate control must be observed while securing the airway with alternative approaches such as fiberoptic intubation. It is important to prevent hypoxia, tachycardia, hypotension, hypertension, and myocardial ischemia. Regardless of the drugs administered before tracheal intubation, however, it must be recognized that an excessive concentration of anesthetic drugs can produce decreases in systemic arterial blood pressure that are as undesirable as hypertension. An important concept for limiting pressor responses elicited by tracheal intubation is to limit the duration of direct laryngoscopy to less than 15 seconds if possible. In addition, the administration of laryngotracheal lidocaine immediately before placement of the tube in the trachea will minimize any additional pressor response.

## Maintenance of Anesthesia

The goal during maintenance of anesthesia is to adjust the concentrations of anesthetics to avoid tachycardia and minimize wide fluctuations in systemic arterial blood pressure (Box 25.8). No single anesthetic technique has been shown to be superior. Combinations of volatile anesthetics with or without nitrous oxide and a narcotic are commonly used. Changes in the concentration of volatile anesthetics allow rapid adjustments in the depth of

IV

anesthesia in response to increases or decreases in systemic arterial blood pressure. Changes in surgical stimulation may lead to changes in arterial blood pressure and heart rate. Additional doses of narcotics, β-adrenergic blockers, and changes in the dose of volatile anesthetics can be used to control hemodynamics. Heart rate control is the most critical element for preventing cardiac morbidity and fatality. Heart rates above 120 beats/min increase mortality rate. Volatile anesthetics are useful for attenuating activity of the sympathetic nervous system, which is responsible for these pressor responses. The ability to rapidly increase the alveolar concentration of sevoflurane (because of its low solubility) makes this volatile anesthetic uniquely efficacious for treating sudden increases in systemic arterial blood pressure (see "Maintenance of Anesthesia" under "Coronary Artery Disease"). Rapid changes in desflurane concentration may lead to tachycardia, hypertension, pulmonary hypertension, and myocardial ischemia and should be avoided.[46] A positive

feedback situation can occur with desflurane anesthetics whereby a surgical stimulus can raise arterial blood pressure, the anesthesia provider rapidly raises the desflurane concentration, which stimulates the sympathetic system causing the arterial blood pressure to increase, which causes the anesthesia provider to further increase the desflurane concentration, which further increases the arterial blood pressure.[46]

A nitrous oxide–opioid technique is also acceptable for the maintenance of anesthesia, but the addition of a volatile anesthetic is often necessary to control undesirable increases in systemic arterial blood pressure, particularly during periods of maximal surgical stimulation. Total intravenous anesthesia (combinations of dexmedetomidine, propofol, narcotics, and benzodiazepines) can also be used with effect. Continuous intravenous infusions of phenylephrine, nitroprusside, nitroglycerin, or esmolol can be used to maintain normotension during the intraoperative period. Combinations of narcotic, benzodiazepine, and inhaled anesthetics are commonly used. Hypotension that occurs during maintenance of anesthesia is often treated by decreasing the concentrations of volatile anesthetics while infusing fluids intravenously to increase intravascular fluid volume. Sympathomimetics, such as ephedrine, or vasoconstrictors such as phenylephrine may be necessary to restore perfusion pressures until the underlying cause of hypotension can be corrected.

The choice of intraoperative monitors for patients with coexisting essential hypertension is influenced by the complexity of the surgery. The ECG is monitored with the goal of recognizing changes suggestive of myocardial ischemia. Invasive monitoring with an intra-arterial pressure monitor is commonly used. Continuous cardiac output monitors with calculation of SVV or PPV can be used to monitor intravascular fluid status as a part of goal-directed therapy. Pulmonary artery catheters may be considered if major surgery is planned and there is evidence preoperatively of left ventricular dysfunction, although there is no evidence that demonstrates improved outcomes with pulmonary artery catheter monitoring. Monitoring with TEE is an alternative to placement of a pulmonary artery catheter.

A regional anesthetic is an excellent choice for patients with multiple medical conditions who are scheduled for peripheral surgery. Whatever the choice of anesthetic, β-adrenegic blockers and sedatives can be used to reduce sympathetic nervous system stimulation. Patients with cardiac disease who are scheduled for elective surgery can have episodes of myocardial ischemia in the days prior to surgery. The night before surgery is stressful, and prophylactic β-adrenergic blockade can reduce the risk of sympathetic stimulation resulting in tachycardia and subsequent myocardial ischemia. There is the erroneous belief that minor surgery causes minor stress. Patients scheduled for ophthalmic surgery, a minor outpatient procedure, commonly have sympathetic stimulation resulting in preoperative hypertension. Prophylactic therapy with β-adrenergic blockers can reduce the preoperative hypertensive episodes and myocardial ischemia. Appropriate dosing of all medications is essential and inappropriate dosing may lead to hypotension, bradycardia, and increased morbidity and mortality rates.[37] All medications have a therapeutic index. Withholding antihypertensive medications may lead to withdrawal phenomena and increase the morbidity and mortality rates.[19,21,32,33]

## Postoperative Management

Hypertension in the early postoperative period is a frequent occurrence in patients with a preoperative diagnosis of essential hypertension. Prophylactic or therapeutic administration of β-adrenergic blockers can reduce these episodes of hypertension and reduce risk of perioperative ischemia and death. If hypertension persists despite β-adrenergic blockers and adequate analgesia, it may be necessary to pharmacologically decrease systemic arterial blood pressure utilizing a continuous intravenous infusion of nitroprusside, nitroglycerin, or intermittent injections of hydralazine (5 to 20 mg IV) or labetalol (0.1 to 0.5 mg/kg IV). Tachycardia in the postoperative period must be actively avoided as it increases morbidity and mortality rates (also see Chapter 39). A heart rate of 120 beats/min raises the risk of postoperative death. Clearly the arterial blood pressure needs to be controlled during the entire perioperative period. The patient needs preoperative, intraoperative, and postoperative hemodynamic and autonomic control to prevent associated cardiac morbidity and death. Anesthesia care for patients with cardiac disease truly needs to be perioperative for optimal outcomes. If medication is needed to control arterial blood pressure and heart rate while at home, the patient will likely need it during surgery and postoperative care. Withdrawal of antihypertensive and anti-ischemic medications in the perioperative period increases cardiac risk.[27,29,30]

## CONGESTIVE HEART FAILURE

Elective surgery should not be performed in patients with untreated CHF unless optimally treated. The preoperative presence of CHF is often associated with significant postoperative morbidity or mortality rates. Cardiology consultation is frequently helpful in patients with congestive failure as consideration of surgical or interventional revascularization and optimization of medical therapy can improve cardiac function. Preoperative initiation of β-adrenergic blockers and vasodilator therapy with angiotensin-converting enzyme inhibitors can improve ventricular function and reduce operative risk. These drugs should be started by physicians with expertise in treating CHF and the doses increased slowly as tolerated over 3 to 6 months as the heart function recovers.

## Management of Anesthesia

When surgery cannot be delayed, however, the drugs and techniques chosen to provide anesthesia must be selected with the goal of minimizing detrimental effects on cardiac output. Optimal cardiac output can be obtained when the impedance of the vasculature (preload and afterload) matches the impedance of the heart and can be achieved by careful preload and afterload management.

Etomidate may be useful for the induction of anesthesia in the presence of CHF because of its limited effect on the sympathetic nervous system. Small doses of volatile anesthetics can maintain anesthesia, but must be used carefully to avoid cardiac depression. In the presence of severe CHF, the use of opioids in large doses as the primary anesthetic in combination with amnestic benzodiazepines (midazolam) may be justified, although no evidence supports this approach over the use of a primary volatile anesthetic combined with narcotics.[52] Positive-pressure ventilation of the lungs may be beneficial by decreasing pulmonary congestion, improving arterial oxygenation, and eliminating the work of breathing. Care must be taken on extubation of patients with CHF as the resumption of negative intrathoracic pressures with spontaneous ventilation can lead to increased filling pressures and worsening heart failure. Invasive monitoring of intra-arterial blood pressure is helpful for hemodynamic management of patients undergoing both regional and general anesthetics. Use of pulmonary artery catheters can be helpful in hemodynamic management, but no evidence exists to suggest that they reduce operative risk or improve outcome. Maintenance of arterial blood pressure with vasoconstrictors (phenylephrine) should precede increasing myocardial contractility with continuous intravenous infusions of inotropic drugs such as epinephrine, dopamine, and dobutamine. The use of β-adrenergic agonists in patients with CHF may decrease the chance of survival and should be used only when necessary.

Regional anesthesia (also see Chapters 17 and 18) should be considered for patients with CHF requiring peripheral or minor surgery. Anesthetics with minimal hemodynamic effects are optimal. If the surgery precludes such a choice, general anesthesia with careful hemodynamic control with intra-arterial pressure monitoring, infusions of vasoconstrictors, and possibly inotropic drugs, with the careful avoidance of tachycardia, should be used.

## HYPERTROPHIC CARDIOMYOPATHY

Hypertrophic cardiomyopathy (idiopathic hypertrophic subaortic stenosis) is characterized by obstruction to left ventricular outflow produced by asymmetric hypertrophy of the intraventricular septal muscle.[73] Associated left ventricular hypertrophy in an attempt to overcome the

> **Box 25.9** Events That Decrease Left Ventricular Outflow Obstruction in the Presence of Hypertrophic Cardiomyopathy
>
> **Decreased Myocardial Contractility**
> - β-Adrenergic blockade (atenolol, metoprolol, propranolol, esmolol)
> - Volatile anesthetic (sevoflurane or isoflurane)
>
> **Increased Preload**
> - Increased intravascular fluid volume
> - Bradycardia (fentanyl or sufentanil)
>
> **Increased Afterload**
> - α-Adrenergic stimulation (phenylephrine infusions)

obstruction may be so massive that the volume of the left ventricular chamber is decreased. Despite these adverse changes, the stroke volume remains normal or increased owing to the hypercontractile state of the myocardium. This disease is often hereditary, and the genetic defect seems to be an increased density of calcium channels manifesting as myocardial hypertrophy.

## Management of Anesthesia

The goal during management of anesthesia for patients with hypertrophic cardiomyopathy is to decrease the pressure gradient across the left ventricular outflow obstruction (Box 25.9). Decreases in myocardial contractility and increases in preload (ventricular volume) and afterload will decrease the magnitude of left ventricular outflow obstruction. Volatile anesthetics are useful for maintenance of anesthesia, providing mild depression of myocardial contractility. Theoretically, isoflurane, desflurane, and sevoflurane would be less ideal choices than halothane because these drugs decrease SVR more than does halothane. Rapid increases in desflurane may cause sympathetic stimulation with tachycardia, hypertension, bronchospasm, and pulmonary hypertension and should be avoided.[46] Primary opioid anesthetics may not be optimal as they do not produce myocardial depression and can decrease SVR. High potency opioids stimulate the vagus nerve, lower heart rate, and can decrease sympathetic stimulation improving hemodynamics. Combinations of volatile drugs (sevoflurane or isoflurane) with an opioid are commonly selected.

Intraoperative hypotension is generally treated with intravenous fluids or an α-agonist such as phenylephrine. Drugs with β-agonist activity are not likely to be used to treat hypotension because any increase in cardiac contractility or heart rate could increase left ventricular outflow obstruction. When hypertension occurs, an increased delivered concentration of isoflurane or sevoflurane can be used. Vasodilators, such as nitroprusside or nitroglycerin, should be used with caution because decreases in SVR can increase left ventricular outflow obstruction.

## PULMONARY HYPERTENSION AND COR PULMONALE

Cor pulmonale is the designation for right ventricular hypertrophy and eventual cardiac dysfunction that occurs secondary to chronic pulmonary hypertension. Elective operations in patients with cor pulmonale should not be performed until any reversible components in the coexisting pulmonary vascular disease have been treated.

## Management of Anesthesia

Goals during management of anesthesia in patients with cor pulmonale are to avoid events or drugs that could increase PVR. Volatile anesthetics are useful for relaxing vascular smooth muscle and attenuating airway responsiveness to stimuli produced by a tracheal tube. Pulmonary vasodilation with prostaglandins (epoprostenol, treprostinil, iloprost, beraprost), endothelin receptor antagonists (bosentan, sitaxentan, ambrisentan), inhaled nitric oxide, inhaled milrinone, type 5 phosphodiesterase inhibitors (sildenafil, vardenafil), or soluble guanylate cyclase activators (cinaciguat, riociguat) have been tried with variable success. Patients with pulmonary hypertension have significant increased risk and should be treated with extreme care. Nitrous oxide may increase PVR and should be avoided.[61] Another disadvantage of nitrous oxide is the associated decrease in the inspired concentration of oxygen necessitated by the administration of this drug.

Intra-arterial pressure monitoring is very helpful for hemodynamic management. Monitoring of pulmonary arterial or right atrial pressure (or both) may be helpful to detect any adverse effect on pulmonary vasculature. TEE monitoring can be very helpful in blood volume management. In severe cor pulmonale, inotropic support with β-agonists can improve cardiac function. Therapy should be chosen based on the hemodynamic problem (volume, SVR, chronotropy, inotropy, and pulmonary hypertension). β-Agonists must be used carefully to avoid myocardial ischemia. In severe right ventricular failure, combinations of β-agonists and phosphodiesterase inhibitors (amrinone or milrinone) can provide synergistic improvements in ventricular function and vasodilation (amrinone or milrinone), thus improving cardiac output. The cyclic guanosine monophosphate–dependent phosphodiesterase inhibitors (sildenafil and vardenafil) can be used to vasodilate the pulmonary vasculature with minimal effects on SVR.

## CARDIAC TAMPONADE

Cardiac tamponade is characterized by (1) decreases in diastolic filling of the ventricles, (2) decreases in stroke volume, and (3) decreases in systemic arterial blood pressure due to increased intrapericardial pressure from

## Box 25.10 Manifestations of Cardiac Tamponade

- Primary diastolic dysfunction from increased pericardial pressure
- Hypotension
- Tachycardia
- Increased systemic vascular resistance
- Low cardiac output
- Equalization of left and right diastolic filling pressures
- Exaggeration of arterial blood pressure variation with respiration
- Fixed and reduced stroke volume (cardiac output and systemic arterial blood pressure dependent on heart rate)
- Failure to respond to volume and multiple inotropes with cardiogenic shock

accumulation of fluid in the pericardial space (Box 25.10). Decreased stroke volume from inadequate ventricular filling results in activation of the sympathetic nervous system (tachycardia, vasoconstriction) as the cardiovascular system attempts to maintain the cardiac output. Cardiac output and systemic arterial blood pressure are maintained only as long as the pressure in the central veins exceeds the right ventricular end-diastolic pressure. Institution of general anesthesia and positive-pressure ventilation of the lungs in the presence of cardiac tamponade can lead to immediate and profound hypotension or death, reflecting anesthetic-induced peripheral vasodilation, direct myocardial depression, and decreased venous return from positive-pressure ventilation. When percutaneous pericardiocentesis cannot be performed using local anesthesia, the induction and maintenance of general anesthesia are extremely dangerous but may be achieved while carefully maintaining spontaneous respiration. Potential adverse effects of increased intrathoracic pressure from controlled respiration on venous return must be taken seriously. If possible, positive-pressure ventilation of the lungs should be avoided until drainage of the pericardial space is imminent. With this in mind, tracheal intubation with topical anesthesia has been suggested.

### Management of Anesthesia

Prior to the induction of general anesthesia in patients with significant cardiac tamponade, the patient should be positioned on the operating room table. Intra-arterial monitoring is helpful if time permits. The chest and abdomen should be prepped and draped for surgery. The surgeons should be scrubbed, gowned, gloved, and at the operating room table ready for incision prior to anesthetic induction. It is optimal if anesthetic induction, intubation, incision, and drainage of the pericardial tamponade can occur in extremely rapid succession (less than 60 seconds). Although continuous intravenous infusions of catecholamines (epinephrine, norepinephrine, dopamine, dobutamine, or isoproterenol) and vasoconstrictors

may be necessary to maintain cardiac output and arterial blood pressure, the primary therapy is pericardial drainage. A common sign of cardiac tamponade is hemodynamic collapse and cardiogenic shock unresponsive to fluids and inotropes. Systolic ventricular function is not the problem; diastolic dysfunction from increased pericardial pressure is the primary problem. Once the pericardium is drained, venous return can enter the heart and hemodynamics will rapidly normalize.

## ANEURYSMS OF THE AORTA

Aneurysms of the aorta most often involve the abdominal aorta but may involve any part including thoracic or abdominal. Most patients are hypertensive, and many have associated atherosclerosis. A dissecting aneurysm denotes a tear in the intima of the aorta that allows blood to enter and penetrate between the walls of the vessel, producing a false lumen. Ultimately, the dissection may reenter the lumen through another tear in the intima or rupture through the adventitia.

Elective repair of an abdominal aneurysm is often recommended when the estimated diameter of the aneurysm is more than 5 cm. The incidence of spontaneous rupture increases dramatically when the size of the aneurysm exceeds this diameter. Extension of the abdominal aneurysm to include the renal arteries occurs in about 5% of patients.

### Management of Anesthesia

All surgery patients with vascular disease should be considered for prophylactic β-adrenergic blocker and statin therapy. Perioperative administration of β-adrenergic blockers reduces perioperative mortality rate 50% to 90%. β-Adrenergic blocking drugs should be started as soon as patients are identified as needing surgery.[6] Perioperative statin use reduces risk an additional 50% over the benefits of β-adrenergic blockers and should be started 30 days preoperatively and continued at least 30 days postoperatively, if not indefinitely.[15]

The surgical approach certainly influences the anesthetic. Endovascular aneurysm repair is less invasive and may require only regional anesthesia, although in prolonged cases general anesthesia is preferred. Open procedures for aortic aneurysm surgery are major procedures and require general anesthesia. All patients undergoing anesthesia for resection of an abdominal aortic aneurysm should have monitoring of intra-arterial pressures. Epidural catheter placement may be helpful for the management of postoperative pain. Continuous cardiac output monitoring with calculation of SVV or PPV can be used to direct goal-directed therapy of volume replacement. The use of pulmonary arterial pressure monitoring is controversial and not supported by improved survival data.[57,58]

**IV**

Patients with coexisting CAD are likely to develop evidence of myocardial ischemia during cross-clamping of the abdominal aorta. TEE may be useful in evaluating the adequacy of intravascular volume replacement and in the recognition of cardiac wall motion abnormalities associated with myocardial ischemia, although no data support its use as a risk reduction strategy. Intraoperatively, myocardial ischemia is treated by decreasing heart rate with β-adrenergic blockers and maintaining systemic arterial blood pressure and filling pressures to acceptable levels by pharmacologic interventions, which may include continuous intravenous infusion of phenylephrine (for hypotension), nitroprusside, or nitroglycerin (for hypertension). Preoperative hydration with a balanced salt solution and prompt intraoperative replacement of blood loss as guided by data obtained from echocardiography or continuous cardiac output devices are considered useful for maintaining intravascular fluid volume and thus renal function. Diuresis is often facilitated by intraoperative administration of a diuretic (mannitol, furosemide, or both) with or without dopamine. Despite these interventions, glomerular filtration rate and renal blood flow are not predictably improved.[74]

Hypotension can accompany unclamping of the abdominal aorta, presumably reflecting sudden decreases in vascular resistance and increases in venous compliance with reperfusion. Systemic arterial blood pressure decreases can be minimized by infusing intravenous fluids prior to cross-clamp release. Gradual removal of the aortic cross-clamp minimizes decreases in systemic arterial blood pressure by allowing time for return of pooled venous blood to the circulation.

## CARDIOPULMONARY BYPASS

Cardiopulmonary bypass (extracorporeal circulation) support is used to stabilize the myocardium reducing motion during coronary artery bypass surgery and allow ascending aortic and intraventricular procedures (valve repair or replacement) (also see Chapter 26). Cardiopulmonary bypass is characterized by gravity drainage of blood from the vena cava into a reservoir, followed by its pumping through a heat exchanger, oxygenator, and filter followed by its return to the arterial system, usually the ascending aorta, by means of a centrifugal or roller pump (Fig. 25.3).[75] In the presence of a competent aortic valve, the heart is excluded from the patient's circulation by either a single venous cannula inserted into the right atrium (see Fig. 25.3) and advanced into the inferior vena cava, or by dual catheters placed into the superior and inferior venae cavae so that all returning blood enters the large cannulas in these vessels. If the aortic valve is not competent, venting of the left ventricle may be necessary (1) through a drain placed from the right superior pulmonary vein into the left ventricle, (2) by aspirating from the antegrade

cardioplegia line placed in the proximal ascending aorta, or (3) via a pulmonary venous drain. Otherwise, retrograde blood flow through the incompetent aortic valve could cause distention of the left ventricle and damage ventricular function. Venting of blood returning via thebesian or bronchial veins may also be necessary. An aortic cross-clamp is placed between the antegrade cardioplegia catheter and the arterial inflow catheter to separate the heart from the circulation and allow cardioplegic arrest. The ventricle should not be overdistended in any situation in which it is not pumping. If the aortic cross-clamp is removed and ventricular contraction has not returned, the ventricle may become overdistended in situations with aortic valve insufficiency. When the heart is isolated from the circulation, total cardiopulmonary bypass is present, and ventilation of the lungs is no longer necessary to maintain oxygenation. However, in any situation where there is a pulsatile pulmonary pressure detected by pulmonary arterial catheter measurement, there is partial pulmonary bypass, and the lungs should be ventilated to avoid pumping desaturated blood systemically. Gravity-dependent venous drainage to the cardiopulmonary bypass machine can be improved by raising the level of the operating table or placing a small vacuum on the cardiotomy reservoir.

The use of extracorporeal circulatory support is dangerous and requires special precautions. Prior to going on cardiopulmonary bypass it is important to review a checklist of required items. Checklists are effective in improving anesthetic care. The checklist prior to going on cardiopulmonary bypass can be recalled by using the mnemonic HADDSUE, pronounced HAD TO SUE, making each item easy to remember (Box 25.11).

### Components of the Cardiopulmonary Bypass Circuit

The bypass pump produces nonpulsatile flow into the patient's aorta by either a centrifugal or roller pump. The centrifugal pump has three disks rotating at 3000 to 4000 rpm that use blood viscosity to pump blood. Centrifugal pumps are superior to roller pumps because they are less traumatic to blood cells, do not pump air bubbles secondary to air being less dense than blood, and are afterload-dependent, avoiding the risk of line rupture with clamping of the arterial inflow circuit. Roller pumps compress the fluid-filled tubing between the roller and curved metal back plate and are able to pump air and can have tube rupture with arterial inflow clamping. The necessary cardiac index delivered by the bypass pump is determined by the patient's body temperature and oxygen consumption. For normothermia or mild hypothermia, a cardiac index of 2 to 4 $L/min/m^2$ is satisfactory, although flows of about half these levels have been used successfully. Low flows have the advantage of less blood trauma and less noncoronary collateral blood flow, which might

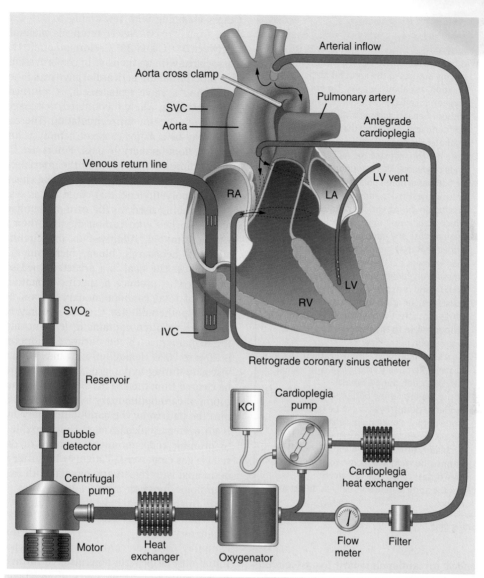

**Fig. 25.3** Schematic diagram of a cardiopulmonary bypass circuit. Blood from cannulas placed through the right atrium (RA) and into the inferior vena cava (IVC) drains by gravity into a reservoir and then is pumped by a centrifugal pump through a heat exchanger, oxygenator, and filter prior to return to the ascending aorta. Blood mixed with cardioplegia solution is pumped alternatively into the proximal ascending aorta or into the coronary sinus. Venting can be from a cannula placed through the right superior pulmonary vein into the left ventricle, or from the ascending aorta antegrade cardioplegia cannula, or the pulmonary artery. *LA*, Left atrium; *LV*, left ventricle; *RV*, right ventricle; *SVC*, superior vena cava.

result in better myocardial protection. Blood is oxygenated by a membrane or bubble oxygenator. Membrane oxygenators use a blood-membrane-gas interface rather than a blood-gas interface and produce less trauma to the blood compared with bubble oxygenators. Because membrane oxygenators cause less trauma to blood components than bubble oxygenators, membrane-based oxygenator systems are the norm. Bubble oxygenators consisted of an oxygenator column, a defoaming section

to remove air bubbles, and an arterial reservoir. They are not commonly used today. With either form of oxygenator $Pa_{O_2}$ is maintained by adjusting the concentration of oxygen into the oxygenator. Air-oxygen mixing may be used to avoid hyperoxia. Carbon dioxide levels are controlled between 35 and 45 mm Hg by controlling the sweep (the total free gas flow through the oxygenator). In the past, carbon dioxide was added to maintain $Pa_{CO_2}$ and pH at levels considered normal for 37° C. Carbon dioxide

| **Box 25.11** Protocol to Initiate Cardiopulmonary Bypass: HADDSUE | |
|---|---|
| Heparin | Was heparin administered? If the surgeon is placing sutures in the aorta for aortic cannulation, ask about heparin. Do not allow a surgeon to initiate cardiopulmonary bypass without heparin administration or alternative profound anticoagulant; the results will immediately be fatal. |
| ACT | Did the heparin increase the ACT to 450 seconds or greater? Were antifibrinolytics given? |
| Drugs | Were additional nondepolarizing muscle relaxants or anesthetics administered to prevent inspiration during venous cannula placement, which could result in gas emboli? |
| Drips | Did you discuss any infusions with the perfusionist that may interfere with hemodynamic management during bypass? Arterial blood pressure on cardiopulmonary bypass depends on flow and resistance. Drugs that affect resistance will affect arterial blood pressure. Drugs that affect venous capacity will reduce venous return to the reservoir and force a reduction in pump flow. |
| Swan | Pull back the pulmonary arterial catheter 5 cm to avoid pulmonary arterial injury or pulmonary infarction during bypass. |
| Urine | Measure the total urine output so that the urine produced during bypass can be tabulated. Urine output can be quite variable during bypass depending on the extracorporeal circulatory prime, volume administered, intrinsic hormonal response to cardiopulmonary bypass, and renal function. |
| Emboli | Check the aortic cannula visually to detect any emboli. |

*ACT,* Activated clotting time.

is no longer added to cardiopulmonary bypass circuits to maintain blood gases. Bypass circuits are flushed with carbon dioxide prior to priming to speed priming and reduce gas emboli in the circuit. Carbon dioxide is also continuously flushed into the pericardial cavity to replace air during bypass in an effort to reduce the significance of gas emboli during bypass. Carbon dioxide is more easily absorbed than the nitrogen in air reducing the duration that gas emboli take to be resorbed.

Heat exchangers are incorporated into bypass circuits to control the patient's body temperature by heating or cooling blood as it circulates. Hot or cold water entering the unit at one end with blood entering at the other provides an efficient countercurrent flow system. Metabolic requirements are decreased about 8% for every degree Celsius decrease in body temperature below 37° C. The optimal temperature management for cardiopulmonary bypass is not entirely clear. Eighteen degrees (18° C) is used prior to circulatory arrest and 28° C is common during aortic

cross-clamping with rewarming to 37° C prior to weaning from bypass. Newer protocols maintain temperature between 31° C and 33° C. Normothermic (37° C) bypass is associated with an increase in cerebrovascular accidents.[76]

Blood from the pericardial cavity and the opened heart, as during a valve replacement, is returned to a cardiotomy reservoir, where it is filtered, defoamed, and pumped to the oxygenator for recirculation. The cardiotomy suction may be a major cause of hemolysis and emboli during cardiopulmonary bypass. Filters are incorporated in the cardiotomy reservoir and the arterial circuit to act as traps for particulate debris (e.g., blood clot, latex, talc, fat, Silastic, polyethylene) that could act as systemic emboli.

The tubing used for the cardiopulmonary bypass system is flushed with carbon dioxide, then filled (primed) with crystalloid. Additives to the circuit may include albumin, hetastarch, blood, bicarbonate, heparin, and antibiotics. The goal is a predetermined solution that is calculated to produce a specific hematocrit with institution of total cardiopulmonary bypass. Because whole body hypothermia (18° C to 28° C) may be utilized, the pump prime often contains little or no blood, such that the hematocrit of blood during cardiopulmonary bypass is 20% to 30%. Hemodilution is important for decreasing viscosity during hypothermia. It is mandatory that all air be cleared from the arterial side of the circuit before institution of cardiopulmonary bypass. Indeed, pumping of air into the patient by the cardiopulmonary bypass machine is an ever-present hazard. Carbon dioxide flushing prior to priming and continuous flushing of the pericardium reduce gas emboli risk. Patients who suffer gas emboli can be treated with hyperbaric oxygen with improvements in neurologic function even 24 hours after embolization.[77] Early treatment may have better results.

Heparin-induced anticoagulation of the patient is mandatory before placement of the venous and aortic cannulas used for cardiopulmonary bypass. The usual initial dose of heparin administered intravenously is 300 to 400 units/kg. The adequacy of anticoagulation is subsequently confirmed by determination of the activated coagulation time, which is typically maintained at greater than 450 seconds during cardiopulmonary bypass (when baseline normal is 90 to 120 seconds).[75]

## Monitoring During Cardiopulmonary Bypass

Institution of cardiopulmonary bypass is often associated with decreases in mean arterial pressure, presumably reflecting the dramatic decreases in viscosity that result from infusion of prime solutions and activation of systemic inflammatory response. In addition, peripheral vasodilation may accompany decreased oxygen delivery that occurs in the early period of hemodilution. Administration of an α-agonist, such as phenylephrine, to increase perfusion pressures to higher than 40 mm Hg in the early period after institution of cardiopulmonary bypass may be recommended on the assumption that perfusion pressure is important for maintenance of cerebral blood flow. The correct arterial blood pressure during bypass is debatable. Lower pressures may reduce cerebral blood flow and reduce emboli load to the brain. Higher pressures may improve cerebral blood flow and reduce watershed infarction, but higher pressures come from higher flows and more emboli per unit time. Pressures below 40 mm Hg are avoided if possible in adults. Pressures higher than 60 mm Hg are used during rewarming. Pressures up to 80 to 90 mm Hg may be used in patients with cerebral vascular disease. Evidence to support these recommendations is limited.

After the initial decrease, mean arterial pressure during cardiopulmonary bypass often begins to increase spontaneously, perhaps reflecting activation of the renin-angiotensin system or sympathetic nervous system. Mean arterial pressures higher than 100 mm Hg can lead to impairment of tissue perfusion as well as the risk of intracranial hemorrhage. Furthermore, noncoronary collateral blood flow is likely to be increased as mean arterial pressure increases, resulting in perfusion of the heart with blood at higher temperatures than desired for optimal cellular protection. Hypertension is often treated by decreasing SVR with volatile anesthetics administered through the oxygenator or the continuous intravenous administration of nitroprusside. Nitroglycerine has reduced effect on cardiopulmonary bypass because its action is predominantly venodilation and arterial pressures during bypass are primarily dependent on SVR.

An increasing central venous pressure with or without facial edema (eyelids and scleras) may reflect improper placement of the vena cava cannula resulting in obstruction to venous drainage. For example, insertion of a cannula too far into the superior vena cava can obstruct the right innominate vein, leading to an increase of cerebral venous pressure with associated cerebral edema. Placement of a cannula too far into the inferior vena cava results in abdominal distention. Confirmatory evidence of misplacement of a vena cava cannula is inadequate venous return from the patient to the cardiopulmonary bypass machine. Prompt withdrawal of the vena cava cannula to a more proximal position should immediately improve venous drainage.

A pulmonary artery catheter detects increases in pulmonary artery pressures caused by malfunction of the left ventricular vent and the associated inadequate decompression of the left ventricle. Persistent left ventricular distention can result in damage to the contractile elements of the myocardium.

Blood gases and pH are monitored frequently during cardiopulmonary bypass. A mixed venous $Po_2$ less than 30 mm Hg associated with metabolic acidosis may indicate inadequate tissue perfusion. Temperature correction of $Paco_2$ and pH is probably not necessary. Urine output may serve as a guide to the adequacy of renal perfusion,

with an output of 1 mL/kg/h being a common expectation. Continuous cerebral oximetry with infrared spectroscopy can detect poor cerebral perfusion and may reduce risk.

During total cardiopulmonary bypass, the lungs are left quiescent with or without moderate continuous positive airway pressure. The best composition of gases in the lungs during this period is unsettled. Continued ventilation of the lungs with oxygen may be appropriate when there is some pulmonary blood flow, as evidenced by a pulsatile pulmonary artery trace. If there is a pulsatile pulmonary arterial pressure or systemic arterial pressure, the lungs should be ventilated because there is only partial cardiopulmonary bypass.

Esophageal, rectal, bladder, and blood temperatures are monitored routinely. Rapid rewarming caused by a high blood-to-body temperature gradient is avoided to prevent gas emboli. Drug-induced vasodilation as produced by a volatile anesthetic or nitroprusside may speed the rewarming process, as reflected by a more rapid approach of the rectal (core) to esophageal (blood) temperature, but should be used carefully. Measurement of urinary bladder temperature may be a superior alternative to monitoring rectal temperature, as bladder temperature may reflect core temperatures better than rectal.

## Myocardial Preservation

The goal of myocardial preservation is to decrease myocardial damage introduced by the period of ischemia associated with cardiopulmonary bypass. This goal is achieved by decreasing myocardial oxygen consumption by infusing cardioplegia solutions containing potassium into the aortic root, which in the presence of a distally cross-clamped aorta, and competent aortic valve ensures diversion of the solution into the coronary arteries. Alternatively, the cardioplegia solution may be administered retrograde through a cannula placed into the coronary sinus. Monitoring of coronary sinus pressures during retrograde administration is used to assess catheter placement. If the pressure at the distal tip of the coronary sinus catheter during cardioplegia administration at 200 mL/min is equal to central venous pressure, the catheter is not in the coronary sinus but is most likely in the right atrium. If the pressure is very high (more than 100 mm Hg), the coronary sinus catheter is up against a vascular wall. If the pressure in the coronary sinus catheter is 40 to 60 mm Hg during a 200 mL/min infusion, the catheter is correctly positioned. Positioning of the coronary sinus catheter should be checked with TEE and manual feel by the surgeon. If the catheter is in too deep, cardioplegia to the right ventricle will be compromised, resulting in poor right ventricular protection. An additional route for infusion of cardioplegia solutions is directly into newly placed bypass grafts.

Potassium in the cardioplegia solution blocks the initial phase of myocardial depolarization, resulting in cessation

IV

of electrical and mechanical activity. The cold solution produces selective hypothermia of the cardiac muscle. At 30° C, the normally contracting heart muscle consumes oxygen at a rate of 8 to 10 mL/100 g/min. Oxygen consumption in the fibrillating ventricle at 22° C is 2 mL/100 g/min. The electromechanically quiet heart at 22° C consumes oxygen at a rate of 0.3 mL/100 g/min. The effectiveness of cold cardioplegia is monitored by measuring heart temperature with a temperature probe placed into the left ventricular muscle plus the absence of any visible electrical activity on the ECG. Cold cardioplegia infusions are supplemented by total-body hypothermia and localized epicardial surface cooling using ice or cold irrigation solutions placed into the pericardial space. Cardioplegia solutions may also contain many additives including blood, insulin, glucose, aspartate, glutamate, calcium, magnesium, nitroglycerin, and superoxide dismutase, at the discretion of the surgeon. None of these additives is definitively better than cold blood cardioplegia with a short cross-clamp time. Adequate myocardial preservation is suggested by good myocardial contractility without the need for inotropic drugs at the conclusion of cardiopulmonary bypass.

A side effect of cardioplegia solutions is an increased incidence of atrioventricular heart block due to intramyocardial hyperkalemia. This heart block usually resolves in 1 to 2 hours and can be treated temporarily by use of an artificial cardiac pacemaker. Intramyocardial hyperkalemia also produces decreased myocardial contractility. Systemic hyperkalemia is likely to occur when coronary sinus blood containing cardioplegia solution is returned to the oxygenator for subsequent circulation. Decreased renal function during cardiopulmonary bypass will also contribute to hyperkalemia. If hyperkalemia persists at the conclusion of cardiopulmonary bypass, regular insulin (10 to 20 units IV) can be given in combination with glucose (25 to 50 mg IV) in an attempt to shift potassium into the cells. The perfusionists can also add crystalloid solutions to the bypass circuit and then use a hemoconcentrator to ultrafiltrate the blood thereby eliminating potassium.

## Management of Anesthesia

Drugs selected for maintenance of anesthesia in patients undergoing cardiopulmonary bypass are influenced by the patient's cardiac disease. Patients with diabetes or those who develop glucose intolerance during surgery should have infusions of insulin with a target of glucose between 120 and 180 mg/dL. Avoidance of hypoglycemia is essential to avoid neurologic injury. Hyperglycemia may lead to increased risk of infections and neurologic sequelae. Infusions of dexmedetomidine are associated with reduced risk of delirium.[53] Institution of cardiopulmonary bypass may produce a sudden dilution of circulating drug concentrations. For this reason, supplemental

anesthetics, such as benzodiazepines or opioids, may be needed. Likewise, skeletal muscle paralysis may be supplemented with additional nondepolarizing neuromuscular blocking drugs. An additional dose of nondepolarizing muscle relaxant should be administered just prior to placement of the venous cannula to avoid inspiratory efforts entraining air. Anesthetic depth can also be increased by volatile anesthetics from vaporizers incorporated into the cardiopulmonary bypass circuit. The effect of hemodilution on drug concentrations is likely to be offset by a decreased need for drugs during hypothermia. Anesthetic requirements seem to be minimal following rewarming to a normal body temperature at the conclusion of cardiopulmonary bypass. Therefore, additional anesthesia is not routinely required during rewarming or the early period after the conclusion of cardiopulmonary bypass. However, additional anesthetic will be needed to maintain tracheal intubation for transfer and postoperative ventilation in the ICU. An intravenous anesthetic infusion (propofol or dexmedetomidine) with minimal hemodynamic effects should be given in the procedure and continued into the ICU. Dexmedetomidine-induced sedation may reduce the risk of postoperative delirium after cardiac surgery.[53]

## Discontinuation of Cardiopulmonary Bypass

Optimal anesthetic care can be achieved with checklists. The checklist for weaning from cardiopulmonary bypass consists of the mnemonic WRMVP (Box 25.12), as in Wide Receiver Most Valuable Player (a wide receiver is an American football position for our non–United States readers):

1. Warm: Is the patient at 37° C?
2. Rhythm: Does the patient have a stable cardiac rhythm?
3. Monitors: Are the monitors turned back on? How about the pulse oximeter? The pulse oximeter is essential postoperatively both as a monitor of arterial oxygen

---

**Box 25.12** Checklist for Weaning From Cardiopulmonary Bypass: WRMVP

| | |
|---|---|
| Warm | Body temperature (37° C) is likely to decrease rapidly after cardiopulmonary bypass if patient is not adequately rewarmed, with resultant metabolic acidosis and poor myocardial contractility. |
| Rhythm | Confirm that the patient has a stable cardiac rhythm. |
| Monitors | Confirm that the monitors are turned on; pulse oximeter is essential for arterial oxygen saturation and cardiac output. |
| Ventilator | Confirm that it is turned on. |
| Perfusion | Confirm heart beating, presence of vasodilation. |

saturation and cardiac output. If the pulse oximeter is not working, it may be that perfusion is inadequate. The pulse oximeter is an excellent low cardiac output alarm.

4. Ventilator: Is the ventilator back on? It is easy to forget this, and rapid desaturation after bypass detected from the pulse oximeter should be quickly identified.

5. Perfusion: Is the heart beating, is the vasculature appropriate for the cardiac function? Very few hearts following cardiopulmonary bypass are adequate to maintain an arterial blood pressure in the face of profound systemic vasodilation. The SVR should be normal (not profoundly vasodilated or constricted). Cardiopulmonary bypass is discontinued when the patient is hemodynamically stable and normothermia has been reestablished. In the absence of adequate rewarming before discontinuation of cardiopulmonary bypass, body temperature is likely to decrease rapidly in the post–cardiopulmonary bypass period, resulting in metabolic acidosis and poor myocardial contractility. When the left side of the heart has been opened, as during valve replacement surgery, it is mandatory to remove all air from the cardiac chambers and pulmonary veins before permitting the heart to eject blood into the aorta. Otherwise, systemic air emboli can occur with disastrous cardiac and central nervous system effects. The presence of air can be checked with TEE. Unrecognized air in the coronary arteries may be a cause of sudden onset of poor myocardial contractility after discontinuation of cardiopulmonary bypass. Air embolization with neurologic defects can be treated with hyperbaric oxygen even 24 hours after surgery with improvements in neurologic outcome.[77] Measurement of cardiac filling pressures, determination of thermodilution cardiac outputs, and calculation of systemic and PVR are helpful for guiding

intravenous fluid replacement and the appropriate selection of drugs in the early post–cardiopulmonary bypass period (Table 25.4). Alternatively, TEE can be used to estimate the adequacy of intravascular fluid volume and myocardial contractility. TEE is also useful for evaluating cardiac valve function and intracardiac blood flow patterns, particularly following surgical repair or replacement.

The most common hemodynamic abnormality after cardiopulmonary bypass is inadequate SVR. It is very difficult to wean the patient from cardiopulmonary bypass with an SVR that is low. SVR can be calculated as follows:

$$\text{Mean arterial pressure (mm Hg)} - \text{central venous pressure (mm Hg)/pump flow (L/min)} \times 80$$

SVR should be between 1200 and 1400 prior to weaning from bypass. The units of SVR are dyne-seconds/centimeters$^5$ (dyn-s/cm$^5$). SVR can be normalized with a vasoconstrictor prior to weaning from cardiopulmonary bypass. The goal should be to match the vascular input impedance to the cardiac output impedance to optimize energy transfer. It is much easier to adjust the vasculature to match the heart than to force the heart to tolerate a dilated vasculature. On occasion, an inotropic drug, such as epinephrine, norepinephrine, dopamine, or dobutamine, is needed. In cases of severe ventricular dysfunction, a combination of drugs (epinephrine or norepinephrine and amrinone or milrinone) with an intra-aortic balloon pump or left ventricular assist device is necessary to maintain optimal cardiac output. The use of combinations of β-agonists and phosphodiesterase inhibitors produces synergistic increases in cardiac function. The vasoconstriction of epinephrine or norepinephrine is counterbalanced by the vasodilation of the

**IV**

**Table 25.4**   Diagnosis and Treatment of Cardiovascular Dysfunction After Cardiopulmonary Bypass

| Systemic Blood Pressure | Atrial Pressure | Cardiac Output | Diagnosis | Therapy |
|---|---|---|---|---|
| Decreased | Decreased | Decreased | Hypovolemia | Administer volume |
| Decreased | Decreased | Increased | Vasodilation Low blood viscosity | Vasoconstrictor Erythrocyte transfusion |
| Decreased | Increased | Decreased | Left ventricular dysfunction | Inotrope Inodilator Vasodilator Mechanical assistance |
| Increased | Increased | Decreased | Vasoconstriction Left ventricular dysfunction | Vasodilator Inotrope |
| Increased | Decreased | Increased | Hyperdynamic | Volatile anesthetic β-Antagonist |

phosphodiesterase inhibitor. Careful measurement of SVR and supplementation with a vasoconstrictor, such as phenylephrine, are frequently needed to maintain a normal SVR. If β-agonists are needed, frequent attention must be given to measurement and control of potassium, glucose, calcium, pH, and the presence of arrhythmias. Gas emboli to the coronary arteries may suddenly and profoundly reduce ventricular function. Posterior papillary muscle dysfunction at the conclusion of cardiopulmonary bypass may result in mitral regurgitation as evidenced by the presence of prominent V waves on the pulmonary artery occlusion pressure tracing. This dysfunction may reflect less than optimal cardioplegic protection of the posterior myocardium, which is most vulnerable to warming effects from blood in the adjacent descending aorta, as well as perfusion with warm blood representing noncoronary collateral circulation. Acute mitral regurgitation can also occur with volume overload from excessive fluid administration; it can be managed simply by the use of reverse Trendelenburg position to reduce venous return to the heart.

A mechanical complement to inotropic support of cardiac output is the intra-aortic balloon pump. The intra-aortic balloon pump (a 25-cm long balloon mounted on a 90-cm stiff plastic catheter) is typically inserted percutaneously through the femoral artery and advanced so that the tip is just distal to the left subclavian artery. The balloon is timed to inflate during diastole to augment diastolic blood pressure and increase the gradient for coronary perfusion improving coronary blood flow. The balloon deflates immediately before systole, thus decreasing afterload and lowering oxygen requirements. Coronary blood flow is increased, with little or no increase in cardiac work, which may result in improvements in cardiac output. Aortic insufficiency may be worsened by intra-aortic balloon inflation. Rapid heart rates and cardiac dysrhythmias interfere with proper balloon timing and optimal augmentation of cardiac output. Temporary ventricular assist can also be provided by catheters with impellers that rely on the Archimedes screw technology. The impeller device comes in two sizes capable of 2.5 or 5.0 L/min flow.

When an adequate systemic arterial blood pressure and cardiac output have been maintained for several minutes, the vena cava cannula is removed and protamine administration is begun to reverse heparin anticoagulation. Protamine administration is dangerous and frequently is associated with hypotension from release of histamine. Occasionally there is severe pulmonary hypertension or even anaphylaxis from protamine administration. Protamine should be administered after a test dose and given slowly to avoid catastrophic hemodyamic collapse. Administration of the vasoconstrictor phenylephrine can be used to maintain arterial blood pressure. In cases of hemodyamic collapse even epinephrine boluses will be inadequate, and return to cardiopulmonary bypass after emergency reheparinization

can be lifesaving. Isophane (NPH) insulin is made with protamine. Diabetics who use NPH insulin may be at increased risk for protamine reactions. Protamine allergic reactions may be reduced with a combination of histamine blockade (H$_1$ [diphenhydramine] and H$_2$ blocker [ranitidine]) and a steroid (hydrocortisone). The aortic cannula is removed after protamine administration is safely concluded. Pharmacologic measures to decrease bleeding include administration of antifibrinolytics (aminocaproic acid, tranexamic acid, and formerly aprotinin) and desmopressin (improves platelet function in patients with von Willebrand disease). Blood loss throughout the procedure as well as the blood in the bypass tubing can be salvaged, washed, and retransfused using "cell saver" devices.

Administration of nitrous oxide after cardiopulmonary bypass is not recommended because this gas could unmask the presence of air in the heart or coronary arteries. For this reason, anesthesia is most often supplemented, when necessary, by the intravenous administration of propofol, dexmedetomidine, opioids, benzodiazepines, or alternatively with low inhaled concentrations of volatile anesthetics. The blood and fluid that remain in the cardiopulmonary bypass circuit are washed and collected into sterile plastic bags as packed cells for possible reinfusion to the patient. High resistance to blood flow in the arm induced by vasoconstriction may result in a falsely low systemic arterial blood pressure reading from the radial artery in the early period after cardiopulmonary bypass. If there is a question of inadequate arterial blood pressure, direct pressure measurement from the ascending aorta can be instantly obtained. Placement of a femoral arterial catheter is needed if there is a gradient between central and radial pressure. Any gradient between central aortic and radial artery blood pressure usually disappears within 60 minutes.

Intravenous anesthetics such as propofol infusions,[78] dexmedetomidine infusions,[53] or opioids and benzodiazepines are continued after bypass and continued into the ICU to provide sedation prior to tracheal extubation. Dexmedetomidine-induced sedation may reduce postoperative delirium after cardiac surgery.[53] The time to tracheal extubation is shortening after cardiopulmonary bypass but some period of time of postoperative intubation is common after leaving the operating room. Once oxygenation is adequate (Pao$_2$ above 80 mm Hg on 40% oxygen), the bleeding is controlled, the patient is awake, and neuromuscular function has recovered, extubation can be considered. There is no benefit from prolonged postoperative ventilation in cardiac surgery.

The large financial cost of cardiac surgery is due in part to the duration of intensive care required for these patients. Improvements in anesthetic, surgical, and perfusion techniques serve to decrease the need for prolonged care of these patients in an ICU. The concept known as "fast track" as applied to cardiac surgical patients includes early postoperative awakening and tracheal extubation.[79]

## Off-Pump Coronary Artery Bypass Graft Surgery

In an effort to minimize postoperative morbidity, CABG surgery may be accomplished in selected patients without institution of cardiopulmonary bypass and in the presence of a spontaneously beating heart and normothermia. Cardiopulmonary bypass using extracorporeal circulatory support was developed because it is difficult to safely produce a high-quality anastomosis between a vessel and a coronary artery while the heart is beating. Off-pump CABG was developed to reduce the sequelae of extracorporeal circulatory support, which may include stroke, global encephalopathy, renal failure, pulmonary injury, and death. Off-pump CABG surgery is limited by several considerations including the quality of the distal anastomosis and long-term graft patency is of primary concern. There are several problems with off-pump CABG or "beating heart" surgery. The first is motion of the coronary artery, making suture placement for the anastomosis difficult. Anticoagulation with heparin is achieved and activated clotting time (ACT) is measured. There is some debate on the appropriate ACT levels of an off-pump CABG with some surgeons using standard doses appropriate for cardiopulmonary bypass (300 to 400 units/kg ACT > 450 s) and others using smaller dose heparin (200 unit/kg). Antifibrinolytics (aprotinin, aminocaproic acid, or tranexamic acid) are sometimes not used if the patient is not going on extracorporeal circulatory support. The ability to immediately go on extracorporeal circulatory support must be available during the conduct of off-pump CABG should the patient have circulatory collapse or cardiac arrest. Blood flow in the target coronary artery is usually stopped by placement of a proximal and distal latex suture, which is lifted up, consequently arresting flow. Alternatively, a silicon stent can be placed in the target coronary artery during production of the anastomosis to maintain coronary flow. The silicon stent is removed just prior to tightening the suture. Stopping the coronary blood flow in the target coronary may cause myocardial ischemia, ventricular arrhythmias, ventricular dysfunction, heart block, hemodynamic collapse, and cardiac arrest. When flow is resumed in the coronary artery, reperfusion arrhythmias may occur. Prophylactic antiarrhythmic therapy should be administered prior to off-pump CABG. Magnesium (2 g IV slowly) combined with lidocaine (100-mg bolus followed by 2 mg/min) infusion works well. Intravenous amiodarone should be used in patients who demonstrate a tendency toward ventricular tachycardia or fibrillation.

The technology for the off-pump CABG was developed in the 1990s and initially stabilized the heart with a retractor that simply pushed on the myocardium while it was lifted into the retractor with stay sutures. This system was difficult to use because ventricular diastolic filling was compromised by external pressure on the heart. The development of a retractor that used a vacuum foot (Octopus) to stabilize the heart eliminated the external pressure on the myocardium and improved ventricular diastolic function during the distal anastomosis. Coronary grafts to the inferior and lateral circulation were difficult to perform because retraction of the heart reduced diastolic filling and caused hemodynamic collapse. The use of suction retractors (Starfish and Urchin) for lateral and anterior displacement of the heart during production of the lateral and inferior anastomosis in combination with steep Trendelenburg positioning greatly stabilized hemodynamics.

Careful cooperation between the cardiac surgeon and cardiac anesthesiologist is essential for off-pump CABG. Surgical positioning must be performed in conjunction with anesthesia. The surgeon must not open the coronary artery for a distal anastomosis without ensuring that the patient will hemodynamically tolerate the 10- to 15-minute anastomosis. Communication between the cardiac surgeon and cardiac anesthesiologist is especially critical during this process. Some surgeons use a 5-minute period of ischemic preconditioning prior to a 5-minute recovery period followed by the anastomosis. The 5-minute preconditioning period can be used to optimize hemodynamics and test to see if the patient will tolerate the anastomosis. Ischemic preconditioning may reduce ischemic injury at the cost of a longer operative time.

Anastomosis of the left internal mammary artery (LIMA) to the left anterior descending (LAD) coronary artery was the first off-pump bypass and is technically the simplest and most important for reducing myocardial ischemia. The LIMA to LAD anastomosis is usually conducted first, which improves coronary blood flow to the LAD circulation. Saphenous vein grafts are then placed to the obtuse marginal (OM) branches off the circumflex artery and finally to the posterior descending artery (PDA), which usually branches from the right coronary artery. Placement of the lateral wall grafts to the obtuse marginal requires shifting the heart to the right, which may be better tolerated by opening the right pleural space and placing lifting-stay sutures into the inferior pericardium. Steep Trendelenburg positioning with right tilt will improve hemodynamics. Intravascular administration of colloid and vasoconstriction with phenylephrine should be used to maintain arterial blood pressure. The ECG amplitude may diminish dramatically making ST segments difficult to observe secondary to myocardial positioning. TEE of the ventricle may be impossible secondary to lifting of the ventricle off the esophagus. Anastomosis to the posterior descending coronary artery can be produced with steep Trendelenburg position, volume loading, and vasoconstriction with phenylephrine. Low cardiac outputs can be tolerated for the brief period of the distal anastomosis. Completion of the proximal aortic anastomosis for the saphenous vein grafts requires placement of a side biter clamp on the ascending aorta.

**IV**

Devices that staple the proximal anastomosis are available and may reduce the use of side biter clamps with less aortic trauma. Arterial blood pressure can be decreased to assist placement of this clamp with increasing inspired concentrations of volatile anesthetics or cardiac manipulation to reduce venous return. Once the distal and proximal anastomoses are complete, any air in the saphenous vein graft must be removed to avoid coronary gas emboli. Removal of the aortic side biter should only be done once any remaining air is removed from the saphenous vein grafts to avoid systemic gas emboli. Heparin anticoagulation should then be carefully reversed with protamine. Protamine reactions, which include hypotension, pulmonary hypertension, and anaphylaxis, are more difficult to treat in off-pump CABG because rapid return to extracorporeal circulatory support will require full reheparinization, bypass circuit priming, followed by proximal aortic cannula and right atrial venous cannula placement. If hypotension occurs following protamine administration, rapid treatment with the vasoconstrictor phenylephrine is frequently needed. Severe reactions to protamine may be treated with intravenous epinephrine, diphenhydramine, $H_2$ blockade, steroids, intravascular fluid administration, and if necessary reheparinization, and initiation of extracorporeal circulatory support. The use of off-pump CABG is becoming less frequent after the publication of the ROOBY (randomized on/off bypass) trial, which showed a reduction in graft patency and poorer outcomes in the off-pump group.[80]

### Management of Anesthesia

Anesthesia for off-pump CABG is very similar to anesthesia for on-pump CABG with a few notable exceptions. Patients for off-pump CABG have similar medical conditions, medical therapies, and requirements for care as those receiving on-pump CABG. All preoperative medications with the exception of oral hypoglycemic agents should be continued in the perioperative period. Patients with diabetes should be managed with intravenous insulin infusions and frequent blood glucose determinations. Coumadin (warfarin) should be stopped at least 7 days prior to an operation. Platelet inhibitors, with the exception of aspirin, should be discontinued preoperatively depending on clearance. Preoperative heparin infusions can be continued into the operating room and discontinued after full heparinization. Preoperative sedation with a benzodiazepine and nasal cannula oxygen is effective at reducing sympathetic stimulation but is rarely used in the current era.

Induction of anesthesia should have the goal to maintain arterial blood pressure within 10% to 20% of baseline. Baseline measurements of heart rate, arterial blood pressure, pulmonary artery pressures, central venous pressures, and cardiac output can be obtained using intra-arterial and pulmonary arterial catheters allowing preinduction optimization of hemodynamics.

If severe pulmonary hypertension or low cardiac output is identified, a discussion of the case with the cardiac surgeon is warranted. An infusion of the vasoconstrictor phenylephrine may be started prior to induction of anesthesia and then titrated to maintain arterial blood pressure. Any intravenous anesthetic can be used to induce anesthesia, but benzodiazepines (midazolam) and narcotics (fentanyl) are common. Sufentanil decreases heart rate more than fentanyl, which may or may not be advantageous. Dexmedetomidine can be used to supplement other drugs and may reduce stress response and postoperative delirium.[53] Etomidate, propofol, and sodium thiopental are also effective for induction of anesthesia, but doses should be reduced in patients at risk for hypotension.

Once anesthetic induction is complete, nondepolarizing muscle relaxants (rocuronium, vecuronium, cisatracurium) or succinylcholine can be used to facilitate tracheal intubation. Bradycardia (heart rates between 45 and 60 beats/min) is helpful during conduct of the distal anastomosis. If reflux is a concern, a modified rapid sequence induction with cricoid pressure is warranted. If the patient is thought to have a difficult airway, the standard difficult airway protocols should be used with special attention to avoid tachycardia and sympathetic stimulation. Intubation of cardiac surgery patients should follow the standard protocols for airway management, the only difference being that the tolerance for tachycardia, hypotension, or hypertension is greatly reduced and myocardial ischemia, ventricular arrhythmias, and hemodynamic collapse are the possible rapid sequelae of complications.

Maintenance of anesthesia is usually with a volatile anesthetic (isoflurane or sevoflurane) in combination with an opioid (fentanyl or sufentanil). Nitrous oxide should be avoided secondary to reduction in $Fio_2$, potential for pulmonary vasoconstriction, and potential to increase the volume of gas emboli. Maintenance infusions of propofol, dexmedetomidine, or remifentanil are also commonly used. If remifentanil is chosen, inadvertent discontinuation of the infusion should be avoided because the metabolism is rapid. Cardiac depression may be greater with remifentanil than fentanyl or sufentanil, making its use more difficult in patients with limited cardiac reserve. Prophylactic antiarrhythmic therapy (lidocaine and magnesium or amiodarone) is appropriate to avoid arrhythmias from manual manipulation of the heart, from ischemia during the distal anastomosis, and upon reperfusion after completion of the anastomosis. Anticoagulation is achieved with heparin and monitored with ACT or heparin assay. Hemodynamic stability during the distal anastomosis is achieved with careful surgical manipulation and retraction of the heart, table positioning, infusions of vasoconstrictors, and volume. Inotropic stimulation with β-agonists has the potential to raise the heart rate, making completion of the distal anastomosis more difficult and lowering the threshold for ventricular arrhythmias. If β-agonists are needed to support cardiac output during conduct of the distal anastomosis, use of extracorporeal circulatory support should be considered. Heparin anticoagulation is reversed with protamine after completion of the proximal and distal anastomoses and is confirmed by measurement of an ACT near baseline (120 to 140 seconds).

The duration and requirements for postoperative ventilation and sedation may be reduced in off-pump CABG and extubation of the trachea should be performed once hemodynamics are stable, bleeding is controlled, oxygen requirements are reduced ($F_{IO_2} = 0.40$ with $P_{O_2}$ more than 80 mm Hg), neuromuscular blockade is reversed, and the patient is awake and breathing spontaneously with the help of continuous positive-pressure ventilation. Postoperative administration of β-adrenergic blockade may reduce the incidence of atrial fibrillation and myocardial ischemia and should be started as soon as hemodynamics will tolerate. Aspirin therapy should be resumed once bleeding is controlled. Discontinuation of anti-ischemic and vasodilator drugs (β-adrenergic blockers, calcium channel blockers, nitrates, and angiotensin inhibitors) should be avoided because withdrawal phenomena may lead to increased morbidity and mortality rates.

Cardiac surgery is continually advancing with hybrid operations, off-pump CABG, minimal access, surgical ventricular restoration, left ventricular assist devices, artificial hearts, and robotic mitral and coronary artery bypass surgery. Vigilance, cooperation, team work, and a very clear understanding of the surgical plans and hemodynamic consequences of procedures are essential to reduce the morbidity and mortality rates of these operations.

## QUESTIONS OF THE DAY

1. How does risk stratification for cardiac disease differ from risk reduction?

2. How have the results of the POISE study impacted recommendations for perioperative cardiac risk reduction therapy?

3. A patient with severe aortic stenosis requires general anesthesia. What are the hemodynamic goals for the patient? What are the risks of hypotension during induction of anesthesia?

4. What is the "magnet mode" of a programmable cardiac pacemaker? Why should the specific magnet mode be known during the perioperative period?

5. A patient with hypertrophic cardiomyopathy develops intraoperative hypotension. What interventions are most likely to be effective?

6. A patient with cardiac tamponade is scheduled for a pericardial window in the operating room. What precautions should be taken before and during anesthesia induction to minimize the chance for cardiac arrest?

7. What are the major components of a cardiopulmonary bypass circuit? What principles are relevant in determining appropriate perfusion pressure during cardiopulmonary bypass?

**IV**

## REFERENCES

1. Mangano DT, Goldman L. Preoperative assessment of patients with known or suspected coronary disease. *N Engl J Med.* 1995;333(26):1750–1756.

2. Mozaffarian D, Benjamin EJ, Go AS, et al. American Heart Association Statistics Committee and Stroke Statistics Subcommittee. Heart disease and stroke statistics–2015 update: a report from the American Heart Association. *Circulation.* 2015;131(4):e29–e322.

3. Mangano DT, Browner WS, Hollenberg M, et al. Long-term cardiac prognosis following noncardiac surgery. The Study of Perioperative Ischemia Research Group. *JAMA.* 1992;268(2):233–239.

4. Mangano DT, Browner WS, Hollenberg M, et al. Association of perioperative myocardial ischemia with cardiac morbidity and mortality in men undergoing noncardiac surgery. The Study of Perioperative Ischemia Research Group. *N Engl J Med.* 1990;323(26):1781–1788.

5. Fleisher LA, Barash PG. Preoperative cardiac evaluation for noncardiac surgery: a functional approach. *Anesth Analg.* 1992;74(4):586–598.

6. Fleisher LA, Fleischmann KE, Auerbach AD, et al. 2014 ACC/AHA guideline on perioperative cardiovascular evaluation and management of patients undergoing noncardiac surgery: executive summary: a report of the American College of Cardiology/American Heart Association Task Force on practice guidelines. Developed in collaboration with the American College of Surgeons, American Society of Anesthesiologists, American Society of Echocardiography, American Society of Nuclear Cardiology, Heart Rhythm Society, Society for Cardiovascular Angiography and Interventions, Society of Cardiovascular Anesthesiologists, and Society of Vascular Medicine Endorsed by the Society of Hospital Medicine. *J Nucl Cardiol.* 2015;22(1):162–215.

7. Mangano DT, London MJ, Tubau JF, et al. Dipyridamole thallium-201 scintigraphy as a preoperative screening test. A reexamination of its predictive potential. Study of Perioperative Ischemia Research Group. *Circulation.* 1991;84(2):493–502.

8. Baron JF, Mundler O, Bertrand M, et al. Dipyridamole-thallium scintigraphy and gated radionuclide angiography to assess cardiac risk before abdominal aortic surgery. *N Engl J Med.* 1994;330(10):663–669.

9. Tarhan S, Moffitt EA, Taylor WF, et al. Myocardial infarction after general anesthesia. *Anesth Analg.* 1977;56(3):455–461.

10. Steen PA, Tinker JH, Tarhan S. Myocardial reinfarction after anesthesia and surgery. *JAMA.* 1978;239(24):2566–2570.

11. Rao TL, Jacobs KH, El-Etr AA. Reinfarction following anesthesia in patients with myocardial infarction. *Anesthesiology.* 1983;59(6):499–505.

12. Shah KB, Kleinman BS, Sami H, et al. Reevaluation of perioperative myocardial infarction in patients with prior myocardial infarction undergoing noncardiac operations. *Anesth Analg.* 1990;71(3):231–235.

13. Landesberg G, Beattie WS, Mosseri M, et al. Perioperative myocardial infarction. *Circulation.* 2009;119(22):2936–2944.

14. Mangano DT, Layug EL, Wallace A, et al. Effect of atenolol on mortality and cardiovascular morbidity after noncardiac surgery. Multicenter Study of Perioperative Ischemia Research Group. [Erratum in *N Engl J Med.* 1997;336(14):1039]. *N Engl J Med.* 1996;335(23):1713–1720.

15. Schouten O, Boersma E, Hoeks SE, et al. Fluvastatin and perioperative events in patients undergoing vascular surgery. *N Engl J Med.* 2009;361(10):980–989.

16. Mangano DT, Layug EL, Wallace A. Effect of atenolol on mortality and cardiovascular morbidity after noncardiac surgery. Multicenter Study of Perioperative Ischemia Research Group. *N Engl J Med.* 1996;335(23):1713–1720.

17. Wallace A, Layug B, Tateo I, et al. Prophylactic atenolol reduces postoperative myocardial ischemia. McSPI Research Group. *Anesthesiology.* 1998;88(1):7–17.

18. Slogoff S, Keats AS, Ott E. Preoperative propranolol therapy and aorto-coronary bypass operation. *JAMA.* 1978;240(14):1487–1490.

19. Mudumbai SC, Takemoto S, Cason BA, et al. Thirty-day mortality risk associated with the postoperative nonresumption of angiotensin-converting enzyme inhibitors: a retrospective study of the Veterans Affairs Healthcare System. *J Hosp Med.* 2014;9(5):289–296.

20. Drenger B, Fontes ML, Miao Y, et al. Investigators of the Ischemia Research and Education Foundation; Multicenter Study of Perioperative Ischemia Research Group. Patterns of use of perioperative angiotensin-converting enzyme inhibitors in coronary artery bypass graft surgery with cardiopulmonary bypass: effects on in-hospital morbidity and mortality. *Circulation.* 2012;126(3):261–269.

21. Lee SM, Takemoto S, Wallace AW. The association between withholding angiotensin receptor blockers in the early postoperative period and 30-day mortality: a cohort study of the Veterans Affairs healthcare system. *Anesthesiology.* 2015;123(2):288–306.

22. Wallace AW. Clonidine and modification of perioperative outcome. *Curr Opin Anaesthesiol.* 2006;19(4):411–417.

23. McFalls EO, Ward HB, Moritz TE. Coronary-artery revascularization before elective major vascular surgery. *N Engl J Med.* 2004;351(27):2795–2804.

24. Kaluza GL, Joseph J, Lee JR, et al. Catastrophic outcomes of noncardiac surgery soon after coronary stenting. *J Am Coll Cardiol.* 2000;35(5):1288–1294.

25. Hueb W, Soares PR, Gersh BJ. The medicine, angioplasty, or surgery study (MASS-II): a randomized, controlled clinical trial of three therapeutic strategies for multivessel coronary artery disease: one-year results. *J Am Coll Cardiol.* 2004;43(10):1743–1751.

26. Shelton RJ, Velavan P, Nikitin NP, et al. Clinical trials update from the American Heart Association meeting: ACORN-CSD, primary care trial of chronic disease management, PEACE, CREATE, SHIELD, A-HeFT, GEMINI, vitamin E meta-analysis, ESCAPE, CARP, and SCD-HeFT cost-effectiveness study. Disparate opinions regarding indications for coronary artery revascularization before elective vascular surgery. Myocardial revascularization before carotid endarterectomy. How to avoid cardiac ischemic events associated with aortic surgery. *Eur J Heart Fail.* 2005;7(1):127–135.

27. Eagle KA, Berger PB, Calkins H, et al. ACC/AHA guideline update for perioperative cardiovascular evaluation for noncardiac surgery—executive summary. A report of the American College of Cardiology/American Heart Association Task Force on Practice Guidelines (Committee to Update the 1996 Guidelines on Perioperative Cardiovascular Evaluation for Noncardiac Surgery). *Anesth Analg.* 2002;94(5):1052–1064.

28. Eagle KA, Berger PB, Calkins H, et al. American College of Cardiology; American Heart Association. ACC/AHA guideline update for perioperative cardiovascular evaluation for noncardiac surgery—executive summary: a report of the American College of Cardiology/American Heart Association Task Force on Practice Guidelines (Committee to Update the 1996 Guidelines on Perioperative Cardiovascular Evaluation for Noncardiac Surgery). *J Am Coll Cardiol.* 2002;39(3):542–553.

29. Fleischmann KE, Beckman JA, Buller CE, et al. 2009 ACCF/AHA focused update on perioperative beta blockade. A report of the American College of Cardiology Foundation/American Heart Association Task Force on Practice Guidelines. *Circulation.* 2009;120(21):2123–2151.

30. Fleisher LA, Beckman JA, Brown KA, et al. ACC/AHA 2006 guideline update on perioperative cardiovascular evaluation for noncardiac surgery: focused update on perioperative beta-blocker therapy: a report of the American College of Cardiology/American Heart Association Task Force on Practice Guidelines (Writing Committee to Update the 2002 Guidelines on Perioperative Cardiovascular Evaluation for Noncardiac Surgery): developed in collaboration with the American Society of Echocardiography, American Society of Nuclear Cardiology, Heart Rhythm Society, Society of Cardiovascular Anesthesiologists, Society for Cardiovascular Angiography and Interventions, and Society for Vascular Medicine and Biology. *Circulation.* 2006;113(22):2662–2674.

31. Gordon AJ, Macpherson DS. Guideline chaos: conflicting recommendations for preoperative cardiac assessment. *Am J Cardiol.* 2003;91(11):1299–1303.

32. Wallace AW, Au S, Cason BA. Association of the pattern of use of perioperative β-blockade and postoperative mortality. *Anesthesiology.* 2010;113(4):794–805.

33. Wallace AW, Au S, Cason BA. Perioperative beta-blockade: atenolol is associated with reduced mortality when compared to metoprolol. *Anesthesiology.* 2011;114(4):824–836.

34. Mangano DT. Aspirin and mortality from coronary bypass surgery. *N Engl J Med.* 2002;347(17):1309–1317.

35. Devereaux PJ, Mrkobrada M, Sessler DI, et al. POISE-2 Investigators. Aspirin in patients undergoing noncardiac surgery. *N Engl J Med.* 2014;370(16):1494–1503.

36. POISE Trial Investigators, Devereaux PJ, Yang H, Guyatt GH, et al. Rationale, design, and organization of the PeriOperative ISchemic Evaluation (POISE) trial: a randomized controlled trial of metoprolol versus placebo in patients undergoing noncardiac surgery. *Am Heart J.* 2006;152(2):223–230.

37. Devereaux PJ, Yang H, Yusuf S, et al. Effects of extended-release metoprolol succinate in patients undergoing non-cardiac surgery (POISE trial): a randomised controlled trial. *Lancet.* 2008;371(9627):1839–1847.

38. Krupski WC, Nehler MR. How to avoid cardiac ischemic events associated with aortic surgery. *Semin Vasc Surg.* 2001;14(4):235–244.

39. Rabbitts JA, Nuttall GA, Brown MJ, et al. Cardiac risk of noncardiac surgery after percutaneous coronary intervention with drug-eluting stents. *Anesthesiology.* 2008;109(4):596–604.

40. Nuttall GA, Brown MJ, Stombaugh JW, et al. Time and cardiac risk of surgery after bare-metal stent percutaneous coronary intervention. *Anesthesiology.* 2008;109(4):588–595.

41. Wallace AW, Galindez D, Salahieh A, et al. Effect of clonidine on cardiovascular morbidity and mortality after noncardiac surgery. *Anesthesiology.* 2004;101(2):284–293.

42. Slogoff S, Keats AS. Does chronic treatment with calcium entry blocking drugs reduce perioperative myocardial ischemia? *Anesthesiology.* 1988;68(5):676–680.

43. Slogoff S, Keats AS. Further observations on perioperative myocardial ischemia. *Anesthesiology.* 1986;65(5):539–542.

44. Wakeling HG, McFall MR, Jenkins CS, et al. Intraoperative oesophageal Doppler guided fluid management shortens postoperative hospital stay after major bowel surgery. *Br J Anaesth.* 2005;95(5):634–642.

45. Ebert TJ, Muzi M, Berens R, et al. Sympathetic responses to induction of anesthesia in humans with propofol or etomidate. *Anesthesiology.* 1992;76(5):725–733.

46. Helman JD, Leung JM, Bellows WH, et al. The risk of myocardial ischemia in patients receiving desflurane versus sufentanil anesthesia for coronary artery bypass graft surgery. The S.P.I. Research Group. *Anesthesiology.* 1992;77(1):47–62.

47. Slogoff S, Keats AS, Dear WE, et al. Steal-prone coronary anatomy and myocardial ischemia associated with four primary anesthetic agents in humans. *Anesth Analg.* 1991;72(1):22–27.

48. Diana P, Tullock WC, Gorcsan J, et al. Myocardial ischemia: a comparison between isoflurane and enflurane in coronary artery bypass patients. *Anesth Analg.* 1993;77(2):221–226.

49. Leung JM, Goehner P, O'Kelly BF, et al. Isoflurane anesthesia and myocardial ischemia: comparative risk versus sufentanil anesthesia in patients undergoing coronary artery bypass graft surgery. The SPI (Study of Perioperative Ischemia) Research Group. *Anesthesiology.* 1991;74(5):838–847.

50. Hanley PJ, Ray J, Brandt U, Daut J. Halothane, isoflurane and sevoflurane inhibit NADH:ubiquinone oxidoreductase (complex I) of cardiac mitochondria. *J Physiol.* 2002;544(Pt 3):687–693.

51. Cason BA, Gamperl AK, Slocum RE, Hickey RF. Anesthetic-induced preconditioning: previous administration of isoflurane decreases myocardial infarct size in rabbits. *Anesthesiology.* 1997;87(5):1182–1190.

52. Slogoff S, Keats AS. Randomized trial of primary anesthetic agents on outcome of coronary artery bypass operations. *Anesthesiology.* 1989;70(2):179–188.

53. Maldonado JR, Wysong A, van der Starre PJ, et al. Dexmedetomidine and the reduction of postoperative delirium after cardiac surgery. *Psychosomatics.* 2009;50(3):206–217.

54. Sandham JD, Hull RD, Brant RF, et al. Canadian Critical Care Clinical Trials Group. A randomized, controlled trial of the use of pulmonary-artery catheters in high-risk surgical patients. *N Engl J Med.* 2003;348(1):5–14.

55. Xu F, Wang Q, Zhang H, et al. Use of pulmonary artery catheter in coronary artery bypass graft. Costs and long-term outcomes. *PLoS One.* 2015;10(2):e0117610.

56. Fontes ML, Bellows W, Ngo L, Mangano DT. Assessment of ventricular function in critically ill patients: limitations of pulmonary artery catheterization. Institutions of the McSPI Research Group. *J Cardiothorac Vasc Anesth.* 1999;13(5):521–527.

57. Practice guidelines for pulmonary artery catheterization. A report by the American Society of Anesthesiologists Task Force on Pulmonary Artery Catheterization. *Anesthesiology.* 1993;78(2):380–394.

58. American Society of Anesthesiologists Task Force on Pulmonary Artery Catheterization. Practice guidelines for pulmonary artery catheterization: an updated report by the American Society of Anesthesiologists Task Force on Pulmonary Artery Catheterization. *Anesthesiology.* 2003;99(4):988–1014.

59. Mangano DT. Dynamic predictors of perioperative risk. Study of Perioperative Ischemia (SPI) Research Group. *J Card Surg.* 1990;5(suppl 3):231–236.

60. Carabello BA, Crawford FA Jr. Valvular heart disease. *N Engl J Med.* 1997;337(1):32–41.

61. Hilgenberg JC, McCammon RL, Stoelting RK. Pulmonary and systemic vascular responses to nitrous oxide in patients with mitral stenosis and pulmonary hypertension. *Anesth Analg.* 1980;59(5):323–326.

62. Greenberg BH, Rahimtoola SH. Vasodilator therapy for valvular heart disease. *JAMA.* 1981;246(3):269–272.

63. Hanson EW, Neerhut RK, Lynch C 3rd. Mitral valve prolapse. *Anesthesiology.* 1996;85(1):178–195.

64. Freed LA, Levy D, Levine RA, et al. Prevalence and clinical outcome of mitral-valve prolapse. *N Engl J Med.* 1999;341(1):1–7.

65. Atlee JL. Perioperative cardiac dysrhythmias: diagnosis and management. *Anesthesiology.* 1997;86(6):1397–1424.

66. Gallagher JD, Weindling SN, Anderson G, Fillinger MP. Effects of sevoflurane on QT interval in a patient with congenital long QT syndrome. *Anesthesiology.* 1998;89(6):1569–1573.

67. Michalets EL, Smith LK, Van Tassel ED. Torsade de pointes resulting from the addition of droperidol to an existing cytochrome P450 drug interaction. *Ann Pharmacother.* 1998;32(7–8):761–765.

68. Guy JM, André-Fouet X, Porte J, et al. Torsades de pointes and prolongation of the duration of QT interval after injection of droperidol. *Ann Cardiol Angeiol (Paris).* 1991;40(9):541–545.

69. Kusumoto FM, Goldschlager N. Cardiac pacing. *N Engl J Med.* 1996;334(2):89–97.

70. Zaidan JR. Pacemakers. *Anesthesiology.* 1984;60(4):319–334.

71. Dagnino J, Prys-Roberts C. Studies of anaesthesia in relation to hypertension. VI: cardiovascular responses to extradural blockade of treated and untreated hypertensive patients. *Br J Anaesth.* 1984;56(10):1065–1073.

72. Nikolov NM, Fontes ML, White WD, et al. Pulse pressure and long-term survival after coronary artery bypass graft surgery. *Anesth Analg.* 2010;110(2):335–340.

73. Spirito P, Seidman CE, McKenna WJ, Maron BJ. The management of hypertrophic cardiomyopathy. *N Engl J Med.* 1997;336(11):775–785.

74. Pass LJ, Eberhart RC, Brown JC, et al. The effect of mannitol and dopamine on the renal response to thoracic aortic cross-clamping. *J Thorac Cardiovasc Surg.* 1988;95(4):608–612.

75. Despotis GJ, Gravlee G, Filos K, Levy J. Anticoagulation monitoring during cardiac surgery: a review of current and emerging techniques. *Anesthesiology.* 1999;91(4):1122–1151.

76. Martin TD, Craver JM, Gott JP, et al. Prospective, randomized trial of retrograde warm blood cardioplegia: myocardial benefit and neurologic threat. *Ann Thorac Surg.* 1994;57(2):298–302. discussion 302–304.

77. Gibson AJ, Davis FM. Hyperbaric oxygen therapy in the treatment of post cardiac surgical strokes—a case series and review of the literature. *Anaesth Intensive Care.* 2010;38(1):175–184.

78. Wahr JA, Plunkett JJ, Ramsay JG, et al. Cardiovascular responses during sedation after coronary revascularization. Incidence of myocardial ischemia and hemodynamic episodes with propofol versus midazolam. Institutions of the McSPI Research Group. *Anesthesiology.* 1996;84(6):1350–1360.

79. Engelman RM, Rousou JA, Flack JE 3rd, et al. Fast-track recovery of the coronary bypass patient. *Ann Thorac Surg.* 1994;58(6):1742–1746.

80. Shroyer AL, Grover FL, Hattler B, et al. Veterans Affairs Randomized On/Off Bypass (ROOBY) Study Group. On-pump versus off-pump coronary-artery bypass surgery. *N Engl J Med.* 2009;361(19):1827–1837.

**IV**

# 26 CONGENITAL HEART DISEASE

Jin J. Huang, Stephen D. Weston, and Scott R. Schulman

Categorization of congenital heart disease (CHD) may be based on distinctive anatomic or physiologic features of the defects (Box 26.1). Sometimes complete comprehension of the anatomic complexities in a patient with CHD may be difficult because of a wide range of anatomic lesions. Fortunately, many lesions share similar pathophysiologic conditions despite their anatomic variations. Understanding these physiologic conditions will lead to successful management of a patient with complex CHD.

## FUNDAMENTAL PATHOPHYSIOLOGY IN CONGENITAL HEART DISEASE

Normally, pulmonary blood flow (Qp) and systemic blood flow (Qs) do not mix, and the entire cardiac output flows sequentially from one circulation to the other. All of the systemic venous return is directed to the pulmonary circulation and, likewise, all of the pulmonary venous return is directed to the systemic arterial circulation. Shunting occurs when a portion of the venous return of one circulation is redirected back to the arterial outflow of the same circulation.[1] This redirected flow occurs when there is an abnormal communication or a defect between two otherwise separate structures. The relative downstream blood pressures of the communicating structures dictate the direction of the shunt flow, whereas the size of the defect determines the amount of shunting. Small defects tend to be *restrictive* with limited flow, and large defects tend to be *nonrestrictive* with unimpaired flow.[1]

### Left-to-Right Shunts

A left-to-right (L → R) shunt occurs when part of the pulmonary venous return is redirected toward the pulmonary

The editors and publisher would like to thank Drs. James E. Baker and Isobel A. Russell for contributing to this chapter in the previous edition of this work. It has provided the framework for much of this chapter.

arterial system.[1] This defect may occur at numerous locations, including the pulmonary veins (anomalous pulmonary venous return), the atrial septum (atrial septal defect), the ventricular septum (ventricular septal defect [VSD]), and at the great vessels (patent ductus arteriosus [PDA]).

The portion of the pulmonary blood flow (Qp) that is redirected toward the pulmonary artery is *recirculated* pulmonary blood flow. The portion of the pulmonary blood flow that is appropriately directed toward the systemic circulation (Qs) is *effective* pulmonary blood flow. Their sum is the total pulmonary blood flow (Qp) (Fig. 26.1).

Typically, CHD lesions with left-to-right (L → R) shunts remain acyanotic lesions. However, pulmonary overflow

can result in pulmonary edema and hypotension. Prolonged hypotension can lead to circulatory shock with multiple organ system failure and lactic acidosis; the long-term effects of pulmonary overflow may be an increase of pulmonary vascular resistance (PVR) and abnormal cardiac chamber dilation. Over time an unrepaired large left-to-right (L → R) shunt can reverse its direction and become a cyanotic lesion. This is known as Eisenmenger physiology.

### Right-to-Left Shunts

A right-to-left (R → L) shunt occurs when a portion of the systemic venous return is redirected to the systemic arterial outflow without first circulating through the lungs. The hallmark of lesions producing a right-to-left shunt is arterial oxygen desaturation. CHD lesions with right-to-left (R → L) shunts are cyanotic lesions. The physiologic effect of a right-to-left (R → L) shunt is arterial oxygen desaturation, because the recirculated oxygen-poor systemic venous blood mixes with the oxygen-rich pulmonary venous blood. The degree of desaturation depends

---

**Box 26.1**  Categorization of Congenital Heart Disease

Acyanotic versus cyanotic—VSD versus TOF
Simple versus complex—ASD versus HLHS
Left-to-right shunt versus right-to-left shunt versus mixing lesions—ASD versus TOF versus HLHS

*ASD,* Atrial septal defect; *HLHS,* hypoplastic left heart syndrome; *TOF,* tetralogy of Fallot; *VSD,* ventricular septal defect.

---

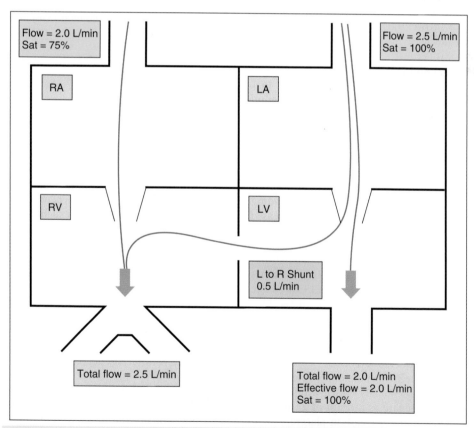

**Fig. 26.1**  Schematic diagram of a ventricular septal defect. A left-to-right shunt occurs at a septal defect with 0.5 L/min flow. Thus, total pulmonary flow is 2.5 L/min, of which the 2 L/min is the effective pulmonary flow; 2 L/min is also the systemic flow (Qs < Qp). *LA,* Left atrium; *LV,* left ventricle; *Qp,* pulmonary flow; *Qs,* systemic flow; *RA,* right atrium; *RV,* right ventricle.

upon the magnitude of right-to-left shunt as well as the degree of desaturation of the systemic venous return.[2]

## Mixing Lesions

Whereas a shunt connotes a communication between pulmonary and systemic venous circulations with *partial* mixing, many forms of CHD result in a *complete* blending of the two. Mixing lesions therefore are conditions in which oxygen content is equilibrated between the two circulations, yielding identical or nearly identical oxygen saturation at both the pulmonary and systemic arterial level.[2]

As with right-to-left shunts, one of the chief characteristics of mixing lesions is systemic arterial oxygen desaturation. The degree of desaturation depends on the flow volume of the two contributing circulations as well as the difference in the individual oxygen saturation. A decrease in pulmonary venous saturation from apnea or atelectasis will decrease the saturation of the final mixed circulation. A decrease in the systemic venous saturation will also cause the final systemic arterial saturation to decrease. Factors that cause a decrease in systemic venous oxygen saturation include fever (increase of systemic oxygen consumption), low cardiac output states (which cause increased oxygen extraction in the microvasculature), and anemia (decrease in systemic oxygen delivery).

### Significance of Qp:Qs Ratio in Mixing Lesions

In CHD with mixing physiology, a Qp:Qs ratio close to 1 will maximize the *effective* component of each circulation and minimize the wasteful *recirculated* component. For Qp:Qs ratio more than 1, preferential flow toward the pulmonary artery increases pulmonary blood flow, resulting in increased oxygen saturation of the mixed blood, but decreases systemic cardiac output and yields less oxygen delivery. For a Qp:Qs ratio less than 1, preferential flow toward the aorta increases systemic blood flow leading to higher systemic perfusion pressure, but the increased output contains blood with lower oxygen saturation and also leads to a decrease in oxygen delivery.

Relative resistance to flow of the two circulations, PVR and systemic vascular resistance (SVR), determines the Qp:Qs ratio. If PVR exceeds SVR, Qs will exceed Qp. Likewise, if SVR exceeds PVR, Qp will exceed Qs. SVR and PVR are both affected by many factors, which are listed in Box 26.2.[3]

### Significance of the Patent Ductus Arteriosus

The ductus arteriosus connects the pulmonary artery to the descending aorta and is functionally closed within 4 days after birth in a healthy neonate as a result of an increase in arterial oxygen tension and decrease in placental prostaglandins (also see Chapter 34). However, mixing lesions with one functional ventricle often require a PDA to supply blood flow to the underdeveloped side. Shunting through the PDA in systole is either left to right (e.g., pulmonary

---

**Box 26.2** Impact of Anesthetic Management on Peripheral and Systemic Vascular Resistance

**Events That Increase Systemic Vascular Resistance**
Light anesthesia
Sympathetic nervous system activation
Administration of α-agonists
Physical manipulations (e.g., compression of the femoral arteries by flexing the hips of infants and small children)

**Events That Decrease Systemic Vascular Resistance**
Deep anesthesia
Administration of vasodilating drugs—nitrates, intravenous and inhaled anesthetics

**Events That Increase Pulmonary Vascular Resistance**
Alveolar hypoxemia (e.g., from low inspired oxygen concentrations)
Hypercapnia
Acidosis
High lung volumes or pressures—tend to collapse pulmonary capillaries
Low lung volumes with atelectasis—tend to collapse larger pulmonary blood vessels
Light anesthesia
Sympathetic nervous system stimulation
Hypothermia

**Events That Decrease Pulmonary Vascular Resistance**
Hyperventilation
Hypocarbia
Alkalosis
Oxygenation
Inhaled nitric oxide
Warmth
Bronchodilators (e.g., albuterol)

---

atresia with intact ventricular septum) or right to left (e.g., hypoplastic left heart syndrome [HLHS]), depending on which side of the heart is hypoplastic. In other words, systemic blood flow is ductal-dependent in certain lesions such as HLHS. For other lesions such as pulmonary atresia the ductus arteriosus is required for pulmonary blood flow.

Ductal shunting during diastole, however, is usually left to right through the PDA because the aorta has a higher resting tone than the pulmonary artery. This means that a large amount of blood can be diverted to the lungs and away from the coronary arteries during diastole. Consequently the myocardium may become ischemic and infarcted because of coronary ischemia. Maneuvers that decrease PVR will cause more pulmonary runoff and exacerbate coronary ischemia.

## Eisenmenger Syndrome

CHD may subject the lungs to abnormal blood flow or pulmonary artery pressure (Box 26.3). Over time, the pulmonary vasculature may undergo a process of remodeling with a gradual increase in PVR that results in pulmonary hypertension, even if the underlying hemodynamic

> **Box 26.3** Defects Resulting in Increased Pulmonary Blood Flow and Pulmonary Artery Pressure Over Time
>
> **Increased Pulmonary Blood Flow**
> Atrial septal defect
> Anomalous pulmonary venous return
>
> **Increased Pulmonary Artery Pressure**
> Ventricular septal defect
> Atrioventricular canal defect
> Aortopulmonary window
> Truncus arteriosus
> Transposition of the great arteries
> Double-inlet left ventricle
> Patent ductus arteriosus

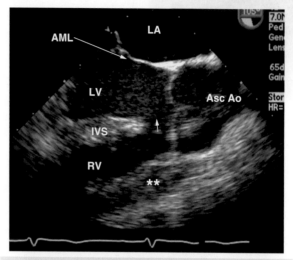

**Fig. 26.2** Transesophageal echocardiogram of an adult with unrepaired tetralogy of Fallot. Note that the aorta is straddling over both ventricles, and a ventricular defect (*short arrow*) is seen immediately below the aortic valve. Right ventricle is hypertrophied (**). *AML*, Anterior mitral leaflet; *Asc Ao*, ascending aorta; *IVS*, interventricular septum; *LA*, left atrium; *LV*, left ventricle; *RV*, right ventricle.

problem is corrected.[3] When pulmonary hypertension becomes irreversible and pulmonary pressure becomes supersystemic, blood is preferentially directed toward the systemic circulation and the direction of the shunt is right to left (R → L) even if the original shunting pattern was left to right (L → R). This condition is called Eisenmenger syndrome and often is a contraindication for surgical correction of the shunt.

## Obstructive Lesions

Obstructive lesions consist mainly of left ventricular outflow track (LVOT) obstructions and coarctation of the aorta.

### Left Ventricular Outflow Track Obstruction

LVOT obstructive lesions account for about 3% to 6% of CHD and can occur at subvalvar, valvar, and supravalvar levels.[4] Valvar aortic stenosis is the most common form of LVOT obstruction in children.[4,5] Bicuspid aortic valve is the most prevalent abnormality in this disease and often leads to clinical manifestations in early adulthood. Subvalvar aortic stenosis encompasses a variety of lesions, which include a thin membrane, thick fibromuscular ridge, diffuse tunnel-like obstruction, and abnormal mitral valve attachments.[6] Supravalvar aortic stenosis (Fig. 26.2) often has an hourglass deformity consisting of a discrete constriction of a thickened ascending aorta at the superior aspect of the sinuses of Valsalva and is often a feature in patients with Williams syndrome.[7]

In utero, critical aortic stenosis can lead to HLHS. Infants with severe aortic stenosis present with heart failure and failure to thrive. Older children with aortic stenosis are rarely symptomatic but will develop left ventricular hypertrophy, premature coronary atherosclerosis, and congestive heart failure over time. Various interventional and surgical approaches are available for aortic stenosis including balloon valvuloplasty, the Ross-Konno procedure, resection of the obstruction, and valve replacement. Timing and type of the surgery depend on the individual case.

### Coarctation of the Aorta

Coarctation of the aorta is a discrete narrowing of the thoracic aorta just distal to the left subclavian artery (Fig. 26.3). It can be an isolated lesion or may be found in conjunction with other lesions such as aortic stenosis and VSDs. Infants with critical coarctation are at risk of developing heart failure and death when the ductus arteriosus closes. Those infants whose circulation is ductal dependent need to continue intravenous prostaglandin $E_1$ infusion to maintain the patency of the ductus arteriosus until surgery. Long-term follow-up of patients with coarctation of the aorta is imperative as there are long-term sequelae in adulthood, including recoarctation, hypertension, aortic aneurysm, coronary artery disease, and stroke.[8] In parturients, preeclampsia can occur in pregnancy, even after successful surgical correction[8] (also see Chapter 33).

## PERIOPERATIVE MANAGEMENT

Surgery for CHD is planned with the cooperative input of a multidisciplinary team that includes surgeons, cardiologists, critical care specialists, and anesthesiologists. Patients require optimal medical care prior to surgery. For the anesthesia provider, understanding the physiology of the cardiac lesion and the subsequent effects of the planned surgical palliative or corrective procedure will lead to successful management of the patient (also see Chapter 13).

**IV**

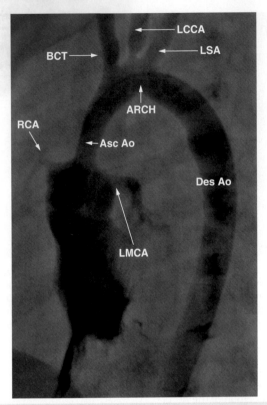

**Fig. 26.3** Angiogram of the aorta during systole showing narrowing of the ascending aorta. This is an example of supravalvular aortic stenosis. The left main coronary artery is dilated and the orifice of the left common carotid artery is stenosed. *Asc Ao,* Ascending aorta; *BCT,* brachiocephalic trunk; *Des Ao,* descending aorta; *LCCA,* left common carotid artery; *LMCA,* left main coronary artery; *LSA,* left subclavian artery; *RCA,* right coronary artery.

## History and Physical Examination

A review of the patient's history includes attention to details that are of importance to pediatric anesthetic care in general, such as pertinent pregnancy details, prematurity, and postnatal course (also see Chapter 34). Patients with CHD frequently have associated syndromes (trisomy 21, DiGeorge syndrome) or evidence of chronic illness (renal dysfunction, pulmonary edema, imbalances in electrolyte and glucose metabolism). Complete review of the patient's preoperative medications and laboratory studies (i.e., complete blood count, electrolytes, coagulation studies, indices of renal and hepatic function) is mandatory.

The anesthesia provider should review the available diagnostic studies such as the echocardiograms (Fig. 26.4) and cardiac catheterization studies (see Fig. 26.2). Magnetic resonance imaging (MRI) will also provide invaluable anatomic details (see Fig. 26.4). Electrocardiograms and chest radiographs are part of the routine preoperative evaluation. Medical and surgical interventions that

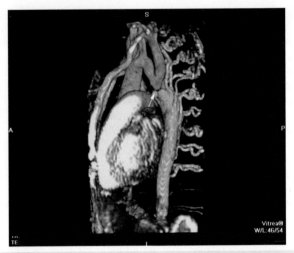

**Fig. 26.4** Three-dimensional magnetic resonance image of a coarctation of aorta (*arrow*). Note the numerous collateral arteries to the descending aorta.

have been instituted previously and any interim change or deterioration in the patient's status are evaluated. Previous sternotomy is a risk factor for increased operative blood loss and cardiac trauma during dissection as a result of adhesions to the sternum and chest wall. Many hospitalized neonates require continuous infusions of inotropic drugs or other medications such as prostaglandin $E_1$ to maintain ductal patency and hemodynamic stability while awaiting surgery.

Physical examination includes an assessment of airway problems (such as might occur in patients with genetic syndromes, e.g., trisomy 21), signs of congestive heart failure (tachypnea, wheezing, dilated neck veins), cyanosis, nutritional status, and any other coexisting conditions. Outpatients who have been scheduled for elective surgery are evaluated the day of surgery for new onset of signs or symptoms of an intercurrent illness such as an upper respiratory tract infection. Inpatients are evaluated for their hospital course along with any developing problems such as an increased white blood cell count, which could indicate the presence of an infectious or inflammatory process.

## Preparation for Surgery

All patients must follow the standard American Society of Anesthesiologists (ASA) guidelines for fasting. Outpatients taking cardiac medications are generally advised to continue therapy up to and including the day of surgery, although preference may vary among anesthesia providers regarding diuretics and angiotensin-converting enzyme inhibitors as well as angiotensin receptor blocking (ARB) drugs. Anticoagulants and antiplatelet medications are usually not given several days before surgery.

## Operating Room Setup

Preparation of the operating room should include readiness of age-appropriate airway equipment, intravenous equipment, and invasive monitors. All intravenous administration sets should be meticulously de-aired to prevent paradoxical arterial embolization of intravenous air bubbles. A warming blanket or surface cooling equipment is made available, and adjustment of the operating room temperature precedes entry of the patient (27° C for small or premature infants and 24° C for older children). Hemodynamic medications are prepared in weight-appropriate dilutions before surgery. Preparation also includes readiness of specialized equipment such as transesophageal echocardiography (TEE) or nitric oxide (iNO) delivery systems.

## Induction of Anesthesia

Induction of anesthesia for patients with CHD may involve either the use of inhaled or intravenous anesthetics (Boxes 26.4 and 26.5). The goal is to execute a smooth anesthetic induction to avoid increased anxiety, crying, coughing, or breath-holding. These events may aggravate unfavorable physiologic effects such as increased right-to-left shunting and dynamic right- or left-sided ventricular outflow tract obstruction in susceptible patients.

The choice of anesthetic and route of delivery are less important than the practitioner's understanding of the hemodynamic effects of a particular drug on the underlying patient physiology. The ability to recognize untoward responses and intervene to correct the problem are hallmarks of the pediatric cardiac anesthesiologist.

### Inhaled Induction of Anesthesia

Awake infants and children without intravenous access are frequently amenable to an inhaled induction of anesthesia. This strategy is typically reserved for those with minimal or well-controlled congestive heart failure because a dose-dependent decrease in myocardial contractility occurs with volatile anesthetics. Sevoflurane is probably the preferred volatile anesthetic because of its lack of pungency and airway irritant effect and the absence of cardiac sensitization to catecholamines.[9] Nitrous oxide may hasten the induction of anesthesia and decrease the necessary concentration of sevoflurane. Concerns regarding the propensity of nitrous oxide to increase PVR have not been substantiated in patients with CHD, but the decrease in fraction of inspired oxygen ($F_{IO_2}$) may impair protection against increased PVR. Because of nitrous oxide's property to expand intravascular air bubbles, its administration is often discontinued shortly after induction of anesthesia.

Placement of a pulse oximetry probe is minimally distressing to an anxious, awake child and provides ample monitoring for the initial stages of an inhaled induction

---

**Box 26.4** Anesthetics Used for Induction of Anesthesia in Congenital Heart Disease

Sevoflurane 1.5%-3.5% (ET)
   Decrease SVR, contractility
   Decrease dose if $N_2O$ used; may cause myocardial depression
Fentanyl 20-50 µg/kg
   Nonsignificant effect on contractility, SVR
   May cause loss of sympathetic tone, bradycardia
   May cause chest wall rigidity with rapid administration or large doses
Sufentanil 5-10 µg/kg
   Similar to fentanyl
Ketamine (IV) 1-2 mg/kg
   Increases HR, increase or no change in SVR, PVR
   Actually a myocardial depressant with sympathetic stimulant properties; may decrease contractility in patients with depleted SNS
   May cause bronchorrhea (prevented with atropine, 20 µg/kg)
Ketamine (IM) 3-5 mg/kg
Etomidate (IV) 0.2-0.3 mg/kg
   Preserves HR, SVR, PVR, contractility
   May inhibit endogenous corticosteroid production; burning pain at the injection site

*BP*, Blood pressure; *CHF*, congestive heart failure; *CO*, cardiac output; *ET*, end-tidal; *HR*, heart rate; *IM*, intramuscular; *IV*, intravenous; *PVR*, pulmonary vascular resistance; *SNS*, sympathetic nervous system; *SVR*, systemic vascular resistance.

---

of anesthesia. Once an adequate stage of anesthesia has been achieved, other noninvasive monitors are placed in a timely fashion. After intravenous access is secured, additional intravenous anesthetics, neuromuscular blocking drugs, and possibly anticholinergics may be given before laryngoscopy and tracheal intubation.

### Intravenous Induction of Anesthesia

Patients with poorly controlled congestive heart failure, moderately impaired ventricular function, significant right-to-left shunting, or complete mixing lesions may benefit from the increased stability afforded by intravenous induction of anesthesia. Frequently, these patients come to the operating room from a critical care setting with intravenous access already in place. Traditionally, intravenous opioids have been used in this setting because they produce little or no myocardial depression and also lack vasodilating properties in both the pulmonary and systemic vascular beds.[9] Other intravenously administered anesthetics that are used in patients with CHD include benzodiazepines, etomidate, and ketamine. Propofol can cause hypotension or increased right-to-left shunting in some patients with right ventricular outflow tract obstruction. In other patients with adequate ventricular function, propofol is tolerated when incrementally administered. Ketamine preserves or augments sympathetic nervous system tone and, in so doing, maintains

IV

**Box 26.5** Common Congenital Cardiac Lesions: Summary of Anesthetic Goals and Induction Strategies

**General Goals and Principles**
- Avoid air entrapment in intravenous and pressure tubing; use meticulous clearing techniques.
- Avoid dehydration; give careful orders regarding NPO status (following ASA guidelines).
- Avoid myocardial depression.
- Maintain sinus rhythm whenever possible.
- Well-sedated, cooperative patient is ideal.
- Premedication is indicated for patients older than 1 year (oral midazolam, 0.5-1 mg/kg).
- Close monitoring after sedation.

**Lesions Characterized by Excessive Pulmonary Blood Flow**

*Atrial Septal Defects*
- Avoid further decreases in pulmonary vascular resistance (hyperventilation, high $F_{IO_2}$).
- Consider early tracheal extubation.

*Ventricular Septal Defects*
- Avoid decreases in pulmonary vascular resistance.
- Avoid excessive myocardial depression, particularly in patients with congestive heart failure—inhaled induction may be rapid.

*Atrioventricular Septal Defects*
- Avoid decreases in pulmonary vascular resistance before cardiopulmonary bypass.
- Prepare to treat pulmonary hypertension (100% oxygen, hyperventilation, alkalinization, deep sedation).
- Have nitric oxide available and ready.
- Inotropic support frequently is required.

*Truncus Arteriosus*
- Neonates are critically ill and require close management of systemic and pulmonary vascular resistance to balance systemic and pulmonary blood flow.
- Addition of carbon dioxide or nitrogen may be needed to decrease $F_{IO_2}$ to 17%.

**Hypoplastic Left Heart Syndrome**
Surgical correction occurs in three stages:
Stage I: Norwood procedure
- Perform ascending aorta and arch reconstruction.
- Perform PDA ligation.
- Construct a reliable pulmonary blood flow source using a Blalock-Taussig shunt or Sano shunt.
- Anesthetic management includes prebypass $PGE_1$ infusion, maintenance of nearly equal pulmonary and systemic blood flow for adequate systemic perfusion, precautions against air embolism, maintenance of anesthesia with intravenous drugs, and postbypass maintenance of a high hematocrit and probably a need for inotropic support.
Stage II: Glenn procedure
- Create a direct connection between the superior vena cava and pulmonary artery.
- Anesthetic management includes maintenance of a high hematocrit, elevation of the head of the bed to facilitate venous drainage, avoidance of central lines to reduce the risk for pulmonary artery thrombus, and recognition that positive-pressure ventilation of the patient's lungs may decrease pulmonary blood flow and cardiac output.
- Mild hypoventilation may increase oxygen saturation.
Stage III: Fontan procedure

- Reroute blood flow from the inferior vena cava into the pulmonary circulation, usually accomplished using an extra-cardiac conduit.
- Preload to the heart is completely passive. Management of patient status after Fontan procedure should focus on maintaining reasonable preload, i.e., passive flow from systemic veins to the pulmonary artery and eventually to the common atrium.
- Poor prognostic factors are high pulmonary vascular resistance, tricuspid regurgitation, and decreased ventricular function.

**Lesions With Inadequate Pulmonary Blood Flow**
*Transposition of the Great Arteries (TGA)*
- $PGE_1$ infusion is maintained before cardiopulmonary bypass.
- Patient may need Rashkind procedure (atrial septectomy) if patent ductus does not provide adequate mixing for survival.
- Manipulate pulmonary vascular resistance before cardiopulmonary bypass.
- Use an opioid-based anesthetic.

*Tetralogy of Fallot (see Fig. 26.2)*
- Adequate preoperative hydration is essential.
- Manipulations are indicated to decrease pulmonary vascular resistance and improve pulmonary blood flow.
- Hypercyanotic episodes are treated by intravenous fluid administration, sedation, and pharmacologically induced increases in systemic vascular resistance (phenylephrine).
- Avoid increases in heart rate, which may worsen infundibular pulmonary stenosis.
- Rate of induction of anesthesia with a volatile anesthetic may be slowed because of a right-to-left shunt.

*Tricuspid Atresia or Pulmonary Atresia With Intact Ventricular Septum*
- Usually the right ventricle is diminutive or hypoplastic.
- Surgical approach involves an aortopulmonary shunt and subsequent Glenn and Fontan procedures.

*Total Anomalous Pulmonary Venous Return*
- Severe cyanosis is treated with high $F_{IO_2}$.
- Avoid systemic acidosis and high hematocrit.

**Obstructive Lesions**
*Coarctation of the Aorta (see Fig. 26.4)*
- Use arterial monitoring in the right arm.
- Use cuffed endotracheal tube to provide adequate ventilation to patients requiring the thoracotomy position.
- Avoid acidosis.

*Aortic Stenosis*
- Avoid tachycardia, dysrhythmias, hypotension.
- Decrease myocardial oxygen demand.
- Maintain preload and afterload.

*Subvalvular Aortic Stenosis*
- Avoid tachycardia, dysrhythmias, hypotension.
- Decrease myocardial oxygen demand.
- Maintain preload and afterload.

*Supravalvular Aortic Stenosis (see Fig. 26.3)*
- Note that this is associated with Williams syndrome.
- Patient may have concomitant pulmonary artery stenosis.
- Avoid tachycardia, dysrhythmias, hypotension.
- Coronary abnormalities are common.
- Avoid acute afterload reduction.

*ASA,* American Society of Anesthesiologists; *$F_{IO_2}$,* inspired oxygen concentration; *NPO,* nil per os (nothing by mouth); *PDA,* patent ductus arteriosus; *$PGE_1$,* prostaglandin $E_1$.

a high degree of circulatory stability. Concern regarding ketamine's propensity to increase PVR has not been substantiated in patients with CHD.[10] Ketamine may be administered intramuscularly to achieve stable induction of anesthesia and allow subsequent vascular cannulation to proceed in an anesthetized patient. Obviously, during the administration of all intravenous drugs, avoidance of air is mandatory. The presence of circulatory mixing or shunting in patients with CHD poses a real risk for paradoxical air embolization should any bubbles reach the central circulation.

## Airway Management (Also See Chapter 16)

The size of the endotracheal tube is individualized according to the age and size of the patient. Administration of a neuromuscular blocking drug will facilitate tracheal intubation (also see Chapter 11). The selection of the drug depends on the patient (age, type of lesion, renal function) and the characteristics of the drug (duration of action, hemodynamic properties, and mode of elimination). Vecuronium and rocuronium have an intermediate duration of action but rocuronium has a faster onset of action than vecuronium. Rocuronium also increases heart rate, which is useful in pediatric patients. Succinylcholine is rarely used in pediatric anesthesia.

The approach to ventilatory management hinges upon how the circulatory system will be affected by changes in PVR in relationship to the SVR. The ventilation strategy should have minimal impact on blood flow across shunts or on tenuously balanced pulmonary-to-systemic flow ratios. Understanding how changes in PVR will affect the physiology of the cardiac lesion will help govern such parameters as $F_{IO_2}$, minute ventilation, use of positive end-expiratory pressure, and peak inspiratory airway pressure.

## Monitoring (Also See Chapter 20)

Invasive monitoring is usually established after induction of anesthesia. Patients undergoing cardiac surgery generally require arterial line placement, as well as some form of central venous access. The cardiac lesion dictates the site for arterial line placement. For example, in a patient who has a Blalock-Taussig shunt (diversion of the subclavian artery to the ipsilateral pulmonary artery), the arterial line is placed contralaterally. Similarly, patients with coarctation of the aorta may have unreliable pressure measurement in the left upper extremity either because of the location of the coarctation or because of aortic cross-clamp placement at or near the left subclavian artery during surgery. The internal jugular vein is a common choice for central pressure monitoring and infusion of medications intraoperatively. Recently, many centers performing neonatal surgical repairs have moved away from the internal jugular approach owing to the risk of central venous catheter thrombosis. For this reason, many surgeons prefer to directly insert a right atrial catheter

intraoperatively before separation from bypass. The catheter is then tunneled through the thorax.

TEE has become an invaluable monitoring tool in the operating room to further delineate anatomy that may not be clearly demonstrated by preoperative transthoracic echocardiography (TTE), to rule out additional defects, and to assess the quality of the repair.

## Blood Tranfusions (Also See Chapter 24)

Many operations for CHD will require blood product administration, and the likelihood increases with smaller infants, lower preoperative hematocrit levels, repeat sternotomy incisions, and long cardiopulmonary bypass (CPB) times. Judgment and experience dictate how much and what type of blood products are made available at the start of surgery. Generally, small infants are allocated blood that is as fresh as possible (less than 5 days of storage) because older blood may become significantly hyperkalemic and develop leftward shifting of the oxygen-hemoglobin dissociation curve. Blood is administered with the use of appropriate filters and warming devices because small infants are particularly susceptible to intraoperative hypothermia and to bradydysrhythmias from boluses of hypothermic blood products. Having packed red blood cells (PRBCs) available in the operating room before the skin incision is appropriate in cases of repeat sternotomy inasmuch as these patients are at risk for severe bleeding from unintentional injury to major cardiac structures. Often, other components of the blood, such as fresh frozen plasma (FFP), platelets, and sometimes cryoprecipitate (CRYO), are administered after weaning from CPB, especially for small infants and complex cases with long CPB time.

## Antifibrinolytic Drugs

Antifibrinolytic drugs can reduce blood loss and transfusion requirements during surgery for CHD. Aminocaproic acid is the preferred drug in our institution, whereas tranexamic acid is used in others. Aprotinin is no longer available for use.[11,12]

## Maintenance of Anesthesia

Typically anesthesia is maintained with a combination of intravenous opioids, benzodiazepines, and volatile anesthetics (doses < 1 minimum alveolar concentration [MAC]), and neuromuscular blocking drugs. Use of a small concentration of a volatile anesthetic minimizes the myocardial depressant effects of the drug while also decreasing the total dose of opioids that would otherwise be necessary to ensure adequate anesthetic depth. Large doses of opioids (fentanyl, 50 to 100 µg/kg intravenously) are often given over the course of an operation.[10,12] These opioids may be administered in divided doses according to judgment of anesthetic depth or in anticipation of noxious surgical stimuli. Alternatively, opioids may be delivered as a continuous intravenous infusion. Patients who are critically ill or who have complex cardiac anomalies may benefit from high-dose opioid techniques so that the hypotensive and myocardial depressant effects of the volatile anesthetics are minimized. In contrast, limited opioid administration (fentanyl <20 µg/kg) in patients with good cardiac reserve undergoing procedures for simple defects (e.g., atrial septal defect, VSD, PDA, coarctation of the aorta) will facilitate early postoperative tracheal extubation.[10] Dexmedetomidine (Precedex) is sometimes used as an anesthetic adjunct. It is infused at rates between 0.2 and 2.0 µg/kg/h. Dexmedetomidine has a tendency to slow the heart rate in some patients and for this reason has not been widely adopted. Nitrous oxide is generally not used for maintenance of anesthesia because of its propensity to expand unintentional intravascular air emboli.

### Monitoring Changes in Shunt Ratios

The potential for significant changes in the circulatory system after anesthetic induction warrants early and possibly repeated analysis of arterial blood gases to allow early correction or refinement of pulmonary ventilation variables, as well as acid-base disorders, before the development of important circulatory derangements. In patients with shunts or mixing lesions, pulse oximetry also provides a continuous monitor of changes in the balance between pulmonary and systemic blood flow or changes in shunt direction or magnitude.

### Anticoagulation

Anticoagulation with unfractionated heparin (3 to 4 mg/kg) delivered intravenously is achieved before cannulation for CPB. The subsequent anticoagulation effect is assessed by measuring the activated clotting time (ACT). Target ACT values may vary with institutional preference, but 480 seconds is typical. Additional heparin is administered if target values are not initially obtained. Heparin concentration assays may also be used instead of or as a supplement to the ACT.

## Cardiopulmonary Bypass

Most procedures for repair of congenital cardiac defects require use of CPB (also see Chapter 25). As with adults, CPB for infants and children entails diversion of systemic venous return to the CPB machine and return of oxygenated blood to the arterial system. Venous blood is drained passively (by gravity) through two venous cannulas, one for each vena cava. The cannulas converge through a Y-connector to a cardiotomy reservoir, which allows rapid administration of blood products, crystalloid and colloid solutions, medications, and blood suctioned from the field by the surgeon ("pump suction"). The cardiotomy reservoir also provides a temporary buffer in the event that venous return is temporarily interrupted. Blood is next conducted to a pump mechanism, which is generally a centrifugal pump. This adjustable pump permits delivery of a specified rate of blood flow to the patient. Generally, flow rates are adjusted to maintain an age-appropriate mean arterial pressure. Blood is then channeled through a membrane oxygenator, which equilibrates the blood with a supply of fresh gas; in this way, oxygen is added and carbon dioxide is removed. The perfusionist controls oxygenation and ventilation by adjusting the blend ($FIO_2$) and flow rate (sweep) of the fresh gas. Modern oxygenator circuits also allow rapid adjustment of blood temperature by running cooled or warmed water through a coil in contact with the blood path. Blood is then conducted back to the patient through tubing connected to a cannula positioned in the ascending aorta. An arterial filter is generally used downstream from the oxygenator to prevent microembolization of debris to the arterial tree.[13]

Complete diversion of venous return to the CPB machine followed by aortic cross-clamping and immediate administration of a cardioplegia solution will yield a still and bloodless heart for the surgeon. Because the act of aortic cross-clamping renders the heart ischemic, the cardioplegia solution has a dual purpose of providing both mechanical quiescence and myocardial protection. As with adults, these effects are achieved through the use of a cold (4° C) hyperkalemic crystalloid solution. Hypothermia and electromechanical arrest each contribute to minimizing myocardial oxygen requirements and lengthening the tolerable period of myocardial ischemia.

### Calculation of Physiologic Variables

The perfusionist and anesthesiologist take into account the patient's size to calculate the necessary flow rate to maintain metabolic function. Equally important is the patient's estimated blood volume because it determines the degree of hemodilution that results when the patient's blood mixes with the obligatory "priming volume" of fluid that occupies the CPB machine's tubing, oxygenator, and cardiotomy reservoir at the onset of CPB. Whereas adult patients frequently have acceptable degrees of anemia as a result of this hemodilution, infants and small children require smaller, shorter tubing and lower-volume cardiotomy reservoirs to minimize this effect. Most infants require some blood product to be mixed with the circuit prime to preserve adequate oxygen-carrying capacity while on CPB. The amount of blood product required is a function of the patient's starting hematocrit, estimated blood volume, circuit prime volume, and the lowest acceptable limit of anemia (institutional and physician preferences vary but are commonly in the range of a hematocrit of 20% to 30%).

### Body Temperature During Cardiopulmonary Bypass

Institutional, surgeon, or anesthesiologist preference also provides the perfusionist with a target patient temperature to be achieved while on CPB. Mild (30° C to 35.5° C) to moderate (25° C to 30° C) systemic hypothermia reduces metabolic oxygen requirements (7% per degree Celsius) and provides protective effects on both cerebral and myocardial tissue.[13] Hypothermia is usually achieved by active cooling of CPB blood with a heat exchange device incorporated in the membrane oxygenator. Active rewarming is initiated toward the end of CPB. Deleterious effects of post-CPB hypothermia may include myocardial ischemia, cardiac dysrhythmias, elevated PVR, coagulation failure, or renal dysfunction.

### Deep Hypothermic Circulatory Arrest

Deep hypothermic circulatory arrest (DHCA) was used in situations in which adequate surgical repair is precluded by CPB cannula placement or by the requirement to repair the aorta at or near the arch.[14-16] Because of adverse outcomes associated with DHCA, many medical centers are using regional low-flow cerebral perfusion via the innominate artery (25 to 50 mL/kg/min) to permit surgical repair in a field unencumbered by CPB cannulas. Cardiac cannulation and active cooling by CPB are required to lower core temperature to approximately 18° C to 20° C. After surgical repair, CPB is reestablished, and the patient is rewarmed and reperfused.

### Weaning From Cardiopulmonary Bypass

Successful weaning from CPB requires close communication between the anesthesiologist, cardiac surgeon, and perfusionist. The surgeon requests the perfusionist to start rewarming at an appropriate point during the surgical procedure. The anesthesiologist commences pulmonary ventilation at the surgeon's request after the endotracheal tube is suctioned. With the patient warm and ventilated, weaning from CPB is initiated.

### Cardiac Rhythm

Ventricular fibrillation can occur after removal of the aortic cross-clamp and reperfusion of the coronary arteries, especially when the hypothermia has not been fully corrected. It may revert spontaneously to a sinus rhythm but often requires electrical defibrillation. Acid-base or electrolyte disorders (hyperkalemia) may contribute to disturbances in cardiac rhythm. Relative bradycardia or atrioventricular node conduction failure can be corrected by means of temporary cardiac pacing. Many patients with good cardiac reserve who have endured relatively short periods (<1.5 hours) of aortic cross-clamping and the attendant myocardial ischemia may be able to separate from CPB without inotropic assistance. Many others will require infusion of inotropic drugs to achieve adequate cardiac output and systemic blood pressure. In particular, those with preexisting myocardial dysfunction, congestive heart failure, or hemodynamic instability are likely to require pharmacologic assistance for successful separation from CPB (Table 26.1). Inotropic drugs commonly utilized include dopamine, milrinone, epinephrine, and calcium.

| Table 26.1 | Common Vasoactive Drugs | |
| --- | --- | --- |
| **Drug** | **Dose Range** | **Comments** |
| Dopamine | 3-20 µg/kg/min | Lower maximum effect than with epinephrine and norepinephrine Tachycardia |
| Epinephrine | 0.02-0.1 µg/kg/min | Drug of choice when maximum inotropic effect is required Strong effect at the medium- to high-dose range Tachycardia |
| Norepinephrine | 0.02-0.1 µg/kg/min | Strong α, β effects, with activity at lower doses than with epinephrine |
| Milrinone | 0.25-1 µg/kg/min | Can lower both PVR and SVR No tachycardia May need α-agonist to prevent hypotension Loading dose typically is 25-50 µg/kg |
| Dobutamine | 1-20 µg/kg/min | Lower maximum effect than with epinephrine and norepinephrine May decrease SVR or BP because of peripheral β2-vasodilation |

*BP*, Blood pressure; *PVR*, pulmonary vascular resistance; *SVR*, systemic vascular resistance.

### Ventilation and Pulmonary Vascular Resistance

The approach to PVR and ventilation of the lungs must be carefully considered before separation from CPB. Patients with simple defects that have been repaired are no longer at risk for shunting and unbalanced Qp:Qs ratios. For this reason, such patients are typically ventilated with 100% inspired oxygen ($F_{IO_2}$ of 1.0) at the time of separation from CPB, with minute ventilation sufficient to avoid respiratory acidosis. Patients with long-standing excessive pulmonary blood flow may have underlying pulmonary hypertension and may be at risk for pulmonary hypertensive crisis at the time of separation from CPB. These patients may benefit from maneuvers that minimize PVR including the application of inhaled nitric oxide (see Box 26.2).

### Presence of a Residual Mixing Lesion

Difficulty arises when a palliative procedure has left the patient with a mixing lesion. This situation is exemplified by surgical treatment of HLHS (Norwood procedure) that results in a single ventricle supplying blood flow to both the pulmonary and systemic circulation (see Box 26.5). In such circumstances, which circulation will be likely to receive

> **Box 26.6** Causes of Difficulty in Separation From Cardiopulmonary Bypass
>
> Inadequate pulmonary blood flow (associated with arterial hypoxemia)
>
> Inadequate systemic blood flow (associated with hypotension and metabolic acidosis)
>
> Valvular dysfunction
>
> Dynamic outflow obstruction (decreases in cardiac output related to hyperdynamic or hypovolemic states)
>
> Decreased systemic vascular resistance (associated with long cardiopulmonary bypass times)
>
> Cardiac rhythm disturbances
>
> Hypovolemia

most of the cardiac output must be anticipated and adjusted so that PVR and SVR tend to yield a balanced circulation. Pulse oximetry is an invaluable tool in this particular situation because a patient with a complete mixing lesion will tend to have systemic oxygen saturation near 80% when the systemic and pulmonary circulations are balanced. Systemic saturation greater than 85% to 90% indicates excessive pulmonary blood flow (possibly with resultant systemic hypoperfusion or hypotension), whereas saturation less than 75% indicates inadequate pulmonary blood flow. The best possible milieu in the setting of the underlying defect must be provided in order to promote satisfactory cardiac output, adequate oxygenation, and a balanced circulation.

### Difficulty in Separation of the Patient From Cardiopulmonary Bypass

Difficulty in separation from CPB may reflect multiple physiologic derangements but most often is due to inadequate pulmonary blood flow or inadequate systemic blood flow (Box 26.6). After separation from CPB, systemic arterial blood pressure, systemic oxygenation, and acid-base status must be closely monitored. Data derived from a central venous or pulmonary artery catheter may be helpful in diagnosing hemodynamic problems. TEE is useful in evaluating the surgical repair of CHD and cardiac function in the period after separation from CPB. In the event that pharmacologic support of cardiac contractility, vascular tone, and management of ventilation fails to achieve circulatory stability, patients may require resumption of CPB support. In some cases, a period of "rest" on CPB allows resolution of cross-clamp–related ischemic ventricular dysfunction, whereas in other situations, revision of the surgical repair may be indicated. If the patient cannot be separated from CPB despite surgical revision and maximal inotropic support, then extracorporeal life support may be instituted and continued until adequate cardiac and pulmonary function is regained.

### Reversal of Heparin-Induced Anticoagulation

After successful weaning from CPB, protamine reverses the anticoagulation effect of heparin and is administered by means of slow intravenous infusion (over at least a 10-minute period). Pediatric patients, although susceptible to some detrimental complications of protamine administration, including anaphylactic, anaphylactoid, hypotensive, or severe pulmonary hypertensive reactions, are often spared these untoward effects more commonly observed in adults.

### Coagulopathy

Although return of the ACT to baseline indicates successful reversal of heparin, there can be residual clinical coagulopathy from coagulation factor or platelet deficiency. Hypothermia and hypocalcemia may contribute to in vivo coagulopathy but will not be reflected in the ACT or other laboratory tests of coagulation. Early measurement of the platelet count, prothrombin time, and partial thromboplastin time will facilitate appropriate blood product therapy in the event that hemostasis is not achieved with protamine. Thromboelastography (TEG) is a test of hemostasis performed on whole blood that examines platelet function and the coagulation pathway (also see Chapter 42). However, its use has not been widely accepted owing to the lack of evidence supporting TEG-guided transfusion therapy as yielding better outcomes than the current transfusion practices.[17] Often the degree of clinical coagulopathy necessitates empirical administration of platelets, FFP, or other factor preparations before the results of any laboratory study become available.

### Blood Component and Intravascular Volume Therapy (Also See Chapter 24)

Blood component and intravascular volume therapy must be administered very carefully to infants because their total intravascular volume is small in comparison to adults. Unless critically hypovolemic, blood product or volume therapy should proceed in aliquots of approximately 5 mL/kg to prevent excessive intravascular volume and possible ventricular dysfunction. Citrated blood products may cause important degrees of hypocalcemia, and calcium replacement may thus be necessary. Dilutional anemia can occur when administering platelet or plasma preparations. Fluid-warming devices prevent the delivery of cold fluid boluses to cardiac conduction tissue, as well as the development of systemic hypothermia.

### Recombinant Activated Factor VII

Recombinant activated factor VII (rFVIIa) is approved by the Food and Drug Administration (FDA) for use in the prevention and treatment of bleeding in patients with hemophilia A or B with inhibitors to factor VIII or IX, factor VII deficiency, or Glanzmann thrombasthenia (also see Chapter 22).[18] Its role in pediatric cardiac surgery is evolving. rFVIIa is appropriate as rescue therapy when conventional hemostatic measures have failed to stop the bleeding after separation from bypass despite conventional therapy. The dose is typically 90 to 120 µg/kg every 2 hours for excessive bleeding. rFVIIa must be used cautiously as there is risk of thromboembolic complications, particularly in patients who have undergone the arterial switch operation for transposition of the great arteries.[19,20]

## POSTOPERATIVE CARE

Children undergoing surgery for CHD are managed in an intensive care setting, where continuous invasive monitoring is possible along with one-to-one nursing care. Mechanical ventilation of the patient's lungs is continued for variable intervals, depending on the type of surgery performed and the overall status of the patient. Sedation is maintained throughout the period of ongoing tracheal intubation. Critical care management entails the continuation of hemodynamic drug infusions and possibly electrical pacing of cardiac rhythm. Early postoperative management frequently involves correction of various electrolyte, glucose, and hematologic parameters. Mediastinal bleeding is assessed frequently. An intense index of suspicion is always maintained for the possible

requirement for revision of the surgical repair, and bedside echocardiography is frequently undertaken in the intensive care unit to clarify hemodynamic problems or abnormal convalescence.

## QUESTIONS OF THE DAY

1. What factors affect the degree of hypoxemia in a patient with a right-to-left shunt?
2. What is the physiologic effect of patent ductus arteriosus (PDA)? What is the significance of the ductus arteriosus in a patient with one functional ventricle?
3. What is Eisenmenger syndrome? What congenital heart defects are associated with its development?
4. A patient with congestive heart disease (CHD) requires arterial line monitoring. What factors influence the choice of monitoring site?
5. In a patient receiving general anesthesia for repair of CHD, what events can increase or decrease pulmonary vascular resistance (PVR)?

## REFERENCES

1. Walker SG. Anesthesia for left-to-right shunt lesions. In: Andropoulos DB, Stayer SA, Russell IA, eds. *Anesthesia for Congenital Heart Disease.* 2nd ed. West Sussex: Wiley-Blackwell; 2010:373–397.
2. Mossad EB, Joglar J. Preoperative evaluation and preparation. In: Andropoulous DB, Stayer SA, Russell IA, Mossad EB, eds. *Anesthesia for Congenital Heart Disease.* 2nd ed. West Sussex: Wiley-Blackwell; 2010:223–243.
3. Fischer LG, Van Aken H, Burkle H. Management of pulmonary hypertension: physiological and pharmacological considerations for anesthesiologists. *Anesth Analg.* 2003;96:1603–1616.
4. Hoffman JI, Kaplan S. The incidence of congenital heart disease. *J Am Coll Cardiol.* 2002;39:1890.
5. Keane JF, Fyler DC. Aortic outflow abnormalities. In: Keane JF, Lock JE, Fyler DC, eds. *Nadas' Pediatric Cardiology.* Philadelphia: Saunders/Elsevier; 2006:581.
6. Newfeld EA, Muster AJ, Paul MH, et al. Discrete subvalvular aortic stenosis in childhood. Study of 51 patients. *Am J Cardiol.* 1976;38(1):53.
7. Collins RT II. Cardiovascular disease in Williams syndrome. *Circulation.* 2013;127(21):2125–2134.
8. Brown ML, Burkhart HM, Connolly HM, et al. Coarctation of aorta: life-

long surveillance is mandatory following surgical repair. *J Am Coll Cardiol.* 2013;62:1020.
9. Russell IA, Miller Hance WC, Gregory G, et al. The safety and efficacy of sevoflurane anesthesia in infants and children with congenital heart disease. *Anesth Analg.* 2001;92(5):1152–1158.
10. Williams GD, Philip BM, Chu LF, et al. Ketamine does not increase pulmonary vascular resistance in children with pulmonary hypertension undergoing sevoflurane anesthesia and spontaneous ventilation. *Anesth Analg.* 2007;105: 1578–1584.
11. Fergusson DA, Hebert PC, Mazer CD, et al. A comparison of aprotinin and lysine analogues in high-risk cardiac surgery. *N Engl J Med.* 2008;358:2319–2331.
12. Duncan HP, Cloote A, Weir PM, et al. Reducing stress responses in the prebypass phase of open heart surgery in infants and young children: a comparison of different fentanyl doses. *Br J Anaesth.* 2000;84:556–564.
13. Vinas M. Extracorporeal circulation. In: Kambam J, ed. *Cardiac Anesthesia for Infants and Children.* St. Louis: Mosby-Year Book; 1994:20–32.
14. Jonas RA. Deep hypothermic circulatory arrest: current status and indications. *Semin Thorac Cardiovasc Surg Pediatr Card Surg Annu.* 2002;5:76–88.

15. Wypij D, Newburger JW, Rappaport LA, et al. The effect of duration of deep hypothermic circulatory arrest in infant heart surgery on late neurodevelopment: the Boston Circulatory Arrest Trial. *J Thorac Cardiovasc Surg.* 2003;126:1397–1403.
16. Hickey PR. Neurologic sequelae associated with deep hypothermic circulatory arrest. *Ann Thorac Surg.* 1998;65:S65–S69. discussion S69–S70, S74–S76.
17. Hunt H, Stanworth S, Curry N, et al. Thromboelastography (TEG) and rotational thromboelastometry (ROTEM) for trauma induced coagulopathy in adult trauma patients with bleeding. *Cochrane Database Syst Rev.* 2015;(2). CD010438.
18. Warren O, Mandal K, Hadjianastassiou V, et al. Recombinant activated factor VII in cardiac surgery: a systemic review. *Ann Thorac Surg.* 2007;83:707–714.
19. Warren OJ, Rogers PL, Watret AL, et al. Defining the role of recombinant activated factor VII in pediatric cardiac surgery: where should we go from here? *Pediatr Crit Care Med.* 2009;10:572–582.
20. Guzzetta NA, Russell IA, Williams GD. Review of the off-label use of recombinant activated factor VII in pediatric surgery patients. *Anesth Analg.* 2012;115(2):364.

IV

# 27 CHRONIC PULMONARY DISEASE AND THORACIC ANESTHESIA

Andrew J. Deacon and Peter D. Slinger

## INTRODUCTION

Chronic respiratory problems include obstructive and restrictive lung diseases, obstructive sleep apnea (OSA), and pulmonary hypertension. Obstructive lung diseases are commonly divided into reactive airway disorders (asthma) and chronic obstructive pulmonary disease (COPD). However, many patients have more than one type of lung disease. Avoiding general anesthesia, if possible, with regional or local anesthesia is usually preferable for patients with chronic respiratory diseases.

The editors and publisher would like to thank Drs. Luca M. Bigatello and Venkatesh Srinivasa for contributing to this chapter in the previous edition of this work. It has served as the foundation for the current chapter.

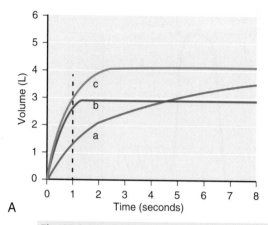
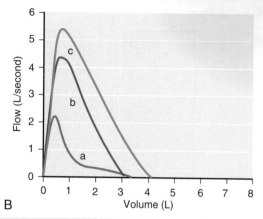

**Fig. 27.1** Simple spirometry patterns in obstructive lung disease (*a*), restrictive lung disease (*b*) and normal patients (*c*). (A) Volume-time curves. The exhaled volume during the first second of a maximal expiratory effort is the forced expiratory volume in 1 second (FEV$_1$). The maximal expired volume is the forced vital capacity (FVC). (B) Flow-volume curves. The maximal flow during a forced expiration is the peak expiratory flow (PEF). (From Patterson GA, Cooper JD, Deslauriers J, et al, eds. *Pearson's Thoracic and Esophageal Surgery*. 3rd ed. Philadelphia: Elsevier; 2008, used with permission.)

## History

Common symptoms elicited in all patients include cough, wheezing, shortness of breath, chest tightness, sputum production, and reduced exercise tolerance. Important components of the history are recent exacerbations, current and previous therapies including hospital admissions, emergency room visits, and tobacco use.

## Physical Examination

Signs of chronic respiratory disease include tachypnea, cyanosis, use of accessory muscles of respiration, and clubbing of the fingers. Of prime importance are the presence of unequal breath sounds, wheezing, and rales during auscultative examination.

## Laboratory Examination

### Chest Imaging
A recent preoperative chest x-ray examination is not required for all patients but should be considered in any patient with a chronic respiratory disease or a patient with a recent change in respiratory symptoms or signs.

### Spirometry
Simple spirometry (expired volume or flow vs. time), forced vital capacity (FVC), and forced expiratory volume in 1 second (FEV$_1$) (Fig. 27.1) are not required in all stable patients but should be ordered if there is any doubt about the severity of disease, such as a recent change in symptoms, if the patient is unable to give a clear history, or if any patient with chronic lung disease is having lung surgery. Full pulmonary function tests (plethysmography)

(Fig. 27.2) including measurement of residual volume (RV), functional residual capacity (FRC), and measurement of the lung diffusing capacity for carbon monoxide (D$_{LCO}$) are only indicated if the diagnosis or severity of the lung disease is unclear from the simple spirometry procedure.

### Gas Exchange
Oxygen saturation (pulse oximetry, Sp$_{O_2}$%) should be documented preoperatively in every patient with a chronic respiratory disease. Arterial blood gases are required preoperatively in patients with moderate or severe chronic respiratory disease who are at risk of requiring postoperative mechanical ventilation (major abdominal, thoracic, cardiac, spine, or neurosurgery) or if symptoms have become more intense.

## ASTHMA

### Clinical Presentation

Asthma is a common form of episodic recurrent lower airway obstruction that affects 3% to 5% of the population. Sixty-five percent of people with asthma become symptomatic before age 5 years.[1] Patients with childhood asthma often become quiescent with time but can have recurrences. Inflammation of the airways is a hallmark of asthma. Steroids (inhaled, oral, or both) are the most effective medications in controlling this inflammation. The inflamed airway is hyperresponsive to irritant stimuli with subsequent bronchospasm and mucous secretions. Bronchospastic stimuli can include allergens, dust, cold air, instrumentation of the airways, and medications (aspirin or histamine-releasing drugs). Asthmatics are at risk for life-threatening bronchospasm during anesthesia

Lung volumes and capacities

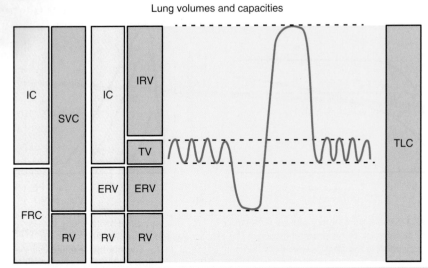

**Fig. 27.2** Complete pulmonary function testing will provide data on lung volumes and capacities to differentiate obstructive from restrictive diseases. *ERV,* Expiratory reserve volume; *FRC,* functional residual capacity; *IC,* inspiratory capacity; *IRV,* inspiratory reserve volume; *RV,* residual volume; *SVC,* slow vital capacity; *TLC,* total lung capacity; *TV,* tidal volume. (Reprinted from Patterson AG, Cooper JD, Deslauriers J, et al, eds. *Pearson's Thoracic and Esophageal Surgery.* 3rd ed. Philadelphia: Elsevier; 2008. p 1168 with permission.)

---

**Box 27.1** Stepwise Therapy for the Treatment of Asthma

1. Inhaled short-acting $\beta_2$-agonists (e.g., salbutamol 100-200 µg prn)
2. Inhaled short-acting $\beta_2$-agonists and inhaled steroids at up to 400 µg/day
3. Step 2 and additional long-acting $\beta_2$-agonist (LABA)
4. Inhaled steroids up to 800 µg/day and LABA/leukotriene receptor antagonist
5. Oral steroids/additional therapy as required reducing steroid use

*prn,* As needed.

if improperly managed, particularly during or recently after a respiratory tract infection. Elective surgery should therefore be delayed at least 6 weeks after a respiratory infection in these patients.

The severity of asthma is defined by the amount of treatment required to control symptoms (Box 27.1). Most patients will be conducting steps 1 or 2 of this treatment protocol. After step 3, when anesthetizing patients extra caution is required. A history of severe or life-threatening exacerbations, or being a patient in intensive care or with endotracheal intubation, is indicative of patients at increased risk of major pulmonary complications. Peak expiratory flow (PEF) rate is a very simple and useful measurement of the severity of asthma. Many patients measure their own PEF to guide their therapy. PEF rates less than 50% of the predicted value (corrected for age/gender/height) indicate severe asthma. A PEF increase of more than 15% after bronchodilator administration suggests inadequate treatment of asthma.

Suppression of the hypothalamic-pituitary-adrenal (HPA) axis may occur with corticosteroid therapy. Adrenal crisis may be precipitated by the stress of surgery. Short courses of oral prednisone used to treat asthma exacerbations can affect HPA function for up to 10 days, but dysfunction is unlikely to be prolonged. Large doses, prolonged therapy (>3 weeks), evening dosing, and continuous (as opposed to alternate day) dosing all increase suppression of the HPA axis and may take up to a year before returning to normal. Inhaled steroids are less likely to cause suppression of HPA axis.

## Management of Anesthesia

The adequacy of asthma control needs to be assessed during preoperative evaluation, and symptoms uncharacteristic of asthma need to be excluded (Table 27.1) (also see Chapter 13). Principles of perioperative management of patients with asthma are outlined in Box 27.2. Volatile anesthetics, particularly sevoflurane,[2] reduce bronchomotor tone and produce a degree of bronchodilation (except desflurane) that may be helpful in patients with obstructive lung disease or bronchoconstriction.[3]

## CHRONIC OBSTRUCTIVE PULMONARY DISEASE

### Clinical Presentation

COPD incorporates three disorders: emphysema, peripheral airways disease, and chronic bronchitis. The $FEV_1$/FVC ratio will be less than 70%, and RV will be increased.

**Table 27.1**   Preoperative Assessment for Asthma

**History Suggestive of Inadequate Asthma Control**
Frequency of symptoms
Use of $\beta_2$-agonist medications/relievers frequently
Hospital attendances
Hospital/intensive care unit (ICU) admissions
Use of oral steroids/high-dose inhaled steroids

| Features Uncharacteristic of Asthma | Differential Diagnosis |
|---|---|
| Unremitting wheeze/stridor | Suggestive of fixed airway obstruction |
| Persisting wet cough/productive cough | Suggestive of suppurative lung disease |
| Wheeze present from birth (rare with asthma) | Tracheomalacia/bronchomalacia |
| A monophonic wheeze loudest over the glottis | Vocal cord dysfunction |

**Box 27.2**  Principles of Perioperative Management of Asthma

- Usual inhalers per normal on day of surgery. Inhaled $\beta_2$-agonists prior to anesthesia.
- Avoid lower airway manipulation (e.g., endotracheal intubation) if possible. Use regional anesthesia, or an LMA/mask for general anesthesia if possible.
- Avoid medications that release histamine (e.g., thiopental, morphine, atracurium).
- Use anesthetic drugs that promote bronchodilation (propofol, ketamine, sevoflurane).
- If instrumentation of the lower airway is necessary, it should be performed after attaining a deep level of general anesthesia to decrease airway reflexes.

LMA, Laryngeal mask airway.

The severity of COPD is assessed by the percent of $FEV_1$: stage I, more than 50% predicted (this category includes both mild and moderate COPD); stage II, 35% to 50%; and stage III, less than 35%.[4] Stage I patients should not have significant dyspnea, hypoxemia, or hypercarbia. Specific complications of COPD to be considered preoperatively are described next.

Carbon Dioxide Retention (Baseline $Paco_2$ > 45 mm Hg)
Many stage II or III COPD patients have an elevated $Paco_2$ at rest. *$CO_2$ retainers* cannot be differentiated from non-retainers on the basis of history, physical examination, or spirometry. When these patients are given supplemental oxygen, their $Paco_2$ values increase because increased inspired oxygen concentrations cause an increase in alveolar dead space owing to a decrease in regional hypoxic pulmonary vasoconstriction and the Haldane effect.[5] However, supplemental oxygen must be administered to these patients to prevent the hypoxemia associated with

the postoperative decrease in FRC. Increased $CO_2$ concentrations above baseline lead to respiratory acidosis, which causes cardiovascular changes (tachycardia, hypotension, and pulmonary vasoconstriction). $Paco_2$ levels more than 80 mm Hg can cause a decreased level of consciousness. The increase in $Paco_2$ in these patients postoperatively should be anticipated and monitored. To identify these patients preoperatively, patients with stage II or III COPD should have an analysis of arterial blood gas performed.

Right Ventricular Dysfunction
Right ventricular dysfunction occurs in up to 50% of patients with severe COPD. Chronic recurrent hypoxemia is the cause of right ventricular dysfunction and subsequent progression to cor pulmonale. Cor pulmonale occurs in 70% of adult COPD patients with an $FEV_1$ less than 0.6 L. Mortality risk in these patients is primarily related to chronic hypoxemia. Administration of oxygen is the only therapy that improves long-term survival and decreases right-sided heart strain associated with COPD. Patients who have a resting $Pao_2$ less than 55 mm Hg should receive supplemental oxygen to maintain $Pao_2$ at 60 to 65 mm Hg at home.

Bullae
Many patients with moderate or severe COPD develop cystic air spaces in the lung parenchyma known as bullae. These bullae will often be asymptomatic unless they occupy more than 50% of the hemithorax, in which case the patient will present with findings of restrictive respiratory disease in addition to their obstructive disease. A bulla is actually a localized loss of structural support tissue in the lung with elastic recoil of surrounding parenchyma. The pressure in a bulla is the mean pressure in the surrounding alveoli averaged over the respiratory cycle. Whenever positive-pressure ventilation is used, the pressure in a bulla will become positive in relation to the adjacent lung tissue and the bulla will expand with the attendant risk of rupture, tension pneumothorax, and bronchopleural fistula. Positive-pressure ventilation can be used safely in patients with bullae, provided the airway pressures are low and adequate expertise and equipment is immediately available to insert a chest drain and obtain lung isolation if necessary. Nitrous oxide will diffuse into a bulla more quickly than the less soluble nitrogen can diffuse out and may lead to rupture of the bulla. The presence of bullae should be ascertained by examination of chest imaging of any patient with COPD preoperatively.

Flow Limitation
Severe COPD patients are often flow limited, even during normal breathing. Flow limitation occurs when any increase in expiratory effort will not produce an increase in flow at that given lung volume. Flow limitation is present in normal patients only during a forced expiratory maneuver and in patients with COPD as a result of the

**IV**

loss of lung elastic recoil. During positive-pressure ventilation this can lead to the development of an intrinsic positive end-expiratory pressure (auto-PEEP). Severely flow-limited patients are at risk of hemodynamic collapse during positive-pressure ventilation owing to dynamic hyperinflation of the lungs leading to obstruction of pulmonary blood flow.

## Perioperative Management

Four treatable complications of COPD must be actively sought and managed at the time of preoperative assessment: atelectasis, bronchospasm, respiratory tract infections, and congestive heart failure. Atelectasis impairs local lung lymphocyte and macrophage function predisposing to infection. Wheezing may be a symptom both of airways obstruction and congestive heart failure. All patients with COPD should receive bronchodilator therapy as guided by their symptoms. If sympathomimetic and anticholinergic bronchodilators provide inadequate therapy, a trial of corticosteroid therapy should be instituted.

COPD patients have fewer postoperative pulmonary complications when intensive chest physiotherapy is initiated preoperatively. Even in patients with severe COPD, exercise tolerance can be improved with physiotherapy[6] at least 1 month or more. Among COPD patients, those with excessive sputum benefit the most from chest physiotherapy. A comprehensive program of pulmonary rehabilitation involving physiotherapy, exercise, nutrition, and education has been shown consistently to improve functional capacity for patients with severe COPD. These programs typically have a duration of several months and are generally not an option in resections for malignancy.

## INTERSTITIAL LUNG DISEASE

Interstitial lung disease (ILD) is a chronic restrictive pulmonary disease (i.e., $FEV_1$ < 70% predicted, $FEV_1$/FVC ratio normal or increased, and RV decreased). Approximately 35% of ILD is attributable to an identifiable cause, such as exposure to inorganic dust, organic antigen, drugs, or radiation. The inciting agent in the remaining 65% of patients is unknown. In many of these patients, the lung is part of an autoimmune disorder.

Elastic recoil of the lungs increases as a consequence of inflammation and fibrosis of the alveolar walls, which results in decreased lung volumes. Early in the disease, patients adapt to smaller tidal volumes by increasing their respiratory rate. As the disease progresses, increased respiratory effort and energy are required to maintain sufficient tidal volumes to prevent alveolar hypoventilation. Uneven disease distribution throughout the lung can cause significant ventilation/perfusion mismatch and is the primary cause of hypoxemia in patients with ILD.

Controlled ventilation via an endotracheal tube is often the most reliable and safest approach to optimizing oxygenation and ventilation in patients with ILD when a general anesthetic is required. The goal of mechanical ventilation in patients with ILD is to maintain adequate ventilation and oxygenation while minimizing the risks of barotrauma and acute lung injury. Potential strategies to minimize airway pressures include the use of long durations of inspiration compared to the duration of expiration ratios (e.g., ratios of 1:1 to 1:1.5), small tidal volumes, and rapid respiratory rates. In contrast to obstructive lung disease, PEEP can be used safely in ILD.

## CYSTIC FIBROSIS

Cystic fibrosis is an autosomal recessive disorder that results in impaired transport of sodium, chloride, and water across epithelial tissue. This leads to exocrine gland malfunction with abnormally viscous secretions, which can cause obstruction of the respiratory tracts, pancreas, biliary system, intestines, and sweat glands. It presents as a mixed obstructive and restrictive lung disease. Inability to clear the thick purulent secretions enhances bacterial growth and, as the disease advances, leads to bronchiectasis.[7] The early mortality of cystic fibrosis is primarily the result of pulmonary complications, including air-trapping, pneumothorax, massive hemoptysis, and respiratory failure. Effective sputum elimination is a key goal in the long-term management of cystic fibrosis. To optimize patients with cystic fibrosis for anesthesia, chest physiotherapy should be performed immediately prior to surgery. Endotracheal intubation with a large endotracheal tube is preferred as it facilitates endobronchial toileting with a suction catheter, bronchoscopy, or both.

## OBSTRUCTIVE SLEEP APNEA

### Clinical Presentation

OSA affects approximately 4% of middle-aged men and 2% of middle-aged women (also see Chapter 50).[8] Obesity is the most important physical characteristic associated with OSA, though OSA may be present in patients with a normal body mass index (BMI) and absent in the obese (also see Chapter 29).

Patients with risk factors (male gender, middle age, BMI > 28 $kg/m^2$, alcohol and sedative use) presenting for surgery should be screened for signs and symptoms of OSA (Box 27.3).

The pathophysiology of airflow obstruction is related primarily to upper airway pharyngeal collapse. Upper airway patency depends on the action of dilator muscles (i.e., tensor palatine, genioglossus muscle, and

**Box 27.3** Clinical Signs and Symptoms Suggestive of Obstructive Sleep Apnea

1. Predisposing clinical characteristics:
   - Body mass index (BMI) ≥ 35 kg/m² (or 95th percentile for age and gender)
   - Neck circumference of ≥17 inches (men) or ≥16 inches (women)
   - Craniofacial abnormalities affecting the airway
   - Anatomic nasal obstruction
   - Tonsils touching or nearly touching in the midline
2. History of apparent airway obstruction during sleep (two or more of the following are present):
   - Frequent snoring
   - Observed pauses in breathing during sleep
   - Awakens from sleep with choking sensation
   - Frequent arousals from sleep
3. Somnolence:
   - Frequent somnolence or fatigue despite adequate "sleep"
   - Falls asleep easily in a nonstimulating environment despite "adequate sleep"

If a patient has signs or symptoms in two or more of the previous categories, there is a significant probability that he or she has obstructive sleep apnea (OSA). The severity of OSA can be determined using a sleep study. In the absence of a sleep study, patients should be treated as though they have moderate sleep apnea unless one of the previous signs or symptoms is severely abnormal (i.e., marked increased BMI) in which case they are classified as having severe sleep apnea.

**Table 27.2**  Determination of Severity of Obstructive Sleep Apnea on the Basis of a Sleep Study

| Adult AHI | Pediatric AHI | OSA Severity | OSA Severity Score |
|---|---|---|---|
| 6-20 | 1-5 | Mild | 1 |
| 21-40 | 6-10 | Moderate | 2 |
| >40 | >10 | Severe | 3 |

*AHI*, Apnea-hypopnea index; *OSA*, obstructive sleep apnea.

of apneic or hypopneic episodes occurring per hour of sleep (Table 27.2).

## Treatment of Obstructive Sleep Apnea

Treatment should include correction of reversible exacerbating factors by means of weight reduction, avoidance of alcohol and sedatives, and nasal decongestants, if needed. Patients with mild OSA can achieve clinical improvement through lifestyle modification. For severe OSA, the three main therapeutic options are continuous positive airway pressure (CPAP), dental appliances, and upper airway surgery.

## Preoperative Evaluation of Patients With Obstructive Sleep Apnea

The goals of the preoperative assessment are to identify anticipated difficulties in airway management (difficult ventilation via a face mask, endotracheal intubation, or both) and coexisting cardiovascular disease. Associated medical conditions should be treated, in as much as possible, prior to elective surgery.

1. *Airway:* Anticipated difficulties with airway management include difficult ventilation via a mask and tracheal intubation.
2. *Respiratory system:* Patients with obesity will have evidence of restrictive lung disease on pulmonary function testing secondary to decreased chest wall compliance.
3. *Cardiovascular system:* Preoperative evaluation should be directed toward the detection of end-organ dysfunction resulting from chronic hypoxemia, hypercarbia, and polycythemia. Systemic hypertension, pulmonary hypertension, and signs of biventricular dysfunction (cor pulmonale and congestive heart failure) should be sought.
4. *Endocrine and gastrointestinal systems:* Fasting blood glucose levels should be sought to screen for type II diabetes. Symptoms of esophageal reflux should lead to aspiration prophylaxis prior to induction of anesthesia. Liver function tests may indicate fatty liver infiltration causing hepatic dysfunction in severe cases.

hyoid muscles). During sleep, laryngeal muscle tone is decreased and apnea occurs when the upper airway collapses. Nonobese patients may develop OSA as a result of adenotonsillar hypertrophy or craniofacial abnormalities (retrognathia). Recurrent episodes of apnea or hypopnea lead to hypoxia, hypercapnia, increased sympathetic stimulation, and arousal from sleep. Patients may develop cardiopulmonary dysfunction manifesting as systemic or pulmonary hypertension and cor pulmonale. Nonrestoration of sleep can lead to cognitive dysfunction manifesting as intellectual impairment and hypersomnolence.

The diagnosis of OSA can be based on clinical impression or a formal sleep study. OSA should be suspected when a patient with predisposing clinical risk factors reports heavy snoring and excessive daytime sleepiness, which are the cardinal features of OSA. OSA is characterized by frequent episodes of apnea or hypopnea during sleep. Apnea is defined as complete cessation of breathing for 10 seconds or more. Hypopnea is defined as more than 50% decrease in ventilation or oxygen desaturation of more than 3% to 4% for 10 seconds or more. It is definitively diagnosed by polysomnography in a sleep laboratory. The severity of OSA is measured by using the apnea-hypopnea index (AHI), which is the number

## Perioperative Management

Patients with OSA are exquisitely sensitive to the respiratory depressant and sedative effects of benzodiazepines and opioids, which can cause upper airway obstruction or apnea. These medications should be withheld preoperatively or used with caution in a monitored environment.

Intraoperative anesthetic concerns in patients with OSA relate to (1) airway management; (2) choice of anesthetic technique; (3) patient positioning; (4) monitoring—inaccurate noninvasive blood pressure measurements and significant underlying cardiorespiratory disease warrant insertion of an arterial line for analysis of arterial blood gas monitoring and beat-to-beat blood pressure measurements; and (5) vascular access—difficult intravenous (IV) access secondary to excess adipose tissue may necessitate central line placement.

Upper airway abnormalities or increased airway adiposity in patients with OSA predisposes them as difficult to adequately ventilate with a bag and mask apparatus following induction of anesthesia. Oral and nasopharyngeal airways should be readily available. Excessive pharyngeal adipose tissue can make exposure of the glottic opening difficult during direct laryngoscopy and endotracheal intubation.

Use of short-acting inhaled (sevoflurane and desflurane) and injected (propofol, remifentanil) drugs are recommended for intraoperative use to minimize postoperative respiratory depression. Nitrous oxide is best avoided in patients with coexisting pulmonary hypertension (also see Chapter 7). Short- to intermediate-acting neuromuscular blocking drugs (also see Chapter 11) can be used for muscle relaxation if required.

The anesthesia provider should consider tracheal extubation with the patient in a semiupright position with an oral or nasopharyngeal airway in place to facilitate spontaneous ventilation. A two-person bag and mask ventilation may be required and possible reintubation of the trachea will be required should acute airway obstruction develop. Administration of supplemental oxygen via a face mask should be provided during transfer of the patient to the postanesthesia care unit (PACU) (also see Chapter 39). CPAP must be available for postoperative use in patients on CPAP or bilevel positive airway pressure (BiPAP) preoperatively.

## Postoperative Management

Multimodal analgesia with nonsteroidal antiinflammatory drugs (NSAIDs), acetaminophen, and regional analgesia aims to minimize opiate analgesia and resultant respiratory depression. CPAP should be reinstituted postoperatively. Surveillance in a high-dependency unit such as the PACU, step-down unit, or intensive care unit (ICU) is prudent for patients with severe OSA (also see Chapter 39).

| Table 27.3 | Scoring Invasiveness of Surgery and Anesthesia | |
|---|---|---|
| **Surgery** | **Anesthesia** | **Invasive Score** |
| Superficial or peripheral | Local infiltration or peripheral nerve block with no sedation | 0 |
| | Moderate sedation Spinal or epidural | 1 |
| | General anesthetic | 2 |
| Major or airway | General anesthetic | 3 |

| Table 27.4 | Scoring of Opioid Requirement |
|---|---|
| **Opioid Requirement** | **Score** |
| None | 0 |
| Low-dose oral | 1 |
| High-dose oral | 2 |
| Parenteral or spinal/epidural | 3 |

**Box 27.4** Determination of Perioperative Obstructive Sleep Apnea Risk Score

OSA Severity Score (1-3)
+
Invasiveness of anesthesia or surgery (1-3)
OR
Postoperative opioid requirement (1-3) (whichever is greater)
If risk score = 4 →increased perioperative risk
If risk score ≥ 5 →significantly increased perioperative risk

OSA, Obstructive sleep apnea.

Postoperative disposition of OSA is influenced by three factors:

1. Severity of the OSA (either by historical information or objective findings of a sleep study) (see Table 27.2)
2. Invasiveness of the surgical procedure and anesthesia (Table 27.3)
3. Predicted postoperative opioid use (Table 27.4)

A patient with increased perioperative risk of airway obstruction and resultant hypoxemia (perioperative OSA risk score greater than 4) should receive continuous oxygen saturation monitoring in either the ICU, a step-down unit, or telemetry unit (Box 27.4) (also see Chapter 41).

## Obesity Hypoventilation Syndrome

Obesity hypoventilation syndrome (OHS) is defined by chronic daytime hypoxemia ($Pao_2$ < 65 mm Hg) and hypoventilation ($Paco_2$ > 45 mm Hg) in an obese patient without coexisting COPD. It is a long-term consequence of OSA. Patients exhibit signs of central sleep apnea (apnea without respiratory efforts). This may culminate in the pickwickian syndrome characterized by obesity, daytime hypersomnolence, hypoxemia, and hypercarbia.

Preoperatively, obese patients should be screened for OHS with pulse oximetry. Patients with oxygen saturation less than 96% warrant analysis of arterial blood gases to assess carbon dioxide retention.

Ultimately, the information obtained from preoperative investigations allows the anesthesia provider to optimize the patient's clinical status prior to elective surgery and plan perioperative care, including arrangements for appropriate postoperative monitoring (i.e., step-down bed, ICU). Interventions may include treatment of coexisting conditions (systemic hypertension, cardiac dysrhythmias, congestive heart failure) and initiation of CPAP. A 2-week period of CPAP therapy is usually quite effective in correcting the abnormal ventilatory drive of patients with OHS.

## PULMONARY HYPERTENSION

### Pathophysiology

Patients with pulmonary hypertension (mean pulmonary artery pressure > 25 mm Hg by catheterization or systolic pulmonary artery pressure > 50 mm Hg on echocardiography)[9] may present for a variety of noncardiac surgical procedures.[10] Patients with pulmonary hypertension are at increased risk of respiratory complications and prolonged intubation after noncardiac surgery.[11]

### Preoperative Evaluation

There are two commonly encountered types of pulmonary hypertension: pulmonary hypertension from left-sided heart disease and pulmonary hypertension from lung disease. Patients who present for noncardiac surgery are more likely to have pulmonary hypertension because of lung disease. Much of what has been learned about anesthesia for patients with pulmonary hypertension owing to lung disease has come from clinical experience in pulmonary endarterectomies[12] and lung transplantation. Avoiding hypotension is the key to managing these patients (Box 27.5).

### Management of Anesthesia

The increased right ventricular transmural and intracavitary pressures associated with pulmonary hypertension

---

> **Box 27.5** Management Principles for Pulmonary Hypertension Secondary to Lung Disease
>
> - Avoid hypotensive and vasodilating anesthetic drugs whenever possible
> - Ketamine does not exacerbate pulmonary hypertension
> - Support mean blood pressure with vasopressors: norepinephrine, phenylephrine, vasopressin
> - Use inhaled pulmonary vasodilators (nitric oxide, prostacyclin) in preference to intravenous vasodilators as needed
> - Use thoracic epidural local anesthetics cautiously and with inotropes as needed
> - Monitor cardiac output if possible

---

may restrict perfusion of the right coronary artery during systole, especially as pulmonary artery pressures approach systemic levels. The impact of pulmonary hypertension on right ventricular dysfunction has several anesthetic implications. The hemodynamic goals are similar to other conditions in which cardiac output is relatively fixed. Care should be taken to avoid physiologic states that will worsen pulmonary hypertension, such as hypoxemia, hypercarbia, acidosis, and hypothermia. Conditions that impair right ventricular filling, such as tachycardia and arrhythmias, are not well tolerated. Ideally, under anesthesia, right ventricular contractility and systemic vascular resistance are maintained or increased while pulmonary vascular resistance is decreased. Ketamine is a useful anesthetic in pulmonary hypertension due to lung disease.[13] Inotropes and inodilators, such as dobutamine and milrinone, may improve hemodynamics in patients with pulmonary hypertension due to left-sided heart disease; however, they decrease systemic vascular tone and tachycardia and can lead to a deterioration in the hemodynamics of patients with pulmonary hypertension due to lung disease. Vasopressors such as phenylephrine, norepinephrine, and vasopressin are commonly used to maintain a systemic blood pressure greater than pulmonary pressures. Vasopressin can increase systemic blood pressure significantly without affecting pulmonary artery pressure in patients with pulmonary hypertension.[14] In patients with severe pulmonary hypertension, selective inhaled pulmonary vasodilators, including nitric oxide (10 to 40 ppm)[15] or nebulized prostaglandins (prostacyclin 50 ng/kg/min),[16] should be considered.

Lumbar epidural analgesia and anesthesia have been used in obstetric patients with pulmonary hypertension,[17] and occasionally thoracic epidural analgesia is used in patients with pulmonary hypertension (also see Chapter 23). Patients with pulmonary hypertension due to lung disease seem to be extremely dependent on tonic cardiac sympathetic innervation for normal hemodynamic stability.[18] These patients will often require a low-dose infusion of inotropes or vasopressors during thoracic epidural local analgesia.

## ANESTHESIA FOR LUNG RESECTION

Thoracic surgery is a relatively young specialty that has been significantly aided by the development of positive-pressure ventilation in the early 1950s, and advanced by the use of double-lumen endobronchial tubes (DLTs) and flexible bronchoscopes. These developments now enable a thoracic anesthesiologist to employ reliable lung isolation allowing surgical access to the thorax and managing anesthesia during one-lung ventilation (OLV).

## Preoperative Assessment for Pulmonary Resection

Preoperative assessment prior to pulmonary resection aims to identify patients at increased risk of perioperative morbidity and mortality in order to focus resources and improve their outcome. Postoperative preservation of respiratory function is proportional to the amount of lung parenchyma preserved. The major causes of perioperative morbidity and mortality risks in the thoracic surgical population are respiratory complications. Major respiratory complications, such as atelectasis, pneumonia, and respiratory failure, occur in 15% to 20% of patients and account for much of the 3% to 4% mortality rate.[19] Objective measures of pulmonary function are required to guide anesthetic management and to transmit information easily between members of the health care team.

### Objective Assessment of Pulmonary Function

No test of respiratory function is adequate as a sole preoperative assessment. Before surgery, respiratory function should be assessed in three related but independent areas: respiratory mechanics, gas exchange, and cardiorespiratory interaction (Fig. 27.3). This "three-legged stool" approach can be used to plan intraoperative and postoperative management.

### Respiratory Mechanics

Of all objective measures obtained via spirometry (e.g., FVC, FEV$_1$, ratio of FEV$_1$:FVC), the FEV$_1$ is most helpful. Spirometry measurements should be expressed as a percent of predicted volume corrected for age, sex, and height (e.g., an FEV$_1$ of 74%). The predicted postoperative FEV$_1$ (ppoFEV$_1$%) is the most effective test for prediction of postthoracotomy respiratory complications.[20] It is calculated as follows:

Eq. 1

$$ppoFEV_1\% = preoperative\ FEV_1\%$$
$$\times (100 - \%\ of\ functional\ tissue\ removed/100)$$

Counting the number of lung segments to be removed allows estimation of the percent of functional lung tissue removed (Fig. 27.4). Patients with a ppoFEV$_1$ of more than 40% are at low risk of postoperative pulmonary complications, whereas those with a ppoFEV$_1$ less than 30% are at high risk.

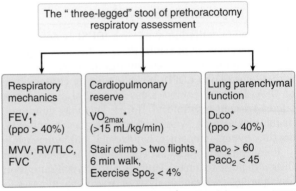

The "three-legged" stool of prethoracotomy respiratory assessment

| Respiratory mechanics | Cardiopulmonary reserve | Lung parenchymal function |
|---|---|---|
| FEV$_1$* (ppo > 40%) | VO$_{2max}$* (>15 mL/kg/min) | D$_{LCO}$* (ppo > 40%) |
| MVV, RV/TLC, FVC | Stair climb > two flights, 6 min walk, Exercise Spo$_2$ < 4% | Pao$_2$ > 60 Paco$_2$ < 45 |

**Fig. 27.3** The three-legged stool of prethoracotomy respiratory assessment. *Most valid test (see text). *D$_{LCO}$*, Lung diffusing capacity for carbon monoxide; *FEV$_1$*, forced expiratory volume in 1 second; *FVC*, forced vital capacity; *MVV*, maximum voluntary ventilation; *Paco$_2$*, partial pressure of carbon dioxide in mm Hg; *Pao$_2$*, partial pressure of oxygen (arterial) in mm Hg; *ppo*, predicted postoperative; *RV*, residual volume; *Spo$_2$*, pulse oximeter saturation; *TLC*, total lung capacity; *VO$_{2max}$*, maximal oxygen consumption. (From Slinger PD, ed. *Principles and Practice of Anesthesia for Thoracic Surgery*. New York: Springer; 2011, used with permission.)

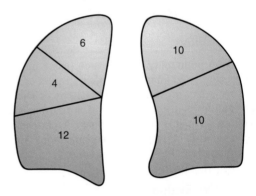

Lung segments
Total subsegments = 42

Example: Right lower lobectomy
postoperative FEV$_1$ decrease = 12/42 (29%)

**Fig. 27.4** The number of subsegments of each lobe is used to calculate the predicted postoperative (ppo) pulmonary function. In this example, after a right lower lobectomy, a patient with a preoperative FEV$_1$ 70% of normal would be expected to have a ppoFEV$_1$ of 70% × (100 − 29/100) = 50%. (From Slinger PD, ed. *Principles and Practice of Anesthesia for Thoracic Surgery*. New York: Springer; 2011, used with permission.)

### Lung Parenchymal Function

Lung parenchymal function refers to the ability of the lung to exchange oxygen and carbon dioxide between the pulmonary vascular bed and the alveoli. Traditionally, analysis of arterial blood gas data such as a partial pressure of oxygen (Pao$_2$) less than 60 mm Hg or a partial pressure of carbon dioxide ($Paco_2$) more than 45 mm Hg has been used as a warning indicator of increased risk of respiratory failure. The most useful indicator of lung parenchymal function is the $D_{LCO}$ obtained during lung function testing. The $D_{LCO}$ correlates with the total functioning surface area of alveolar-capillary interface. The corrected $D_{LCO}$ can be used to calculate a predicted postresection (ppo) value using the same calculation as $FEV_1$ (see Eq. 1). Like $FEV_1$, a ppo $D_{LCO}$ greater than 40% correlates with low risk of postoperative pulmonary complications.[21]

## Cardiopulmonary Interaction

The final step in assessment of respiratory function is the assessment of cardiopulmonary interaction. Formal laboratory exercise testing is the gold standard[22] with the maximal oxygen consumption ($\dot{V}O_{2max}$) being the most useful predictor of postthoracotomy outcome. The risks of morbidity and mortality are increased if the $\dot{V}O_{2max}$ is less than 15 mL/kg/min. Complete laboratory exercise testing is expensive and not available to all centers. Several alternatives are valid surrogate tests for prethoracotomy assessment (outlined in Fig. 27.3).

## Ventilation-Perfusion Scintigraphy

Prediction of postresection pulmonary function can be further refined by assessment of the preoperative contribution of the lung or lobe to be resected using ventilation/perfusion scintigraphy ($\dot{V}/\dot{Q}$ scan). If the lung to be resected is minimally functional, this will modify the ppoFEV$_1$.

## Preoperative Cardiac Assessment

Cardiac complications are the second most common cause of perioperative morbidity and death in the thoracic surgical population. Intrathoracic surgery is considered a risk factor for major adverse cardiac events by the American College of Cardiology and American Heart Association.[23] Further, dysrhythmia occurs in 12% to 44% of patients following thoracic or esophageal surgery, the majority of which is atrial fibrillation.[24] The onset of atrial fibrillation occurs most commonly on postoperative days 2 and 3, with the risk reverting to the patient's baseline risk by week 6. Risk factors for postoperative atrial fibrillation include male sex, older age, magnitude of lung or esophagus resected, history of congestive cardiac failure, concomitant lung disease, and length of procedure. It may be reasonable to give high-risk patients (e.g., older patients undergoing pneumonectomy) prophylactic diltiazem to decrease the incidence of postoperative atrial fibrillation.

## Smoking Cessation

Pulmonary complications are reduced in patients undergoing lung resection who cease smoking perioperatively, regardless of the timing of cessation prior to surgery.[25] The patient should be encouraged to stop smoking at the

---

**Box 27.6** Anesthetic Considerations in Patients With Lung Cancer (the Four Ms)

| | |
|---|---|
| **M**ass effects | Obstructive pneumonia, lung abscess, superior vena cava syndrome, tracheobronchial distortion, Pancoast syndrome, recurrent laryngeal nerve or phrenic nerve paresis, chest wall or mediastinal extension |
| **M**etabolic abnormalities | Lambert-Eaton syndrome, hypercalcemia, hyponatremia, Cushing syndrome |
| **M**etastases | Particularly to brain, bone, liver, adrenal gland |
| **M**edications | Chemotherapy drugs, pulmonary toxicity (bleomycin, mitomycin), cardiac toxicity (doxorubicin), renal toxicity (cisplatin) |

---

preoperative assessment as patients may be more receptive to the message at this time.

## Assessment of the Patient With Lung Cancer

Patients undergoing lung resection for malignancy should be assessed for the four Ms: *m*ass effects, *m*etabolic abnormalities, *m*etastases, and *m*edications. These considerations are outlined in Box 27.6.

## Indications for Lung Isolation

Lung isolation techniques are designed to:

- Allow OLV and therefore surgical access to the thorax and adjacent structures, such as for lung resection, mediastinal, cardiac, vascular, esophageal, and spinal surgery;
- Control ventilation, such as a patient with a bronchopleural fistula;
- Prevent contralateral lung soiling, such as pulmonary hemorrhage, bronchopleural fistula, and whole lung lavage;
- Allow for differential patterns of ventilation in patients with unilateral lung injury.

## Options for Lung Isolation

There are several options to facilitate selective ventilation of one lung. These include DLTs (Fig. 27.5), bronchial blockers (BBs) placed through a single-lumen endotracheal tube (SLT) (see Fig. 27.11), and a single-lumen tube (standard endotracheal tube or endobronchial tube) placed directly into a bronchus. The advantages and disadvantages of each device are listed in Table 27.5.

## Airway Anatomy

In order to place a device for lung isolation, the anesthesia provider must appreciate the bronchial anatomy (Fig. 27.6). Without this knowledge it is easy to place a device

**IV**

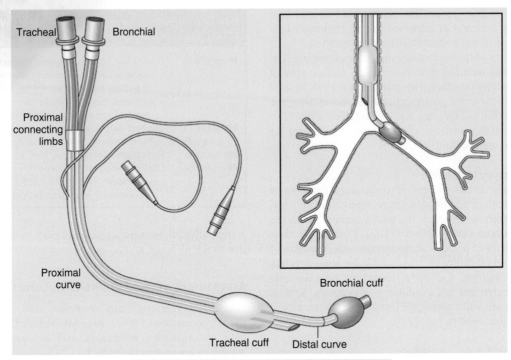

**Fig. 27.5** Left-sided double-lumen endobronchial tube.

**Table 27.5**  Options for Lung Isolation

| Option | Advantages | Disadvantages |
|---|---|---|
| Double-lumen tube | Easy to place successfully<br>Repositioning rarely required<br>Bronchoscopy to isolated lung<br>Suction to isolated lung<br>CPAP easily applied<br>Can alternate one-lung ventilation to either lung easily<br>Placement possible if bronchoscopy not available | Size selection more difficult<br>Difficult to place in patients with difficult airways or abnormal tracheas<br>Not optimal for postoperative ventilation<br>Potential laryngeal and bronchial trauma |
| Bronchial blockers | Size selection rarely an issue<br>Easily added to regular ETT<br>Allows ventilation during placement<br>Easier placement in patients with difficult airways and in children<br>Postoperative two-lung ventilation easy by withdrawing blocker<br>Selective lobar isolation possible<br>CPAP to isolated lung possible | More time required to position<br>Repositioning required more often<br>Bronchoscope essential for positioning<br>Limited right-lung isolation due to RUL anatomy<br>Bronchoscopy to isolated lung impossible<br>Minimal suction to isolated lung<br>Difficult to alternate one-lung ventilation to either lung |
| Endobronchial tube | Easier placement in patients with difficult airways<br>Short cuff designed for lung isolation | Bronchoscopy necessary for placement<br>Does not allow for bronchoscopy, suctioning, or CPAP to isolated lung<br>Difficult one-lung ventilation to right lung |
| Endotracheal tube advanced into bronchus | Easier placement in patients with difficult airways | Bronchoscopy necessary for placement<br>Does not allow for bronchoscopy, suctioning, or CPAP to isolated lung<br>Cuff not designed for lung isolation<br>Extremely difficult one-lung ventilation to right lung |

*CPAP*, Continuous positive airway pressure; *ETT*, endotracheal tube; *RUL*, right upper lobe of lung.

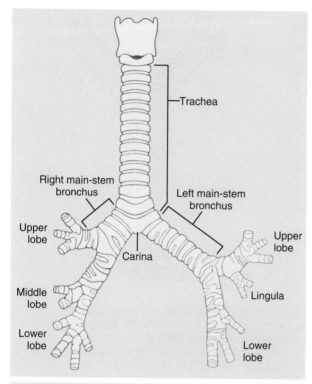

**Fig. 27.6** Tracheobronchial anatomy. Right main bronchus is typically 1.5 to 2 cm. Left main bronchus is typically 4.5 to 5 cm.

| Table 27.6 | Selection of Double-Lumen Tube Size Based on Adult Patient's Sex and Height | |
|---|---|---|
| **Sex** | **Height (cm)** | **Size of Double-lumen Tube (Fr)** |
| Female | <160 (63 in) | 35 |
| | >160 | 37 |
| Male | <170 (67 in) | 39 |
| | >170 | 41 |

*Note:* For females of short stature (<152 cm or 60 in), consider 32-Fr double-lumen tube. For males of short stature (<160 cm) consider 37-Fr double-lumen tube.

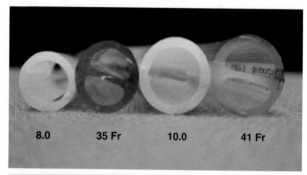

| 8.0 | 35 Fr | 10.0 | 41 Fr |

**Fig. 27.7** Photograph of the cut cross sections of several single-lumen tubes and double-lumen tubes illustrating comparative size. (Courtesy of Professor Jerome Klafta, Department of Anesthesia and Critical Care, University of Chicago.)

incorrectly and difficult to recognize and troubleshoot malposition.[26]

Salient aspects of the bronchial anatomy include the following:

- Carina: bifurcation is "sharp" with no further divisions seen in the left or right lumen
- Right main bronchus: typically 1.5 to 2 cm
- Right upper lobe: the only trifurcation within the tracheobronchial tree, aberrant take-off at or above carina in 1 in 250 patients
- Left main bronchus: typically 4.5 to 5 cm
- Lower lobes: can be identified bilaterally as the longitudinal fibers of the trachealis muscle descend into them

For a more detailed description of bronchial anatomy please see the online bronchoscopy simulator.[27]

### Sizing a Double-Lumen Endobronchial Tube

There is no consensus as to the optimal method to size a DLT. An ideally sized DLT should have a bronchial external diameter 1 to 2 mm smaller than the bronchial diameter in order to fit the deflated bronchial cuff. Chest x-ray images may be used to assist DLT selection.[28] The authors' preference is a simplified method based on

patient sex and height (Table 27.6). A further important step prior to placement is to check a chest radiograph, or ideally a computed tomography (CT) chest coronal slice, to exclude aberrant anatomy, such as endoluminal obstruction, significant tracheal deviation, or aberrant right upper lobe take-off. It is important to appreciate that compared to SLTs, DLTs have a large external diameter and should not be advanced against resistance (Fig. 27.7).

### Methods of Insertion of a Left-Sided Double-Lumen Tube

Two techniques are commonly used when inserting a left-sided DLT. One is a blind technique: the endobronchial lumen of the DLT is passed through the glottis by laryngoscopy and the DLT then turned 90 degrees counterclockwise and advanced until resistance is felt (Fig. 27.8). Blind insertion alone results in malposition in approximately 35% of cases, and, therefore, confirmation of position with a flexible bronchoscope is important.[29,30]

The alternative technique involves direct vision with the use of a flexible bronchoscope. The tip of the endobronchial lumen is passed through the glottis, the DLT is rotated 90 degrees counterclockwise, and

IV

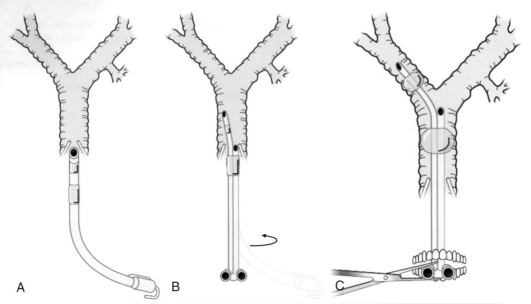

**Fig. 27.8** Blind method for placement of a left-sided double-lumen tube. (A) The double-lumen tube is passed with laryngoscopy beyond the vocal cords. (B) The double-lumen tube is rotated 90 degrees counterclockwise. (C) The double-lumen tube is advanced to an appropriate depth (generally 27 to 29 cm marking at the level of the teeth). (From Campos JH. How to achieve successful lung separation. *SAJAA*. 2008;14:22-26.)

the DLT is advanced so the tracheal cuff is just past the glottis. A flexible bronchoscope is then inserted into the endobronchial lumen to its opening, and the DLT and bronchoscope advanced simultaneously into the correct bronchus. Alternatively the bronchoscope may be advanced through the endobronchial lumen and into the left main bronchus, with the DLT advanced over it.

## Positioning a Left-Sided Double-Lumen Tube

Correct positioning of a DLT is important to avoid ventilation of the collapsed lung, which may obscure the surgeon's field, and to avoid partial collapse of the ventilated lung resulting in hypoxemia. Auscultation alone is unreliable for confirmation of DLT placement. It is still useful as it will increase the anesthesia provider's index of suspicion regarding malposition prior to bronchoscopy, because troubleshooting an incorrectly placed DLT can be confusing to the inexperienced.[26] Both auscultation and bronchoscopy should be used when a DLT is initially placed and again after the patient is repositioned.

Bronchoscopy using a pediatric bronchoscope (≥3.5 mm diameter) is first performed through the tracheal lumen to ensure the endobronchial portion of the DLT is in the left bronchus and the blue endobronchial cuff is approximately 5 mm below the tracheal carina (Fig. 27.9). The right upper lobe take-off should be identified at this time to confirm anatomic landmarks. The bronchoscope is removed and reinserted into the

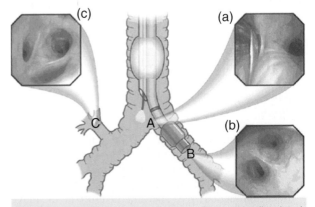

**Fig. 27.9** Bronchoscopic examination of an optimally placed Mallinckrodt left-sided double-lumen tube. (*a*) The bronchoscope is passed through the tracheal lumen, and the edge of the endobronchial cuff is seen 5 mm below tracheal carina. A white line marker is seen above the tracheal carina. (*b*) The bronchoscope is advanced through the endobronchial lumen, and a clear view of the left bronchial bifurcation (left upper and left lower bronchi) is seen. (*c*) A clear view of the right upper lobe bronchus and its three orifices confirms this is the right side. (From Campos JH. Update on tracheobronchial anatomy and flexible fiberoptic bronchoscopy in thoracic anesthesia. *Curr Opin Anaesthesiol.* 2009;22:4-10.)

bronchial lumen, ensuring both the left upper and lower lobes can be seen. Both lobes must be identified to ensure distal migration of the endobronchial lumen has not led to insertion into the left lower lobe and occlusion of the left upper lobe.

**Box 27.7** Indications for a Right-Sided Double-Lumen Tube

Distorted anatomy of the entrance of the left main bronchus
- External or intraluminal tumor compression
- Descending thoracic aortic aneurysm
- Site of surgery involving the left main bronchus
- Left lung transplantation
- Left-sided tracheobronchial disruption
- Left-sided pneumonectomy[a]
- Left-sided sleeve resection

[a]It is possible to manage a left pneumonectomy with a left-sided double-lumen tube (DLT) or bronchial blocker, but the DLT or blocker will have to be withdrawn before stapling the left main bronchus.

## Right-Sided Double-Lumen Tube Indications

Although a left-sided DLT is used most frequently for thoracic procedures, there are specific clinical situations in which the use of a right-sided DLT is indicated (Box 27.7). A right-sided DLT incorporates a modified cuff and slot in the endobronchial lumen that allows ventilation of the right upper lobe (Fig. 27.10). Tracheobronchial anatomy must be checked prior to insertion of the right-sided DLT (CT scan or bronchoscopy) to confirm normal positioning of the right upper lobe orifice.

## Positioning a Bronchial Blocker

The method of insertion of a BB depends on the blocker's design. Three commercially available BBs are shown in Fig. 27.11. The unifying principle of a BB is that it is inserted within an SLT and advanced into the left or right main bronchus or, less commonly, into a lobe. The cuff of the BB is inflated to obstruct the lumen (Fig. 27.12) allowing lung isolation, and a small channel within the blocker may be used to apply suction to the lung, intermittently insufflate oxygen, and apply PEEP. An adaptor attaches to the SLT allowing insertion of a BB or flexible bronchoscope and attachment to the anesthetic circuit. The advantages and disadvantages of BBs compared to other methods of lung isolation are listed in Table 27.5.

## Physiologic Considerations of One-Lung Ventilation in the Lateral Position

Initiation of OLV with an open chest in the lateral position (also see Chapter 19) exposes physiologic changes that improve ventilation and perfusion matching compared to two-lung ventilation (TLV) with a closed chest. Perfusion to the nonventilated, nondependent lung is decreased from hypoxic pulmonary vasoconstriction and gravity, thereby favoring perfusion of the dependent, ventilated lung and decreasing shunt (Fig. 27.13). Changes in cardiac output can have varying effects, but typically shunt

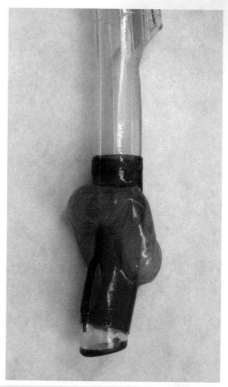

**Fig. 27.10** A Mallinckrodt right-sided double-lumen tube. Note the modified cuff allowing right-lung isolation and slot in the endobronchial lumen allowing ventilation of the right upper lobe. (Courtesy of Dr. Andrew Deacon, Department of Anesthesia, The Canberra Hospital, Australia.)

IV

is lowest (and arterial $P_{O_2}$ is greatest) at a "normal" cardiac output during OLV.[31,32]

Ventilation of the nondependent lung is stopped by virtue of lung isolation. The compliance of the dependent lung decreases owing to the cephalad shift of the diaphragm after induction of anesthesia and muscle relaxation, mediastinal shift following opening of the chest, and surgical pushing and manipulation of the mediastinum. This decrease in compliance and FRC can be improved with the application of PEEP. PEEP (5 to 10 cm $H_2O$) to the dependent lung also helps to reduce blood flow to the nondependent lung as pulmonary vascular resistance is lowest at FRC (Fig. 27.14). Excessive PEEP may increase pulmonary vascular resistance, thereby increasing blood flow to the nondependent lung and worsening shunt.

## Conduct of Anesthesia

Any anesthetic technique that provides safe and stable general anesthesia can be used for thoracic surgery. Although volatile anesthetics impair hypoxic pulmonary vasoconstriction, they do so only at a minimum alveolar

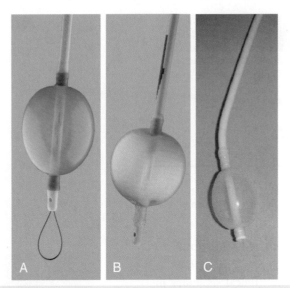

**Fig. 27.11** Three commercially available endobronchial blockers. (A) The Arndt endobronchial blocker (Cook Critical Care, Bloomington, IN). (B) The Cohen Flexitip blocker (Cook Critical Care, Bloomington, IN). (C) The Fuji Uniblocker (Fuji Systems Corporation, Tokyo, Japan).

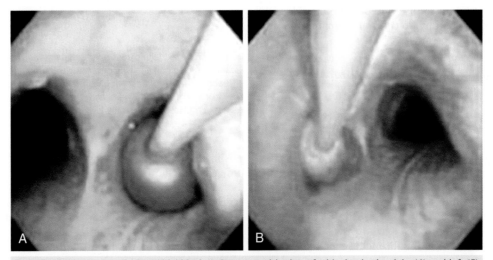

**Fig. 27.12** Placement of a bronchial blocker. Correct positioning of a blocker in the right (*A*) and left (*B*) main bronchi as seen through a bronchoscope in the trachea just above the carina. (From Campos JH. How to achieve successful lung separation. *SAJAA.* 2008;14:22-26.)

concentration (MAC) greater than routine use and there is no clear advantage of a propofol total intravenous anesthetic compared to a volatile anesthetic in terms of shunt fraction or hypoxemia.[33-35]

The majority of thoracic surgical procedures are of moderate duration (2 to 4 hours) and performed in the lateral position with an open hemithorax and OLV. Further, the surgeon is operating in close proximity to important structures, such as the heart and great vessels, and access to the patient is limited after lateral positioning.

Thus, the risk-benefit ratio for intraoperative monitoring favors being overly invasive at the outset.

Choice of monitoring should be guided by a knowledge of which complications are likely to occur (Table 27.7). An intra-arterial catheter allows hemodynamic monitoring and analysis of arterial blood gases. It is the authors' practice to place intra-arterial catheters in all but the most simple thoracic cases (e.g., wedge resection) being performed on patients without comorbid disease. Central venous catheters allow vasoactive agents to be infused, assisting

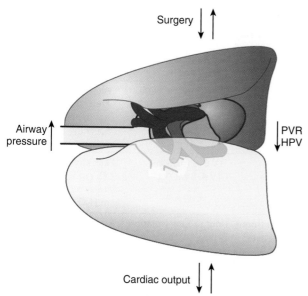

**Fig. 27.13** Factors affecting distribution of pulmonary blood flow during one-lung ventilation. Hypoxic pulmonary vasoconstriction (HPV) and the collapse of the nonventilated lung, which increases pulmonary vascular resistance (PVR), tend to redistribute blood flow toward the ventilated lung. The airway pressure gradient between the ventilated and nonventilated thoraces tends to encourage blood flow to the nonventilated lung. Surgery and cardiac output can have variable effects, either increasing or decreasing the proportional flow to the ventilated lung.

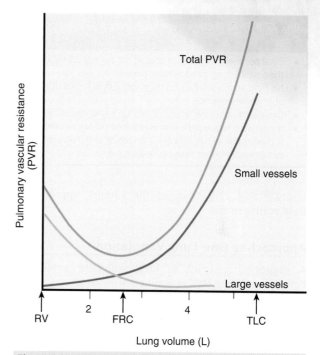

**Fig. 27.14** The relationship between pulmonary vascular resistance (PVR) and lung volume. PVR is lowest at functional residual capacity (FRC) and increases as the lung volume decreases toward residual volume (RV), caused primarily by an increase in resistance of large pulmonary vessels. PVR also increases as lung volume increases above FRC toward total lung capacity (TLC) as a result of an increase in resistance of small interalveolar vessels.

IV

hemodynamic stability in patients who are at risk of intraoperative hemorrhage or postoperative hypervolemia, such as for pneumonectomy, complex procedures, and redo-thoracotomy. The open hemithorax provides a large surface area for evaporative cooling, therefore devices to measure and maintain patient normothermia are required.

Another useful monitor during OLV is continuous spirometry. Available on most modern ventilators, this allows for continuous monitoring of inspiratory and expiratory volumes, pressures, and flows. Attention to the difference between the inspired and expired volumes during OLV may indicate an air leak and loss of lung isolation (>30 mL/breath). During TLV after lung resection, this difference correlates to an air leak through the lung parenchyma. The development of gas trapping in patients with obstructive lung disease is indicated by persistent end-expiratory flow.

## Approach to Intravenous Fluid Management

Intravenous fluid administration is aimed at maintaining euvolemia, that is, replacement of intravascular volume deficits and maintenance only. A positive fluid balance in excess of 3 to 4 L in the first 24 hours has been associated with postpneumonectomy acute lung

| Table 27.7 | Intraoperative Complications That Occur With Increased Frequency During Thoracotomy |
|---|---|
| **Complication** | **Cause** |
| Hypoxemia | Intrapulmonary shunt during one-lung ventilation |
| Sudden hypotension | Surgical compression of the heart or great vessels |
| Sudden changes in ventilating pressure or volume | Movement of endobronchial tube/blocker, air leak |
| Arrhythmia | Mechanical irritation of the heart |
| Bronchospasm | Direct airway stimulation, increased frequency of reactive airways disease |
| Hemorrhage | Surgical blood loss from great vessels or inflamed pleura |
| Hypothermia | Heat loss from open hemithorax |

**Box 27.8** Fluid Management for Pulmonary Resection Surgery

- Total positive fluid balance should not exceed 20 mL/kg in the first 24-hour perioperative period.
- No fluid administration for third space fluid losses during pulmonary resection.
- Urine output greater than 0.5 mL/kg/h is unnecessary.
- If increased tissue perfusion is required postoperatively, it is advisable to use invasive monitoring and inotropes/vasopressors rather than cause fluid overload.

injury.[36] Box 27.8 describes the authors' approach to fluid management.

## Approach to One-Lung Ventilation

A suggested approach to lung protective ventilation before and during OLV is outlined in Table 27.8.

## Prediction of Intraoperative Hypoxia

There are many patient-, surgical-, and position-related factors that can be used to predict which patients are at risk of hypoxemia during OLV. These factors are outlined in Box 27.9.

## Management of Hypoxia During One-Lung Ventilation

Less than 5% of patients develop hypoxia during OLV.[37] Although there is no consensus as to the lowest acceptable $Spo_2$ or $Po_2$ during OLV, an $Spo_2$ less than 94% typically indicates a problem. A stepwise plan for management of this complication is shown in Table 27.9. The most common cause of desaturation during OLV is DLT malposition (i.e., the DLT has advanced and is occluding the upper lobe)[37] and should therefore be investigated with a bronchoscope.

## Conclusion of Surgery

A suggested plan for tracheal extubation at the conclusion of lung resection is outlined in Fig. 27.15. A prerequisite for extubation of the trachea is a patient who is alert, warm, and comfortable (AWaC).

## Pain Management

Posterolateral thoracotomy is one of the most painful surgical incisions. Improvements in analgesic techniques over the last 30 years have contributed to a decrease in postoperative mortality rate for these procedures.[38] No single analgesic technique can block the multiple sensory afferents that transmit nociceptive stimuli after thoracotomy (thoracic and cervical, vagus, and phrenic nerves); therefore, analgesia should be multimodal. The optimal

**Table 27.8** A Suggested Approach to One-Lung Ventilation

| Parameter | Suggested Application | Explanation |
|---|---|---|
| $Fio_2$ | Induction and early maintenance $Fio_2$ 1.0 Decrease $Fio_2$ during OLV if tolerated | Aids absorption atelectasis in nondependent lung, speeding lung collapse |
| Tidal volume | TLV 6-8 mL/kg OLV 4-6 mL/kg[a] | Peak airway pressure <35 cm $H_2O$, plateau airway pressure <25 cm $H_2O$ |
| Recruitment maneuver | Prior to lung isolation During OLV as needed | Reverses atelectasis in ventilated lung improving $Po_2$ during OLV[a] |
| Positive end-expiratory pressure | Routine PEEP 5-10 cm to dependent lung | No PEEP in patients with obstructive disease |
| Respiratory rate | Respiratory rate 12-16 breaths/min | May be higher if required |
| $Pco_2$ | Permissive hypercapnia during OLV | Aim to keep pH ≥7.20 |
| Mode | Volume or pressure controlled | Pressure control for patients at risk of lung injury, such as bullae, preexisting lung disease, pneumonectomy, lung transplantation |

*OLV*, One-lung ventilation; *PEEP*, positive end-expiratory pressure; *TLV*, two-lung ventilation.
[a]Unzueta C, Tusman G, Suarez-Sipmann F, et al. Alveolar recruitment improves ventilation during thoracic surgery: a randomized controlled trial. Br J Anaesth. 2012;108:517–524.

**Box 27.9** Factors That Correlate With an Increased Risk of Desaturation During One-Lung Ventilation

- Higher percentage of ventilation or perfusion to the operative lung on preoperative $\dot{V}/\dot{Q}$ scan
- Poor $Pao_2$ during two-lung ventilation, particularly in the lateral position intraoperatively
- Right-sided thoracotomy
- Normal preoperative spirometry ($FEV_1$ or FVC) or restrictive lung disease
- Supine position during one-lung ventilation

*FEV₁*, Forced expiratory volume in 1 second; *FVC*, functional residual capacity; *Pao₂*, partial pressure of oxygen (arterial); *$\dot{V}/\dot{Q}$*, ventilation/perfusion ratio.

| Table 27.9 | Management of Hypoxemia During One-Lung Ventilation |

| Management | Notes |
| --- | --- |
| $F_{IO_2}$ 1.0 | If not already done |
| Check DLT position via bronchoscope | Bronchial lumen may be too deep, occluding upper lobe bronchus |
| Optimize cardiac output | High or low cardiac output may contribute to hypoxia<br>Decrease volatile anesthesia to <1 MAC |
| Recruitment maneuver to dependent (ventilated) lung + application of PEEP 5-10 cm $H_2O$ if not already applied (except in patients with emphysematous disease) | Reverse atelectasis in dependent lung<br>Recruitment of ventilated lung will transiently increase blood flow and therefore shunt to the operative lung |
| Passive $O_2$ insufflation to operative lung | Suction catheter inserted into DLT connected to $O_2$ 1-2 L/min<br>More effective if lung partially reinflated prior to oxygenation |
| Partial recruitment maneuver to operative lung followed by CPAP 1-5 cm $H_2O$ | Nondependent (operative) lung will be partially inflated, obscuring surgical access during VATS<br>Aim to use the lowest PEEP possible |
| Lobar $O_2$ insufflation using bronchoscope | $O_2$ connected to working port of bronchoscope, $O_2$ intermittently insufflated during period of OLV |
| Lobar collapse using a bronchial blocker if possible | Isolation only of the lobe to be operated on |
| Intermittent reinflation of lung | |
| Temporary occlusion of pulmonary artery | |

*Note:* This table only discusses management specific to the gradual onset of hypoxemia during one-lung ventilation and is listed from least intrusive to most intrusive to surgical access. Sudden and severe hypoxemia should be managed by informing the surgeon of the problem, reinflation of the isolated lung provided it is safe to do so, and two-lung ventilation while attempting to identify and manage the cause.
*CPAP,* Continuous positive airway pressure; *DLT,* double-lumen tube; *MAC,* minimum alveolar concentration; *OLV,* one-lung ventilation; *PEEP,* positive end-expiratory pressure; *VATS,* video-assisted thoracic surgery.

IV

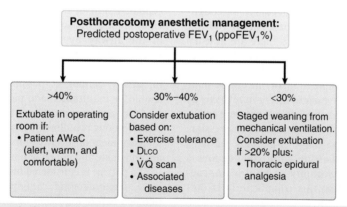

**Fig. 27.15** Anesthetic management guided by preoperative assessment and the amount of functioning lung tissue removed during surgery. *DLCO,* Lung diffusing capacity for carbon monoxide; *FEV₁,* forced expiratory volume in 1 second; *V/Q,* ventilation/perfusion. (From Slinger PD, ed. *Principles and Practice of Anesthesia for Thoracic Surgery.* New York: Springer; 2011, used with permission.)

choice is based on patient factors (contraindications, preferences), surgical factors (type of incision), and system factors (available equipment, monitoring, nursing support, institutional familiarity with techniques). The ideal postthoracotomy analgesic technique includes opioids, antiinflammatory agents, and regional anesthesia (also see Chapter 40).

## MEDIASTINOSCOPY

Mediastinoscopy to stage lung cancer prior to resection has been largely superseded by endobronchial ultrasound-guided transbronchial needle aspiration (EBUS),[39] which may aid in the diagnosis of anterior and superior mediastinal masses.

**Box 27.10** Anesthetic Management of Mediastinoscopy Hemorrhage

1. Stop surgery and pack the wound. There is a serious risk that the patient will approach the point of hemodynamic collapse if the surgery-anesthesia team does not realize soon enough that there is a problem.
2. Begin resuscitation and call for help, both anesthetic and surgical.
3. Obtain large-bore intravenous access in the lower limbs.
4. Place an arterial line (if not placed at induction).
5. Obtain crossmatched blood in the operating room.
6. Place a double-lumen tube or bronchial blocker if the surgeon thinks thoracotomy is a possibility.
7. Once the patient is stabilized and all preparations are made, the surgeon can reexplore the surgical incision.
8. Convert to sternotomy or thoracotomy if indicated.

**Table 27.10** Management of Potentially Life-Threatening Complications of Mediastinal Masses

| Complication | Options for Management |
|---|---|
| Airway obstruction | Maintenance of spontaneous ventilation, avoidance of muscle relaxants<br>Awake fiberoptic intubation with single-lumen endotracheal or endobronchial tube placed distal to the obstruction<br>Patient repositioning: optimal position determined preinduction based on patient's symptoms<br>Rigid bronchoscopy and ventilation distal to the obstruction; experienced bronchoscopist and equipment in the room at induction |
| Cardiovascular collapse | Lower limb intravenous access (large-bore IV with or without central line)<br>Patient repositioning<br>Elective cardiopulmonary bypass preinduction in extreme cases |

The most common surgical approach is via a small (2 to 3 cm) midline, transverse incision superior to the suprasternal notch. Surgical access is limited, and there are many structures that may be compressed or transected, such as trachea and bronchi, pleura, great vessels (particularly the innominate artery and vein), lymphatic vessels, phrenic and recurrent laryngeal nerves, and esophagus.

Any anesthetic technique can be used for mediastinoscopy. Although local anesthesia can be used for cooperative and motivated patients with relatively superficial lesions, general anesthesia with an SLT is typical. It is important the patient be still, as movement or coughing may result in surgical complications. An arterial line probably should not be inserted unless there are unusual patient or surgical factors. It is useful to monitor the pulse in the right hand (pulse oximeter, arterial line, anesthesia provider's finger) as compression of the innominate artery supplying blood to the carotid artery may occur by the mediastinoscope. A noninvasive blood pressure cuff is placed on the left arm to confirm innominate compression.

Massive mediastinal hemorrhage is perhaps the most feared complication of mediastinoscopy and requires a median sternotomy or thoracotomy to control. A suggested approach to managing this complication is outlined in Box 27.10.

## MEDIASTINAL MASSES

Patients with mediastinal masses, particularly anterior and superior masses, present unique problems for anesthesia care. Mediastinal masses may cause obstruction of major airways distal to an endotracheal tube and major vascular structures, such as main pulmonary arteries, atria, and superior vena cava. Patients who are symptomatic or have significant compression of these vital structures visible on CT scans are likely to be at high risk of life-threatening respiratory or cardiovascular collapse.

Anesthetic deaths occur mainly in children because of the more compressible cartilaginous airway and difficulty in obtaining a history of positional symptoms.

General anesthesia is potentially dangerous for a patient with a mediastinal mass for several reasons. General anesthesia leads to a decrease in lung volume with cephalad shift of the diaphragm and relaxation of bronchial smooth muscle, resulting in more compressibility of the airway by the overlying mass. Further, muscle relaxant–induced paralysis leads to a loss of the normal transpleural pressure gradient and a subsequent decrease in airway caliber. If possible, spontaneous ventilation should be maintained and paralysis avoided.

A suggested approach to the management of potential complications is outlined in Table 27.10. Flow-volume loops for assessment of severity of intrathoracic airway obstruction are unreliable and not recommended for decision making.[40,41]

If a patient is considered high risk for cardiovascular collapse, femorofemoral cardiopulmonary bypass should be initiated before induction of anesthesia as there is insufficient time for this to be started after cardiovascular collapse.

## QUESTIONS OF THE DAY

1. A patient with chronic obstructive pulmonary disease (COPD) is scheduled for surgery. What treatable complications of COPD should be addressed during the preoperative evaluation?
2. A patient with obstructive sleep apnea (OSA) requires abdominal surgery. What steps can be taken to decrease the risk of postoperative respiratory depression or airway obstruction?

3. A patient is undergoing medical evaluation before resection of a lung mass. What tests should be performed to predict the risks of postoperative pulmonary complications?

4. What bronchoscopic findings confirm proper placement of a left-sided double-lumen tube?

5. A patient who is undergoing one-lung ventilation (OLV) during lung resection gradually develops hypoxemia over a 20-minute period. What steps should be taken to terminate the evolving hypoxia?

6. A patient presents for resection of a mediastinal mass. What patient factors are associated with increased risk of respiratory or cardiovascular collapse during surgery? If airway obstruction develops after induction of anesthesia, what are the next steps in management of a patient with such a mass?

## REFERENCES

1. Fanta CH. Asthma. *N Engl J Med.* 2009;360:1002–1014.
2. Rooke GA, Choi JH, Bishop MJ. The effect of isoflurane, halothane, sevoflurane, and thiopental/nitrous oxide on respiratory system resistance after tracheal intubation. *Anesthesiology.* 1997;86:1294–1299.
3. Goff MJ, Arain SR, Ficke DJ, et al. Absence of bronchodilation during desflurane anesthesia: a comparison to sevoflurane and thiopental. *Anesthesiology.* 2000;93:404–408.
4. Rennard SI. Chronic obstructive pulmonary disease: definition, clinical manifestations, diagnosis, and staging. In: Stoller JK, ed. *UpToDate.* Waltham, MA: UpToDate; 2015. Accessed July 29, 2015.
5. Wilson FA, Heunks L. Oxygen induced hypercapnia in COPD: myths and facts. *Crit Care.* 2012;16:323–328.
6. Morano M, Araujo A, Nascimento F, et al. Preoperative pulmonary rehabilitation versus chest physical therapy in patients undergoing lung cancer resection. *Arch Phys Med Rehab.* 2013;94:53–58.
7. Huffmayer J, Littlewood K, Nemergut E. Perioperative management of the adult with cystic fibrosis. *Anesth Analg.* 2009;109:1949–1961.
8. Olsen E, Chung F, Seet E. Surgical risk and the preoperative evaluation and management of adults with obstructive sleep apnea. In: Jones S, Collop N, eds. *UpToDate.* Waltham, MA: UpToDate; 2014. Accessed July 29, 2015.
9. Galie N, Hoeper MM, Humbert H, et al. Guidelines for the diagnosis and treatment of pulmonary hypertension. *Eur Heart J.* 2009;30:2493–2537.
10. Pilkington SA, Taboada D, Martinez G. Pulmonary hypertension and its management in patients undergoing non-cardiac surgery. *Anaesthesia.* 2015;70:56–70.
11. Lai HC, Lai HC, Wang KY, et al. Severe pulmonary hypertension complicates postoperative outcome of non-cardiac surgery. *Br J Anaesth.* 2007;99(2):184–190.
12. Banks DA, Pretorius GV, Kerr KM, Manecke GR. Pulmonary endarterectomy: part II. Operation, anesthetic management, and postoperative care. *Semin Cardiothorac Vasc Anesth.* 2014;18(4):331–340.
13. Maxwell BG, Jackson E. Role of ketamine in the management of pulmonary hypertension and right ventricular failure. *J Cardiothorac Vasc Anesth.* 2012;26:e24.
14. Currigan DA, Hughes RJA, Wright CE, et al. Vasoconstrictor responses to vasopressor agents in human pulmonary and radial arteries. *Anesthesiology.* 2014;121:930–936.
15. Wauthy P, Abdel Kafi S, Mooi WJ, et al. Inhaled nitric oxide versus prostacyclin in chronic shunt-induced pulmonary hypertension. *J Thorac Cardiovasc Surg.* 2003;126(5):1434–1441.
16. Jerath A, Srinivas C, Vegas A, et al. The successful management of severe protamine-induced pulmonary hypertension using inhaled prostacyclin. *Anesth Analg.* 2010;110:365–369.
17. Smelickerdstadt KG, Cramb R, Morison DH. Pulmonary hypertension and pregnancy: a series of eight cases. *Can J Anesth.* 1994;41:502–512.
18. Missant C, Claus P, Rex S, Wouters PF. Differential effects of lumbar and thoracic epidural anesthesia on the haemodynamic response to acute right ventricular pressure overload. *Br J Anaesth.* 2009;104:143.
19. Licker M, Widikker I, Robert J, et al. Operative mortality and respiratory complications after lung resection for cancer: impact of chronic obstructive pulmonary disease and time trends. *Ann Thorac Surg.* 2006;81:1830–1837.
20. Lim E, Baldwin D, Beckles M, et al. British Thoracic Society; Society for Cardiothoracic Surgery in Great Britain and Ireland. Guidelines on the radical management of patients with lung cancer. *Thorax.* 2010;65(suppl 3):iii1–iii27.
21. Spiro SG, Gould MK, Colice GK. Initial evaluation of the patient with lung cancer. ACCP evidence-based clinical practice guidelines (2nd edition). *Chest.* 2007;132:149S–160S.
22. Weisman IM. Cardiopulmonary exercise testing in the preoperative assessment for lung resection surgery. *Semin Thorac Cardiovasc Surg.* 2001;13:116–125.
23. Fleisher LA, Fleishmann KE, Auerbach AD, et al. 2014 ACC/AHA guideline on perioperative cardiovascular evaluation and management of patients undergoing noncardiac surgery. *J Am Coll Cardiol.* 2014;64(22):e77–e137.
24. Fernando HC, Jaklitsch MT, Walsh GL, et al. The society of thoracic surgeons practice guideline on prophylaxis and management of atrial fibrillation associated with general thoracic surgery: executive summary. *Ann Thorac Surg.* 2011;92:1144–1152.
25. Mason DP, Subramanian S, Nowicki ER, et al. Impact of smoking cessation before resection of lung cancer: a society of thoracic surgeons general thoracic surgery database study. *Ann Thorac Surg.* 2009;88:362–371.
26. Campos JH, Hallam EA, Van Natta T, et al. Devices for lung isolation used by anesthesiologists with limited thoracic experience: comparison of double-lumen endotracheal tube, Univent torque control blocker, and Arndt wire-guided endobronchial blocker. *Anesthesiology.* 2006;104(2):261–266.
27. Toronto General Hospital Department of Anesthesia. Perioperative Interactive Education. http://pie.med.utoronto.ca/VB/.
28. Brodsky JB, Macario A, Mark JB. Tracheal diameter predicts double-lumen tube size: a method for selecting left double lumen tubes. *Anesth Analg.* 1996;82:861–864.
29. Klein U, Karzai W, Bloos F, et al. Role of fiberoptic bronchoscopy in conjunction with the use of double-lumen tubes for thoracic anesthesia: a prospective study. *Anesthesiology.* 1998;88:346–350.
30. de Bellis M, Accardo R, Di Maio M, et al. Is flexible bronchoscopy necessary to confirm the position of double-lumen tubes before thoracic surgery? *Eur J Cardiothorac Surg.* 2011;40:912–918.
31. Slinger P, Scott WA. Arterial oxygenation during one-lung ventilation. A comparison of enflurane and isoflurane. *Anesthesiology.* 1995;82:940–946.
32. Russell WJ, James MF. The effects on arterial haemoglobin oxygenation saturation and on shunt of increasing cardi-

IV

ac output with dopamine or dobutamine during one-lung ventilation. *Anaesth Intensive Care.* 2004;32:644–648.

33. Beck DH, Doepfmer UR, Sinemus C, et al. Effects of sevoflurane and propofol on pulmonary shunt fraction during one lung ventilation for thoracic surgery. *Br J Anaesth.* 2001;86:38–43.

34. Pruszkowski O, Dalibon N, Moutafis M, et al. Effects of propofol vs sevoflurane on arterial oxygenation during one-lung ventilation. *Br J Anaesth.* 2007;98:539–544.

35. Von Dossow V, Welte M, Zaune U, et al. Thoracic epidural anesthesia combined with general anesthesia: the preferred anesthetic technique for thoracic surgery. *Anesth Analg.* 2001;92:848–854.

36. Licker M, de Perrot M, Spiliopoulos A, et al. Risk factors for acute lung injury after thoracic surgery for lung cancer. *Anesth Analg.* 2003;97:1558–1565.

37. Brodsky JB, Lemmens JM. Left double-lumen tubes: clinical experience with 1,170 patients. *J Cardiothorac Vasc Anesth.* 2003;17:289–298.

38. Licker M, Widikker I, Robert J, et al. Operative mortality and respiratory complications after lung resection for cancer: impact of chronic obstructive pulmonary disease and time trends. *Ann Thorac Surg.* 2006;81:1830–1837.

39. Czarnecka A, Yasufuku K. Endobronchial ultrasound-guided transbronchial needle aspiration for staging patients with lung cancer with clinical N0 disease. *Ann Am Thorac Soc.* 2015;12(3):297–299.

40. Vander Els NJ, Sorhage F, Bach AM, et al. Abnormal flow volume loops in patients with intrathoracic Hodgkin's disease. *Chest.* 2000;117(5):1256–1261.

41. Hnatiuk OW, Corcoran PC, Sierra P. Spirometry in surgery for anterior mediastinal masses. *Chest.* 2001;120:1152–1156.

# 28 RENAL, LIVER, AND BILIARY TRACT DISEASE

## Anup Pamnani and Vinod Malhotra

## RENAL DISEASE

Normal renal function is important for the excretion of anesthetics and medications, maintaining fluid and acid-base balance, and regulating hemoglobin levels in the perioperative period.

Renal disease is quite prevalent in patients presenting for surgery and is associated with increased likelihood of poor postoperative outcomes. Even mild renal dysfunction is associated with a more likely risk of postoperative complications.[1]

Multiple preoperative risk factors have also been identified that predict renal dysfunction in the postoperative period (Box 28.1).[2,3]

### Renal Blood Flow

Although the kidneys represent only 0.5% of total body weight, their blood flow is equivalent to about 20% of cardiac output. Approximately two thirds of renal blood flow is distributed to the renal cortex. Renal blood flow and the glomerular filtration rate (GFR) remain relatively constant at renal arterial blood pressures in the range of 80 to 180 mm Hg (Fig. 28.1). Being able to maintain renal blood flow at a constant rate independent of changes in perfusion pressure is known as autoregulation. It is achieved by adjustment of afferent arteriolar tone, which alters the resistance to blood flow. Autoregulation protects the glomerular capillaries from hypertension during acute hypertensive episodes and maintains GFR and renal tubule function during modest decreases in arterial blood pressure. When mean arterial blood pressure is outside the autoregulatory range, renal blood flow becomes pressure dependent. Autoregulation is reset by chronic hypertension and may be abolished in the diabetic kidney.

Renal blood flow is also strongly influenced by the activity of the sympathetic nervous system and by release of renin and other hormones. Sympathetic nervous

**Box 28.1** Predictors of Postoperative Acute Kidney Injury

- Preexisting chronic kidney disease
- Advanced age
- Emergent surgery
- Liver disease
- High-risk surgery
- Body mass index > 32
- Peripheral vascular occlusive disease
- Chronic obstructive pulmonary disease

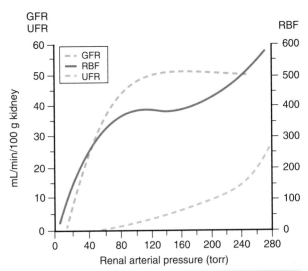

**Fig. 28.1** Autoregulation of renal blood flow (RBF) and the glomerular filtration rate (GFR). The relationships between RBF, GFR, and urine flow rate (UFR) and mean renal arterial pressure in dogs are shown as renal arterial pressure is varied from 20 to 280 mm Hg. Autoregulation of RBF and GFR is observed between about 80 mm Hg and 180 mm Hg. (Redrawn from Hemmings HC. Anesthetics, adjuvants and drugs and the kidney. In Malhotra V, ed. *Anesthesia for Renal and Genitourinary Surgery*. New York: McGraw-Hill; 1996:18.)

system stimulation can produce renal vasoconstriction and a marked decrease in renal blood flow even if systemic blood pressure is within the autoregulatory range. Any decrease in renal blood flow will initiate the release of renin, which can further decrease renal blood flow.

## Glomerular Filtration Rate

GFR reflects glomerular function and is a measure of the ability of the glomerular membrane to allow filtration. About 90% of the fluid filtered at the glomeruli is reabsorbed from renal tubules into peritubular capillaries and thus returned to the circulation (Fig. 28.2). Normal GFR is approximately 125 mL/min and is very dependent on glomerular filtration pressure (GFP). GFP, in turn, is a function of renal artery pressure, afferent and efferent arteriolar tone, and glomerular oncotic

pressure. Hydrostatic pressure within the glomerular capillaries is about 50 mm Hg. This pressure forces water and other low-molecular-weight substances such as electrolytes through the glomerular capillaries into Bowman space. Plasma oncotic pressure is about 25 mm Hg at the afferent arteriole and with filtration increases to about 35 mm Hg at the efferent arteriole. Despite a relatively low net filtration pressure, the glomerular capillaries are able to filter plasma at a rate equivalent to about 125 mL/min. GFR is reduced by significantly decreased mean arterial pressure or renal blood flow. Afferent arteriolar constriction decreases GFR by decreasing glomerular flow. Conversely, afferent arteriolar dilation and mild efferent vasoconstriction increase GFP and GFR.

## Humoral Mediators of Renal Function

### Renin-Angiotensin-Aldosterone System

Renin is a proteolytic enzyme secreted by the juxtaglomerular apparatus of the kidneys in response to (1) sympathetic nervous system stimulation, (2) decreased renal perfusion pressure, and (3) decreases in the delivery of sodium to the distal convoluted renal tubules. Renin acts on angiotensinogen (a circulating globulin in plasma) to form angiotensin I. Angiotensin I is converted in the lungs by angiotensin-converting enzyme to angiotensin II. Angiotensin II, a potent vasoconstrictor, stimulates the release of aldosterone from the adrenal cortex. It selectively increases efferent renal arteriolar tone at low levels and causes afferent arteriolar constriction at higher levels. Aldosterone, in turn, stimulates reabsorption of sodium and water in the distal tubule and collecting ducts.

### Prostaglandins

Prostaglandins are produced in the renal medulla via the enzymes phospholipase $A_2$ and cyclooxygenase and released in response to sympathetic nervous system stimulation, hypotension, and increased levels of angiotensin II. During periods of hemodynamic instability, prostaglandins act to modulate the effects of arginine vasopressin (AVP), the renin-angiotensin system, and norepinephrine by vasodilating juxtamedullary vessels and maintaining cortical blood flow.

### Arginine Vasopressin

Previously known as antidiuretic hormone, AVP regulates osmolality and diuresis. Although secreted in the supraoptic and paraventricular nuclei in the hypothalamus, it exerts significant effects on the renal collecting system. AVP actions are concentrated on collecting duct $V_2$ receptors to increase membrane permeability and facilitate water reabsorption. The overall effect of AVP is to decrease serum osmolality and increase urine osmolality.

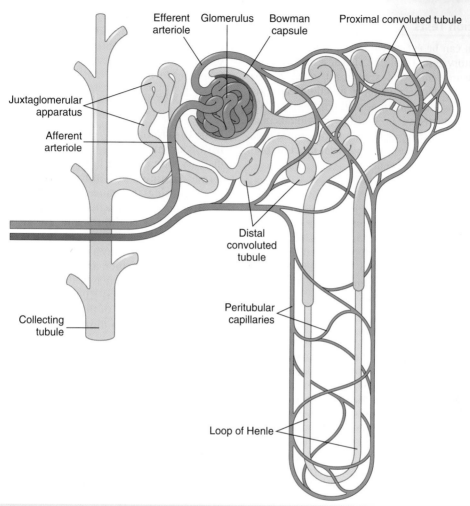

**Fig. 28.2** Anatomy of a nephron. The glomerulus is formed by the invaginated and blind end of the nephron known as *Bowman capsule*. Hydrostatic pressure in these capillaries causes water and low-molecular-weight substances to filter through the glomerulus. Glomerular filtrate travels along the renal tubule (proximal convoluted tubule, loop of Henle, distal convoluted tubule), during which most of its water and various amounts of solutes are reabsorbed from the renal tubular lumen into peritubular capillaries. The remaining glomerular filtrate becomes urine.

Atrial Natriuretic Peptide

Atrial natriuretic peptide (ANP) is secreted when stretch receptors in the atria of the heart, and other organs, are stimulated by increased intravascular volume. ANP acts by relaxing vascular smooth muscle to cause vasodilation, inhibiting the renin-angiotensin system, and stimulating diuresis and natriuresis. The net effect of ANP is to decrease systemic blood pressure and intravascular volume.

## Drug Clearance

Excretion of drugs or their metabolites into urine depends on three mechanisms: (1) glomerular filtration, (2) active secretion by the renal tubules, and (3) passive reabsorption by the tubules. The glomerular filtration of small molecules characteristic of anesthetic drugs depends on the GFR and the fractional plasma protein binding. Drugs that are highly protein bound will be inefficiently filtered at the glomerulus. Nonionized acidic and basic compounds undergo passive reabsorption by backdiffusion in the proximal and distal renal tubules. Ionized forms of these weak acids and bases, on the other hand, are trapped within renal tubules, accounting for increased renal elimination by either alkalinization or acidification of urine. Conjugation of drugs in the liver to water-soluble metabolites is another mechanism by which renal excretion of substances is achieved.

## Renal Function Tests

Renal function can be evaluated preoperatively by using several laboratory tests (Table 28.1). These tests are not sensitive measurements, and significant renal disease (more than a 50% decrease in renal function) can exist while laboratory values remain normal. Furthermore, the normal values established in healthy individuals may not be adjusted for age or applicable during anesthesia. Trends are more useful for evaluating renal function than a single laboratory measurement.

### Serum Creatinine

Serum creatinine concentration, which reflects the balance between creatinine production by muscle and its renal excretion, is often used as a marker of GFR. In contrast to blood urea nitrogen (BUN) concentration, serum creatinine level is not influenced by protein metabolism or the rate of fluid flow through renal tubules. It is, however, influenced by skeletal muscle mass. Furthermore, increases in serum creatinine are not typically noted until GFR has declined by at least 50%. Thus, increased creatinine level may serve as a late marker of renal injury. For example, elderly patients, with known decreases in GFR, frequently display normal serum creatinine concentrations because of decreased creatinine production as a consequence of the decrease in skeletal muscle mass. Indeed, mild increases in the serum creatinine concentration in elderly patients may suggest significant renal disease. Likewise, in patients with chronic renal failure, serum creatinine concentrations may not accurately reflect the GFR because of (1) decreased creatinine production, (2) the presence of decreased skeletal muscle mass, or (3) nonrenal (gastrointestinal tract) excretion of creatinine. GFR can be estimated from serum creatinine by a variety of methods including the following formula:

$$GFR = (140 - age) \times weight\ (in\ kg)/(serum\ creatinine \times 72)$$

### Blood Urea Nitrogen

BUN concentrations, which are normally 10 to 20 mg/dL, vary with changes in GFR. The relationship between serum creatinine and BUN levels is particularly useful in diagnosing the cause of renal failure. Like serum creatinine, increases in BUN level are frequently a late sign of renal injury and are affected by dietary intake, coexisting illnesses, and intravascular fluid volume. For example, high-protein diets or gastrointestinal bleeding can increase the production of urea and thereby result in increased BUN concentrations (azotemia) despite a normal GFR. Other causes of increased BUN concentrations in the presence of normal GFR are increased catabolism during febrile illnesses and dehydration. Conversely, BUN concentrations can remain normal in the presence of low-protein diets despite decreases in GFR.

Increased BUN concentrations relative to serum creatinine in the presence of dehydration likely reflect increased urea absorption due to decreased urinary flow through the renal tubules, which results in a BUN-creatinine ratio more than 20. Although BUN concentration is susceptible to multiple extraneous influences, values more than 50 mg/dL inevitably reflect a decreased GFR.

### Creatinine Clearance

Creatinine clearance (normal, 110 to 150 mL/min) is a measurement of the ability of the glomeruli to excrete creatinine into urine for a given serum creatinine concentration. Because clearance does not depend on corrections for age or the presence of a steady state, measurement of GFR is more reliable than the serum BUN or creatinine values. The principal disadvantage of this test, however, is the need for timed (2 hours may be as acceptable as 24 hours) urine collections. Creatinine clearance (CrCl) and by proxy GFR can be calculated from the formula

$$GFR = CrCl = Ucr \times V/Pcr$$

where Ucr is urine creatinine, Pcr is plasma creatinine drawn at midpoint of the timed collection, and V is urinary flow rate.

### Proteinuria

Small amounts of protein are normally filtered through glomerular capillaries and then reabsorbed in the proximal convoluted tubules. Proteinuria (excretion of more than 150 mg of protein per day) is most likely due to

| **Table 28.1** | Tests Used for Evaluation of Renal Function | |
|---|---|---|
| **Test** | **Normal Value** | **Factors That Influence Interpretation** |
| **Test of Glomerular Filtration** | | |
| Blood urea nitrogen | 8-20 mg/dL | Dehydration<br>Variable protein intake<br>Gastrointestinal bleeding<br>Catabolism |
| Serum creatinine | 0.5-1.2 mg/dL | Age<br>Skeletal muscle mass<br>Catabolism |
| Creatinine clearance | 120 mL/min | Accurate urine volume measurement |
| **Tests of Tubular Function** | | |
| Urine specific gravity | 1.003-1.030 | All are affected by dehydration, solutes, filtrates, proteins, diuretics, dehydration, drugs, and extremes of age |
| Urine osmolality | 350-500 mOsm | |
| Urine sodium | 20-40 mEq | |

abnormally high filtration rather than impaired reabsorption by the renal tubules. Intermittent proteinuria occasionally occurs in healthy individuals when standing and disappears when supine. Other nonrenal causes of proteinuria include exercise, fever, and congestive heart failure.

### Urine Indices

Measurement of urine osmolality and urinary sodium and calculation of the fractional excretion of sodium can help differentiate between prerenal and renal tubular causes of azotemia.

### Newer Tests of Renal Function

Several new markers of renal function have recently been identified. Serum cystatin C, a ubiquitous protein that is exclusively excreted by glomerular filtration, is less influenced by variations in muscle mass and nutrition than creatinine. It may better predict risk of death and end-stage renal disease (ESRD) across diverse populations.[4]

Other biomarkers such as $N$-acetyl-$\beta$-D-glucosaminidase, kidney injury molecule-1, and interleukin 18 are promising in the early detection of kidney injury. These biomarkers may have a role in the future in reducing morbidity and mortality rates associated with kidney injury in the perioperative setting.[5]

## Pharmacology of Diuretics

### Thiazide Diuretics

Thiazide diuretics (hydrochlorothiazide, chlorthalidone) are generally administered for the treatment of essential hypertension and for mobilization of the edema fluid that is associated with renal, hepatic, or cardiac dysfunction. Diuresis occurs as a result of the inhibition of reabsorption of sodium and chloride ions from the early distal renal tubules. Side effects associated with diuretic-induced hypokalemia may include (1) skeletal muscle weakness, (2) increased risk for digitalis toxicity, and (3) enhancement of nondepolarizing neuromuscular blocking drugs (Table 28.2).

**Table 28.2**  Side Effects of Diuretics

| Diuretic Class | Hypokalemic, Hypochloremic Metabolic Alkalosis | Hyperkalemia | Hyperglycemia |
| --- | --- | --- | --- |
| Thiazide diuretics | Yes | No | Yes |
| Loop diuretics | Yes | No | Minimal |
| Osmotic diuretics | No | No | No |
| Aldosterone antagonists | No | Yes | No |

### Loop Diuretics

Loop diuretics (ethacrynic acid, furosemide, bumetanide) inhibit the reabsorption of sodium and chloride and augment the secretion of potassium, primarily in the loop of Henle. Intravenous administration of these drugs produces a diuretic response within minutes. Chronic administration of loop diuretics may result in hypochloremic, hypokalemic metabolic alkalosis and, in rare instances, deafness.[6]

### Osmotic Diuretics

The most frequently administered osmotic diuretic is the six-carbon sugar mannitol. Mannitol produces diuresis because it is filtered by the glomeruli and not reabsorbed within the renal tubules. This leads to increased osmolarity of the renal tubule fluid and associated excretion of water.

Mannitol increases fluid movement from intracellular spaces into extracellular spaces such that intravascular fluid volume expands acutely. This redistribution of fluid from intracellular to extracellular compartments decreases brain size and intracranial pressure (also see Chapter 30). Mannitol may further diminish intracranial pressure by decreasing the rate of cerebrospinal fluid formation.

### Aldosterone Antagonists

Spironolactone blocks the renal tubular effects of aldosterone and offsets the loss of potassium from administration of thiazide diuretics. Ascites and peripheral edema secondary to cirrhosis of the liver is often treated with spironolactone. The most serious toxic effect of spironolactone is hyperkalemia. Serum potassium concentration should be monitored closely in patients taking spironolactone.

### Dopamine and Fenoldopam

Dopamine dilates renal arterioles via its agonist action at the DA1 receptor, leading to increased renal blood flow and GFR. Treatment with low-dose dopamine (0.5 to 3 µg/kg/min) may increase urine output but yet not alter the course of renal failure. In addition, dose-dependent side effects of dopamine include tachydysrhythmias, pulmonary shunting, and tissue ischemia (gastrointestinal tract, digits).[7,8]

Fenoldopam, a dopamine analog, also possesses DA1 agonist activity but lacks the adrenergic activity of dopamine. It also increases renal blood flow and GFR, which may help the treatment of acute kidney injury. Yet its role in the treatment of renal failure is unclear. It is currently approved for short-term parenteral treatment of severe hypertension.[9]

## Pathophysiology of End-Stage Renal Disease

ESRD causes profound physiologic changes that affect several organs (Box 28.2 and Table 28.3).

IV

**Box 28.2** Changes Characteristic of Chronic Renal Disease

- Anemia
- Decreased ejection fraction
- Decreased platelet adhesiveness
- Hyperkalemia
- Unpredictable intravascular fluid volume
- Metabolic acidosis
- Systemic hypertension
- Pericardial effusion
- Decreased sympathetic nervous system activity

**Table 28.3** Stages of Chronic Renal Failure

| Stage | Glomerular Filtration Rate (mL/min/1.73 m$^2$) |
|---|---|
| 1 | >90 |
| 2 | 60-89 |
| 3 | 30-59 |
| 4 | 15-29 |
| 5 | <15 |

Cardiovascular Disease

Cardiovascular disease is the predominant cause of death in patients with ESRD. Acute myocardial infarction, cardiac arrest of unknown cause, cardiac dysrhythmias, and cardiomyopathy account for more than 50% of deaths in patients receiving dialysis. Hypertension commonly exists in patients with ESRD. This systemic hypertension can be severe and refractory to antihypertensive therapy. Hypervolemia and excess activation of the renin-angiotensin-aldosterone system are the most common causes.

Additionally, the accumulation of uremic toxins and metabolic acids may contribute to poor myocardial performance. Yet, the presence of ESRD with significantly depressed cardiac function does not necessarily contraindicate renal transplantation because cardiac ventricular function often improves after transplantation.

Uremia causes changes in lipid metabolism that lead to increased concentrations of serum triglycerides and reduced levels of protective high-density lipoproteins. Thus, ESRD accelerates the progression of atherosclerosis. Pericardial disease and cardiac dysrhythmias can also be encountered in patients with ESRD. Pericardial effusions typically resolve when patients are adequately dialyzed.

Metabolic Disease

Many patients with ESRD also have diabetes mellitus. Kidney failure as a result of diabetes develops in nearly 30% to 40% of patients with ESRD and accounts for 30% of those on the waiting list for kidney transplantation. In fact, nephropathy develops in nearly 60% of insulin-dependent diabetic patients. Patients with ESRD and diabetes have a more likely risk of cardiovascular problems than do patients with renal failure alone.[10]

Once patients are unable to excrete their dietary fluid and electrolyte loads, abnormalities in plasma electrolyte concentrations (sodium, potassium, calcium, magnesium, and phosphate) can develop. The most life-threatening electrolyte abnormality is hyperkalemia.

Anemia and Abnormal Coagulation

Patients with renal failure generally display a normochromic, normocytic anemia because of decreased erythropoiesis and retained toxins that are secondary to renal failure. Treatment with recombinant erythropoietin can frequently increase hemoglobin concentrations. Symptoms of fatigue are reduced and both cerebral and cardiac function are improved. Occasionally, recombinant erythropoietin therapy may exacerbate preexisting essential hypertension. Patients with renal failure may also display uremia-induced defects in platelet function.

## Management of Anesthesia in Patients With End-Stage Renal Disease

General anesthesia with tracheal intubation provides acceptable hemodynamics, excellent skeletal muscle relaxation, and a predictable depth of anesthesia in patients with ESRD who are undergoing major operations. Patients with advanced stages of comorbid conditions may require more extensive monitoring, such as continuous monitoring of systemic blood pressure and perhaps central venous pressure. Large variations in arterial blood pressure may occur with hypotension being more likely than hypertension during maintenance of anesthesia. This is especially the case if the patient has recently been hemodialyzed in preparation for the surgical procedure. Those with the most severe comorbid conditions, such as symptomatic coronary artery disease or a history of congestive heart failure, may benefit from monitoring with a pulmonary artery catheter or transesophageal echocardiography (TEE).

The status of hemodialysis shunts or fistulas should be monitored and documented (e.g., presence of a palpable thrill) during positioning and intraoperatively to confirm continued patency. Peripheral lines and arterial blood pressure monitoring cuffs should not be placed in proximity to such implanted vascular access devices.

Normal saline (NS) is often given instead of lactated Ringer solution for intravascular fluid resuscitation in patients with ESRD. The rationale is the hypothesized risk of hyperkalemia from potassium contained in lactated Ringer solution. Yet this conclusion has not been proved to be likely. For example, a prospective randomized double-blind clinical trial comparing the two intraoperative fluid therapies in ESRD patients undergoing renal transplantation has shown more hyperkalemia and greater degree of acidosis with NS than lactated Ringer solution.[11]

Patients with uremia and other comorbid conditions (e.g., diabetes mellitus) are at an increased risk for aspiration of gastric contents during induction of anesthesia. The use of a rapid-sequence induction of anesthesia technique may be indicated in such patients. Succinylcholine is not contraindicated in patients with ESRD. The increase in serum potassium concentration after a large dose of succinylcholine is approximately 0.6 mEq/L for patients both with and without ESRD. This increase can be tolerated without imposing a significant cardiac risk, even if initial (i.e., preanesthetic) serum potassium concentration is more than 5 mEq/L.

Several strategies have achieved adequate heart rate and arterial blood pressure control during induction of anesthesia. Moderate to large doses of opioids, such as fentanyl, can blunt the response to laryngoscopy. However, systemic blood pressure is frequently more difficult to maintain after induction of anesthesia, and hypotension may require treatment with vasoconstrictors. The short-acting β-adrenergic blocker esmolol can blunt the hemodynamic response to tracheal intubation and is ideally suited for patients with an adequate ejection fraction.

Drugs or their metabolites that depend on renal elimination (pancuronium, vecuronium, morphine, meperidine) should be used cautiously or avoided. Cisatracurium is a good choice as most of it is metabolized by spontaneous Hoffman degradation, which makes its duration of action independent of liver or kidney function. The elimination half-life of rocuronium is increased because of increased volume of distribution with no change in clearance. Mivacurium is metabolized by plasma cholinesterase but its action may be prolonged by 10 to 15 minutes as a result of reduced cholinesterase activity in these patients (also see Chapter 11). Because morphine has long-acting renally excreted metabolites such as morphine-6-glucuronide, alternative opioid choices are preferred (e.g., fentanyl, sufentanil, alfentanil, remifentanil).

Appropriate choices of inhaled anesthetics include desflurane, isoflurane, and sevoflurane. The metabolism of sevoflurane to inorganic fluoride has been implicated in experimental studies of renal toxicity, although no controlled human studies are available to indicate either safety concerns or danger when using sevoflurane in the setting of ESRD.

## Differential Diagnosis and Management of Perioperative Oliguria

### Prerenal Oliguria

Prerenal oliguria is characterized by the excretion of concentrated urine that contains minimal amounts of sodium (Table 28.4). Excretion of highly concentrated and sodium-poor urine confirms that renal tubular function is intact and reflects an attempt by

| Table 28.4 | Oliguria Versus Acute Tubular Necrosis: Preoperative Differential Diagnosis | |
|---|---|---|
| **Diagnostic Feature** | **Prerenal Oliguria** | **Acute Tubular Necrosis** |
| Fractional excretion of sodium | <1% | >3% |
| Urine specific gravity | >1.015 | 1.01-1.015 |
| Urine sodium (mEq/L) | <40 | >40 |
| Urine osmolality (mOsm/L) | >400 | <400 |
| Causes | Decreased renal blood flow (hypotension, hypovolemia, decreased cardiac output) | Renal ischemia, nephrotoxins, free hemoglobin or myoglobin |

the kidneys to conserve sodium and restore intravascular fluid volume in response to decreased renal blood flow. The decreased renal blood flow most likely reflects an acute decrease in intravascular fluid volume or decreased cardiac output. Other causes of decreased renal blood flow are sepsis, liver failure, and congestive heart failure.[11]

The initial management of patients with perioperative oliguria is influenced by their risk for the development of acute renal failure. A brisk diuresis in response to an intravascular fluid challenge suggests that an acute decrease in intravascular fluid volume is the cause of the prerenal oliguria. When intravascular fluid replacement does not result in increased urine output, intrinsic renal disease or hemodynamic causes should be considered. Prompt recognition and treatment of prerenal oliguria is critical as prolonged severe ischemia can lead to necrosis of renal tubules and convert reversible injury to irreversible intrarenal disease.

Administration of diuretics to maintain or stimulate urine flow in the perioperative period is controversial. One theory is that prevention of renal tubule urine stasis with diuretics can prevent prerenal oliguria from progressing to acute tubular necrosis. Nevertheless, urine output that is enhanced by the administration of a diuretic does not necessarily predict postoperative renal function. There is no evidence that drug-induced diuresis (dopamine, furosemide, mannitol) in the presence of reduced cardiac output or hypovolemia, or both, protects renal function. In fact, a recent meta-analysis of clinical trials did not find any interventions (e.g., diuretics, dopamine and its analogs, calcium channel blockers, angiotensin-converting enzyme inhibitors, specific hydration fluids, N-acetylcysteine, ANP, or erythropoietin) that can reduce the risk of perioperative renal failure.[12]

**IV**

**Table 28.5** Liver Function Tests With Normal Values

| Test | Normal Values[a] |
| --- | --- |
| Albumin | 3.5-5.5 g/dL |
| Bilirubin | 0.3-1.1 mg/dL |
| Unconjugated bilirubin (indirect reacting) | 0.2-0.7 mg/dL |
| Conjugated bilirubin (direct reacting) | 0.1-0.4 mg/dL |
| Aspartate aminotransferase (i.e., SGOT) | 10-40 U/mL |
| Alanine aminotransferase (i.e., SGPT) | 5-35 U/mL |
| Alkaline phosphatase | 10-30 U/mL |
| Prothrombin time | 12-14 s |

[a]Normal values for each individual laboratory should be considered in interpreting liver function test results.
*SGOT,* Serum glutamic-oxaloacetic (acid) transaminase; *SGPT,* serum glumate-pyruvate transaminase.

### Intrinsic Renal Disease

Acute tubular necrosis, glomerulonephritis, and acute interstitial nephritis are intrinsic renal causes of oliguria. In contrast to oliguria secondary to hypovolemia, the urine of patients with acute tubular necrosis is poorly concentrated and contains excessive amounts of sodium (Table 28.5). Intrinsic renal disease is the most severe of the different forms of oliguria and is typically the hardest to reverse.

### Postrenal Oliguria

An obstruction that is distal to the renal collecting system usually involves a mechanical problem such as a blood clot in the ureter, bladder, or urethra. Surgical ligation, renal calculi, and edema are other postrenal causes of low urine output. Another common postrenal cause is bladder catheter obstruction. Postrenal oliguria is frequently reversible once the source of the obstruction is removed.[13]

## LIVER DISEASE

The liver is responsible for the production of essential plasma proteins, the metabolism and detoxification of drugs and deleterious xenobiotics, the absorption of critical nutrients, and carbohydrate metabolism. Impaired liver function affects nearly every organ system in the body.

### Hepatic Blood Flow

The liver is unique in that it receives a dual afferent blood supply that is equal to about 25% of cardiac output (Fig. 28.3). Approximately 70% of hepatic blood flow is supplied by the portal vein with the remainder supplied by the hepatic artery. Under normal conditions, each blood vessel contributes roughly 50% to the liver's

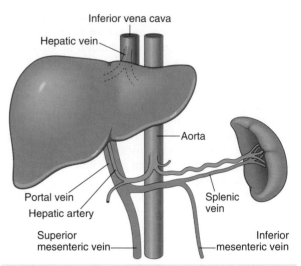

**Fig. 28.3** Schematic depiction of the dual afferent blood supply to the liver provided by the portal vein and hepatic artery. About 70% of hepatic blood flow is via the portal vein, with the remainder via the hepatic artery. Total hepatic blood flow is directly proportional to perfusion pressure across the liver and inversely related to splanchnic vascular resistance. Cirrhosis of the liver increases resistance to blood flow through the portal vein and decreases hepatic blood flow.

oxygen supply. Portal vein flow is not regulated and is susceptible to systemic hypotension and decreases in cardiac output.

### Intrinsic Determinants of Hepatic Blood Flow

Reduction in portal flow (up to a 50% reduction) is compensated by modulating hepatic artery tone to maintain perfusion to the liver. This is primarily mediated via the hepatic arterial buffer response, which reciprocally varies hepatic arterial blood flow to changes in portal flow mediated by adenosine. The response is stimulated by low pH and $O_2$ content and increased $P_{CO_2}$. Volatile anesthetics and cirrhosis of the liver attenuate this reciprocal relationship and render the liver vulnerable to ischemia.

### Extrinsic Determinants of Hepatic Blood Flow

Hepatic perfusion pressure (mean arterial or portal vein pressure minus hepatic vein pressure) and splanchnic vascular resistance determine hepatic blood flow. The splanchnic vessels receive vasomotor innervation from the sympathetic nervous system. Splanchnic nerve stimulation (pain, arterial hypoxemia, surgical stress) increases splanchnic vascular resistance and decreases hepatic blood flow.

Surgical stimulation and the proximity of the operative site to the liver are important determinants of the magnitude of the decrease in hepatic blood flow seen during general anesthesia. β-Adrenergic receptor blockers such as propranolol are associated with decreases in hepatic blood flow. Positive-pressure ventilation of the lungs, congestive heart failure, and administration of excessive intravascular fluid cause increased central venous pressure, resulting in increased hepatic venous pressure, which effectively decreases hepatic perfusion pressure and blood flow.

## Glucose Homeostasis

The liver is the main organ for the storage and release of glucose. Hepatocytes extract glucose via an insulin-mediated mechanism, where it can be stored as glycogen. Glucagon-mediated catabolism of glycogen (glycogenolysis) releases glucose back into the systemic circulation for maintenance of euglycemia. Surgical stress, starvation, and sympathetic nervous system activation stimulate glycogen depolymerization to glucose. When glycogen stores are depleted hepatic gluconeogenesis from substrates such as lactate, glycerol, and certain amino acids restores blood glucose levels.

## Coagulation

Hepatocytes are responsible for the synthesis of the majority of procoagulant proteins as well as regulators such as proteins C and S and antithrombin III. An important exception to this is factor VIII, which is partially produced in endothelial cells. Vitamin K, which is absorbed by bile secretion into the gastrointestinal tract, plays an important role in catalysis of some of the procoagulant proteins to produce factors II, VII, IX, and X. Laboratory studies such as prothrombin time (international normalized ratio [INR]), partial thromboplastin time (PTT), and fibrinogen levels can be used to evaluate impaired coagulation and hepatic function. Impaired laboratory studies reflect significant hepatic dysfunction because most coagulation factors maintain function at up to 20% to 30% of their normal levels.

## Drug Metabolism

Hepatic drug metabolism is characterized by the conversion of lipid-soluble drugs to more water-soluble forms to facilitate renal excretion, transformation to pharmacologically less active substances, and excretion in bile.

Three major pathways are utilized to accomplish these goals. Phase 1 metabolism involves an increase in polarity of drugs via cytochrome P and mixed function oxidases. Phase 2 metabolism involves conjugation of metabolites to water-soluble substrates. Phase 3 elimination relies on energy-dependent excretion of drugs into bile. Chronic liver disease may interfere with the metabolism of drugs because of the decreased number of enzyme-containing hepatocytes or the decreased hepatic blood flow that typically accompanies cirrhosis of the liver. Prolonged elimination half-times for morphine, alfentanil, diazepam, lidocaine, pancuronium, and vecuronium occur in patients with cirrhosis of the liver. Likewise, chronic drug therapy can inhibit hepatic enzymes and inhibit metabolism of anesthetic drugs leading to higher circulating blood levels. Conversely, enzyme induction, particularly of cytochrome P isoforms, can also occur as a response to chronic therapy with drugs such as phenytoin, isoniazid, and rifampin or as a result of alcohol abuse. Induction of hepatic enzymes can increase metabolism of administered anesthetic and therapeutic drugs, thereby reducing plasma levels.

## Heme Metabolism

Although fetal erythrocyte production occurs exclusively in the liver, hepatic hematopoiesis accounts for only 20% of adult heme synthesis with the remainder produced in the bone marrow. Heme synthesis occurs from glycine and succinyl coenzyme A (CoA) through a reaction catalyzed by aminolevulinic acid (ALA) synthase. ALA synthase is the rate-limiting step in the heme synthesis pathway and is regulated by feedback inhibition by its end product heme. Porphyrias are rare genetic diseases characterized by interruption of feedback inhibition of ALA synthase.

Heme degradation, primarily by the reticuloendothelial system, results in formation of bilirubin as an end product. Formed bilirubin is then bound to plasma albumin for transport to the liver, where it is extracted and conjugated for secretion into canalicular bile. The majority of bilirubin excretion occurs in the gut, although a small portion is recirculated to the liver via the enterohepatic circulation. This accounts for the small amount of bilirubin conjugates present in blood. Conjugated bilirubin is water soluble and about 10% is excreted in the urine.

## Cholesterol and Lipid Metabolism

The liver stores dietary fat as triglycerides, cholesterol, and phospholipids and releases free fatty acids via triglyceride hydrolysis. In addition, the liver synthesizes free fatty acids from glucose, lipids, and protein. The liver also plays an important role in regulation of cholesterol uptake, metabolism, and transport. Bile salts, the end product of cholesterol synthesis, serve as regulators of lipid metabolism. Elimination of cholesterol is achieved by biliary secretion and by excretion of bile acids.

## Protein Metabolism

The liver plays a vital role in protein metabolism. Numerous biologically active proteins including albumin, cytokines, hormones, and coagulation factors are manufactured in the liver. In addition, nonessential amino acid synthesis can also occur in hepatocytes when necessary.

IV

Protein degradation is another important function of the liver. The urea (Krebs) cycle is utilized by hepatocytes to convert the end products of amino acid degradation, such as ammonia and other nitrogenous waste products, to urea, which is readily excreted by the kidney. Severe hepatic dysfunction, such as that which occurs in end-stage liver disease (ESLD), leads to accumulation of ammonia in the serum resulting in hepatic encephalopathy (HE).

## Pathophysiology of End-Stage Liver Disease

### Cardiovascular Complications

Severe parenchymal disease that has advanced to the point of cirrhosis usually results in a hyperdynamic circulation. Hemodynamic measurements generally reveal normal to low systemic blood pressure, increased cardiac output, and decreased systemic vascular resistance. Decreased systemic vascular resistance is a result of vasodilation and abnormal anatomic and physiologic shunting. Physiologic shunting is the passage of blood from the arterial to the venous side of the circulation without effectively traversing a capillary bed. Abnormal blood vessels, such as those seen in the skin as spider angiomas, represent an anatomic shunt.[14,15]

### Portal Hypertension

High resistance to blood flow through the liver, a hallmark of ESLD, causes an accumulation of blood in the vascular beds that are immediately upstream of the liver. Vessels draining the esophagus, stomach, spleen, and intestines dilate and hypertrophy, which leads to the development of splenomegaly and esophageal, gastric, and intra-abdominal varices. Symptoms of portal hypertension include anorexia, nausea, ascites, esophageal varices, spider nevi, and HE. It is central to the pathogenesis of a variety of complications associated with ESLD including massive hemorrhage, increased susceptibility to infection, renal failure, and mental status changes.

### Pulmonary Complications

ESLD is associated with the hepatopulmonary syndrome and portopulmonary hypertension. Hepatopulmonary syndrome develops as a result of intrapulmonary arteriovenous communications that are not ventilated, impairment of hypoxic pulmonary vasoconstriction, atelectasis, and restrictive pulmonary disease secondary to ascites and pleural effusion. Arterial hypoxemia, secondary to the hepatopulmonary syndrome, may improve somewhat with supplemental oxygen in the early stages of the disease, but oxygen may not be effective with disease progression.

Portopulmonary hypertension is an increase in intrapulmonary vascular pressure in patients with portal hypertension. The cause is not well established. This syndrome occurs in less than 5% of patients, including the liver transplant population. Nevertheless, these patients are at increased risk for acute right-sided heart failure if physiologic conditions that increase pulmonary vascular resistance (acidosis, arterial hypoxemia, hypercapnia) occur during anesthesia. Hepatic hydrothorax, defined as pleural effusions occurring in the absence of cardiopulmonary disease, can also occur in up to 10% of cirrhotic patients. In some patients, the pleural effusions from hepatic hydrothorax are large enough to impair oxygenation.

### Hepatic Encephalopathy

Altered mental state is a frequent complication of both acute and chronic liver failure with a clinically variable presentation ranging from minor changes in brain function to deep coma. The cause of this complex neuropsychiatric syndrome is multifactorial. The serum concentrations of many chemicals, which are normally filtered by the healthy liver and are present in higher concentrations with hepatic dysfunction, likely play an important role. Ammonia is heavily implicated as a precipitating factor of episodes of HE. Other etiologic factors include disruption of the blood-brain barrier, increased central nervous system inhibitory neurotransmission, and altered cerebral energy metabolism. The reversibility of symptoms of HE with administration of flumazenil supports an important role for the GABA (γ-aminobutyric acid) receptor activation in HE pathogenesis. It is also important to rule out other causes of altered mental status in the patient with liver disease, such as intracranial bleeding or masses, hypoglycemia, or a postictal state. As effective treatments for many of the putative etiologic factors in HE do not yet exist, current treatment still revolves around reducing the production and absorption of the ammonia. Typically, neomycin (to reduce ammonia production by urease-producing bacteria) and the administration of lactulose (to reduce ammonia absorption) are employed.[16]

### Impaired Drug Binding

When liver disease is so severe that albumin production is decreased, fewer sites are available for drug binding. This limited availability can increase levels of the unbound, pharmacologically active fraction of drugs, such as thiopental and alfentanil. Increased drug sensitivity as a result of decreased protein binding is most likely to be manifested when plasma albumin concentrations are lower than 2.5 g/dL.

### Ascites

Ascites is a common complication of cirrhosis affecting up to 50% of cirrhotic patients. The development of ascites is associated with significant morbidity and heralds the end stages of cirrhosis. Complications associated with ascites include marked abdominal distention (leading to atelectasis and restrictive pulmonary disease), spontaneous bacterial peritonitis, and circulatory instability due to compression of the inferior vena cava and right atrium. Although the exact mechanism of ascites is unclear, excess sodium retention by the kidney, decreased oncotic pressure due to hypoalbuminemia, and portal hypertension appear to play a central role. Initial therapy includes restriction of fluid administration, reduction of sodium intake, and administration of diuretics. In severe cases, abdominal paracentesis can be effective at transiently reducing abdominal distention and restoring hemodynamic stability.[17,18] Some patients with refractory ascites are candidates for transjugular intrahepatic portosystemic shunt (TIPS), an interventional radiologic procedure to place a stent between a branch of the hepatic vein and portal vein (also see Chapter 38).

### Renal Dysfunction and Hepatorenal Syndrome

Renal dysfunction can develop in a significant portion of patients with cirrhosis. A variety of etiologic factors including diuretic therapy, reduced intravascular volume secondary to ascites or gastrointestinal hemorrhage, nephrotoxic drugs, and sepsis can provoke acute renal failure and ultimately acute tubular necrosis in cirrhotic patients.

In the absence of obvious factors precipitating renal failure, the hepatorenal syndrome (HRS) can be diagnosed. HRS is characterized by intense renal vasoconstriction as an end-stage response to decreased effective arterial blood volume. Type 1 HRS, typically presenting as rapidly progressing prerenal failure, is associated with a poor prognosis in the absence of therapeutic intervention. Conversely, type 2 HRS presents with a milder degree of renal dysfunction. Treatment with octreotide, glucagon, and midodrine have shown some promise at reversing type 1 HRS.[19,20]

## Effects of Anesthesia and Surgery on the Liver

### Impact of Anesthetics on Hepatic Blood Flow

Inhaled anesthetics and regional anesthesia both typically decrease hepatic blood flow 20% to 30% in the absence of surgical stimulation. These changes reflect drug- or technique-induced effects on hepatic perfusion pressure or splanchnic vascular resistance, or both. For example, reduced hepatic blood flow from volatile anesthetics, as well as regional anesthesia (T5 sensory level), is likely due to decreased hepatic perfusion pressure. Autoregulation (increased hepatic artery blood flow offsetting decreases in portal vein blood flow) of hepatic blood flow may be best maintained with isoflurane. However, hepatic blood flow during the administration of desflurane and sevoflurane is maintained by a similar mechanism.

### Volatile Anesthetic-Induced Hepatic Dysfunction

A rare, but life-threatening form of hepatic dysfunction may reflect an immune-mediated hepatotoxicity caused by halothane. Two patterns of hepatic injury have occurred with use of halothane. A mild form occurs in up to 20% of patients and is associated with minimal sequelae. A rare fulminant form is associated with a fatality rate of 50% to 70%. Risk factors for development of this condition include prior exposure to halothane, age older than 40 years, obesity, and female gender. Isoflurane and desflurane are also capable of causing hepatic dysfunction, but the incidence of hepatitis after exposure to these volatile anesthetics is extremely rare, mainly because of the decreased magnitude of metabolism in comparison to halothane. Given its rare incidence and the disappearance of halothane in modern clinical practice in North America, volatile anesthetic–induced hepatic dysfunction remains a diagnosis of exclusion in the patient presenting with hepatitis in the perioperative period.[20,21]

## Management of Anesthesia in Patients With End-Stage Liver Disease

### Preoperative Evaluation of Liver Disease

Liver function tests (Table 28.6) detect the presence of liver disease preoperatively and establish the diagnosis when postoperative liver dysfunction occurs. The Child-Pugh and Model for End-Stage Liver Disease (MELD) scores are two methods of evaluating severity of liver dysfunction (Table 28.7). Patients with Child-Pugh class C liver dysfunction or MELD score greater than 14 have an increased risk for perioperative morbidity and death. Morbidity and mortality rates after elective operations are more frequent in patients with preexisting cirrhosis of the liver than in patients

**Table 28.6** Child-Pugh Classification System and MELD Score Formula for Liver Disease

| Finding | Child-Pugh Score A | B | C |
|---|---|---|---|
| Serum bilirubin (mg/dL) | <2.0 | 2.0-3.0 | >3.0 |
| Serum albumin (g/dL) | >3.5 | 2.8-3.5 | <2.8 |
| Prothrombin time (seconds prolonged) | 1-4 s | 4-6 s | >6 s |
| Ascites | None | Slight | Moderate |
| Encephalopathy | None | Minimal | Advanced |

**MELD (Model for End-Stage Liver Disease) Score Formula**

MELD score = $(0.957 \times \log_e [\text{serum creatinine (mg/dL)}] + 0.378 \times \log_e [\text{total serum bilirubin (mg/dL)}] + 1.120 \times \log_e [\text{INR}]) \times 10$

Minimum for all values is 1.
Maximum value for creatinine is 4.

**Table 28.7** Classification and Causes of Postoperative Liver Dysfunction

| Diagnostic Feature | Prehepatic | Intrahepatic | Posthepatic |
|---|---|---|---|
| Bilirubin | Increased (unconjugated fraction) | Increased (conjugated fraction) | Increased (conjugated fraction) |
| Aminotransferase enzymes | No change | Markedly increased | Normal to slightly increased |
| Alkaline phosphatase | No change | No change to slightly increased | Markedly increased |
| Prothrombin time | No change | Prolonged | No change to prolonged |
| Albumin | No change | Decreased | No change to decreased |
| Causes | Hemolysis<br>Hematoma reabsorption<br>Bilirubin overload from whole blood | Viruses<br>Drugs<br>Sepsis<br>Arterial hypoxemia<br>Congestive heart failure<br>Cirrhosis | Stones<br>Cancer<br>Sepsis |

undergoing similar operations but in the absence of liver disease.[20,21]

Unfortunately, liver function tests are rarely specific. Postoperative liver dysfunction is more likely in the presence of coexisting liver disease. Furthermore, the large reserve of the liver means that considerable hepatic damage can be present before liver function test results become altered. Indeed, cirrhosis of the liver may cause little alteration in liver function. It may take additional stressors, such as anesthesia and surgery, to reveal the underlying liver disease. Inadequate hepatocyte function during anesthesia and surgery can be manifested as metabolic acidosis intraoperatively.

### Intraoperative Management

Most major operations in patients with significant liver disease involve the use of general anesthesia. Regional techniques can be considered in selected patients who have normal coagulation values.

The magnitude of the operation determines the extent of invasive monitoring that is required. Major operations during which blood loss is likely require continuous means of monitoring arterial blood pressure (arterial line) and filling pressure (central venous line). Patients with significant comorbid conditions (including cardiac diseases) undergoing procedures involving large anticipated blood loss may require placement of a pulmonary artery catheter.

Correction of severe coagulopathy before vascular line placement should be considered. Ultrasound guidance may minimize the risk of complications related to vascular access. Communication with the blood bank (also see Chapter 24) before surgery is crucial to ensure adequate availability of red blood cells, platelets, and clotting factors, including fresh frozen plasma and cryoprecipitate. In patients with esophageal varices, the risk of bleeding from insertion of a TEE probe is increased.

### Induction and Maintenance of Anesthesia

Most patients have well-preserved cardiac function and no significant systemic or pulmonary hypertension. Induction of anesthesia can be achieved with an intravenous anesthetic such as propofol, thiopental, or etomidate, along with opioids and short- or intermediate-acting neuromuscular blocking drugs. Intravenous anesthetics have minimal impact on hepatic blood flow provided arterial blood pressure is adequately maintained. Thus, arterial blood pressure should be preserved and sympathetic stimulation avoided, which also has an adverse effect on hepatic blood flow. A rapid-sequence or modified rapid-sequence induction of anesthesia is warranted if patients have significant ascites or delayed gastric emptying. Hypotension after induction of anesthesia occurs commonly as a result of the low systemic vascular resistance and relative hypovolemia. This can usually be treated with small doses of vasoconstrictors such as phenylephrine. With the exception of halothane, all volatile anesthetics are suitable for patients with severe liver disease. No optimal anesthetic technique has been established for the maintenance of anesthesia.

### Management of Coagulopathy

Traditionally, surgical blood loss and coagulopathy have been managed by administering blood products either by clinical judgment alone, if bleeding is rapid, or guided by conventional laboratory tests (e.g., PTT, INR, platelet count), if bleeding is controlled (also see Chapter 24). Standard laboratory testing, however, can be slow to yield results and does not provide information about the qualitative aspects of clot formation.

Advances in point-of-care coagulation technology, such as rotational thromboelastometry and platelet function analysis, however, allow the clinician to rapidly diagnose and manage coagulopathy associated with ESLD in the perioperative setting. Additional information, unavailable through conventional laboratory tests, such as clot strength, platelet function, and hyperfibrinolysis, can be assessed rapidly at the bedside with these newer techniques.[22]

The introduction of various factor concentrate therapies, such as prothrombin complex concentrate and fibrinogen concentrate, into clinical practice may also play a significant role in blood product management in patients with ESLD. Hemostatic algorithms that utilize point-of-care coagulation testing and factor concentrate-based therapy are showing considerable promise in the management of patients with coagulopathy related to liver disease.[23]

## Postoperative Jaundice

Halothane or other volatile anesthetics are often implicated as the cause of postoperative jaundice, but there are many other and probably more likely causes (see Table 28.7). A surgical cause of postoperative jaundice is likely if the operation involved the liver or biliary tract. Similarly, multiple blood transfusions and resorption of surgical hematoma can lead to jaundice in the perioperative period. Drugs, including antibiotics, and other metabolic or infectious causes such as sepsis, must also be considered in the differential diagnosis of postoperative jaundice.

## Management of Anesthesia in Intoxicated Patients

Acutely intoxicated patients require less anesthetic because there is an additive depressant effect between alcohol and anesthetics. Lower minimum alveolar concentration (MAC) levels in the acutely intoxicated patient may also reduce the amount of volatile anesthetic needed to maintain anesthesia. Intoxicated patients are more vulnerable to regurgitation of gastric contents and aspiration pneumonia because alcohol slows gastric emptying and decreases the tone of the lower esophageal sphincter.

## Alcohol Withdrawal Syndrome

Initial symptoms of alcohol withdrawal, including agitation, tachycardia, and signs of increased sympathetic stimulation, may be subtle and mistaken for other common perioperative complications such as pain and delirium. However, a history of chronic alcohol use should always prompt consideration of this entity in the differential diagnosis and prophylactic benzodiazepine treatment may be promptly initiated. Manifestations of severe alcohol withdrawal syndrome (delirium tremens) usually appear 48 to 72 hours after cessation of drinking. This syndrome represents a medical emergency. Such patients may manifest tremulousness and hallucinations. There is significantly increased activity of the sympathetic nervous system with subsequent catecholamine release, leading to diaphoresis, hyperpyrexia, cardiac dysrhythmias, and hemodynamic instability. In some patients, grand mal seizures may be the first indication of alcohol withdrawal syndrome. When seizures occur, hypoglycemia and other possible causes, including brain injury, should also be ruled out.

### Treatment

Treatment of delirium tremens must be aggressive and typically consists of benzodiazepine administration at regular intervals. A β-antagonist (propranolol or esmolol) can be used to control the heart rate. If mental status declines significantly, airway protection may be achieved by endotracheal intubation. Correction of fluid, electrolyte (magnesium, potassium), and metabolic (thiamine) derangements is important. Despite aggressive treatment, mortality rate from delirium tremens is about 10%. Death is often due to hemodynamic instability, cardiac dysrhythmias, or seizures.[24]

## DISEASES OF THE BILIARY TRACT

Gallstones are reported to be present in 10% of men and 20% of women between 55 and 65 years of age. These patients usually have normal liver function test results, except for increased serum bilirubin or alkaline phosphatase concentrations due to choledocholithiasis (common bile duct stone) or chronic cholangitis. Gilbert syndrome, a benign disorder causing elevation in unconjugated bilirubin, is one of the most common causes of jaundice and may occasionally be mistaken for postoperative hepatobiliary dysfunction. Conversely, Dubin-Johnson and Rotor syndromes are congenital disorders leading to elevated conjugated bilirubin levels that can be exacerbated by surgery.

## Management of Anesthesia

Anesthesia for cholecystectomy or exploration of the common bile duct, or both, is influenced by the effect of the drugs used for anesthesia on intraluminal pressure in the biliary tract. Specifically, opioids can produce spasm of the choledochoduodenal sphincter, which increases common bile duct pressure. Such spasm may impair the passage of contrast medium into the duodenum and erroneously suggest the need for sphincteroplasty or the presence of common bile duct stones. However, opioids have been used in many instances without adverse effect, which emphasizes the fact that not all patients respond to opioids with choledochoduodenal sphincter spasm. Treatment of biliary spasm includes naloxone, glucagon, and nitroglycerin.

### Laparoscopic Cholecystectomy
Anesthetic considerations for laparoscopic cholecystectomy are similar to those for other laparoscopic

IV

495

procedures.[24] For example, insufflation of the abdominal cavity (pneumoperitoneum) with carbon dioxide introduced through a needle placed via a supraumbilical incision results in increased intra-abdominal pressure that may interfere with ventilation of the lungs and venous return. During laparoscopic cholecystectomy, placement of the patient in the reverse Trendelenburg position favors movement of the abdominal contents away from the operative site and may facilitate mechanical ventilation of the lungs. This position, however, may further interfere with venous return. Generous intravascular fluid replacement during laparoscopic cholecystectomy may facilitate recovery from this type of surgery.[25]

Monitoring end-tidal carbon dioxide concentrations during laparoscopic abdominal surgical procedures is useful because of the unpredictability of systemic absorption of the carbon dioxide used to create the pneumoperitoneum. Intraoperative decompression of the stomach with a nasogastric or orogastric tube may decrease the risk for visceral puncture at the time of needle insertion and may subsequently improve laparoscopic visualization. Administration of nitrous oxide during laparoscopic cholecystectomy has typically not been recommended because of the possibility that it could expand bowel gas volume, causing interference with surgical working conditions and the theoretical possibility that diffusion into the abdominal cavity could support combustion.[26] Loss of hemostasis or injury to the hepatic artery or liver may require prompt intervention via a conventional laparotomy incision.

## QUESTIONS OF THE DAY

1. What are the humoral mediators of renal function? What are their effects on the cardiovascular system?
2. What are the complications of administering thiazide, loop, and osmotic diuretics?
3. What is the differential diagnosis of prerenal and postrenal oliguria?
4. What are the physiologic changes associated with end-stage liver disease (ESLD)?
5. What is the differential diagnosis of postoperative jaundice?
6. What are the effects of carbon dioxide insufflation in the abdominal cavity during laparoscopic biliary surgery?

## REFERENCES

1. Mooney JF, Chow CK, Hillis GS. Perioperative renal function and surgical outcome. *Curr Opin Anesthesiol.* 2014;27:195–200.
2. Kheterpal S, Tremper KK, Egnlesbe MJ, et al. Predictors of postoperative acute renal failure after noncardiac surgery in patients with previously normal renal function. *Anesthesiology.* 2007;107:892–902.
3. Hoste E, Clermont G, Kersten A, et al. RIFLE criteria for acute kidney injury are associated with hospital mortality in critically ill patients: a cohort analysis. *Crit Care.* 2006;10:R73.
4. Shlipak MG, Coresh J, Gansevoort RT. Cystatin C versus creatinine for kidney function-based risk. *N Engl J Med.* 2013;369:2457–2459.
5. Mårtensson J, Martling CR, Bell M. Novel biomarkers of acute kidney injury and failure: clinical applicability. *Br J Anaesth.* 2012;109(6):843–850.
6. Sica DA. Diuretic use in renal disease. *Nat Rev Nephrol.* 2011;8:100–109.
7. ANZICS Clinical Trials Group. Low-dose dopamine in patients with early renal dysfunction: a placebo-controlled randomized trial. *Lancet.* 2000;356:2139–2143.
8. Friedrich JO, Adhikari N, Herridge MS, et al. Meta-analysis: low dose dopamine increases urine output but does not prevent renal dysfunction or death. *Ann Intern Med.* 2005;142:510–524.
9. Landoni G, Biondi-Zoccai GG, Tumlin JA, et al. Beneficial impact of fenoldopam in critically ill patients with or at risk for acute renal failure: a meta-analysis of randomized clinical trials. *Am J Kidney Dis.* 2007;49:56–68.
10. Jones DR, Lee HT. Perioperative renal protection. *Best Pract Res Clin Anaesthesiol.* 2008;22:193–208.
11. O'Malley CM, Frumento RJ, Hardy MA, et al. A randomized, double-blind comparison of lactated Ringer's solution and 0.9% NaCl during renal transplantation. *Anesth Analg.* 2005;100:1518–1524.
12. Zacharias M, Mugawar M, Herbison GP, et al. Interventions for protecting renal function in the perioperative period. *Cochrane Database Syst Rev.* 2013;(9):CD003590.
13. Sear JW. Kidney dysfunction in the postoperative period. *Br J Anaesth.* 2005;95:20–32.
14. Kiamanesh D, Rumley J, Moitra VK. Monitoring and managing hepatic disease in anaesthesia. *Br J Anaesth.* 2013;111(suppl 1):i50–i61.
15. Moller S, Henriksen JH. Cardiovascular complications of cirrhosis. *Gut.* 2008;57:268–278.
16. Sundaram V, Shaikh OS. Hepatic encephalopathy: pathophysiology and emerging therapies. *Med Clin North Am.* 2009;93:819–836.
17. Gines P, Cardenas A, Arroyo V, et al. Management of cirrhosis and ascites. *N Engl J Med.* 2004;350:1646–1654.
18. Schuppan D, Afdhal NH. Liver cirrhosis. *Lancet.* 2008;371:838–851.
19. Gines P, Schrier RW. Renal failure in cirrhosis. *N Engl J Med.* 2009;361:1279–1290.
20. Hoetzel A, Ryan H, Schmidt R. Anesthetic considerations for the patient with liver disease. *Curr Opin Anaesthesiol.* 2012;25:340–347.
21. Muilenburg DJ, Singh A, Torzilli G, et al. Surgery in the patient with liver disease. *Anesthesiol Clin.* 2009;27:721–737.
22. Mallett SV. Clinical utility of viscoelastic tests of coagulation (TEG/ROTEM) in patients with liver disease and during liver transplantation. *Semin Thromb Hemost.* 2015;41(5):527–537.
23. Theusinger OM, Stein P, Levy JH. Point of care and factor concentrate-based coagulation algorithms. *Transfus Med Hemother.* 2015;42(2):115–121.
24. Kosten TR, O'Connor PG. Management of drug and alcohol withdrawal. *N Engl J Med.* 2003;348:1786–1795.
25. Gerges FJ, Kanazi GE, Jabbour-Khoury SI. Anesthesia for laparoscopy: a review. *J Clin Anesth.* 2006;18:67–78.
26. Diemunsch PA, Torp KD, Van Dorsselaer T, Mutter D. Nitrous oxide fraction in the carbon dioxide pneumoperitoneum during laparoscopy under general inhaled anesthesia in pigs. *Anesth Analg.* 2000;90:k951–k953.

# 29 NUTRITIONAL, GASTROINTESTINAL, AND ENDOCRINE DISEASE

Amy C. Robertson and William R. Furman

## NUTRITIONAL DISORDERS

### Morbid Obesity

Approximately 1.9 billion people worldwide are considered overweight, which is defined as a body mass index (BMI, weight in kg/height in m$^2$) between 25 to 30.[1] A desirable BMI is 18 to 25. The Centers for Disease Control and Prevention report that approximately 34% of U.S. adults older than 20 years of age are overweight and 35% are obese (BMI 30 to 40).[2] Morbid obesity is defined by a BMI of 40 or more. Superobesity (BMI ≥ 50) and super-superobesity (BMI ≥ 60) are an increasingly frequent health care challenge.[3]

The morbidity associated with obesity can affect virtually any part of the body and may account for 2.5 million deaths per year. Pulmonary manifestations of obesity include a reduced functional residual capacity (with rapidly decreasing oxygen saturations during apnea), restrictive lung disease, and obstructive sleep apnea. Hypertension, stroke, and right-sided heart failure are associated with morbid obesity, as are colon and breast cancer. Increased intra-abdominal pressure may predispose to hiatal hernias and gastroesophageal reflux. Skeletal diseases are also common, including back pain and osteoarthritis, particularly affecting the knees. Endocrine abnormalities may lead to reproductive hormonal imbalances and impaired fertility, and these patients may also be at increased risk for depression and other psychological illnesses.[4]

The combination of specific complications of obesity is called the *metabolic syndrome*. The metabolic syndrome has six components: abdominal obesity, atherogenic dyslipidemia, hypertension, insulin resistance (glucose intolerance), a proinflammatory state, and a prothrombotic

The editors and publisher would like to thank Dr. Steven Hyman for contributing to the chapter on this topic in the prior edition of this work.

state. The metabolic syndrome is diagnosed by the presence of three of the five following factors: abdominal obesity, increased triglycerides, low high-density lipids, hypertension, and increased fasting blood glucose concentrations. The diagnosis and treatment are important because obesity alone predicts approximately 25% of all new-onset cardiovascular disease.[5]

The pathophysiology of morbid obesity is multifactorial and involves genetic, environmental, metabolic, and psychosocial factors. Caloric consumption is important, but the urge to eat (or overeat) can be modulated by hormones or inflammation. Treatment must be multifaceted; weight loss is not as easy as simply not eating because fasting releases several orexigenic (appetite-stimulating) hormones.[6,7]

### Perioperative Considerations (Also See Chapter 13)

In the 1970s, fasted obese patients were asserted to have larger, more acidic gastric fluid volumes than nonobese patients and therefore at increased risk for pulmonary aspiration of injurious gastric contents.[8] Actually, just the opposite may be true. Nondiabetic obese patients may have a smaller volume of gastric contents with a higher pH than do lean nondiabetic patients.[9]

The care of obese patients presents several logistical issues because of their size and shape. These issues include intravenous (IV) access, noninvasive blood pressure monitoring, positioning, endotracheal intubation, and emergence techniques. Because of the amount of subcutaneous fat, insertion of a peripheral IV line may be difficult. As a result, central venous catheterization may be required for access, independent of the nature of the surgical procedure. Noninvasive blood pressure monitoring may be made difficult by the conical shape of the upper arm. Most arterial blood pressure cuffs are designed for a more cylindrical profile and may not remain in position or function correctly on a cone-shaped arm. Practical options in this situation include utilizing the forearm or inserting an arterial catheter for arterial blood pressure monitoring.

An obese patient may be wider than the horizontal surface of the operating table, and the table must be able to support the patient's weight and be able to move into positions required by the surgeon. If extreme angles of tilt are needed, the patient must be well secured and potential pressure points must be addressed.

Induction of anesthesia may be complicated by a rapid decrease of blood oxygen saturation because of a smaller functional residual capacity. Reverse Trendelenburg position (head up) can reduce atelectasis in dependent areas of the lung and may also move chest and breast tissue caudally, allowing easier access to the mouth for endotracheal intubation. Obesity may increase the risk of a difficult laryngeal intubation, especially in patients with a Mallampati airway classification score of III-IV, obstructive sleep apnea, reduced mobility of the cervical spine, and large neck circumference.[10,11]

No anesthetic drug has a distinct advantage in the obese patient, but emergence can be prolonged because elimination of some anesthetics from adipose tissues is slow. Obese patients are at risk of developing postoperative hypoxemia from atelectasis and hypercarbia due to airway obstruction. Noninvasive ventilator support in the recovery room may improve oxygenation.[12]

### Bariatric Surgery

Surgical treatment of obesity was first described in 1954 with the creation of the jejunoileal bypass (JIB). The JIB was a malabsorptive operation that was used to treat many conditions ranging from hyperlipidemia and atherosclerosis to obesity. The JIB was abandoned by the 1980s because of unacceptable complications, including uveitis, kidney dysfunction, intestinal bacterial overgrowth, and liver damage.[13]

Subsequent operations were directed toward restriction of the intestinal tract with the goal of weight loss through decreased intake. Examples of commonly performed restrictive operations are the gastric bypass, gastric sleeve, and adjustable gastric band. Because of lower early postoperative morbidity and mortality rates, laparoscopic procedures are now preferred as compared to open bariatric procedures.[14] In the United States, the number of bariatric operations peaked in 2004 and has since plateaued. Use of the laparoscopic approach to bariatric surgery accounts for more than 90% of bariatric operations. In-hospital mortality rate is estimated at 0.1%.[15]

Most people who undergo bariatric procedures are morbidly obese (BMI ≥ 40), but surgical weight loss is more effective than conventional medical therapy if BMI is as low as 30.[16] Patients generally have improvements in their quality of life and a reduction in comorbid conditions and cardiovascular events (myocardial infarction and stroke).[17] Bariatric surgery improves several conditions such as hypertension, diabetes, and obstructive sleep apnea.

Appetite and insulin-regulating hormonal function may be changed by bariatric surgery, thus promoting weight loss. Ghrelin, an orexigenic hormone secreted by the gastric fundus and proximal small intestine, is increased in the face of nonsurgical weight loss, but ghrelin levels are either unchanged or decreased after bariatric procedures. Several other intestinal hormones that regulate appetite and glucose metabolism are affected more favorably by bariatric surgery than by fasting. These hormones include glucagon-like peptide-1 (GLP-1), glucose-dependent insulinotropic peptide, and peptide YY, which are all secreted by the gastrointestinal tract in response to food.[18]

## Malnutrition

Malnutrition occurs when caloric requirements exceed intake. Decreased intake, impaired absorption, or increased metabolic rate may cause profound malnutrition in a very short time. Malnutrition may be present when weight loss of 10% to 20% occurs during a short period of time, when weight is less than 90% of ideal body weight, or when BMI is less than 18.5. Healthy patients may quickly become malnourished after an episode of trauma or acute illness.

Critically ill patients develop malnutrition if they are not properly fed. Feeding may take place enterally, through an enteric feeding tube, or parenterally, through an IV catheter. The preferred method of nutritional replacement usually is enteral nutrition because it maintains the absorptive villi of the gastrointestinal tract and reduces pathologic bacterial transfer across the gastrointestinal mucosa and into the bloodstream. Improved outcomes, including decreased infectious complications and fewer ventilator and intensive care unit days, have been demonstrated.[19] Long-term feeding usually requires a gastrostomy or jejunostomy tube. Postpyloric placement is frequently preferred because it is believed to reduce the potential for regurgitation and aspiration of gastric contents. However, the risk of vomiting and aspiration of gastric contents is not significantly different between postpyloric and gastric tube feeding.[20] In patients who have pancreatitis, jejunal placement helps avoid stimulation of pancreatic enzyme secretions.

IV feeding (total parenteral nutrition, or TPN) is required when the gastrointestinal tract is not functional. Peripheral parenteral nutrition may be used for brief periods, but long-term alimentation requires central venous access. TPN lacks the beneficial effects of enteral feeding on the gut and carries risks of catheter sepsis, thrombosis, hyperglycemia, iatrogenic hypoglycemia (from insulin added to the feeding solution in response to hyperglycemia), and the development of fatty liver.

### Perioperative Considerations

Acute nutritional replacement in a malnourished patient may cause a refeeding syndrome, characterized by increased ATP (adenosine triphosphate) production and metabolic rate. Increased ATP production may cause a significant decrease in plasma phosphate, leading to respiratory and cardiac failure. An increased metabolic rate may cause a significant increase in $CO_2$ production, leading to respiratory acidosis. The refeeding syndrome can be avoided by slowly increasing the nutritional intake toward caloric goals.

In the perioperative setting malnourished patients may have muscular (including respiratory) weakness and may be immunocompromised. For severely malnourished patients, TPN or enteral feeding should be administered for 7 to 10 days prior to an elective surgical procedure as it takes several days to achieve goal-feeding levels.

An important clinical issue commonly arises for enterally fed critically ill patients (such as burn and trauma patients) who require a surgical procedure. A decision must be made regarding how long to fast such a patient prior to induction of anesthesia. The risk of pulmonary aspiration of gastric contents must be weighed against the benefit of continuing to keep the nutritional intake at the patient's goal level. Nutrition probably should be continued as long as possible. A short fast (45 minutes) from nutritional administration is reasonable when the feeding tube is located beyond the ligament of Treitz.[21] When TPN is in use, insulin is typically part of the infusion, and therefore blood glucose monitoring should be performed for procedures longer than 2 hours in duration.

## GASTROINTESTINAL DISEASE

### Inflammatory Bowel Disease

Inflammatory bowel disease (IBD) affects an estimated 1.4 million Americans and results from an aberrant response by the bowel mucosal immune system to normal luminal flora.[22] IBD is divided into two categories: ulcerative colitis (UC) and Crohn disease (CD). UC is restricted to the large intestine and manifests itself as inflammation and loss of colonic mucosa. CD can affect any part of the digestive tract and may cause transmural inflammation leading to abscesses or granulomatous disease. Although they are distinct entities, differentiation between the two diseases may be difficult when CD manifests itself by only affecting the colon.

The trigger for the activation of the immune system in IBD is multifactorial. Because of a genetic basis, there is an increased risk in close family members. Caucasian patients are more likely to develop IBD than other patients. Jewish patients have a more frequent risk for CD. In addition, several environmental factors including smoking, appendectomy, antibiotics, oral contraceptives, and nonsteroidal antiinflammatory drugs (NSAIDs) are associated with increased risk. Diagnosis may be suspected based on symptoms of chronic abdominal pain, fever, and diarrhea and is confirmed by endoscopy and biopsy.[23]

Although the primary mode of therapy is nonoperative, 60% to 70% of patients with IBD require surgical treatment at some point. Reasons include complications of the disease (fistulas, strictures, or toxic megacolon), complications of surgery (small bowel obstruction due to postoperative scarring), cancer prevention (colectomy in the case of UC), plus other reasons unrelated to the intestinal disease.[24]

### Perioperative Considerations

CD and UC are chronic diseases that are typically managed by using up to six different classes of medications: antidiarrheal, antiinflammatory, immunosuppressant, antibiotic, anti-TNF (tumor necrosis factor), and other investigational

**IV**

drugs. Patients who are taking steroids should continue to do so prior to surgery and may require supplementation in anticipation of adrenal insufficiency.

Specific anesthetics are neither preferred nor contraindicated for patients with IBD, but certain of their medications may have anesthetic implications. In general, potential interactions between anesthetic and antineoplastic drugs are not clear. Cyclosporine increases the minimum alveolar concentration (MAC) of volatile anesthetics.[25] Azathioprine has phosphodiesterase effects and may partially antagonize nondepolarizing neuromuscular blocking drugs. Cyclosporine and infliximab may enhance the potency of the nondepolarizing neuromuscular blocking drugs.[26] The clinical consequence of these interactions is minimal.

## Gastroesophageal Reflux Disease

Gastroesophageal reflux disease (GERD) is defined as the retrograde movement of gastric contents through the lower esophageal sphincter (LES) into the esophagus. The pathophysiology of GERD involves impaired esophageal motility, LES, and gastric motility.[27] Retrograde movement of gastric contents past both the LES and the upper esophageal sphincter into the pharynx can lead to pulmonary aspiration of gastric acid and particulate matter.

GERD is an extremely common syndrome. The prevalence of GERD—defined as at least weekly heartburn or regurgitation, or both—in the United States is 18% to 28%.[28] Besides heartburn, the most common symptoms are noncardiac chest pain, dysphagia, pharyngitis, cough, asthma, hoarseness, laryngitis, sinusitis, and dental erosions.

Reflux occurs when the LES is incompetent or when LES pressure (LESP) is less than intra-abdominal (or intragastric) pressure. GERD can occur as a result of esophageal dysmotility or a hiatal hernia. In a patient with a hiatal hernia, the LES may be displaced cephalad into the thoracic cavity so that it loses the diaphragmatic contribution to LES function. The diaphragm can also obstruct the esophagus. GERD is associated with other conditions, including pregnancy, obesity, obstructive sleep apnea, gastric hypersecretion, gastric outlet obstruction, gastric neuropathy, and increased intra-abdominal pressure. The risk of pulmonary aspiration of gastric contents during induction of anesthesia in patients with GERD or the previously mentioned predisposing factors is not well established. In contrast, increased intra-abdominal (gastric) pressure and pregnancy are important risk factors. Significant GERD occurs with at least 30% to 50% of pregnant women. The mechanism is primarily a progesterone-mediated relaxation of LES tone, but there also may be contributions from delayed gastric emptying, impaired LES due to increased intra-abdominal pressure from the enlarging gravid uterus, and decreased bowel transit.[29]

Initial management of GERD usually consists of a combination of lifestyle modifications and drug therapy using medications that are moderately effective and have limited side effects. Lifestyle management includes elevating the head of the bed, eating food high in lean protein, and avoiding smoking, coffee, and foods and drugs known to relax the LES. Antacids and mucoprotective drugs may relieve symptoms. If not, further medical management includes drugs that are prokinetic and reduce gastric acid secretion.

Prokinetics minimize contact time of gastric contents with the esophagus by blocking dopamine or serotonin (5-HT [5-hydroxytryptamine]) receptors. Metoclopramide (a 5-HT receptor antagonist) can produce choreoathetosis and other extrapyramidal side effects. Histamine ($H_2$) receptor blockers decrease gastric acid secretion by gastric parietal cells; however, they may increase the production of gastrin and decrease LESP. In some patients, particularly the elderly (also see Chapter 35), $H_2$ receptor blocking drugs may cause adverse central nervous system side effects including confusion, agitation, and psychosis. Proton pump inhibitors (PPIs) are the most potent therapy for severe erosive esophagitis. Omeprazole may inhibit the metabolism and elimination of warfarin, digoxin, phenytoin, and benzodiazepines.[30]

### Perioperative Considerations (Also See Chapter 13)

The customary approach to induction of general anesthesia in the patient at risk for pulmonary aspiration of gastric acid is the rapid-sequence induction (RSI) using cricoid pressure (CP) to obstruct any potential flow of gastric contents into the pharynx and trachea (also see Chapter 14). The putative benefits of the RSI and CP remain controversial. CP can be ineffective, especially if not properly applied, and can have undesired side effects including potentially increasing the risk of regurgitation and failed tracheal intubation. Furthermore, improperly performed CP sometimes might not effectively align the cricoid and esophagus with the solid cervical spine underneath. CP is not a benign procedure and can be associated

| Table 29.1 | Categories of Patients at Risk From Inappropriately Applied Cricoid Pressure |
|---|---|
| **Patient Group at Risk** | **Reason** |
| Elderly | Esophageal rupture, laryngeal obstruction |
| Children | Laryngeal obstruction |
| Parturient | May require more pressure |
| Laryngeal trauma | May require surgical repair after cricoid pressure |
| Cervical spine trauma | May displace an unstable cervical spine |
| Difficult airway | May worsen visualization |

Modified from Brimacombe JR, Berry AM. Cricoid pressure. *Can J Anaesth.* 1997;44:414-425.

with several complications (Table 29.1). In addition, complications are more likely in the elderly, children, pregnant women, patients with cervical injury, and patients with a difficult airway and when there is difficulty palpating the cricoid cartilage.[31]

Surgical management of symptomatic reflux disease may be treated with an antireflux operation—most commonly the Nissen fundoplication in adults. This operation is typically performed laparoscopically. The Nissen fundoplication consists of reducing the herniated stomach, repairing the diaphragmatic defect, and performing a gastric wrap to prevent the stomach and LES from retracting into the thorax. Hypertension, bradycardia, high mean airway pressures, and desaturation are potential intraoperative complications and are a consequence of pneumoperitoneum and increased intra-abdominal pressure. Important postoperative events include discomfort from carbon dioxide gas accumulation under the diaphragm and postoperative nausea and vomiting. Subcutaneous air may also appear in the neck and chest. This is benign and self-limited because $CO_2$ gas is rapidly reabsorbed by the body. Nausea and vomiting are more serious complications associated with esophageal surgery because vomiting can lead to esophageal rupture.[32]

## ENDOCRINE DISORDERS

### Diabetes Mellitus

Between 1990 and 2010, the number of adults with a diagnosis of diabetes more than tripled from 6.5 million to 20.7 million. Diabetes mellitus, a disease that complicates most organ systems, is characterized by increased blood glucose concentrations due to a relative lack of endogenous insulin.[33] Previously, diabetes was classified in terms of insulin requirement (insulin-dependent versus non–insulin-dependent), but this system has proved less satisfactory because nearly all diabetics develop a need for insulin at some point. The current classification labels patients as having either type 1 (T1DM) or type 2 (T2DM) diabetes. T1DM is typically characterized by the absence of insulin production from the pancreas, whereas T2DM involves a relative lack of insulin plus resistance to endogenous insulin.

Blood glucose control is required in both types, but T1DM always requires insulin to prevent hyperglycemia, ketoacidosis, and other complications. Type 2 diabetics may require insulin, but often only require oral hypoglycemic drugs, weight loss, or dietary management. T1DM is commonly heralded at an early age by a dramatic episode of ketoacidosis. The onset of T2DM usually is more insidious. Type 2 diabetics constitute the majority and, unlike type 1 diabetics, are often overweight. Dietary control and weight loss are important in T2DM, but the cornerstone of management of both types is pharmacologic.[34]

Effectiveness of glucose control is monitored by measuring glycated hemoglobin ($HbA_{1c}$) levels. During hyperglycemia, glucose can permanently combine with hemoglobin in erythrocytes and form $HbA_{1c}$. Because erythrocytes normally have a 120-day life span, $HbA_{1c}$ levels give an indication of how well the diabetes is being controlled over time. Normal $HbA_{1c}$ levels are less than 6%, and risk of complications from diabetes increases with higher $HbA_{1c}$ levels.[35]

Insulin is categorized as rapid, intermediate, or long acting. In the outpatient setting it is usually given by subcutaneous injection. For T1DM, intensive therapy consisting of three or more injections per day of basal and prandial insulin or continuous subcutaneous insulin infusion is imperative for improved glycemic control and prevention of ketoacidosis. Metformin is the preferred initial pharmacologic therapy for T2DM. Metformin reduces glucose load by decreasing hepatic production. If non-insulin monotherapy does not achieve target $HbA_{1c}$, the addition of a second oral agent, GLP-1 receptor agonist, or insulin is recommended.[34]

Complications are common in long-standing diabetes and result largely from microangiopathy and macroangiopathy. Diabetes is a well-recognized risk factor for large- and small-vessel coronary artery disease and was originally advanced as an indication for perioperative β-adrenergic blockade.[36] Diabetes in young and middle-aged adults is the leading cause of renal failure requiring hemodialysis. Diabetic retinopathy is characterized by a spectrum of lesions within the retina and is the leading cause of blindness among adults 20 to 74 years old. More than half of all individuals with diabetes eventually develop neuropathy, with a lifetime risk of one or more lower extremity amputations estimated to be 15%. Autonomic neuropathy occurs in 20% to 40% of patients with long-standing diabetes, particularly those with peripheral sensory neuropathy, renal failure, or systemic hypertension. Cardiac autonomic neuropathy may mask angina pectoris and obscure the presence of coronary artery disease. Gastroparesis, which may cause delayed gastric emptying, is a sign of autonomic neuropathy affecting the vagus nerves.[37]

#### Perioperative Considerations

A patient with well-controlled diabetes may not require special treatment before and during surgery, although reducing the morning dose of insulin by 30% to 50% in order to prevent hypoglycemia because of fasting is common and reasonable. Sulfonylurea drugs may be continued until the evening before surgery; however, these drugs may also produce hypoglycemia in the absence of morning caloric intake, so they should not be taken the morning of surgery.[38] (See Chapter 13, medications section for additional recommendations on perioperative insulin management.)

Recommendations regarding biguanides such as metformin have recently changed. The first biguanide introduced, phenformin, was associated with lactic acidosis and was eventually replaced in clinical use by metformin. In the 1990s, a common recommendation was made for metformin to be discontinued 48 hours preoperatively to avoid risk of fatal lactic acidosis. This initial recommendation was based on individual case reports but was questioned by a subsequent meta-analysis.[39]

Perioperative hyperglycemia may result from many causes including stress-induced neuroendocrine changes, exogenous glucose administration, and a patient's underlying metabolic state. Preoperative measurement of blood glucose is usually performed prior to anesthesia; however, the desired intraoperative glucose level is not well established. Perioperative concerns include the risks of diabetic ketoacidosis, severe dehydration and coma related to the hyperosmolar hyperglycemic nonketotic state, the adverse effect of hyperglycemia on neurologic outcome after cerebral ischemia, and the increased risk of surgical wound infection. The optimal level of glucose control in the perioperative and critical care setting remains controversial. Attempts to maintain glucose levels of 81 to 108 mg/dL in critically ill patients resulted in higher rates of cardiovascular mortality and severe hypoglycemia compared to those patients in whom the level was controlled in the range below 180 mg/dL.[40-42]

## Hyperthyroidism and Thyroid Storm

Hyperthyroidism, or thyrotoxicosis, is characterized by increasing circulating levels of unbound thyroid hormones triiodothyronine ($T_3$) and tetraiodothyronine (thyroxine, or $T_4$). The most common cause is Graves disease, an autoimmune condition in which thyrotropin receptor antibodies continuously mimic the effect of thyroid-stimulating hormone (TSH). However, it may also be caused by the following:[43]

- Toxic multinodular goiter
- Thyroiditis
- β-Human chorionic gonadotropin–mediated hyperthyroidism—gestational hyperthyroidism, choriocarcinoma, hydatidiform mole
- Struma ovarii, which is the presence of thyroid tissue in an ovarian teratoma
- The administration of iodinated contrast dye to a susceptible patient
- Drug-induced by amiodarone (which can lead to both hypo- and hyperthyroidism), lithium, interferon-α
- TSH secreting pituitary adenoma

The principal signs and symptoms of hyperthyroidism are cardiac, neurologic, and constitutional. Thyroid hormone increases cardiac sensitivity to catecholamines, resulting in hypertension and tachyarrhythmias. Other signs of severe hyperthyroidism include high-output congestive heart failure or angina, even in the absence of coronary plaques. Tremor, hyperreflexia, and irritability are common neurologic manifestations. Periodic paralysis, characterized by hypokalemia and proximal muscle weakness, may also occur. Fever and heat intolerance are common. Gastrointestinal symptoms include nausea, vomiting, and diarrhea as well as hepatic dysfunction and jaundice. Diagnosis is confirmed by demonstrating increased thyroid hormone levels in blood.[44]

Thyroid storm is characterized by worsening of the signs and symptoms of thyrotoxicosis, including severe cardiac dysfunction, hyperglycemia, hypercalcemia, hyperbilirubinemia, altered mental status, seizures, and coma. Thyroid storm may be triggered in a thyrotoxic patient by any of several stresses:[45]

- Infection
- Stroke
- Trauma, especially to the thyroid gland
- Thyroid and nonthyroid surgery
- Diabetic ketoacidosis
- Drugs: pseudoephedrine, aspirin, excess iodine intake, contrast dye, amiodarone
- Incorrect antithyroid drug discontinuation
- Metastatic thyroid cancer

The distinction between thyrotoxicosis and thyroid storm is one of degree, with thyroid storm being the most severe form of the disorder. All hyperthyroid patients are at risk to develop thyroid storm, which is a life-threatening emergent clinical syndrome that has approximately 30% mortality rate in spite of treatment. For this reason, the general rule regarding surgery in the setting of thyrotoxicosis or thyroid storm is to undertake only that which cannot be delayed until control of thyroid hormone secretion and effect has been accomplished, either with medical management or through ablation of the thyroid using radioiodine.

### Perioperative Considerations

The initial medical treatment for hyperthyroidism is to reduce thyroid hormone synthesis. This is accomplished by administration of a thioamide such as propylthiouracil (PTU) or methimazole (MMI). PTU and MMI inhibit thyroid peroxidase (TPO), the enzyme that catalyzes the incorporation of iodide into thyroglobulin to produce $T_3$ and $T_4$. At least an hour after giving the thioamide, large doses of stable iodide may be given. This step takes advantage of a paradoxic effect, called the *Wolff-Chaikoff effect*. Rather than catalyze additional incorporation of iodide into thyroglobulin, as might be expected, large amounts of iodide suppress gene transcription of TPO, further reducing the gland's capacity to produce and release hormone. This benefit is temporary, lasting about a week.

In addition, especially in cases of thyroid storm, administration of β-adrenergic blockers reduces adrenergic symptoms. Propranolol is the β-blocker traditionally selected because it also inhibits peripheral conversion of $T_4$ to the more potent hormone $T_3$; however, other β-adrenergic blockers such as atenolol, metoprolol, and esmolol have been used and are not contraindicated.[46] Corticosteroids can treat the relative adrenal insufficiency that results from accelerated metabolism in the context of thyroid storm. Cortisol levels tend to be in the normal range in these patients, but they should be higher to be appropriate to the level of stress. Plasmapheresis has been utilized as an adjunct method to reduce circulating thyroid hormone levels by removing $T_3$ and $T_4$ from the bloodstream.[47]

The goal of anesthesia is to avoid an increase in heart rate or sympathetic activation. Conversely, anesthetics and techniques that reduce or blunt sympathetic activity are usually favored. Ketamine would not be ideal to induce anesthesia or provide analgesia. Rather, fentanyl and its congeners would be favored for analgesia. Isoflurane, sevoflurane, and desflurane would all be useful for maintenance of general anesthesia, with the warning that high inspiratory concentrations of desflurane might not be advantageous. Regional anesthesia, when practical, might also be efficacious in avoiding sympathetic activation. Intraoperative thyroid storm may be difficult to distinguish from malignant hyperthermia. Dantrolene is beneficial in either situation and should be considered if there is suspicion of either condition.

## Hypothyroidism

Hypothyroidism is characterized by decreased circulating levels of unbound thyroid hormones $T_3$ and $T_4$. Hypothyroidism may be congenital (cretinism) or acquired. The most common acquired cause in adults is Hashimoto thyroiditis, a chronic autoimmune disease characterized by progressive destruction of the thyroid gland. Medical or surgical treatment of hyperthyroidism may lead to iatrogenic hypothyroidism. Hypothyroidism after radioactive iodine treatment of hyperthyroidism occurs in at least 50% of patients within 10 years after treatment. Secondary hypothyroidism may occur as a consequence of hypothalamic or pituitary disease or after surgery on these structures. The absence of dietary iodine causes hypothyroidism and an enlarged gland ("endemic goiter").[48]

The onset of hypothyroidism usually is insidious, and the symptoms are often nonspecific. Adults may have easy fatigability, lethargy, weakness, and weight gain. The skin is usually dry and the hair brittle. In severe cases, myxedema develops and is characterized by a reduced cardiac output, attenuated deep tendon reflexes, and nonpitting pretibial edema. Untreated, hypothyroidism may progress to include electrolyte disturbance, hypoventilation, hypothermia, and coma.

Hypothyroidism may be either overt or subclinical. Overt hypothyroidism is diagnosed by measuring low $T_3$

and $T_4$ levels in blood. Primary hypothyroidism is characterized by low $T_3$ and $T_4$ levels but an elevated TSH. In secondary hypothyroidism, all thyroid-related hormones are reduced. Subclinical hypothyroidism, manifested by an increased serum concentration of TSH in combination with a normal free $T_4$, is present in about 5% to 8% of the American population, with a prevalence of more than 13% in otherwise healthy elderly patients, especially women.[49]

Hypothyroidism is treated with oral administration of synthetic levothyroxine, 75 to 150 µg/day. Thyroid replacement is initiated slowly because acute cardiac ischemia can develop in patients with coronary artery disease from the sudden increase in myocardial oxygen demand as the metabolism and cardiac output increase. Although IV thyroid replacement therapy is available, its use is limited to severe presentations such as myxedema coma.[48]

### Perioperative Considerations

Asymptomatic mild to moderate hypothyroidism does not increase the risk of perioperative morbidity. Mildly hypothyroid patients do not possess unusual sensitivity to inhaled anesthetics, sedatives, or narcotics. Symptomatic or severe hypothyroidism in contrast should necessitate surgical delay for thyroid hormone replacement until the neurologic and cardiovascular abnormalities have resolved.

## Thyroid Surgery

The most important perioperative considerations related to thyroid surgery involve physical or functional airway obstruction from tracheal compression or damage to the recurrent laryngeal nerves. Airway management is one of the primary challenges for providing safe anesthetic care to patients undergoing thyroidectomy. The potential issues are whether goiters predict difficult bag-mask ventilation, difficult laryngoscopy, and difficult endotracheal intubation. Tracheal compression may lead to the symptoms of dyspnea, wheezing, obstructive sleep apnea, or cough. Patients with thyroid enlargement should be evaluated prior to surgery for evidence of tracheal compression or deviation. Review of available computed tomography scans may reveal the size of the goiter and the resultant alteration of anatomy.[50]

There is a question as to whether tracheal compression or deviation has an impact on outcome. A prospective study reported the incidence of difficult endotracheal intubation in euthyroid patients undergoing a thyroidectomy as 5%; however, the cause of the airway difficulty was not related to the thyroid. Rather, the usual anatomic factors that predict a difficult airway in the general population were the predictors in this patient group. Independent risk factors of difficult intubation were cancerous goiter and Cormack grade III or IV view

**IV**

at laryngoscopy.[51] In the presence of a cancerous goiter, tracheal invasion and tissue infiltration with associated fibrosis may reduce the mobility of laryngeal structures and impede the laryngoscopy view of the glottic opening. In patients with severe tracheal compression causing stridor, intubation of the trachea with the patient awake may be the method of choice to limit the risk of complete airway obstruction after spontaneous ventilation has been ablated. The surgical team should be prepared and ready to perform an emergent tracheotomy or rigid bronchoscopy if necessary.[52]

An important aspect of the anesthetic technique is directed at preventing coughing during emergence as a means of reducing the risk of postoperative hemorrhage. Various methods have been proposed as ways to minimize cough during emergence, including extubation during deep anesthesia and administration of the potent short-acting narcotic remifentanil, the $\alpha_2$-agonist dexmedetomidine, or lidocaine. However, no single method has been proved superior.[53,54]

Postextubation airway compromise following thyroid surgery can result from an expanding wound hematoma, vocal cord dysfunction due to recurrent laryngeal nerve injury, or tracheomalacia. In the past, it was common practice to attempt to perform a direct laryngoscopy after extubation in order to confirm that both vocal cords moved normally. Many practitioners found it difficult to execute this maneuver at exactly the moment when the patient could tolerate laryngoscopy and demonstrate vocal cord mobility. This practice has not been validated as a predictor of postoperative vocal cord dysfunction and is not commonly recommended today.

Unilateral laryngeal nerve injuries from thyroid surgery produce voice impairment but are not a threat to airway function. Bilateral recurrent laryngeal nerve injury, in contrast, compromises the function of the posterior cricoarytenoid muscles, which are the muscles responsible for separating the cords during breathing. This can lead to life-threatening inspiratory airway obstruction that can only be relieved by intubation or tracheostomy. In such patients, the paralyzed vocal cords do not abduct during the respiratory cycle, and may appear apposed in the midline when seen during direct laryngoscopy.

Some surgeons request the use of a laryngeal nerve monitoring endotracheal tube during thyroid surgery as a putative safety measure to prevent inadvertent injury to the laryngeal nerves. These specialized endotracheal tubes have electrodes that are positioned in the immediate vicinity of the vocal cords and send an electromyographic signal to a receiver whenever the vocal cords contract. As a result, if the surgeon stimulates a laryngeal nerve either by retracting it or by using an electrocautery close to it, an audible signal provides a warning.[55]

## Pheochromocytoma and Paraganglioma

Tumor overproduction of any of the adrenal medullary hormones dopamine, norepinephrine, and epinephrine results in hypertension and tachycardia plus cardiovascular hyperresponsiveness to noxious stimulation. The cells that produce these hormones are of neural crest origin. When the tumor arises in the adrenal medulla, it is called a *pheochromocytoma*; when it arises from ganglia of the sympathetic nervous system, it is called a *paraganglioma*. The biologic behavior is the same in either case. Life-threatening hypertensive crises and tachyarrhythmias may occur, especially during surgery on a previously undiagnosed patient. Pheochromocytoma often goes unrecognized because its symptoms (headache, palpitations, sweating) are nonspecific and as many as 8% are asymptomatic. These tumors are relatively rare (approximate prevalence is 1 in 2000 in the general population) and are diagnosed in less than 1% of patients with hypertension.[56]

Hypertension probably occurs because arteriolar smooth muscle has been exposed to norepinephrine, the neurotransmitter for sympathetic nervous system mediated vasoconstriction. According to this theory, tumor-secreted norepinephrine bathes the synapses directly. But if this were true, the production of norepinephrine by the sympathetic nerves should be suppressed and sympathetic nervous system activity should not be able to regulate arterial blood pressure; instead the circulating hormones would do so. This theory has prompted the practice of preoperative $\alpha$-adrenergic blockade with phenoxybenzamine prior to tumor resection. It also may be the basis for the unproven beliefs that blood catecholamine levels correlate with arterial blood pressure values and that hypertension occurs when the surgeon manipulates the tumor because this manipulation squeezes hormones out of the tumor and into the bloodstream.

Other interpretations are likely. Catecholamine levels do not correlate with the time or magnitude of increases in arterial blood pressure value,[57] and clinical experience is that 2 weeks of preoperative treatment with nonselective $\alpha$-adrenergic blockade is commonly ineffective for prevention of intraoperative hypertension. An alternative approach to preoperative preparation should be considered. Hypertension, if present, may be controlled prior to surgery with any of a variety of drugs, and once arterial blood pressure is under reasonable control, the tumor is resected. There is, however, no basis to expect that arterial blood pressure and heart rate lability during the surgery can be entirely prevented, no matter what pretreatment is administered.[58]

An alternate theory of why adrenergic receptor blockade is not fully effective is that chronic catecholamine exposure amplifies the sympathetic nervous system's responses to all forms of physical stimulation. These responses would include hypertension and tachycardia from laryngoscopy and any surgical manipulations. Such hemodynamic responses may be seen in any patient, but the effect may be exaggerated under the influence of high catecholamine levels. Such a theory is supported by animal data suggesting that, despite chronic catecholamine excess, sympathetic nerves remain active and continue to release mediators that influence or even control blood pressure. The failure of competitive receptor blockade might be explained by the ability of the sympathetic nervous system to overwhelm the competitive blockade by releasing norepinephrine in quantities that are much greater than normal.[59]

### Perioperative Considerations

In theory, the nonspecific α-blocking drug phenoxybenzamine should not be chosen because it has $\alpha_2$-blocking properties. Because $\alpha_2$-agonists generally produce bradycardia, sedation, and decreased arterial blood pressure, blocking the $\alpha_2$-receptor should increase arterial blood pressure and heart rate, which would not be the intended therapeutic result. Nevertheless, phenoxybenzamine is often recommended. For the chronic treatment of patients with unresectable catecholamine-secreting tumors, its long pharmacologic half-life is desirable. However, phenoxybenzamine is very expensive, and many less costly alternatives exist for preoperative blood pressure control. The $\alpha_1$-selective blockers (prazosin, doxazosin, terazosin), calcium channel blockers, angiotensin-converting enzyme (ACE) inhibitors and angiotensin receptor blockers, β-adrenergic blockers, and $\alpha_2$-agonists all have been used with beneficial result prior to adrenalectomy. Intraoperative infusions of vasodilators and esmolol still may be required to treat hypertension or tachycardia. Infusions of magnesium and the $\alpha_2$-agonist dexmedetomidine may be useful as well.[60]

## Multiple Endocrine Neoplasia and Neuroendocrine Tumors

The two groups of multiple endocrine neoplasia (MEN) syndromes were originally called *Wermer syndrome* and *Sipple syndrome* but are now known as *MEN type 1* (MEN1) and *MEN type 2* (MEN2), respectively.

### MEN1

This syndrome includes the triad of tumors of the pancreas, pituitary, and parathyroid glands and is inherited as an autosomal dominant trait. Parathyroid tumors, resulting in primary hyperparathyroidism, are the most common feature of MEN1 and occur in approximately 95% of MEN1 patients. All four parathyroid glands usually are removed surgically because all are involved by the disease.

Pancreatic tumors in MEN1 patients are usually adenomas that secrete an excess of a specific hormone. Gastrin secretion is most common, occurring in approximately 40%, but insulin, glucagon, vasoactive intestinal polypeptide, and pancreatic polypeptide secreting tumors are seen. Pituitary tumors most commonly secrete prolactin (60%) or growth hormone (25%). A small number secrete adrenocorticotropic hormone (ACTH), with the balance being nonfunctioning adenomas. Other tumors in MEN1 include adrenocortical adenomas, carcinoids and neuroendocrine tumors, lipomas, angiofibromas, and collagenomas.[61] There are no specific anesthetic implications of MEN1.

### MEN2

Medullary (solid) thyroid carcinomas (MTCs) are a component of two endocrine syndromes, which are now called *MEN2A* and *MEN2B*. MEN2A accounts for 80% of hereditary MTC syndromes. In addition to MTC, up to 50% of patients with MEN2A develop pheochromocytomas and up to 30% develop hyperparathyroidism. MEN2B accounts for 5% of hereditary MTCs and includes mucosal neuromas, pheochromocytoma, and MTC. These patients may have a marfanoid habitus, ocular abnormalities (enlarged corneal nerves, conjunctivitis sicca, and the inability to cry tears), and musculoskeletal manifestations (bowing of the extremities and slipped capital femoral epiphysis). Unlike patients with MEN1, they do not develop parathyroid adenomas. A third subtype of MEN2 is characterized only by familial MTC. All the MEN2 subtypes are autosomal dominant conditions caused by germline activating mutations in the *RET* proto-oncogene on chromosome 10.[62] The anesthetic implications of MEN2 are related to its components and associated conditions. Von Hippel-Lindau disease, which may include cerebellar tumors, is associated with MEN2 and pheochromocytomas.[63] MTC, which accounts for only 5% of all thyroid tumors, is commonly malignant and is the most common cause of death in MEN2 patients. A patient of any age with MTC is therefore likely to undergo thyroidectomy and may be at risk to have an undiagnosed pheochromocytoma at the time of surgery.

### Neuroendocrine Tumors

Carcinoid and neuroendocrine tumors arise from dispersed cells of neural crest embryologic origin. The normal function of these cells is to synthesize serotonin from the essential amino acid tryptophan. When these tumors arise in the midgut, they are called *carcinoid tumors*. When they arise elsewhere in the body, they are called *neuroendocrine tumors*.

The biochemical behavior of these tumors is to overproduce serotonin in preference to the normal products of tryptophan metabolism, including niacin (vitamin $B_3$). In rare instances, patients may therefore develop symptomatic niacin deficiency (pellagra), but this is rare. Most commonly, midgut carcinoid tumors are asymptomatic until they cause bowel obstruction or appendicitis because their venous drainage is via the portal vein to

**IV**

the liver, which detoxifies the excess serotonin they produce. When the tumors arise outside the drainage field of the hepatic portal venous system, or when metastatic disease has replaced so much of the liver as to compromise hepatic synthetic function, systemic symptoms of serotonin excess occur. This is known as the *carcinoid syndrome* and is characterized by diarrhea, flushing, palpitations, and bronchoconstriction. Medical management with octreotide may help ameliorate these symptoms.[64]

### Perioperative Considerations

The direct hemodynamic effects of serotonin usually are not problematic in the context of perioperative anesthetic care, and an escalation of hemodynamic monitoring is seldom required as a consequence of the endocrine activity of the tumor. However, certain medications can trigger mediator release resulting in labile arterial blood pressure. Drugs that trigger mediator release include opioids (particularly meperidine and morphine), neuromuscular blockers (atracurium, mivacurium, and d-tubocurarine), epinephrine, norepinephrine, and dopamine (also see Chapters 9 and 11).

Among those with carcinoid syndrome, approximately 50% develop carcinoid heart disease, which typically causes abnormalities of the right side of the heart. Echocardiography should be considered as a diagnostic tool. Right-sided heart failure, due to the sclerosing effect of serotonin on the tricuspid and pulmonary valves, ultimately may be the cause of death in 50% of patients with the carcinoid syndrome.[65]

## Adrenal Insufficiency and Steroid Replacement

The principal hormones secreted by the adrenal cortex are cortisol and aldosterone. Cortisol production is stimulated by blood concentrations of pituitary ACTH, which is in turn secreted in response to hypothalamic corticotropin-releasing hormone (CRH). Stress stimulates the hypothalamus to release CRH, and blood cortisol levels exert negative feedback influence on the production of both CRH and ACTH. Chronic insufficient cortisol production and secretion, with or without aldosterone insufficiency, is referred to as *Addison syndrome*.[66]

The symptoms of chronic adrenal insufficiency are nonspecific. They include fatigue, malaise, lethargy, weight loss, anorexia, arthralgias, myalgias, nausea, vomiting, abdominal pain, diarrhea, and fever. In primary adrenocortical insufficiency, due to nonfunction of the adrenal glands, hyponatremia and hyperkalemia resulting from concomitant aldosterone deficiency may occur. In secondary or tertiary insufficiency, due to failure of the hypothalamus or pituitary to stimulate the adrenal glands, or when cortisol production is suppressed by exogenously administered steroid medications, aldosterone production is unimpaired. This is because the stimulus for aldosterone production is the renin-angiotensin system. In developed countries, 80% to 90% of cases of primary adrenal insufficiency are caused by autoimmune adrenalitis, which can be isolated (40%) or part of an autoimmune polyendocrinopathy syndrome (60%). Less common causes of primary chronic adrenal insufficiency are malignant (metastatic cancer, commonly from lung or breast) and infectious (such as tuberculosis).[67]

Cortisol maintains homeostasis of the cardiovascular system, especially in the presence of stress. It maintains vascular tone, endothelial integrity, and the distribution of total body water in the vascular compartment. It reduces vascular permeability and it potentiates the vasoconstrictor effects of catecholamines. When cortisol levels are deficient, systemic vascular resistance and myocardial contractility are decreased.

The term *acute adrenal failure*, or *Addisonian crisis*, refers to circulatory shock due to cortisol deficiency. It generally occurs in the presence of primary adrenal insufficiency with a superimposed acute stress such as trauma, surgery, or infection and is characterized by hypovolemic shock with myocardial and vascular unresponsiveness to catecholamines. Treatment usually requires the IV infusion of several liters of isotonic saline and corticosteroid administration. In an adult, 100 mg of IV cortisol (or the equivalent every 6 to 8 hours) usually reverses the pathophysiology within the first day of treatment. Orally administered drugs can be started in 1 to 4 days.[67] The equivalent doses of these drugs are expressed using hydrocortisone, the synthetic form of cortisol, with 100 mg as the standard for comparison (Table 29.2).[68]

Critical illness–related corticosteroid insufficiency (CIRCI) applies to clinical situations in which 100 to 300 mg/day of IV hydrocortisone eliminates a preexisting need for vasopressors.[69] The implication is that the patient may not meet traditional criteria for adrenocortical dysfunction, but the adrenal response to critical illness and other stresses is inadequate. Prior steroid treatment is a potential cause of this condition. Signs and symptoms may include unexplained vasopressor-dependent refractory hypotension, a discrepancy between the anticipated

| Table 29.2 | Relative Equivalent Potencies of Common Corticosteroid Drugs | | |
|---|---|---|---|
| Agent | Equivalent Dose (mg) | Relative Potency | Duration (h) |
| Hydrocortisone | 100 | 1 | 8-12 |
| Cortisone | 125 | 0.8 | 8-12 |
| Prednisone; prednisolone | 25 | 4 | 12-36 |
| Methylprednisolone | 20 | 5 | 12-36 |
| Dexamethasone | 4 | 30 | 36-72 |

severity of the patient's disease and the present state of the patient, high fever without apparent cause or not responding to antibiotics, hypoglycemia, hyponatremia, hyperkalemia, neutropenia, and eosinophilia.

### Perioperative Considerations

Etomidate (also see Chapter 8) is a relatively noncardio-vascular depressant anesthetic that can suppress adrenocortical function. This is a significant but transient effect (<24 hours) even after a single dose of the drug. It can be clinically significant in the setting of CIRCI. Perhaps an anesthetic can be developed with the advantages of etomidate but without its adrenal suppressing effects.[70]

Steroid replacement for the patient who has received exogenous steroids and may have adrenal insufficiency should be adequate but not excessive. The proper dose of replacement steroids is based on surgical research in primates showing that 10 times the normal cortisol production rate was not superior to simply replacing the normal daily production of cortisol.

Stress dose steroid administration during the perioperative period remains controversial (also see Chapter 13). Steroid-induced adrenal suppression is highly variable, and its duration is unpredictable (days to perhaps years). Daily cortisol production rate is between 20 and 30 mg/day. In the past, the recommended approach had been to begin at the time of surgery with a dose between one and five times the daily production (no more than 100 to 150 mg of cortisol equivalent) per day and administer tapered replacement over 48 to 72 hours. However, a recent Cochrane review found only two randomized control trials assessing stress dose of steroids. These studies reported that endogenously produced steroid combined with exogenous steroid administration (i.e., daily dose) is adequate in the perioperative period. The authors concluded that the recommendations on the use of additional corticosteroids for surgical patients receiving preoperative steroids have not been adequately investigated.[66]

## Pituitary Apoplexy

Acute pituitary hemorrhage, swelling, and infarction (pituitary apoplexy) is an exception to the general rule that adrenal crisis is not usually associated with secondary adrenal hypofunction. Pituitary apoplexy is a potentially life-threatening condition that can lead to sudden total loss of all anterior and posterior pituitary hormonal secretion and severe hypoglycemia, hypotension, central nervous system hemorrhage, cerebral edema, and loss of vision (often bitemporal hemianopia).

Two well-known causes of spontaneous pituitary apoplexy are infarction of a large pituitary adenoma and postpartum hypotensive pituitary necrosis (Sheehan syndrome). Other associations include diabetes, hypertension, sickle cell anemia, and acute shock. Acute pituitary hemorrhage into an unsuspected pituitary adenoma has also been reported following cardiopulmonary bypass.[71]

Signs and symptoms of pituitary apoplexy include severe headache, meningeal irritation, bitemporal hemianopia, ophthalmoplegia, cardiovascular collapse, and loss of consciousness. Computed tomography or magnetic resonance imaging most often confirms the diagnosis. Corticosteroid replacement is the first line of treatment, both for the resulting adrenal insufficiency and for brain swelling. If there is significant visual loss or mental status alteration, acute surgical decompression may be required.[72]

## Cushing Syndrome

Cushing syndrome is characterized by elevated cortisol levels in the blood. Primary Cushing syndrome is independent of pituitary ACTH secretion, whereas secondary and tertiary disease is due to increased circulating levels of ACTH or an ACTH-like substance produced by a tumor. The primary condition is usually due to a hyperfunctioning adrenal gland or adenoma. The term *Cushing disease* usually refers to one specific form of secondary Cushing syndrome, that of adrenocortical hyperfunction due to excess production of ACTH by a pituitary adenoma, which accounts for 80% of Cushing syndrome patients. The remainder of the patients with secondary or tertiary Cushing syndrome have abnormal ACTH production from ectopic sources such as primary or metastatic cancers of the lung (usually small cell), thyroid, or prostate; tumors of the pancreas; or intrathoracic neuroendocrine tumors and have an increased ACTH as a result of hypothalamic oversecretion of CRH. Cushing syndrome may also be caused by exogenous administration of cortisol-like medications or synthetic ACTH.

Patients with Cushing syndrome are often recognizable by a physical appearance that consists of rounding of the face, truncal obesity and thin extremities, an upper thoracic fat pad or "buffalo hump," purple abdominal striae, and thinning of the skin. The physiologic effects of chronic elevated corticosteroid levels include weight gain, hypertension, hypercoagulability, muscular weakness, glucose intolerance, gonadal dysfunction, and osteoporosis. Biochemical diagnosis is made by measuring an elevated 24-hour urinary free cortisol.[73]

There is no definitive medical treatment for Cushing syndrome. Effective treatment requires removal of the source of the increased hormone production, followed by corticosteroid replacement therapy if necessary. Anesthetic management of patients with Cushing syndrome may have associated differences as compared to normal patients. For example, they may be more susceptible to the effects of neuromuscular blocking drugs and resultant unanticipated postoperative respiratory

IV

failure (also see Chapter 11), even after laparoscopic surgery.[74]

## QUESTIONS OF THE DAY

1. A morbidly obese patient presents for surgery. What logistical problems may be present during patient positioning and monitoring of vital signs? How can these potential problems be addressed?

2. In a patient at risk for aspiration of gastric contents, what is the potential benefit of cricoid pressure during rapid-sequence induction of anesthesia? What are the risks of inappropriately applied cricoid pressure?

3. A patient with type 2 diabetes mellitus presents on the day of surgery with a serum glucose level of 290 mg/dL. Is additional information needed? What are the risks of proceeding with surgery with this degree of hyperglycemia?

4. A patient develops respiratory distress in the postanesthesia care unit after thyroid surgery. What are the initial steps in management of the patient? What are the potential causes?

5. What are the options for preoperative arterial blood pressure control in a patient with a pheochromocytoma? What medications can be given intraoperatively to treat an episode of severe hypertension in a patient with a pheochromocytoma?

6. What is the rationale for perioperative intravenous steroid administration for a patient who may have adrenal insufficiency? What is the appropriate hydrocortisone dose in this setting?

## REFERENCES

1. World Health Organization (WHO). Obesity and Overweight Fact Sheet. 2015. Accessed August 3, 2015. http://www.who.int/mediacentre/factsheets/fs311/en/.

2. Centers for Disease Control and Prevention (CDC). Prevalence of Overweight, Obesity, and Extreme Obesity Among Adults: United States, 1960–1962 Through 2011–2012. September 2014. http://www.cdc.gov/nchs/data/hestat/obesity_adult_11_12/.htm. Accessed August 3, 2015.

3. Colquitt JL, Pickett K, Loveman E, Frampton GK. Surgery for weight loss in adults. *Cochrane Database Syst Rev.* 2014;(8):CD003641.

4. Jensen MD, Ryan DH, Apovian CM, et al. 2013 AHA/ACC/TOS guideline for the management of overweight and obesity in adults: a report of the American College of Cardiology/American Heart Association Task Force on Practice Guidelines and The Obesity Society. *Circulation.* 2014;129(25 suppl 2): S102–S138.

5. Grundy SM, Brewer HB, Cleeman JI, et al. Definition of metabolic syndrome: report of the National Heart, Lung, and Blood Institute/American Heart Association conference on scientific issues related to definition. *Circulation.* 2004;109:433–438.

6. Peterli R, Steinert RE, Woelnerhanssen B, et al. Metabolic and hormonal changes after laparoscopic Roux-en-Y gastric bypass and sleeve gastrectomy: a randomized, prospective trial. *Obes Surg.* 2012;22:740–748.

7. Illán-Gómez F, Gonzálvez-Ortega M, Orea-Soler I, et al. Obesity and inflammation: change in adiponectin, C-reactive protein, tumour necrosis factor-alpha and interleukin-6 after bariatric surgery. *Obes Surg.* 2012;22:950–955.

8. Vaughan RW, Bauer S, Wise L. Volume and pH of gastric juice in obese patients. *Anesthesiology.* 1975;43:686–689.

9. Harter RL, Kelly WB, Kramer MG, et al. A comparison of the volume and pH of gastric contents of obese and lean surgical patients. *Anesth Analg.* 1998;86:147–152.

10. De Jong A, Molinari N, Pouzeratte Y, et al. Difficult intubation in obese patients: incidence, risk factors, and complications in the operating theatre and in intensive care units. *Br J Anaesth.* 2015;114:297–306.

11. Brodsky JB, Lemmens HJ, Brock-Utne JG, et al. Morbid obesity and tracheal intubation. *Anesth Analg.* 2002;94: 732–736.

12. Hodgson LE, Murphy PB, Hart N. Respiratory management of the obese patient undergoing surgery. *J Thorac Dis.* 2015;7:943–952.

13. Baker MT. The history and evolution of bariatric surgical procedures. *Surg Clin North Am.* 2011;91:1181–1201.

14. Mechanick JI, Youdim A, Jones DB, et al. Clinical practice guidelines for the perioperative nutritional, metabolic, and nonsurgical support of the bariatric surgery patient—2013 update: cosponsored by American Association of Clinical Endocrinologists, The Obesity Society, and American Society for Metabolic & Bariatric Surgery. *Obesity (Silver Spring).* 2013;21(suppl 1): S1–S27.

15. Nguyen NT, Masoomi H, Magno CP, et al. Trends in use of bariatric surgery, 2003-2008. *J Am Coll Surg.* 2011;213:261–266.

16. Varela JE, Frey W. Perioperative outcomes of laparoscopic adjustable gastric banding in mildly obese (BMI < 35 kg/m$^2$) compared to severely obese. *Obes Surg.* 2011;21:421–425.

17. Sjöström L, Peltonen M, Jacobson P, et al. Bariatric surgery and long-term cardiovascular events. *JAMA.* 2012;307:56–65.

18. Martínez-Moreno JM, Garciacaballero M. Influences of the diabetes surgery on pancreatic β-cells mass. *Nutr Hosp.* 2013;28(suppl 2):88–94.

19. Correia MI, Hegazi RA, Higashiguchi T, et al. Evidence-based recommendations for addressing malnutrition in health care: an updated strategy from the feed M.E. Global Study Group. *J Am Med Dir Assoc.* 2014;15(8):544–550.

20. Jiyong J, Tiancha H, Huiqin W, Jingfen J. Effect of gastric versus post-pyloric feeding on the incidence of pneumonia in critically ill patients: observations from traditional and Bayesian random-effects meta-analysis. *Clin Nutr.* 2013;32:8–15.

21. Pousman RM, Pepper C, Pandharipande P, et al. Feasibility of implementing a reduced fasting protocol for critically ill trauma patients undergoing operative and nonoperative procedures. *JPEN J Parenter Enteral Nutr.* 2009;33(2): 176–180.

22. Park KT, Bass D. Inflammatory bowel disease-attributable costs and cost-effective strategies in the United States: a review. *Inflamm Bowel Dis.* 2011;17:1603–1609.

23. Sobczak M, Fabisiak A, Murawska N, et al. Current overview of extrinsic and intrinsic factors in etiology and progression of inflammatory bowel diseases. *Pharmacol Rep.* 2014;66:766–775.

24. Mowat C, Cole A, Windsor A, et al. Guidelines for the management of inflammatory bowel disease in adults. *Gut.* 2011;60:571–607.

25. Niemann CU, Stabernack C, Serkova N, et al. Cyclosporine can increase isoflurane MAC. *Anesth Analg.* 2002;95:930–934.

26. Kumar A, Auron M, Aneja A, et al. Inflammatory bowel disease: perioperative pharmacological considerations. *Mayo Clin Proc.* 2011;86:748–757.

27. Mikami DJ, Murayama KM. Physiology and pathogenesis of gastroesophageal reflux disease. *Surg Clin North Am.* 2015;95:515–525.

28. El-Serag HB, Sweet S, Winchester CC, Dent J. Update on the epidemiology of gastro-oesophageal reflux disease: a systematic review. *Gut.* 2014;63:871–880.

29. Phupong V, Hanprasertpong T. Interventions for heartburn in pregnancy. *Cochrane Database Syst Rev.* 2015;(9):CD011379.

30. Gaumnitz EA. Pharmacologic treatment of GERD. In: Meyer KC, Raghu G, eds. *Gastroesophageal Reflux and the Lung.* New York: Springer; 2012:227–247.

31. Salem MR, Khorasani A, Saatee S, et al. Gastric tubes and airway management in patients at risk of aspiration: history, current concepts, and proposal of an algorithm. *Anesth Analg.* 2014;118:569–579.

32. Samra T, Sharma S. Incidence and severity of adverse events in laparoscopic Nissen fundoplication: an anesthesiologist's perspective. *Anaesth Pain Intensive Care.* 2013;17:233–237.

33. Gregg EW, Li Y, Wang J, et al. Changes in diabetes-related complications in the United States, 1990-2010. *N Engl J Med.* 2014;370:1514–1523.

34. American Diabetes Association. Standards of medical care in diabetes–2013. *Diabetes Care.* 2013;36(suppl 1):S11–S66.

35. Inzucchi SE. Diagnosis of diabetes. *N Engl J Med.* 2012;367:542–550.

36. Fox CS, Golden SH, Anderson C, et al. Update on Prevention of Cardiovascular Disease in Adults With Type 2 Diabetes Mellitus in Light of Recent Evidence: a Scientific Statement From the American Heart Association and the American Diabetes Association. *Circulation.* 2015;132(8):691–718.

37. Forbes JM, Cooper ME. Mechanisms of diabetic complications. *Physiol Rev.* 2013;93:137–188.

38. Kadoi Y. Anesthetic considerations in diabetic patients. Part I: preoperative considerations of patients with diabetes mellitus. *J Anesth.* 2010;24: 739–747.

39. Salpeter SR, Greyber E, Pasternak GA, Salpeter EE. Risk of fatal and nonfatal lactic acidosis with metformin use in type 2 diabetes mellitus. *Cochrane Database Syst Rev.* 2010; (4):CD002967.

40. Akhtar S, Barash PG, Inzucchi SE. Scientific principles and clinical implications of perioperative glucose regulation and control. *Anesth Analg.* 2010;110:478–497.

41. Lipshutz AK, Gropper MA. Perioperative glycemic control: an evidence-based review. *Anesthesiology.* 2009;110(2): 408–421.

42. NICE-SUGAR Study Investigators Finfer S, Chittock DR, Su SY, et al. Intensive versus conventional glucose control in critically ill patients. *N Engl J Med.* 2009;360(13):1283–1297.

43. Vaidya B, Pearce SH. Diagnosis and management of thyrotoxicosis. *BMJ.* 2014;349: g5128.

44. Bahn Chair RS, Burch HB, Cooper DS, et al. Hyperthyroidism and other causes of thyrotoxicosis: management guidelines of the American Thyroid Association and American Association of Clinical Endocrinologists. *Thyroid.* 2011;21:593–646.

45. Chiha M, Samarasinghe S, Kabaker AS. Thyroid storm: an updated review. *J Intensive Care Med.* 2015;30:131–140.

46. Kohl BA, Schwartz S. How to manage perioperative endocrine insufficiency. *Anesthesiol Clin.* 2010;28:139–155.

47. Bajwa SJ, Kaur G. Endocrinopathies: the current and changing perspectives in anesthesia practice. *Indian J Endocrinol Metab.* 2015;19(4):462–469.

48. Almandoz JP, Gharib H. Hypothyroidism: etiology, diagnosis, and management. *Med Clin North Am.* 2012;96:203–221.

49. Garber JR, Cobin RH, Gharib H, et al. Clinical practice guidelines for hypothyroidism in adults: cosponsored by the American Association of Clinical Endocrinologists and the American Thyroid Association. *Thyroid.* 2012;22:1200–1235.

50. Barker P, Mason RA, Thorpe MH. Computerised axial tomography of the trachea. A useful investigation when a retrosternal goitre causes symptomatic tracheal compression. *Anaesthesia.* 1991;46:195–198.

51. Bouaggad A, Nejmi SE, Bouderka MA, Abbassi O. Prediction of difficult tracheal intubation in thyroid surgery. *Anesth Analg.* 2004;99:603–606.

52. Bacuzzi A, Dionigi G, Del Bosco A, et al. Anaesthesia for thyroid surgery: perioperative management. *Int J Surg.* 2008;6(suppl 1):S82–S85.

53. Park JS, Kim KJ, Lee JH, et al. A randomized comparison of remifentanil target-controlled infusion versus dexmedetomidine single-dose administration: a better method for smooth recovery from general sevoflurane anesthesia. *Am J Ther.* 2016;23(3):e690–e696.

54. Lee JH, Koo BN, Jeong JJ, et al. Differential effects of lidocaine and remifentanil on response to the tracheal tube during emergence from general anaesthesia. *Br J Anaesth.* 2011;106:410–415.

55. Bajwa SJ, Sehgal V. Anesthesia and thyroid surgery: the never ending challenges. *Indian J Endocrinol Metab.* 2013;17(2):228–234.

56. Hodin R, Lubitz C, Phitayakorn R, Stephen A. Diagnosis and management of pheochromocytoma. *Curr Probl Surg.* 2014;51:151–187.

57. Bravo EL, Tarazi RC, Gifford RW, Stewart BH. Circulating and urinary catecholamines in pheochromocytoma. Diagnostic and pathophysiologic implications. *N Engl J Med.* 1979;301:682–686.

58. Lenders JW, Duh QY, Eisenhofer G, et al. Endocrine Society. Pheochromocytoma and paraganglioma: an endocrine society clinical practice guideline. *J Clin Endocrinol Metab.* 2014;99(6):1915–1942.

59. Martucci VL, Pacak K. Pheochromocytoma and paraganglioma: diagnosis, genetics, management, and treatment. *Curr Probl Cancer.* 2014;38:7–41.

60. Phitayakorn R, McHenry CR. Perioperative considerations in patients with adrenal tumors. *J Surg Oncol.* 2012;106:604–610.

61. Thakker RV, Newey PJ, Walls GV, et al. Clinical practice guidelines for multiple endocrine neoplasia type 1 (MEN1). *J Clin Endocrinol Metab.* 2012;97:2990–3011.

62. Wells SA, Pacini F, Robinson BG, Santoro M. Multiple endocrine neoplasia type 2 and familial medullary thyroid carcinoma: an update. *J Clin Endocrinol Metab.* 2013;98:3149–3164.

63. Maher ER, Neumann HP, Richard S. von Hippel-Lindau disease: a clinical and scientific review. *Eur J Hum Genet.* 2011;19:617–623.

64. Mancuso K, Mancuso K, Kaye AD, et al. Carcinoid syndrome and perioperative anesthetic considerations. *J Clin Anesth.* 2011;23:329–341.

65. Patel C, Mathur M, Escarcega RO, Bove AA. Carcinoid heart disease: current understanding and future directions. *Am Heart J.* 2014;167:789–795.

66. Yong SL, Coulthard P, Wrzosek A. Supplemental perioperative steroids for surgical patients with adrenal insufficiency. *Cochrane Database Syst Rev.* 2012;(12):CD005367.

67. Charmandari E, Nicolaides NC, Chrousos GP. Adrenal insufficiency. *Lancet.* 2014;383:2152–2167.

68. Liu D, Ahmet A, Ward L. A practical guide to the monitoring and management of the complications of systemic corticosteroid therapy. *Allergy Asthma Clin Immunol.* 2013;9(1):30.

IV

69. Marik PE, Pastores SM, Annane D, et al. Recommendations for the diagnosis and management of corticosteroid insufficiency in critically ill adult patients: consensus statements from an international task force by the American College of Critical Care Medicine. *Crit Care Med.* 2008;36(6):1937–1949.

70. Cotten JF, Husain SS, Forman SA, et al. Methoxycarbonyl-etomidate: a novel rapidly metabolized and ultra-short-acting etomidate analogue that does not produce prolonged adrenocortical suppression. *Anesthesiology.* 2009;111:240–249.

71. Levy E, Korach A, Merin G, et al. Pituitary apoplexy and CABG: should we change our strategy? *Ann Thorac Surg.* 2007;84:1388–1390.

72. Singh TD, Valizadeh N, Meyer FB, et al. Management and outcomes of pituitary apoplexy. *J Neurosurg.* 2015;122:1450–1457.

73. van der Pas R, de Herder WW, Hofland LJ, Feelders RA. New developments in the medical treatment of Cushing's syndrome. *Endocr Relat Cancer.* 2012;19:R205–R223.

74. Kissane NA, Cendan JC. Patients with Cushing's syndrome are care-intensive even in the era of laparoscopic adrenalectomy. *Am Surg.* 2009;75:279–283.

# 30 CENTRAL NERVOUS SYSTEM DISEASE

## Lingzhong Meng and Alana Flexman

The central nervous system (CNS) deserves special consideration in the perioperative setting for several reasons. First, many CNS diseases, such as intracranial tumors or aneurysms, are amenable to surgical treatment. Second, many patients presenting for non-neurologic procedures have concurrent CNS diseases such as prior stroke or Parkinson disease. Third, the CNS is metabolically active with little oxygen reserve and is therefore sensitive to ischemia and hypoxia even for very brief periods of time. The latter is especially important in patients with increased vulnerability to complications from cerebrovascular insufficiency or other flow-relevant abnormalities. This chapter discusses the relevant knowledge base and clinical care needed when taking care of patients with CNS diseases in the perioperative setting.

## NEUROANATOMY

Conceptually, the cranium is divided into supratentorial and infratentorial compartments. The supratentorial compartment contains the cerebral hemispheres and diencephalon (thalamus and hypothalamus), whereas the brainstem and cerebellum make up the infratentorial compartment. In addition, intracranial lesions may be classified as either intra-axial or extra-axial, within or outside the brain parenchyma, respectively. The location of an intracranial lesion has important implications on the anesthetic considerations for that patient and determines the patient's position during surgery. The location of intra-axial mass lesions is particularly relevant, as some lesions may place eloquent areas such as the language centers and motor cortex of the brain at risk. In this case, functional preservation during surgery becomes critically important.

The editors and publisher would like to thank Drs. Lundy Campbell and Michael Gropper for contributing to this chapter in the previous edition of this work. It has served as the foundation for the current chapter.

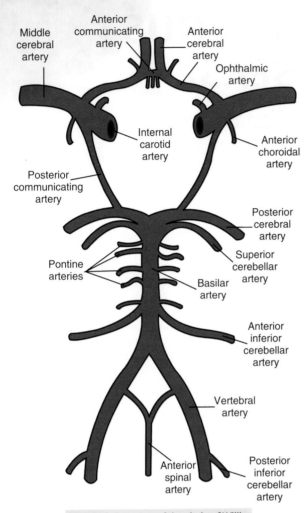

**Fig. 30.1** Anatomy of the circle of Willis.

The arterial blood supply to the brain is through the left and right internal carotid arteries (anterior circulation) and the vertebrobasilar system (posterior circulation). Anastomoses between these vessels form the circle of Willis (Fig. 30.1) and create a collateral blood supply to protect against focal ischemia. However, this ring is not complete in all patients; approximately 20% of the population has an abnormal circulation, implying that the collateralization may not be complete. The clinical significance of an abnormal circle of Willis may depend on the pattern of the abnormality and the coexisting cerebrovascular diseases.

There are 12 pairs of intracranial nerves. It is important to understand the distribution and the sensorimotor and autonomic function of each nerve for the following reasons. First, some neurosurgery procedures may jeopardize specific intracranial nerves during surgery; for example, resection of acoustic neuroma may injure the vestibulocochlear nerve. Second, some of the intracranial nerves are monitored intraoperatively to facilitate timely

detection of reversible injury and theoretically prevent permanent deficit. Both somatosensory and motor evoked potentials are frequently monitored intraoperatively. The anatomy of the sensorimotor cortex and pathways is also important for the anesthesia provider to understand.

The anatomic and functional integrity of the blood-brain barrier has important clinical implications. The blood-brain barrier is composed of capillary endothelial cells with tight junctions that prevent free passage of macromolecules or proteins. In contrast, lipid-soluble substances (carbon dioxide, oxygen, anesthetic drugs) cross the blood-brain barrier easily. The blood-brain barrier may be disrupted by acute systemic hypertension, trauma, infection, arterial hypoxemia, severe hypercapnia, tumors, or sustained seizure activity. Osmotic pharmacologic therapy for intracranial hypertension or the need for intraprocedural brain relaxation relies on an intact blood-brain barrier in order to move the free water from the brain parenchyma to the intravascular space.

## NEUROPHYSIOLOGY

### Regulation of Cerebral Blood Flow

Normal cerebral blood flow (CBF) is approximately 50 mL/100 g/min and represents 12% to 15% of total cardiac output. The brain, albeit being 2% of the total body weight, receives a disproportionately large share of cardiac output because of its high metabolic rate and inability to store energy. Some of the important factors or physiologic processes that regulate CBF include (1) cerebral metabolic rate via neurovascular coupling, (2) cerebral perfusion pressure (CPP) via cerebral autoregulation, (3) arterial blood carbon dioxide and oxygen partial pressure ($Paco_2$ and $Pao_2$, respectively) via cerebrovascular reactivity, (4) sympathetic nervous activity, (5) cardiac output, and (6) some anesthetic drugs. Different regulatory mechanisms may exert distinctive effects on CBF, which are integrated at the level of cerebral resistance arteries/arterioles to determine the CBF.[1,2]

### Cerebral Metabolic Rate and Neurovascular Coupling

Cerebral metabolic rate of oxygen ($CMRO_2$) is often used as an index of the cerebral metabolic activity. $CMRO_2$ and CBF are closely related—an increase or decrease in $CMRO_2$ results in a proportional increase or decrease in CBF. This is named neurovascular coupling or cerebral metabolism-flow coupling. In the perioperative setting, $CMRO_2$ can be reduced by hypothermia and most intravenous anesthetic drugs, which produce a coupled reduction in CBF in healthy brains. CBF decreases 7% for every 1° C decrease in body temperature below 37° C.[3] In contrast, $CMRO_2$ and CBF may be dramatically increased by seizure activity.

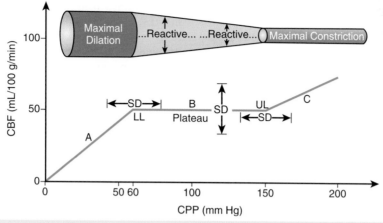

**Fig. 30.2** Cerebral autoregulation describes the relationship between cerebral blood flow (CBF) and cerebral perfusion pressure (CPP). The three key elements of an autoregulation curve are the lower limit (LL), the upper limit (UL), and the plateau. The cerebrovascular reactivity is also illustrated. CBF remains stable in the CPP range between the lower and upper limits and is pressure passive outside this range. As described in the text, there is significant variation among individual patients. *SD*, Standard deviation. (From Meng L, Gelb AW. Regulation of cerebral autoregulation by carbon dioxide. *Anesthesiology.* 2015;122:196-205.)

## Cerebral Perfusion Pressure and Cerebral Autoregulation

CPP is the difference between mean arterial pressure (MAP) and intracranial pressure (ICP) or central venous pressure. How CPP affects CBF is determined by cerebral autoregulation, which maintains a stable CBF during a fluctuating CPP as a result of cerebral vasoconstriction or vasodilation in response to an increase or decrease in CPP, respectively.[1] That is, the simultaneous and proportionate changes in CPP and cerebrovascular resistance due to cerebrovascular pressure reactivity lead to a stable CBF. However, as static cerebral autoregulation takes minutes to take effect, a rapid increase or decrease in MAP may cause a brief period of cerebral hyperperfusion or hypoperfusion, respectively.[4]

The cerebral autoregulation curve has three portions: the plateau, the lower limit, and the upper limit (Fig. 30.2). The lower limit is the CPP level below which the CBF decreases linearly with a decreasing CPP. In contrast, the upper limit is the CPP level above which the CBF increases linearly with an increasing CPP. The plateau is the CPP range between the lower and upper limits where CBF remains stable (approximately 50 mL/100 g/min). The frequently quoted limits of autoregulation are a lower limit of 60 mm Hg and an upper limit of 150 mm Hg. However, although these numbers may apply to young and healthy humans, they may not apply in patients with various medical and surgical comorbid conditions.[1] For example, chronic uncontrolled hypertension or sympathetic stimulation shifts the autoregulatory curve to the right. If this is the case, then a higher minimum CPP will be required to maintain an adequate CBF.

Cerebral autoregulation may be impaired or even abolished following traumatic brain injury and intracranial surgery. As a result, CBF becomes pressure passive, implying that it no longer remains stable across the autoregulatory CPP range and instead changes linearly with changes in CPP. Severe hypercapnia, often as a result of hypoventilation, can also impair cerebral autoregulation. Higher inhaled anesthetic concentrations are potent cerebral vasodilators and impair autoregulation. In contrast, intravenous anesthetic drugs do not disrupt this regulatory mechanism. In circumstances when cerebral autoregulation is impaired, the CPP should be carefully controlled because a change in CPP also changes CBF owing to the loss of autoregulatory capability.

## Cerebrovascular Paco$_2$ and Pao$_2$ Reactivity

Both Paco$_2$ and Pao$_2$ are powerful modulators of CBF and can cause a robust cerebrovascular Paco$_2$- and Pao$_2$-induced reactivity. Changes in Paco$_2$ produce corresponding and same directional changes in CBF when Paco$_2$ is between 20 and 80 mm Hg (Fig. 30.3). CBF increases or decreases approximately 1 mL/100 g/min or 2% for every 1 mm Hg increase or decrease in Paco$_2$ from 40 mm Hg. Such changes in CBF reflect the effect of carbon dioxide–mediated alterations in perivascular pH that leads to cerebral arteriolar dilation or constriction. The Paco$_2$-related change in CBF only lasts for about 6 to 8 hours owing to the compensatory change in bicarbonate ($HCO_3^-$) concentration. Both extreme hyperventilation and hypoventilation should be avoided as they can cause cerebral hypoperfusion and hyperperfusion, respectively. Prolonged aggressive hyperventilation following traumatic brain injury is associated with poorer neurologic outcome.[5] In contrast, decreases in Pao$_2$ less than a threshold value of about 50 mm Hg result in an exponential increase in CBF (see Fig. 30.3), likely a compensatory mechanism to maintain cerebral oxygen delivery (cerebral oxygen delivery = arterial blood oxygen content × CBF).

IV

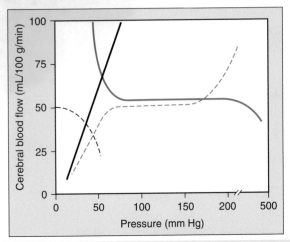

**Fig. 30.3** Schematic depiction of the impact of intracranial pressure *(dashed black line)*, Pao$_2$ *(solid red line)*, Paco$_2$ *(solid black line)*, and cerebral perfusion pressure (mean arterial pressure minus intracranial pressure or central venous pressure, whichever is greater) *(dashed red line)* on cerebral blood flow.

## Effects of Anesthetics on Cerebral Blood Flow

Intravenously administered anesthetic drugs such as propofol and thiopental cause simultaneous reductions of CMRO$_2$ and CBF. The effect of intravenous anesthetics on CBF is attributed to neurovascular coupling, that is, the decrease in CMRO$_2$ leads to a corresponding decrease in CBF. The effects of ketamine on cerebrovascular physiology have been variable, which likely reflects different research study conditions.[6] When ketamine is given on its own without control of ventilation, there is an increase in Paco$_2$, CBF, and ICP. However, when ketamine is given in the presence of another sedative or anesthetic drug in patients whose ventilation is controlled, these effects are not noted. Because of this controversy, however, ketamine is usually avoided in patients with known intracranial disease.

Benzodiazepines and opioids decrease CMRO$_2$ and CBF, analogous to propofol and thiopental, although to a lesser extent. However, associated respiratory depression and increase in Paco$_2$ may produce the opposite effect. Opioids should be cautiously given to patients with intracranial disease because of their (1) depressant effects on consciousness, (2) production of miosis, and (3) depression of ventilation with associated increases in ICP from increased Paco$_2$.

$\alpha_2$-Agonists (clonidine and dexmedetomidine) are unique sedatives in that they do not cause significant respiratory depression. They decrease arterial blood pressure, CPP, and CBF with minimal effects on ICP. $\alpha_2$-Agonists can be used intraoperatively to reduce the dose of other anesthetic drugs and analgesics, or postoperatively as sedatives and to attenuate postoperative hypertension and tachycardia.

In contrast to intravenous anesthetics, volatile anesthetics are potent cerebral vasodilators. When administered during normocapnia at concentrations higher than 0.5 minimal alveolar concentration (MAC), desflurane, sevoflurane, and isoflurane rapidly produce cerebral vasodilation and result in dose-dependent increases in CBF even though CMRO$_2$ is decreased. Therefore, volatile anesthetics produce divergent changes in CMRO$_2$ and CBF that are distinct from those of intravenous anesthetics. When used in isolation, nitrous oxide increases CBF and possibly CMRO$_2$, however, these effects are attenuated by the coadministration of other anesthetics.

## INTRACRANIAL PRESSURE

### Determinants of ICP and the Compensation for an Increased ICP

The intracranial compartment normally contains three components: (1) brain matter, (2) cerebrospinal fluid, and (3) blood. Increases in any of these components or the addition of a pathologic lesion (e.g., tumor) can result in an elevated ICP, defined as a sustained increase of ICP higher than 15 mm Hg. Marked increases in ICP can decrease CPP and thereby CBF to the point of causing cerebral ischemia. However, there is a mechanism that restores ICP to normal in the face of an expanding component. This mechanism is accomplished via compensatory reduction of other intracranial components, including the translocation of cerebrospinal fluid from intracranial space to extracranial space. At the moment when this compensatory mechanism is exhausted, ICP starts to increase and cerebral blood vessels are eventually compressed (Fig. 30.4). CBF must be differentiated from cerebral blood volume (CBV) because the former represents flow whereas the latter applies to the intracranial blood volume. These two terms are related but not interchangeable. The treatment of intracranial hypertension is primarily via the reduction of various intracranial components (Box 30.1).

### Effect of Anesthetics on Intracranial Pressure

Most intravenously administered anesthetics reduce CBF, which is associated with a decrease in ICP. The effect of ketamine is controversial and has been discussed previously. These drugs should be considered in patients whose ICP is abnormally increased. However, large doses of propofol or thiopental may decrease systemic blood pressure and CPP. An increased frequency of excitatory peaks on the electroencephalogram (EEG) of patients receiving etomidate, as compared with thiopental, suggests etomidate should be administered with caution to patients with a history of epilepsy, especially considering that seizure increases CMRO$_2$, CBF, and ICP as a consequence.[7] Opioids and benzodiazepines reduce ICP

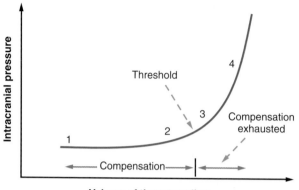

**Fig. 30.4** Graph of the effect of an expanding intracranial component on intracranial pressure (ICP). As the volume of an intracranial component increases from point 1 to point 2 on the curve, ICP remains relatively stable owing to the compensatory mechanisms including the translocation of cerebrospinal fluid from the intracranial space into the spinal subarachnoid space. Between points 1 and 2, the volumetric sum of all intracranial components remains relatively constant. Patients with intracranial tumors who are between point 1 and point 2 on the curve are unlikely to manifest clinical symptoms of increased ICP. The compensation ability is exhausted on the rising portion of the curve (point 3) when a small volumetric increase of the expanding intracranial component leads to a noticeable increase of ICP. Clinical signs and symptoms attributable to increased ICP are likely at this stage. Additional increases in intracranial volume at this point, as produced by increased cerebral blood flow secondary to hypercapnia or inhaled anesthesia, can precipitate abrupt further increases in ICP (point 4).

**Box 30.1** Methods to Decrease Intracranial Pressure

**Cerebral Blood Volume Reduction**
*Decrease Cerebral Blood Flow*
  Intravenous anesthetic drugs are preferred
  Decrease $CMRO_2$ (propofol, barbiturates)
  Employ hyperventilation
  Avoid cerebral vasodilators
  Avoid extreme hypertension

*Increase Venous Outflow*
  Elevate head
  Avoid constriction at the neck
  Avoid PEEP and excessive airway pressure

**Cerebrospinal Fluid Reduction**
External ventricular drain
Lumbar drain
Head elevation (translocation of intracranial cerebrospinal fluid)
Acetazolamide (Diamox)

**Cerebral Edema Reduction**
Osmotic therapy (mannitol, hypertonic saline)
Furosemide (Lasix)
Prevention of ischemia and secondary edema
Dexamethasone to reduce peritumoral vasogenic edema

**Resection of Space-Occupying Lesions**
**Decompressive Craniectomy**

$CMRO_2$, Cerebral metabolic rate of oxygen; *PEEP*, positive end-expiratory pressure.

IV

through reductions in $CMRO_2$ and CBF although this benefit will be offset if respiratory depression and an increase in $Paco_2$ occur.

As discussed previously, volatile anesthetic drugs are cerebral vasodilators and produce dose-dependent increases in ICP that parallel the increases in CBF and CBV. Hyperventilation to decrease $Paco_2$ to less than 35 mm Hg attenuates the tendency for volatile anesthetics to increase ICP. In patients undergoing craniotomy for supratentorial tumors with evidence of a midline shift, neither isoflurane nor desflurane significantly affected lumbar CSF pressure when moderate hypocapnia ($Paco_2$ of 30 mm Hg) was maintained.[8] However, these inhaled anesthetics are better avoided in patients with exhausted ICP-compensating mechanisms as evidenced by increased ICP, abnormal mental status, or imaging studies.

Neuromuscular blocking drugs (also see Chapter 11) do not usually affect ICP unless they induce release of histamine or hypotension. Histamine can cause cerebral vasodilation leading to an increase in ICP. Succinylcholine may increase ICP through increases in CBF although this is not well documented.[9] Because CBF is coupled to $CMRO_2$, a decrease in $CMRO_2$ leads to a decrease in

CBF and thus facilitates the management of intracranial hypertension. Therefore, in patients refractory to initial treatment of intracranial hypertension, a deep level of anesthesia, such as propofol-induced burst suppression or barbiturate coma, can be an alternative option.

## NEUROPROTECTION

Many anesthetics have been proposed as neuroprotectants based on their potential to reduce cerebral metabolic rate and excitotoxicity during periods of oxygen deprivation. Many anesthetics, including volatile anesthetics, barbiturates, propofol, and xenon, can provide neuroprotection in animals; convincing human data are lacking. Hypothermia may provide cerebral protection during acute injury. Several animal studies have shown that decreasing body temperature reduces ischemic injury. However, several large prospective, randomized trials of hypothermia in aneurysm surgery and traumatic brain injury have failed to demonstrate such benefit.[3] Yet, cooling patients with return of spontaneous circulation after cardiac arrest improved neurologic outcome in a randomized controlled trial,[10] although a more recent trial contradicted these findings.[11] In contrast, hyperthermia worsens ischemic injury and should be avoided in patients vulnerable to cerebral ischemia.

## NEUROPHYSIOLOGIC MONITORING

Neurophysiologic monitoring is employed during various neurologic surgeries with increasing frequency because of minimal risk to patients and the potential to reduce intraprocedural neurologic injuries. An understanding of the effects of anesthetics on various monitoring modalities, including the EEG, somatosensory and motor evoked potentials, and intracranial nerve monitoring, is especially critical in neuroanesthesia. The monitoring techniques can be transcranial, direct cortical, or subcortical in approach. Different monitoring modalities often require different anesthetic regimens to preserve the quality of monitoring. Electrocorticography (ECoG) is frequently used during neurologic surgery (also see Chapter 20) to identify epileptic foci or activity (afterdischarge) during epilepsy surgery or surgery with intraoperative stimulation mapping. ECoG is sensitive to anesthetic drugs that change the seizure threshold (e.g., benzodiazepines, propofol, and volatile anesthetics).

## ANESTHESIA FOR NEUROSURGERY

### Preoperative Assessment

Patients presenting for neurosurgical procedures can have a wide range of signs and symptoms (also see Chapter 13). Patients with intracranial mass lesions may present with seizures, altered levels of consciousness, headaches, cranial nerve abnormalities, and motor or sensory deficits. Aneurysms and arteriovenous malformations (AVMs) can present with a severe ("thunderclap") headache if ruptured and focal deficits or visual impairment from compression of the optic chiasm when unruptured. Some neurosurgical patients are asymptomatic and present with an incidental finding.

Evidence of increased ICP should be elicited during the preoperative visit. Clinical signs may be consistent with but do not reliably indicate the level of ICP (Box 30.2). Imaging may reveal a midline shift, encroachment of expanding brain on cerebral ventricles, cerebral edema, hydrocephalus, or any combination of these signs. In symptomatic patients, preoperative medications that cause sedation or depression of ventilation are usually avoided. Drug-induced depression of ventilation can lead to increased $Paco_2$ and subsequent increases in CBF and ICP. In alert patients, small doses of benzodiazepines may provide a useful degree of anxiolysis.

Medications the patient takes should be noted, especially antiepileptic drugs (e.g., levetiracetam), drugs used to reduce peritumoral vasogenic edema (e.g., dexamethasone), and drugs used to reduce brain free water (e.g., mannitol, hypertonic saline). In addition, it is important to note antihypertensive drugs, drugs used for blood glucose control, drugs for chronic pain, and anticoagulants. Abnormal laboratory results should be investigated

---

**Box 30.2** Preoperative Evidence of Increased Intracranial Pressure

Positional headache
Nausea and vomiting
Hypertension and bradycardia
Altered level of consciousness
Altered patterns of breathing
Papilledema

---

and corrected if clinically indicated. Coagulation profile including platelet count and international normalized ratio (INR) and other studies, such as echocardiography, brain magnetic resonance imaging, computed tomography, and angiography, should be reviewed. The side of the brain lesion, left versus right, should be specifically noted.

### Monitoring

In addition to standard monitors, continuous monitoring of systemic blood pressure via a peripheral arterial catheter is recommended. The advantages of invasive arterial blood pressure monitoring include the ability to continuously assess CPP and intravascular volume via indexes such as systolic pressure variation and pulse pressure variation. In addition, these catheters allow analysis of arterial blood gases especially the $Paco_2$. Central venous catheters are not routinely used; however, exceptions include difficult peripheral venous access and the potential need for massive blood transfusion (also see Chapter 24). Measurement of the exhaled carbon dioxide concentration (capnography) is used to adjust mechanical ventilation or assess spontaneous breathing if the airway is not instrumented. The electrocardiogram (ECG) allows prompt detection of cardiac dysrhythmias caused by surgical stimulation of brainstem or intracranial nerves. Neuromuscular blockade is monitored with a peripheral nerve stimulator (also see Chapter 11). Because of the length of these surgical procedures and the use of diuretics, a bladder catheter is often necessary and helps in guiding intravenous fluid therapy. A continuous monitor of ICP is helpful but rarely used after the bone flap is removed and the dura is opened. There are two types of ICP monitors that are inserted by neurosurgeons. The intraventricular catheter or external ventricular device (EVD) permits direct measurement of ICP and drainage of CSF. The subarachnoid or subdural bolt is placed through a burr hole and can be inserted quickly in an emergency setting, but it does not allow for CSF drainage (also see Chapter 20).

### Induction of Anesthesia

The goal of induction of anesthesia is to achieve a sufficient level of anesthesia to blunt the stimulation of direct laryngoscopy and tracheal intubation without compromising cerebral perfusion by increasing ICP or decreasing MAP. Intravenous induction of anesthesia with propofol, 1.5 to 3 mg/kg, thiopental, 3 to 6 mg/kg, or etomidate, 0.2 to 0.5 mg/kg, produces reliable and prompt onset of unconsciousness and is unlikely to adversely increase ICP. However, the specific dose depends on the patient's age, physical condition, and comorbid conditions in addition to the patient's response to the drug initially administered. Hemodynamic support with sympathomimetic drugs, such as phenylephrine and ephedrine, may be necessary, and such drugs should be readily available, especially in cases in which CPP may already be compromised. A nondepolarizing neuromuscular blocking drug or succinylcholine is used to facilitate tracheal intubation, mechanical ventilation of the lungs, and patient positioning on the operating table (also see Chapters 10 and 19). Increases in ICP may occur after the administration of succinylcholine, but the extent of the increase is usually short-lived and clinically inconsequential.[9] The trachea is intubated ideally after a peripheral nerve stimulator confirms the establishment of skeletal muscle paralysis so that coughing is avoided, which may result in marked increases in ICP. Injection of additional intravenous doses of propofol, thiopental, opioids, or lidocaine 1 to 2 minutes before initiating direct laryngoscopy may be effective in attenuating the increase in systemic blood pressure and ICP that can accompany tracheal intubation.

## Positioning

The head of the operating table is frequently turned 90 to 180 degrees away from the anesthesia workstation during intracranial procedures (also see Chapter 19). Typically, the anesthesia provider will have limited access to the patient's head, so the endotracheal tube should be safely secured prior to draping. The breathing circuit, monitor cables, and intravenous and intra-arterial lines should be organized in order to facilitate trouble shooting and avoid cumbersome tangling.

Resection of supratentorial tumors and intracranial vascular lesions is typically accomplished with the patient in supine, semilateral, or lateral position. Resection of posterior fossa/infratentorial tumors frequently requires placement of the patient in prone or sitting position. The sitting position facilitates surgical exposure of posterior fossa tumors, but because of the frequent risk of venous air embolism (>25% incidence), the prone position is often used instead. Other risks associated with the sitting position include upper airway edema as a result of venous obstruction from excessive cervical flexion and quadriplegia from spinal cord compression and ischemia, especially in the presence of preexisting cervical stenosis. An alternative approach is the "park bench position" in which the patient is placed in a lateral position but rolled slightly forward with the head further rotated to "look" at the floor. This position allows the surgeon full access to

the posterior fossa and minimizes the risk for venous air embolism (also see Chapter 19).

Extreme rotation, flexion, and extension of the head and neck should be avoided, especially in patients with cervical spine diseases or elderly patients with arthritis or osteoporosis. Twisting, stretching, and compression of the neck vascular structures should also be avoided. A chest roll is frequently used in patients positioned in lateral or in park bench position, but not semilateral. Pressure points should be adequately padded to avoid compression injury. The body weight should be supported at multiple points, not a single point, in an even distribution fashion. Slight flexion of elbows and knees is recommended. The eyelids are closed shut and covered by transparent and waterproof film dressing to avoid scratching and chemical injury to the eyes from preparatory solutions. A soft but effective bite block is recommended to prevent soft tissue injury due to an intraoperative seizure or various motor stimulations due to monitoring. The mechanisms of preventing patients from slipping should be instituted intraoperatively if the operating table is to be tilted at the surgeon's request. A patient's tolerance and ease of airway instrumentation should also be taken into consideration during positioning for any procedure that is to be done under monitored anesthesia care such as deep brain stimulator placement or awake craniotomy.

A special consideration during neurologic surgery is the application of a head frame using three pins (Mayfield head clamp). Caution must be exercised to avoid bucking or movement during the placement and removal of the head frame and while the patient is fixed in the frame to avoid injury to the patient. Additional doses of propofol, or opioids, or both, are frequently administered right before the head frame placement to blunt the hemodynamic fluctuation. Local anesthesia injection at the site of pin insertion will also reduce the painful response to Mayfield head clamp placement.

## Maintenance of Anesthesia

After tracheal intubation, measures should be taken to minimize increases in ICP and optimize CPP. Maintenance of anesthesia is often achieved with a combination of opioid (either bolus or infusion), continuous infusion of propofol, and inhalation of a volatile anesthetic with or without nitrous oxide. Volatile anesthetic drugs must be used carefully because of their ability to increase ICP. Nevertheless, at low concentrations, volatile anesthetics (<0.5 MAC) are useful for blunting the increases in systemic blood pressure evoked by surgical stimulation. The choice of anesthetic drugs should also take into account the neurophysiologic monitoring being used because certain drugs (e.g., volatile anesthetics, nitrous oxide, neuromuscular blocking drugs) will impede neurophysiologic monitors such as motor or somatosensory evoked potentials.

**IV**

Direct-acting vasodilating drugs (hydralazine, nitroprusside, nitroglycerin, calcium channel blockers) may increase CBF and ICP despite causing simultaneous decreases in systemic blood pressure; therefore, use of these drugs, particularly before the dura is open, is not encouraged. On the contrary, sympathomimetic drugs such as phenylephrine or norepinephrine are often infused to maintain an ideal CPP.

Movement, coughing, or reacting to the presence of the tracheal tube during intracranial procedures is avoided because these responses can lead to increases in ICP, bleeding into the operative site, and a brain that bulges into the operative site and makes surgical exposure difficult. Thus, maintenance of an adequate depth of anesthesia is important. Skeletal muscle paralysis is often used to provide added insurance against movement or coughing. However, continuous administration of muscle relaxants is not possible in cases in which motor function monitoring is applied (e.g., either evoked potential, or direct cortical or subcortical stimulation).

## Intracranial Pressure Reduction and Brain Relaxation

ICP reduction and brain relaxation are related but distinctive concepts. The former is a pressure concept used in the absence of craniectomy and the latter is more a volume concept used during craniotomy indicating the size relationship between the intracranial components and capacity. Osmotic drugs such as mannitol (0.25 to 1 g/kg intravenously) or 3% hypertonic saline are frequently administered to reduce cerebral water content and decrease ICP before craniectomy, and to improve brain relaxation after craniectomy. The onset of action is 5 to 10 minutes, maximum effects are seen in 20 to 30 minutes, and its effects last for about 2 to 4 hours. However, if administered rapidly, mannitol can also cause peripheral vasodilation (hypotension) and short-term intravascular volume expansion, which could result in increased ICP and intravascular volume overload. Acute mannitol toxicity, as manifested by hyponatremia, high measured serum osmolality, and a gap between the measured and calculated serum osmolality of more than 10 mOsm/kg, can also occur when large doses of the drug (2 to 3 g/kg intravenously) are given. Furosemide (0.5 to 1 mg/kg intravenously) is often used to decrease brain water and ICP and is likely synergistic with mannitol in decreasing ICP. However, hypovolemia secondary to diuresis can decrease the preload and cardiac output that may do more harm than good in terms of tissue perfusion. Intermittent intravenous injections of thiopental or propofol may also be effective in decreasing ICP. When possible, the patient should be in a head-up position to avoid constriction around the neck, which may impair venous drainage. Other useful measures include hyperventilation, discontinuing the administration of volatile anesthetic drugs, and cerebrospinal fluid drainage.

## Ventilation Adjustment

After tracheal intubation, ventilation of the lungs is controlled at a rate and tidal volume sufficient to maintain $Paco_2$ between 30 and 35 mm Hg. There is no evidence of additional therapeutic benefit when $Paco_2$ is decreased below this range.

Whether a smaller tidal volume is lung protective during neurologic procedures is not clear. Use of positive end-expiratory pressure (PEEP) is not encouraged because it could impair cerebral venous drainage and increase ICP, but it can usually be counteracted by elevating the head 10 to 15 cm above the level of the chest. Hypoventilation is not indicated because hypercapnia causes cerebral vasodilation, increases CBF and ICP, and impairs cerebral autoregulation.[1] Overall, eucapnia probably should be maintained during intracranial surgery, and relative hyperventilation should be used only as a temporizing measure.

## Intravascular Fluid Management

Maintaining euvolemia is recommended. Dextrose solutions are not recommended because they are rapidly distributed throughout body water and, if blood glucose concentrations decrease more rapidly than brain glucose concentrations, water crosses the blood-brain barrier and cerebral edema results. Furthermore, hyperglycemia augments ischemic neuronal cell damage by promoting neuronal lactate production, which worsens cellular injury. Therefore, crystalloid solutions such as normal saline, Plasma-Lyte, and lactated Ringer solution are recommended. Colloids such as 5% albumin are also an acceptable replacement fluid, but no improvement in outcome has been shown (also see Chapter 23).

## Postoperative Care

On awakening from anesthesia, coughing or straining by the patient should be avoided because these responses could increase the possibility of intracranial hemorrhage or edema formation (also see Chapter 39). A prior intravenous bolus of lidocaine, opioid, or both may help decrease the likelihood of coughing during tracheal extubation. Low-rate remifentanil infusion can facilitate a smooth emergence. Postoperatively, early and frequent neurologic assessment and adequate analgesia are important. Delayed return of consciousness or neurologic deterioration in the postoperative period should be carefully monitored and evaluated by computed tomography or magnetic resonance imaging. Intracranial hemorrhage and stroke should be detected as soon as possible. Tension pneumocephalus as a cause of neurologic deterioration is a consideration. The postoperative stress response and resulting hyperdynamic events (hypertension, tachycardia) are attenuated with the use of hemodynamically active drugs and opioids. Labetalol is commonly used to treat hypertension based on its ability to reduce MAP without cerebral vasodilation.

## Venous Air Embolism

Neurosurgery that requires significant elevation of the head is associated with an increased risk for venous air embolism.[12] Not only is the operative site above the level of the heart but the venous sinuses in the cut edge of bone or dura may not collapse when transected. Air enters the pulmonary circulation and becomes trapped in the small vessels, thereby causing an acute increase in dead space. Massive air embolism may cause air to enter and be trapped in the right ventricle and lead to acute right ventricular failure. Microvascular bubbles may also cause reflex bronchoconstriction and activate the release of endothelial mediators causing pulmonary edema. Death is usually due to cardiovascular collapse and arterial hypoxemia. Air may reach the coronary and cerebral circulations (paradoxic air embolism) by crossing a patent foramen ovale (a probe-patent foramen ovale is present in 20% to 30% of adults) and result in myocardial infarction or stroke. Furthermore, transpulmonary passage of venous air is possible in the absence of a patent foramen ovale.

Transesophageal echocardiography is the most sensitive method to detect air embolism, but it is invasive and cumbersome. A precordial Doppler ultrasound transducer placed over the right side of the heart (over the second or third intercostal space to the right of the sternum to maximize audible signals from the right atrium) is the next most sensitive method (detects amounts of air as small as 0.25 mL) and a practical noninvasive indicator of the presence of intracardiac air. A sudden decrease in end-tidal concentrations of carbon dioxide reflects increased dead space secondary to continued ventilation of alveoli no longer being perfused because of obstruction of their vascular supply by air bubbles. An increased end-tidal nitrogen concentration may reflect nitrogen from venous air embolism if the inspired oxygen concentration is higher than that of room air but this is rarely available. Aspiration of air through a correctly positioned central venous catheter can also be used to diagnose air embolism. In this regard, a right atrial catheter with the tip positioned at the junction of the superior vena cava and the right atrium may provide the most rapid aspiration of air. During controlled ventilation of the lungs, sudden attempts (gasps) by patients to initiate spontaneous breaths may be the first indication of the occurrence of venous air embolism. Hypotension, tachycardia, cardiac dysrhythmias, cyanosis, and a "mill wheel" murmur are late signs of venous air embolism. A pulmonary artery catheter may provide additional evidence that venous air embolism has occurred because of abrupt increases in pulmonary artery pressure. Additional signs in patients who are not receiving general anesthesia include chest pain and coughing.

The surgeon should be notified immediately whenever a venous air embolism is suspected. Venous air embolism is treated by (1) irrigation of the operative site with fluid, as well as the application of occlusive material to all bone edges so that sites of venous air entry are occluded; (2) placement of the patient in a head-down position; (3) gentle compression of the internal jugular veins; (4) provision of 100% of inspired oxygen concentration; and (5) supportive care of hemodynamic derangements. If nitrous oxide is being administered, it should be promptly discontinued to avoid the risk of increasing the size of venous air bubbles because of diffusion of this gas into the air bubbles. Despite the logic of PEEP to decrease entrainment of air, the efficacy of this maneuver has not been confirmed. Furthermore, PEEP could reverse the pressure gradient between the left and right atria and predispose to passage of air across a patent foramen ovale.

## COMMON CLINICAL CASES

### Intracranial Mass Lesions

Intracranial mass lesions (Box 30.3), especially primary brain tumors, occur most often in patients 40 to 60 years

---

**Box 30.3** Management of Anesthesia for Patients With Intracranial Masses

**Preoperative**
- Avoid sedatives and opioids if ICP is elevated.
- Standard anxiolytics can be given if ICP is not elevated.

**Monitors**
*Supratentorial Masses*
- Standard ASA monitors, arterial line, Foley catheter are used.

*Infratentorial Masses—Depending on Positioning*
- Prone or park bench position: Standard ASA monitors, arterial line, Foley catheter are adequate.
- Sitting position (associated with frequency of VAE): Standard monitors plus central venous catheter, precordial Doppler, or TEE are required.

**Induction**
- Deep anesthesia and skeletal muscle paralysis are obtained before direct laryngoscopy/tracheal intubation to avoid increasing ICP while maintaining CPP.

**Maintenance**
- Minimize ICP and maintain adequate CPP.
- Opioid plus propofol and/or volatile anesthetic with or without nitrous oxide.
- Avoid intraoperative muscle relaxant if motor function is tested/mapped.
- Mannitol (0.25-1 g/kg IV) also can be given.
- Maintain euvolemia.
- Eucapnia if normal ICP; temporary hyperventilation for a tight brain only.

**Postoperative**
- Avoid coughing, straining, and systemic hypertension during tracheal extubation.
- Rapid awakening allows early neurologic assessment.

*ASA*, American Society of Anesthesiologists; *CPP*, cerebral perfusion pressure; *ICP*, intracranial pressure; *IV*, intravenous; *TEE*, transesophageal echocardiography; *VAE*, venous air embolism.

IV

of age, and the initial signs and symptoms may or may not reflect increases in ICP. Headache and seizures that appear in a previously asymptomatic adult suggest the presence of an intracranial tumor, and such tumors are usually confirmed by computed tomography or magnetic resonance imaging. Avoidance of abrupt increases in ICP is an important anesthetic goal when managing patients with intracranial tumors.

The sitting position for posterior fossa masses has several additional considerations. The arterial line transducer should be positioned no lower than the external ear canal level in order to facilitate the assessment of CPP. A properly positioned central venous catheter and precordial Doppler should be used given the high incidence of venous air embolism. Adequate hydration is warranted to compensate for the intravascular volume pooling in the lower extremities. Posterior fossa operations have the potential of stimulating or injuring vital brainstem respiratory and circulatory centers and result in intraoperative hemodynamic fluctuations and postoperative ventilation abnormalities. The cranial nerves can also be stimulated or affected, which can lead to intraoperative dysrhythmias and postoperative impairment of protective airway reflexes. Postoperatively, the airway needs to be assessed as to whether the patient will be able to maintain and protect the airway or whether tracheal intubation and ventilation should be continued in the intensive care unit.

## Intracranial Aneurysms

Intracranial aneurysms (Box 30.4) are the most common cause of intracranial hemorrhage. They occur in 2% to 4% of the population, with 1% to 2% rupturing per year. Although aneurysms may be found incidentally or appear as a slowly enlarging mass, they are most frequently manifested as hemorrhage together with a sudden, severe headache, nausea, vomiting, focal neurologic signs, and decreased level of consciousness. Major complications of aneurysmal rupture include death, rebleeding, and vasospasm. Definitive treatment may include either endovascular coiling or surgical clipping via craniectomy. Short- to medium-term outcomes are similar in patients treated surgically versus endovascular insertion of platinum coils, although the long-term benefits of one technique over the other continues to be debated.[13] Some patients are unsuitable candidates for endovascular coiling because of the anatomy and location of their aneurysms; in these cases, surgical clipping is needed.

Early treatment is advocated for prevention of rebleeding, but surgery may be associated with more technical difficulty because of a swollen inflamed brain, whereas delaying treatment increases the risk for rebleeding. Cerebral vasospasm is generally manifested clinically 3 to 5 days after subarachnoid hemorrhage (SAH) and is the foremost cause of morbidity and death. Transcranial Doppler and cerebral arteriography can detect cerebral

---

**Box 30.4** Anesthetic Management of Patients With Intracranial Aneurysms

**Preoperative**
- Neurologic evaluation is performed to look for evidence of increased intracranial pressure and vasospasm.
- Electrocardiogram changes are often present.
- HHH therapy is indicated if vasospasm is present.
- Calcium channel blockers.

**Induction**
- Avoid increases in systemic blood pressure.
- Maintain cerebral perfusion pressure to avoid ischemia.

**Maintenance**
- Opioid plus propofol and/or volatile anesthetic is recommended regimen.
- Mannitol (0.25-1 g/kg IV) also can be given.
- Maintain normal to increased systemic blood pressure to avoid ischemia during surgical retraction and temporary clipping.
- Maintain euvolemia.
- Maintain eucapnia; avoid unnecessary hyperventilation.
- Burst-suppression and mild hypothermia can be considered.

**Postoperative**
- Maintain normal to increased systemic blood pressure.
- Early awakening is recommended to facilitate neurologic assessment.
- HHH therapy is given as needed.

*HHH,* Hypervolemia, hypertension, hemodilution; *IV,* intravenous.

---

vasospasm before clinical symptoms (worsening headache, neurologic deterioration, loss of consciousness) occur. Treatment of vasospasm often includes "triple H" therapy (hypervolemia, hypertension, hemodilution), which consists of intravenous administration of fluids or inotropic drugs, or both. The intravenous administration of a calcium channel blocker, nimodipine, decreases the morbidity and mortality risks from vasospasm. Other treatment modalities include selective intra-arterial injection of vasodilators and balloon dilation (angioplasty) of the affected arterial segments using interventional radiology approaches.

Other complications of SAH include seizures (10%), acute and chronic hydrocephalus, and intracerebral hematoma. Changes on the ECG (T-wave inversions, U waves, ST-segment depressions, prolonged QT interval, and rarely Q waves) and mild elevation of cardiac enzymes are frequent but do not usually correlate with significant myocardial dysfunction or poor outcome. Hyponatremia is commonly seen after SAH. Significant electrolyte and acid-base abnormalities or hemodynamic derangements should be corrected if present, and a cardiac workup should ensue if Q waves are seen on the ECG.

The anesthetic care for intracranial aneurysm clipping is designed to (1) prevent sudden increases in systemic arterial blood pressure, which would increase the aneurysm's transmural pressure and could result in rupture or rebleeding, and (2) facilitate surgical exposure and access to the aneurysm (see Box 30.4). Induction and maintenance of anesthesia must be designed to minimize the hypertensive responses evoked by noxious stimulation, such as direct laryngoscopy and placing the patient's head in immobilizing pins. Conversely, CPP must be maintained to prevent ischemia during surgical retraction or temporary vessel occlusion, or as a result of vasospasm.

Hemodynamic control is important during dissection of the aneurysm to prevent intraoperative rupture. Temporary occlusive clips applied to the major feeding artery of the aneurysm can create regional hypotension without the need for systemic hypotension and its inherent risks on multiple organ systems. As a result, normal or even increased systemic arterial blood pressure should be instituted to facilitate perfusion through collateral circulations. In addition to maintaining collateral cerebral circulations via systemic relative hypertension, drugs such as propofol or thiopental may be administered, via either boluses or high-rate infusion to the point of burst-suppression on electroencephalography monitoring, in the hope that they can provide some protection from cerebral ischemia. Occasionally, hypothermic circulatory arrest may be used for very large complex aneurysms. Nonetheless, convincing outcome evidence of these maneuvers is lacking.

The patient's trachea is generally extubated at the completion of surgery unless there is significant neurologic impairment or other intraoperative complications. Measures to prevent vasospasm and seizures while maintaining adequate CPP should be continued during care of these patients postoperatively.

## Arteriovenous Malformations

The incidence of AVMs in the general population and the annual rate of rupture is similar to aneurysms at 2% to 4% and 2%, respectively. Up to 10% of patients diagnosed with an AVM have an associated aneurysm.[14] Risk of hemorrhage is related to the anatomic features of the AVM including size and characteristics of the feeding arteries. These patients may be treated several ways: expectantly, open resection, endovascular embolization, or stereotactic radiosurgery (Gamma Knife). Preoperative embolization is frequently employed to reduce blood loss and facilitate surgical resection.

Anesthesia for resection or embolization of AVMs is similar to that of aneurysms with a few distinct considerations. Because of their flow characteristics (low-pressure, high-flow shunts), AVMs are unlikely to rupture during acute systemic hypertension, such as during laryngoscopy. Despite this, hypertension should still be avoided during induction of anesthesia, given the frequent rate of associated aneurysms. Finally, anesthesia for intracranial AVM resection must include preparation for massive, persistent blood loss and postoperative cerebral swelling.

---

**Box 30.5** Management of Anesthesia for Patients With Carotid Stenosis

**Preoperative**
- Neurologic examination is indicated to look for preoperative deficits.
- Screen for associated CAD.
- Anxiolytics may be useful.

**Monitors**
- Standard ASA monitors, arterial line, Foley catheter are used.
- Cerebral ischemia monitoring depends on institutional and individual practitioner's preference.

**Induction**
- Avoid increases in mean arterial pressure or heart rate if CAD is suspected.
- Maintain adequate CPP.

**Maintenance**
- Maintain adequate CPP (baseline to 20% above) during carotid clamping.
- Opioid plus propofol and/or volatile anesthetic can be used with or without nitrous oxide.
- Close intraoperative monitoring for cerebral ischemia during carotid clamping by keeping the patient awake or based on various monitoring modalities.

**Postoperative**
- Avoid coughing, straining, and systemic hypertension during tracheal extubation.
- Rapid awakening allows early neurologic assessment.
- Monitor for hyperperfusion syndrome and airway compromise.

*ASA*, American Society of Anesthesiologists; *CAD*, coronary artery disease; *CPP*, cerebral perfusion pressure.

## Carotid Disease

Stroke can result in severe disability and death. Atherosclerotic stenosis of the carotid artery is an important cause of stroke. Despite the technical advancement and increasing adoption of carotid artery stenting (CAS), carotid endarterectomy (CEA) remains the "gold standard" in treating symptomatic carotid disease (Box 30.5).[15] Although the perioperative risk of stroke and death (approximately 4% to 7%) must be taken into account, CEA may be beneficial in asymptomatic patients as well.[16] Data suggest that early CEA (<30 days after symptom onset) is optimal given the presence of unstable atherosclerotic plaque.[17]

Preoperative assessment of patients undergoing CEA should focus on assessment of perioperative risk of cardiac ischemia as these patients typically have atherosclerotic disease. Either general or regional anesthesia (deep and superficial cervical plexus block) may be used for this procedure. Regional anesthesia may permit a more accurate intraoperative assessment of the patient's neurologic status and more stable hemodynamic profile, but it requires a cooperative and motionless patient. Current analysis of the literature suggests that outcomes are

IV

similar whether CEA is performed under regional or general anesthesia.[18]

Goals of anesthesia for CEA include (1) prevention of cerebral ischemia through maintenance of adequate CPP and (2) prevention of myocardial ischemia through avoidance of acute increases in arterial blood pressure and heart rate. Invasive hemodynamic monitoring with an arterial catheter is indicated to ensure adequate CPP. This is especially important during intraoperative clamping of the carotid artery. The anesthesia provider should ensure that the MAP is maintained above the patient's baseline pressure (within 20%) to ensure adequate collateral flow through the circle of Willis. Hypocarbia should be avoided given the risk of cerebral vasoconstriction and ischemia. Many methods have been employed to detect intraoperative cerebral ischemia and need for shunting during clamping including EEG, evoked potentials, transcranial Doppler, cerebral oximetry, and stump pressure, although none has been shown to definitively improve outcome.

Postoperative complications include cardiovascular ischemia and neurologic deficits secondary to intraoperative emboli. Hypertension should be avoided because it may lead to complications such as neck hematoma with airway compromise or hyperperfusion syndrome (ipsilateral headache, seizure, focal neurologic signs in the absence of cerebral ischemia).

## QUESTIONS OF THE DAY

1. What is the relationship between cerebral perfusion pressure and cerebral blood flow? How does the relationship change when the cerebral perfusion pressure is above and below the limits of autoregulation? What disease processes can impair normal cerebral autoregulation?

2. How do $Pa_{CO_2}$ and $Pa_{O_2}$ affect cerebral blood flow? How long do the $Pa_{CO_2}$-related changes in cerebral blood flow last, and what is the mechanism for this phenomenon?

3. How do different intravenous anesthetics (e.g., benzodiazepines, opioids, propofol, ketamine) and inhaled anesthetics affect cerebral blood flow and cerebral metabolic rate?

4. Draw a diagram of the relationship between intracranial volume and intracranial pressure in the adult. What components of the intracranial compartment can be manipulated to effect a reduction in intracranial pressure?

5. A patient is undergoing craniotomy for removal of brain mass. After craniectomy and dural opening, the surgeon notes "brain swelling" in the operative field. What steps can be taken to promote brain relaxation?

6. What are the goals of anesthesia care for a patient undergoing intracranial aneurysm clipping? What complications of subarachnoid hemorrhage may develop in the perioperative period?

7. What are the manifestations of venous air embolism in a patient undergoing craniotomy during general anesthesia? What are the appropriate steps in management?

8. What are the goals of intraoperative anesthesia management for a patient undergoing carotid endarterectomy? What complications should be anticipated after surgery?

## REFERENCES

1. Meng L, Gelb AW. Regulation of cerebral autoregulation by carbon dioxide. *Anesthesiology*. 2015;122:196–205.
2. Meng L, Hou W, Chui J, et al. Cardiac output and cerebral blood flow: the integrated regulation of brain perfusion in adult humans. *Anesthesiology*. 2015;123(5):1198–1208.
3. Polderman KH. Mechanism of action, physiological effects and complications of hypothermia. *Crit Care Med*. 2009;37:S186–S202.
4. Dagal A, Lam AM. Cerebral autoregulation and anesthesia. *Curr Opin Anaesthesiol*. 2009;22:547–552.
5. Brain Trauma Foundation; American Association of Neurological Surgeons; Congress of Neurological Surgeons. Guidelines for the management of severe traumatic brain injury. *J Neurotrauma*. 2007;24(suppl 1):S1–S106.
6. Albanese J, Arnaud S, Rey M, et al. Ketamine decreases intracranial pressure and electroencephalographic activity in traumatic brain injury patients during propofol sedation. *Anesthesiology*. 1997;87:1328–1334.
7. Reddy RV, Moorthy SS, Dierdorf SF, et al. Excitatory effects and electroencephalographic correlation of etomidate, thiopental, methohexital and propofol. *Anesth Analg*. 1993;77:1008–1011.
8. Muzzi D, Losasso T, Dietz N, et al. The effect of desflurane and isoflurane on cerebrospinal fluid pressure in humans with supratentorial mass lesions. *Anesthesiology*. 1992;76:720–724.
9. Kovarik WD, Mayberg TS, Lam AM, et al. Succinylcholine does not change intracranial pressure, cerebral blood flow velocity, or the electroencephalogram in patients with neurologic injury. *Anesth Analg*. 1994;78:469–473.
10. Bernard SA, Gray TW, Buist MD, et al. Treatment of comatose survivors of out of hospital cardiac arrest with induced hypothermia. *N Engl J Med*. 2002;346:557–563.
11. Nielsen N, Wetterslev J, Cronberg T, et al. Targeted temperature management at 33 degrees C versus 36 degrees C after cardiac arrest. *N Engl J Med*. 2013;369:2197–2206.
12. Muth CM, Shank ES. Gas embolism. *N Engl J Med*. 2000;342:476–482.

13. Thomas AJ, Ogilvy CS. ISAT: equipoise in treatment of ruptured cerebral aneurysms? *Lancet.* 2015;385:666–668.

14. Olgilvy CS, Stieg PE, Awak I, et al. Recommendations for the management of intracranial arteriovenous malformations. *Circulation.* 2001;103:2644–2657.

15. Kolkert JL, Meerwaldt R, Geelkerken RH, et al. Endarterectomy or carotid artery stenting: the quest continues part two. *Am J Surg.* 2015;209:403–412.

16. Raman G, Moorthy D, Hadar N, et al. Management strategies for asymptomatic carotid stenosis: a systematic review and meta-analysis. *Ann Intern Med.* 2013;158:676–685.

17. Rerkasem K, Rothwell PM. Systematic review of the operative risks of carotid endarterectomy for recently symptomatic stenosis in relation to the timing of surgery. *Stroke.* 2009;40:e564–e572.

18. GALA Trial Collaborative Group; Lewis SC, Warlow CP, Bodenham AR, et al. General anaesthesia versus local anaesthesia for carotid surgery (GALA): a multicentre, randomised controlled trial. *Lancet.* 2008;372(9656):2132–2142.

IV

# 31 OPHTHALMOLOGY AND OTOLARYNGOLOGY

## Steven Gayer and Howard D. Palte

In addition to the usual anesthetic issues, surgical procedures of the head and neck present unique anesthetic challenges. Isolation from the surgical field physically places the anesthesia provider at a distance from the airway and hampers access to the patient. In addition to common anesthetic problems, the region's extensive parasympathetic innervations predispose patients to intraoperative bradycardia and asystole. Ophthalmic and otolaryngologic procedures require smooth induction of and emergence from anesthesia. This is especially important because coughing and "bucking" increase venous and intraocular pressure, which may negatively impact surgical outcome.

## OPHTHALMOLOGY

Ophthalmic procedures are among the most commonly performed surgical procedures worldwide. More than 2 million cataract operations are performed nationally each year. Most eye procedures are considered an uncommon risk for perioperative complications; however, ophthalmic patients are often at greater risk during surgery because typically they include the elderly (also see Chapter 35), who frequently have multiple concomitant medical issues, or pediatric patients (also see Chapter 34), who may be premature or have associated syndromes.[1] Additionally, most operations are conducted on an ambulatory basis (also see Chapter 37), emphasizing the importance of preoperative evaluation (also see Chapter 13).

Most ophthalmologic procedures are performed via monitored anesthesia care (MAC) and some form of regional or topical eye anesthetic.[2] Aside from intraoperative analgesia and akinesia, advantages of ophthalmic regional blocks include suppression of the oculocardiac reflex (OCR) and provision of postoperative pain management. An understanding of regional block techniques and management of their complications is requisite. General anesthesia is reserved for operations of prolonged duration, more invasive orbital procedures, and for patients unable to remain relatively still such as neonates, infants, and children (also see Chapter 34).

Anesthetic drugs and maneuvers may affect ocular dynamics and surgical outcomes, and ophthalmic medications can cause adverse anesthesia reactions or may significantly impact systemic physiology. Appreciation of factors affecting intraocular pressure (IOP) and vigilance vis-à-vis the OCR are critical.

## Intraocular Pressure

Adequate pressure within the eye serves to maintain refracting surfaces, corneal contour, and functionally correct vision. IOP is primarily derived from a balance between aqueous humor production and drainage. Aqueous humor is actively secreted from the posterior chamber's ciliary body and flows through the pupil into the anterior chamber where it is admixed with aqueous passively produced by blood vessels on the iris's forward surface. After washing over the avascular lens and corneal endothelium, aqueous humor filters through the spongy trabecular meshwork into the canal of Schlemm tubules at the base of the cornea. From there, it exits the eye into episcleral veins and ultimately to the superior vena cava and right atrium. Therefore, any obstruction of venous return from the eye to the right side of the heart can increase IOP. Lesser factors that influence IOP include force transmitted to the globe by contraction of the orbicularis oculi or extraocular muscles as well as hardening of the lens, vitreous, and sclera that can occur with aging (also see Chapter 35).

IOP ranges between 10 and 22 mm Hg in the intact normal eye. Typically, there is a 2 to 5 mm Hg diurnal variation. Small transient changes occur with each cardiac contraction as well as with eyelid closure, mydriasis, and postural changes. These changes are normal and have no bearing on the intact eye. A sustained increase in IOP during anesthesia, however, has the potential to produce acute glaucoma, retinal ischemia, hemorrhage, and permanent visual loss.

### Factors That Influence Intraocular Pressure

Venous congestion resulting from obstruction at any point from the episcleral veins to the right atrium may cause substantive increase of IOP. Prior to induction of anesthesia, Trendelenburg positioning or presence of a tight cervical collar can increase intraocular blood volume, dilate orbital vessels, and inhibit aqueous drainage. Straining, retching, or coughing during induction of anesthesia will markedly increase venous pressure and can readily precipitate an increase in IOP of 40 mm Hg or more. Should this occur while the globe is open during surgery, such as during corneal transplant, loss of vitreous, hemorrhage, and expulsion of eye contents

may lead to permanent damage to the eye or even blindness. Arterial hypertension can transiently increase IOP, but has much less impact than perturbations of venous drainage. External compression on the globe by a tightly applied face mask, laryngoscopy, and tracheal intubation also elevate IOP, but placement of a supraglottic airway has minimal impact. Hypoxemia and hypoventilation can increase IOP. Hyperventilation and hypothermia have the opposite effect.

### Anesthetic Drugs and Intraocular Pressure

Inhaled and most intravenous anesthetics produce dose-related reductions in IOP. Although the exact mechanisms are not known, IOP is probably reduced by a combination of central nervous system depression, diminished aqueous humor production, enhanced aqueous outflow, and relaxation of extraocular muscles. There is controversy surrounding the effect of ketamine on IOP. Although ketamine may not increase IOP, it does cause rotatory nystagmus and blepharospasm, making it a less than ideal anesthetic for eye surgery.

In the absence of alveolar hypoventilation, nondepolarizing neuromuscular blocking drugs decrease IOP via relaxation of the extraocular muscles. In contrast, succinylcholine produces an increase of about 9 mm Hg in 1 to 4 minutes after intravenous administration with a subsequent diminution to baseline within 7 minutes. The increase in IOP is probably due to several mechanisms, including tonic contraction of extraocular muscles, relaxation of orbital smooth muscle, choroidal vascular dilation, and aqueous outflow-impeding cycloplegia. Pretreatment with a small dose of a nondepolarizing neuromuscular blocking drug, lidocaine, β-blocker, or acetazolamide may attenuate the increase in IOP associated with induction of anesthesia with succinylcholine, direct laryngoscopy, and endotracheal intubation. However, this approach for induction of anesthesia is rarely used.

## Ophthalmic Medications

Systemic absorption of topical ophthalmic drugs from either the conjunctiva or via drainage through the nasolacrimal duct onto the nasal mucosa can produce untoward side effects. These drops include acetylcholine, anticholinesterases, cyclopentolate, epinephrine, phenylephrine, and timolol (Table 31.1). Phospholine iodide (echothiophate) is a miosis-inducing anticholinesterase that profoundly interferes with metabolism of succinylcholine. Prolonged paralysis following a single dose of succinylcholine may ensue. Phenylephrine drops are available in concentrations of 2.5% and 10%. Systemic absorption via the nasolacrimal duct of 10% phenylephrine drops can induce transient malignant hypertension. Parenteral administration of a long-acting antihypertensive drug may result in untoward

IV

**Table 31.1** Drugs Administered to Ophthalmic Surgery Patients

| Ophthalmic Indication | Drug | Mechanism of Action | Systemic Effect |
|---|---|---|---|
| Miosis | Acetylcholine | Cholinergic agonist | Bronchospasm, bradycardia, hypotension |
| Glaucoma (increased intraocular pressure) | Acetazolamide<br>Echothiophate | Carbonic anhydrase inhibitor<br>Irreversible cholinesterase inhibitor | Diuresis, hypokalemic metabolic acidosis<br>Prolongation of succinylcholine's effects<br>Reduction in plasma cholinesterase activity up to 3-7 weeks after discontinuation<br>Bradycardia, bronchospasm |
| | Timolol | β-Adrenergic antagonist | Atropine-resistant bradycardia, bronchospasm, exacerbation of congestive heart failure; possible exacerbation of myasthenia gravis |
| Mydriasis, ophthalmic capillary decongestion | Atropine | Anticholinergic | Central anticholinergic syndrome (*mad as a hatter*, delirium, agitation; *hot as a hare*, fever; *red as a beet*, flushing; *dry as a bone*, xerostomia, anhidrosis)<br>Blurred vision (cycloplegia, photophobia) |
| | Cyclopentolate<br>Epinephrine | Anticholinergic<br>α-, β-Adrenergic agonist | Disorientation, psychosis, convulsions, dysarthria<br>Hypertension, tachycardia, cardiac dysrhythmias; epinephrine paradoxically leads to decreased intraocular pressure and can also be used for glaucoma |
| | Phenylephrine | α-Adrenergic agonist, direct-acting vasopressor | Hypertension (1 drop, or 0.05 mL, of a 10% solution contains 5 mg of phenylephrine) |
| | Scopolamine | Anticholinergic | Central anticholinergic syndrome (see atropine earlier) |

hypotension following resolution of the short-acting phenylephrine. Some systemic ophthalmic drugs, such as glycerol, mannitol, and acetazolamide, may also produce untoward side effects.

## Oculocardiac Reflex

The OCR is a sudden profound decrease in heart rate in response to traction on the extraocular muscles or external pressure on the globe. There is a wide range of reported incidence, varying from approximately 15% to 80%. This reflex occurs more commonly in young patients. The reflex arc has a trigeminal nerve afferent limb that generates an efferent vagal response that may precipitate a variety of dysrhythmias including junctional or sinus bradycardia, atrioventricular block, ventricular bigeminy, multifocal premature ventricular contractions, ventricular tachycardia, and asystole.

The OCR is most often encountered during strabismus surgery but can occur during any type of ophthalmic surgery. OCR may also occur while performing an eye regional anesthetic nerve block. Hypercarbia, hypoxemia, and light planes of anesthetic depth augment the incidence and severity of OCR.

Prompt removal of the instigating surgical stimulus frequently results in rapid recovery. Unrelenting tension may induce cardiac arrest, so heart rate must be continuously monitored during eye regional block and surgery. At the first sign of dysrhythmia, surgery must stop and all pressure on the eye or traction on eye muscles discontinued. The ventilatory status and depth of anesthesia should be reassessed. The reflex may extinguish itself after a few minutes; it also can be abated by administration of a parasympatholytic drug such as atropine or glycopyrrolate. The OCR can also be eradicated by inserting a regional anesthetic eye block, thereby abolishing its afferent arc. Paradoxically, placement of a regional block can induce the OCR.

The prophylactic use of intramuscular anticholinergics for adult ophthalmic surgery patients is not effective. In fact, tachycardia following atropine or glycopyrrolate may have significant consequence for geriatric patients with history of cardiac disease (also see Chapter 25). In children (also see Chapter 34), who are more dependent on heart rate to maintain cardiac output, prophylactic intravenous administration of atropine (0.01 to 0.02 mg/kg) or glycopyrrolate may be prudent just prior to commencing eye surgery.

## Preoperative Assessment

Patients having eye surgery are often at the extremes of age—ranging from premature babies with retinopathy to the elderly. Hence, special age-related considerations such as altered pharmacokinetics and pharmacodynamics apply (also see Chapters 13 and 35). The elderly, pediatric patients with various syndromes, and premature infants frequently have multiple comorbid conditions. Preoperative evaluation is vital, but routine laboratory testing is not appropriate. For cataract surgery in particular, routine testing is associated with a significant increase in health care spending.[3] Physician assessment and judgment determine the need for indicated laboratory testing.[4] Cessation of antiplatelet/anticoagulant drugs prior to eye surgery is controversial.[5] The risk of intraocular bleeding versus the risk of perioperative stroke, myocardial ischemia, and deep venous thrombosis must be assessed.[6]

One of the most important preoperative assessments is the likelihood of patient movement during surgery. Inability to remain supine and relatively still during intraocular surgery with MAC result in eye injury and have devastating long-term visual consequences.[7]

## Anesthetic Options

Anesthetic options for most ophthalmic procedures include general anesthesia, retrobulbar (intraconal) block, peribulbar (extraconal) anesthesia, sub-Tenon block, and topical analgesia (see Box 31.1). Often, there is minimal exposure to regional anesthetic eye block techniques during anesthesia training, creating a reluctance to perform such blocks. Professional societies dedicated to teaching safe ophthalmic regional anesthesia can provide valuable instruction.[8] Site of surgery errors is more common for eye procedures than all other surgeries (except dental and digital). Of prime importance is confirmation of the correct eye (i.e., right versus left) immediately prior to anesthesia and surgery.

### Needle-Based Ophthalmic Regional Anesthesia

The anatomic foundation of needle-based eye blocks rests upon the concept of the orbital cone. This structure consists of the four ocular rectus muscles extending from their origin at the apex of the orbit to the globe anteriorly. These muscles and their surrounding connective tissue form a compartment behind the globe akin to the brachial plexus sheath in the axilla.

A retrobulbar block is performed by inserting a steeply angled needle from the inferotemporal orbital rim into this muscle cone such that the tip of the needle is behind

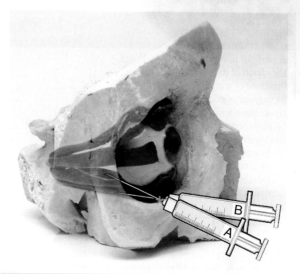

**Fig. 31.1** Needle-based regional anesthesia for ophthalmic surgery. (A) An intraconal (retrobulbar) block is placed deeper and is more steeply angled. (B) An extraconal (peribulbar) block is shallower and minimally angled. Asterisk indicates needle entry point. A portion of the lateral orbital rim is removed. (Model courtesy of Dr. Roy Hamilton.)

(retro) the globe (bulbar).[9] A more descriptive term is intraconal block (Fig. 31.1).[10] Injection of a small volume of local anesthetics into this compartment will produce rapid onset of akinesia and analgesia.

The boundary separating the intraconal from extraconal space is porous, and thus local anesthetics injected outside the muscle cone diffuse inwardly. A peribulbar block can be achieved by directing a minimally angled needle to a shallow depth such that the tip remains outside the cone (see Fig. 31.1). This extraconal block is theoretically safer because the needle is not directed toward the apex of the orbit; hence the needle tip is ultimately situated further from key intraorbital structures. This distance minimizes the potential for optic nerve trauma, optic nerve sheath injection, orbital epidural, and brainstem anesthesia. Complications of needle-based eye blocks are listed in Box 31.2. Because extraconal block local anesthetics are injected at a farther distance from the nerves, larger volumes and more time for diffusion of the local anesthetic are needed. Thus, intraconal versus extraconal anesthesia is somewhat analogous to subarachnoid versus epidural anesthesia in terms of volume, onset, and density of block.

Altered physiologic status following an ophthalmic anesthetic block has important implications. Differential diagnosis includes oversedation, brainstem anesthesia, and intravascular injection of local anesthetic (Table 31.2). Abrupt onset of seizure activity is characteristic of intravascular injection. Convulsions are typically of brief and limited duration. Brainstem anesthesia

IV

**Box 31.2** Complications of Regional Anesthesia for Ophthalmic Surgery

Superficial or retrobulbar hemorrhage
Elicitation of the oculocardiac reflex
Puncture of the globe
Intraocular injection
Optic nerve trauma
Seizures (intravenous injection of local anesthetic solution)
Brainstem anesthesia (spread of local anesthetic to the brainstem causing delayed-onset loss of consciousness, respiratory depression, paralysis of the contralateral extraocular muscles)
Central retinal artery occlusion
Blindness

**Table 31.2** Differential Diagnosis of Altered Physiologic Status After Regional Anesthesia for Ophthalmic Surgery

| Alteration | Oversedation | Brainstem Anesthesia | Intravascular Injection |
|---|---|---|---|
| Loss of consciousness | ± | + | + |
| Apnea | ± | + | ± |
| Cardiac instability | ± | + | ± |
| Seizure activity | Ø | Ø | + |
| Contralateral mydriasis | Ø | ± | Ø |
| Contralateral eye block | Ø | ± | Ø |

+, Likely; ±, may or may not be present; Ø, not present.

may have a gradual latency of onset and persist for 10 to 40 minutes, or longer. Patients must be continuously monitored following anesthetic eye blocks for signs of oversedation, brainstem anesthesia, and intravascular absorption of local anesthetics.

Branches of the facial nerve that innervate the eyelid's orbicularis oculi muscle are blocked by the larger volume of local anesthetic used with extraconal injection. This prevents eyelid squeezing and is a distinct advantage during corneal transplantation. An intraconal block requires a separate facial nerve injection to limit blepharospasm.

Cannula-Based Ophthalmic Regional Anesthesia
Ophthalmic anesthesia can also be achieved by instilling local anesthetics through a blunt cannula into the space between the globe's rigid sclera and sub-Tenon capsule (Fig. 31.2).[11] The capsule consists of fascia that envelops the eye, providing a smooth friction-free interface in which to rotate. Anteriorly, it originates near the limbal margin where it is fused to the conjunctiva. As the capsule extends posteriorly, it surrounds the eye, with portions reflected onto the extraocular muscles. Local anesthetics injected into the sub-Tenon space block cranial and ciliary nerves that penetrate the capsule as well as the optic nerve posteriorly.

## Anesthesia Management of Specific Ophthalmic Procedures

### Retina Surgery
The globe's posterior inner wall is lined by the retina, sensory tissue that converts incoming light into neural output and, ultimately, vision. The densely packed macula near its center provides fine detailed vision. Perfusion comes from the choroid layer situated between the sclera and the retina. The retina may break or detach from the choroid leading to ischemia and compromised vision. Diabetics and people with myopia are at particular risk. Surgical options include combinations of scleral buckle, vitrectomy, laser, cryotherapy, and injection of intravitreal gas.

Preoperative evaluation of patients with diabetes and coexisting comorbid conditions (also see Chapter 13) is important, and appropriate changes should be made to ensure that these patients are in optimal medical condition for surgery. Sudden death during retina surgery can occur due to venous air embolism introduced into the choroid blood flow during the air/fluid exchange portion of vitrectomy. Retina surgery is often prolonged and associated with more extensive manipulation of the eye, therefore requiring general anesthesia or dense regional anesthetic block with MAC. Perfluorocarbons such as sulfur hexafluoride (SF6) and $C_3F_8$ are inert, relatively insoluble gases that are injected to internally tamponade the retina onto the choroid. Resorption can take 10 to 28 days depending on which drug is selected. As nitrous oxide is over 100-fold more diffusible than SF6, it can expand the size of the gas bubble, increase IOP, and potentially cause retinal ischemia and permanent loss of vision.[12] Nitrous oxide should be discontinued 20 minutes prior to gas injection or omitted altogether.

### Glaucoma
Glaucoma is commonly characterized as a sustained increase in IOP that leads to diminished perfusion of the optic nerve and eventual loss of vision. Various forms of glaucoma exist, each presenting with differing degrees of IOP variation. Terminology can be confusing, resulting in several classifications: acquired versus congenital, high-IOP versus normal-pressure, acute versus chronic, and open- versus narrow- or closed-angle. Angle-closure (acute) glaucoma occurs when the angle between the iris and cornea narrows and obstructs outflow. Open-angle (chronic) glaucoma results from sclerosis of trabecular

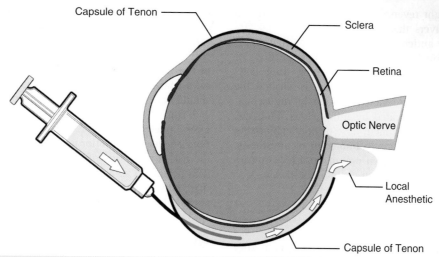

**Fig. 31.2** Sub-Tenon block. Local anesthetic is infused via a cannula into the potential space between Capsule of Tenon and the sclera, ultimately arriving at the optic nerve.

meshwork and impaired aqueous drainage. Outflow is improved with constriction of the pupil by miotic drugs. Administration of atropine drops into the eye produce mydriasis and are contraindicated. Intravenous atropine on the other hand is minimally absorbed by the eye and should be used when indicated during anesthesia. Infantile glaucoma may readily progress to blindness, making early surgery more urgent. Congenital glaucoma is often a component of many syndromes, several of which have important anesthesia implications.

Many adult glaucoma procedures can be managed with regional anesthesia and MAC. General anesthesia is a requisite for pediatric glaucoma cases. Anesthesia implications include (1) avoiding mydriasis by continuing all miotic drops, (2) understanding the interactions of antiglaucoma medications and anesthetics (see Table 31.1), and (3) preventing increases in IOP associated with induction, maintenance, and emergence from anesthesia.

### Strabismus Surgery
Strabismus surgery is performed to correct misalignment of extraocular muscles and realign the visual axis. Most patients are pediatric (also see Chapter 34). Special considerations include (1) frequent incidence of intraoperative OCR, (2) potential increased risk for malignant hyperthermia, and (3) marked prevalence of postoperative nausea and vomiting (PONV).

### Nausea and Vomiting
The incidence of PONV following strabismus surgery varies widely but has been quoted as high as 85% (also see Chapter 39). PONV is the most common reason for pediatric inpatient admission after outpatient surgery and is probably a vagal-mediated response to surgical manipulation of extraocular muscles. Multimodal antiemetics with differing mechanisms of action may be more effective than individual medications for those patients at most risk of PONV following eye surgery.

### Malignant Hyperthermia
Strabismus is a neuromuscular disorder that can be associated with other myopathies. The frequency of masseter muscle spasm after succinylcholine is fourfold greater than baseline. Suspect malignant hyperthermia if hypertension, tachycardia, hypercarbia, and increasing temperature occur.

### Traumatic Eye Injuries
Eye injury occurs as a result of penetrating or blunt trauma. The anesthesia plan must balance specific risks. Increased IOP due to a tightly applied face mask, laryngoscopy, and endotracheal intubation, or due to coughing or bucking, can cause extrusion of globe contents and jeopardize vision. Additionally, in emergency situations, the patient may be nonfasting and at risk of aspiration of gastric contents upon induction of general anesthesia. Control of the airway can be achieved with a rapid-sequence induction of anesthesia including succinylcholine; however, succinylcholine can also cause a transient increase in IOP.[13] Awake endotracheal intubation may be appropriate for patients with difficult airways; however, the resultant increases in IOP can be disastrous. The risks of succinylcholine or awake intubation on IOP must be weighed against the dangers imposed by a full stomach or difficult airway.

The anesthesia provider should ask the ophthalmologist if the operative repair can be delayed until the stomach is considered safe. If not, then proceed after careful evaluation to rule out other issues. Administer appropriate drugs to decrease gastric acidity and volume. Place

IV

the patient in slight reverse Trendelenburg position and avoid any maneuvers that may increase IOP. If no airway problems are anticipated, consider a modified rapid-sequence induction of anesthesia with a large dose of a nondepolarizing neuromuscular blocking drug (e.g., rocuronium, 1.0 mg/kg). If succinylcholine is selected, the IOP and systemic hypertension following laryngoscopy/intubation can be moderated by intravenous lidocaine, opioids, or a small pretreatment dose of nondepolarizing neuromuscular blocker prior to induction of anesthesia. Regional anesthesia may be an option for select injuries and patients at greater risk from general anesthesia.[14]

## Postoperative Eye Issues

### Corneal Abrasion
The most common cause of postoperative eye pain after general anesthesia is corneal abrasion. It manifests with conjunctivitis, tearing, and foreign body sensation. Damage may be mechanically incurred by dangling ID tags, the anesthesia mask, drapes, and other objects. During general anesthesia, abrasion may also occur because of the loss of the blink reflex, the drying effects of exposure to air, and diminished tear production. Preventive measures include gently taping the eyelids shut during mask ventilation, endotracheal intubation, and thereafter. Ointments may cause allergic reaction or blurred postemergence vision. Protective goggles may be best. Antibiotic ointment and patching the eye usually result in healing of corneal abrasions within a day or two.

### Acute Glaucoma
Acute glaucoma is also painful. Presence of a mydriatic pupil may be diagnostic. This is an urgent matter calling for consult with an ophthalmologist. Intravenous mannitol or acetazolamide can decrease IOP and relieve pain.

### Postoperative Visual Loss
Painless loss of vision after surgery may be due to ischemic optic neuropathy (ION) or brain injury. Both are rare events. Risk is more frequent with spine surgery in the prone position and cardiac surgery.[15] Consultation with an ophthalmologist is mandatory as early funduscopic examination may aid in diagnosis.

## OTOLARYNGOLOGY

Ear, nose, and throat (ENT) surgery can make the airway fairly inaccessible and is commonly referred to as *field avoidance*. Preoperative planning with the surgeon and nursing staff is essential.[16] There is a distinct possibility of encountering a difficult airway because of anatomic factors, surgical issues, or underlying disease. Attention should be directed to the establishment and firm anchoring of an endotracheal airway. The endotracheal tube

(ETT) should be manually supported during patient repositioning such as turning of the head because movement can result in endobronchial intubation, tube occlusion, cuff leaks, disconnections, or even frank dislodgement of the ETT and inadvertent extubation. Prior to surgical preparation or placement of drapes, the neck position should be reassessed, and susceptible pressure points padded. During surgery, the airway may be compromised by often undetected bleeding, edema, or surgical manipulation. The use of posterior pharyngeal packs can minimize the risk of aspiration of gastric contents. Operating room (OR) personnel should be alerted to their placement, and there must be confirmation of the complete removal of all packs prior to extubation of the trachea.

## Special Considerations for Head and Neck Surgery

### The Difficult Airway (Also See Chapter 16)
All airway concerns should be addressed with surgical colleagues prior to patient entry into the OR. Supplementary equipment must be readied in anticipation of a possible difficult airway, and expert assistance should be immediately available. Modified techniques to secure the airway include use of videolaryngoscopy, fiberoptic bronchoscopy, or even performance of a tracheostomy under local anesthesia. The placement of tracheal retention sutures with tracheostomy can facilitate recapture of airway access should it become compromised during or after surgery. Procedures within the airway can produce significant edema resulting in acute obstruction. In the postoperative period these patients may need to remain tracheally intubated, or, if extubated, they may require treatment with humidified oxygen or nebulized bronchodilators.

### Laryngospasm
The laryngospasm reflex is mediated through vagal stimulation of the superior laryngeal nerve. Abrupt intense, prolonged closure of the larynx with compromise of ventilation can occur upon instrumentation of the endolarynx, with blood or foreign body presence, and with inadequate depth of anesthesia. If the airway is completely obstructed, the anesthesia provider may be unable to ventilate the patient despite an adequate mask fit. The ensuing hypercarbia, hypoxia, and acidosis elicit an autonomic sympathetic response producing hypertension and tachycardia. A temporal reduction in brainstem firing to the superior laryngeal nerve eventually causes relaxation of the vocal cords. In small children even brief laryngospasm is particularly perilous as peripheral oxygen saturation decreases precipitously as a result of a small functional residual capacity and relatively high cardiac output (also see Chapter 34). Prompt recognition and intervention are essential. Treatment modalities include the administration of 100% oxygen via positive-pressure

face mask ventilation, placement of an oral/nasal airway, and deepening of anesthesia with intravenously administered anesthetics. Small doses of succinylcholine (0.25 to 0.5 mg/kg) and tracheal intubation may be necessary in refractory cases. The likelihood of encountering laryngospasm may be reduced with use of intravenous or topical lidocaine (4% lidocaine spray) prior to laryngoscopy and endotracheal intubation.

## Upper Respiratory Infections

Patients, especially children, scheduled for elective ENT surgery may present with an unresolved upper respiratory infection (URI) predisposing to airway hyperreactivity. They are at enhanced risk of intraoperative breath-holding, desaturation, and postoperative croup.[17] Postponing surgery for uncomplicated pediatric URI is controversial and may not be required for brief nonairway ENT procedures such as myringotomy and tube placement (also see Chapter 34).

## Epistaxis

After massive epistaxis, patients are often anxious, hypovolemic, and hypertensive. Rehydration and reassurance are essential. Because blood is being continuously swallowed, these patients are considered at high risk for regurgitation and aspiration of gastric contents and are managed accordingly. A large-bore peripheral intravenous cannula is vital because some blood loss is occult, and hypotension or continued hemorrhage is likely after induction of anesthesia.

## Obstructive Sleep Apnea (Also See Chapter 13)

Obstructive sleep apnea (OSA) is characterized by upper airway obstruction and disordered breathing patterns during sleep. Symptoms include snoring, headache, sleep disturbance, daytime somnolence, and personality changes. Polysomnography (sleep study) establishes the diagnosis and severity of the disorder but is not routinely performed. Pediatric patients may have behavior and growth disturbances as well as poor school performance (also see Chapter 34). Patients are often obese with short, thick necks and large tongues. These factors contribute to difficult airway management during mask ventilation, direct laryngoscopy, tracheal intubation, and extubation.[18] Patients with OSA are exquisitely sensitive to the effects of hypnotics and narcotics and may require prolonged recovery room stay.

## Airway Fires

Airway fires are a direct patient hazard and source of medical litigation. Three elements are needed for the creation of a fire in the OR:

1. Heat/source of ignition (laser or electrosurgical unit)
2. Fuel (paper drapes, ETT, or gauze swabs)
3. Oxidizer ($O_2$, air, or $N_2O$)

The danger of an airway fire is not limited to general anesthesia. It may also occur during face and neck procedures conducted under MAC because electrocautery is used in close proximity to an open source of oxygen, such as nasal cannula.[19]

## Anesthesia Management of Specific Otolaryngology Procedures

### Ear Surgery

There are several points to consider for anesthesia and ear surgery:

#### Nitrous Oxide

Nitrous oxide is more soluble than nitrogen in blood and diffuses into air-filled cavities quicker than nitrogen diffuses out. The ensuing increased middle ear pressure may be problematic, including potential dislodgement of tympanoplasty grafts. Furthermore, acute discontinuation of high concentrations of nitrous oxide markedly decreases cavity pressure and may cause serous otitis. Nitrous oxide should be avoided or used in moderate concentration (<50%) and discontinued approximately 15 to 30 minutes prior to graft application.

#### Facial Nerve Monitoring

The surgeon may elect to use a facial nerve monitor to prevent accidental incision of facial nerve branches during surgery. Complete paralysis by neuromuscular blocking drugs can inhibit facial nerve monitor function. The use of neuromuscular blocking drugs should be curtailed to small doses or to only succinylcholine. Also, use of a neuromuscular monitor can be used to confirm a response to train-of-four stimulation of a peripheral nerve and absence of full paralysis prior to surgical dissection in the middle ear (also see Chapter 11).

#### Epinephrine

Epinephrine is frequently injected during ear microsurgery to decrease bleeding and improve the visual field. Systemic uptake may precipitate tachydysrhythmias. Hence, epinephrine concentration should be limited to a 1:200,000 solution.[20] Other means to control bleeding include moderate reverse Trendelenburg (head-up) positioning to decrease venous congestion and the use of volatile anesthetics to decrease systolic arterial blood pressures within an acceptable range. The use of vasoactive drugs and controlled hypotension is controversial.

#### Emergence

Head and neck manipulation during the application of bandages at the conclusion of surgery produces movement of the ETT and airway irritation. Coughing and bucking increase venous pressure, which can lead to graft disruption or acute bleeding. In the patient with an

IV

uncomplicated airway, extubation of the trachea at a deep plane of anesthesia may be beneficial.

### Postoperative Nausea and Vomiting (Also See Chapter 39)

As a result of manipulation of the vestibular apparatus, PONV is common after middle ear surgery. Factors that may exacerbate PONV include anesthetic technique (use of nitrous oxide and narcotics), inadequate rehydration, and postoperative movement. The extent of prophylactic measures taken to prevent PONV is guided by a graded risk analysis.[21] Prophylactic interventions may include use of one or more antiemetics including corticosteroid, 5-$HT_3$-receptor antagonist, neurokinin-1 receptor antagonist, scopolamine patch, low-dose propofol, and gastric decompression. Scopolamine may cause confusion and probably should not be used in geriatric patients.

### Myringotomy and Tube Insertion

Myringotomy and tube insertion is performed for children with disorders of the middle ear who have a history of repeated ear infections with unsatisfactory response to antibiotic therapy. There may be residual inflammation of the middle ear and upper airway irritability. An inhaled induction and maintenance of anesthesia with ventilation via a face mask is preferred for this brief procedure. Postoperative pain is minimal, so premedication may not be needed and may result in residual postoperative sedative effects (also see Chapter 34).

### Tonsillectomy and Adenoidectomy

Most patients undergoing this procedure are young and healthy. Common surgical perioperative issues include airway obstruction, bleeding, cardiac arrhythmias, and croup (postextubation airway edema). Patients frequently have obstruction of the upper airway, which only becomes apparent during sleep (OSA). In general, a comprehensive history and physical examination are sufficient for a preoperative workup, but any history of sleep-disordered breathing, obesity, or a bleeding diathesis warrants further investigation. Sedative premedication is best avoided for children with OSA, obesity, intermittent airway obstruction, or significant tonsil hypertrophy.

In young children, an inhaled induction of anesthesia is preferred because preoperative establishment of an intravenous line may be difficult or traumatic. An intravenous line can be started once the child is anesthetized. Loss of pharyngeal muscle tone upon induction of anesthesia may lead to airway obstruction. Continuous positive airway pressure may relieve the problem. Placement of a cuffed preformed curved oral ETT optimizes field visualization and decreases the likelihood of accidental extubation of the trachea (Fig. 31.3). An air leak at 20 cm $H_2O$ peak airway pressure reduces the probability of tissue edema, a critical factor for pediatric patients who have narrower airway diameters than adults. A precordial stethoscope is useful to monitor breath sounds because

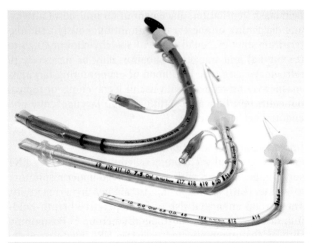

**Fig. 31.3** Armored and cuffed preformed curved oral endotracheal tubes.

ETT dislodgement can occur with movement of the head or mouth gag. The supraglottic area is occasionally packed with gauze to protect against aspiration. Prior to extubation of the trachea, the pack must be removed and the stomach should be decompressed. Tracheal extubation can be performed when the child is fully awake and actively responsive. Some anesthesia providers perform tracheal extubation when the patient is still anesthetized in order to minimize coughing and laryngospasm related to the presence of the ETT.

Intravenous dexamethasone may decrease edema and postoperative pain as well as PONV. Postoperative airway obstruction can occur for a variety of reasons ranging from secretions or blood on the vocal cords to a retained pharyngeal pack. Airway obstruction occasionally produces negative-pressure pulmonary edema. This manifests when the patient breathes against a closed glottis creating a marked negative intrathoracic pressure. This pressure is transmitted to interstitial tissue and promotes flow of fluid from the pulmonary circulation into the alveoli. Young children (younger than 4 years old) are susceptible to airway obstruction as late as 24 hours postoperatively and may benefit from prolonged postoperative monitoring.

### Bleeding Tonsils After Tonsillectomy and Adenoidectomy

The family's expectation is that a patient undergoing tonsillectomy will have a complete and uncomplicated procedure and anesthesia. Yet, serious complications can occur. Hemorrhage after tonsillectomy normally occurs within a few hours of surgery and presents with expectoration of red blood, repeated swallowing, tachycardia, and PONV.[22] Blood loss is often underestimated because it is mostly swallowed. Intravenous fluid administration is critical prior to corrective urgent surgery. Patients are considered to have a full stomach, so precautions are taken during induction of anesthesia to avert regurgitation and pulmonary aspiration of blood and gastric contents. Features of a rapid-sequence induction of anesthesia include application of cricoid pressure (Sellick maneuver) until correct ETT positioning is confirmed, administration of intravenous anesthetics and neuromuscular blocking drugs in quick succession, and presence of a working suction catheter at the head of the table.

### Epiglottitis (Also See Chapter 34)

Acute epiglottitis is an infectious disease caused by *Haemophilus influenzae* type B, most often affecting children between 2 and 7 years of age.[23] There is often a history of sudden onset of fever and dysphagia. Symptomatic progression from pharyngitis to airway obstruction and respiratory failure can be rapid (within hours). The child with epiglottitis appears agitated, drools, and leans forward holding the head in an extended position. Exhaustion may result from labored breathing against an almost fully occluded airway.

Direct visualization of the glottis should not be attempted because stimulation of the patient and struggling may result in complete airway obstruction. Anesthesia commences only when all emergency airway equipment is open and readied, with a surgeon adept at rigid bronchoscopy and tracheostomy present. An inhaled induction of anesthesia maintaining spontaneous ventilation is preferred. Atropine may be given to avoid bradycardia and to dry secretions. The edematous airway necessitates use of a small ETT. Because the degree of airway narrowing is unpredictable a range of ETT sizes should be available. In the event of any difficulty, the surgeon should intervene and secure the airway with a rigid bronchoscope or establish a surgical airway.

### Foreign Body in Airway

Tracheal aspiration of a foreign body is an emergency, especially in the pediatric population (also see Chapter 34). Clinical manifestations include sudden dyspnea, dry cough, hoarseness, and wheezing. Mutual cooperation between the anesthesia provider and surgeon is vital to avoid inadvertent distal displacement of the foreign body and complete airway obstruction.

Removal of the foreign body is achieved either via direct laryngoscopy or rigid bronchoscopy, without application of positive airway pressure.[24] The surgeon should be present and ready to perform emergency cricothyrotomy or tracheostomy in the event of complete airway occlusion. Total intravenous anesthesia maintaining spontaneous respiration avoids exposing OR personnel to volatile anesthetics. Postoperatively, the patient should breathe humidified oxygen and remain under close observation for airway edema.

### Nasal and Sinus Surgery

Nasal surgery is performed for either cosmetic or functional purposes. Common surgical operations include polypectomy, septoplasty, functional endoscopic sinus surgery, and rhinoplasty. Patients having nasal surgery often also have significant nasal passage obstruction, which may hinder ventilation via face mask. Furthermore, nasal polyps are associated with allergy and reactive airway disease. The nose's rich vascular supply can result in substantial intraoperative blood loss that may be undetected as blood trickles backward into the pharynx. Many nasal procedures can be performed under regional anesthesia and sedation.

The anterior ethmoidal and sphenopalatine branches of the trigeminal nerve provide sensory innervation to the nasal septum and lateral walls. Topical anesthesia is achieved by packing the nose with 4% cocaine pledgets, which are left in situ for 15 minutes. The advantages of using cocaine include production of topical anesthesia, vasoconstriction of vascular tissue, and shrinking of the mucosa. Because cocaine's disadvantages include altered sensorium and deleterious cardiovascular effects, it is frequently replaced by a "pseudococaine" solution of a different local anesthetic mixed with a vasoconstrictor.[25] Anesthesia can be supplemented by submucosal local anesthetic infiltration. When general anesthesia is chosen, the airway should be secured with a cuffed ETT. A posterior pharyngeal pack can prevent aspiration of gastric contents and decrease PONV due to swallowed blood. Extubation of the trachea should be performed only on return of protective airway reflexes.

### Endoscopic Surgery

Endoscopy includes esophagoscopy, bronchoscopy, laryngoscopy, and microlaryngoscopy (with or without laser surgery). Airway evaluation is performed for a variety of pathologic conditions, ranging from foreign body, gastroesophageal reflux, and papillomatosis to tumors or tracheal stenosis. The compromised and symptomatic airway needs careful preoperative assessment. Airway issues should be discussed with the surgeon, and preoperative investigations such as analysis of arterial blood gases, flow-volume loops, radiographic studies, or magnetic resonance imaging may be warranted.

A proactive airway management plan is necessary. Consideration must be given to a fiberoptic endotracheal intubation in an unsedated patient if doubts exist about the efficacy of successful mask ventilation and direct laryngoscopy. Sedative premedication should be cautiously considered in the presence of upper airway obstruction. Administration of an anticholinergic drug will diminish secretions and facilitate airway visualization. If the patient exhibits stridor or inspiratory retractions, airway obstruction probably exists. Although rarely done, a tracheostomy under local anesthesia can be performed.

Techniques can be employed to provide oxygenation and ventilation during endoscopy. The trachea can be intubated with a small-diameter pediatric ETT, but these

IV

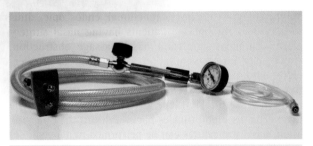

**Fig. 31.4** Sanders injector apparatus uses high-flow oxygen insufflations through a small-gauge catheter placed in the trachea.

tubes are frequently too short for use in adults and offer high resistance to flow. Because an ETT impairs visualization of the posterior commissure, a technique using high-flow oxygen insufflations through a small-gauge catheter placed in the trachea is useful (Fig. 31.4).[26] Another alternative is a manual jet ventilator, which attaches to a side port of the laryngoscope. High-pressure oxygen (30 to 50 psi) is delivered during inspiration and concomitantly entrains air into the trachea via the Venturi effect. This technique carries risk of pneumothorax and pneumomediastinum from rupture of alveolar blebs.

An adequate degree of masseter relaxation is required for introduction of a suspension laryngoscope by the endoscopist. Even though a succinylcholine infusion provides the necessary relaxation, a phase II neuromuscular blockade can result, which often cannot be rapidly terminated (also see Chapter 11).

## Laser Surgery

Laser (light amplification by stimulated emission of radiation) surgery affords precision in targeting lesions, provides hemostasis, causes minimal tissue edema, and promotes rapid healing. Its physical properties depend on the medium used to create the beam. Laser is used in the treatment of vocal cord papillomas, laryngeal webs, and resection of subglottic occlusive tissue. The use of a small-diameter ETT is necessary for maximum exposure.[27] Laser energy can cause retinal damage, and can produce a laser plume of toxic fumes, which has potential to transmit disease. An efficient smoke evacuator and special masks are necessary because small particles are readily inhaled. The patient's eyes should be taped, and OR personnel must wear protective eyeglasses.

The greatest danger during laser surgery is ETT fire (also see Chapter 48), as described earlier, so suitable precautions should be taken (Box 31.3). Flexible stainless steel laser-resistant tubes are available for the specific type of laser employed (Fig. 31.5). In order to dissipate heat and detect cuff rupture, the tube cuff should be filled with saline and an indicator dye. Although polyvinylchloride tubes are flammable, they may be modified with a metallic tape wrap. Nonetheless, they may retain a risk of ignition and can reflect the laser beam onto nontargeted

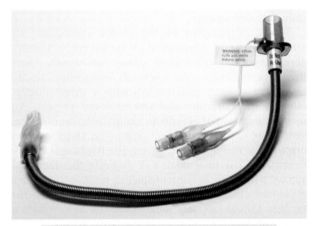

**Fig. 31.5** Laser endotracheal tube—stainless steel.

tissue. The tissue adjacent to the surgical field should be protected with moist packing. Postoperatively, patients should be monitored for laryngeal edema.

## Neck Dissection Surgery

Neck dissection may be complete, modified, or functional. Anatomically, the structures principally involved are (1) the sternocleidomastoid muscle, (2) cranial nerve XI, and (3) the internal and external jugular veins and carotid artery. Frequently, neck dissection is performed for removal of a tumor and may also involve partial or total glossectomy. Patients with such tumors may have a history of tobacco and alcohol abuse. Pulmonary disease is likely and is an indication for a preoperative pulmonary evaluation.

In many cases, the neck dissection may be bilateral, and a tracheostomy may be performed to maintain a patent airway. Upper airway management may be difficult in these patients, especially if there is a history of radiation treatment of the larynx and pharynx or if a mass is present in the oral cavity. Neuromuscular

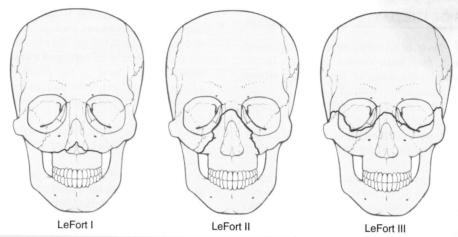

LeFort I          LeFort II          LeFort III

**Fig. 31.6** Facial injuries and the LeFort fracture classification. (From Myer CM. Trauma of the larynx and craniofacial structures: airway implications. *Paediatr Anaesth.* 2004;14:103-106, used with permission.)

blocking drugs are avoided or the dose is markedly decreased if neuromonitoring is used. Traction or pressure on the carotid sinus can provoke prolongation of the QT interval, bradydysrhythmias, and even asystole. Treatment consists of early detection, cessation of surgical stimulus, and administration of atropine. The carotid sinus reflex can be blocked with local anesthetic infiltration. During dissection, open veins carry risk of venous air embolism.

### Postoperative Complications

In the postoperative period the anesthesia provider should be aware of potential nerve injuries. Damage to the recurrent laryngeal nerve can cause vocal cord dysfunction and, if bilateral, results in airway obstruction. The phrenic nerve also traverses through the operative field, and injury to it can result in paralysis of the ipsilateral hemidiaphragm. Pneumothorax can also occur in the postoperative period. Excessive coughing or agitation can result in hematoma formation and airway compromise. If tracheostomy is not performed as part of the procedure, the patient should be monitored closely for signs of laryngeal or upper airway obstruction (also see Chapter 39).

### Thyroid and Parathyroid Surgery

Thyroid storm may be encountered in a patient who has inadequately controlled hyperthyroidism. It manifests with signs of massive catecholamine release including tachycardia, hypertension, and diaphoresis. Intraoperative anesthesia considerations again focus on airway management. Surgical manipulation of the head and neck can occlude a standard ETT, so an armored ETT may be beneficial (see Fig. 31.3). Airway obstruction after thyroid or parathyroid surgery can be caused by bleeding from the operative site compressing the trachea. Emergency measures include prompt incision and opening of the wound to release the accumulated hematoma. Surgical trauma to one or both recurrent laryngeal nerves can manifest as postextubation hoarseness or stridor. Some surgeons use electromyography (EMG) to monitor recurrent laryngeal nerve integrity, using a special ETT and EMG monitor. Parathyroid injury or removal may cause hypocalcemia with clinical signs of tetany, cardiac dysrhythmias, and laryngospasm.

### Parotid Surgery

The parotid gland may be excised in toto or surgery may be limited to the superficial portion of the gland. Because the parotid is traversed by the facial nerve, nerve function can be monitored with a facial nerve monitor in order to circumvent surgical trauma.[28] The facial nerve may need to be sacrificed during radical parotidectomy and reconstructed with a graft from the contralateral greater auricular nerve (branch of the superficial cervical plexus). Nasotracheal intubation is appropriate if a mandibular resection is planned.

### Facial Trauma

Facial fractures are characterized by the LeFort classification of maxilla fractures (Fig. 31.6).[29] A LeFort I fracture extends across the lower portion of the maxilla but does not continue up into the medial canthal region. A LeFort II fracture also extends across the maxilla, but at a more cephalad level, and it continues upward to the medial canthal region. A LeFort III fracture is a high-level transverse fracture above the malar bone and through the orbits. It is characterized by complete separation of the maxilla from the craniofacial skeleton. Orotracheal intubation is necessary when intranasal damage is a possibility. In orthognathic surgery, LeFort fractures are created for cosmetic repair.

IV

## QUESTIONS OF THE DAY

1. What are the effects of different airway management techniques (e.g., face mask ventilation, direct laryngoscopy, tracheal intubation, or supraglottic airway placement) on intraocular pressure?

2. What are the potential systemic side effects of ophthalmic medications?

3. What are the clinical manifestations of the oculocardiac reflex (OCR)? What are the options for managing OCR?

4. A patient who received a retrobulbar block prior to eye surgery develops decreased level of consciousness. What are the potential causes, and what is the appropriate management?

5. A patient is undergoing retinal surgery with general anesthesia. The surgeon plans injection of an intravitreal gas bubble. What are the anesthetic implications?

6. An adult patient who sustained a traumatic eye injury requires urgent surgery. The patient recently ingested a large meal. What are the options for anesthesia management that address both the risk of aspiration and visual loss?

7. What measures can be taken to reduce the risk of airway fire during laser surgery of the vocal cords and trachea?

8. A patient is undergoing neck dissection and laryngectomy. What are the implications for intraoperative anesthesia management? What postoperative complications should be anticipated?

## REFERENCES

1. Gayer S, Zuleta J. Perioperative management of the elderly undergoing eye surgery. *Clin Geriatr Med.* 2008;24(4):687–700.

2. Vann MA, Ogunnaike BO, Joshi GP. Sedation and anesthesia care for ophthalmologic surgery during local/regional anesthesia. *Anesthesiology.* 2007;107(3):502–508.

3. Chen CL, Lin GA, Bardach NS, et al. Preoperative medical testing in Medicare patients undergoing cataract surgery. *N Engl J Med.* 2015;372(16):1530–1538.

4. Schein OD, Katz J, Bass EB, et al. The value of routine preoperative medical testing before cataract surgery. Study of Medical Testing for Cataract Surgery. *N Engl J Med.* 2000;342:168–175.

5. Katz J, Feldman MA, Bass EB, et al. Risks and benefits of anticoagulant and antiplatelet medication use before cataract surgery. *Ophthalmology.* 2003;110(9):1784–1788.

6. McClellan AJ, Flynn Jr HW, Gayer S. The use of perioperative antithrombotic agents in posterior segment ocular surgery. *Am J Ophthalmol.* 2014;158(5):858–859.

7. Bhananker SM, Posner FW, Cheney KL, et al. Injury and liability associated with monitored anesthesia care. A closed claims analysis. *Anesthesiology.* 2006;104(2):228–234.

8. Ophthalmic Anesthesia Society. www.eyeanesthesia.org.

9. Fanning GL. Orbital regional anesthesia. *Ophthalmol Clin North Am.* 2006;19(2):221–232.

10. Gayer S. Ophthalmic anesthesia: more than meets the eye. *ASA Refresher Courses in Anesthesiology.* 2006;34(5):55–63.

11. Kumar CM, Dodds C. Sub-Tenon's anesthesia. *Ophthalmol Clin North Am.* 2006;19(2):209–219.

12. Wolf GL, Capuano C, Hartung J. Nitrous oxide increases intraocular pressure after intravitreal sulfur hexafluoride injection. *Anesthesiology.* 1983;59:547–548.

13. Vachon CA, Warner DO, Bacon DR. Succinylcholine and the open globe. Tracing the teaching. *Anesthesiology.* 2003;99:220–223.

14. Gayer S. Rethinking anesthesia strategies for patients with traumatic eye injuries: alternatives to general anesthesia. *Curr Anaesth Crit Care.* 2006;17:191–196.

15. Shen Y, Drum M, Roth S. The prevalence of perioperative visual loss in the United States: a 10 year study from 1996 to 2005 of spinal, orthopedic, cardiac, and general surgery. *Anesth Analg.* 2009;109(5):1534–1545.

16. Satloff RT, Brown AC. Special equipment in the operating room for otolaryngology–head and neck surgery. *Otolaryngol Clin North Am.* 1981;14:669–686.

17. Tait AR, Malviya S, Voepel-Lewis T, et al. Risk factors for perioperative adverse respiratory events in children with upper respiratory tract infections. *Anesthesiology.* 2001;95:299–306.

18. Gross JB, Bachenberg KL, Benumof JL, et al. Practice guidelines for the perioperative management of patients with obstructive sleep apnea: a report by the American Society of Anesthesiologists (ASA) Task Force on Perioperative Management of patients with obstructive sleep apnea. *Anesthesiology.* 2006;104(5):1081–1093.

19. American Society of Anesthesiologists Task Force on Operating Room Fires; Caplan RA, Barker SJ, Connis RT, et al. Practice advisory for the prevention and management of operating room fires. *Anesthesiology.* 2008;108(5):786–801.

20. Dunlevy TM, O'Malley TP, Postma GN. Optimal concentration of epinephrine for vasoconstriction in neck surgery. *Laryngoscope.* 1996;106:1412–1414.

21. Apfel CC, Laara E, Koivuranta M, et al. A simplified risk score for predicting postoperative nausea and vomiting: conclusions from cross-validations between two centers. *Anesthesiology.* 1999;91:693–700.

22. Randall DA, Hoffer ME. Complications of tonsillectomy and adenoidectomy. *Otolaryngol Head Neck Surg.* 1998;118:61–68.

23. Tanner K, Fitzsimmons G, Carrol ED, et al. Haemophilus influenzae type b epiglottitis as a cause of acute upper airways obstruction in children. *BMJ.* 2002;325:1099–1100.

24. Lam HC, Woo JK, van Hasselt CA. Management of ingested foreign bodies: a retrospective review of 5240 patients. *J Laryngol Otol.* 2001;115:954–957.

25. Lange RA, Cigarroa RG, Yancy Jr CW, et al. Cocaine-induced coronary-artery vasoconstriction. *N Engl J Med.* 1989;321:1557–1562.

26. Rajagopalan R, Smith F, Ramachandran PR. Anaesthesia for microlaryngoscopy and definitive surgery. *Can Anaesth Soc J.* 1972;19:83–86.

27. Rampil IJ. Anesthetic considerations for laser surgery. *Anesth Analg.* 1992;74:424–435.

28. Terrell JE, Kileny PR, Yian C, et al. Clinical outcome of continuous facial nerve monitoring during primary parotidectomy. *Arch Otolaryngol Head Neck Surg.* 1997;123:1081–1087.

29. Myer CM. Trauma of the larynx and craniofacial structures, airway implications. *Paediatr Anaesth.* 2004;14:103–106.

# 32 ORTHOPEDIC SURGERY

## Andrew D. Rosenberg and Mitchell H. Marshall

## RHEUMATOLOGIC DISORDERS

Patients with rheumatoid arthritis (RA) and other rheumatologic disorders, such as ankylosing spondylitis, present for orthopedic surgery related to their disease state. Knowledge of these diseases and their underlying medical issues is essential for optimal anesthetic and perioperative management.

### Rheumatoid Arthritis

RA is a chronic inflammatory disease that initially destroys joints and adjacent connective tissue and then progresses to a systemic disease affecting major organ systems (Fig. 32.1). Implicated predisposing causes include genetic (over 100 gene loci have been identified), environmental, bacterial, viral, and hormonal factors.[1-5] The role of T cells, autoimmunity, and inflammatory mediators are important in the progression of RA and may serve as sites for potential new treatments.[2-5]

Systemic manifestations of RA are widespread. They may include pulmonary involvement with interstitial fibrosis and cysts with honeycombing, gastritis, and ulcers from aspirin and other analgesics, neuropathy, muscle wasting, vasculitis, and anemia. Ultimately the anatomy of the airway is damaged and altered in patients with RA.[2-5]

#### Airway and Cervical Spine Changes

The patient must be carefully evaluated for both complexity and risks of endotracheal intubation. For example, the airway may be difficult to visualize when attempting intubation. Furthermore, the performance of maneuvers to intubate the trachea may result in an increased risk

The editors and publisher would like to thank Dr. Thomas J.J. Blanck for contributing to this chapter in the previous edition of this work. It has provided the framework for much of this chapter.

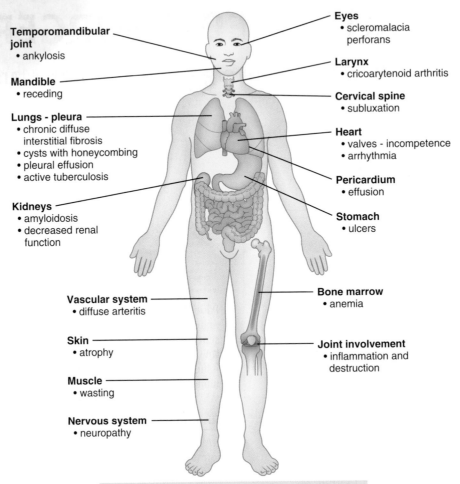

**Fig. 32.1** Systemic manifestations of rheumatoid arthritis.

of cervical spine injury. Many airway abnormalities may occur in patients with RA. Normal mouth opening may be decreased as a result of temporomandibular arthritis. This difficulty may be compounded by the presence of a hypoplastic mandible, which may fuse early in patients with juvenile RA. This results in the noticeable overbite in some patients with RA.[2-5]

As with other joints, the cricoarytenoid joint may be affected. Cricoarytenoid arthritis may result in shortness of breath and snoring. Patients with RA have been misdiagnosed as having sleep apnea as a result of this condition.[6] Patients with cricoarytenoid arthritis may present with stridor during inspiration, which may occur in the postanesthesia care unit (PACU) after surgery while recovering from anesthesia. Acute subluxation of the cricoarytenoid joint as a result of tracheal intubation can cause stridor as well, and it is not responsive to administration of racemic epinephrine.[3]

The cervical spine is abnormal in as many as 80% of patients with RA. Subluxation and unrestricted motion of the cervical spine can lead to impingement of the spinal cord and its injury.[7] Three anatomic areas of the cervical spine may become involved, resulting in atlantoaxial subluxation, subaxial subluxation, or superior migration of the odontoid (Fig. 32.2).

Atlantoaxial Subluxation
Atlantoaxial subluxation is the abnormal movement of the C1 cervical vertebra (the atlas) on C2 (the axis). Normally, the transverse axial ligament (TAL) holds the odontoid process, also referred to as the *dens*, which is the superior projection of the vertebra of C2, in place directly behind the anterior arch of C1 (Fig. 32.3A). With an intact TAL, as the cervical spine is flexed and extended, the odontoid moves with the cervical arch of C1 and the movement between the two is minimal. With destruction of the TAL by RA, movement of the dens is no longer restricted. As the neck is flexed and extended, the C1 vertebra can sublux on the C2 vertebra as the dens and C1 cervical spine no longer move together (Fig. 32.3B). This can result in impingement of the spinal cord, placing it at risk for damage. Subluxation of C1 on C2, referred to as *atlantoaxial subluxation*, can be quantified by a measurement

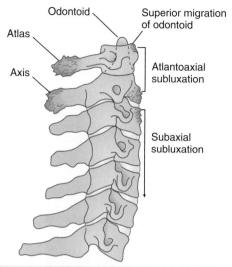

Fig. 32.2 Sites of potential involvement of rheumatoid arthritis in the cervical spine.

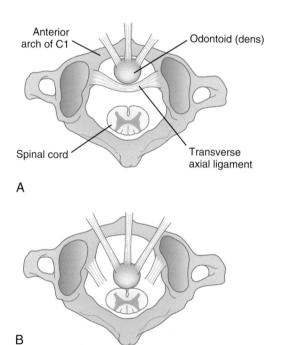

A

B

Fig. 32.3 (A) Cross-sectional view demonstrating intact TAL (transverse axial ligament) holding odontoid in place against the anterior arch of C1 vertebra. (B) Rupture of TAL may result in spinal cord impingement.

made between the back of the anterior arch of C1 and the front of the dens or odontoid. This distance is referred to as the *atlas-dens interval* (ADI). Flexion and extension radiographs of the cervical spine are obtained in order to determine the distance between the atlas and dens and the degree of subluxation (Fig. 32.4). If the ADI is 4 mm

or more, atlantoaxial instability is present, the amount of subluxation is considered significant, and the patient is considered to be at risk for spinal cord injury. Because the ring of the cervical arch is an enclosed space, as the ADI increases, the safe area for the cord (SAC), that area left within the arch of C1, decreases and motion can lead to impingement of the cord. In a situation in which the TAL is disrupted, extension of the head minimizes the ADI and increases the SAC, whereas flexion increases the ADI (Fig. 32.5) and decreases the SAC, making flexion a more frequent risk position. However, as RA affects more than just the TAL, all neck movements in patients with RA have to be evaluated carefully and extension of the neck can also lead to problems. Although uncommon, asymptomatic patients can have ADI measurements as high as 8 mm to 10 mm. These asymptomatic patients are able to compensate for their cervical spine instability with use of local musculature while awake, but this is not possible when anesthetized. Therefore, neck motion should be minimized after administration of sedation or general anesthesia in patients with atlantoaxial subluxation.[2-5,7-10]

### Subaxial Subluxation

Subluxation of 15% or more of one cervical vertebra on another below the level of the axis (C2) is referred to as *subaxial subluxation*. This can result in significant spinal cord impingement and neurologic symptoms. The C5-C6 level is the most common area for subaxial subluxation.[9,10] As a result, neck motion can increase impingement and result in spinal cord injury. Therefore, minimal motion of the cervical spine is recommended in patients with this condition.

### Superior Migration of the Odontoid

Inflammation and bone destruction can result in cervical spine collapse in patients with RA. Not all areas of the cervical spine are equally affected in any given patient. For example, if the odontoid is spared, cervical spine collapse may actually result in an intact odontoid process projecting up through the foramen magnum and into the skull. The odontoid can impinge on the brainstem and patients may suffer neurologic symptoms including quadriparesis or paralysis (Fig. 32.6). This pathologic anatomic condition is referred to as *superior migration of the odontoid*. The odontoid needs to be removed in order to decompress the spinal cord and brainstem. A complicated operative procedure, a transoral odontoidectomy, may accomplish this and involves an incision in the posterior pharyngeal wall, followed by removal of the arch of C1 and then removal of the odontoid, or pannus, or both, which is causing the neurologic symptoms. With completion of the transoral portion of the procedure, the cervical spine is very unstable, necessitating a posterior spinal fusion.

### The Trachea in Rheumatoid Arthritis

Although the cervical spine is affected by RA and may collapse from bone destruction, the trachea is usually

IV

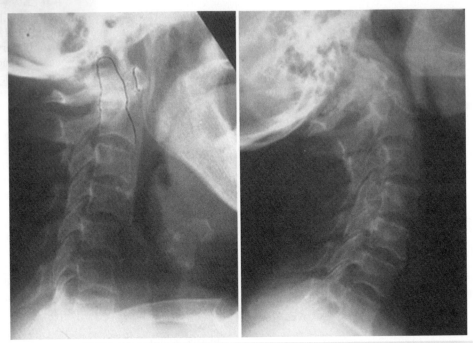

**Fig. 32.4** Radiographs of cervical spine in flexion and extension. Note significant atlantoaxial instability with flexion in left panel where odontoid and arch of C1 are outlined. Note contrast in right panel where in extension odontoid and arch of C1 are in close proximity.

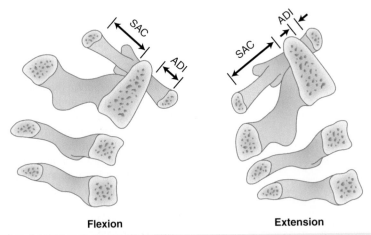

Flexion                                         Extension

**Fig. 32.5** Flexion and extension views demonstrating how flexion increases the ADI (atlas-dens interval) and decreases the SAC (safe area for the spinal cord). In extension the ADI is decreased and the SAC is increased.

spared. This results in the trachea twisting in a characteristic manner as the cervical spine collapses, only serving to increase the difficulty of intubating these patients.[9] Tracheal intubation aids such as a fiberoptic bronchoscope, Glidescope, Airtraq, or intubating laryngeal mask airway (LMA) should be available for assistance in intubating these patients should it be needed (also see Chapter 16).

## Ankylosing Spondylitis

Ankylosing spondylitis is an inflammatory rheumatologic disorder in which repetitive minute bone fractures followed by healing results in the characteristic bamboo spine, disease of the sacroiliac joint, fusion of the posterior elements of the spinal column, and fixed neck flexion that is characteristic in this patient population. There is an association between ankylosing spondylitis and HLA-B27,

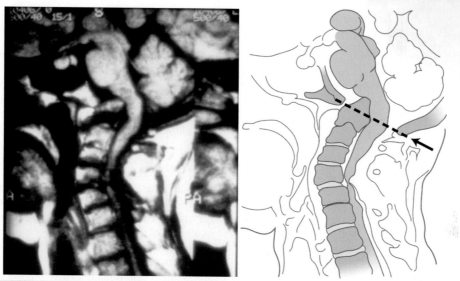

**Fig. 32.6** Magnetic resonance image (MRI) and reconstruction demonstrating superior migration of the odontoid through the foramen magnum and impingement on medulla and pons. Also note subaxial subluxation. (MRI courtesy of Malcolm Dobrow, MD.)

although most HLA-B27 positive patients are not affected with the disease. Patients also develop thoracic and costochondral involvement, which may result in a rapid shallow breathing pattern.[3,11] The cervical spine becomes rigid, and direct laryngoscopy and airway manipulation should be performed only after careful assessment. A tracheal intubation assist device can help secure the airway. Return of the neck to the neutral position via cervical spine surgery involves removal of all the bony elements of the posterior portion of the spine followed by extension of the head back into a neutral position. This is a very complicated and dangerous procedure, especially at the time when the neck is extended back to the neutral position, which relies on spinal cord monitoring to assess neurologic function as the spine is manipulated.

## SPINE SURGERY

Posterior spinal fusion, scoliosis correction, and combined anteroposterior spine procedures may be long, complex operations associated with significant blood loss, marked fluid shifts, and major hemodynamic alterations. These factors necessitate adequate patient preparation for the perioperative period including a detailed preoperative evaluation (also see Chapter 13), anticipation regarding perioperative intravenous fluid administration, and appropriate monitoring requirements. Some patients have underlying neuromuscular disorders that could influence the timing of tracheal extubation. Preoperative pulmonary function testing will facilitate clinical decisions in this patient population. Appropriate size and number of

intravenous catheters, as well as hemodynamic and neurologic monitoring needs, should be determined. In addition, the blood bank needs to be advised that significant blood loss can occur requiring rapid administration of blood and blood products (also see Chapter 24).

Anterior spine surgery may be performed via abdominal or thoracic approaches. Thoracic surgery may involve open thoracotomy or thoracoscopic techniques. Preoperative discussion with the surgeon is crucial to determine the surgical approach, as there may be a need to provide lung isolation and one-lung ventilation. High thoracic and thoracoscopic procedures frequently require one-lung ventilation to ensure adequate visualization (also see Chapter 27). This can be accomplished with the use of a double-lumen or a bronchial blocker tube.

If the procedure is a combined anteroposterior procedure, a double-lumen endotracheal tube (ETT) can be used for the anterior component with the tube exchanged for a single-lumen ETT for the posterior portion of the surgery. Although double-lumen ETTs provide value in facilitating surgical exposure, they can also create risks, such as difficult intraoperative exchange of the double-lumen ETT to a single-lumen ETT. Reintubation of the trachea can become difficult, owing to airway edema, and may be traumatic. Alternatively, a bronchial blocker can be used with a single-lumen ETT (Fig. 32.7) (also see Chapter 27).[4,12]

Advantages of the bronchial blocker include avoiding the need to change the tube between different stages of the procedure or at the end of the surgery. Deflating the cuff and withdrawing the catheter back into its casing and recapping the proximal end returns the ETT to its single-lumen tube characteristics. If extubation of the trachea at

IV

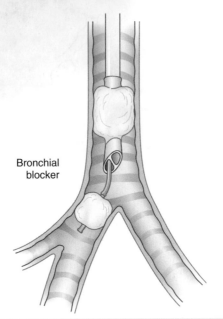

Bronchial
blocker

**Fig. 32.7** Depiction of how a bronchial blocker is placed to isolate lung for one-lung ventilation.

the end of the surgical procedure is not indicated, the ETT does not have to be changed at the end of the operation, thereby avoiding the possibility of changing an ETT in the presence of potentially significant airway edema or difficult endotracheal intubation. The PACU or intensive care unit staff needs to be properly educated as to the various ports of the bronchial blocker.[3,4,12]

Some surgeons are using $CO_2$ insufflation as the sole means of moving the lung away from the surgical field, even in high thoracic spine surgical procedures. This allows for the use of a single-lumen ETT for the entire procedure, bypassing the need for either a double-lumen tube or a bronchial blocker.

## Anesthetic Technique

The anesthetic technique is geared to provide anesthesia and analgesia for the procedure while avoiding drugs that may interfere with acquisition of the waveforms required for perioperative neurologic evaluation of the spine. Nitrous oxide/oxygen or air/oxygen are used in combination with opioids and an infusion of propofol or dexmedetomidine. If somatosensory evoked potentials (SSEPs) alone are being monitored, an inhaled anesthetic, equivalent to a small percentage (typically < 50%) of 1 MAC (minimum alveolar concentration), can be administered. Volatile anesthetics may interfere with signal acquisition in patients monitored with transcranial motor evoked potentials (TCMEPs) and may have to be discontinued, if used at all, if adequate signals cannot be obtained. Although neuromuscular blockade may be used to facilitate tracheal intubation, paralysis

should not be maintained if TCMEPs are being continuously monitored. If the patient is having pedicle screws placed, then the neuromuscular blockade needs to be terminated before the electromyograms (EMGs) are obtained so that testing can be properly performed. A small dose of ketamine, either as a bolus or continuous infusion, can be given in the perioperative period as an additional pain relief modality to provide analgesia for major surgery including spine surgery (also see Chapter 8).[13,14]

## Awareness

Intraoperative awareness is a concern for patients and physicians (also see Chapter 47). Patients undergoing spine surgery may be at increased risk for intraoperative awareness as a result of the requirement that the anesthetic techniques administered to them be modified to allow for adequate intraoperative neurophysiologic monitoring waveforms to assess spinal cord function. Therefore, the use of brain function monitoring in these patients may help avoid intraoperative awareness. However, this is not a standard and, as noted in the Practice Advisory for Intraoperative Awareness and Brain Function Monitoring,[15] a decision should be made on a case-by-case basis by the individual practitioner for selected patients (e.g., light anesthesia). There was a consensus in the advisory that brain function monitoring is not routinely indicated for patients undergoing general anesthesia as the "general applicability of these monitors in the prevention of intraoperative awareness had not been established." In fact, Avidan and associates demonstrated that awareness is not decreased with use of brain function monitoring.[16] The need for brain monitoring is still not clear.

## Blood Conservation During Spine Surgery

Methods to decrease blood loss in spine surgery patients include predonation, hemodilution, wound infiltration with a dilute epinephrine solution, hypotensive anesthetic techniques, use of cell salvage devices, positioning to diminish venous pressure, careful surgical hemostasis, and administration of antifibrinolytics (also see Chapter 24). Medications that have been employed to decrease blood loss during spine surgery include the antifibrinolytics aprotinin, tranexamic acid, and ε-aminocaproic acid. Aprotinin, a serine protease inhibitor, effectively decreases blood loss in cardiac patients and has also been demonstrated to be efficacious in patients undergoing spine surgery.[17-19] The synthetic lysine analogs tranexamic acid and ε-aminocaproic acid have also been employed in spine surgery as well as in patients undergoing orthopedic joint replacement surgery.[19] Tranexamic acid can be administered by an initial bolus injection of 10 mg/kg over 30 minutes followed by a continuous infusion of 1 mg/kg/h, although other regimens may be used. Tranexamic acid may alternatively be given topically or intra-articularly in appropriate patients.

Although apparently ε-aminocaproic acid can be helpful, a meta-analysis of the use of antifibrinolytics in orthopedic patients demonstrated that although both aprotinin and tranexamic acid are effective in decreasing blood loss, the data were not sufficient to demonstrate efficacy with ε-aminocaproic acid.[18] However, the negative side effects of aprotinin in cardiac patients include (1) increased risk of myocardial infarction (MI) or heart failure by approximately 55%, nearly double the risk of stroke; (2) increased long-term risk of mortality; and (3) a more frequent death rate in patients receiving aprotinin as demonstrated in a study over a 5-year period comparing aprotinin and lysine analogs in high-risk cardiac surgery. The study was terminated early and resulted in relabeling and ultimately withdrawing aprotinin from the market so that it is no longer available.[20-22]

## Positioning

Spine surgery is often performed with the patient in the prone position (also see Chapter 19). Careful positioning is crucial to avoid patient injury. Movement to the prone position should be performed in a carefully coordinated manner with the surgical team. The neck should not be hyperextended or hyperflexed but placed in the neutral position and the ETT is positioned so that it is not kinked. Contact areas are padded, and the face and eyes are protected. Prolonged prone positioning has resulted in pressure ulcers on the face, especially the chin and forehead, and other areas. When possible, periodic repositioning of the head during prolonged procedures may minimize the risk of such injuries. Direct pressure on the eye can result in visual loss. Pressure and stretch on nerves are avoided by proper padding and avoiding any extension over 90 degrees. The abdomen needs to be hanging free to avoid increased venous pressure and thereby increased venous bleeding. The prone position alters pulmonary dynamics, so pulmonary function must be reassessed in this position.

## Intraoperative Spinal Cord Monitoring

Monitoring spinal cord function is an important component of major surgical procedures involving distraction and rotation of the spine such as occur with major anteroposterior spinal fusions and scoliosis surgery (also see Chapter 20). Spinal cord monitoring is employed in order to detect and hopefully reverse, in a timely manner, any adverse effects noted during the operative period. Spinal cord monitoring may include use of SSEPs, motor evoked potentials (MEPs) including TCMEPs, EMGs, or a wake-up test. The anesthetic technique must be adjusted appropriately when spinal cord monitoring is employed. Some anesthetics interfere with acquisition of the waveforms that are obtained intraoperatively and utilized to analyze spinal cord integrity.

SSEPs are sensory evoked potential waves generated in the cerebral cortex that result from sensory stimuli caused by repetitive peripheral nerve stimulation in the extremities that propagate up through the dorsum or sensory portion of the spinal cord and into the brain. These waveforms are then detected via electrodes placed over the scalp. Specific areas on the scalp coincide with the brain's sensory areas for the upper and lower extremities and proper signal acquisition obtained over these sites indicates an intact sensory or dorsal portion of the spinal cord. The SSEP waveform generated from multiple repetitive stimulations is analyzed for its latency and amplitude (Fig. 32.8). An increase in latency of more than 10% or a decrease in amplitude of 60% or more, as well as inability to obtain a proper waveform or signal, may be indicative of spinal cord dysfunction or disruption. Many factors can alter waveforms unrelated to surgery. They should be properly detected and eliminated. Surgically unrelated causes may include hypotension, hypothermia, high concentrations of volatile anesthetics, benzodiazepines, hyper- or hypocarbia, and anemia. Only a small concentration of volatile anesthetic (typically 1% to 2% desflurane) should be employed when SSEP monitoring is used. Midazolam and other benzodiazepines are avoided because they may interfere with obtaining a waveform. Some anesthesia providers avoid nitrous oxide and use a combination of air in oxygen.[3-5,13,14]

Surgically related conditions resulting in loss of SSEPs include direct injury or trauma to the cord or impairment of blood supply. Distraction, rotation, excessive bleeding, and severing or clamping of arterial blood supply can result in ischemia to the cord and neurologic injury. Unlike direct injury, which is demonstrated immediately by changes in SSEPs, ischemia may take time, up to half an hour or longer, to manifest itself. Some areas of the spinal cord are more vulnerable and therefore more prone to ischemia as their blood supply is dependent on watershed blood flow. Surgical intervention as a result of either direct contact or stretching may impair blood supply and thus render the cord ischemic.[23] Once a significant change in SSEPs or other monitor is noted, specific maneuvers should be used such as releasing the rotation and distraction of the spine if it has occurred. In addition, as a result of distraction there may be insufficient blood supply to the spine, and therefore, the mean arterial blood pressure should be increased in an effort to restore adequate blood flow. All variables such as hemoglobin, temperature, $CO_2$, and arterial blood pressure should be considered. Once these are all evaluated, a wake-up test (see following discussion) may be necessary if the waveforms do not improve.

### Transcranial Motor Evoked Potentials

As SSEP monitoring only helps determine adequate status of the dorsal or sensory portion of the spinal cord, a method to monitor the motor or ventral aspect of the

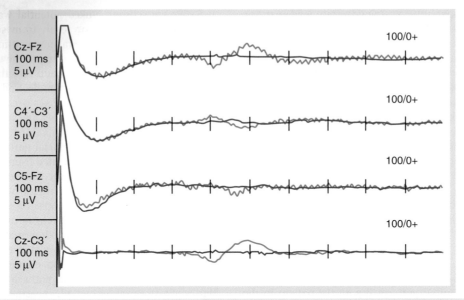

**Fig. 32.8** Somatosensory evoked potentials (SSEPs) of tibial nerve demonstrating loss of SSEP waveform. Note how the newly acquired waveforms *(purple)* are flattened when compared to baseline tracings *(red)* as amplitude of tracings are decreased and latency increased. Tracings returned to normal after retraction of cauda equina was released. (Courtesy of Department of Neurophysiology, NYU Hospital for Joint Diseases.)

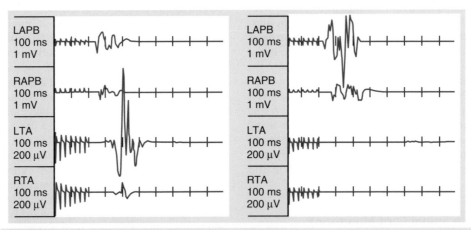

**Fig. 32.9** Normal transcranial motor evoked potentials *(left)* and loss of waveform *(right lower two panels)* indicating possible neurologic issue with motor component of spinal cord. (Courtesy of Department of Neurophysiology, NYU Hospital for Joint Diseases.)

spinal cord became necessary.[24] Initially this was provided via neurogenic MEPs, but these waveforms could be obtained only while the surgical incision was open and the spinous processes available for insertion of electrodes. Thus, some vulnerable operative time periods remained unmonitored. TCMEPs allow for monitoring the patient's motor pathways throughout the entire procedure. Stimulation over the motor cortex of the brain generates a waveform, which is propagated down the motor pathways and detected distally in the arm or leg.

This stimulation results in a characteristic waveform (Fig. 32.9). Loss of the wave may be indicative of neurologic injury (see Fig. 32.9). As with SSEP waveforms, loss of the tracings requires the following steps: an evaluation to determine the cause, attention to physiologic variables, intervention to increase arterial blood pressure, and possibly a wake-up test as well.[25]

In order to generate TCMEPs, the patient cannot have a residual neuromuscular blockade (also see Chapter 11). Importantly, it should be understood that the electric current causing the stimulus over the motor cortex also stimulates muscles directly in the area of the electrodes placed in the scalp—the masseter muscle and muscles of mastication. This muscle contraction may result in a strong bite, which can potentially injure the tongue, lip, and ETT. Instances of significant tongue lacerations and damage to ETTs can occur and potentially develop into emergency situations, especially with the patient in the prone position (also see Chapter 19).[26] The tongue should not protrude through the teeth. Placing a bite block made of tongue depressors and gauze in the back of the mouth along the teeth line bilaterally will help prevent injury. In the prone (face-down) position, any motion may allow for the tongue to slip and fall between the teeth, rendering it vulnerable to laceration. Each stimulus is associated with a masseter muscle contraction so the patient is at risk as long as waveforms are being generated.[25,26]

## Electromyograms

After pedicle screw placement, the surgeon may request EMGs to determine if the screw is in close proximity to a nerve root, as this can result in neurologic problems. An electric current is sent through the screw, and EMGs are measured distally. If a low milliampere (mA) current can stimulate the nerve root, then the screw is too close to the nerve root. Therefore, in general, a current greater than 7 mA is sent to generate a response to know that screws are not too close to nerve roots. For accurate muscle EMGs, residual neuromuscular blockade must be terminated or reversed (also see Chapter 11).

## Wake-Up Test

The wake-up test was traditionally utilized to assess spinal cord integrity in many scoliosis cases. Development of sophisticated spinal cord monitoring is now standard in many hospitals, and the wake-up test is generally reserved for those situations in which monitoring is unobtainable or a significant intraoperative change in spinal cord monitoring waveforms is noted. During the wake-up test the anesthetic is discontinued and the patient is asked to move the extremities. Potential complications of this approach include increased bleeding, venous air embolism, and even inadvertent extubation of the trachea in the prone position with the wound exposed. The wake-up test is performed as follows: Turn off all inhaled anesthetics, reverse any neuromuscular blocking drug-induced paralysis, and stop infusions such as dexmedetomidine, propofol, or ketamine. If spontaneous respirations do not begin, inject naloxone, 0.04 mg at a time, to reverse any residual narcotic effect. The patient's head should be held to reduce the risk of self-extubation of the trachea. Prior to assessing lower extremity function, confirm upper extremity function. This can be accomplished by having the patient squeeze an observer's hand. Patient compliance denotes adequate recovery from general anesthesia. Then, while someone is observing the feet, ask the patient

to wiggle his or her toes. A rapid-acting anesthetic such as propofol should be ready to be administered as soon as the assessment is complete, so the patient can rapidly be reanesthetized. If the wake-up test is not successful in demonstrating adequate motor movement, further surgical intervention may be warranted and the patient may require transport to the radiology suite for additional imaging studies.[3,5,27]

### Conclusion of the Case

At the conclusion of the operation, the patient is placed in the supine position. All lines and tubes are secured so that intravenous line, arterial line, and airway access are not lost at this crucial time. Carefully reassess the patient for hemodynamic status, intravascular volume status, hematocrit, blood loss, degree of fluid and blood replacement, temperature, and the potential for airway edema. Premature extubation of the trachea must be avoided. Also, facial edema, respiratory effort, the amount of pain medication, and the presence of splinting and pain should be evaluated prior to extubating the trachea. After the decision is made to extubate the trachea, or not, the patient may be properly transported to the PACU. Supplemental oxygen should be utilized in the PACU. Electrolytes, hemoglobin, and clotting studies should be ordered as indicated.

Postoperative pain management (also see Chapter 40) may prove complicated after spine surgery as some patients may be taking significant amounts of pain medications, particularly opioids, prior to surgery. For these patients as well as for narcotic-naïve patients, a perioperative pain management plan can be developed and incorporated in the patient's care plan. In fact, the pain management pathway should consider utilizing preoperative oral pain medications, intraoperative infusion of pain medications, and use of postoperative medications to supply a multimodal pain regimen with the goal of maximizing pain relief while considering methods to decrease narcotic related respiratory depression. Applying individual consideration to a standard pain pathway, preoperative pain medications may include acetaminophen, gabapentin, or other antiinflammatory pain medications. Patient-controlled analgesia (PCA) may be effective postoperatively, with the dose tailored to the patient's needs. Some centers utilize ketamine as an analgesic adjunct, either intraoperatively or postoperatively. The use of nonsteroidal antiinflammatory drugs (NSAIDs), such as ketorolac, needs careful consideration as it will interfere with bone formation and therefore should be avoided in patients who just underwent spinal fusion.[28] NSAIDs can be considered on an individual basis when bone healing is not a factor, with cautionary consideration of cardiac-related issues resulting from their administration. Other oral medications are helpful in the perioperative period and may be considered for administration preoperatively and postoperatively. These drugs may include

**IV**

acetaminophen, anticonvulsants (e.g., gabapentin and pregabalin), antispasmodics that work at the spinal cord level (e.g., baclofen, tizanidine), antiinflammatory medications, and opioids. Intravenous acetaminophen is an excellent addition to the pain management regimen in patients who are nil per os, or nothing by mouth (NPO).

## Vision Loss

Postoperative visual loss (POVL) is a rare but potentially devastating complication occurring in patients undergoing spine surgery (also see Chapters 19 and 31).[29-36] Although its cause is unclear, patients having prolonged spine surgery (>6 hours) in the prone position who have large blood loss (>1 L) are particularly at risk.[29] Yet, patients with small blood loss and short procedures also have had visual loss. Perioperative factors such as anemia, hypotension, prolonged surgery, blood loss, increased venous pressure from positioning in the prone position, edema, a compartment syndrome within the orbit, and resistance to blood flow such as direct pressure on the eye, as well as systemic diseases such as diabetes, hypertension, and vascular disease have all been considered possible etiologic factors.[29-36]

Ischemic optic neuropathy (ION) is a major cause of POVL. Variations in blood supply to the optic nerve may play a role in the development of ION including reliance on a watershed blood supply to critical areas of the optic nerve. The head-down position allows edema to develop in the orbit and this increase in venous pressure may impact arterial blood flow. Ocular perfusion pressure (OPP), or the blood pressure supplying blood flow to the optic nerve, is a function of the mean arterial pressure (MAP) and intraocular pressure (IOP) such that OPP = MAP − IOP. Increases in IOP or decreases in MAP can have a negative impact on OPP.[12] Increases in IOP can decrease OPP and lead to ischemia, and the prone position is associated with increases in IOP.[31]

A visual loss registry has been established by the American Society of Anesthesiologists (ASA) to facilitate establishing the cause of POVL.[30] An ASA Practice Advisory points to ION as the most likely cause of POVL (Box 32.1).[29-36] In a published report of 93 cases reported in the POVL registry, 83 resulted from ION, with the remainder attributed to central retinal artery occlusion (CRAO). CRAO may be embolic in nature or the result of direct pressure on the eyeball and tends to be unilateral. Most patients in the registry were healthy and placed in the prone position for spine surgery. Blood loss more than 1 L and procedures of 6 hours or longer were present in 96% of cases. Fifty-five of the POVL cases were bilateral, with 47 having total visual loss. The registry publication reveals that blood loss in patients with POVL varied widely with a mean of 2 L but ranged from 0.1 to 25 L.[30,34,35] The advisory and registry publications promote a preoperative discussion with the patient and some suggest staged spine procedures for prolonged surgeries.[30,34,35]

---

**Box 32.1** Summary of the ASA Practice Advisory

- There is a subset of patients who undergo spine procedures in the prone position and are at increased risk for perioperative visual loss. Patients who may be at increased risk are those having long procedures or substantial blood loss or both.
- Consider informing high-risk patients that there is a small, unpredictable risk of perioperative visual loss.
- The use of deliberate hypotensive techniques during spine surgery is not associated with perioperative visual loss.
- In patients who have substantial blood loss, colloids should be administered in addition to crystalloids to maintain intravascular volume.
- There is no apparent transfusion "trigger" that would eliminate the risk of perioperative visual loss related to anemia.
- When positioning high-risk patients, the head should be level with or higher than the heart when possible. In addition, when possible, the head should be maintained in a neutral forward position (e.g., without significant neck flexion, extension, lateral flexion, or rotation).
- Staged spine procedures should be considered in high-risk patients.

*ASA,* American Society of Anesthesiologists.
From American Society of Anesthesiologists Task Force on Perioperative Visual Loss. Practice advisory for perioperative visual loss associated with spine surgery: an updated report by the American Society of Anesthesiologists Task Force on Perioperative Visual Loss. *Anesthesiology.* 2012;116(2):274-285.

---

A study comparing 80 patients who suffered ION reported in the registry publication with matched control subjects revealed more insight concerning risk. An increased incidence of ION was noted in patients with the following risk factors: males, obese patients, patients who underwent surgery on a Wilson frame, longer anesthesia time, cases with larger blood loss, and those who received a smaller percentage of colloid.[37]

## SURGERY IN THE SITTING POSITION

Shoulder surgery is frequently performed with patients in the sitting, or "beach chair," position with the head and upper torso elevated 30 to 90 degrees from the supine position (also see Chapter 19). Anesthesia in this position is associated with rare but significant and devastating neurologic complications including stroke, ischemic brain injury, and vegetative states.[38,39] The cause is a decrease in cerebral perfusion pressure resulting in insufficient blood supply to the brain. This is due to the arterial blood pressure gradient that develops between the heart and brain in this position. For each centimeter of head elevation above the level of the heart, there is a decrease in arterial blood pressure of 0.77 mm Hg. Therefore, arterial blood pressure measured at the level of the heart is not the blood and perfusion pressure at the brain.

Measurements obtained at the level of the heart must be recalculated. A 20-cm height differential is not uncommon, which calculates to approximately a 15 to 16 mm Hg gradient. A convenient point for measuring height difference between the heart and brain is the external auditory meatus, which is at the same level as the circle of Willis (COW). Even so, there is still a significant amount of brain tissue above this level. If arterial blood pressure decreases, or the surgeon's request for significant hypotensive anesthesia is followed, cerebral hypotension and therefore a significantly diminished cerebral perfusion pressure may occur at the level of the COW and the brain. Therefore, significant hypotension should be avoided in these patients especially those elderly, hypertensive patients whose autoregulatory curve is undoubtedly compromised (also see Chapter 35).

## FRACTURED HIP

Hip fractures occur frequently in elderly patients who often also suffer from multiple preexisting medical conditions or comorbid conditions. Factors predisposing to fracture include medical comorbid conditions, osteoporosis, lower limb dysfunction, visual impairment, increasing age, Parkinson disease, previous fracture, stroke, female gender, dementia, institutionalized patients, excess alcohol or caffeine consumption, cold climate, and use of psychotropic medications.[40] Mortality rates can range up to 14% to 36% in the first year after fracture.[40] Medical status affects morbidity and mortality risks. One example is the number of preexisting comorbid conditions from which the patient suffers. For example, the presence of four to six comorbid conditions is associated with increased mortality rate when compared to patients with fewer comorbid conditions.[41] Roche and associates in studying 2448 patients reported that the presence of three or more comorbid conditions was a strong preoperative risk factor with the postoperative development of chest infection or heart failure being associated with high mortality rate.[42] White and associates reported that ASA physical status classification I and II patients had mortality rates equal to age-matched control subjects, but ASA physical status classification III and IV patients had higher mortality rates (49% vs. 8%) after hip fracture.[43]

Generally, when significant comorbid conditions that need correction exist, patients benefit from delay in surgery while their medical status is improved. Mortality rate in high-risk patients was decreased from 29% to 2.9% in one study when time was taken to correct physiologic abnormalities.[44] This benefit was also demonstrated by Kenzora and coworkers, who noted a higher mortality rate (34% vs. 6.9%) in patients who went immediately into surgery as compared to those who were delayed 2 to 5 days to improve their medical status.[41] Moran and

colleagues, in a study of 2660 hip fracture patients with an overall mortality rate of 9% at 30 days, 19% at 90 days, and 30% at 12 months, noted that healthy patients did well as long as surgery was performed within 4 days.[45] Patients with comorbid conditions had a nearly 2.5 times increased mortality rate at 30 days as compared to healthy patients. Also, patients admitted to the hospital immediately after fracture did better than those admitted more than a day later.[45] Shiga and associates noted that operative delay over 48 hours after admission was associated with increased mortality rate and suggested that undue delay may be harmful to patients, especially young or low-risk patients.[46]

Preoperative evaluation (also see Chapter 13) is especially important. The diagnosis of a recent MI illustrates how these evaluations have changed. Previously, surgery was delayed up to 6 months following an MI, but now, the tendency is to risk-stratify patients based on the severity of their MI to determine wait time until surgery.[47] The recent MI needs to be evaluated on a risk-benefit ratio comparing the risk of surgery after a recent MI with the negative side effects of keeping a patient bed bound with its attendant risks of pneumonia, pulmonary embolism, pain, loss of ability to walk, and decubitus ulcers. Factors to consider are the extent of the MI, additional myocardium that may be at risk, presence of postinfarction angina, and presence of congestive heart failure (CHF). Although ongoing angina or the presence of CHF may preclude early surgery, a small subendocardial MI with minimal increase in cardiac enzymes and normal echocardiogram and stress test would allow consideration for an earlier intervention. A fractured hip usually prevents the patient from undergoing a normal exercise stress test. Therefore, if indicated, a pharmacologic stress test may be needed.

### Anesthetic Technique

A long-standing issue is whether one anesthetic technique, general or regional, is associated with better outcomes in patients undergoing hip fracture repair. In general, the data accumulated over many years and many different studies have not documented a clear advantage of one technique over another.[3,5,48,49] Therefore, choice of spinal or general anesthesia should be made on a case-by-case basis taking the patient's specific medical issues into consideration. The pros and cons of both spinal and general anesthesia must be considered when choosing the technique for a given patient (also see Chapter 14). General anesthesia, although easy to administer, does not provide any thromboembolic protection for the patient that may be provided by a regional technique.[3,5] In what may prove to be a clearer elucidation of whether anesthetic technique (neuraxial or general anesthesia) affects outcome in hip fracture patients, a 2012 retrospective study involving 18,158 hip fracture patients revealed

IV

that use of regional anesthesia resulted in lower mortality rates and fewer pulmonary complications in patients with intertrochanteric hip fractures but not in those patients suffering femoral neck fractures.[50]

The anesthetic provider should consider the type of fracture when preparing for surgery. Intertrochanteric fractures are associated with larger blood losses and longer operations, because a plate and screw are inserted, than intracapsular fractures that may be repaired with cannulated screws or a hemiarthroplasty depending on the viability of the femoral head.

Advantages of regional anesthesia, such as provided by a spinal anesthetic, are that (1) it avoids endotracheal intubation and airway manipulation and the medications that need to be administered to accomplish this, (2) it decreases the total amount of systemic medication the patient receives throughout the procedure, and (3) it may play a role in decreasing the risk of thromboembolism. The vasodilatory effect of the spinal anesthetic may help the patient with CHF. However, intravascular fluid still should be given cautiously because CHF may worsen as the intravascular vasodilatory effect of the spinal recedes.[3,5]

Preoperatively, intravascular volume status is a concern as fractures can result in significant blood loss, and a spinal anesthetic in the presence of hypovolemia can result in profound hypotension. An additional concern is the amount of time the patient must lay on the fracture table, especially in the elderly, as even small amounts of sedation can result in significant respiratory depression.

Peripheral nerve blocks including lumbar plexus, femoral, and lateral femoral cutaneous nerve (LFCN) blocks may also be used in selected situations. Chayen and coworkers demonstrated the effectiveness of lumbar plexus blocks in fractured hip patients.[51] This block can be performed with the nerve stimulator technique or the use of ultrasound guidance. Fracture repair requiring only cannulated pins may be performed with combined femoral and LFCN blocks. The femoral nerve block provides analgesia in the region of the hip, and the LFCN block will anesthetize the region of cannulated pin insertion located on the lateral aspect of the thigh. An LFCN block is performed by administering a fan of local anesthetic in a cephalad direction from a point 1 cm medial and inferior to the anterior superior iliac spine. The LFCN is a sensory nerve and therefore not amenable to location with a nerve stimulator. Alternatively, the nerve can be blocked using ultrasound guidance.

Intraoperative considerations for patients undergoing fractured hip repair include proper positioning and padding on the fracture table, maintaining adequate intravascular volume status as blood is lost, and adequately maintaining body temperature. Observation for hemodynamic alterations, and other unanticipated responses in the elderly patient, is especially important as the procedure progresses.

At the conclusion of the surgery, reassess hemodynamic status, ensuring that the patient has received adequate blood and fluid replacement. Determine if the dose of narcotic the patient received is going to have a prolonged effect, thereby resulting in respiratory depression once the patient is extubated. Check for hypothermia and anemia, and evaluate the patient's end-tidal $CO_2$ as the elderly can be slow to awaken and can easily hypoventilate as a result of the opioids they received. Once the trachea is extubated, administer supplemental oxygen. The dose and frequency of pain medication should be determined cautiously as increased circulation time and the cumulative effect of administered opioids may become evident when not expected.

## TOTAL JOINT REPLACEMENT

Total hip, knee, and shoulder replacements are frequently performed in patients suffering from osteoarthritis, rheumatologic disorders, and trauma. Operations may include replacement of an entire joint, partial joint replacement, replacement of individual components, or resurfacing procedures. Major concerns include the patient's age, concurrent medical conditions, blood loss, proper positioning and padding, hemodynamic variations during the procedure, the response to methylmethacrylate cement (MMC), and the risk of fat and pulmonary emboli.

### Total Hip Replacement

Total hip replacements (THRs) are performed with patients traditionally in either the supine or lateral decubitus position. A relatively new approach, the anterior approach to the hip, is frequently performed with the patient in the supine position on a special operating room table. Using this technique, selected patients are candidates for same-day hip replacement. In the supine position, the arm that is on the same side as the hip needs to be flexed away from the side. In the lateral position an axillary roll is placed just caudal to the axilla to protect the axillary artery and brachial plexus from compression (also see Chapter 19). Patients having procedures in the lateral position also have a lateral positioner placed to stabilize their pelvis. The positioner can push abdominal contents cephalad and interfere with respiratory function.

A THR may have MMC used to secure the prosthesis. Younger patients tend to receive noncemented joint replacements. The use of MMC is associated with cardiopulmonary side effects such as hypoxia, bronchoconstriction, hypotension, cardiovascular collapse, and even death. The cause for the systemic reaction to MMC may result from the liquid MMC monomer itself, which is used in producing the cement for cementing the prosthesis, or may be due to air, fat, or bone marrow elements being forced into circulation. The higher the liquid content of the liquid monomer in the mix with the polymer MMC at the time of insertion, which occurs from not adequately mixing or not waiting long enough for mixing to occur, the more frequently side effects are noted.[3,4,52] High-risk patients include those who are hypovolemic at the time of cementing, those who are hypertensive, and those with significant preexisting cardiac disease.[3,43,44]

Transesophageal echocardiographic evaluation (also see Chapter 25) of cardiac structure and function during reaming and cementing does indicate MMC and fat emboli flow centrally to the heart from the surgical site.[52] If a patient has a patent foramen ovale, these emboli can theoretically cross the patent foramen into the left ventricle and then move into the arterial circulation. If the patient has a probe-patent foramen ovale, an increase in pulmonary pressures as a result of bronchoconstriction may occur. MMC, for example, can increase right atrial pressure and shunt blood flow directly across the probe-patent foramen ovale. Many patients may have a decreased $Pa_{O_2}$ during the reaming and cementing process intraoperatively. An increase in the $F_{I_{O_2}}$ of 1.0 may be necessary.

At the conclusion of surgery, the patient is transferred to the PACU. Supplemental oxygen is administered, and a hemoglobin count should be considered. Further testing is based upon the patient's underlying medical condition. A postoperative pain management plan should be considered preoperatively (also see Chapter 40). Pain pathways are utilized at some medical centers that include preoperative oral medications. More comprehensive protocols to optimize management for same-day procedures are also being utilized. They may include recommendations for intravascular fluid management, dosing of spinal anesthetics, and medications to promote bladder contractility. For inpatients, postoperative pain management may include epidural infusion with epidural PCA, intravenous PCA, oral medications, or peripheral nerve block including lumbar plexus block. The postoperative pain management the patient receives may be influenced by the thromboembolism prophylaxis administered (also see Chapter 40).

## Total Knee Replacements and Tourniquets

Total knee replacements (TKRs) are frequently performed with a tourniquet in place to provide a bloodless surgical field. The tourniquet should be carefully placed on the upper thigh over appropriate padding. The leg may be wrapped with an Esmarch elastic bandage to help exsanguinate the limb prior to tourniquet inflation. In the lower extremity, the tourniquet is inflated to approximately 100 mm Hg above the systolic blood pressure, as this will prevent arterial blood from entering the exsanguinated limb.[3,4,53]

As tourniquets render the limb ischemic, there is a limit to inflation time before the ischemia can result in permanent limb damage. The safe upper limit of ischemia time is about 2 hours. The surgeon should be informed of tourniquet inflation time at 1 hour and then as the tourniquet approaches the 2-hour limit so it can be deflated in a timely manner. If the total tourniquet time will exceed the 2-hour limit, the tourniquet should be deflated at 2 hours for a period of at least 15 to 20 minutes before it is reinflated. This will allow for the "wash-out" of acidic metabolites from the ischemic limb as the limb is reperfused with oxygenated blood. Recirculation of the ischemic limb with release of the tourniquet is noted by a decrease in arterial blood pressure and an increase in end-tidal $CO_2$ as the acid products recirculate.[3] The hypotension usually responds to intravascular fluid administration and vasopressors if necessary.[3,53]

Pain is noted as the duration of tourniquet inflation time increases, manifesting itself as an increase in arterial blood pressure and heart rate. Overaggressively treating the increase in arterial blood pressure with opioids and other medications can result in hypotension after the tourniquet is released. Animal models have determined the pain to occur as result of C-fiber firing. A regional block proximal to the tourniquet can prevent C-fibers from firing.[3,53,54]

Complications noted with tourniquet use include nerve damage, vessel damage (especially in patients with atherosclerosis), pulmonary embolism, and skin damage. Skin injury may be due to the antiseptic prep solution if it is allowed to seep under the tourniquet and tourniquet padding at the time of skin prep causing a chemical burn. Additional concerns at the time of tourniquet deflation are pulmonary embolism and a decrease in core temperature as the isolated extremity is reperfused.[3,47,48]

After deflating the tourniquet, the surgical field should be observed for evidence of bleeding. Occasionally the tourniquet is deflated at the tourniquet control box but there is no bleeding because the tubing to the tourniquet is kinked. This is a significant complication as the tourniquet is effectively still inflated and the patient is then at risk for prolonged tourniquet inflation time, limb ischemia, and complications. One method to help ensure tourniquet deflation is to disconnect the tubing from the tourniquet box and observe the incision for bleeding, which is an indicator of tourniquet deflation.

TKRs are frequently performed under regional anesthesia with intravenous sedation. As a tourniquet is used during the operation, in the operating room blood loss is usually not significant. However, if much blood loss occurs into drains in the PACU, hypotension may result. Some surgeons do not deflate the tourniquet until the wound is closed and the dressing is on the patient. In this situation blood loss is usually less but there is a risk of postoperative bleeding.[55]

Debate exists as to whether bilateral TKRs should be performed in one setting. Many patients have undergone bilateral TKRs in one day or during one hospital admission.[56-59] If bilateral TKRs are scheduled, they should be performed after careful patient selection. Many institutions have guidelines delineating those patients felt to be acceptable candidates for bilateral procedures based on comorbid conditions and ASA physical status. Intraoperatively, the anesthesia provider should be aware that drainage from the first total joint will be occurring into the wound drainage system, which may be "under the drapes," and if bleeding is significant, hypotension can occur for what might be "unrecognized" reasons.

TKR patients have more postoperative pain than patients receiving THR. A postoperative pain management plan should be delineated to address anticipated pain. This plan may include oral and intravenous pain medications as well as nerve blocks. Preoperative oral pain medications such as acetaminophen, gabapentin, or NSAIDs (with cardiovascular risk considered) are employed by some as part of a total knee pain pathway. With early ambulation becoming popular, even as early as in the PACU, there is a need to provide adequate pain relief for mobilization. Peripheral nerve blocks, such as a femoral or an adductor canal block, can supply such pain relief.[60] The adductor canal block potentially spares motor components of the femoral nerve preserving motor strength in the femoral nerve distribution. It is not clear that use of femoral or adductor canal blocks result in a more frequent incidence of falls.[61] Postoperative pain relief may also include PCA, continuous infusions through catheters, individual nerve blocks of the lower extremities, and intravenous or oral medications. The use of intravenous dexamethasone administered at the time of a peripheral nerve block prolongs the block's duration, which may be useful in this setting.[62] Some surgeons are using "off-label" periarticular infiltrations of liposomal bupivacaine in the operating room, in lieu of peripheral nerve blocks, to achieve extended postoperative analgesia. Evidence of efficacy of this technique is pending.[63]

## Deep Venous Thrombosis and Thromboembolism Prophylaxis

The need for, and technique of, perioperative deep venous thrombosis (DVT) prophylaxis varies by surgeon and institution. Thromboembolism management should be coordinated with the anesthesia providers. Options for DVT prophylaxis include warfarin, low-molecular-weight heparin (LMWH), sequential compression boots, and aspirin. Although guidelines do exist as to which medications to use, the choice of DVT thromboprophylaxis is still variable. The surgeon's choice and timing of DVT prophylaxis will influence the choice of technique: general, spinal, combined spinal and epidural, epidural, peripheral block, or nerve block and catheter. At issue is concern that catheter manipulation while a patient is anticoagulated will result in bleeding, and if the catheter is in the epidural space, its removal can potentially result in epidural bleeding, epidural hematoma formation, and paralysis. Once an epidural hematoma develops, the catheter must be removed expeditiously before irreversible paralysis occurs. Although epidural hematomas classically present with severe pain and onset of numbness and weakness, in patients receiving epidural infusions of local anesthetics, these classic symptoms may be masked.

After introduction of the LMWH, enoxaparin in the United States, the incidence of epidural hematomas increased. This did not occur to the same extent in Europe, where a once-daily dosing schedule was employed in comparison to the twice-daily administration in the United States. Epidural hematoma formation probably resulted from a number of factors including performance of neuraxial anesthesia or removal of epidural catheters while the anticoagulation effect of LMWH was still present, the use of multiple medications at the same time that have anticoagulation properties, or the lack of attention to dosing schedule. This prompted a warning from the Food and Drug Administration (FDA) noting "reports of epidural or spinal hematomas with concurrent use of low molecular weight heparin and spinal/epidural anesthesia or spinal puncture." Consensus statements from the American Society of Regional Anesthesia and Pain Medicine (ASRA) addressed the issue.[64-66] Recommendations, recently updated by the FDA, include waiting at least 12 hours before neuraxial needle placement in a patient who received a preoperative dose of enoxaparin; waiting 4 hours (increased from the previous 2-hour waiting period) prior to dosing enoxaparin after an epidural catheter is removed; patients receiving warfarin should have their catheter removed only when the international normalized ratio (INR) is less than 1.5. Other anticoagulants and antiplatelet medications should be avoided when LMWH is being used and an epidural catheter is in place.[64-67]

The potent antiplatelet effect of clopidogrel also places a patient at an increased risk for a neuraxial hematoma should a spinal or epidural anesthetic be performed while its effect is present. Current recommendations in the *ASRA Practice Advisory, Anticoagulation*, 3rd edition, 2010, suggest that clopidogrel be discontinued for 7 days prior to performing a neuraxial block. However, the article quotes labeling as recommending this while the *Physicians' Desk Reference* (PDR) section for clopidogrel actually recommends that for elective surgery it only be discontinued for 5 days.[65] The Executive Summary for the Anesthetic Management of the Patient Receiving Antiplatelet Medication, as part of the 3rd edition, states, "On the basis of labeling and surgical reviews, the suggested time interval between discontinuation of thienopyridine therapy and neuraxial blockade is 14 days for ticlopidine and 7 days for clopidogrel. If a neuraxial block is indicated between 5 and 7 days of discontinuation of clopidogrel, normalization of platelet function should be documented."[66] In patients who need to be maintained on clopidogrel or have not discontinued it for an adequate time period, other anesthesia techniques should be considered. The guidelines for some of the antiplatelet medications will probably undergo revision as physicians gain experience with the use of medications such as clopidogrel in the perioperative period.

## QUESTIONS OF THE DAY

1. A patient with rheumatoid arthritis presents for hip surgery. What are the changes in the airway and cervical spine that may be present? What is the appropriate evaluation, and what is the potential impact on airway management?

2. What methods can be used to decrease blood loss during extensive, multilevel spinal fusion surgery?

3. What tests can be used to monitor the integrity of spinal cord pathways during spine surgery? How do commonly used anesthetic medications (e.g., inhaled anesthetics, propofol, opioids, benzodiazepines, neuromuscular blocking drugs) impact commonly used monitoring techniques?

4. What are the advantages and disadvantages of regional anesthesia techniques for an elderly patient who requires hip fracture repair? What neuraxial or peripheral regional blocks would be appropriate for the patient?

5. What are the options for providing postoperative analgesia to a patient scheduled to undergo total knee replacement?

6. How should the use of low molecular weight heparin influence the choice of epidural anesthesia for a patient undergoing total hip arthroplasty?

## REFERENCES

1. Okada Y, Wu D, Trynka G, et al. Genetics of rheumatoid arthritis contributes to biology and drug discovery. *Nature.* 2014;506(7488):376–381.

2. Rheumatoid arthritis: epidemiology, pathology and pathogenesis. In: Klippel JH, Crofford LJ, Stone JH, Weyland CM, eds. *Primer on the Rheumatic Diseases.* 12th ed. Atlanta, GA: Arthritis Foundation; 2001:209–232. Chap. 9.

3. Bernstein RL, Rosenberg AD. *Manual of Orthopedic Anesthesia and Related Pain Syndromes.* New York: Churchill Livingstone; 1993.

4. Rosenberg AD. Current issues in the anesthetic treatment of the patient for orthopedic surgery. *ASA Refresher Courses in Anesthesiology.* 2004;32:169–178.

5. Rosenberg AD. Anesthesia for major orthopedic surgery. *ASA Refresher Courses in Anesthesiology.* 1997;25:131–144.

6. Bienenstock H, Ehrlich GE, Freyberg RH. Rheumatoid arthritis of the cricoarytenoid joint: a clinicopathological study. *Arthritis Rheum.* 1963;6:48–63.

7. Skues MA, Welchew EA. Anaesthesia and rheumatoid arthritis. *Anaesthesia.* 1993;48:989–997.

8. Steel HH. Anatomical and mechanical considerations of the atlantoaxial articulations. *J Bone Joint Surg Am.* 1968;50:1481–1490.

9. Keenan MA, Stiles CM, Kaufman RL. Acquired laryngeal deviation associated with cervical spine disease in erosive polyarticular arthritis. Use of the fiberoptic bronchoscope in rheumatic disease. *Anesthesiology.* 1983;58:441–449.

10. Macarthur A, Kleiman S. Rheumatoid cervical joint disease—a challenge to the anesthetist. *Can J Anaesth.* 1993;40(2):154–159.

11. Seronegative spondyloarthropathies, ankylosing spondylitis. In: Klippel JH, Crofford LJ, Stone JH, Weyland CM, eds. *Primer on the Rheumatic Diseases.* 12th ed. Atlanta, GA: Arthritis Foundation; 2001:250–254. Chap. 11C.

12. Rosenberg AD. Annual Meeting 58th Refresher Course Lectures and Basic Science Review RCL American Society of Anesthesiology. *Anesthesiology.* 2007;119.

13. Zakine J, Samarcq D, Lorne E, et al. Postoperative ketamine administration decreases morphine consumption in major abdominal surgery: a prospective, randomized, double-blind, controlled study. *Anesth Analg.* 2008;106(6):1856–1861.

14. Subramaniam K, Subramaniam B, Steinbrook RA. Ketamine as adjuvant analgesic to opioids: a quantitative and qualitative systematic review. *Anesth Analg.* 2004;99:482–495.

15. American Society of Anesthesiologists Task Force on Intraoperative Awareness. Practice advisory for intraoperative awareness and brain function monitoring: a report by the American Society of Anesthesiologists Task Force on Intraoperative Awareness. *Anesthesiology.* 2006;104:847–864.

16. Avidan MS, Zhang L, Burnside BA, et al. Anesthesia awareness and the bispectral index. *N Engl J Med.* 2008;358:1097–1108.

17. Urban MK, Jules-Elysee K, Urquhart B, et al. The efficacy of antifibrinolytics in the reduction of blood loss during complex adult reconstructive spine surgery. *Spine (Phila Pa 1976).* 2001;26:1152–1156.

18. Zufferey P, Merquiol F, Laporte S, et al. Do antifibrinolytics reduce allogeneic blood in orthopedic surgery? *Anesthesiology.* 2006;105(5):1034–1046.

19. Neilipovitz DT, Murto K, Hall L, et al. A randomized trial of tranexamic acid to reduce blood transfusion for scoliosis surgery. *Anesth Analg.* 2001;93:82–87.

20. Mangano DT, Tudor IC, Dietzel C, et al. The risk associated with aprotinin in cardiac surgery. *N Engl J Med.* 2006;354:353–365.

21. Mangano DT, Miao Y, Vuylsteke A, et al. Mortality associated with aprotinin during 5 years following coronary bypass graft surgery. *JAMA.* 2007;297:471–479.

22. Fergusson DA, Hebert PC, Mazer CD, et al. A comparison of aprotinin and lysine analogues in high-risk cardiac surgery. *N Engl J Med.* 2008;358:2319–2331.

23. Pasternak BM, Boyd DP, Ellis FH. Spinal cord injury after procedures on the aorta. *Surg Gynecol Obstet.* 1972;135:29–34.

24. Owen JH, Laschinger J, Bridwell K, et al. Sensitivity and specificity of somatosensory and neurogenic motor evoked potentials in animals and humans. *Spine (Phila Pa 1976).* 1988;13(10):1111–1118.

25. Hilibrand AS, Schwartz DM, Sethuraman V, et al. Comparison of transcranial electric motor and somatosensory evoked potential monitoring during cervical spine surgery. *J Bone Joint Surg Am.* 2004;86:1248–1253.

26. MacDonald D. Intraoperative motor evoked potential monitoring: overview and update. *J Clin Monit Comput.* 2006;20(5):347–377.

27. Vauzelle C, Stagnara P, Jouvinroux P. Functional monitoring of spinal cord activity during spinal surgery. *Clin Orthop Relat Res.* 1973;93:173–178.

28. Glassman SD, Rose SM, Dimar JR, et al. The effect of postoperative nonsteroidal antiinflammatory drug administration on spinal fusion. *Spine (Phila Pa 1976).* 1998;23:834–838.

29. Williams EL. Postoperative blindness. *Anesthiol Clin North Am.* 2002;20:605–622.

IV

30. Lee L, Roth S, Posner K, et al. The American Society of Anesthesiologists Postoperative Visual Loss Registry: analysis of 93 spine surgery cases with postoperative visual loss. *Anesthesiology*. 2006;105(4):652–659.

31. Cheng MA, Todorov A, Tempelhoff R, et al. The effect of prone positioning on intraocular pressure in anesthetized patients. *Anesthesiology*. 2001;95:1351–1355.

32. Lee L, Lam A. Unilateral blindness after position lumbar spine surgery. *Anesthesiology*. 2001;95:793–795.

33. Roth S, Barach P. Postoperative visual loss: still no answers—yet. *Anesthesiology*. 2001;95:575–577.

34. Warner MA. Postoperative visual loss: experts, data and practice. *Anesthesiology*. 2006;105:641–642.

35. American Society of Anesthesiologists Task Force on Perioperative Visual Loss. Practice advisory for perioperative visual loss associated with spine surgery: an updated report by the American Society of Anesthesiologists Task Force on Perioperative Visual Loss. *Anesthesiology*. 2012;116(2):274–285.

36. Roth S. Perioperative Visual Loss: what do we know, what can we do? *Br J Anaesth*. 2009;103(suppl):i31–i40.

37. The Postoperative Visual Loss Study Group. Risk factors associated with ischemic optic neuropathy after spine surgery. *Anesthesiology*. 2012;116(1):15–24.

38. Pohl A, Cullen DJ. Cerebral ischemia during shoulder surgery in the upright position: a case series. *J Clin Anesth*. 2005;17:463–469.

39. Cullen DJ, Kirby RB. Beach chair position may decrease cerebral perfusion pressure. Catastrophic outcomes have occurred. *APSF Newsl*. 2007;22(2):25.

40. Zuckerman J. Hip fracture. *N Engl J Med*. 1996;334:1519–1525.

41. Kenzora JE, McCarthy RE, Lowell JD, et al. Hip fracture mortality: relation to age, treatment, preoperative illness, time of surgery, and complications. *Clin Orthop Relat Res*. 1984;186:45–56.

42. Roche JJ, Wenn RT, Sahota O, et al. Effect of comorbidities and postoperative complications on mortality after hip fracture in elderly people: prospective observational cohort study. *BMJ*. 2005;331(7529):1374.

43. White BL, Fisher WD, Laurin CA. Rate of mortality for elderly patients after fracture of the hip in the 1980s. *J Bone Joint Surg Am*. 1987;69(9):1335–1340.

44. Schultz RJ, Whitfield GF, LaMura JJ, et al. The role of physiologic monitoring in patients with fractures of the hip. *J Trauma*. 1985;25:309–316.

45. Moran CG, Wenn RT, Sikand M, et al. Early mortality after hip fracture: is delay before surgery important? *J Bone Joint Surg Am*. 2005;87:483–489.

46. Shiga T, Wajimaa Z, Ohe Y. Is operative delay associated with increased mortality of hip fracture patients? Systematic review, meta-analysis, and meta-regression. *Can J Anaesth*. 2008;55:146–154.

47. Shah KB, Kleinman BS, Sami H, et al. Reevaluation of perioperative myocardial infarction in patients with prior myocardial infarction undergoing noncardiac operations. *Anesth Analg*. 1990;71:231–235.

48. Valentin N, Lomholt B, Jensen JS, et al. Spinal or general anaesthesia for surgery of the fractured hip? A prospective study of mortality in 578 patients. *Br J Anaesth*. 1986;58:284–291.

49. Davis FM, Woolner DF, Frampton C, et al. Prospective multi-centre trial of mortality following general or spinal anesthesia for hip fracture surgery in the elderly. *Br J Anaesth*. 1987;59:1080–1088.

50. Neuman MD, Silber JH, Elkassabany NM, et al. Comparative effectiveness of regional versus general anesthesia for hip fracture surgery in adults. *Anesthesiology*. 2012;117:72–92.

51. Chayen D, Nathan H, Chayen M. The psoas compartment block. *Anesthesiology*. 1976;45:95–99.

52. Donaldson AJ, Thompson HE, Harper NJ, Kenny NW. Bone cement implantation syndrome. *Br J Anaesth*. 2009;102(1):12–22.

53. Odinsson A, Finsen V. Tourniquet use and its complications in Norway. *J Bone Joint Surg*. 2006;88:1090–1092.

54. Chabel C, Russell LC, Lee R. Tourniquet-induced limb ischemia: a neurophysiologic animal model. *Anesthesiology*. 1990;71:1038–1044.

55. Rama KR, Apsingi S, Poovali S, et al. Timing of tourniquet release in knee arthroplasty. Meta-analysis of randomized, controlled trials. *J Bone Joint Surg Am*. 2007;89:699–705.

56. Memtsoudis SG, Ma Y, Gonzalez Della Valle A, et al. Perioperative outcomes after unilateral and bilateral total knee arthroplasty. *Anesthesiology*. 2009;111:1206–1216.

57. Chan WC, Musonda P, Cooper AS, et al. One-stage versus two-stage bilateral unicompartmental knee replacement: a comparison of immediate post-operative complications. *J Bone Joint Surg*. 2009;91:1305–1309.

58. Ritter MA, Harty LD, Davis KE, et al. Simultaneous bilateral, staged bilateral, and unilateral total knee arthroplasty: a survival analysis. *J Bone Joint Surg Am*. 2003;85:1532–1537.

59. Restrepo C, Parvizi J, Dietrich T, et al. Safety of simulataneous bilateral total knee arthroplasty. A meta-analysis. *J Bone Joint Surg Am*. 2007;89:1220–1226.

60. Kim DH, Lin Y, Goytizolo EA, et al. Adductor canal block versus femoral nerve block for total knee arthroplasy. *Anesthesiology*. 2104;120:540–555.

61. Memtsoudis AG, Danninger T, Rasul R, et al. Inpatient falls after total knee arthroplasty. The role of anesthesia type and peripheral nerve blocks. *Anesthesiology*. 2014;120:551–563.

62. Abdallah FW, Johnson J, Chan V, et al. Intravenous dexamethasone and perineural dexamethasone similarly prolong the duration of analgesia after supraclavicular block: a randomized, triple arm, double blind, placebo-controlled trial. *Reg Anesth Pain Med*. 2015;40(2):125–132.

63. Surdam JW, Licini DJ, Baynes NT, Arce BR. The use of exparil to manage postoperative pain in unilateral total knee replacement. *J Arthroplasty*. 2015;30(2):325–329.

64. Horlocker TT, Wedel DJ, Benzon H, et al. Regional anesthesia in the anticoagulated patient: defining the risks (the second ASRA Consensus Conference on Neuraxial Anesthesia and Anticoagulation). *Reg Anesth Pain Med*. 2003;28:172–197.

65. Horlocker TT, Wedel D, Rowlingson JC, et al. Regional anesthesia in the patient receiving antithrombotic or thrombolytic therapy: American Society of Regional Anesthesia and Pain Medicine Evidence-Based Guidelines (Third Edition). *Reg Anesth Pain Med*. 2010;35(1):64–101.

66. Horlocker TT, Wedel DJ, Rowlingson JC, Enneking FK. Executive summary: regional anesthesia in the patient receiving antithrombotic or thrombolytic therapy: American Society of Regional Anesthesia and Pain Medicine Evidence-Based Guidelines (Third Edition). *Reg Anesth Pain Med*. 2010;35(1):102–105.

67. Food and Drug Administration. FDA Drug Safety Communication: updated recommendations to decrease risk of spinal column bleeding and paralysis in patients on low molecular weight heparins. Nov. 6, 2013. http://www.fda.gov/Drugs/DrugSafety/ucm373595.htm.

# 33 OBSTETRICS

## Jennifer M. Lucero and Mark D. Rollins

**EVALUATION OF THE NEONATE AND NEONATAL RESUSCITATION**
Cardiopulmonary Resuscitation

**QUESTIONS OF THE DAY**

Providing peripartum analgesia and anesthesia requires an understanding of the physiologic changes during pregnancy and labor; the effects of anesthetics on the mother, fetus, and neonate; and the benefits and risks associated with various anesthetic techniques. The course of labor and delivery and knowledge of high-risk maternal conditions must be clearly understood. These conditions require the ability to provide several analgesic and anesthetic techniques. Lastly, proper training and organization need to exist for potential obstetric emergencies and complications requiring immediate intervention, such as fetal distress and maternal hemorrhage.

## PHYSIOLOGIC CHANGES IN PREGNANT WOMEN

During pregnancy, labor, and delivery, women undergo significant changes in anatomy and physiology as a result of (1) altered hormonal activity; (2) biochemical changes associated with increasing metabolic demands of a growing fetus, placenta, and uterus; and (3) mechanical displacement by an enlarging uterus.[1,2]

### Cardiovascular System Changes

Changes in the cardiovascular system during pregnancy can be summarized as (1) an increase in intravascular fluid volume; (2) an increase in cardiac output; (3) a decrease in systemic vascular resistance; and (4) the presence of supine aortocaval compression (Table 33.1).

#### Intravascular Fluid and Hematology

Maternal intravascular fluid volume begins to increase in the first trimester. At term, plasma volume increases about 50% above the nonpregnant state, whereas the erythrocyte volume increases only about 25%. This disproportionate increase in plasma volume accounts for the relative anemia of pregnancy. Yet, the hemoglobin normally remains at 11 g/dL or more. This expanded intravascular fluid volume of 1000 to 1500 mL at term offsets the 300 to 500 mL blood loss that accompanies vaginal delivery and the average 800 to 1000 mL blood loss that accompanies cesarean delivery. In addition, the contracted uterus following delivery

**Table 33.1** Changes in the Cardiovascular System During Pregnancy

| System Parameter | Value at Term Compared With Nonpregnant Value |
|---|---|
| **Cardiovascular System** | |
| Intravascular fluid volume | Increased 35%-45% |
| Plasma volume | Increased 45%-55% |
| Erythrocyte volume | Increased 20%-30% |
| Cardiac output | Increased 40%-50% |
| Stroke volume | Increased 25%-30% |
| Heart rate | Increased 15%-25% |
| Peripheral circulation | |
| Systemic vascular resistance | Decreased 20% |
| Pulmonary vascular resistance | Decreased 35% |
| Central venous pressure | No change |
| Pulmonary capillary wedge pressure | No change |
| Femoral venous pressure | Increased 15%-50% |
| **Pulmonary System** | |
| Minute ventilation | Increased 45%-50% |
| Tidal volume | Increased 40%-45% |
| Breathing frequency | Increased 0-15% |
| Lung volumes | |
| Expiratory reserve volume | Decreased 20%-25% |
| Residual volume | Decreased 15%-20% |
| Functional residual capacity | Decreased 20% |
| Vital capacity | No change |
| Total lung capacity | Decreased 0-5% |
| Arterial blood gases and pH | |
| $Pao_2$ | Normal or slightly increased |
| $Paco_2$ | Decreased 10 mm Hg |
| pH | No change or minimal alkalosis |
| Oxygen consumption | Increased 20% |

Data from Cheek TG, Gutsche BB. Maternal physiologic alterations. In Hughes SC, Levinson G, Rosen MA, Shnider SM, eds. *Shnider and Levinson's Anesthesia for Obstetrics.* 4th ed. Philadelphia: Lippincott Williams & Wilkins; 2002:3-18; and Gaiser R. Physiologic changes of pregnancy. In Chestnut DH, Polley LS, Tsen LC, Wong CA, eds. *Chestnut's Obstetric Anesthesia: Principles and Practice.* 4th ed. Philadelphia: Elsevier; 2009:15-36.

causes a form of *autotransfusion*, often in excess of 500 mL of blood.

The total plasma protein concentration is decreased as a result of the dilutional effect of the increased intravascular fluid volume. Pregnancy is a hypercoagulable state with concentration increases in factors I, VII,

VIII, IX, X, and XII and decreases in factors XI, XIII, and antithrombin III. This results in an approximately 20% decrease in prothrombin time (PT) and partial thromboplastin time (PTT). Platelet count may remain normal or decrease 10% by term, and leukocytosis is common.

## Cardiac Output
Cardiac output increases by about 35% by the end of the first trimester and increases to about 50% above baseline by the third trimester because of increases in both stroke volume (25% to 30%) and heart rate (15% to 25%). Additional increases of 10% to 25% in cardiac output occur with the onset of labor during the first stage and 40% in the second stage. The largest increase occurs immediately after delivery, when cardiac output is increased by as much as 80% above prelabor values. This presents a unique postpartum risk for patients with cardiac disease, such as fixed valvular stenosis. Cardiac output decreases within the first hours after delivery and reaches prelabor values about 48 hours postpartum. It then decreases substantially toward prepregnant values by 2 weeks postpartum.

## Systemic Vascular Resistance
Although cardiac output and plasma volume increase, arterial blood pressure decreases in an uncomplicated pregnancy secondary to a 20% reduction in systemic vascular resistance at term. Systolic, mean, and diastolic blood pressure may all decrease 5% to 20% by 20 weeks of gestational age and gradually increase slightly toward prepregnant values as the pregnancy progresses further. There is no change in central venous pressure during pregnancy despite the increased plasma volume because of an increase in venous capacitance.

## Aortocaval Compression
When supine, the gravid uterus can compress the aorta and vena cava. Compression of the vena cava can decrease preload, cardiac output, and systemic blood pressure (Fig. 33.1). At term, the inferior vena cava is almost completely occluded in the supine position, with venous return of blood from the lower extremities through the epidural, azygos, and vertebral veins. In addition, significant aortoiliac artery compression occurs in 15% to 20% of pregnant women. Nearly 15% of pregnant women at term experience significant hypotension in the supine position. Diaphoresis, nausea, vomiting, and changes in cerebration often accompany the hypotension. This constellation of symptoms is termed *supine hypotension syndrome*. Vena cava compression decreases cardiac output 10% to 20% and may also contribute to lower extremity venous stasis and thereby result in ankle edema, varices, and increased risk of venous thrombosis.

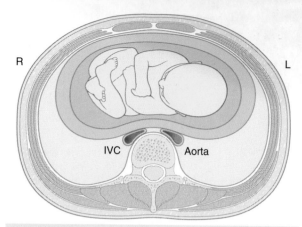

**Fig. 33.1** Schematic diagram showing compression of the inferior vena cava (IVC) and abdominal aorta by the gravid uterus in the supine position.

## Echocardiography Changes
There are significant changes in echocardiography during pregnancy.[3] The heart is displaced anteriorly and leftward. Right-sided chambers increase in size by 20% and left-sided chambers increase in size by 10% to 12% with an associated left ventricular eccentric hypertrophy and increase in ejection fraction. Mitral, tricuspid, and pulmonary valve annuli diameters increase, but the aortic annulus remains the same. Tricuspid and pulmonary valve regurgitation is common, and about 1 in 4 women has mitral regurgitation. In addition, small insignificant pericardial effusions may be present during pregnancy.

## Compensatory Responses and Risks
In the supine position, significant arterial hypotension is uncommon because the patient compensates for a decrease in preload by reflex increases in systemic vascular resistance. This compensatory increase in systemic vascular resistance is impaired by regional anesthetic techniques. Consequently, supine positioning is avoided during neuraxial anesthetic administration in the second and third trimesters. Significant lateral tilt is frequently used during labor analgesia and cesarean deliveries to reduce hypotension and preserve fetal circulation by displacing the gravid uterus leftward and off the inferior vena cava (Fig. 33.2). Left uterine displacement can be accomplished by placing the patient in a left lateral position or by elevation of the right hip 10 to 15 cm with a blanket, wedge, or table tilt.

The gravid uterus can also compress the lower abdominal aorta. Arterial hypotension can then occur in the lower extremities, which accounts for systemic blood pressure measurements in the arms not reflective of this decrease. Aortocaval compression decreases uterine and placental blood flow. Even with a healthy uteroplacental unit, prolonged maternal hypotension (more than 25% decrease for an average patient) for longer than 10 to

IV

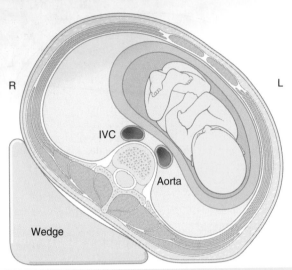

**Fig. 33.2** Schematic diagram depicting left uterine displacement by elevation of the right hip with a wedge. This position deflects the gravid uterus off the inferior vena cava (IVC) and aorta.

15 minutes can significantly decrease uterine blood flow (UBF) and lead to progressive fetal acidosis.

The increased venous pressure distal to the level of vena caval compression serves to divert blood return from the lower half of the body via the paravertebral venous plexuses to the azygos vein. Flow from the azygos vein enters the superior vena cava, and cardiac venous return is maintained. Dilation of the epidural veins may increase the rate of unintentional intravascular placement of the epidural catheter. This could lead to accidental intravascular injection of the local anesthetic solution, which can have profound effects on the cardiovascular system and central nervous system (CNS) with potential for complete hemodynamic collapse, seizures, and death. A *test dose* is administered before dosing an epidural catheter in order to decrease the likelihood of an unintended intravascular placement before initiating neuraxial blockade. This technique is described later in the section "Epidural Analgesia" (also see Chapter 17).

## Pulmonary System Changes

The most significant changes in the pulmonary system during pregnancy include alterations in (1) the upper airway, (2) minute ventilation, (3) arterial oxygenation, and (4) lung volumes (see Table 33.1).

### Upper Airway (Also See Chapter 16)

During pregnancy there is significant capillary engorgement of the mucosal lining of the upper respiratory tract and increased tissue friability. As a result, instrumentation of the upper airway is more likely to cause obstruction from tissue edema and bleeding. Additional care is needed during suctioning, placement of airways (avoid nasal instrumentation if possible), direct laryngoscopy, and intubation. It may be prudent to select a smaller cuffed tracheal tube (6.0 to 6.5 mm internal diameter) because the vocal cords and arytenoids are often edematous. The presence of preeclampsia, upper respiratory tract infections, and active pushing with associated increased venous pressure further exacerbate airway tissue edema making both endotracheal intubation and subsequent ventilation more challenging. In addition, the weight gain associated with pregnancy, particularly in women of short stature or with coexisting obesity (also see Chapter 29), can result in difficulty placing the laryngoscope because of a shorter neck and increased breast tissue.

### Minute Ventilation and Oxygenation

Minute ventilation is increased about 50% above prepregnant levels during the first trimester and is maintained for the remainder of the pregnancy. This increased minute ventilation is achieved primarily by an increase in tidal volumes, with small increases in the respiratory rate (see Table 33.1). Increased circulating levels of progesterone and increased $CO_2$ production are the likely stimulus for the increased minute ventilation. Resting maternal $Pa_{CO_2}$ decreases from 40 mm Hg to approximately 30 mm Hg during the first trimester as a reflection of the increased minute ventilation. Arterial pH, however, remains only mildly alkalotic (7.42 to 7.44) because of increased renal excretion of bicarbonate ions ($HCO^{3-}$ of approximately 20 to 21 mEq/L at term).

Early in gestation, maternal $Pa_{O_2}$ while breathing room air is normally above 100 mm Hg because of the presence of hyperventilation and the associated decrease in alveolar $CO_2$. Later, $Pa_{O_2}$ becomes normal or even slightly decreased, most likely reflecting airway closure and intrapulmonary shunt. Maternal hemoglobin is shifted to the right with the $P_{50}$ increasing from 27 to approximately 30 mm Hg.

At term, oxygen consumption is increased by 20%. The added work of labor results in further increases in both minute ventilation and oxygen consumption. During labor, oxygen consumption increases above prelabor rates by 40% during the first stage and 75% during the second stage. The pain of labor can result in severe hyperventilation causing $Pa_{CO_2}$ to decrease below 20 mm Hg. This pain-associated hyperventilation and alkalosis can be attenuated by neuraxial analgesic techniques.

### Lung Volumes

The expiratory reserve volume (ERV) and residual lung volume (RV), in contrast to the early appearance of increased minute ventilation, do not begin to change until about the third month of pregnancy (see Table 33.1). With increasing enlargement of the uterus, the diaphragm is forced cephalad, which is primarily responsible for the 20% decrease in functional residual capacity (FRC) present at term. This change is created by approximately equal decreases in the ERV and RV. As a result, FRC can be smaller than closing capacity for many small airways and may cause atelectasis in the supine position. Vital capacity is not significantly changed with pregnancy. The combination of increased minute ventilation and decreased FRC results in a more rapid rate at which changes in the alveolar concentration of inhaled anesthetics can be achieved. Respiratory measures of $FEV_1$, $FEV_1/FVC$ (forced vital capacity), and closing capacity do not change significantly with pregnancy.

### Anesthetic Implications

During induction of general anesthesia in a pregnant patient, $Pa_{O_2}$ decreases much more rapidly than in a nonpregnant patient because of decreased oxygen reserve (decreased FRC) and increased oxygen uptake (increased metabolic rate). For these reasons, the administration of supplemental oxygen or preoxygenation prior to general anesthesia is especially critical for patient safety. The pregnant patient should breathe oxygen for 3 minutes before any period of anticipated apnea (such as induction of anesthesia) or take four maximal breaths over the 30 seconds just prior to induction of anesthesia if emergent general anesthesia is needed. In addition, the increased airway edema makes both ventilation and intubation more difficult and further increases the potential for complications and morbidity.

## Gastrointestinal Changes

Gastrointestinal changes during pregnancy make women beyond 20 weeks gestation vulnerable to regurgitation, aspiration of gastric contents, and the development of acid pneumonitis. Displacement of the stomach and pylorus cephalad by the enlarged uterus repositions the intra-abdominal portion of the esophagus into the thorax and decreases the competence of the esophageal sphincter. Increased progesterone and estrogen levels of pregnancy further reduce esophageal sphincter tone. During vaginal delivery, gastric pressure is increased by both the gravid uterus and the lithotomy position. Gastrin, which is secreted by the placenta, stimulates gastric hydrogen ion secretion such that the pH of gastric fluid is predictably low in pregnant women. For these reasons, gastric fluid reflux into the esophagus with subsequent esophagitis (heartburn) is common and increases with the pregnancy gestational age. In addition, gastric emptying is delayed with the onset of labor or administration of opioids, further increasing the risk of aspiration.

### Anesthetic Implications

Regardless of the time interval since the ingestion of food, women in labor must be treated as having a full stomach and an increased risk for pulmonary aspiration of gastric contents. This includes the routine use of nonparticulate antacids, rapid sequence induction, cricoid pressure, and cuffed endotracheal intubation as part of the general anesthesia induction sequence in a pregnant woman after approximately 20 weeks gestational age. Pain, anxiety, and opioids administered during labor can further slow gastric emptying beyond an already prolonged transit time. Epidural analgesia using local anesthetics does not delay gastric emptying, but using epidural boluses of fentanyl does.[4] The low pH of aspirated gastric fluid is important in the production and severity of acid pneumonitis and is the basis for the administration of antacids to pregnant women before induction of anesthesia. Current American Society of Anesthesiologists (ASA) guidelines[5] recommend the "timely administration of oral nonparticulate antacids, intravenous (IV) $H_2$-receptor antagonists, and/or metoclopramide for aspiration prophylaxis" prior to the induction of anesthesia in pregnant women. Nonparticulate antacids such as sodium citrate (30 mL) work rapidly. Metoclopramide can significantly decrease gastric volume in as little as 15 minutes, although gastric hypomotility associated with prior opioid administration reduces the effectiveness of metoclopramide.[6] $H_2$-receptor antagonists increase gastric fluid pH in pregnant women approximately 1 hour after administration without producing adverse effects. Antacids plus $H_2$-antagonists are better than antacids alone in decreasing gastric acidity.[7]

## Nervous System Changes

Volatile anesthetic requirements (minimum alveolar concentration, or MAC) decrease up to 40% during pregnancy in animal studies[8] and 28% in humans[9] within the first trimester of pregnancy. However, an electroencephalographic monitoring study illustrated that the anesthetic effects of sevoflurane on the brain are similar in pregnant and nonpregnant women.[10] Consequently the magnitude and mechanism of the decreased anesthetic requirement remains uncertain. A clinical implication of this decreased MAC is that alveolar anesthetic concentrations that would not routinely produce unconsciousness may approximate anesthetizing concentrations in pregnant women. Judicious administration of anesthetics that depress the CNS is required to prevent unintended impairment of upper airway reflexes and add to the already increased risk of aspiration of gastric contents.

Pregnant patients are more sensitive to the local anesthetics used during neuraxial blockade. There is a decrease in local anesthetic dose needed for epidural or spinal anesthesia in pregnant women at term. The observation of decreased neuraxial local anesthetic doses as early as the first trimester suggests a role for both anatomic and biochemical changes. This decreased requirement is occurring before significant aortocaval compression and decreases in the volume of the epidural space from dilated veins. Although this increased sensitivity is likely based on hormonal changes, mechanical changes may also be involved. Engorgement of epidural

IV

veins as intra-abdominal pressure increases with progressive enlargement of the uterus results in a decrease in both the size of the epidural space and volume of cerebrospinal fluid (CSF) in the subarachnoid space. The decreased volume of these spaces facilitates the spread of local anesthetics. Yet, the CSF pressure itself does not increase with pregnancy.

### Renal Changes

Renal blood flow and the glomerular filtration rate are increased about 50% to 60% by the third month of pregnancy and do not return to prepregnant levels until 3 months postpartum. Therefore, the normal upper limits in blood urea nitrogen and serum creatinine concentrations are decreased about 50% in pregnant women. There is decreased tubular resorption of both protein and glucose, and excretion of them in the urine is common. In a 24-hour urine collection, findings of less than 300 mg protein or 10 g glucose are considered the upper limits of normal in pregnancy.

### Hepatic Changes

Liver blood flow does not change significantly with pregnancy. Plasma protein concentrations are reduced during pregnancy, and decreased serum albumin levels can increase free blood levels of highly protein-bound drugs. Slightly increased liver function tests are common in the third trimester. Plasma cholinesterase (pseudocholinesterase) activity is decreased about 25% to 30% from the tenth week of gestation up to 6 weeks postpartum. Yet, this decreased activity is likely not sufficient to prolong the neuromuscular blockade of succinylcholine. In addition, incomplete gallbladder emptying and changes in bile composition increase the risk of gallbladder disease during pregnancy. Even without underlying pathologic abnormality, alkaline phosphatase levels double during pregnancy from placental production.

## PHYSIOLOGY OF THE UTEROPLACENTAL CIRCULATION

The placenta is the interface of maternal and fetal tissue for the purpose of physiologic exchange. Maternal blood is delivered to the uterus and placenta by two uterine arteries. Nutrient-rich and waste-free blood is transferred from the placenta to the fetus through a single umbilical vein and fetal blood returns to interface with the maternal circulation via two umbilical arteries.

### Uterine Blood Flow

UBF increases throughout gestation from about 100 mL/min before pregnancy to 700 mL/min (about 10% of cardiac output) at term gestation. About 80% of the UBF perfuses the intervillous space (placenta) and 20% supports the myometrium. The uterine vasculature has limited autoregulation and remains essentially maximally dilated under normal pregnancy conditions. UBF decreases because of either reduced uterine perfusion pressure or increased umbilical arterial resistance. Decreased perfusion pressure can result from systemic hypotension secondary to hypovolemia, aortocaval compression, or decreased systemic resistance from either general or neuraxial anesthesia. UBF also decreases with increased uterine venous pressure. This can result from vena caval compression (supine position), prolonged or frequent uterine contractions, or significant abdominal musculature contraction (Valsalva maneuver during pushing). Additionally, extreme hypocapnia ($Paco_2 < 20$ mm Hg) associated with hyperventilation secondary to labor pain can reduce UBF to the point of fetal hypoxemia and acidosis.

Epidural or spinal anesthesia does not alter UBF as long as maternal hypotension is avoided. Endogenous catecholamines induced by stress or pain and exogenous vasopressors have the capability of increasing uterine arterial resistance and decreasing UBF. The use of phenylephrine ($\alpha$-adrenergic agonist) to correct maternal hypotension does not influence fetal well-being. Although ephedrine is safe to use to correct maternal hypotension, phenylephrine administration results in less fetal acidosis and base deficit as shown in clinical trials.[11-13] Although further work is needed to confirm the safety and efficacy of norepinephrine as a vasopressor in obstetric patients before routine clinical use, a 2015 study comparing norepinephrine and phenylephrine for arterial blood pressure maintenance during cesarean delivery noted norepinephrine was associated with a more rapid maternal heart rate and increased cardiac output.[14]

### Placental Exchange

Transfer of oxygen from the mother to the fetus is dependent on a variety of factors including the ratio of maternal UBF to fetal umbilical blood flow, the oxygen partial pressure gradient, the respective hemoglobin concentrations and affinities, the placental diffusing capacity, and the acid-base status of the fetal and maternal blood (Bohr effect). The fetal oxyhemoglobin dissociation curve is left-shifted (greater oxygen affinity) whereas the maternal hemoglobin binding curve is right-shifted (decreased oxygen affinity), resulting in facilitated oxygen transfer to the fetus. The fetal $Pao_2$ is normally 40 mm Hg and never more than 60 mm Hg even if the mother is breathing 100% oxygen.[15] This is because the placental exchange to the fetus from the mother represents venous rather than arterial blood. Carbon dioxide readily crosses the placenta and is not limited by diffusion but rather flow.

Placental exchange of most drugs and other substances less than 1000 Da occurs principally by diffusion from the maternal circulation to the fetus and vice versa. Diffusion of a substance across the placenta to the fetus depends on maternal-to-fetal concentration gradients, maternal protein binding, molecular weight, lipid solubility, and the degree of ionization of that substance. Minimizing the maternal blood concentration of a drug is the most important method of limiting the amount that ultimately reaches the fetus.

The large molecular weight and poor lipid solubility of nondepolarizing neuromuscular blocking drugs result in the limited ability of these drugs to cross the placenta (also see Chapter 11). Succinylcholine has a low molecular weight but is highly ionized and therefore does not readily cross the placenta. Thus, during administration of a general anesthetic for cesarean delivery, the fetus/neonate is not paralyzed. Additionally, both heparin and glycopyrrolate have significantly limited placental transfer. Placental transfer of barbiturates, local anesthetics, and opioids is facilitated by the relatively low molecular weights of these substances. In general, drugs that readily cross the blood-brain barrier also cross the placenta.

## Fetal Uptake

Fetal uptake of a substance that crosses the placenta is affected by the lower pH (0.1 unit) of fetal blood compared to maternal. The lower fetal pH means that weakly basic drugs (local anesthetics, opioids) that cross the placenta in the nonionized form will become ionized in the fetal circulation. Because an ionized drug cannot readily cross the placenta and return to the maternal circulation, this drug will accumulate in the fetal blood against a concentration gradient. Therefore, in an acidotic fetus, larger concentrations of local anesthetic can accumulate (ion trapping), especially during periods of fetal distress. Increased concentrations of local anesthetics in the fetus can result in decreased neonatal neuromuscular tone. If direct maternal intravascular local anesthetic injection occurs, significant fetal toxicity can result in bradycardia, ventricular arrhythmia, acidosis, and severe cardiac depression. Placental transfer and fetal uptake of specific analgesic and anesthetic drugs are detailed in the upcoming sections on "Methods of Labor Analgesia" and "Anesthesia for Cesarean Delivery."

## Characteristics of the Fetal Circulation

The fetal circulation helps protect vital fetal organs from exposure to large concentrations of drugs initially present in umbilical venous blood. For example, about 75% of umbilical venous blood initially passes through the fetal liver, such that significant portions of many drugs are metabolized before reaching the fetal arterial circulation for delivery to the heart and brain. Despite decreased liver enzyme activity in comparison to adults, fetal/neonatal enzyme systems still can metabolize most drugs.

Moreover, drugs in the portion of umbilical venous blood that enter the inferior vena cava via the ductus venosus will be diluted by drug-free blood returning from the lower extremities and pelvic viscera of the fetus. These circulatory characteristics decrease the fetal plasma drug concentrations compared to maternal following an IV drug bolus.

## STAGES OF LABOR

It is important to understand the stages of labor and when labor can become dysfunctional, resulting in more intervention from the obstetrician. Obstetrics can be predictably unpredictable. A patient may adopt a particular birth plan only to have it change at the outset of labor or after many hours. Labor can occur spontaneously or be induced based on maternal or fetal indications. What constitutes normal labor progress has been more precisely defined.[16,17] Ideally these changes will prevent cesarean deliveries in the first stage of labor (active stage arrest) when the woman is not yet in active labor.

Labor is a continuous process divided into three stages. The *first stage* refers to the onset of labor until the cervix is fully dilated. The first stage is further divided into two phases: latent phase and active phase. The latent phase can persist for many hours and in some cases days. Active phase begins at the point when the rate of cervical dilation increases. This usually occurs between 5 to 6 cm dilation. The *second stage* of labor begins when the cervix is fully dilated and ends when the neonate is born. This stage is referred to as the "pushing and expulsion" stage. Once the neonate is delivered the *third and final stage* begins and is completed when the placenta is delivered. If progression of labor through the stages is halted or delayed, there is concern for dysfunctional labor and potential for obstetric intervention.

If a woman's cervix fails to dilate or dilates slowly in the active phase (first stage of labor) despite pharmacologic interventions, this is considered an active phase arrest and will result in a cesarean delivery. Arrest of descent occurs during the second stage of labor, when the neonate is unable to deliver vaginally. The mode of delivery depends on what pelvic level the arrest of descent occurs and the position of the neonatal head. If the neonate is low enough in the pelvis, the obstetrician can perform an instrumented vaginal delivery (also known as an *operative vaginal delivery*) via vacuum or forceps. If the neonate remains too high in the pelvis, then the woman will need to undergo a cesarean delivery. In addition, the fetal condition can dictate a change in labor course and delivery mode based on the fetal heart rate (FHR) tracing.

The anesthesia provider can be consulted at any time throughout the labor to aid in a safe delivery. The labor course, mode of delivery, and maternal comorbid conditions should all be considered in determining which analgesic or anesthetic technique is most appropriate.

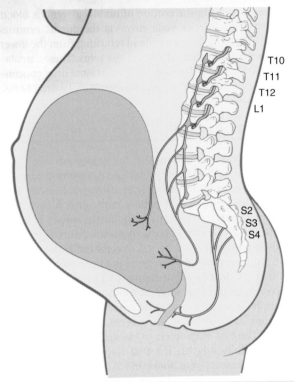

T10
T11
T12
L1

S2
S3
S4

**Fig. 33.3** Schematic diagram of pain pathways during pregnancy. Visceral pain during the first stage of labor is due to uterine contraction and cervical dilation. Afferent sensory fibers from the uterus and cervix travel with sympathetic nerve fibers and enter the spinal cord at T10-L1. Somatic afferents from the vagina and perineum travel via the pudendal nerve to levels S2-S4.

## ANATOMY OF LABOR PAIN

Contraction of the uterus, dilatation of the cervix, and distention of the perineum cause pain during labor and delivery. Somatic and visceral afferent sensory fibers from the uterus and cervix travel with sympathetic nerve fibers to the spinal cord (Fig. 33.3). During the first stage of labor (cervical dilation), the majority of painful stimuli are the result of afferent nerve impulses from the lower uterine segment and cervix, with contributions from the uterine body causing visceral pain (poorly localized, diffused, and usually described as a dull but intense aching). These fibers pass through the paracervical tissue and course with the hypogastric nerves and the sympathetic chain to the dorsal root ganglia of levels T10 to L1. During the second stage of labor (pushing and expulsion), afferents innervating the vagina and perineum cause somatic pain (well localized and described as sharp). These somatic impulses travel primarily via the pudendal nerve to dorsal root ganglia of levels S2 to S4. Pain during this stage is also caused by distention and tissue ischemia of the vagina, perineum, and pelvic floor muscles. Pain is associated with descent of the fetus into the pelvis

and delivery. Neuraxial analgesic techniques that block levels T10 to L1 during the first stage of labor must be extended to include S2 to S4 for efficacy during the second stage of labor.

Labor pain can have significant physiologic effects on the mother, fetus, and the course of labor. Pain stimulates the sympathetic nervous system, increases plasma catecholamine levels, creates reflex maternal tachycardia and hypertension, and can reduce UBF. In addition, changes in uterine activity can occur with the rapid decrease in plasma epinephrine concentrations associated with onset of neuraxial analgesia. Oscillations in epinephrine can cause many uterine effects ranging from a transient period of uterine tachysystole (extremely frequent uterine contractions) to a period of uterine quiescence. Alternatively, these epinephrine changes can convert dysfunctional uterine activity patterns associated with poorly progressive cervical dilation to more regular patterns associated with normal cervical dilation.[18]

## METHODS OF LABOR ANALGESIA

### Nonpharmacologic Techniques

A variety of nonpharmacologic techniques for labor analgesia exist. Although data are limited, acupuncture, acupressure, transcutaneous electrical nerve stimulation, relaxation, and massage all demonstrate a modest analgesic benefit.[19] Other techniques such as hypnosis and intradermal water injections do not show significant benefit beyond control. Most nonpharmacologic techniques seem to reduce labor pain perception but lack the rigorous scientific methodology for useful comparison of these techniques to pharmacologic methods. A woman's satisfaction with labor and delivery may not be directly associated with analgesic efficacy. A meta-analysis reviewing the effectiveness of a support individual (e.g., doula, family member) noted that women with a support individual used less pharmacologic analgesia, had a decreased length of labor, were more likely to have a vaginal birth, and were less likely to have negative feelings about childbirth.[20]

### Systemic Medications

Systemic analgesics are utilized on labor and delivery, but normally limited by bolus dose, dosing interval, and 24-hour cumulative dose. Although the use of systemic opioid analgesics is quite common, the use of sedatives, anxiolytics, and dissociative drugs is rare. The potential for maternal sedation, respiratory compromise, loss of airway protection, and proximity to time of delivery dictate judicious use of systemic opioids. For women who are in early spontaneous labor or beginning induction of labor, systemic opioid analgesia can be especially beneficial.

## Opioids (Also See Chapter 9)

Although there are individual differences among opioids, all readily cross the placental barrier and exert neonatal effects in typical clinical doses, including decreased FHR variability and dose-related neonatal respiratory depression. All opioids can have maternal side effects, including nausea, vomiting, pruritus, and decreased stomach emptying.

*Meperidine* is one of the most frequently used opioids worldwide likely secondary to cost, availability, and easy administration. It can be administered in doses of 12.5 to 25 mg IV or 25 to 50 mg intramuscularly. Maternal half-life of meperidine is 2 to 3 hours with half-life in the fetus and newborn significantly greater (13 to 23 hours) and more variable. In addition, meperidine is metabolized to an active metabolite (normeperidine) that can significantly accumulate after repeated doses. With increased dosing and shortened time interval between dose and delivery, neonatal risks of decreased Apgar scores, lowered oxygen saturation, and prolonged time to sustained respiration are more likely.[21]

*Morphine* was used more frequently in the past, but currently is rarely used. Like meperidine it has an active metabolite (morphine-6-glucuronide) and a prolonged duration of analgesia; the half-life is longer in neonates compared to adults, and it produces significant maternal sedation. In latent labor, obstetric providers may use intramuscular morphine combined with phenergan for analgesia, sedation, and rest, termed *morphine sleep*. This produces analgesia for approximately 2.5 to 6 hours with an onset of 10 to 20 minutes and does not appear to affect maternal or neonatal morbidity.[22]

*Fentanyl* is commonly used for labor analgesia. It has a short duration and no active metabolites. When given in small IV doses of 50 to 100 μg in an hour, there are no significant differences in neonatal Apgar scores and respiratory effort compared to newborns of mothers not receiving fentanyl.[23,24]

*Remifentanil* patient-controlled analgesia (PCA) may be considered for women who have contraindications to neuraxial blockade. Although labor pain improved with remifentanil, a randomized controlled trial comparing epidural analgesia to remifentanil PCA had overall pain scores that were smaller in the epidural group.[25] More sedation and hemoglobin desaturation were noted during remifentanil analgesia, but there was no difference between groups in fetal and neonatal outcomes. A more recent (2015) equivalence trial performed between remifentanil PCA and epidural analgesia found remifentanil was inferior to epidural analgesia for satisfaction of pain relief and pain relief scores.[26] Because remifentanil has potential for significant maternal respiratory depression, its use should remain under close supervision of an anesthesiologist.

## Nitrous Oxide

Inhaled nitrous oxide ($N_2O$) has been used for decades for labor analgesia and recently has increased in use within the United States. Nitrous oxide is typically inhaled intermittently in a fixed mixture of 50% $N_2O$ with 50% oxygen. It provides satisfactory analgesia in some women but is inferior to epidural analgesia. The side effects are mild with nausea, dizziness, and drowsiness among the most common.[27] Without coadministration of opioids, it is safe and does not result in hypoxia, unconsciousness, or loss of protective airway reflexes.[28] Maternal cardiovascular and respiratory depression are minimal and uterine contractility is not affected. In addition, newborn Apgar scores from mothers using nitrous oxide in labor are similar to those from mothers using other labor pain management methods or no analgesia. When delivered with appropriate scavenging equipment there does not appear to be concern regarding occupational exposure. Despite its historical use, rigorous scientific studies are lacking to further assess its overall efficacy, safety, and long-term effects on the fetus and newborn.[29]

## Neuraxial (Regional) Analgesia

Neuraxial analgesia (e.g., epidural, spinal, combined spinal-epidural [CSE]) is currently the most widely used method of labor analgesia in the United States. Placement of paracervical and pudendal blocks for analgesia is rare. Neuraxial analgesia typically involves the administration of local anesthetics, and often the coadministration of opioid analgesics. In addition, adjuvant drugs such as epinephrine and clonidine decrease the dose of local anesthetics or opioids required for analgesia.[30,31] However, given that the FDA (Food and Drug Administration) issued a black box warning regarding the possibility of significant hypotension with neuraxial clonidine in obstetrics, caution should be used.

### Local Anesthetics

The ester-linked local anesthetics (e.g., 2-chloroprocaine, procaine, tetracaine) are rapidly metabolized by plasma cholinesterase, decreasing the risk of maternal toxicity and placental drug transfer. Amide-linked local anesthetics (e.g., lidocaine, bupivacaine, ropivacaine) are degraded by P-450 enzymes in the liver. Bupivacaine and ropivacaine are the most commonly used local anesthetics for labor analgesia, and both are extremely safe when appropriately dosed for epidural or intrathecal administration. An accidental, large intravascular dose of any local anesthetic can result in significant maternal morbidity (seizures, loss of consciousness, severe arrhythmias, and cardiovascular collapse) or fatality and the potential for fetal accumulation (ion trapping); see discussion under "Physiology of Uteroplacental Circulation." Immediate recognition and treatment is essential (see "Systemic Toxicity and Excessive Blockade").

**IV**

### Neuraxial Opioids (Also See Chapter 9)

Neuraxial opioids are commonly used in obstetric anesthesia. Lipid-soluble opioids such as fentanyl and sufentanil are frequently used to augment the neuraxial analgesia of local anesthetics. The administration of opioids alone in the epidural space can provide moderate analgesia, but they are not as effective as dilute solutions of local anesthetic. Intrathecal opioids are more potent than epidural or systemic administration but are of limited duration (<2 hours) and also less effective than using neuraxial local anesthetics. Coadministration of opioids with local anesthetics prolongs and improves the quality of analgesia and has local anesthetic-sparing effects. The addition of neuraxial opioids is associated with dose-related maternal side effects including pruritus, sedation, and nausea. In addition, administration of intrathecal opioids can result in fetal bradycardia independent of hypotension.[32] The mechanism for fetal bradycardia is unclear but may result from uterine hyperactivity following the rapid onset of analgesia.

## NEURAXIAL TECHNIQUES

Neuraxial techniques represent the most effective form of labor analgesia and achieve the highest rates of maternal satisfaction.[33] The patient remains awake and alert without sedative side effects, maternal catecholamine concentrations are reduced, hyperventilation is avoided, cooperation and capacity to participate actively during labor are facilitated, and excellent, predictable analgesia can be achieved, superior to the analgesia provided by all other techniques. However, a delay in providing neuraxial pain relief, inadequate analgesia, or poorly communicating information about neuraxial labor analgesia can contribute to a negative childbirth experience (also see Chapter 17).[34]

### Preoperative Assessment

Prior to initiation of any neuraxial blockade, anesthesia providers should assess the patient's pregnancy and health history; perform a focused physical examination; discuss the risks, benefits, and alternatives; and obtain consent (also see Chapter 13). In otherwise healthy women, routine laboratory tests are not required.[5] Resuscitation equipment and drugs must be immediately available to manage serious complications secondary to initiation of epidural or spinal blocks (see "Contraindications of Neuraxial Anesthesia" and "Complications of Regional Anesthesia"). During initiation of the neuraxial blockade, mother and fetus are closely monitored (maternal vital signs and FHR monitoring). Current recommendations allow otherwise healthy laboring women to have modest amounts of clear liquids. However, in complicated labors (e.g., by morbid obesity, difficult airway, concerning fetal status), the decision to restrict oral intake should be determined by the individual anesthesia provider.[5]

### Timing and Placement of Epidural

The decision of when to place an epidural was previously controversial over the concern of adversely affecting the progress of labor. Current ASA and American College of Obstetricians and Gynecologists (ACOG) guidelines recommend that a maternal request for labor pain relief is sufficient justification for epidural placement, and the decision should not depend on an arbitrary cervical dilation.[5,35] Randomized controlled clinical trials comparing patients receiving either systemic opioids or neuraxial analgesia in early labor (both spontaneous and induced) demonstrated no difference in rates of cesarean delivery.[36,37] A Cochrane review based on studies dating up to 2011 that compared neuraxial and systemic opioid labor analgesia noted no difference in rates of cesarean delivery, but women with neuraxial analgesia did have an increased rate of instrumented vaginal delivery.[38,39] Neuraxial analgesia is associated with a prolonged second stage of labor, and the mean duration of the second stage is approximately 20 minutes longer with epidural labor analgesia.[38] A 2015 clinical trial found no difference between epidurals dosed with fentanyl alone versus local anesthetic suggesting a prolonged second stage is not a result of decreased pushing effort secondary to local analgesia.[40] This increase in the second stage is not harmful to the infant or mother, and as long as the fetal status is reassuring and there is ongoing progress toward delivery, the duration of the second stage does not require intervention.[41]

### Epidural Technique

Epidural analgesia is a catheter-based technique used to provide continuous pain relief during labor (also see Chapter 17). The technique involves insertion of a specialized needle (Tuohy) between vertebral spinous processes in the back, into the epidural space (Fig. 33.4). This needle has a slightly curved blunt tip to minimize dural puncture. The woman can either be in the sitting or lateral position based on both the experience of the anesthetic provider and optimal exposure to critical anatomic landmarks. Based on ASA task force recommendations regarding neuraxial infectious complications, aseptic techniques should always be used during placement of neuraxial needles and catheters, including (1) removal of jewelry (e.g., rings and watches), handwashing, and wearing of caps, masks, and sterile gloves; (2) use of individual packets of antiseptics for skin preparation; (3) use of chlorhexidine (preferred) or povidone-iodine (preferably with alcohol) for skin preparation, allowing for adequate

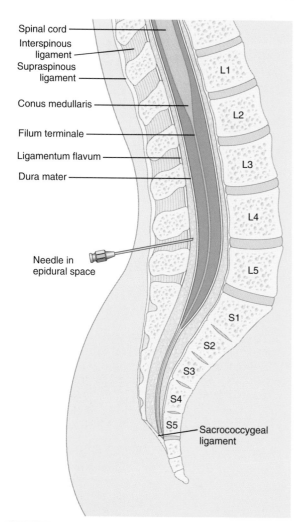

Spinal cord
Interspinous ligament
Supraspinous ligament
Conus medullaris
Filum terminale
Ligamentum flavum
Dura mater
L1
L2
L3
L4
L5
Needle in epidural space
S1
S2
S3
S4
S5
Sacrococcygeal ligament

**Fig. 33.4** Schematic diagram of lumbosacral anatomy showing needle placement for epidural block.

epidural space, and the needle is removed. The catheter is secure and used for intermittent or continuous injections. Once the catheter is in place, analgesia is achieved by administration of local anesthetics, or opioids, or both (see earlier discussion), and maintained throughout the course of labor and delivery. The catheter can also be used for instrumented or cesarean delivery as well as administration of morphine for postoperative analgesia, when necessary.

## Combined Spinal-Epidural Technique

The CSE technique follows the epidural technique as described, but after the loss of resistance a spinal needle (24- to 27-gauge, pencil-point needle) is inserted into the epidural needle, using a needle through needle procedure. Once CSF is visualized, an intrathecal dose of local anesthetic and opioid is administered. The spinal needle is removed and the epidural catheter is threaded as described with the epidural technique. The benefits of the CSE include quicker onset of analgesia and no motor blockade if opioids alone are placed intrathecally. A systematic review of CSE versus epidural literature found no major difference in maternal benefit or fetal risks but an increased rate of analgesia onset and maternal pruritus with the CSE technique.[43]

## Epidural and Combined Spinal-Epidural Dosing and Delivery Techniques

During labor, an epidural catheter allows continuous infusion of local anesthetic with or without opioid drugs. In addition, anesthesia providers can bolus the catheter with either the same or a more concentrated solution of local anesthetic. Programmable infusion pumps allow a patient-controlled epidural analgesia (PCEA) method of delivering the chosen anesthetic mixture with or without a background infusion. Compared to a continuous infusion alone, a PCEA method of delivery allows for fewer medical personnel, decreased motor block, improved patient satisfaction, and lower local anesthetic consumption.[5,44] Adding a background infusion to PCEA further improves labor analgesia, reduces the need for clinician boluses, and does not increase maternal or neonatal adverse events. However, there is not enough current evidence to determine if adding a continuous background infusion to a PCEA affects the length of labor and need for operative delivery.[5,44] Programmed intermittent epidural bolus (PIEB) is a more recent method of administering automated fixed epidural boluses at scheduled intervals. PIEB can be used alone or with a PCEA technique. Use of PIEB may slightly reduce local anesthetic usage, improve maternal satisfaction, and decrease the need for rescue boluses.[45,46] Concentrations of labor epidural local anesthetics have decreased over time because dense motor blockade may adversely affect

IV

drying time; (4) sterile draping of the patient; and (5) use of sterile occlusive dressings at the catheter insertion site.[42] The needle is normally inserted between L2 and L4. The needle traverses the skin and subcutaneous tissues, supraspinous ligament, interspinous ligament, and the ligamentum flavum and is advanced into the epidural space (Fig. 33.5). The tip of the Tuohy needle should not penetrate the dura, which forms the boundary between the intrathecal or subarachnoid space and the epidural space. To locate the epidural space, a tactile technique called *loss of resistance* is used. The tactile resistance noted with pressure on the plunger of an air- or saline-filled syringe dramatically decreases as the tip of the needle is advanced through the ligamentum flavum (dense resistance) into the epidural space (no resistance), which has an average depth of approximately 5 cm from the skin. Once the needle is properly positioned, a catheter is inserted through the needle. The catheter remains in the

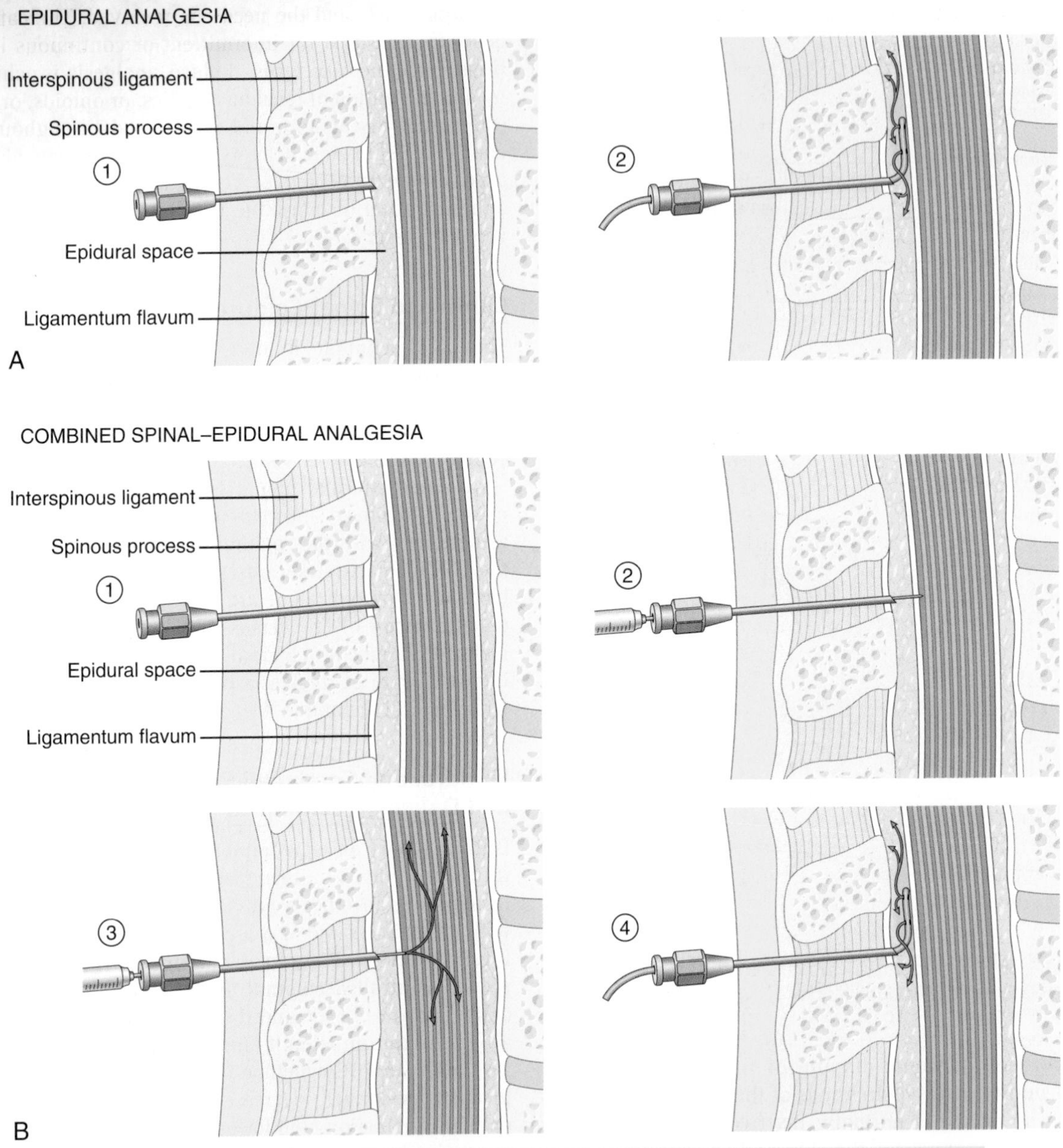

**Fig. 33.5** Technique of epidural and combined spinal-epidural analgesia. (A) Epidural catheter placement for labor analgesia: (1) The desired epidural space L2-L4 is identified. Following infiltration with local anesthetic a Tuohy needle is seated in the intervertebral ligaments. A syringe is connected to the epidural needle for confirmation of degree of resistance using constant or periodic pressure on the plunger. As the needle tip is passed from the high resistance of the ligamentum flavum to the low resistance in the epidural space, a sudden loss of resistance is recognized by the anesthesia provider and advancement is stopped. (2) An epidural catheter is advanced through the needle into the space. Analgesic medications are administered through the catheter following a test dose. (B) Combined spinal-epidural analgesia: (1) Following Tuohy needle placement into the epidural space, (2) a spinal needle (24- to 26-gauge) is introduced through the epidural needle into the subarachnoid space. (3) Proper placement is confirmed by free flow of the cerebrospinal fluid. A bolus of local anesthetic or opioid is administered through the spinal needle. (4) Following spinal needle removal, an epidural catheter is advanced through the Tuohy needle into the epidural space. The epidural catheter can be used for continuation of labor analgesia. (From Eltzschig HK, Lieberman ES, Camann WR. Regional anesthesia and analgesia for labor and delivery. *N Engl J Med.* 2003;348:319-332, used with permission.)

vaginal delivery rate. Typical maintenance infusion concentrations for epidural bupivacaine (0.04% to 0.125%) or ropivacaine (0.0625% to 0.2%) are both effective. Opioids such as fentanyl (2 µg/mL) or sufentanil (0.2 µg/mL) may be added to the infusion mixture to augment analgesia and decrease local anesthetic requirements, but they increase the side effects of pruritus, nausea, and sedation in a dose-dependent manner. Bolus administration of opioids can also be administered through the epidural catheter with typical doses of fentanyl 50 to 100 µg or sufentanil 5 to 10 µg to improve analgesia. Dilute concentrations of epinephrine (1:300,000 to 1:800,000) can also be added to the epidural mixture to augment analgesia.

For CSEs the initial intrathecal dose can include an opioid, local anesthetic, or a combination of the two. Typical intrathecal doses for opioids are fentanyl (10 to 20 µg) or sufentanil (1.5 to 5 µg), and local anesthetic doses include bupivacaine (1.25 to 3.5 mg) and ropivacaine (2 to 5 mg). Use of large-dose opioids (e.g., sufentanil 7.5 µg) is associated with increased risk of fetal bradycardia and severe pruritus even without the presence of hypotension.[32] Prior to initiation of the epidural, a *test dose* should be performed to evaluate the possibility of unintended IV or intrathecal catheter placement. Commonly, 3 mL of 1.5% lidocaine containing 1:200,000 epinephrine is used. Increases in heart rate and arterial blood pressure more than 20% above baseline (intravascular placement) or rapid analgesia and lower extremity motor block (intrathecal placement) indicate epidural catheter misplacement. Whenever a bolus is administered in the epidural for initiation or breakthrough pain, it is recommended to administer the anesthetic mixture incrementally through the epidural catheter while monitoring maternal arterial blood pressure and FHR continuously.

Instrumented vaginal delivery may become necessary for arrest of descent and fetal indications. Use of forceps often requires a denser block with perineal anesthesia. Supplementation with 5 to 10 mL of epidural lidocaine (1% to 2%) or 2-chloroprocaine (2% to 3%) may be needed.

## Spinal Labor Analgesia

Spinal analgesia can be administered just before vaginal delivery. This technique is useful for advanced second-stage analgesia, instrumented (forceps/vacuum) delivery, evaluation/evacuation of retained placenta, or repair of high-degree perineal lacerations. Placement of spinal block (3 to 5 mg bupivacaine with or without 10 to 20 µg of fentanyl) allows the rapid onset of analgesia. This dose is significantly less than that needed for a cesarean delivery. The duration of this type of spinal analgesia is approximately 60 to 90 minutes. A 24- to 27-gauge pencil-point spinal needle is selected to reduce the risk of post–dural puncture headache. If anesthesia is primarily needed for perineal laceration repair, the patient may be left in the sitting position for a few additional minutes following use of hyperbaric local anesthetic in order to concentrate the sensory block in the perineal region (saddle block). A true saddle block anesthetic does not produce complete uterine pain relief because the afferent fibers (extending to T10) from the uterus are not blocked.

## CONTRAINDICATIONS OF NEURAXIAL ANESTHESIA

Certain conditions contraindicate neuraxial procedures. They include (1) patient refusal, (2) infection at the needle insertion site, (3) significant coagulopathy, (4) hypovolemic shock, (5) increased intracranial pressure from mass lesion, and (6) inadequate resources or provider expertise. Other conditions such as systemic infection, neurologic disease, and mild coagulopathies are relative contraindications that should be evaluated on a case-by-case basis using current guidelines.[47,48] Human immunodeficiency virus (HIV) and hepatitis infection are not contraindications to neuraxial technique in pregnant women.

## COMPLICATIONS OF REGIONAL ANESTHESIA

The retrospective rates of inadequate epidural analgesia or inadequate CSE analgesia requiring catheter replacement were 7% and 3%, respectively, at a U.S. academic center.[49] The rate of accidental dural puncture during epidural catheter placement is approximately 1% to 2%, and about half of these punctures result in a severe headache, which is typically managed with analgesics, hydration, rest, caffeine, or blood patch if necessary. Other potential side effects from neuraxial blockade include pruritus, nausea, shivering, urinary retention, motor weakness, low back soreness, and a prolonged block. More serious complications of meningitis, epidural hematoma, and nerve or spinal cord injury are extremely rare. A 2014 multicenter database analysis of 257,000 obstetric patients examined rates of serious neurologic events.[50] The rate of epidural abscess or meningitis was 1:63,000, epidural hematoma was 1:251,000, and high neuraxial block 1:4300. A 2006 meta-analysis of 1.37 million women receiving labor epidurals noted rates of deep epidural infections 1:145,000, epidural hematoma 1:168,000, and persistent neurologic injury remaining longer than 1 year at 1:240,000 (also see Chapter 17).[51]

### Systemic Toxicity and Excessive Blockade

Infrequent but occasionally life-threatening complications can result from administration of neuraxial anesthesia. The most serious complications are from accidental IV or intrathecal injections of local anesthetics. An unintended bolus of IV local anesthetic causes dose-dependent consequences ranging from minor side

**IV**

effects (e.g., tinnitus, perioral tingling, mild arterial blood pressure, and heart rate changes) to major complications (seizures, loss of consciousness, severe arrhythmias, cardiovascular collapse). The severity depends on the dose, type of local anesthetic, and preexisting condition of the patient. Bupivacaine has greater affinity for sodium channels than lidocaine and dissociates more slowly. In addition, its high protein affinity makes cardiac resuscitation more difficult and prolonged. Measures that minimize the likelihood of accidental intravascular injection include careful aspiration of the catheter before injection, test dosing, and incremental administration of therapeutic doses. Successful resuscitation and support of the mother will reestablish UBF. This will provide adequate fetal oxygenation and allow time for excretion of local anesthetic from the fetus. The neonate has an extremely limited ability to metabolize local anesthetics and may have prolonged convulsions if emergent delivery is required.

A high spinal (total spinal) block can result from an unrecognized epidural catheter placed subdural, migration of the catheter during its use, or an overdose of local anesthetic in the epidural space (i.e., high epidural). Both high spinal blocks and high epidural blocks can result in severe maternal hypotension, bradycardia, loss of consciousness, and blockade of the motor nerves to the respiratory muscles.

### Treatment

Treatment of complications resulting from both intravascular injection and high spinal block are directed at restoring maternal and fetal oxygenation, ventilation, and circulation. Intubation, vasopressors, fluids, and advanced cardiac life support (ACLS) algorithms are often required. Changes to ACLS guidelines for pregnancy include use of manual left uterine displacement (rather than tilt) to relieve aortocaval compression, avoidance of lower extremity vessels for drug delivery, and no modifications to pharmacologic or defibrillation protocol except removal of fetal and uterine monitors prior to shock, unless it would delay the intervention.[52,53] If a local anesthetic overdose occurs, consider use of a 20% IV lipid emulsion to bind the drug and decrease toxicity.[54] In any situation of maternal cardiac arrest with unsuccessful return of spontaneous circulation, the fetus should be emergently delivered if the mother is not resuscitated within 4 minutes of the arrest. This guideline for emergent cesarean delivery increases the chances of survival for both the mother and neonate. In addition, the use of checklists and simulation can improve performance during the rare but critical events.

### Hypotension

Hypotension (decrease in systolic blood pressure > 20%) secondary to sympathetic blockade is the most common complication of neuraxial blockade for labor analgesia with rates of approximately 14%.[43] Prophylactic measures include left uterine displacement and hydration. Although

a standard for timing, amount, and hydration fluid remains controversial, all agree dehydration should be avoided. Prehydration with up to 1 L IV crystalloid does not appear to significantly decrease rates of hypotension from small-dose labor epidurals.[55] Although IV fluid preloading may be used to reduce the frequency of maternal hypotension after spinal anesthesia, there is no consistently significant difference in hypotension following spinal anesthesia if a preload or co-load of either IV crystalloid or colloid is administered.[5,56,57] Treatment of hypotension consists of further uterine displacement, IV fluids, and vasopressor administration. Either phenylephrine or ephedrine can be used to treat hypotension. Although ephedrine (primarily β-adrenergic) was historically used, more recent data confirm that (1) a phenylephrine (primarily α-adrenergic) infusion at the time of spinal placement is effective at preventing hypotension; (2) compared with ephedrine, phenylephrine is associated with less placental transfer and fetal acidosis; and (3) phenylephrine is now widely considered the vasopressor of choice for treating maternal hypotension.[12,58] However, significant decreases in maternal heart rate below baseline signify a decrease in cardiac output, and consequently both heart rate and arterial blood pressure should be considered when choosing vasopressor drugs to manage maternal hypotension.[58,59] If treated promptly, transient maternal hypotension does not lead to fetal depression or neonatal morbidity.

### Increased Core Temperature

An increase in core maternal body temperature and fever are associated with labor epidural analgesia (also see Chapter 20). Only about 20% of women who receive epidural labor analgesia develop a fever and the remaining 80% have no increase in core body temperature.[60] Although the cause of the maternal temperature rise remains uncertain, an association with noninfectious inflammation mediated by proinflammatory cytokines is a likely cause. This increase in maternal temperature is not associated with a change in white blood cell count or with an infectious process, and treatment is not necessary.[60] In addition, the fever associated with epidural labor analgesia does not increase the incidence of neonatal sepsis and need not affect neonatal septic workup. Although some studies note no effect on fetal well-being, other studies suggest maternal temperatures greater than 38° C are associated with adverse neonatal outcomes including seizures, hypotonia, and need for a period of assisted ventilation.[60,61]

## OTHER NERVE BLOCKS FOR LABOR

### Paracervical Block

A paracervical block is infrequently used to provide pain relief during the first stage of labor. The technique consists of submucosal administration of local anesthetic immediately lateral and posterior to the uterocervical junction, which blocks transmission of pain impulses at the paracervical ganglion. Complications from systemic absorption can occur as well as the possibility of direct fetal trauma or injection. Paracervical block is associated with a 15% rate of fetal bradycardia.[62] The mechanism of this phenomenon is unclear, and close fetal monitoring is warranted. The fetal bradycardia is usually limited to less than 15 minutes, and treatment is mainly supportive.

## Pudendal Block

A pudendal block is infrequently used to provide pain relief during the second stage of labor at the time of delivery. In most medical centers this technique is used when neuraxial techniques are unavailable. The obstetrician guides a sheathed needle through the vaginal mucosa and sacrospinous ligament just medial and posterior to the ischial spine. Local anesthesia injection around the pudendal nerve blocks sensation of the lower vagina and perineum. Although the technique provides analgesia for vaginal delivery or uncomplicated instrumented vaginal delivery, the rate of failure is high.[63] Complications in addition to failure include systemic local anesthetic toxicity, ischiorectal or vaginal hematoma, and, rarely, fetal injection of local anesthetic.

## ANESTHESIA FOR CESAREAN DELIVERY

The majority of cesarean deliveries are performed with neuraxial anesthesia. Use of regional anesthesia (1) avoids the risks of maternal aspiration of gastric contents and difficult airway management associated with general anesthesia, (2) allows less anesthetic exposure to the neonate, (3) has the benefit of an awake mother, and (4) allows placement of neuraxial opioids to decrease postoperative pain. Sometimes the severity of the fetal condition and emergent nature of the situation (e.g., fetal bradycardia or uterine rupture) necessitate the use of general anesthesia because of its rapidity and reliability. Other times it is required when regional anesthesia is contraindicated (e.g., coagulopathy or severe hemorrhage). In addition to its rapid and dependable onset, benefits of general anesthesia over regional include a secure airway, controlled ventilation, and potential for less hemodynamic instability. Current ASA guidelines[5] recommend the "timely administration of oral nonparticulate antacids, IV $H_2$-receptor antagonists, and/or metoclopramide for aspiration prophylaxis" prior to the induction of general anesthesia in pregnant women. In emergent situations, an oral nonparticulate antacid may be most appropriate.

## Spinal Anesthesia

For a pregnant patient without an epidural catheter, spinal anesthesia is the most common regional anesthetic technique used for cesarean delivery (also see Chapter 17). The block is technically easier than an epidural anesthetic, is more rapid in onset, does not carry the risk of systemic drug toxicity owing to the smaller dose, and is more reliable in providing surgical anesthesia from the midthoracic level to the sacrum. The incidence of post–dural puncture headache has become low (<1%) with the introduction of smaller diameter, noncutting, pencil-point spinal needles. However, maternal hypotension is more likely and more profound with spinal anesthesia than with epidural anesthesia because the onset of sympathectomy is more rapid (see previous section on "Hypotension"). Spinal anesthesia can be used safely for patients with preeclampsia. A typical spinal anesthetic could consist of bupivacaine (10 to 15 mg) with preservative-free morphine (50 to 200 µg) added to decrease postoperative pain. Many other combinations of local anesthetics and opioids are also used. A hyperbaric solution of local anesthetic is often used to facilitate anatomic and gravitational control of the block distribution. The medication will flow with the spinal curvature to a position near T4. The duration of a single-shot spinal anesthetic is variable but normally provides adequate surgical anesthesia for 90 minutes. A continuous spinal anesthetic technique with deliberate catheter placement approximately 3 cm subdural is a rarely used alternative, but sometimes is chosen in cases of accidental dural puncture during attempts to place an epidural catheter. This allows the advantage of a titratable, reliable, dense anesthetic, but it carries the risks of high spinal block if the intrathecal catheter is mistaken for an epidural catheter or the provider is unfamiliar with the technique. The rates of rare complications such as meningitis or neurologic impairment from local anesthetic toxicity with use of a spinal catheter may be more frequent than those for the other neuraxial techniques but remain unknown. Leaving the spinal catheter in place for 24 hours may decrease the risk of post–dural puncture headache.[64]

## Epidural Anesthesia

Epidural anesthesia is an excellent choice for surgical anesthesia when an indwelling, functioning epidural catheter has been placed for labor analgesia (also see Chapter 17). It allows titration to the desired level of anesthesia and ability to extend the block time if needed. It is also ideal for patients who cannot tolerate the sudden onset of sympathectomy, such as some patients with severe cardiac disease. Some disadvantages include a slower onset compared to spinal anesthesia and a greater risk of maternal systemic drug toxicity. The volume and concentration of local anesthetic drugs used for surgical anesthesia are larger than those used for labor analgesia; however, the technique of catheter placement, test dosing, and potential complications are similar. A standard dosing regimen for epidural anesthesia for cesarean delivery could include approximately 15 to 20 mL of

IV

2% lidocaine or 3% 2-chloroprocaine in divided doses. For urgent cesarean deliveries, 3% 2-chloroprocaine is often selected because it has the most rapid onset of any epidural local anesthetic. Compared to lidocaine, 2-chloroprocaine diminishes both the efficacy and duration of epidural morphine administered for postoperative analgesia.[65] Addition of epinephrine (1:200,000) or fentanyl (50 to 100 µg) can enhance the intensity and duration of the block. Typically, the anesthesia provider attempts to provide sensory anesthesia from the T4 level to the sacrum. Epidural block failure rates for cesarean delivery following use of a labor epidural are known to be greater in the urgent setting compared to elective cases and range between 1.7% and 19.8%.[66] In some cases conversion to general endotracheal anesthesia may be required. Epidural morphine (1.5 to 3 mg) is typically administered near the end of the procedure to decrease postoperative pain for up to 24 hours.

## Combined Spinal-Epidural Anesthesia

In selected circumstances, use of a CSE technique offers the advantage of a spinal anesthetic with rapid, reliable onset of a dense block, as well as the ability to administer additional local anesthetic through the epidural catheter. This allows titration of the block level or extension of the block duration if the procedure lasts for a longer period. One disadvantage is the delay in verification of a functioning epidural catheter.

## General Anesthesia

General anesthesia is used in obstetric practice for cesarean delivery, typically when neuraxial anesthesia is contraindicated or for emergencies because of its rapid and predictable action. Based on data from 1997 through 2002, the relative risk of general anesthesia is 1.7 times that of neuraxial anesthesia. Approximately two thirds of the deaths associated with general anesthesia were caused by intubation failure or induction problems.[67] Appropriate airway examination, preparation, and familiarity with techniques and an algorithm for the difficult airway are critical for providing a safe anesthetic (Fig. 33.6). A multi-institutional database of adverse obstetric anesthesia events indicates that current rates of failed intubation are approximately 1:533, although none of the 10 failed obstetric intubations in the database resulted in maternal fatality.[50] The sequence of events for inducing general anesthesia for cesarean delivery are detailed in Box 33.1.

After administration of a nonparticulate antacid, preoxygenation, and confirmation of surgical readiness, a rapid-sequence induction is typically performed and a cuffed endotracheal tube placed. Surgical incision is made after confirmation of tracheal intubation and adequate ventilation. Anesthesia is maintained by administration of a combination of a volatile anesthetic, as well as benzodiazepines,

opioid analgesics, propofol, nitrous oxide, and additional muscle relaxant if needed. During typical general anesthesia for cesarean delivery, opioids and benzodiazepines are administered after the baby is delivered to avoid placental transfer of these drugs to the neonate. Prior to delivery of the baby, the primary anesthetic for the incision and delivery is the induction agent, as there is little time for uptake and distribution of the inhaled anesthetic into either the mother or fetus. If intubation attempts fail, the cesarean delivery may proceed if the anesthesia provider communicates that she or he can reliably ventilate the mother with either face mask or laryngeal mask airway[68] (see Fig. 33.6). Halogenated anesthetics are often partially replaced with other anesthetics following delivery to decrease uterine atony. They may be entirely replaced with maintenance anesthetics that do not affect uterine tone (e.g., total intravenous anesthesia [TIVA] with propofol and opioids) to further reduce the risk of uterine atony.

### Drugs for Induction of General Anesthesia (Also See Chapter 7)

A number of drugs are used by anesthesia providers to rapidly induce general anesthesia.

#### Propofol

This highly lipid-soluble drug results in rapid onset of action that renders the patient unconscious within approximately 30 seconds. It is preservative free and must be drawn up only hours before use, decreases the incidence of nausea and vomiting, and is currently not a controlled substance. Propofol administration has no significant effect on neonatal behavior scores with induction doses (2.5 mg/kg), but larger doses (9 mg/kg) are associated with newborn depression.

#### Etomidate

Like propofol, etomidate has a rapid onset of action because its high lipid solubility and rapid hydrolysis result in a relatively short duration of action. Unlike propofol, at typical induction doses (0.3 mg/kg) etomidate has minimal effects on the cardiovascular system, but it is painful on injection, can cause involuntary muscle tremors, has higher rates of nausea and vomiting, and can increase the risk of seizures in patients with decreased thresholds.

#### Ketamine

Ketamine produces a rapid onset of anesthesia, but unlike propofol, ketamine's sympathomimetic characteristics increase arterial pressure, heart rate, and cardiac output through central stimulation of the sympathetic nervous system, making it an ideal choice for a pregnant woman in hemodynamic compromise. Doses above those appropriate for induction of general anesthesia (1 to 1.5 mg/kg) can increase uterine tone, reduce uterine arterial perfusion, and lower seizure threshold. In low doses (0.25 mg/kg), ketamine has profound analgesic effects, unlike

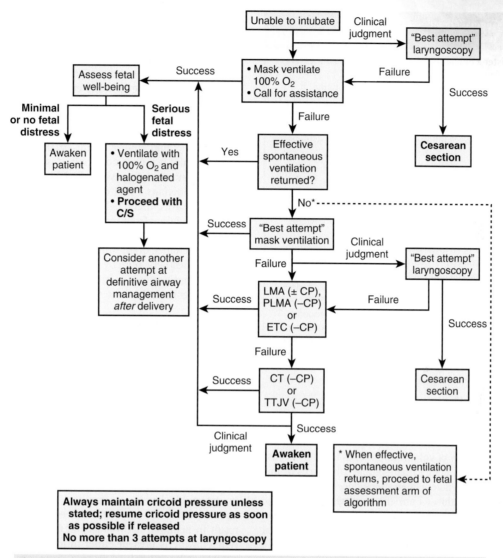

**Fig. 33.6** Algorithm for difficult airway management with failed intubation in obstetrics. *CP*, Cricoid pressure; *C/S*, cesarean section; *CT*, cricothyrotomy; *ETC*, esophageal tracheal combitube; *LMA*, laryngeal mask airway; *PLMA*, ProSeal laryngeal mask airway (Laryngeal Mask Company, Henley-on-Thames, England); *TTJV*, transtracheal jet ventilation. (From Hughes S, Levinson G, Rosen M, Shnider SM, eds. *Shnider and Levinson's Anesthesia for Obstetrics.* 4th ed. Philadelphia: Lippincott; 2002, used with permission.)

barbiturates, but has been associated with undesirable psychomimetic side effects (bad dreams), which can be lessened by coadministration of benzodiazepines. Both ketamine and etomidate are considered appropriate for induction of anesthesia in a pregnant woman who is actively hemorrhaging, has uncertain blood volume, and is at risk for profound hypotension.

### Anxiolytics
*Diazepam* is used in obstetrics, but it will readily cross the placenta and yield roughly equal maternal and fetal blood levels. Because neonates have a limited ability to excrete

the active metabolites, use of diazepam has been associated with neonatal respiratory depression. *Midazolam* is a shorter acting anxiolytic but also rapidly crosses the placenta, and large induction doses have been associated with profound neonatal hypotonia. Anxiolytic use has been controversial; however, in specific obstetric situations, lower doses may be beneficial keeping in mind their amnestic properties.

### Maintenance of Anesthesia
Maintenance of anesthesia for cesarean delivery often includes the inhalation of a low concentration (<0.75 MAC) of volatile anesthetic. The volatile anesthetic is an important

- Administer a nonparticulate oral antacid (sodium citrate) prior to induction of anesthesia
- Place standard monitors and maintain left uterine displacement
- Start an infusion of crystalloid solution through a large-bore intravenous catheter
- Preoxygenate for 3 minutes, or four maximal breaths over 30 seconds
- When the surgeon is ready and patient prepped, an assistant should apply cricoid pressure (and maintain until the position of the endotracheal tube is verified)[a]
- Administer induction drug and paralytic in rapid sequence, wait 30 to 60 seconds, and then initiate direct laryngoscopy for endotracheal intubation
- After confiming endotracheal tube placement, communicate to surgeon to proceed with incision
- Administer oxygen and a volatile anesthetic
- After delivery, anesthesia may be maintained by administering a combination of a halogenated drug (< 0.75 MAC), as well as benzodiazepines, opioid analgesics, propofol, nitrous oxide, and additional muscle relaxant as needed
- Extubate the trachea when the patient is fully awake and strong

[a]Not all agree that cricoid pressure is efficacious or required in every patient.

component of general anesthesia because the incidence of maternal recall is increased with emergent cesarean delivery. Placental transfer of volatile anesthetics is rapid because they are nonionized, highly lipid-soluble substances of low molecular weight. Fetal concentrations depend on the concentration and duration of anesthetic administered to the mother. During a typical general anesthetic for cesarean delivery, opioids are administered after the baby is delivered to avoid placental transfer to the neonate.

There may be confusion regarding the presence of fetal distress, the use of general anesthesia, and subsequent delivery of a depressed neonate. A depressed fetus is likely to be associated with a depressed neonate, and general anesthesia is selected because it is the most rapidly acting and reliable anesthetic technique to allow cesarean delivery. A Cochrane review of 16 studies comparing neuraxial blockade versus general anesthesia in otherwise uncomplicated cesarean deliveries found that "No significant difference was seen in terms of neonatal Apgar scores of 6 or less and of 4 or less at one and five minutes or the need for neonatal resuscitation."[69] The authors concluded that there was no evidence to show that neuraxial anesthesia was superior to general anesthesia for neonatal outcome. The induction to delivery interval is not as important to neonatal outcome as the interval from uterine incision to delivery, when UBF is compromised and fetal asphyxia may occur. A lengthy duration between induction to delivery may result in a lightly anesthetized, but not an

asphyxiated neonate. If excessive concentrations of volatile anesthetics are administered for prolonged periods, neonatal effects of these drugs, as evidenced by flaccidity, cardiorespiratory depression, and decreased tone, may be anticipated. It is important to recognize that if neonatal depression is due to transfer of anesthetic drugs, the infant is merely anesthetized and should respond easily to simple treatment measures such as assisted ventilation of the lungs to facilitate elimination of the volatile anesthetic. Rapid improvement of the infant should be expected, and if it does not occur, it is important to search for other causes of depression. For these reasons, it is critical that clinicians experienced with neonatal ventilation are present at cesarean deliveries under general anesthesia in which the time from incision to delivery may be longer, or if maternal condition necessitates an atypical induction and maintenance of anesthesia. A discussion of the operative and anesthetic plan by the neonatologist, obstetrician, and anesthesia provider is crucial for optimizing the outcome of neonates in these situations.

## Neuromuscular Blocking Drugs (Also See Chapter 11)

*Succinylcholine* (1 to 1.5 mg/kg IV) remains the neuromuscular blocking drug of choice for obstetric anesthesia because of its rapid onset (30 to 45 seconds) and short duration of action. Because it is highly ionized and poorly lipid soluble, only small amounts cross the placenta. It is normally hydrolyzed in maternal blood by the enzyme pseudocholinesterase and does not generally interfere with fetal neuromuscular activity. Although pseudocholinesterase activity is decreased in pregnancy, neuromuscular blockade by succinylcholine is not significantly prolonged. If large doses are given (2 to 3 mg/kg) it results in detectable levels in umbilical cord blood. However, extreme doses (10 mg/kg) are needed for the transfer to result in neonatal neuromuscular blockade. If the hydrolytic enzyme is present either in low concentration or in a genetically determined atypical form, prolonged maternal paralysis can occur and the return of neuromuscular strength should always be determined before additional muscle relaxants are given or extubation of the trachea.

*Rocuronium* is an acceptable alternative to succinylcholine. It provides adequate tracheal intubating conditions in approximately 90 seconds at doses of 0.6 mg/kg and under 60 seconds at doses of 1.2 mg/kg. Unlike succinylcholine, it has a much longer duration of action, decreasing maternal safety in the event the anesthesia provider is unable to intubate the trachea or ventilate the patient. Uterine smooth muscle is not affected by neuromuscular blockade. The blockade can be terminated by administration of neostigmine. Under normal circumstances, the poorly lipid-soluble, highly ionized, nondepolarizing neuromuscular blockers (i.e., rocuronium, vecuronium, cisatracurium, pancuronium) do not cross the placenta in amounts significant enough to cause neonatal muscle weakness. This placental impermeability is only relative and when large doses are given over long periods, neonatal neuromuscular blockade can occur. A paralyzed neonate will have normal cardiovascular function and good color but no spontaneous ventilatory movements, no reflex responses, and skeletal muscle flaccidity. Treatment consists of respiratory support until the neonate excretes the drug, which may take up to 48 hours. Antagonism of nondepolarizing neuromuscular blocking drugs with cholinesterase inhibitors may be attempted, but adequate respiratory support is the mainstay of treatment.

## ABNORMAL PRESENTATIONS AND MULTIPLE BIRTHS

### Multiple Gestations

The United States is seeing an increase in multiple gestations with the expanded use of artificial reproductive technologies. Twin pregnancy accounts for 3.4% of the live births in 2013.[70] The vast majority of multiple gestations are twin (97% to 98%). Higher order multiples account for 0.1% to 0.2% of the births. Multiple pregnancies account for a significant risk to both the mother and the fetuses. Antepartum complications may develop in up to 80% of the multiple gestations. These complications include a higher rate of preterm labor, preeclampsia, gestational diabetes, preterm premature rupture of membranes, intrauterine growth restriction, and intrauterine fetal demise. Pregnancies with multiple gestations account for 9% to 12% of the perinatal deaths.[71] A 2013 randomized control trial showed that planned cesarean delivery did not decrease risk of fetal or neonatal death compared to a planned vaginal delivery.[72] The majority of twin pregnancies are vertex-vertex positioning of the fetuses. If the second twin is breech, it is important to discuss the mode of delivery with the obstetricians. If vaginal delivery is attempted, an emergent cesarean delivery might be required if (1) the second twin changes position after delivery of the first twin or (2) there is fetal bradycardia in the second twin. In cases of vaginal delivery, women are strongly advised to undergo placement of an epidural to facilitate delivery and extraction of the second twin. In cases of breech extraction of the second twin, the epidural provides both analgesia and optimal perineal relaxation during the delivery of the fetal head of the second twin. Relaxation of the uterus improves delivery conditions of the second twin and reduces the risk of head entrapment. This is best achieved by using drugs that provide quick uterine relaxation (e.g., IV nitroglycerin). The obstetrician may need to perform an instrumented delivery of the second twin. At the late second stage of delivery a more concentrated local anesthetic will optimize the perineal anesthesia and relaxation during this critical portion of the delivery. At this time, the potential for head entrapment or fetal bradycardia is highest and a denser block allows for possible transition to cesarean delivery.

## Abnormal Presentations

### Breech Presentation

Singleton breech presentation occurs in about 3% to 4% of all pregnancies. External cephalic version (ECV) has a mean success rate of approximately 60%. The procedure involves rotating the fetus via external palpation and pressure of the fetal parts. Ultrasound and FHR monitoring are useful in assessing position and fetal distress during this procedure. Throughout the ECV, maternal relaxation of abdominal muscles is beneficial. Neuraxial analgesia reduces pain and may improve success of the ECV.[73] The risks of ECV include placental abruption, fetal bradycardia, and rupture of membranes. These risks are low, but the anesthesia provider should be immediately available if an ECV is being performed in case an urgent or emergent cesarean delivery is needed.

Few medical centers perform singleton vaginal breech delivery. Only recently (2006) have obstetric practice guidelines allowed individual obstetricians the flexibility of performing these deliveries based on their experience and comfort level.[74] Institutions offering a singleton vaginal breech delivery should have clear guidelines for performing the procedure. Women should undergo pelvimetry, an ultrasound to determine fetal weight, and counseling by the obstetrician to review the risks of the procedure. The patient is strongly encouraged to have an epidural placed during labor as the anesthetic management and risks are similar to a breech extraction of the second twin.

### Shoulder Dystocia

A shoulder dystocia is an obstetric emergency. The diagnosis is made after the delivery of the fetal head when further expulsion of the infant is prevented by impaction of the fetal shoulders with the maternal pelvis. It occurs in approximately 1% to 1.5% of all deliveries. Risk factors include macrosomia, diabetes, obesity, history of dystocia, labor induction, and instrumented delivery. Among deliveries with shoulder dystocia, the risk of postpartum hemorrhage is increased 11% and fourth-degree laceration increased 3.8%.[75] Once shoulder dystocia is diagnosed by the obstetrician, a set of maneuvers are performed to deliver the infant. Fetal pH declines 0.04 unit/min between delivery of the head and trunk. Cases of shoulder dystocia 7 minutes or longer have a significant increase in risk of neonatal brain injury. The final maneuver in a failed shoulder dystocia delivery requires pushing the fetus back up and proceeding to emergent cesarean delivery. Among the fetal injuries and sequelae of shoulder dystocia are brachial plexus injury, neurologic injury from asphyxia, and broken clavicle. Often these neurologic injuries improve over time with roughly less than 10% resulting in permanent Erb palsy. The average perinatal mortality rate is estimated at 0.4% to 0.5% of deliveries complicated by shoulder dystocia.[75]

IV

# HYPERTENSIVE DISORDERS OF PREGNANCY

The clinical spectrum of hypertensive diseases during pregnancy has varying maternal and fetal effects. The definition of hypertensive disorders in pregnancy were updated and changed in 2013.[76] Hypertensive disorders in pregnancy have been classified into four types: (1) preeclampsia-eclampsia, (2) chronic hypertension, (3) chronic hypertension with superimposed preeclampsia, and (4) gestational hypertension. *Gestational hypertension* is new-onset increased arterial blood pressures occurring after 20 weeks of gestation most often near term with the cause unclear, but with the need for increased surveillance during pregnancy. If the increased blood pressure persists through 12 weeks postpartum, the patient is considered a *chronic hypertensive. Chronic hypertension* is elevated blood pressures predating pregnancy or occurring prior to 20 weeks of gestation. These women are at more frequent risk for developing superimposed preeclampsia.

## Preeclampsia

Preeclampsia is a pregnancy-specific disorder with a multisystem involvement that has increased 30% over the past decade and affects 7.5% of pregnancies worldwide and between 2% and 5% of pregnant women in the United States.[77] Risk factors include primigravida, chronic hypertension, gestational/preexisting diabetes, obesity, preeclamptic family history, multiple gestation, and use of assisted reproductive technology. Preeclampsia is a systemic disease affecting every organ system with both maternal and fetal manifestations. Current diagnostic criteria are detailed in Boxes 33.2 and 33.3, which define preeclampsia into two distinct categories: (1) preeclampsia and (2) preeclampsia with severe features. The term *mild preeclampsia* has been removed and the requirement of proteinuria is no longer necessary to make the diagnosis of preeclampsia. A subcategory of severe preeclampsia is *HELLP syndrome*, which is a constellation of *h*emolysis, *e*levated *l*iver enzymes, and *l*ow *p*latelet count. Eclampsia (presence of seizures) in a patient with the diagnosis of preeclampsia is rare. In 10% to 15% of eclamptics, symptoms of preeclampsia were not previously detected.

Preeclampsia begins with the pathogenic maternal/fetal interface. During placental formation there is failure of complete trophoblast cell invasion of the uterine spiral arteries. The failure of spiral artery remodeling creates decreased placental perfusion, which may ultimately lead to early placental hypoxia. Ultimately there is upregulation of cytokines and inflammatory factors as seen in sepsis.[78]

Currently, the treatment of maternal symptoms of preeclampsia is delivery. If the pregnancy is remote from term in the presence of preeclampsia with severe features,

---

**Box 33.2** Criteria for Preeclampsia

**Blood Pressure**
- Greater than or equal to 140 mm Hg systolic or greater than or equal to 90 mm Hg diastolic on two occasions at least 4 hours apart after 20 weeks of gestation in a patient with a previously normal arterial blood pressure
- Greater than or equal to 160 mm Hg systolic or greater than or equal to 110 mm Hg diastolic, hypertension can be confirmed within a short interval (minutes) to facilitate timely antihypertensive therapy

AND
- Greater than or equal to 300 mg protein per 24-hour urine collection (or this amount extrapolated from a timed collection)

OR
- Protein/creatinine ratio greater than or equal to 0.3*
- Dipstick reading of 1+ (used only if other quantitative methods not available)

OR IN THE ABSENCE OF PROTEINURIA, NEW-ONSET HYPERTENSION WITH NEW ONSET OF ANY OF THE FOLLOWING:
- Thrombocytopenia: platelet count less than 100,000/μL
- Renal insufficiency: serum creatinine concentrations greater than 1.1 mg/dL or doubling of serum creatinine concentration in absence of other renal disease
- Impaired liver function: elevated blood concentrations of liver transaminases to twice normal concentration
- Cerebral or visual disturbances
- Pulmonary edema or cyanosis

*Each measured as mg/dL.

---

**Box 33.3** Criteria for Preeclampsia With Severe Features

Systolic blood pressure of 160 mm Hg or higher, or diastolic blood pressure of 110 mm Hg or higher on two occasions at least 4 hours apart while the patient is on bed rest (unless antihypertensive therapy is initiated before this time)
Thrombocytopenia (platelet count less than 100,000/μL)
Impaired liver function as indicated by abnormally elevated blood concentrations of liver enzymes (to twice normal concentration), severe persistent right upper quadrant or epigastric pain unresponsive to medication and not accounted for by alternative diagnoses, or both
Progressive renal insufficiency (serum creatinine concentration greater than 1.1 mg/dL or a doubling of the serum creatinine concentration in the absence of other renal disease)
Pulmonary edema
New-onset cerebral or visual disturbances

Boxes 33.2 and 33.3 from American College of Obstetricians and Gynecologists; Task Force on Hypertension in Pregnancy. Hypertension in pregnancy. Report of the American College of Obstetricians and Gynecologists' Task Force on Hypertension in Pregnancy. *Obstet Gynecol.* 2013;122:1122-1131.

---

a determination must be made whether to deliver or expectantly manage. This requires repeated evaluation of the mother and fetus. It is critical for the anesthesia provider on labor and delivery to be aware of these patients and their clinical course, as they can rapidly deteriorate and can require urgent or emergent delivery. Even remote from pregnancy, preeclampsia and gestational hypertension are associated with biologic changes that confer an increased future risk of cardiovascular disease and stroke.[79,80]

## Management

Normally, invasive monitoring is not required and central venous lines may increase risk without known benefit. However, in certain cases of severe preeclampsia and HELLP an invasive pressure line and central venous catheter may be beneficial. These clinical situations might include (1) management of labile hypertension, (2) need for frequent blood gas/laboratory studies (severe pulmonary edema), (3) need for rapid central acting vasoactive medications, or (4) estimation of intravascular volume status (oliguria).[81] The use of judicious administration of fluids to sustain or augment intravascular volume before initiation of neuraxial blockade may be necessary.

## Magnesium

Magnesium sulfate is used for seizure prophylaxis in preeclamptic women. Although a magnesium sulfate infusion reduces seizure rates in women with preeclampsia with severe features, new guidelines do not recommend administering magnesium sulfate to preeclamptic women without severe features.[76] Magnesium reduces CNS irritability by decreasing activity at the neuromuscular junction. Consequently, it can potentiate the action of both depolarizing and nondepolarizing muscle relaxants. Magnesium sulfate also provides uterine and smooth muscle relaxation. Based on the new guidelines magnesium sulfate should be continued intrapartum, including during cesarean delivery and until 24 hours postpartum. Magnesium toxicity is important to consider in preeclamptic women with worsening renal function and oliguria, as it is renally excreted. Women are monitored for magnesium toxicity with evaluation of deep tendon reflexes, respiratory depression, and neurologic compromise. The infusion usually is administered by loading 4 to 6 g over 20 to 30 minutes with a continued magnesium sulfate infusion of 1 g/h until 12 to 24 hours after delivery. The therapeutic range for seizure prophylaxis is between 6 to 8 mg/dL. Loss of deep tendon reflexes occurs at 10 mg/dL with prolonged PQ intervals and widening QRS complex on the electrocardiogram (ECG). Respiratory arrest occurs at 15 to 20 mg/dL, and asystole occurs when the level exceeds 20 to 25 mg/dL. If toxicity occurs, IV calcium chloride (500 mg) or calcium gluconate (1 g) should be administered.

## Antihypertensives

During the intrapartum management of preeclampsia, women often have additional elevations in arterial blood pressure from pain. Arterial blood pressure management may require antihypertensives. Current guidelines recommend treating systolic blood pressure greater than 160 mm Hg for prevention of intracerebral hemorrhage.[76] Initial therapy normally includes IV labetalol and hydralazine; however, without IV access oral nifedipine can be considered.[82] In refractory severe hypertension, nitroglycerin and sodium nitroprusside may be used in the acute situation with appropriate invasive monitoring. Evaluation of maternal arterial blood pressure and FHR are important as drug-induced decreases in maternal perfusion pressure can result in uteroplacental insufficiency and fetal bradycardia.

## Neuraxial Analgesia Considerations

The ACOG considers neuraxial analgesia the preferred analgesic method for labor in preeclamptic patients, but careful titration of the local anesthetic is needed to prevent the reduction in uteroplacental perfusion pressure.[76] Although a routine platelet count is not necessary in otherwise healthy laboring women, for women with preeclampsia, a thorough evaluation of the patient's current hematologic status should be performed. The anesthesia provider should verify hemoglobin and platelet levels prior to placement of any neuraxial block given the potential for thrombocytopenia in severe preeclampsia and HELLP. A specific platelet count predictive of neuraxial anesthetic complications has not been determined, but a stable platelet count of 75 to 80 × $10^9$/L has been suggested as a reasonable minimum platelet level for neuraxial techniques, assuming no additional contraindications to neuraxial anesthesia exist.[79,83] Regardless, the risk-benefit ratio of neuraxial block placement should be frankly discussed with the patient given the risks of epidural hematoma compared to other anesthetic and analgesic alternatives. Care should be taken before epidural catheter removal, as platelet levels often decrease further after delivery. Bleeding time has not been demonstrated to be of clinical value. If hypotension occurs following initiation of neuraxial analgesia, prompt but judicious titration of phenylephrine or ephedrine should be administered, understanding that the patient with preeclampsia may have hypersensitivity to catecholamines.

Given the potential for placental insufficiency with preeclampsia, the anesthesia provider must be prepared for urgent delivery. Exaggerated upper airway edema is frequent in preeclamptics and increases the risk of difficult intubation if an emergent general anesthetic is required. Endotracheal intubation may produce further hypertension during laryngoscopy and a small amount of nitroglycerin (2 µg/kg) or esmolol (1.5 mg/kg) can be beneficial when administered with propofol for induction.[84] If there is concern for a difficult airway, appropriate alternatives such as video laryngoscopy at the outset should be considered. Postpartum uterine atony is more common with magnesium sulfate infusion and accentuated if an inhaled anesthetic is administered. Pitocin and prostaglandins are safe for uterine atony, but methylergonovine (methergine) is relatively contraindicated because it can precipitate hypertensive crisis.

## HEMORRHAGE IN PREGNANT WOMEN

Hemorrhage in pregnant women remains a significant cause of maternal fatality. Placenta previa, abruptio placentae, and uterine rupture are the major causes of bleeding and uncontrolled hemorrhage during the third trimester and labor. Postpartum hemorrhage occurs in 3% to 5% of all vaginal deliveries and is typically due to uterine atony, retained placenta, placenta accreta, or lacerations involving the cervix or vagina. Common problems identified with hemorrhages leading to significant morbidity and mortality risks in obstetrics include (1) poor quantification of blood loss, (2) unrecognized associated risk factors for hemorrhage, (3) delayed initiation of treatment, and (4) inadequate readiness and resources including inadequate transfusion of appropriate blood products in a massive hemorrhage situation.[85]

### Placenta Previa

Placenta previa results from an abnormal uterine implantation of the placenta in front of the presenting fetus. The incidence is approximately 1 in 200 pregnancies. Risk factors include advanced age, multiparity, assisted reproductive techniques, prior hysterotomy, and prior placenta previa. Historically, the classic presentation of placenta previa is painless vaginal bleeding that typically occurs preterm in the third trimester. However, most previas are now diagnosed antenatally by ultrasonography. A trial of labor is acceptable if the placenta edge is further than 2 cm from the internal os. If the placenta is within 1 cm, the patient should undergo cesarean delivery. For placentas that lie between 1 cm and 2 cm from the cervical os, the optimal management remains uncertain and delivery management is currently individualized.[86] Neuraxial anesthesia is an appropriate choice if there is no active bleeding or hypovolemia. The use of two large-bore IV lines with fluid warmers and availability of invasive monitoring is suggested with cesarean delivery for rapid infusion of fluids or blood products given the increased risk of placenta accreta with known previa.[87]

### Massive Hemorrhage

For emergency situations with active hemorrhage, general anesthesia may be required. *Ketamine* (1 to 1.5 mg/kg) or *etomidate* (0.3 mg/kg) IV are useful drugs for induction of anesthesia. If a massive hemorrhage occurs, activation of a massive transfusion protocol with aggressive use of fresh frozen plasma, platelets, and fibrinogen in addition to packed red blood cells may be needed for transfusion in ratios similar to those used for a trauma resuscitation, as a dilutional coagulopathy can quickly result in such a situation.[88] In these cases of uncontrolled rapid hemorrhage, there is often insufficient time to wait for the return of laboratory studies before transfusion of appropriate blood products. Although numerous randomized controlled trials conclude that the use of tranexamic acid significantly decreases postpartum blood loss,[89] these studies do not adequately address questions on safety and efficacy of empiric tranexamic acid use at the time of hemorrhage recognition. An ongoing multicenter randomized controlled trial enrolling 20,000 patients with postpartum hemorrhage (the WOMAN trial) is currently investigating the use of tranexamic acid on a composite end point of maternal death or hysterectomy.[90] Neonates delivered from pregnant women in hemorrhagic shock are likely to be acidotic and hypovolemic and may need resuscitation. If hemorrhage is not controlled with standard pharmacologic measures, the obstetric team can consider (1) uterine artery ligation, (2) B-Lynch sutures, (3) an intrauterine balloon, (4) use of arterial embolization by interventional radiology if the patient is stable for transport, or (5) hysterectomy.

### Abruptio Placentae

Abruptio placentae is separation of the placenta from the uterine wall after 20 weeks of gestation but before delivery. The incidence is approximately 0.4 to 1 in 100 pregnancies. Risk factors include advanced age, hypertension, trauma, smoking, cocaine use, chorioamnionitis, premature rupture of membranes, placenta previa, and history of prior abruption. Placental abruption is associated with 10% to 20% of all perinatal deaths, and although maternal death is rare, maternal mortality rate is increased sevenfold.[91] When the separation involves only the placental margin, the escaping blood can appear as vaginal bleeding often associated with uterine tenderness. Alternatively, large volumes of blood loss (>2 L) can remain entirely concealed in the uterus. Chronic bleeding and clotting between the uterus and placenta can cause maternal disseminated intravascular coagulopathy (DIC). Ultrasound is specific if abruption is noted but has poor sensitivity, and a normal examination does not exclude abruption. Definitive treatment of abruptio placentae is to deliver the pregnancy. The anesthetic plan is based on both the delivery urgency and the abruption severity. If there are no signs of maternal hypovolemia, active bleeding, clotting abnormalities, or fetal distress, epidural analgesia can be used for labor and vaginal delivery. However, severe hemorrhage necessitates emergency cesarean delivery and the use of a general anesthetic similar to that described for placenta previa. It is predictable that neonates born under these circumstances will be acidotic and hypovolemic.

## Uterine Rupture

Uterine rupture is poorly defined and includes cases ranging from scar dehiscence to those with catastrophic uterine wall rupture. In addition to prior uterine scar, uterine rupture is associated with rapid spontaneous delivery, motor vehicle trauma, trauma from instrumented vaginal delivery, large or malpositioned fetus, and excessive oxytocin stimulation. Following a single prior cesarean delivery with a low transverse incision, a trial of labor after cesarean (TOLAC) is associated with a 1% or less incidence of uterine rupture.[92] Spontaneous rupture of an unscarred uterus is far more rare. The presentation is variable with no finding being 100% sensitive but may include fetal bradycardia, persistent abdominal pain, vaginal bleeding, cessation of contractions, loss of station, and breakthrough pain with epidural analgesia. Abdominal pain is not always a diagnostic finding, and continuous FHR monitoring indicating deceleration currently represents the most common sign associated with uterine rupture.[93] Neuraxial labor analgesia may be used as part of TOLAC and should not be expected to mask signs and symptoms of uterine rupture. Immediate evaluation, aggressive resuscitation, and general anesthesia for emergent cesarean delivery are normally required for management. Often uterine repair by the obstetrician can occur following cesarean delivery if a minor scar dehiscence is present, but hysterectomy is needed for most cases of uterine wall rupture of an unscarred uterus. When vaginal birth is planned after a previous cesarean delivery, it is recommended that "TOLAC be undertaken in facilities with staff immediately available to provide emergency care"[93] should a uterine rupture occur. Appropriate staffing considerations include obstetric, anesthesia, pediatric, and nursing personnel.

## Retained Placenta

Retained placenta occurs in about 2% to 3% of all vaginal deliveries and usually necessitates manual exploration of the uterus. If epidural analgesia was not used for vaginal delivery, manual removal of the placenta may be initially attempted with analgesia provided by IV administration of opioids or the inhalation of nitrous oxide. If uterine relaxation is necessary for placenta removal, boluses of IV nitroglycerin (200 µg) are normally effective but have not been shown to reduce the need for manual uterine extraction. Additionally relocation to the operating room and placement of neuraxial analgesia may be beneficial for thorough evaluation. Induction of general anesthesia with endotracheal intubation and administration of a volatile anesthetic to provide uterine relaxation are not typically necessary. An effort to obtain accurate blood loss is critical in determining an appropriate anesthetic and resuscitation plan as retained placenta is associated with an increased risk of postpartum hemorrhage and need for transfusion.[94]

## Uterine Atony

Uterine atony is a common cause of postpartum hemorrhage and can occur immediately after delivery or several hours later. Risk factors for postpartum uterine atony include retained products, long labor, high parity, macrosomia, polyhydramnios, excessive oxytocin augmentation, and chorioamnionitis. A 2013 systematic literature review noted that active management of the third stage (placental delivery) reduced postpartum hemorrhage without increasing risk of retained placenta.[95] Following bimanual massage, uterine atony is initially treated with IV oxytocin. The amount of oxytocin used to prevent postpartum hemorrhage is highly variable. One common approach uses continuous oxytocin infusion of 20 to 40 IU diluted in up to 1 L of crystalloid administered after delivery as a wide open IV infusion. Another protocol uses bolus of IV oxytocin 3 IU at a time in an effort to reduce the overall oxytocin dose required to prevent postpartum hemorrhage. No differences in the uterine tone, maternal hemodynamics, side effects, or blood loss were observed between these different methods of oxytocin dosing.[96] Although a dilute solution of oxytocin typically exerts minimal cardiovascular effects, rapid IV injection of even 3 to 5 IU is associated with tachycardia, vasodilation, and hypotension and should be administered over 30 seconds or more.[96] Periodic communication between the anesthesia and obstetric teams is key in rapidly assessing whether oxytocin is effective or whether additional types of uterotonics should be administered. Methylergonovine (0.2 mg IM) is an ergot derivative that can be given to improve uterine tone. Methylergonovine can cause significant vasoconstriction and is relatively contraindicated in patients with preeclampsia, pulmonary hypertension, or ischemic cardiac disease. The prostaglandin $F_{2\alpha}$ (0.25 mg IM) is another uterotonic used to treat atony. It is associated with nausea, tachycardia, pulmonary hypertension, desaturation, and bronchospasm. It should be avoided in asthmatics. Prostaglandin $E_1$ (600 µg oral/sublingual/rectal) is also effective in treating atony. It has no significant cardiac effects, but may cause hyperthermia. If postpartum hemorrhage is not controlled with these initial methods, more invasive techniques and blood product transfusion will be needed urgently (previously described in the section "Massive Hemorrhage").

## Placenta Accreta

Placental implantation beyond the endometrium gives rise to (1) *placenta accreta vera*, which is implantation and adherence onto the myometrium; (2) *placenta increta*, which is implantation into the myometrium; and (3) *placenta percreta*, which is penetration through the full thickness of the myometrium (Fig. 33.7). With placenta percreta, implantations may occur onto bowel, bladder, ovaries, or other pelvic organs and vessels. Any of these placental implantations can produce a markedly

IV

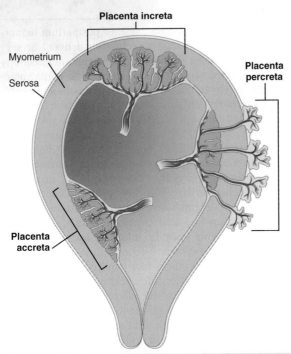

**Fig. 33.7** Classification of placenta accreta based on the degree of penetration of myometrium. (From Kamani AAS, Gambling DR, Chritlaw J, et al. Anesthetic management of patients with placenta accreta. *Can J Anaesth*. 1987;34:613-617, used with permission.)

adherent placenta that cannot be removed without tearing the myometrium and producing a life-threatening severe hemorrhage.

These abnormal placental implantations occur more frequently in association with placenta previa. The rate of placenta accreta disorders has increased nearly 60-fold over the past 50 years, and it currently occurs in approximately 1 in 533 pregnancies.[97] Recent (2015) studies note ultrasonography diagnosis of placenta accreta to have a positive predictive value of only 68% and a diagnostic sensitivity of 55% with a negative predictive value of 98% and specificity of 88%.[97] Consequently, anesthetic management should not be exclusively guided by antepartum ultrasound results. In patients with placenta previa and no previous cesarean delivery, the incidence of accreta is approximately 3%. However, the risk of placenta accreta associated with placenta previa increases with the number of previous cesarean deliveries. With one previous uterine incision, the incidence of placenta accreta has been reported to be 11%, and with two previous uterine incisions the rate is 40%, and with three or more prior uterine incisions the incidence rises to above 60%.[87]

In patients with both placenta previa and accreta, massive and rapid intraoperative blood loss is common with reported median blood loss ranging from 2000 to 5000 mL, and in some, substantially more. Coagulopathies develop in approximately 20% of these patients, and a significant proportion require hysterectomies. Placenta accreta is not reliably diagnosed until the uterus is open. The anesthesia provider must keep in mind this possibility and be prepared to treat sudden massive blood loss. The choice of anesthetic technique can be individualized by case and provider while keeping this possibility in mind. For patients with a preoperative diagnosis, or high suspicion, preparations for massive hemorrhage are needed and intraoperative cell salvage should be considered.[98]

## AMNIOTIC FLUID EMBOLISM

The incidence of amniotic fluid embolism (AFE) is currently estimated between 1 and 6 cases per 100,000 deliveries.[50,99] Clinical features of AFE include the sudden onset of hypotension, fetal distress, respiratory distress, hypoxia, DIC, cardiopulmonary arrest, and altered mental status. These signs must be differentiated from other more common disorders of pregnancy and delivery. AFE can occur during labor, delivery, or uterine surgery or in the immediate postpartum period. The exact cause and pathogenesis of AFE remain uncertain, but it is believed to be a type of anaphylactoid or hypersensitivity reaction to some component of the amniotic fluid. The diagnosis of AFE is a clinical diagnosis of exclusion. Although in the past it had been believed that aspirating amniotic fluid debris such as fetal squamous cells from the maternal pulmonary circulation was diagnostic, it has since been determined that fetal cells are present in the circulation of all pregnant women and no diagnostic laboratory test for AFE currently exists. Conditions that mimic AFE include venous air embolism, pulmonary thromboembolism, acute hemorrhage (i.e., uterine rupture, abruption, accreta), peripartum cardiomyopathy, sepsis, anaphylaxis, local anesthetic toxicity, high spinal block, and inhalation of gastric contents. Treatment of AFE is supportive and directed toward cardiopulmonary resuscitation with inotropic support, transfusion, and correction of hypoxemia. Endotracheal intubation and mechanical support of ventilation are almost always required. Rapid onset of coagulopathy may occur and result in life-threatening hemorrhage. Definitive diagnosis is extremely difficult or impossible, even with postmortem examination.

## ANESTHESIA FOR NONOBSTETRIC SURGERY DURING PREGNANCY

The overall incidence of nonobstetric surgery during pregnancy is 1% to 2%, with trauma, appendicitis, and cholecystitis being the most frequent causes.[100],[101] In addition to management of maternal awareness, hemodynamics, and respiration and taking into account the physiologic changes of pregnancy as described before, anesthesia management objectives for pregnant women undergoing nonobstetric surgery include prevention of intrauterine fetal hypoxia and acidosis. There is concern for spontaneous abortion with procedures early in pregnancy and premature labor with surgery later in pregnancy. Elective procedures should always be delayed until after pregnancy. A pregnant woman should never be denied an indicated surgical procedure; however, nonurgent operations are delayed until after the first trimester in order to minimize teratogenic effects on the fetus by avoiding this period of significant organogenesis. Second trimester is considered the optimal time for intervention as the risk of preterm labor is lowest. In the case of acutely urgent surgical procedures, their timing should mimic that of nonpregnant patients. A 2015 database comparison between women who had surgery during pregnancy and a matched cohort noted that although there were more emergencies during surgery in pregnancy, there was no difference in rates of mortality or morbidity.[102]

For operations that are necessary during pregnancy, the anesthesia provider should (1) determine an anesthetic plan that optimizes the maternal and fetal condition; (2) consult an obstetrician and perinatologist in order to optimize plans for unexpected events; (3) determine a plan for fetal monitoring if appropriate; and (4) discuss a plan in the event of a cesarean delivery or maternal arrest. According to ACOG, when nonobstetric surgery is planned, the "surgery should be done at an institution with neonatal and pediatric services; an obstetric provider with cesarean delivery privileges should be readily available; and a qualified individual should be readily available to interpret the FHR."[103] There is no evidence that a regional anesthetic technique is better than using general anesthesia for nonobstetric surgery during pregnancy, and there is some retrospective evidence that use of regional techniques for abdominal surgery may result in higher rates of preterm labor compared to general anesthesia.[104]

## Avoidance of Teratogenic Drugs

There is always the possibility that anesthesia will be unknowingly administered to patients with an early undiagnosed pregnancy. For this reason, ASA guidelines recommend, "pregnancy testing may be offered to female patients of childbearing age and for whom the result would alter the patient's management."[105] Routine pregnancy testing before elective surgery for women of childbearing age remains controversial. Most drugs, including anesthetics, have been demonstrated to be teratogenic in at least one animal species. In humans,

the critical period of organogenesis is between 15 and 56 days of gestation. No currently used anesthetic drugs have been shown to have any teratogenic effects in humans when using standard concentrations at any gestational age,[103] with the exception of cocaine. The FDA has recently stopped using categories A-D and X in favor of new labeling that describes what is actually known and recommended for use of each drug during pregnancy.[106] Neurodegeneration and widespread apoptosis following exposure to anesthetics has been clearly established in developing animals, and a few studies demonstrate cognitive impairment in adult animals after neonatal anesthetic exposure. The effects of anesthetic exposure in young children remain unknown; however, some but not all studies suggest that neurocognitive deficits could occur in infants and toddlers[107] (also see Chapter 12).

## Avoidance of Intrauterine Fetal Hypoxia and Acidosis

Avoidance of decreased UBF and oxygenation is critical to fetal well-being. The development of intrauterine fetal hypoxia and acidosis is minimized by avoiding maternal hypotension with left uterine displacement after the 20th week of gestation, as well as by preventing arterial hypoxemia and excessive changes in $Paco_2$ because both hypercapnia and hypocapnia result in reduced uterine blood flow and fetal acidosis. High inspired concentrations of oxygen do not increase the risk for in utero retrolental fibroplasia (retinopathy) because the high oxygen consumption of the placenta plus the uneven distribution of maternal and fetal blood flow in the placenta prevent fetal $Pao_2$ from exceeding 60 mm Hg (even if maternal $Pao_2$ exceeds 500 mm Hg).[15]

FHR monitoring via Doppler is possible at 16 to 18 weeks of gestational age, but variability as a marker of well-being is not established until 25 to 27 weeks of gestation. ACOG states that "the decision to use fetal monitoring should be individualized and, if used, should be based on gestational age, type of surgery, and facilities available."[103] The greatest value of fetal monitoring is that by displaying fetal compromise, it allows further optimization of the maternal and fetal condition. Currently there is no evidence for the efficacy of FHR monitoring. In addition, interpretation is difficult as most anesthetics reduce FHR variability, placement and signal acquisition may be challenging, and a trained person is needed to interpret the FHR tracing strip.

## Prevention of Preterm Labor

The underlying disease requiring surgery, and not the anesthetic technique, has been associated with an increased risk for preterm delivery. Intra-abdominal procedures have more risk than minor peripheral procedures.

IV

After successful completion of surgery, both the FHR and maternal uterine activity should be monitored. Preterm labor can be treated with tocolytics (e.g., nifedipine or indomethacin) in consultation with an obstetrician. Although magnesium sulfate does not demonstrate efficacy as a tocolytic, in situations when there is concern for preterm delivery, administration of magnesium sulfate can reduce the risk of cerebral palsy.[108] In addition, maternal corticosteroid administration is recommended for concern of preterm delivery prior to 32 weeks to decrease neonatal morbidity.[108] Postoperative analgesics can alter the perception of contractions, stressing the need for external monitoring.

## Management of Anesthesia

Elective surgery for pregnant women should be deferred until after delivery. When surgery is necessary, it is best to delay the operation until the second trimester. Before proceeding, a plan for fetal monitoring, potential maternal arrest, and implications of an urgent cesarean delivery should be discussed with an obstetrician and perinatologist. When feasible, neuraxial anesthetic techniques should be considered given appropriate provider experience and circumstance as they limit fetal drug exposure and maternal risks associated with general anesthesia. When a general anesthetic is chosen, aspiration prophylaxis and left uterine displacement should be used. Induction technique should be similar to that for cesarean delivery under general anesthesia as previously discussed. Eucarbia should be maintained (30 mm Hg end-tidal $CO_2$) as well as adequate uterine perfusion with fluids and appropriate use of vasopressors such as phenylephrine. Regardless of the anesthetic technique selected, it is recommended that inhaled concentrations of oxygen be at least 50%. Postoperatively, deep venous thrombosis prophylaxis should be instituted, FHR and uterine activity monitored (often at least 24 hours), and a plan for postoperative analgesia determined.

## Laparoscopic Surgery

Laparoscopy is considered safe during any trimester, and the indications for its use are the same as for nonpregnant patients.[109] Trimester does not influence the laparoscopic surgical complication rate, and conversion to an open approach is low (1%), with a slightly higher fetal loss rate, but lower preterm delivery rate was noted compared to open approaches.[110] Most investigations comparing laparoscopic to open techniques note no significant difference in fetal or maternal outcomes. If a laparoscopic technique is used, in addition to considerations discussed earlier, end-tidal $CO_2$ should be monitored throughout surgery and low pneumoperitoneum pressures (10 to 15 mm Hg) should be used if feasible.

# DIAGNOSIS AND MANAGEMENT OF FETAL DISTRESS

The evolution of FHR monitoring began with the question, How do we detect hypoxia and metabolic acidosis in the fetus? Intrapartum fetal monitoring was designed to detect hypoxia in labor and allow the clinicians to intervene prior to acidosis and long-term fetal CNS damage. The fetal brain responds to peripheral and central stimuli, including (1) chemoreceptors, (2) baroreceptors, and (3) direct effects of metabolic changes within the CNS. FHR monitoring was developed as a crude, nonspecific method of tracking fetal oxygenation and distress. Excellent external FHR monitors are available, but it is often necessary to apply an internal fetal scalp electrode to obtain accurate continuous FHR monitoring.

## Key Evaluation Components

Based on a 2008 National Institutes of Health (NIH) report, the assessment of FHR interpretation involves evaluation of (1) uterine contractions, (2) baseline FHR, (3) baseline FHR variability, (4) presence of accelerations, (5) periodic or episodic decelerations, and (6) changes or trends of FHR patterns over time.[111]

### Uterine Contractions

Uterine contractions can be monitored externally or internally. External monitors only relay contraction frequency, but internal monitoring allows for both frequency and measurement of intrauterine pressure (in Montevideo units). Uterine activity and definitions are detailed in Box 33.4. If a tonic contraction or period of tachysystole occurs during labor, treatment with IV nitroglycerin can briefly relax the uterus and restore

---

**Box 33.4** Uterine Activity Terminology

- Normal: ≤5 contractions in 10 minutes, averaged over a 30-minute window
- Tachysystole: >5 contractions in 10 minutes, averaged over a 30-minute window
- Characteristics of uterine contractions: tachysystole should be always qualified as to presence or absence of associated fetal heart rate decelerations.
  - Tachysystole applies to either spontaneous or stimulated labor. The clinical response to tachysystole may differ depending on whether contractions are spontaneous or stimulated.
- Hyperstimulation and hypercontractility are not defined and should be abandoned.

Data from Macones GA, Hankins GD, Spong CY, et al. The 2008 National Institute of Child Health and Human Development workshop report on electronic fetal monitoring: update on definitions, interpretation, and research guidelines. *J Obstet Gynecol Neonatal Nurs.* 2008;37(5):510-515.

fetal perfusion. In addition, the obstetrician can administer subcutaneous terbutaline.

### Baseline Fetal Heart Rate

Baseline FHR is determined by approximating the mean FHR rounded to increments of 5 beats/min during a 10-minute window excluding accelerations, decelerations, and periods of marked FHR variability (change > 25 beats/min). Abnormal baseline includes bradycardia (<110 beats/min) and tachycardia (>160 beats/min).

### Variability

Baseline variability is also determined by examining fluctuations that are irregular in amplitude and frequency during a 10-minute window excluding accelerations and decelerations. Variability is classified as follows:

Absent FHR variability: amplitude range undetectable

Minimal FHR variability: amplitude range greater than undetectable and 5 beats/min or less

Moderate FHR variability: amplitude range 6 beats/min to 25 beats/min.

Marked FHR variability: amplitude range above 25 beats/min

### Accelerations

An acceleration is an abrupt increase in FHR defined as an increase from the acceleration onset to the peak in less than 30 seconds. In addition, the peak must be 15 beats/min or more and last 15 seconds or longer from the onset to return. Before 32 weeks of gestation, accelerations are defined as having a peak of 10 or more beats/min and a duration of 10 seconds or longer.

### Decelerations

Decelerations are classified as variable or late based on specific criteria described here and displayed in Box 33.5 and Fig. 33.8. A prolonged deceleration is present when there is a visually apparent decrease in the FHR from the baseline that is greater than or equal to 15 beats/min, lasting 2 minutes or longer.

*Late decelerations* are a result of uteroplacental insufficiency causing relative fetal brain hypoxia during a contraction. The change results in sympathetic response and increased peripheral vascular resistance, elevating the fetal blood pressure, which is detected by the fetal baroreceptors and results in slowing in the FHR. This response is termed a *reflex* late deceleration. A second type of late deceleration is caused by myocardial depression in the presence of worsening hypoxia. A moderate drop in FHR indicates some uteroplacental insufficiency; however, a more severe drop in the FHR can indicate near total insufficiency. The term *early* deceleration is controversial. Although many texts associate it with head compression, it is more likely a variant of the reflex late deceleration that mirrors the uterine contraction and is considered benign but might evolve into a more typical late deceleration.[112] *Variable decelerations* are generally synonymous with umbilical cord compression. An ominous sinusoidal FHR pattern is defined as having a smooth sine wave–like pattern with a cycle frequency of 3 to 5/min that persists for 20 or more minutes and can be associated with placental abruption.[111]

It is generally accepted that minimal to undetectable FHR variability in the presence of decelerations is associated with fetal acidemia. Severe decelerations (<70 beats/min for >60 sec) are associated with fetal acidemia and are extremely ominous with the absence of variability.[113]

The FHR tracing is a nonspecific assessment of fetal acidosis and should be interpreted over the course of time in relation to the clinical context and fetal and maternal factors. A normal fetus will experience episodes of hypoxia during labor and tolerate these periods without long-term neurologic sequelae.

## Fetal Heart Rate Categories

A three-tiered FHR classification system (Box 33.5) is currently used for a more general fetal assessment.[114] This evaluation system may move between categories over time. A *Category I* FHR tracing is considered normal,

---

**Box 33.5** Fetal Heart Rate (FHR) Tracing Criteria for Decelerations

| Category | Color | Description |
|---|---|---|
| I | Green | No acidemia |
| IIa | Blue | No central fetal acidemia (adequate oxygen) |
| IIb | Yellow | No central fetal acidemia, but FHR pattern suggests intermittent reductions in $O_2$ which may result in fetal $O_2$ debt |
| IIc | Orange | Fetus potentially on verge of decompensation |
| III | Red | Evidence of actual or impending damaging fetal asphyxia |

*Category I.* An FHR tracing with normal baseline rate (110-160 beats/min), moderate FHR variability, absence of late or variable decelerations, and possible presence of early decelerations.

*Category II.* Everything not included in Categories I and III. Most authorities believe that this category needs to be subdivided into three further subcategories, based on the severity of the periodic changes (IIb) and then reduction of FHR variability (IIc).

*Category III.* An FHR tracing with absent FHR variability, recurrent decelerations or bradycardia, or a sinusoidal pattern.

Data from Macones GA, Hankins GD, Spong CY, et al. The 2008 National Institute of Child Health and Human Development workshop report on electronic fetal monitoring: update on definitions, interpretation, and research guidelines. *J Obstet Gynecol Neonatal Nurs.* 2008;37(5):510-515; and Parer JT, Ikeda T. A framework for standardized management of intrapartum fetal heart rate patterns. *Am J Obstet Gynecol.* July 2007;197(1):e1-6.

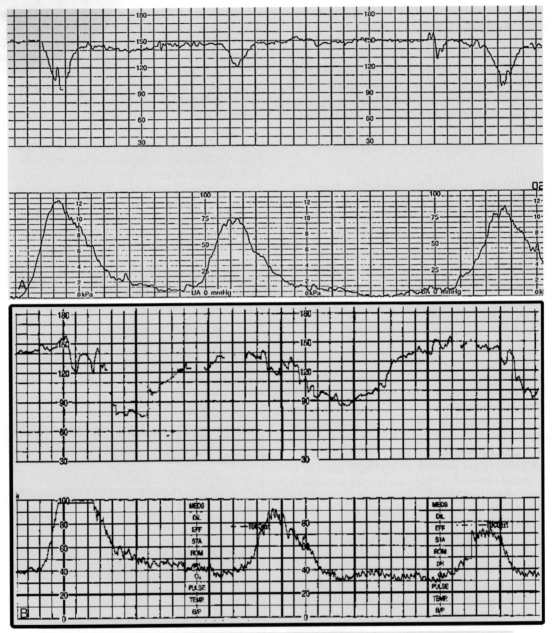

**Fig. 33.8** Fetal heart rate decelerations. (A) Variable deceleration with minimal variability. (B) Late deceleration with minimal variability.

predicts a normal fetal acid-base state at the time of observation, and no specific management is required. To qualify as Category 1, all of the following criteria must be present: (1) baseline FHR of 110 to 160 beats/min; (2) moderate baseline FHR variability; (3) no late or variable decelerations; (4) early decelerations may be present or absent; and (5) accelerations may be present or absent.

A *Category II* FHR tracing is considered indeterminate and includes all tracings not in category I or III. Examples

include fetal tachycardia, prolonged decelerations more than 2 minutes but less than 10 minutes, and recurrent late decelerations with moderate baseline variability. Category II tracings require continued monitoring and reevaluation in light of the entire clinical picture.

A *Category III* FHR tracing is considered abnormal and is associated with an abnormal fetal acid-base state. Category III tracings include either (1) a sinusoidal FHR pattern, or (2) absent FHR variability with recurrent late decelerations, recurrent variable decelerations, or bradycardia. These tracings require prompt patient evaluation and efforts to improve the fetal condition such as intrauterine resuscitation with change in maternal position, treatment of hypotension, use of supplemental oxygen, and treatment of tachysystole if present. If the FHR tracing does not improve, expeditious delivery should proceed.

## EVALUATION OF THE NEONATE AND NEONATAL RESUSCITATION

The transition from fetal to neonate life involves major physiologic changes in the pulmonary and circulatory systems. The importance of the intrapartum and antepartum events can predict how safe and successful the transition to neonate will be. As a measure of fetal assessment, analysis of umbilical cord blood gases is performed at delivery. Typical values are shown in Table 33.2.

Assessment of neonates immediately after birth is important to promptly identify depressed infants who require active resuscitation. The Apgar score assigns a numerical value (0, 1, or 2) to five vital signs measured or observed at 1, 5, and 10 minutes after delivery (Table 33.3). It has not been surpassed as a method of facilitating recognition and guiding resuscitation management of a newborn. Approximately 10% of newborns need some assistance to begin breathing and less than 1% require advanced cardiopulmonary resuscitation that includes chest compressions of resuscitation medications.[115] Most newborns (with Apgar ≥ 8) require little treatment other than suctioning of the nose and mouth, tactile stimulation to promote breathing, and avoiding hypothermia. The neonate's skin should be wiped dry and the baby placed on a radiantly heated bed, covered with warm blankets, or placed in skin-to-skin contact with mother. Apgar scores of 10 are rare because the acrocyanosis persists in a normal newborn well past 5 minutes of life.

### Cardiopulmonary Resuscitation

Management of neonates in the delivery room is implemented in 30-second evaluations and interventions as detailed in Fig. 33.9. At delivery, once the infant is placed under a radiant warmer and drying and stimulation have occurred, the first 30-second evaluation begins based on 2015 neonatal resuscitation guidelines.[115] This evaluation takes into account gestational age and starts with the determination of tone, breathing, or crying. If breathing and crying do not occur, then clearing of the airway (mouth, then nose) and repeated stimulation should be performed while maintaining euthermia; this is the next 30-second evaluation. Evaluation for apnea, gasping, and heart rate occur with determination

| Table 33.2 | Normal Blood Gas Values of Umbilical Artery and Vein | |
|---|---|---|
| Measurement | Mean Artery Value | Mean Vein Value |
| pH | 7.27 | 7.34 |
| $P_{CO_2}$ (mm Hg) | 50 | 40 |
| $P_{O_2}$ (mm Hg) | 20 | 30 |
| Bicarbonate (mEq/L) | 23 | 21 |
| Base excess (mEq/L) | −3.6 | −2.6 |

Data derived from Thorp JA, Rushing RS. Umbilical cord blood gas analysis. *Obstet Gynecol Clin North Am*. 1999;26(4):695-709.

| Table 33.3 | Evaluation of a Neonate With Apgar Score | | |
|---|---|---|---|
| Criterion | 2 | 1 | 0 |
| Heart rate (beats/min) | >100 | <100 | Absent |
| Breathing | Irregular, crying | Slow | Absent |
| Reflex irritability | Cry | Grimace | No response |
| Muscle tone | Active | Flexion of the extremities | Limp |
| Color | Pink | Body pink, extremities cyanotic | Cyanotic |

of the 1-minute Apgar score and possible intervention with positive-pressure ventilation (PPV) assistance and placement of pulse oximetry and ECG monitoring. In the event of a heart rate below 100 beats/min, PPV efficacy should be evaluated by checking for chest movement, optimizing PPV delivery, and consideration of need for intubation or laryngeal mask airway (LMA) placement. If the heart rate drops below 60 beats/min, then chest compressions, intubation, and ventilation with 100% oxygen should commence with ECG monitoring and preparation for umbilical vein cannulation. Based on the 2015 guidelines, it is reasonable to initiate resuscitation with air and add supplemental oxygen titrated to achieve the preductal oxygen saturation approximating the expected value of healthy infants (see Fig. 33.9). In addition, these guidelines endorse use of 100% oxygen in situations in which chest compressions are required. Infants older than 36 weeks of gestation assessed to have moderate to severe hypoxic-ischemic encephalopathy should be enrolled in a therapeutic hypothermia protocol (also see Chapter 45).

IV

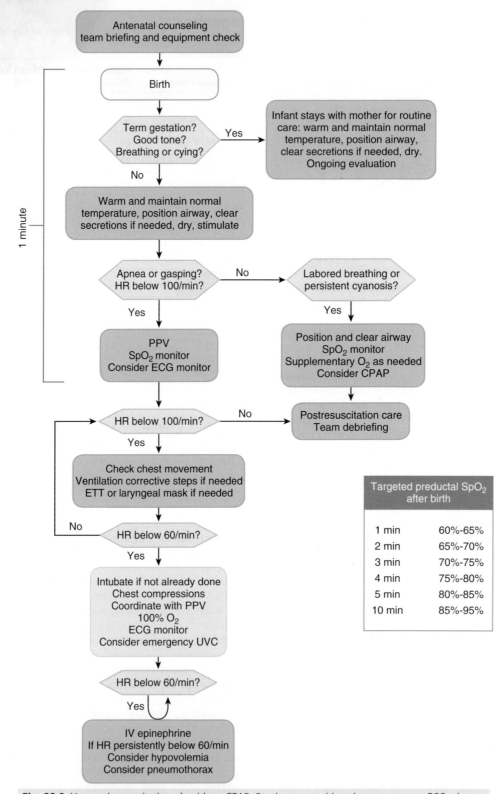

**Fig. 33.9** Neonatal resuscitation algorithm. *CPAP,* Continuous positive airway pressure; *ECG,* electrocardiogram; *ETT,* endotracheal tube; *HR,* heart rate; *IV,* intravenous; *PPV,* positive-pressure ventilation; *UVC,* umbilical vein cannulation. (Based on figure from Wyckoff MH, Aziz K, Escobedo M, et al. Neonatal Resuscitation: 2015 American Heart Association Guidelines Update for Cardiopulmonary Resuscitation and Emergency Cardiovascular Care. *Circulation.* 2015;132(18 suppl 2):S543-S560.)

If meconium is present, an individual skilled in endotracheal intubation should be present at the time of birth. If the infant is vigorous with good respiratory effort and muscle tone following delivery, no significant intervention is needed, but if poor muscle tone and inadequate breathing efforts are present, resuscitation should commence and PPV initiated if the infant is not breathing or the heart rate is less than 100 beats/min.[115] Routine intubation for tracheal suction in this setting is no longer suggested, but instead emphasis should be on initiating ventilation within the first minute of life in the non-breathing or ineffectively breathing infant by clearing the airway and use of PPV.

### Epinephrine

Epinephrine is indicated in the event the heart rate continues to stay below 60 beats/min despite PPV, chest compressions, or immediately if asystole is present. The dose is 0.1 to 0.3 mL/kg of a 1:10,000 IV solution given rapidly. The dose may be repeated every 3 to 5 minutes, if necessary.

### Hypovolemia

In certain circumstances blood loss in the neonate may lead to hypovolemia, such as placental abruption, placenta previa, or vasa previa, although arrest secondary to hypovolemia is rare. Volume expansion should be instituted in a newborn who appears to have suffered blood loss or is in hypovolemic shock and has not responded to other resuscitation measures discussed previously. Blood or isotonic crystalloid (in 10 mL/kg aliquots) may be administered in the delivery room.

### Glucose

During deliveries when the newborn is suspected to have severe asphyxia, intrauterine growth restriction, or maternal diabetes, hypoglycemia should be suspected. During the resuscitation, a heel stick can determine the blood glucose level.

### Naloxone

Naloxone is no longer recommended for use in newborns in the delivery room. Should the newborn manifest respiratory depression in the delivery room, appropriate ventilation should be maintained until the neonate is transported to the intensive care nursery. Continued stabilization and evaluation can be performed in the nursery and administration of naloxone considered once the mother's history is reviewed to evaluate for prenatal exposure to chronic opioids.

## QUESTIONS OF THE DAY

1. How do the following cardiovascular parameters change during pregnancy: blood volume, stroke volume, heart rate, systemic vascular resistance, central venous pressure, femoral venous pressure?
2. What are the expected arterial blood gas values (pH, $Paco_2$, and $Pao_2$) in a pregnant woman at term? What is the mechanism for the differences from the nonpregnant state?
3. What nerves mediate pain during the first stage of labor? Where does pain originate during the second stage of labor? If neuraxial analgesia is used during labor and delivery, what spinal levels should be targeted for the first and second stages?
4. A primigravid patient in early labor is considering options for analgesia. She asks you whether epidural analgesia will prolong her labor or increase the chance for a cesarean section. How would you respond?
5. Describe the 3-tier system of fetal heart rate monitoring and how the further separation of the category II into IIa, IIb, and IIc has improved management and assessment.
6. What are the key changes in the definition and management of preeclampsia beginning in 2013?
7. What is the clinical definition of preeclampsia? What additional criteria define preeclampsia with severe features?
8. What are the most common causes of maternal hemorrhage during the third trimester and labor? What factors can lead to increased risk of morbidity and mortality with massive hemorrhage in the obstetric patient?
9. Immediately after delivery, a neonate with meconium-stained amniotic fluid has good respiratory effort and muscle tone. What interventions should be done next? If the neonate had poor respiratory effort, what would be the next steps in management?

IV

# REFERENCES

1. Cheek TG, Gutsche BB. Maternal physiologic alterations. In: Hughes SC, Levinson G, Rosen MA, Shnider SM, eds. *Shnider and Levinson's Anesthesia for Obstetrics.* 4th ed. Philadelphia: Lippincott Williams & Wilkins; 2002:3–18.

2. Gaiser R. Physiologic changes of pregnancy. In: Chestnut DH, Polley LS, Tsen LC, Wong CA, eds. *Chestnut's Obstetric Anesthesia: Principles and Practice.* 4th ed. Philadelphia: Elsevier; 2009:15–36.

3. Ain DL, Narula J, Sengupta PP. Cardiovascular imaging and diagnostic procedures in pregnancy. *Cardiol Clin.* 2012;30:331–341.

4. Ewah B, Yau K, King M, et al. Effect of epidural opioids on gastric emptying in labour. *Int J Obstet Anesth.* 1993;2:125–128.

5. Practice Guidelines for Obstetric Anesthesia. An Updated Report by the American Society of Anesthesiologists Task Force on Obstetric Anesthesia and the Society for Obstetric Anesthesia and Perinatology. *Anesthesiology.* 2016;124:270–300.

6. Hey VM, Ostick DG, Mazumder JK, Lord WD. Pethidine, metoclopramide and the gastro-oesophageal sphincter. A study in healthy volunteers. *Anaesthesia.* 1981;36:173–176.

7. Paranjothy S, Griffiths JD, Broughton HK, et al. Interventions at caesarean section for reducing the risk of aspiration pneumonitis. *Cochrane Database Syst Rev.* 2010;1:CD004943.

8. Palahniuk RJ, Shnider SM, Eger EI 2nd. Pregnancy decreases the requirement for inhaled anesthetic agents. *Anesthesiology.* 1974;41:82–83.

9. Gin T, Chan MT. Decreased minimum alveolar concentration of isoflurane in pregnant humans. *Anesthesiology.* 1994;81:829–832.

10. Ueyama H, Hagihira S, Takashina M, et al. Pregnancy does not enhance volatile anesthetic sensitivity on the brain: an electroencephalographic analysis study. *Anesthesiology.* 2010;113:577–584.

11. Lee A, Ngan Kee WD, Gin T. A quantitative, systematic review of randomized controlled trials of ephedrine versus phenylephrine for the management of hypotension during spinal anesthesia for cesarean delivery. *Anesth Analg.* 2002;94:920–926.

12. Ngan Kee WD, Khaw KS, Tan PE, et al. Placental transfer and fetal metabolic effects of phenylephrine and ephedrine during spinal anesthesia for cesarean delivery. *Anesthesiology.* 2009;111:506–512.

13. Smiley RM. Burden of proof. *Anesthesiology.* 2009;111:470–472.

14. Ngan Kee WD, Lee SW, Ng FF, et al. Randomized double-blinded comparison of norepinephrine and phenylephrine for maintenance of blood pressure during spinal anesthesia for cesarean delivery. *Anesthesiology.* 2015;122:736–745.

15. Haydon ML, Gorenberg DM, Nageotte MP, et al. The effect of maternal oxygen administration on fetal pulse oximetry during labor in fetuses with nonreassuring fetal heart rate patterns. *Am J Obstet Gynecol.* 2006;195:735–738.

16. Zhang J, Landy HJ, Branch DW, et al. Consortium on Safe Labor. Contemporary patterns of spontaneous labor with normal neonatal outcomes. *Obstet Gynecol.* 2010;116(6):1281–1287.

17. Laughon SK, Branch DW, Beaver J, Zhang J. Changes in labor patterns over 50 years. *Am J Obstet Gynecol.* 2012;206(5):419. e1-e9.

18. Leighton BL, Halpern SH, Wilson DB. Lumbar sympathetic blocks speed early and second stage induced labor in nulliparous women. *Anesthesiology.* 1999;90:1039–1046.

19. Arendt KW, Tessmer-Tuck JA. Nonpharmacologic labor analgesia. *Clin Perinatol.* 2013;40:351–371.

20. Hodnett ED, Gates S, Hofmeyr GJ, Sakala C. Continuous support for women during childbirth. *Cochrane Database Syst Rev.* 2012;(10):CD003766.

21. Nissen E, Widstrom AM, Lilja G, et al. Effects of routinely given pethidine during labour on infants' developing breastfeeding behaviour. Effects of dose-delivery time interval and various concentrations of pethidine/norpethidine in cord plasma. *Acta Paediatr.* 1997;86:201–208.

22. Mackeen AD, Fehnel E, Berghella V, Klein T. Morphine sleep in pregnancy. *Am J Perinatol.* 2014;31:85–90.

23. Rayburn W, Rathke A, Leuschen MP, et al. Fentanyl citrate analgesia during labor. *Am J Obstet Gynecol.* 1989;161:202–206.

24. Fleet J, Belan I, Jones MJ, et al. A comparison of fentanyl with pethidine for pain relief during childbirth: a randomised controlled trial. *Br J Obstet Gynaecol.* 2015;122:983–992.

25. Volmanen P, Sarvela J, Akural EI, et al. Intravenous remifentanil vs. epidural levobupivacaine with fentanyl for pain relief in early labour: a randomised, controlled, double-blinded study. *Acta Anaesthesiol Scand.* 2008;52:249–255.

26. Freeman LM, Bloemenkamp KW, Franssen MT, et al. Patient controlled analgesia with remifentanil versus epidural analgesia in labour: randomised multicentre equivalence trial. *BMJ.* 2015;350:h846.

27. Likis FE, Andrews JC, Collins MR, et al. Nitrous oxide for the management of labor pain: a systematic review. *Anesth Analg.* 2014;118:153–167.

28. Yentis MY, Cohen SE. Inhalational analgesia and anesthesia for labor and vaginal delivery. In: Hughes SC, Levinson G, Rosen MA, Shnider SM, eds. *Shnider and Levinson's Anesthesia for Obstetrics.* 4th ed. Philadelphia: Lippincott Williams & Wilkins; 2002:189–197.

29. King TL, Wong CA. Nitrous oxide for labor pain: is it a laughing matter? *Anesth Analg.* 2014;118:12–14.

30. Polley LS, Columb MO, Naughton NN, et al. Effect of epidural epinephrine on the minimum local analgesic concentration of epidural bupivacaine in labor. *Anesthesiology.* 2002;96:1123–1128.

31. Aveline C, El Metaoua S, Masmoudi A, et al. The effect of clonidine on the minimum local analgesic concentration of epidural ropivacaine during labor. *Anesth Analg.* 2002;95:735–740.

32. Van de Velde M. Neuraxial analgesia and fetal bradycardia. *Curr Opin Anaesthesiol.* 2005;18:253–256.

33. Declercq ER, Sakala C, Corry MP, Applebaum S. Listening to Mothers II: report of the Second National U.S. Survey of Women's Childbearing Experiences: conducted January-February 2006 for Childbirth Connection by Harris Interactive(R) in partnership with Lamaze International. *J Perinat Educ.* 2007;16(4):15–17.

34. Attanasio L, Kozhimannil KB, Jou J, et al. Women's experiences with neuraxial labor analgesia in the Listening to Mothers II Survey: a content analysis of open-ended responses. *Anesth Analg.* 2015;121:974–980.

35. American College of Obstetricians and Gynecologists Committee on Obstetric Practice. ACOG committee opinion No. 339: analgesia and cesarean delivery rates. *Obstet Gynecol.* 2006;107(6):1487–1488.

36. Wong CA, Scavone BM, Peaceman AM, et al. The risk of cesarean delivery with neuraxial analgesia given early versus late in labor. *N Engl J Med.* 2005;352:655–665.

37. Sng BL, Leong WL, Zeng Y, et al. Early versus late initiation of epidural analgesia for labour. *Cochrane Database Syst Rev.* 2014;(10):CD007238.

38. Anim-Somuah M, Smyth RM, Jones L. Epidural versus non-epidural or no analgesia in labour. *Cochrane Database Syst Rev.* 2011;(12):CD000331.

39. Wassen MM, Smits LJ, Scheepers HC, et al. Routine labour epidural analgesia versus labour analgesia on request: a randomised non-inferiority trial. *Br J Obstet Gynaecol.* 2015;122:344–350.

40. Craig MG, Grant EN, Tao W, et al. A randomized control trial of bupiv-

acaine and fentanyl versus fentanyl-only for epidural analgesia during the second stage of labor. *Anesthesiology.* 2015;122:172–177.

41. American College of Obstetricians and Gynecologists Committee on Practice Bulletins–Obstetrics. ACOG Practice Bulletin No. 49, December 2003: dystocia and augmentation of labor. *Obstet Gynecol.* 2003;102(6):1445–1454.

42. American Society of Anesthesiologists task force on infectious complications associated with neuraxial techniques. Practice advisory for the prevention, diagnosis, and management of infectious complications associated with neuraxial techniques: a report by the American Society of Anesthesiologists task force on infectious complications associated with neuraxial techniques. *Anesthesiology.* 2010;112(3):530–545.

43. Simmons SW, Taghizadeh N, Dennis AT, et al. Combined spinal-epidural versus epidural analgesia in labour. *Cochrane Database Syst Rev.* 2012;(10):CD003401.

44. Heesen M, Bohmer J, Klohr S, et al. The effect of adding a background infusion to patient-controlled epidural labor analgesia on labor, maternal, and neonatal outcomes: a systematic review and meta-analysis. *Anesth Analg.* 2015;121:149–158.

45. McKenzie CP, Cobb B, Riley ET, Carvalho B. Programmed intermittent epidural boluses for maintenance of labor analgesia: an impact study. *Int J Obstet Anesth.* 2016;26:32–38.

46. George RB, Allen TK, Habib AS. Intermittent epidural bolus compared with continuous epidural infusions for labor analgesia: a systematic review and meta-analysis. *Anesth Analg.* 2013;116:133–144.

47. Horlocker TT, Wedel DJ, Rowlinson JC, et al. Regional anesthesia in the patient receiving antithrombotic or thrombolytic therapy: American Society of Regional Anesthesia and Pain Medicine Evidence-Based Guidelines (Third Edition). *Reg Anesth Pain Med.* 2010;35(1):64–101.

48. Neal JM, Barrington MJ, Brull R, et al. The Second ASRA Practice Advisory on Neurologic Complications Associated With Regional Anesthesia and Pain Medicine: executive summary 2015. *Reg Anesth Pain Med.* 2015;40(5):401–430.

49. Pan PH, Bogard TD, Owen MD. Incidence and characteristics of failures in obstetric neuraxial analgesia and anesthesia: a retrospective analysis of 19,259 deliveries. *Int J Obstet Anesth.* 2004;13:227–233.

50. D'Angelo R, Smiley RM, Riley ET, Segal S. Serious complications related to obstetric anesthesia: the serious complication repository project of the Society

for Obstetric Anesthesia and Perinatology. *Anesthesiology.* 2014;120:1505–1512.

51. Ruppen W, Derry S, McQuay H, Moore RA. Incidence of epidural hematoma, infection, and neurologic injury in obstetric patients with epidural analgesia/anesthesia. *Anesthesiology.* 2006;105(2):394–399.

52. Lipman S, Cohen S, Einav S, et al. Society for Obstetric Anesthesia and Perinatology. The Society for Obstetric Anesthesia and Perinatology consensus statement on the management of cardiac arrest in pregnancy. *Anesth Analg.* 2014;118(5):1003–1016.

53. Jeejeebhoy FM, Zelop CM, Lipman S, et al. American Heart Association Emergency Cardiovascular Care Committee, Council on Cardiopulmonary, Critical Care, Perioperative and Resuscitation, Council on Cardiovascular Diseases in the Young, and Council on Clinical Cardiology. Cardiac Arrest in Pregnancy: a scientific statement from the American Heart Association. *Circulation.* 2015;132(18):1747–1773.

54. Neal JM, Mulroy MF, Weinberg GL. American Society of Regional Anesthesia and Pain Medicine. American Society of Regional Anesthesia and Pain Medicine checklist for managing local anesthetic systemic toxicity: 2012 version. *Reg Anesth Pain Med.* 2012;37(1):16–18.

55. Hofmeyr G, Cyna A, Middleton P. Prophylactic intravenous preloading for regional analgesia in labour. *Cochrane Database Syst Rev.* 2004;(4):CD000175.

56. Tawfik MM, Hayes SM, Jacoub FY, et al. Comparison between colloid preload and crystalloid co-load in cesarean section under spinal anesthesia: a randomized controlled trial. *Int J Obstet Anesth.* 2014;23:317–323.

57. Banerjee A, Stocche RM, Angle P, Halpern SH. Preload or coload for spinal anesthesia for elective cesarean delivery: a meta-analysis. *Can J Anaesth.* 2010;57:24–31.

58. Butwick AJ, Columb MO, Carvalho B. Preventing spinal hypotension during Caesarean delivery: what is the latest? *Br J Anaesth.* 2015;114:183–186.

59. Dyer RA, Reed AR, van Dyk D, et al. Hemodynamic effects of ephedrine, phenylephrine, and the coadministration of phenylephrine with oxytocin during spinal anesthesia for elective cesarean delivery. *Anesthesiology.* 2009;111:753–765.

60. Arendt KW, Segal BS. The association between epidural labor analgesia and maternal fever. *Clin Perinatol.* 2013;40:385–398.

61. Greenwell EA, Wyshak G, Ringer SA, et al. Intrapartum temperature elevation, epidural use, and adverse outcome in term infants. *Pediatrics.* 2012;129:e447–e454.

62. Rosen MA. Paracervical block for labor analgesia: a brief historic review. *Am J Obstet Gynecol.* 2002;186:S127–S130.

63. Nikpoor P, Bain E. Analgesia for forceps delivery. *Cochrane Database Syst Rev.* 2013;(9):CD008878.

64. Ayad S, Demian Y, Narouze SN, Tetzlaff JE. Subarachnoid catheter placement after wet tap for analgesia in labor: influence on the risk of headache in obstetric patients. *Reg Anesth Pain Med.* 2003;28:512–515.

65. Toledo P, McCarthy RJ, Ebarvia MJ, et al. The interaction between epidural 2-chloroprocaine and morphine: a randomized controlled trial of the effect of drug administration timing on the efficacy of morphine analgesia. *Anesth Analg.* 2009;109:168–173.

66. Carvalho B. Failed epidural top-up for cesarean delivery for failure to progress in labor: the case against single-shot spinal anesthesia. *Int J Obstet Anesth.* 2012;21:357–359.

67. Hawkins JL, Chang J, Palmer SK, et al. Anesthesia-related maternal mortality in the United States: 1979-2002. *Obstet Gynecol.* 2011;117:69–74.

68. American Society of Anesthesiologists Task Force on Obstetric Anesthesia. Practice guidelines for obstetric anesthesia: an updated report by the American Society of Anesthesiologists Task Force on Obstetric Anesthesia. *Anesthesiology.* 2007;106(4):843–863.

69. Afolabi BB, Lesi FE. Regional versus general anaesthesia for caesarean section. *Cochrane Database Syst Rev.* 2012;(10):CD004350.

70. March of Dimes Foundation. PeriStats website; 2016. www.marchofdimes.org/peristats. Accessed May 17, 2016.

71. Norwitz ER, Edusa V, Park JS. Maternal physiology and complications of multiple pregnancy. *Semin Perinatol.* 2005;29:338–348.

72. Barrett JF, Hannah ME, Hutton EK, et al. Twin Birth Study Collaborative Group. A randomized trial of planned cesarean or vaginal delivery for twin pregnancy. *N Engl J Med.* 2013;369(14):1295–1305.

73. Khaw KS, Lee SW, Ngan Kee WD, et al. Randomized trial of anaesthetic interventions in external cephalic version for breech presentation. *Br J Anaesth.* 2015;114:944–950.

74. American College of Obstetricians and Gynecologists. Committee on Obstetric Practice. ACOG committee opinion No. 340: mode of term singleton breech delivery. *Obstet Gynecol.* 2006;108(1):235–237.

75. Dajani NK, Magann EF. Complications of shoulder dystocia. *Semin Perinatol.* 2014;38:201–204.

76. American College of Obstetricians and Gynecologists; Task Force on Hypertension in Pregnancy. Hyperten-

in pregnancy. Report of the American College of Obstetricians and Gynecologists' Task Force on Hypertension in Pregnancy. *Obstet Gynecol.* 2013;122(5):1122–1131.

77. Ananth CV, Keyes KM, Wapner RJ. Pre-eclampsia rates in the United States, 1980-2010: age-period-cohort analysis. *BMJ.* 2013;347:f6564.

78. Davidge ST, de Groot CJM, Taylor RN. Endothelial cell dysfunction. In: Taylor RN, Roberts JM, Cunningham FG, Lindheimer MD, eds. *Chesley's Hypertensive Disorders in Pregnancy.* 4th ed. San Diego: Elsevier; 2015:181–207.

79. Leffert LR. What's new in obstetric anesthesia? Focus on preeclampsia. *Int J Obstet Anesth.* 2015;24(3):264–271.

80. Mannisto T, Mendola P, Vaarasmaki M, et al. Elevated blood pressure in pregnancy and subsequent chronic disease risk. *Circulation.* 2013;127:681–690.

81. Report of the National High Blood Pressure Education Program Working Group on High Blood Pressure in Pregnancy. *Am J Obstet Gynecol.* 2000;183(1):S1–S22.

82. Committee on Obstetric Practice. Committee opinion No. 623: emergent therapy for acute-onset, severe hypertension during pregnancy and the postpartum period. *Obstet Gynecol.* 2015;125(2):521–525.

83. Green L, Machin SJ. Managing anticoagulated patients during neuraxial anaesthesia. *Br J Haematol.* 2010;149:195–208.

84. Pant M, Fong R, Scavone B. Prevention of peri-induction hypertension in preeclamptic patients: a focused review. *Anesth Analg.* 2014;119:1350–1356.

85. Scavone BM, Main EK. The National Partnership for Maternal Safety: a call to action for anesthesiologists. *Anesth Analg.* 2015;121:14–16.

86. Silver RM. Abnormal placentation: placenta previa, vasa previa, and placenta accreta. *Obstet Gynecol.* 2015;126(3):654–668.

87. Silver RM, Landon MB, Rouse DJ, et al. Maternal morbidity associated with multiple repeat cesarean deliveries. *Obstet Gynecol.* 2006;107:1226–1232.

88. Butwick AJ, Goodnough LT. Transfusion and coagulation management in major obstetric hemorrhage. *Curr Opin Anaesthesiol.* 2015;28:275–284.

89. Simonazzi G, Bisulli M, Saccone G, et al. Tranexamic acid for preventing postpartum blood loss after cesarean delivery: a systematic review and meta-analysis of randomized controlled trials. *Acta Obstet Gynecol Scand.* 2016; 95:28–37.

90. Shakur H, Elbourne D, Gulmezoglu M, et al. The WOMAN Trial (World Maternal Antifibrinolytic Trial): tranexamic acid for the treatment of postpartum haemorrhage: an international randomised, double blind placebo controlled trial. *Trials.* 2010;11:40.

91. Tikkanen M. Placental abruption: epidemiology, risk factors and consequences. *Acta Obstet Gynecol Scand.* 2011;90:140–149.

92. Holmgren CM. Uterine rupture associated with VBAC. *Clin Obstet Gynecol.* 2012;55:978–987.

93. American College of Obstetricians and Gynecologists. ACOG Practice Bulletin No. 115: vaginal birth after previous cesarean delivery. *Obstet Gynecol.* 2010;116(2 Pt 1):450–463.

94. Endler M, Grunewald C, Saltvedt S. Epidemiology of retained placenta: oxytocin as an independent risk factor. *Obstet Gynecol.* 2012;119:801–809.

95. Westhoff G, Cotter AM, Tolosa JE. Prophylactic oxytocin for the third stage of labour to prevent postpartum haemorrhage. *Cochrane Database Syst Rev.* 2013;(10):CD001808.

96. Kovacheva VP, Soens MA, Tsen LC. A randomized, double-blinded trial of a "rule of threes" algorithm versus continuous infusion of oxytocin during elective cesarean delivery. *Anesthesiology.* 2015;123(1):92–100.

97. Silver RM, Barbour KD. Placenta accreta spectrum: accreta, increta, and percreta. *Obstet Gynecol Clin North Am.* 2015;42:381–402.

98. Goucher H, Wong CA, Patel SK, Toledo P. Cell salvage in obstetrics. *Anesth Analg.* 2015;121(2):465–468.

99. Ito F, Akasaka J, Koike N, et al. Incidence, diagnosis and pathophysiology of amniotic fluid embolism. *J Obstet Gynaecol.* 2014;34:580–584.

100. Heesen M, Klimek M. Nonobstetric anesthesia during pregnancy. *Curr Opin Anaesthesiol.* 2016;29(3):297–303.

101. Lucia A, Dantoni SE. Trauma management of the pregnant patient. *Crit Care Clin.* 2016;32:109–117.

102. Moore HB, Juarez-Colunga E, Bronsert M, et al. Effect of pregnancy on adverse outcomes after general surgery. *JAMA Surg.* 2015;150(7):637–643.

103. ACOG Committee on Obstetric Practice. ACOG committee opinion No. 474: nonobstetric surgery during pregnancy. *Obstet Gynecol.* 2011;117(2 Pt 1):420–421.

104. Hong JY. Adnexal mass surgery and anesthesia during pregnancy: a 10-year retrospective review. *Int J Obstet Anesth.* 2006;15:212–216.

105. Committee on Standards and Practice Parameters, Apfelbaum JL, Connis RT, Nickinovich DG, American Society of Anesthesiologists Task Force on Preanesthesia Evaluation, Pasternak LR, Arens JF, Caplan RA, et al. Practice advisory for preanesthesia evaluation: an updated report by the American Society of Anesthesiologists Task Force on Preanesthesia Evaluation. *Anesthesiology.* 2012;116(3):522–538.

106. Carvalho B, Wong CA. Drug labeling in the practice of obstetric anesthesia. *Am J Obstet Gynecol.* 2015;212:24–27.

107. Rappaport BA, Suresh S, Hertz S, et al. Anesthetic neurotoxicity–clinical implications of animal models. *N Engl J Med.* 2015;372:796–797.

108. Locatelli A, Consonni S, Ghidini A. Preterm labor: approach to decreasing complications of prematurity. *Obstet Gynecol Clin North Am.* 2015;42:255–274.

109. Soper NJ. SAGES' guidelines for diagnosis, treatment, and use of laparoscopy for surgical problems during pregnancy. *Surg Endosc.* 2011;25:3477–3478.

110. Walsh CA, Tang T, Walsh SR. Laparoscopic versus open appendicectomy in pregnancy: a systematic review. *Int J Surg.* 2008;6:339–344.

111. Macones GA, Hankins GD, Spong CY, et al. The 2008 National Institute of Child Health and Human Development workshop report on electronic fetal monitoring: update on definitions, interpretation, and research guidelines. *J Obstet Gynecol Neonatal Nurs.* 2008;37:510–515.

112. Parer JT. Fetal heart rate patterns: basic and variant. In: Parer JT, ed. *Handbook of Fetal Heart Rate Monitoring.* 2nd ed. Philadelphia: WB Saunders; 1997:145–195.

113. Parer JT, King T, Flanders S, et al. Fetal acidemia and electronic fetal heart rate patterns: is there evidence of an association? *J Matern Fetal Neonatal Med.* 2006;19:289–294.

114. American College of Obstetricians and Gynecologists. ACOG Practice Bulletin No. 106: intrapartum fetal heart rate monitoring: nomenclature, interpretation, and general management principles. *Obstet Gynecol.* 2009;114(1):192–202.

115. Wyckoff MH, Aziz K, Escobedo MB, et al. Part 13: neonatal resuscitation: 2015 American Heart Association Guidelines Update for Cardiopulmonary Resuscitation and Emergency Cardiovascular Care. *Circulation.* 2015;132(18 suppl 2):S543–S560.

# 34 PEDIATRICS

Erin A. Gottlieb and Dean B. Andropoulos

Providing anesthetic care for infants and children poses unique challenges because of the profound differences in physiology, pharmacokinetics, and pharmacodynamics of anesthetic drugs, and the wide variety of procedures that these patients undergo, which are often very different from the adult population. The developmental physiology, pharmacology, fluid and transfusion therapy, and airway management in pediatric anesthesia will be defined. Anesthetic considerations and techniques in pediatric patients, especially in neonates, who are the most unique group of pediatric patients, will be reviewed. The new field of fetal surgery will be addressed, and finally, the growing area of anesthesia in remote locations for pediatric patients and anesthetic neurotoxicity in the developing brain will be discussed briefly.

## DEVELOPMENTAL PHYSIOLOGY

### Respiratory System

#### Lung Development
Lung development begins in the fourth week of gestation, but extrauterine survival becomes possible only when terminal air sacs begin to form and the capillary network surrounding them is sufficient for pulmonary gas exchange around the 26th week. Alveolar formation begins by the 36th postconceptual week, but most alveoli form postnatally. Type II pneumocytes begin producing surfactant around the 24th week of gestation, and production of this mixture of phospholipids and surfactant proteins is critical for reducing surface tension and facilitating the inflation of alveoli.

#### Chest Wall and Respiratory Muscles
The ribs extend from the vertebral column horizontally in infants compared to a caudad angle in adults. This configuration renders the accessory muscles of respiration ineffective in infants. The rib cage also tends to move inward during inspiration because of the high cartilage content in the ribs of neonates and infants. This paradoxic chest wall movement occurs commonly under general anesthesia and is due to decreased tone of the intercostal muscles and upper airway obstruction. The diaphragm increases its work to maintain tidal volume, which can lead to fatigue.

The mature diaphragm has a low content of type I (slow twitch, high oxidative capacity) muscle fibers. Prior to 37 weeks' postconceptual age, less than 10% of the diaphragmatic fibers are type I. A term infant has approximately 25% type I fibers, and an adult has approximately 50%. This means that the diaphragm is more likely to become fatigued in premature and term infants, leading to earlier respiratory failure.

Chest wall compliance decreases throughout childhood and adolescence owing to the ossification of the ribs and development of thoracic muscle mass. The elastic recoil pressure of the lung increases throughout this time from an increase in pulmonary elastic fibers.

### Respiratory Variables
There are some major differences in static lung volumes and respiratory variables between children of different ages and adults (also see Chapter 5). Table 34.1 illustrates the major differences in these and other variables between infants and adults. Total lung capacity (TLC) is much larger per kilogram in adults compared with infants. This is largely due to the relative efficiency and strength of adult muscles of inspiration and effort.

Functional residual capacity (FRC) is similar on a per kilogram basis among age groups. However, the mechanical reasons for this similarity differ. The FRC in adults is defined as the volume at which passive elastic forces of the chest wall are balanced by the recoil of the lung. This is the volume at end exhalation. In infants, both the elastic recoil of the chest and the recoil pressure of the lung are very small. This would predict an FRC of about 10% of TLC. However, the FRC is about 40% of TLC owing to a prolongation of the expiratory time constant by a process known as *laryngeal braking.*

In an apneic infant, the lung volume is smaller than the FRC. Thus, an apneic infant has a disproportionately smaller store of intrapulmonary oxygen than an adult, and hypoxemia will develop rapidly if the airway is poorly maintained.

In infants, the closing capacity (CC) is larger than the FRC, so during exhalation, small airways start to collapse and trap air. In adults, the closing capacity is smaller than the FRC.

### Factors Affecting Respiration
In both infants and adults, $Pa_{O_2}$, $Pa_{CO_2}$, and pH control ventilation. An increase in $Pa_{CO_2}$ increases minute ventilation by increasing respiratory rate and tidal volume. This response to hypercapnia is not enhanced by hypoxemia. In fact, hypoxia may depress the hypercapnic ventilatory response.

High inspired oxygen concentrations depress newborn respiratory drive, and low inspired oxygen concentrations stimulate it. However, continued hypoxia will eventually lead to respiratory depression. Hypoglycemia, anemia, and hypothermia also decrease respiratory drive.

Metabolic demand drives minute ventilation. As oxygen consumption increases, alveolar minute ventilation increases. Although tidal volume also increases, the increase in respiratory rate is the predominant variable that increases minute ventilation in infants.

### Breathing Patterns
Normal newborn breathing is periodic. There are pauses of less than 10 seconds and periods of increased respiratory activity. Periodic breathing is different from apnea, a ventilatory pause associated with desaturation and bradycardia. Apnea is associated with prematurity and is treated with respiratory stimulants and with tactile stimulation such as stroking or rocking. Postoperative apnea in

**Table 34.1**  Age-Dependent Respiratory Variables

| Variable | Units | Neonate | 6 mo | 12 mo | 3 yr | 5 yr | 9 yr | 12 yr | Adult |
|---|---|---|---|---|---|---|---|---|---|
| Approx. weight | kg | 3 | 7 | 10 | 15 | 19 | 30 | 50 | 70 |
| Respiratory rate | breaths/min | 50 ± 10 | 30 ± 5 | 24 ± 6 | 24 ± 6 | 23 ± 5 | 20 ± 5 | 18 ± 5 | 12 ± 3 |
| Tidal volume | mL | 21 | 45 | 78 | 112 | 170 | 230 | 480 | 575 |
| | mL/kg | 6-8 | 6-8 | 6-8 | 6-8 | 7-8 | 7-8 | 7-8 | 6-7 |
| Minute ventilation | mL/min | 1050 | 1350 | 1780 | 2460 | 4000 | | 6200 | 6400 |
| | mL/kg/min | 350 | 193 | 178 | 164 | 210 | | 124 | 91 |
| Alveolar ventilation | mL/min | 665 | | 1245 | 1760 | 1800 | | 3000 | 3100 |
| | mL/kg/min | 222 | 125 | 117 | 95 | 60 | 44 | | |
| Dead space/tidal volume ratio | | 0.3 | 0.3 | 0.3 | 0.3 | 0.3 | 0.3 | 0.3 | 0.3 |
| Oxygen consumption | mL/kg/min | 6-8 | | | | | | | 3-4 |
| Vital capacity | mL | 120 | | | 870 | 1160 | | 3100 | 4000 |
| | mL/kg | 40 | | | 58 | 61 | | 62 | 57 |
| Functional residual capacity | mL | 80 | | | 490 | 680 | | 1970 | 3000 |
| | mL/kg | 27 | | | 33 | 36 | | 39 | 43 |
| Total lung capacity | mL | 160 | | | 1100 | 1500 | | 4000 | 6000 |
| | mL/kg | 53 | | | 73 | 79 | | 80 | 86 |
| Closing volume as percentage of vital capacity | % | | | | | 20 | | 8 | 4 |
| Number of alveoli | Saccules × $10^6$ | 30 | 112 | 129 | 257 | 280 | | | 300 |
| Specific compliance | $C_L$/FRC:mL/cm $H_2O$/L | 0.04 | 0.038 | | | 0.06 | | | 0.05 |
| Specific conductance of small airways | mL/s/cm $H_2O$/g | 0.02 | | 3.1 | 1.7 | 1.2 | | 8.2 | 13.4 |
| Hematocrit | % | 55 ± 7 | 37 ± 3 | 35 ± 2.5 | 40 ± 3 | 40 ± 2 | 40 ± 2 | 42 ± 2 | 43-48 |
| Arterial pH | pH units | 7.30-7.40 | | 7.35-7.45 | | | | | 7.35-7.45 |
| $Paco_2$ | mm Hg | 30-35 | | 30-40 | | | | | 30-40 |
| $Pao_2$ | mm Hg | 60-90 | | 80-100 | | | | | 80-100 |

Modified and reproduced with permission from O'Rourke PP, Crone RK. The respiratory system. In Gregory GA, ed. *Gregory's Pediatric Anesthesia*. 2nd ed. New York: Churchill Livingstone: 1989:63-91.

former premature infants is an important consideration in the planning of outpatient surgery.

## Cardiovascular System

### Fetal Circulation

The fetal circulation is characterized by (1) increased pulmonary vascular resistance (PVR) with very little pulmonary blood flow, (2) decreased systemic vascular resistance (SVR) with the placenta as the major low resistance vascular bed, and (3) right-to-left blood flow through the ductus arteriosus and foramen ovale (Fig. 34.1). At birth, three events change the circulation into its postnatal configuration. First, alveolar oxygen concentration increases, and alveolar carbon dioxide concentration decreases with the expansion of the lungs. This results in a decrease in PVR. Second, the low resistance placental bed is removed from the circulation when the umbilical cord is clamped. This results in an increase in SVR. The decrease in PVR leads to an increase in pulmonary blood

IV

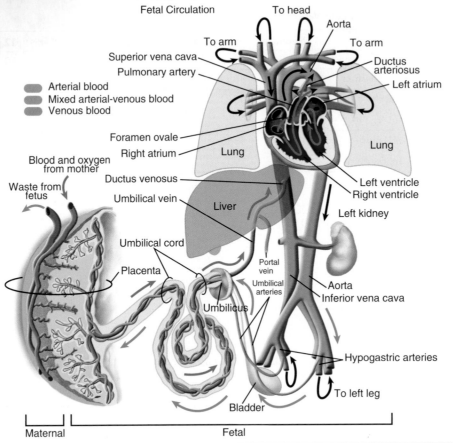

**Fig. 34.1** Course of the fetal circulation in late gestation. Note the selective blood flow patterns across the foramen ovale and the ductus arteriosus. (Greeley WJ, Cripe CC, Nathan AT. Anesthesia for pediatric cardiac surgery. In Miller RD, ed. Miller's Anesthesia Vol 2. 8th ed. Philadelphia: Saunders; 2015:2799-2853.)

flow and therefore an increase in blood return to the left side of the heart. The increase in left atrial pressure functionally closes the foramen ovale.

The three fetal channels that close after birth are the ductus arteriosus, ductus venosus, and foramen ovale. The ductus arteriosus is functionally closed in 98% of neonates at 4 days of life. It constricts because of an increase in arterial oxygen tension and a decrease in prostaglandins released from the placenta. Later, the constricted duct becomes fibrotic becoming the ligamentum arteriosum. The ductus venosus closes with the clamping of the umbilical vein. The portal pressure decreases, and the ductus venosus closes. Via the ductus venosus, an umbilical venous catheter enters the inferior vena cava and becomes a true central venous catheter. The foramen ovale is patent in many infants and is probe patent in 30% of adults.

If pulmonary artery vasoconstriction occurs in the first few days of life as a result of hypoxemia, acidosis, or pulmonary hypertension, blood can shunt right to left through the previously functionally closed foramen ovale or the ductus arteriosus, resulting in profound hypoxemia and acidosis. This is termed *persistent fetal circulation* and can be life threatening. Treatment is directed toward decreasing PVR.

### The Neonatal Myocardium

The neonatal myocardium is characterized by poorly organized myocytes that contain fewer contractile elements than the adult myocardium, in which the myocytes are well organized in a parallel arrangement. The sarcoplasmic reticulum in the neonatal heart is immature with disorganized T-tubules. The neonatal myocardium depends heavily on the concentration of free ionized calcium for contractility. Transfusion of blood products to neonates may cause hypocalcemia and depressed cardiac function, which can be treated with calcium administration (also see Chapter 24).

| | Normal Range | |
|---|---|---|
| **Age Group** | **Heart Rate (beats/min)** | **Systolic Blood Pressure[a] (mm Hg)** |
| Neonate (<30 days) | 120-160 | 60-75 |
| 1-6 months | 110-140 | 65-85 |
| 6-12 months | 100-140 | 70-90 |
| 1-2 years | 90-130 | 75-95 |
| 3-5 years | 80-120 | 80-100 |
| 6-8 years | 75-115 | 85-105 |
| 9-12 years | 70-110 | 90-115 |
| 13-16 years | 60-110 | 95-120 |
| >16 years | 60-100 | 100-125 |

**Table 34.2** Normal Heart Rate and Systolic Blood Pressure as Functions of Age

[a]As measured using oscillometric blood pressure device.

Although the stroke volume of neonates is usually fixed and the cardiac output usually increases by increasing heart rate only, the neonate can increase stroke volume up to a point according to the Frank-Starling relationship if the afterload is kept low.[1]

### Autonomic Innervation of the Heart

The parasympathetic nervous system predominates early in life, while the sympathetic nervous system is still developing. This imbalance is clinically relevant and can be seen as marked bradycardia or even asystole during laryngoscopy, orogastric tube placement, or tracheal suctioning in the neonate or infant. Many anesthesia providers will pretreat with an anticholinergic, atropine or glycopyrrolate, prior to airway instrumentation.

### Newborn Cardiovascular Assessment

The newborn cardiovascular examination should focus on the hemodynamics, including heart rate and arterial blood pressure (in all extremities) and oxygen saturation measurements. Other parts of the examination include capillary refill, peripheral pulses, respiratory status, and the possible presence of a murmur or third or fourth heart sound on auscultation. Urine output trends should be assessed. Analysis of arterial, venous, or capillary blood gases should be performed if acidosis is suspected. If performed, results of a chest radiograph, electrocardiogram, or echocardiogram should be reviewed. Normal cardiovascular variables are displayed in Table 34.2.

## The Renal System

Postnatally, the kidneys replace the placenta in maintaining metabolic homeostasis. The glomerular filtration rate (GFR) is 15% to 30% of adult values at birth and increases to 50% at 5 to 10 days of life. Adult values are reached by 1 year of age. The low GFR affects the neonate's ability to excrete sodium, water loads, and some drugs. Tubular function develops after 34 weeks of gestation. The tubules are immature and have a reduced threshold at which bicarbonate is no longer completely reabsorbed by the kidney. This is associated with the inability of young infants to respond to an acid load and the slightly reduced values of pH (7.37) and plasma bicarbonate (22 mEq/L). Infants also have decreased concentrating ability and a low level of production and excretion of urea. Blood urea nitrogen (BUN) remains normal because less urea is being produced. Creatinine immediately postnatally equals the maternal value and decreases in the first 48 hours to levels of 0.5 mEq/L or less if renal function is normal.

## The Hematologic System

The blood volume in the newborn ranges from 82 to 93 mL/kg for the term newborn to 90 to 105 mL/kg for the preterm newborn. After the first year of life, blood volume declines to approximately 70 to 80 mL/kg. The normal newborn hemoglobin is 14 to 20 g/dL. Fetal hemoglobin (HgF) makes up 70% to 80% of the hemoglobin at birth. HgF has a higher affinity for oxygen than does adult hemoglobin. The higher affinity of HgF for oxygen shifts the oxyhemoglobin dissociation curve to the left. The $P_{50}$ of HgF is 18 to 20 mm Hg, and the $P_{50}$ of adult hemoglobin is 27 mm Hg. The difference in $P_{50}$ between the two types of hemoglobin facilitates the uptake of oxygen by the fetus at the placental interface.

The physiologic nadir in hemoglobin occurs at 9 to 12 weeks of life and is 10 to 11 g/dL in the term infant. The decreased hemoglobin values do not affect oxygen delivery because of a shift in the oxyhemoglobin dissociation curve to the right. The rightward shift is caused by an increase in 2,3-diphosphoglycerate (2,3-DPG) and the replacement of HgF by adult hemoglobin and facilitates the unloading of oxygen in the tissues. The hemoglobin concentration stabilizes at 11.5 to 12 g/dL until 2 years of age, after which it increases gradually to adult values during puberty.

At birth, the vitamin K–dependent coagulation factors (II, VII, IX, X) are present at 20% to 60% of adult levels. This may lead to a prolonged prothrombin time. It can take several weeks for these factors to reach normal values owing to synthesis in an immature liver. Prophylactic intramuscular (IM) vitamin K is given to all newborns. In addition, maternal ingestion of some drugs including anticonvulsants and warfarin can cause vitamin K deficiency in the newborn.

IV

## PHARMACOLOGIC DIFFERENCES

### Pharmacokinetics

Protein binding of drugs is different between infants and adults. Some of this difference is due to a lower concentration of serum protein/albumin in younger children. There is also a lower affinity of protein-bound drugs for serum proteins in neonates compared with adults. With decreased protein binding, the concentration of free drug is increased, resulting in an increase in drug effect. The effect of decreased protein binding is most apparent in highly protein-bound drugs such as phenytoin, bupivacaine, barbiturates, and diazepam (also see Chapter 4).

The difference in body composition also has an effect on pharmacokinetics. Preterm and term neonates have a larger percentage of total body water compared with older children and adults. This is reflected in an increase in the volume of distribution (Vd). A larger initial dose of drug is needed to reach the same therapeutic serum level and pharmacologic effect when the Vd is increased. Larger initial doses are required for digoxin, succinylcholine, and antibiotics in neonates. Fentanyl is an important example of a commonly used anesthetic in neonates that requires larger initial doses. Also, neonates and infants may be more sensitive to the effects of certain drugs and need lower serum blood levels to achieve the same effects. Medications should be given slowly and titrated to predetermined effects.

There is also a decreased percentage of fat and muscle in small infants compared with older children and adults. Drugs that rely on redistribution to these tissues for the termination of clinical effects may last longer in small infants. Thiopental and propofol, for example, depend on redistribution for awakening after a single dose.

### Hepatic Metabolism

Hepatic metabolism of drugs changes lipid-soluble, pharmacologically active drugs into usually inactive, nonlipid-soluble drugs for excretion. The activity of most hepatic enzymes is reduced in neonates, as is blood flow to the liver. This can result in a longer duration of effect of some pharmacologic drugs. Again, fentanyl is an important example. Hepatic metabolism of drugs approximates 50% of adult values at birth in a full-term neonate, rapidly increases during the first month of life to near adult values, and is fully mature by 1 or 2 years of age.

### Renal Excretion

Neonatal kidneys become more efficient with age. Owing to immature glomerular and tubular function, drugs that depend on the kidney for excretion such as aminoglycosides have prolonged elimination half-times in neonates. Glomerular and tubular function is nearly mature at 20 postnatal weeks and is fully mature at 2 years.

### Pharmacology of Inhaled Anesthetics

$F_A/F_I$ is the ratio of concentration of alveolar ($F_A$) to inspired ($F_I$) anesthetic. At the beginning of an inhaled induction of anesthesia, $F_A$ is zero, and $F_I$ is large. As the $F_A/F_I$ increases toward 1, induction of anesthesia occurs. The $F_A/F_I$ ratio increases more rapidly in neonates compared to adults, which means that anesthesia can be induced more rapidly than in adults.[2] There is a larger alveolar ventilation to FRC ratio ($V_A$/FRC) in neonates compared to adults and thus a more rapid increase in $F_A/F_I$. The ratio is 5:1 in neonates and 1.5:1 in adults (also see Chapter 7).

Infants and small children may have an increased cardiac output during an inhaled induction via a mask because of preoperative anxiety. Increased cardiac output is associated with increased pulmonary blood flow and higher uptake of anesthetic from the lungs, which decreases $F_A$ and slows the increase in $F_A/F_I$. Therefore, as a result of uptake, the rate of anesthetic induction would slow down. However, the increased cardiac output also increases anesthetic delivery to the vessel-rich group (VRG), and the partial pressure of anesthetic in the VRG equilibrates with $F_A$. The partial pressure of anesthetic in the venous blood approaches the partial pressure in the alveoli and speeds the increase in $F_A/F_I$.

In neonates, there are also reduced tissue/blood solubility and reduced blood/gas solubility. Blood solubility of the higher solubility inhaled anesthetics (isoflurane) is 18% lower in neonates. Therefore, there is less uptake from the alveoli, and the increase in $F_A/F_I$ is more rapid. The blood solubility of the less soluble inhaled anesthetics, such as sevoflurane and desflurane, does not differ between infants and adults, and $F_A/F_I$ does not increase as rapidly. The reduced tissue solubility of isoflurane also contributes to a more rapid increase in $F_A/F_I$ in neonates compared with adults.

#### Effect of Shunt on an Inhaled Induction of Anesthesia (Also See Chapter 26)

Left-to-right shunts are mostly intracardiac (ventricular or atrial septal defects) and are associated with increased pulmonary blood flow. These have no real effect on the rate at which induction of anesthesia occurs. Right-to-left shunts involve a portion of the systemic venous return that bypasses gas exchange in the lungs and is circulated systemically. Right-to-left shunts can be either intracardiac (tetralogy of Fallot) or intrapulmonary (endobronchial intubation, atelectasis). Right-to-left shunts slow the rise in $F_A/F_I$ and delay induction of anesthesia. This is more pronounced with less soluble anesthetics such as sevoflurane and desflurane.

### Minimum Alveolar Concentration

Minimum alveolar concentration (MAC) varies with age. The MAC of inhaled anesthetic drugs is highest in infants 1 to 6 months old. The MAC is 30% less in full-term neonates for isoflurane and desflurane. Sevoflurane MAC at term is the same as at age 1 month.[2] The presence and degree of prematurity decrease MAC. This may be due to immaturity of the central nervous system or neurohumoral factors. Cerebral palsy and developmental delay also reduce the MAC by 25%.

## FLUIDS AND ELECTROLYTES

### Intraoperative Fluid Administration

Intravenous (IV) fluid given to children in the operating room serves one of four purposes: replacement of a deficit, maintenance fluids, balancing ongoing losses, and treatment of hypovolemia (also see Chapter 23). Although hypotonic solutions such as 0.2% normal saline with added dextrose and potassium are often used outside the operating room for maintenance fluid administration, generally, nonglucose-containing isotonic solutions are given in the operating room in order to avoid hyponatremia and abnormalities of serum potassium concentrations. Lactated Ringer solution and Plasma-Lyte A are the most commonly used isotonic solutions in pediatric patients. Administration of 5% albumin is the most common colloid used in pediatric patients, but disagreement exists as to the efficacy of this therapy versus isotonic crystalloid administration.

#### Replacement of Preoperative Fluid Deficits

The preoperative deficit is the number of hours that a patient has had no oral intake or has been nil per os (NPO) multiplied by the hourly maintenance fluid requirement of the patient (Table 34.3). Generally, 50% of the deficit is replaced in the first hour of anesthesia, and the remaining 50% is replaced during the following 2 hours.[3]

Patients presenting for emergency surgery may have larger fluid deficits from vomiting, fever, third-space fluid loss, or blood loss that needs to be taken into account. The use of warmed fluids should be considered to avoid hypothermia with administration of large amounts of intravascular volume replacement.

#### Maintenance Fluids

The hourly maintenance rate should be calculated using the *"4-2-1 rule"* and should be administered in the form of isotonic solution throughout the case.

#### Ongoing Fluid Losses

Ongoing losses can be characterized as whole blood loss, third-space loss, and evaporation. When blood or colloid is used to replace blood loss, a ratio of 1:1 is used. When crystalloid is used to replace blood loss, a ratio of 3:1 is used. Third-space and evaporative losses vary with the invasiveness of the procedure from noninvasive such as a strabismus repair to very invasive such as an exploratory laparotomy for necrotizing enterocolitis (NEC) (see Table 34.3). Third-space losses can be replaced with isotonic crystalloid.

#### Treatment of Hypovolemia

Intravascular volume can be monitored in pediatric patients by assessing the hemodynamic variables for the age group. Tachycardia and decreased arterial blood pressure suggest hypovolemia. Monitoring of urine output or central venous pressure can provide other information about intravascular

| **Table 34.3** Fluid Replacement in Children | | |
|---|---|---|
| | **Fluid Requirements** | |
| **Basis for Replacement** | **Hourly** | **24 Hours** |
| **Maintenance** | | |
| Weight (kg) | | |
| <10 | 4 mL/kg | 100 mL/kg |
| 11-20 | 40 mL + 2 mL/kg >10 kg | 1000 mL + 50 mL/kg >10 kg |
| >20 | 60 mL + 1 mL/kg >20 kg | 1500 mL + 20 mL/kg >20 kg |
| **Replacement of Ongoing Losses**[a] | | |
| Type of surgery | | |
| Noninvasive (e.g., inguinal hernia repair, clubfoot repair) | 0-2 mL/kg/h | |
| Mildly invasive (e.g., ureteral reimplantation) | 2-4 mL/kg/h | |
| Moderately invasive (e.g., elective bowel reanastomosis) | 4-8 mL/kg/h | |
| Significantly invasive (e.g., bowel resection for necrotizing enterocolitis) | ≥10 mL/kg/h | |

[a]Replacement for ongoing losses with crystalloid must always be integrated with the patient's current cardiorespiratory status, status as evaluated during the surgical procedure, estimated blood loss with plans for blood product replacement, and baseline medical problems.

IV

volume status. If hypovolemia is suspected, a 10 to 20 mL/kg bolus of crystalloid or colloid can be given.

## Glucose Administration

Glucose-containing solutions should not be used routinely in pediatric patients intraoperatively.[3] They should not be used to replace intravascular fluid deficits, third-space losses, or blood loss. In children older than 1 year of age, the stress and catecholamine release associated with surgery usually prevent hypoglycemia. Glucose is commonly given to patients who are younger than 1 year of age or less than 10 kg. Pediatric patients at greater risk for developing hypoglycemia include premature and term neonates and any patient who is critically ill or who has hepatic dysfunction. Patients receiving total parenteral nutrition with high dextrose concentrations preoperatively can either be continued on a reduced rate of the same infusion or can be converted to a 5% or 10% dextrose-containing infusion to maintain the administration of glucose. An infusion pump should be used for high-concentration dextrose solutions to avoid bolus administration. Blood glucose concentration should be monitored closely in patients with risk of glucose instability.

## TRANSFUSION THERAPY

### Maximum Allowable Blood Loss

Before anesthesia, the maximum allowable blood loss (MABL) should be calculated for a given case and to prepare for possible transfusion of red blood cells (also see Chapter 24). The estimated blood volume (EBV) is dependent on the age of the child and hematocrit (Hct):

$$\text{MABL} = \text{EBV} \times (\text{patient Hct} - \text{minimum acceptable Hct})/\text{patient Hct}$$

Initial treatment for blood loss is to maintain intravascular volume by administering crystalloid or colloid solution. When the Hct reaches the threshold, red blood cells should be transfused. The minimum acceptable Hct depends on patient age and comorbid conditions. For example, a higher Hct (e.g., 30% to 45%) is desired in patients with congenital heart disease, those with significant pulmonary disease, and infants with apnea and bradycardia, or tachypnea and tachycardia.

### Transfusion of Blood Products

#### Packed Red Blood Cells

Transfusion of 10 to 15 mL/kg of packed red blood cells (PRBCs) should increase the hemoglobin concentration by 2 to 3 g/dL. The estimated volume of transfusion of PRBCs should be predicted in advance in order to split units of cells in the blood bank into 10 to 15 mL/kg aliquots. This reduces the waste of a residual unit when only 60 mL, for example, is required for transfusion. It also allows the blood bank to reserve the remaining unit for later administration to the same patient, reducing multiple donor exposure for the patient.

Special processing of PRBCs including leukocyte reduction and irradiation is warranted in some settings, including young infants less than 4 months of age and immunosuppressed or transplant patients. Leukocyte reduction is achieved by removing white blood cells by filtration to a maximum concentration of $5 \times 10^6$ leukocytes per PRBC unit. White blood cells are responsible for febrile, nonhemolytic transfusion reactions, human leukocyte antigen (HLA) allosensitization, and transmission of cytomegalovirus.

Irradiation of blood products is necessary to reduce the risk of transfusion-associated graft-versus-host disease, a potentially fatal condition in which transfused lymphocytes engraft and proliferate in the bone marrow of the recipient. Irradiated blood should be given to immunocompromised children and to children with normal immunity who share an HLA haplotype with the donor. For this reason, all directed donor blood from family members is irradiated.

#### Platelets

Platelet concentrates are either derived from whole blood or collected by apheresis. They are suspended in plasma, which contains coagulation factors. Administration of 5 to 10 mL/kg of platelet concentrate should increase the platelet count by 50,000/dL to 100,000/dL. Indications for platelet transfusion are dependent on platelet number, function, and the presence or absence of bleeding. Platelets are a cellular component of blood and may require irradiation using the same criteria noted earlier for PRBCs.

#### Fresh Frozen Plasma

Fresh frozen plasma (FFP) is administered to correct coagulopathy due to insufficient coagulation factors. It contains all coagulation factors and regulatory proteins. Administration of 10 to 15 mL/kg will increase factor levels by 15% to 20%. Prothrombin complex concentrates are derived from human plasma and contain vitamin K-dependent coagulation factors. The use of these agents has been described as a substitute for FFP for emergent reversal of anticoagulation and for the treatment of coagulopathy after cardiopulmonary bypass surgery.[3a,3b,3c]

#### Cryoprecipitate and Fibrinogen Concentrate

Cryoprecipitate and fibrinogen concentrate are sources of fibrinogen for replacement. Cryoprecipitate is primarily used as a source of fibrinogen, factor VIII, and factor XIII. It is ideal for administration to infants because of high levels of these factors in a small volume. Administration of 1 unit (10 to 20 mL) for every 5 kg to a maximum of 4 units is usually adequate for correcting coagulopathy due to insufficient fibrinogen. Fibrinogen concentrate is a plasma-derived source of fibrinogen. It is increasingly being used for fibrinogen replacement in pediatric cardiac surgery and other complex pediatric surgeries, including craniosynostosis and scoliosis repair. Rotational thromboelastometry is often used to guide replacement.[4-6]

## Antifibrinolytics

Antifibrinolytics include aprotinin, a serine protease inhibitor, and tranexamic acid and ε-aminocaproic acid, lysine analogs. These drugs can decrease bleeding and the transfusion requirements during pediatric cardiac, spine, and cranial reconstructive surgery. Aprotinin is not available for use at this time owing to concerns about adverse effects in adults.

## Recombinant Factor VIIa

Recombinant factor VIIa is indicated for the treatment and prevention of bleeding in patients with factor VII deficiency and hemophiliacs with inhibitors to factors VIII and IX. Over the last 10 years, there have been multiple reports of off-label use of the drug in nonhemophiliac pediatric patients in a variety of situations including postcardiopulmonary bypass bleeding and trauma with a reduction in transfusion of blood products and normalization of coagulation studies. Concerns remain about the potential for thromboembolic complications.[7]

## PEDIATRIC AIRWAY

### Airway Assessment

There is no valid airway assessment in children that is similar to the Mallampati classification in adults. Children are often uncooperative with examination. Care should be taken to inspect for micrognathia, midface hypoplasia, limited mouth opening or cervical mobility, and other craniofacial anomalies that can predict difficult laryngoscopy. The patient and parents should be questioned about the presence of loose teeth or orthodontic appliances that may be dislodged or broken during airway manipulation (also see Chapter 16).

### Airway Management Techniques

Airway management techniques in children are similar to those in adult patients, although the anatomy differs. Infants and young children have larger craniums and thus it is unnecessary to place a pillow under the occiput to achieve the "sniffing position" for airway management. The tongue is often relatively large in young infants and can more easily obstruct the airway. The cricoid ring is the narrowest part of the airway of the infant and young child, instead of the laryngeal aperture at the vocal cords as in adults. However, recent magnetic resonance imaging (MRI) and bronchoscopic data indicate that the pediatric airway is cylindrical, and the narrowest part is the glottis, as in adults.[8] The larynx is positioned relatively higher, at C4 in the neonate rather than C6 as in the adult. The epiglottis is omega-shaped and soft in the infant, rather than U-shaped and stiff in the adult. Management of the airway using a face mask is more common in children. An appropriately sized mask should be selected, and care should be taken to optimally position the patient to avoid airway obstruction. If obstruction is encountered, continuous positive airway pressure of 5 to 10 cm $H_2O$ or an oral airway can be introduced to restore airway patency.

Supraglottic airway (SGA) devices are also made in pediatric sizes and can be used for routine cases or as part of a difficult airway algorithm. SGA devices allow the patient to breathe spontaneously with no upper airway obstruction and without instrumentation of the trachea. They can also be used with pressure control mechanical ventilation safely in children. A 2014 meta-analysis found that the use of the laryngeal mask during pediatric anesthesia was associated with a decreased incidence of respiratory complications including desaturation, laryngospasm, cough, and breath-holding compared with tracheal intubation.[9]

Endotracheal tubes are used for a large percentage of anesthetics in children. Historically, uncuffed tubes were the standard of care in children younger than 8 years of age because of concerns about subglottic stenosis and postextubation stridor. However, with the introduction of endotracheal tubes with high-volume–low-pressure cuffs, some studies suggest that there is no increased risk of airway edema with cuffed tubes and that the use of cuffed tubes may decrease the number of laryngoscopies and intubations due to inappropriate tube size. As a result of innovation in material and design, cuffs are now very thin and do not enlarge the outer diameter of the tube, and downsizing the inner diameter tube size to compensate for the bulk of the cuff is no longer recommended.[10] A comparison of classic sizing for uncuffed and cuffed tubes and the new recommendations for cuffed tubes is displayed in Table 34.4.

### Difficult Pediatric Airway

The difficult airway in children can be challenging because of lack of patient cooperation in most age groups, which makes awake endotracheal intubation virtually impossible. Most techniques are performed under deep sedation or general anesthesia. A difficult airway should be anticipated in patients with craniofacial abnormalities or syndromes including Pierre Robin, Treacher Collins, and Goldenhar syndromes. A plan for management of the airway and equipment should be prepared.

Anesthesia can be induced intravenously or via inhalation. Adequacy of ventilation via a mask should be determined. At this point, the airway can be visualized or managed with a variety of airway adjuncts including the optical stylet, videolaryngoscope, flexible fiberoptic bronchoscope, and the SGA, all of which are made in one or more pediatric sizes.[11] The SGA can be used as the primary airway management for the case, or as a backup plan if

**IV**

**Table 34.4** Oral Endotracheal Tube (ETT) Size for Age

| Age Group | Uncuffed ETT Size (ID mm) | Cuffed ETT Size (ID mm) |
|---|---|---|
| Preterm | 2.5-3.0 | NA |
| Term | 3.0-3.5 | 3.0-3.5 |
| 1-6 months | 3.5 | 3.5 |
| 7-12 months | 4.0 | 3.5-4.0 |
| 1-2 years | 4.5 | 4.0-4.5 |
| 3-4 years | 4.5-5.0 | 4.5 |
| 5-6 years | 5.0-5.5 | 4.5-5.0 |
| 7-8 years | NA | 5.0-5.5 |
| 9-10 years | NA | 5.5-6.0 |
| 11-12 years | NA | 6.0-6.5 |
| 13-14 years | NA | 6.5-7.0 |
| 14+ years | NA | 7.0-7.5 |

Depth of insertion:
Multiplying the ID of the ETT by 3 yields the proper depth of insertion to the lips, in cm. *Example:* 4.0 mm ETT × 3 = 12 cm for depth of insertion.

*ID,* Inner diameter.

tracheal intubation is required, either by temporarily securing the airway, or as a conduit through which an endotracheal tube can be placed.[12] Prenatally diagnosed difficult airways (e.g., large cystic hygroma) are occasionally delivered as an ex utero intrapartum therapy (EXIT) procedure during which the fetus is partially delivered via cesarean section and the airway is secured while oxygenation is achieved via placental exchange (see later discussion).

## ANESTHETIC CONSIDERATIONS

### Preoperative Evaluation and Preparation

The preoperative evaluation of a pediatric patient differs from that of an adult for many reasons (also see Chapter 13). Age and weight of the child are extremely important as equipment such as laryngoscopes, endotracheal tubes, masks, and IV fluid setups are based on the age and size of the child. Drugs are commonly dosed based on weight, and accuracy is critical to avoid under- and overdosage. A history of prematurity is important, including the gestational age at which the patient was delivered and any sequelae of prematurity such as cerebral palsy, chronic lung disease and apnea, and bradycardia. If the child has a genetic or dysmorphic syndrome, distinguishing features should be reviewed for potential impact on the anesthetic including craniofacial or cervical spine abnormalities that may lead to a difficult endotracheal intubation.

Previous anesthetic history should be reviewed. A history of sleep-disordered breathing (obstructive sleep apnea), heralded by obstructed breathing or loud snoring during sleep, may be associated with difficult face mask ventilation and higher sensitivity to opioid-induced respiratory depression.

The family should be questioned about risk factors for malignant hyperthermia (MH) including family history of MH, patient history of MH, and congenital myopathies such as central core disease or King-Denborough syndrome. The parents should also be questioned about the presence of muscular dystrophies. Although possibly not associated with true MH, exposure to succinylcholine and inhaled anesthetics can result in hyperkalemia and rhabdomyolysis in patients with muscular dystrophy, and a nontriggering anesthetic (e.g., propofol) should be used.

A review of systems should be performed, and any pertinent positive findings should be explored. The patient and parent should be questioned about the presence or recent history of congestion, cough, fever, vomiting, or diarrhea, which may impact the decision to proceed with an elective procedure. Vital signs, including heart rate, respiratory rate, temperature, and arterial blood pressure, should be measured. Use of a pulse oximeter can be used to screen for occult cardiac or pulmonary disease.

Physical examination should include a general assessment of the patient's growth and development. The airway should be examined as thoroughly as possible with attention to craniofacial abnormalities, presence of micrognathia, and tonsillar size. The heart and lungs should be auscultated to evaluate for murmurs and wheezing or decreased breath sounds. The patient should be examined for any signs of infectious process including rhinorrhea, tonsillar exudate, fever, and cough. Extremities should be examined for potential sites for IV access.

### Preoperative Laboratory Testing

Routine preoperative laboratory testing for healthy children undergoing outpatient surgery is not indicated except in the case of urine pregnancy testing (UPT) (see later discussion). However, preoperative testing may be indicated in children with organ system dysfunction. For example, BUN, creatinine, and potassium levels should be tested preoperatively in patients with renal disease. Hemoglobin should be measured in former premature infants at risk for anemia having procedures associated with significant blood loss. Radiologic examination is not routinely performed. However, if recent radiographs, computed tomography (CT) scans, or MRIs are available, they should be reviewed. If echocardiogram results or subspecialist notes are available, they should also be reviewed.

Preoperative UPT of pediatric patients is a controversial topic. Adolescent females are unlikely to admit that they are sexually active or if there is a chance that they might be pregnant. Parents are reluctant to believe that their child might be pregnant. Asking the parent and child about the possibility of pregnancy can be uncomfortable for all parties. For these reasons, most hospitals have a policy on preoperative UPT and will test all female patients beginning at menarche, or at an arbitrary age (e.g., 10 years old). Occasionally, a UPT will be positive, and there must be a process for verification. There must also be a process for revealing the results to the patient and parents and for counseling, based on local institutional considerations and individual state law.[13]

### Recent Upper Respiratory Tract Infection

The presence or recent history of upper respiratory tract infection (URI) is another controversial topic. Whereas cancellations for URI were quite common in the past, the present view is that the risks associated with anesthetizing a child with URI are manageable with little morbidity. Still, there is a slightly increased risk of airway hyperreactivity with associated bronchospasm, laryngospasm, and postoperative arterial desaturation due to atelectasis. Parents should be questioned about the presence of a URI. The patient should be examined for nasal congestion, cough, wheezing, and fever, and if a decision is made to proceed with the anesthetic, care should be taken to minimize risk of an adverse respiratory event.[14] Signs of lower respiratory tract infection (productive cough, fever, rales, wheezing, rhonchi, diminished or absent breath sounds) require cancellation of elective surgery. Practical considerations usually result in minor surgery being performed in the face of URI, especially ear, nose, and throat (ENT) procedures when URI is frequent and the surgery will often decrease the frequency of these infections. Elective major surgery (i.e., intra-abdominal, intrathoracic, cardiac) is usually postponed for 2 to 6 weeks.

### Preoperative Fasting Guidelines

It is difficult for both the parents and the patient to keep a child NPO for an extended period of time, and fasting can lead to significant perioperative distress for the child and family. However, adherence to fasting guidelines minimizes the risk of aspiration of gastric contents. In the absence of bowel obstruction, gastroesophageal reflux, or other conditions leading to delayed gastric emptying, NPO guidelines in children are as follows: Solid foods are allowed until 6 to 8 hours before anesthesia; milk, fortified breast milk, and infant formula until 6 hours before; unfortified breast milk until 4 hours before; and clear liquids until 2 hours before anesthesia.[15] Forethought in scheduling and giving preoperative instructions about NPO times can minimize the time without oral intake, and children who are scheduled later in the day are often able to ingest clear liquids until 2 hours prior to the beginning of the anesthetic.

### Premedication

Both parental and patient anxiety can lead to significant perioperative stress and dissatisfaction. Attempts should be made to allay anxiety during the preoperative interview. If it appears that the family and child are significantly anxious, premedication may be required to calm and sedate the child. This may, in turn, improve parental anxiety.

The most widely used premedication in North America is midazolam. It can be administered via oral, intranasal, rectal, and IM routes. Midazolam 0.5 to 0.75 mg/kg, provides adequate anxiolysis and sedation approximately 20 minutes after oral administration. Rarely, a child will experience a paradoxic reaction to midazolam characterized by agitation. Diazepam and lorazepam are most often used in older children and also produce sedation and amnesia.

Ketamine, a phencyclidine derivative, can also be used as an oral, nasal, rectal, or IM premedication. It produces sedation, amnesia, and analgesia, but it is also associated with excessive salivation, nystagmus, postoperative nausea and vomiting (PONV), and hallucinations. It does not depress airway reflexes, and airway tone is preserved. IM ketamine may be administered to agitated or developmentally delayed children who refuse to breathe via a mask or accept drugs for premedication.

The $\alpha_2$-agonist clonidine, given orally, provides preoperative sedation that is similar to that produced by benzodiazepines. It acts centrally and peripherally to decrease arterial blood pressure. Anesthetic requirements are decreased so that a lower concentration of volatile anesthetic is required to produce the same effect. Clonidine does not cause airway obstruction and reduces requirements for postoperative pain medication. Clonidine has a longer onset of effect than most other drugs used for premedication and must be given at least 1 hour prior to the anesthetic. This reduces clonidine's utility in most busy, rapid case turnover settings.

Dexmedetomidine, another $\alpha_2$-agonist, is becoming increasingly popular as a premedication. Though its onset is slightly longer than that of midazolam, it produces satisfactory sedation for parental separation and acceptance of breathing via a mask when given intranasally at a dose of 1 to 2 µg/kg. It also reduces the requirement for rescue analgesia and the incidence of postoperative agitation, delirium, and shivering.[16]

Parental presence at induction of anesthesia (PPIA) is another technique used to allay both patient and parental anxiety. The parent accompanies the child to either the operating room or an induction room for the induction of anesthesia. It can be comforting for both the parent and child. However, occasionally PPIA increases parental anxiety and can lead to increased patient anxiety and physiologic changes in the parent, including syncope. The temperament of both the child and the parent should be considered prior to the suggestion of PPIA.[17] A recent

**IV**

Cochrane review of nonpharmacologic interventions for assisting anesthetic induction in children concluded that PPIA is not useful. Other nonpharmacologic techniques, including low-sensory stimulation environment, hand-held video games, and behavioral intervention, are more likely to reduce anxiety and improve patient cooperation during induction of anesthesia.[18]

## Perioperative Considerations

### Thermoregulation and Heat Loss

Because of a larger surface area to weight ratio, small infants tend to lose heat more rapidly than adults when placed in a cold environment, by both radiation and convection. Small infants are unable to shiver and rely on nonshivering thermogenesis by metabolizing brown fat for heat production. Heat loss can also be limited by thermoregulatory vasoconstriction. The warming of the operating room environment and the use of radiant warmers, warmed IV fluids, airway humidification, and forced air warming can help to preserve normothermia in children.

Perioperative hyperthermia may be due to infection, inflammatory states, or overzealous warming. Hyperthermia is a late sign in MH; the first signs are usually tachycardia, hypercarbia, and acidosis.

### Monitoring

Standard American Society of Anesthesiologists monitors include electrocardiography (ECG), blood pressure monitoring, pulse oximetry, and capnography, and they should be utilized in every pediatric anesthetic. A nerve stimulator is recommended for monitoring neuromuscular blockade. The continuous auscultation of breath sounds via esophageal or precordial stethoscope is also recommended, but some surveys demonstrate that this monitor is being utilized less in favor of other monitors.[19] The monitoring of temperature is mandatory to detect MH or, more commonly, hypothermia.

Invasive arterial blood pressure and central venous pressure monitoring are indicated for invasive surgery and with significant cardiopulmonary comorbid conditions. Monitoring cerebral oxygenation via near-infrared spectroscopy can be helpful during cardiac surgery and other cases in which cerebral perfusion may be compromised. Monitoring of processed electroencephalogram is also available for children to estimate anesthetic depth, although there is some controversy over the reliability of this modality in children.[20,13]

### Routes of Induction of Anesthesia

General anesthesia can be induced via inhalation or through the administration of IV or IM drugs in children. An inhaled induction of anesthesia with sevoflurane in oxygen with or without nitrous oxide is a common method used in children because it does not require IV

access. The child is taken to the operating or induction room, monitors are placed, and a face mask is applied. The concentration of inhaled anesthetic should be increased slowly in a cooperative child. As induction progresses, the child will usually pass through stage 2, the excitement phase. During this phase, coughing, vomiting, involuntary movement, and laryngospasm are possible. Attention should be devoted to the adequacy of the mask airway and the extent of obstruction. After the patient has passed through stage 2, an IV catheter can be placed. If laryngospasm occurs prior to placement of the peripheral IV catheter, treatment with continuous positive airway pressure or IM succinylcholine may be required.

IV induction is selected in children who already have IV access, who request an IV induction, or for whom an IV induction is indicated (full stomach, persistent gastroesophageal reflux disease, significant potential for cardiopulmonary compromise). In some medical centers, a peripheral IV catheter is placed in all children presenting for surgery. The most common induction anesthetic in children is propofol 2 to 3 mg/kg. Neuromuscular blockade, usually rocuronium 0.6 to 1.2 mg/kg, or vecuronium 0.08 to 0.1 mg/kg, is often used to facilitate tracheal intubation, particularly in older children. Intubation of the trachea without muscle relaxation, facilitated by a bolus of propofol 1 to 1.5 mg/kg after induction of anesthesia with sevoflurane, is a common approach in infants and young children without significant cardiopulmonary disease.

IM induction of anesthesia is used most commonly in developmentally delayed or severely uncooperative children, and can be achieved with IM administration of ketamine (5 mg/kg). IM atropine or glycopyrrolate can be administered with the ketamine to decrease excess salivation. An IM ketamine induction may also be utilized in burned children with poor peripheral veins and a difficult airway because of extensive scarring for whom an inhaled induction of anesthesia may result in loss of both airway tone and the ability to ventilate the lungs via a mask.

### Maintenance of Anesthesia

Anesthesia is maintained with inhaled anesthetic or IV administration of drugs or a combination of the two. A muscle relaxant can be used to facilitate operative exposure. However, neuromuscular blockade is probably used less frequently in children than in adults (also see Chapter 11).

### Emergence

In pediatric anesthetic practice, the decision to extubate the trachea while deeply anesthetized, or after emergence, must be made on a case-by-case basis. In some circumstances, children are allowed to regain their airway reflexes and are extubated "awake." However, extubation during deep anesthesia and emergence without an endotracheal tube in place is a common practice in pediatric anesthesia. Advantages to waiting to extubate the trachea until the patient is awake include the ability to protect against aspiration of stomach contents or blood/secretions from the airway, and the relative safety of passing through stage 2 with an endotracheal tube in place. Advantages of extubation during deep anesthesia include no coughing or straining against suture lines or incisions and removal of the endotracheal tube before it leads to airway reactivity, both of which lead to a smoother emergence. The child then emerges in the operating room or in the recovery room, and meticulous attention is needed to ensure that laryngospasm or airway obstruction does not go undetected during or after transfer to the postanesthesia care unit (PACU).

### Pain Management (Also See Chapter 40)

Analgesic drugs used for pain control in children include acetaminophen, nonsteroidal antiinflammatory drugs (NSAIDs), and opioids, and they can be administered by an oral, IM, or IV route. The most common opioids used in pediatric anesthesia are fentanyl and morphine. Side effects include sedation, respiratory depression, pruritus, and nausea/vomiting.

IV acetaminophen is now available and is a useful addition to systemic opioids in perioperative pain management. It is critical that perioperative acetaminophen administration is communicated between all providers and parents and documented on the medical record to prevent duplicate dosing and hepatotoxicity.

NSAIDs, including ketorolac, can be associated with platelet dysfunction, gastrointestinal bleeding, and renal dysfunction. Therefore, patient comorbid conditions should be considered such as renal impairment and risk of bleeding (tonsillectomy, cardiac surgery) prior to administration of NSAIDs for pain control. Advantages of acetaminophen and NSAIDs include lack of excessive sedation and respiratory depression, common side effects of opioids.

### Regional Anesthesia (Also See Chapters 17 and 18)

Regional anesthesia for intraoperative and postoperative pain control provides excellent analgesia with minimal side effects and decreases the requirement for opioid and nonopioid pain relievers. The single-shot caudal injection with local anesthetic is most commonly used for surgery at or below the level of the umbilicus. Alternatively, a catheter can be advanced into the caudal epidural space for delivery of an infusion of local anesthetic, which can be continued into the postoperative period. In children younger than 5 years of age, the catheter can usually be advanced to any spinal level and deliver local anesthetic to the associated dermatomes. In addition, the epidural space can be accessed relatively easily from the lumbar or thoracic level with subsequent placement of a catheter.

Other commonly performed regional blocks include brachial plexus, ilioinguinal nerve, femoral nerve, lateral femoral cutaneous nerve, sciatic and popliteal nerve, ankle, and penile blocks. These blocks are performed using landmark technique supplemented by ultrasound guidance; a peripheral nerve stimulator is also occasionally used by many anesthesiologists.

When performing regional blocks in children, the child is commonly receiving a general anesthetic, and therefore unable to communicate the elicitation of a paresthesia or extreme pain on injection, which indicates a possible perineural injection. For this reason, guidance with ultrasound is widely assumed to increase safety of peripheral nerve blocks in children.

Spinal anesthesia has also been used as the sole anesthetic or in combination with a general anesthetic for a variety of cases. The technique gained popularity as an alternative to general anesthesia in former preterm infants having inguinal hernia repair who were high risk for perioperative apnea. Spinal anesthesia has also been used in older infants and children with and without increased risk for a general anesthetic.[21]

## The Postanesthesia Care Unit

### Airway Monitoring

The PACU is a critical phase of the perioperative experience where a number of problems may be encountered (also see Chapter 39). Many patients are transferred deeply anesthetized without an endotracheal tube from the operating room and will emerge from general anesthesia in the PACU. Transport from the operating room to PACU must be carefully monitored to detect hypoventilation or airway obstruction; many institutions require supplemental oxygen administration and even pulse oximetry during transport. As the patient regains airway reflexes, there is an increased risk for airway obstruction. The airway must be monitored closely for signs of obstruction, laryngospasm, and hypoxemia, and a self-inflating or Jackson-Rees style ventilating circuit and mask must be available to provide oxygen, continuous positive airway pressure, and ventilation. In addition, succinylcholine should be available. The airway should also be monitored for stridor/postintubation croup due to swelling. Treatment with dexamethasone, humidified oxygen, or nebulized racemic epinephrine may be warranted. Patients should also be monitored closely for apnea and hypoventilation in the recovery area.

### Postoperative Nausea and Vomiting (Also See Chapter 39)

PONV is ranked by parents as the most unwanted side effect from anesthesia. A recent study identified four risk factors that predict PONV in children: age 3 years and older, strabismus surgery, duration of surgery, and previous history of postoperative vomiting in the patient or in a parent or sibling. If the patient has a high risk of PONV, avoiding opioids and nitrous oxide and the prophylactic

IV

administration of antiemetics will decrease the incidence of PONV. Two-drug pharmacologic prophylaxis with ondansetron and dexamethasone has an expected relative risk reduction for PONV of approximately 80%.[22]

### Emergence Agitation and Delirium

Emergence agitation and delirium is another issue frequently encountered in the PACU that is troublesome to families, recovery room nurses, and anesthesia care providers. It is often encountered after sevoflurane or desflurane. The incidence is the most frequent after sevoflurane. The Pediatric Anesthesia Emergence Delirium (PAED) scale was developed to assist in the diagnosis of emergence delirium. Though many drugs including propofol, fentanyl, clonidine, and dexmedetomidine may decrease the incidence of emergence delirium, only low-dose ketamine and nalbuphine decrease the incidence without prolonging emergence.

### Pain Control (Also See Chapter 40)

The adequacy of pain control must be assessed frequently for pediatric patients of all ages from neonates to adolescents. The patients are recovering from a wide spectrum of procedures with differing amounts of associated pain. The children may be preverbal, nonverbal, or developmentally delayed and unable to communicate their pain level. There are several scales for assessing pain in children, including the FLACC (face, legs, activity, cry, consolability) and Wong-Baker Faces Pain Scale, along with evaluating vital signs. However, pain can be confused with anxiety, emergence delirium, and anger in children. Opioids can be titrated to effectively treat moderate to severe postoperative pain. NSAIDs or acetaminophen can also be administered, and if an epidural catheter is in place, it can be assessed for functionality and redosed.

### Discharge Criteria

PACUs are often structured in two stages. Patients are transferred from the operating room directly to first stage of recovery where the airway is assessed continuously and acute postoperative pain and PONV are treated. After the patient is awake with a stable airway and pain under control, he/she may be moved to a second stage to complete recovery. The modified Aldrete scoring system is the most frequently used scoring system to determine discharge readiness. In the outpatient setting, patients may go directly from the operating room to second stage recovery, known as *fast tracking* (also see Chapter 37).

### Behavioral Recovery

Children can develop maladaptive behavioral changes after surgery including sleep and eating disturbances, separation anxiety, new-onset enuresis, and other behavioral issues. Parental anxiety, parental presence at induction, parental presence in the PACU, and the use of premedication have been shown to influence the incidence of these behavioral changes. Most of these behavioral changes do not persist beyond 3 days postoperatively. However, avoidance of negative behavior changes is associated with higher patient/parent satisfaction and a better overall perioperative experience.[17]

## MEDICAL AND SURGICAL DISEASES AFFECTING THE NEONATE

### Necrotizing Enterocolitis

NEC is a common surgical emergency in the neonate. This condition is primarily seen in premature infants, with over 90% of affected patients born before 36 weeks of gestation. The incidence of NEC among premature and low-birth-weight infants is 3% to 7% and is inversely proportional to gestational age. From 20% to 40% of infants with NEC will require surgery, with a surgical mortality rate of 23% to 36%.[23]

Pathophysiology of NEC involves intestinal mucosal ischemic injury secondary to reduced mesenteric blood flow, often in conjunction with a patent ductus arteriosus (PDA) with its resultant "steal" of blood flow away from the systemic circulation. Bacterial infection is also an important component, and signs of abdominal sepsis are prominent. Ischemia, infection, and inflammation may result in full-thickness necrosis of small intestine, particularly in the ileocolic region, with resultant intestinal perforation.

### Clinical Manifestations

The patient presenting for surgery for NEC is most often a preterm infant, with other complications of prematurity such as respiratory distress syndrome, PDA, a history of birth asphyxia, or other cardiorespiratory instability. Clinical signs include abdominal distention, bloody stools, dilated intestinal loops and pneumatosis intestinalis on abdominal radiograph, temperature instability, and signs of sepsis including thrombocytopenia, hemodynamic instability, and disseminated intravascular coagulopathy (DIC). Intestinal perforation is evident on abdominal radiography and is a surgical emergency; these patients are often critically ill or unstable with hypotension, DIC, metabolic acidosis, and worsening respiratory status.

### Medical and Surgical Treatment

Initial treatment of NEC without intestinal perforation or other signs of extensive bowel necrosis is usually medical, with broad-spectrum antibiotics, gastric decompression, serial abdominal examination and radiographs, and careful monitoring for signs of cardiorespiratory decompensation. Originally, surgery for NEC with perforation was by laparotomy, resection of necrotic intestine, and creation of ostomies. This necessitated later reconstructive surgery and often resulted in resection of extensive lengths of small intestine, resulting in short-gut syndrome. In more recent years, primary peritoneal drainage, whereby a small incision is made and a surgical drain is left in place, has gained popularity for smaller, sicker infants, who may then have definitive surgery later when their medical condition has improved. Some patients may not require further treatment at all, and survival using this more conservative approach is comparable in many series.[23]

## Management of Anesthesia

Surgery for NEC is most often emergent, and preoperative preparation should focus on assessment and correction of intravascular fluid and electrolyte abnormalities, hemodynamic and respiratory instability, providing broad-spectrum antibiotics, and correcting coagulation abnormalities. Surgery for NEC can be performed at the bedside in the neonatal intensive care unit (NICU), necessitating a mobile surgical and anesthesia team and equipment. Most patients are already tracheally intubated. Monitoring often includes a peripheral arterial catheter; umbilical artery catheters are often removed because of concern over further mesenteric ischemia. Central venous access is often desirable, but attempts to secure invasive monitors should not delay emergent surgery.

Anesthesia with synthetic opioids such as fentanyl is the regimen best tolerated in the critically unstable neonate. Doses are titrated, starting at 2 to 5 μg/kg, but additional doses are added to provide 20 to 50 μg/kg fentanyl if tolerated. Volatile anesthetics are often not tolerated owing to vasodilatory effects, and small doses of benzodiazepines such as midazolam 0.05 to 0.1 mg/kg, or ketamine 0.5 mg/kg, may be added. Muscle relaxation with rocuronium, vecuronium, or another nondepolarizing neuromuscular blocking drug, is necessary. Because of large fluid losses from exposed intestine undergoing resection, IV fluid requirements are often very large, at 10 to 20 mL/kg/h, and 5% albumin, PRBCs, FFP, and platelets are often infused in the face of DIC and significant blood loss. Inotropic support in the form of dopamine, 5 to 10 μg/kg/min, or epinephrine, 0.03 to 0.05 μg/kg/min, is often needed and should be instituted early, rather than infusing excessive amounts of IV fluid to maintain blood pressure in unstable patients. Calcium chloride or gluconate bolus is often necessary to maintain normal ionized calcium levels to preserve myocardial contractility and vascular tone, particularly with infusion of significant volumes of citrated blood products. Frequent analysis of arterial blood gases to measure acid-base status and oxygenation, as well as serum electrolytes, glucose, ionized calcium, and lactate, is often desirable to direct therapy. Mechanical ventilation is adjusted to maintain $Pao_2$ 50 to 70 mm Hg and $Spo_2$ 90% to 95% in the premature infant; however, in the extremely ill patient it is preferable to maintain somewhat higher oxygen tensions to allow for a margin of safety. Hemoglobin should be maintained at 10 to 15 g/dL to preserve oxygen-carrying capacity. Temperature management is critical, and these surgeries are often performed on the patient's overhead warming bed. The operating room temperature must be 85° F to 90° F or higher, and forced air warming as well as warmed blood products must be used in an effort to maintain core temperature at 36° C or higher. Postoperatively, mechanical ventilation, inotropic and fluid support, and antibiotics are continued, and a full report of the operation and anesthetic is given to the NICU team.

## Abdominal Wall Defects: Gastroschisis and Omphalocele

Gastroschisis is an abdominal wall defect whereby the intestines protrude, usually to the right of the umbilical cord, without a covering sac, with the umbilical cord not part of the defect (Fig. 34.2).[24] These infants most often do not have associated congenital or chromosomal anomalies. An omphalocele is a midline defect with the intestines covered by a peritoneal sac and the umbilical cord incorporated into the defect (Fig. 34.3). These neonates frequently have other associated anomalies.

### Medical and Surgical Treatment

These diagnoses may be made prenatally, and presurgical management includes covering the exposed bowel with plastic or other synthetic material, attention to fluid replacement, and prevention of volvulus and bowel ischemia. Nasogastric decompression is important to minimize fluid and air accumulation. The size of the defects vary greatly; formerly even large defects were candidates for primary surgical reduction of the viscera and fascial closure, as this was thought to prevent later intestinal complications. However, with excessive increases in intra-abdominal pressure, an abdominal

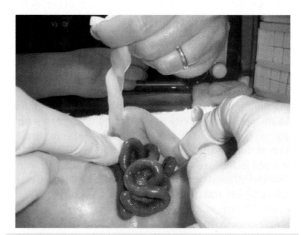

Fig. 34.2 Gastroschisis. Note position to right of umbilical cord, which is not included in the defect. It is also not covered with a peritoneal sac. (From Marven S, Owen A. Contemporary postnatal surgical management strategies for congenital abdominal wall defects. *Semin Pediatr Surg.* 2008;17:224, used with permission.)

IV

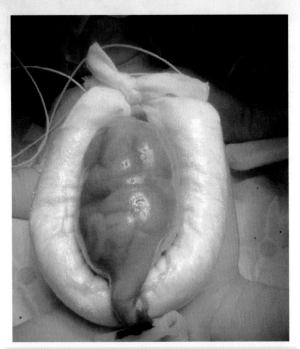

**Fig. 34.3** A giant omphalocele supported with dressing collar. Note the midline position, covering with peritoneal sac, and inclusion of the umbilical cord. (From Marven S, Owen A. Contemporary postnatal surgical management strategies for congenital abdominal wall defects. *Semin Pediatr Surg.* 2008;17:223, used with permission.)

compartment syndrome can arise resulting in intestinal ischemia and renal failure. In addition, the sudden increase in intra-abdominal pressure may lead to increased ventilatory requirements, often necessitating days of sedation, muscle relaxation, and careful monitoring of ventilatory and hemodynamic status. Now a staged approach is often used, which involves containing the viscera in a Silastic silo with its edges sutured to the peritoneum around the defect. Then, using gravity, compression of the bowel, traction, and expansion of the abdominal cavity, the viscera are gradually reduced into the peritoneal cavity over a period of days to weeks. Surgical closure of the peritoneum and skin are undertaken at the end of this period. Some small to moderate-sized defects can be managed with a similar staged reduction strategy, with the peritoneum and skin defects healing by secondary intention.

### Management of Anesthesia

Because of the modern staged approach, the challenges of providing anesthesia for a one-stage reduction and closure are rarely encountered. Still, the initial surgery is often to suture the Silastic silo and partially reduce the viscera. Preoperative preparation includes maintaining adequate fluid replacement to account for losses from the exposed viscera. These infants may be premature but are often full term and have a stable cardiorespiratory status. The general considerations noted earlier for NEC surgery concerning temperature management and fluid replacement apply to surgery for abdominal wall defects. Induction of anesthesia and tracheal intubation can be accomplished with a variety of drugs with precautions to prevent aspiration of gastric contents. The umbilical vessels are not available, so secure large-bore venous access should be obtained, and possibly arterial catheter monitoring for patients with very large defects or unstable cardiorespiratory status. IV fluid replacement of 10 to 20 mL/kg/h is important, along with administration of 5% or 10% dextrose at maintenance rates. Anesthesia can be maintained with volatile anesthetics, benzodiazepines, and opioids, with the dose depending on plans for tracheal extubation at the end of the procedure. If the primary procedure is silo placement without primary reduction, the tracheas of full-term infants can often be extubated at the end of the procedure, and subsequent reductions can be done at the bedside with small-dose sedation. The final fascial and skin closure will require a full general anesthetic. If a full reduction and closure of a major defect is planned, arterial and central venous pressure monitoring are important, along with bladder catheterization and careful management of cardiorespiratory status. This often requires significant increases in positive end-expiratory pressure, additional fluid administration, and inotropic support with dopamine, as well as prolonged postoperative ventilation, sedation, and muscle relaxation.

## Tracheoesophageal Fistula

Tracheoesophageal fistula (TEF) is seen in five different anatomic configurations (Fig. 34.4), with the most common being type C, with esophageal atresia, and a distal TEF. Diagnosis is made when the neonate experiences choking and cyanosis when attempting oral feeds. The chest and abdominal radiograph reveal inability to pass an orogastric tube, which lodges in the blind esophageal pouch, and the presence of gas-filled intestines from the distal TEF. Infants with TEF often have other anomalies, and many have VACTERL association (V, vertebral defects; A, imperforate anus; C, cardiac defects; TE, tracheoesophageal fistula; R, renal anomalies; L, limb anomalies). A thorough evaluation for these additional defects, especially cardiac, should be undertaken in these infants. The severity of illness can be mild (e.g., feeding difficulties in a full-term neonate with no respiratory distress), but some patients are critically ill. Severe respiratory failure can result from continuous aspiration of gastric contents via the distal TEF, exacerbated by respiratory distress syndrome as well as massive abdominal distention from filling of the stomach with gas from the TEF. Patients at more frequent risk of perioperative morbidity and

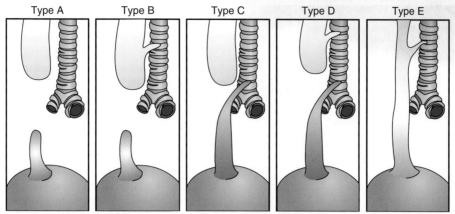

**Fig. 34.4** Classification of tracheoesophageal anomalies in descending order of incidence. Type A (8%) is esophageal atresia without a tracheoesophageal fistula. Type B (1%) is esophageal atresia with a proximal tracheoesophageal fistula. Type C (86%) is esophageal atresia with a distal tracheoesophageal fistula. Type D (1%) is esophageal atresia with both proximal and distal tracheoesophageal fistulas. Type E (4%) is an H-type fistula without esophageal atresia. (From Gross RE. Artesia of the esophagus. *The Surgery of Infancy and Childhood.* Philadelphia: WB Saunders; 1953:75-102.)

mortality include those with complex congenital heart disease, weight less than 2 kg, poor pulmonary compliance, or large pericarinal fistulas, and those scheduled for thoracoscopic repair.[25]

## Surgical Approaches

Earlier approaches were usually staged, often first performing a gastrostomy under local anesthesia to decompress the stomach and allow some recovery of pulmonary function. Then, a right thoracotomy would be performed to ligate the TEF, and possibly to reconstruct the esophageal atresia. Other approaches included a cervical esophagostomy to drain the upper esophageal pouch and prevent aspiration. In recent years, the staged approach has largely been abandoned. In the current era, a one-stage ligation of the TEF with primary esophageal repair, without a gastrostomy, is the preferred strategy in about 80% to 90% of patients.[26] Critically ill premature infants may still require gastrostomy before thoracotomy and TEF ligation, and if the gap between esophageal segments is too long, gastrostomy followed by esophageal dilation and stretching may be required after the initial thoracotomy. Outcomes of neonatal TEF surgery vary; the critically ill premature infant or neonate with multiple anomalies has a higher mortality and morbidity rate; the full-term neonate without other problems has an operative survival rate approaching 100%.

## Anesthetic Management

The critically ill neonate with high ventilation pressures and gastric distention will emergently undergo anesthesia for right thoracotomy and ligation of the TEF. These infants may present in extremis owing to a large TEF with most of the tidal volume being lost through the TEF,

severely compromising pulmonary ventilation. Manual ventilation, inotropic support, sodium bicarbonate, and vasoactive bolus drugs such as epinephrine and atropine may be needed until the TEF is ligated and the stomach decompressed. More commonly the trachea is intubated and there are varying degrees of difficulty with ventilation. After the patient is transported carefully to the operating room, anesthesia is carefully induced with the administration of IV or inhaled anesthetics and muscle relaxants. The patient is then positioned for right thoracotomy. An arterial catheter is essential for monitoring of arterial blood pressure and gas exchange. Very careful attention is paid to adequacy of ventilation during the entire case, as the endotracheal tube may migrate into the TEF and preclude ventilation. End-tidal $CO_2$, careful observation of lung inflation and chest movement, and a precordial stethoscope in the left axillary area are important monitors. Periods of difficult ventilation and hypoxemia during lung retraction and TEF ligation should be expected. Normally, after the TEF is ligated, ventilation improves dramatically.

In the patient whose trachea is not intubated, awake tracheal intubation was classically considered to be the best technique, but in the modern era this is rarely practiced. Instead, either IV or inhaled induction of anesthesia, with muscle relaxation, can be achieved after suctioning the upper esophageal pouch and administration of oxygen. Then, an endotracheal tube is passed into the distal trachea, and gentle positive-pressure ventilation is accomplished with careful assessment of effectiveness of ventilation. Endotracheal tube migration into the TEF should be suspected with ventilation difficulties. Bronchoscopy is performed in some centers to assess the size and position of the TEF before surgery and to properly position the endotracheal tube; only in the presence of a

IV

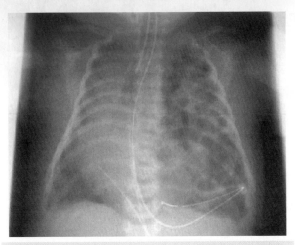

**Fig. 34.5** Left-sided congenital diaphragmatic hernia. Note bowel loops filling the left hemithorax, and nasogastric tube in the stomach, which is also herniated through the defect. The heart is shifted to the right side of the chest. (From de Buys Roessingh AS, Dinh-Xuan A. Congenital diaphragmatic hernia: current status and review of the literature. *Eur J Pediatr.* 2009;168:398, used with permission.)

large TEF (>3 mm) located near the carina is there likely to be difficulty with ventilation.[27] After ligation of the TEF, the esophagus is usually repaired primarily. Some centers are performing TEF repair via the video-assisted thoracoscopy approach, which itself can cause difficulty with ventilation secondary to the $CO_2$ insufflation. Although it is possible to extubate the trachea in the operating room in a vigorous full-term infant without complications, a more prudent approach is to leave the trachea intubated to allow adequate analgesic administration in the NICU. If the patient requires reintubation, the subsequent airway manipulation could disrupt the esophageal repair. A nasogastric tube is placed by the surgeon in the operating room for early gastric decompression and feeding.

## Congenital Diaphragmatic Hernia

Congenital diaphragmatic hernia (CDH) is a defect in the diaphragm evident early in gestation, which results in the herniation of the intestines, spleen, and sometimes stomach or liver, into the thorax. Most commonly, this is on the left side through the foramen of Bochdalek, and results in severe restriction of lung development (Fig. 34.5). This lesion is often diagnosed prenatally, and with significant defects the neonate presents with respiratory failure, requiring mechanical ventilation. These neonates present with a scaphoid abdomen, bowel sounds in the chest, and respiratory distress, and cyanosis of varying degrees. Pulmonary hypertension from lung hypoplasia and immediate postnatal elevation in PVR cause right-to-left shunting through patent foramen ovale and ductus arteriosus, often resulting in severe

cyanosis from persistent fetal circulation. In these cases, surgical treatment, which consists of an abdominal or thoracoabdominal incision to reduce the viscera into the abdominal cavity and repair the diaphragm either primarily or with a synthetic mesh material, must be delayed while therapy is instituted to stabilize the medical condition of the infant. Laparoscopic repair has also been described. High-frequency oscillatory ventilation (HFOV) to improve gas exchange in hypoplastic lungs, inhaled nitric oxide (iNO) to treat the pulmonary hypertension, or extracorporeal membrane oxygenation (ECMO) to stabilize the cardiorespiratory status in the most severely affected neonates may be necessary. Surgical repair is then undertaken several days later, sometimes while on ECMO, which results in reduction of the abdominal viscera but does not solve the problem of lung hypoplasia and pulmonary hypertension, which may require days or weeks of support until they improve sufficiently.[28]

### Management of Anesthesia

These infants are often critically ill. Transport to the operating room is achieved carefully. HFOV may need to be transitioned to conventional ventilation as surgery with HFOV may not be possible. iNO should be continued throughout the operating room course. Anesthesia is provided with large-dose synthetic opioids such as fentanyl, 25 to 50 µg/kg or more, to provide analgesia and blunt the pulmonary hypertensive response to painful stimuli. Volatile anesthetics are often not tolerated, so small doses of benzodiazepines or ketamine can provide amnesia. Monitoring of arterial and central venous pressures via umbilical route is essential, and inotropic support with dopamine or epinephrine is continued. Frequent arterial blood gases are analyzed and changes in ventilation are made to maximize oxygenation, reduce $Paco_2$, and increase pH to lower pulmonary artery pressures. After left thoracoabdominal incision at the costal margin, the abdominal contents are reduced out of the thorax, which may acutely improve ventilation. The diaphragm is reconstructed with a synthetic mesh material. Manual ventilation or ventilation with an ICU ventilator may be necessary throughout the case as standard anesthesia machine ventilators are often not capable of delivering the high inspired gas flows and small tidal volumes necessary to ventilate such patients. The patient is transported back to the NICU where HFOV may need to be reinstated and iNO should be continued.

The most severely ill neonates with CDH receive ECMO support, and surgery may be done while on ECMO, which is problematic because of bleeding secondary to heparinization. Adequate blood products, including PRBCs, platelets, and FFP, must be available if the repair is done on ECMO. Anesthesia is provided with high-dose opioids, benzodiazepines, or ketamine.

## Patent Ductus Arteriosus

The PDA is most often seen in the premature neonate and can result in pulmonary edema, reduced ventilatory compliance, and ventilator dependence worsened by concurrent respiratory distress syndrome or pneumonia (also see Chapter 26). The PDA may prevent weaning from the ventilator and result in secondary complications such as feeding intolerance or NEC. Clinical presentation includes persistent pulmonary edema, bounding pulses and wide pulse pressure from diastolic runoff from the aorta to the pulmonary artery through the PDA, and sometimes hypotension and cardiac failure from the large left-to-right shunt via the PDA, requiring inotropic support. Diagnosis is made with transthoracic echocardiography. Attempts at medical closure with indomethacin may be successful, but this therapy may adversely effect renal and platelet function, and this is important to evaluate if the neonate presenting for surgery has recently failed medical therapy.[29]

### Management of Anesthesia

The patient is often a small premature neonate weighing 500 to 1000 g, is ventilator dependent, and may be hemodynamically unstable. Surgery may be done at the bedside in the NICU in some medical centers. Transport to the operating room must be done carefully with continuous monitoring. Anesthesia is normally provided with synthetic opioids such as fentanyl, 25 to 50 μg/kg, muscle relaxation with a nondepolarizing drug, and small doses of benzodiazepines or ketamine, as volatile anesthetics are usually not tolerated. Arterial monitoring is useful for frequent assessment of hemodynamics and arterial blood gases. A left thoracotomy is done, and the PDA is approached via a retropleural dissection. Careful monitoring of ventilation with visual inspection, capnography, and a precordial or esophageal stethoscope is performed as ventilation is easily compromised. Because of the risk of worsening retinopathy of prematurity (ROP), target $Pao_2$ is normally 50 to 80 mm Hg and $Spo_2$ 90% to 95%, so high inspired $Fio_2$ is avoided unless absolutely necessary. Because the PDA is often larger than the descending thoracic aorta, monitoring with a pulse oximeter and blood pressure cuff on the lower extremity is important to ensure that the surgeon identifies and ligates the correct structure. The PDA can be ligated with sutures or surgical clips. PRBÇs must be immediately available in case there is bleeding from damage to the paper-thin PDA. Maintenance of normothermia and provision of glucose is critically important during PDA ligation in the premature infant. Most infants will remain mechanically ventilated for some period of time after PDA ligation.

In contrast to the premature infant with otherwise normal cardiac anatomy in whom the PDA must be closed, infants with congenital heart disease may be dependent on the PDA to provide pulmonary blood flow in the case of pulmonary atresia or stenosis, or systemic blood flow in the case of hypoplasia of left-sided cardiac structures such as severe coarctation of the aorta or hypoplastic left-sided heart syndrome. Prostaglandin $E_1$ is infused in these cases at 0.025 to 0.05 μg/kg/min and must be maintained until a stable source of pulmonary blood flow is established via surgical or transcatheter intervention.

## Retinopathy of Prematurity

ROP is a vasoproliferative disease affecting premature or low-birth-weight infants. Five stages of ROP exist, and in stages 4 and 5, retinal detachment occurs, which can result in permanent visual loss.[30] The pathophysiology is complex, with the more premature infants at higher risk, but one of the main causes is excessive oxygen tensions in the vessels of the retina, accompanied by wide swings in oxygen tension such as those seen in cardiopulmonary instability with ventilated premature infants with respiratory distress syndrome, PDA, sepsis, apnea/bradycardia, and other problems associated with prematurity. Thus, $Spo_2$ is maintained at 88% to 93% in many premature infants, with resulting oxygen tensions of 50 to 70 mm Hg targeted. Excessive oxygen tensions, as may be seen with general endotracheal anesthesia, are to be avoided, even if short-lived. The challenge for the anesthesia provider caring for such infants is to manage oxygenation with these restrictions in mind.

Premature infants hospitalized in the NICU receive regular retinal examinations, and if high-risk type I or greater ROP is diagnosed, urgent surgical therapy is undertaken within 24 to 72 hours to maximize visual outcomes. This often results in the urgent scheduling of treatment during evening and weekend hours. Retinal ablative therapy with indirect laser photocoagulation of proliferating vessels in one or both eyes is the treatment of choice. Cryotherapy may also be used, and at more severe stages a vitrectomy may be required.

### Management of Anesthesia

Because of the urgent or emergent nature of ROP surgery, the patient may not have feeding withheld. If the patient is still ventilated, any anesthetic technique, usually in conjunction with muscle relaxation, may be used. If the patient is not ventilated, any technique for induction, followed by muscle relaxation and endotracheal intubation, may be used. As these cases may last several hours, especially with extensive disease in both eyes, attention must be paid to patient temperature and provision of glucose during the surgery. Because of the often prolonged nature of the anesthetic, the risk of postanesthetic apnea in the premature infant, and the eye discomfort necessitating analgesia after the procedure, mechanical ventilation should be controlled after ROP surgery for 12 to 24 hours. Regardless of airway management after surgery, the patient must be carefully monitored in the NICU setting for postanesthetic problems.

## Myelomeningocele

Myelomeningocele is a developmental defect of the neural tube, resulting in an open neural placode covered only by a thin membrane and cerebrospinal fluid. The defect is often diagnosed prenatally, varies in size, and may be located in the thoracolumbar, or lumbosacral spine areas. The most common presentation is a lumbosacral myelomeningocele in a full-term infant. Preoperatively, it is critical not to allow the sac covering the spinal defect to rupture, which will result in a frequent risk of meningitis. These infants are nursed prone, with a moist gauze covering the defect. Surgery is scheduled emergently and consists of dissection of nerve roots and covering the defect with fascia and skin. In addition, over 75% of infants have hydrocephalus and many have Arnold-Chiari malformation of the spinal cord and brainstem and will require a ventriculoperitoneal shunt, usually done after the initial repair. Long-term outcome depends on early repair to prevent infection and level of spinal cord dysfunction.[31]

### Management of Anesthesia

Great care must be taken to prevent rupture of the sac covering the myelomeningocele during transport and positioning for induction of anesthesia and surgery. The infant cannot lie directly supine for this reason. Anesthetic induction and endotracheal intubation can be performed with the infant in the left lateral decubitus position. An alternative approach is to carefully place the infant supine in a doughnut-shaped padded foam bolster so that the myelomeningocele defect is in the center but not touching the operating room bed. After confirmation of endotracheal tube position, the infant is positioned prone for surgery. Any technique can be used for induction and maintenance of anesthesia, but the surgeon usually performs the repair under the microscope and requests that no muscle relaxant be used during the repair portion of the surgery so that motor function can be assessed. In addition, as patients with myelomeningocele repair at birth are at highest risk for developing latex allergy, all surgical gloves and all other materials in contact with the patient must be latex free. After surgery the trachea can be extubated, using the same positioning techniques as for intubation. The patient then is turned prone and is kept in this position in which the infant will be nursed for several days.

## Pyloric Stenosis

Pyloric stenosis is hypertrophy of the pyloric muscle leading to a gastric outlet obstruction. A typical presentation is a young infant between 2 and 8 weeks of age with persistent projectile vomiting. This results in weight loss, dehydration, and electrolyte imbalance consisting of a hypochloremic, hypokalemic metabolic alkalosis from loss of hydrogen and chloride ions from stomach contents. These infants may develop severe dehydration, lethargy, poor skin turgor, sunken eyes and fontanel, poor urine output, and plasma chloride concentrations as low as 65 to 70 mEq/dL. Diagnosis is by clinical history; there is a 5:1 male predominance, and average age at presentation is 5 to 6 weeks. An olive-shaped and -sized mass may be palpable in the epigastrium; definitive diagnosis is made by ultrasound. Repair of pyloric stenosis is *not* a surgical emergency; the patient must be rehydrated, starting with a bolus of 10 to 20 mL/kg of normal saline or lactated Ringer solution, and then more than maintenance IV fluids usually consisting of 5% dextrose in half normal saline with potassium chloride. The fluid and electrolyte status is followed carefully and laboratory values rechecked periodically. When the patient has been rehydrated to a normal vascular volume and normal or near-normal electrolytes, the patient is ready for surgery. This preparation may require 12 to 72 hours, depending on the severity at presentation.[32]

### Management of Anesthesia

After adequate rehydration the patient is brought to the operating room, and gastric contents are evacuated with a large-bore orogastric suction catheter before induction of anesthesia. Although awake tracheal intubation was the preferred technique in the past, this is rarely practiced in the modern era. After adequately breathing 100% oxygen, the patient is administered an IV induction of anesthesia with propofol 2 to 2.5 mg/kg, which is preferable to short-acting barbiturates because of its shorter terminal half-life. Cricoid pressure is applied, and paralysis is achieved with succinylcholine 1 to 2 mg/kg (after pretreatment with atropine), or preferably, a nondepolarizing muscle relaxant such as rocuronium. A modified rapid-sequence technique, with rapid small tidal volume via mask ventilation through cricoid pressure, is utilized to prevent arterial desaturation in a young infant whose oxygen consumption is two to three times that of the adult. After successful confirmation of tracheal intubation, maintenance of anesthesia proceeds with a volatile anesthetic. Opioids are best avoided because of the risk of postanesthetic apnea in pyloric stenosis, and instead local anesthetic infiltration of the incision by the surgeon, and rectal acetaminophen are utilized for postoperative analgesia. Surgery proceeds either via small open epigastric incision, or via laparoscopy with $CO_2$ insufflation of the abdomen. After conclusion of the surgery a nasogastric tube may be left in place. The trachea is extubated after reversal of nondepolarizing muscle relaxant and full return of airway reflexes and a regular breathing pattern without pauses or apnea. Because of the metabolic alkalosis seen in many pyloric stenosis patients, cerebrospinal fluid pH may be increased, causing a reduction in respiratory drive, which is not corrected for 12 to 48 hours. This, in conjunction with respiratory drive that may not be fully mature until 44 weeks' postconceptual age, may place even full-term infants undergoing pyloromyotomy at risk for postanesthetic apnea. These patients should be monitored for 12 to 24 hours after anesthesia for this complication.[33]

## SPECIAL ANESTHETIC CONSIDERATIONS

### Anesthesia for the Former Premature Infant

Many former premature infants present for surgery, either during their initial hospitalization, or later as outpatients. The most common procedures include inguinal herniorrhaphy, circumcision, eye examination, and strabismus surgery. Although many infants have recovered well without sequelae, many have chronic conditions such as bronchopulmonary dysplasia (need for supplemental oxygen beyond 30 days of life after a diagnosis of respiratory distress syndrome), apnea and bradycardia, anemia, hydrocephalus from intraventricular hemorrhage, visual disturbances, and developmental delay. The infant's postconceptual age is important; an infant born at 28 weeks' gestation who presents at 12 weeks for surgery is now 40 weeks' postconceptual age and is equivalent in many respects to only a full-term infant, not an infant at 3 months of age. The major risk in this regard is postanesthetic apnea, which in some cases is fatal. The risk of postanesthetic apnea increases with increasing prematurity at birth and younger age at the time of the anesthetic.[34] Although the time at which the risk of apnea is eliminated is not clear, 50 weeks' postconceptual age or less is commonly used as the cutoff point for admitting former premature infants for 24 hours of apnea monitoring after receiving an anesthetic.

### Anesthesia for Remote Locations

Anesthesia and sedation for diagnostic and therapeutic procedures are increasing for children in locations remote from the operating room, and the clinical complexity of the patients requiring care is also increasing (also see Chapter 38). These procedures include MRI and CT scans, interventional radiology procedures, bone marrow aspirations, gastrointestinal endoscopy, auditory brainstem evoked response testing, and cardiac catheterization. Techniques vary widely and include moderate or deep sedation, general anesthesia with IV drugs, volatile anesthetics with mask or laryngeal mask airway, or full general endotracheal intubation anesthesia. Frequently used anesthetics include propofol, ketamine, barbiturates, benzodiazepines, and opioids. The central $\alpha_2$-agonist dexmedetomidine is increasingly being used

for nonpainful diagnostic studies such as MRI.[35] The same standards for preoperative evaluation, monitoring, and recovery must be maintained for anesthesia in remote locations to ensure safety in this environment.[36]

### Ex-Utero Intrapartum Therapy Procedure and Fetal Surgery

The EXIT procedure was first performed in 1989. The purpose is to secure the neonatal airway while the fetus is still being oxygenated via the placenta. The mother is placed under general anesthesia, a hysterotomy is made, and the fetus is partially delivered. This strategy can be used to oxygenate the fetus while the airway is secured by direct laryngoscopy, rigid bronchoscopy, or tracheostomy while on placental bypass. Indications include large neck masses, congenital airway obstruction, and previous tracheal occlusion for CDH. The EXIT procedure has also been used for patients with fetal anomalies in whom neonatal resuscitation may be difficult, including large thoracic masses, CDH, unilateral pulmonary agenesis, and some complex cardiac lesions. Maintenance of placental bypass provides time to establish IV access and an airway, give resuscitative drugs, and cannulate for ECMO when necessary in a controlled manner.[37]

Fetal interventions have been performed as open midgestational (hysterotomy-based) procedures involving exteriorization and replacement of the fetus and as minimally invasive procedures assisted by fetoscopy, ultrasound, and echocardiography. An open approach has been used to treat myelomeningocele, congenital cystic adenomatoid malformation, and sacrococcygeal teratoma with varied success. Minimally invasive approaches have been taken to treat CDH, bladder outlet obstruction, hypoplastic left heart syndrome, and twin-twin transfusion syndrome, among others.

Open midgestational procedures and EXIT procedures are usually performed with maternal general anesthesia, and minimally invasive procedures can be performed with maternal local, sedation, regional, general, or combined regional and general techniques. General anesthesia with inhaled anesthetic provides anesthesia to both the mother and the fetus, and a high concentration volatile anesthetic (2 MAC) can be used to provide uterine relaxation. Anesthetic and resuscitative drugs can then be given directly to the fetus via an IM, IV, intracardiac, or intra-amniotic route. For minimally invasive procedures, it is important to discuss the need for fetal immobility preoperatively. For some fetal cardiac procedures, general anesthesia is required for the mother, and fentanyl, vecuronium, and atropine must be delivered directly to the fetus for safety reasons.

A preoperative plan should be made for intrauterine fetal resuscitation in advance. Maternal interventions

**IV**

including left lateral positioning, oxygen delivery, and blood pressure augmentation with volume or vasopressor administration can facilitate fetal resuscitation. Atropine, epinephrine, calcium gluconate, sodium bicarbonate, and PRBCs can be delivered to the fetus, and cardiac compressions and drainage of pericardial effusions can be carried out.[38,39]

## Anesthetic Neurotoxicity and Neuroprotection in the Developing Brain

Neonatal rodent models of prolonged anesthesia with γ-aminobutyric acid agonists (isoflurane, midazolam, propofol) or N-methyl-D-aspartate antagonists (ketamine) produce accelerated apoptosis, or programmed cell death, of neurons in the developing brain.[40] This data raised concern that commonly used anesthetic drugs could be having similar effects in the developing human brain, generating intense interest and a number of new research avenues to determine if this effect applies to human neonates and infants. Criticism of the animal studies includes the fact that most were conducted in the absence of a surgical stimulus, and that the exposure periods were quite prolonged compared to the corresponding exposure of a human infant during anesthesia and surgery. Other animal models have demonstrated that anesthetics such as ketamine and desflurane are neuroprotective in animal models that include surgery or painful stimuli. Current studies investigating the effects of anesthetic exposure early in life include (1) the GAS study examining neurocognitive performance after either a general or spinal anesthetic during infancy; (2) the PANDA (Pediatric Anesthesia & Neurodevelopment Assessment) study comparing neurocognitive performance in sibling cohorts in which one sibling had an anesthetic exposure before 3 years of age; and (3) the MASK study comparing neurocognitive performance in children exposed to anesthesia before 3 years of age compared to those without an exposure.[41] Currently there is insufficient evidence to change the current approach to anesthesia in the infant (also see Chapter 12).

## QUESTIONS OF THE DAY

1. How does the functional residual capacity (FRC) differ in the infant compared to the adult? How does the oxygen consumption differ? Why do infants develop hypoxemia more rapidly after onset of apnea?

2. What are the major differences between the fetal circulation and the normal postnatal circulatory system? What events can contribute to development of "persistent fetal circulation" in the neonate?

3. How does the minimum alveolar concentration (MAC) vary with patient age? What is the effect of prematurity on MAC?

4. Which pediatric patients are at increased risk of developing hypoglycemia and should receive glucose-containing intravenous fluids intraoperatively?

5. A pediatric patient with a recent upper respiratory infection presents for surgery. What thought process should be followed to determine whether the procedure should be postponed?

6. What types of regional anesthesia are appropriate for infants having surgery below the level of the umbilicus?

7. What is the most common electrolyte abnormality in an infant with pyloric stenosis? What is the appropriate fluid therapy prior to surgery?

8. A former premature infant presents for elective strabismus surgery. What criteria should be used to determine whether the patient should be admitted after surgery for apnea monitoring?

## REFERENCES

1. Andropoulos DB. Physiology and molecular biology of the developing circulation. In: Andropoulos DB, ed. *Anesthesia for Congenital Heart Disease.* 2nd ed. Oxford, UK: Wiley Blackwell; 2010:55–76.
2. Lerman J. Inhalation agents in pediatric anaesthesia—an update. *Curr Opin Anaesthesiol.* 2007;20:221–226.
3. Bailey AG, McNaull PP, Jooste E, et al. Perioperative crystalloid and colloid fluid management in children: where are we and how did we get here? *Anesth Analg.* 2010;110:375–390.
3a. Navaratnam M, Ng A, Williams GD, et al. Perioperative management of pediatric en-bloc combined heart-liver transplants: a case series review. *Pediatr Anesth.* 2016;26:976–986.
3b. Adams CB, Vollman KE, Leventhal EL, Acquiato NM. Emergent pediatric anticoagulation reversal using a 4-factor prothrombin complex concentrate. *Am J Emerg Med.* 2016;34:1182.e1–2.
3c. Jooste EH, Machovec KA, Einhorn LM, et al. 3-Factor prothrombin complex concentrates in infants with refractory bleeding after cardiac surgery. *J Cardiothorac Vasc Anesth.* 2016;30:1627–1631.
4. Haas T, Spielmann N, Dillier C, et al. Higher fibrinogen concentrations for reduction of transfusion requirements during major paediatric surgery: a pro-spective randomized trial. *Br J Anaesth.* 2015;115:234–243.
5. Galas FR, de Almeida JP, Fukushima JT, et al. Hemostatic effects of fibrinogen concentrate compared with cryoprecipitate after cardiac surgery: a randomized pilot trial. *J Thorac Cardiovasc Surg.* 2014;148:1647–1655.
6. Romlin B, Wahlander H, Berggren H, et al. Intraoperative thromboelastometry is associated with reduced transfusion prevalence in pediatric cardiac surgery. *Anesth Analg.* 2011;112:30–36.
7. Alten JA, Benner K, Green K, et al. Pediatric off-label use of recombinant factor VIIa. *Pediatrics.* 2009;123:1066–1072.

8. Dalal PG, Murray D, Messner AH, et al. Pediatric laryngeal dimensions: an age-based analysis. *Anesth Analg.* 2009;108:1475–1479.

9. Luce V, Harkouk H, Brasher C, et al. Supraglottic airway devices vs tracheal intubation in children: a quantitative meta-analysis of respiratory complications. *Paediatr Anaesth.* 2014;24:1088–1098.

10. Salgo B, Schmitz A, Henze G, et al. Evaluation of a new recommendation for improved cuffed tracheal tube size selection in infants and small children. *Acta Anaesthesiol Scand.* 2006;50:557–561.

11. Fiadjoe J, Stricker P. Pediatric difficult airway management: current devices and techniques. *Anesthesiol Clin.* 2009;27:185–195.

12. Jagannathan N, Sequera-Ramos L, Sohn L, et al. Elective use of supraglottic airway devices for primary airway management in children with difficult airways. *Br J Anaesth.* 2014;112:742–748.

13. Wheeler M, Coté CJ. Preoperative pregnancy testing in a tertiary care children's hospital: a medico-legal conundrum. *J Clin Anesth.* 1999;11:56–63.

14. Tait AR, Malviya S. Anesthesia for the child with an upper respiratory tract infection: still a dilemma? *Anesth Analg.* 2005;100:59–65.

15. Practice guidelines for preoperative fasting and the use of pharmacologic agents to reduce the risk of pulmonary aspiration. application to healthy patients undergoing elective procedures: a report by the American Society of Anesthesiologists Task Force on Preoperative Fasting. *Anesthesiology.* 1999;90(3):896–905.

16. Sun Y, Lu Y, Huang Y, et al. Is dexmedetomidine superior to midazolam as a premedication in children? A meta-analysis of randomized controlled trials. *Paediatr Anaesth.* 2014;24:863–874.

17. Sadhasivam S, Cohen LL, Szabova A, et al. Real-time assessment of perioperative behaviors and prediction of perioperative outcomes. *Anesth Analg.* 2009;108:822–826.

18. Mayande A, Cyna AM, Yip P, et al. Non-pharmacological interventions for assisting the induction of anaesthesia in children (review). *Cochrane Database Syst Rev.* 2015;(7):CD006447.

19. Watson A, Visram A. Survey of the use of oesophageal and precordial stethoscopes in current paediatric anaesthetic practice. *Paediatr Anaesth.* 2001;11:437–442.

20. Davidson AJ. Monitoring the anaesthetic depth in children—an update. *Curr Opin Anaesthesiol.* 2007;20:236–243.

21. Tobias JD. Spinal anaesthesia in infants and children. *Paediatr Anaesth.* 2000;10:5–16.

22. Engelman E, Salengros JC, Barvais L. How much does pharmacologic prophylaxis reduce postoperative vomiting in children? Calculation of prophylaxis effectiveness and expected incidence of vomiting under treatment using Bayesian meta-analysis. *Anesthesiology.* 2008;109:1023–1035.

23. Henry MC, Moss RL. Neonatal necrotizing enterocolitis. *Semin Pediatr Surg.* 2008;17:98–109.

24. Marven S, Owen A. Contemporary postnatal surgical management strategies for congenital abdominal wall defects. *Semin Pediatr Surg.* 2008;17:222–235.

25. Broemling N, Campbell F. Anesthetic management of congenital tracheoesophageal fistula. *Paediatr Anaesth.* 2011;21:1092–1099.

26. Orford J, Cass DT, Glasson MJ. Advances in the treatment of oesophageal atresia over three decades: the 1970s and the 1990s. *Pediatr Surg Int.* 2004;20(6):402–407.

27. Andropoulos DB, Rowe RW, Betts JM. Anaesthetic and surgical airway management during tracheo-oesophageal fistula repair. *Paediatr Anaesth.* 1998;8:313–319.

28. de Buys Roessingh AS, Dinh-Xuan A. Congenital diaphragmatic hernia: current status and review of the literature. *Eur J Pediatr.* 2009;168:393–406.

29. Malviya MN, Ohlsson A, Shah SS. Surgical versus medical treatment with cyclooxygenase inhibitors for symptomatic patent ductus arteriosus in preterm infants (review). *Cochrane Database Syst Rev.* 2013;(3):CD003951.

30. Sylvester CL. Retinopathy of prematurity. *Semin Ophthalmol.* 2008:23:318–323.

31. Thompson DN. Postnatal management and outcome for neural tube defects including spina bifida and encephalocoeles. *Prenat Diagn.* 2009;29:412–419.

32. Bissonnette B, Sullivan PJ. Pyloric stenosis. *Can J Anaesth.* 1991;38:668–676.

33. Andropoulos DB, Heard MB, Johnson KL, et al. Postanesthetic apnea in full-term infants after pyloromyotomy. *Anesthesiology.* 1994;80:216–219.

34. Coté CJ, Zaslavsky A, Downes JJ, et al. Postoperative apnea in former preterm infants after inguinal herniorrhaphy: a combined analysis. *Anesthesiology.* 1995;82(4):809–822.

35. Mason KP. Sedation trends in the 21st century: the transition to dexmedetomidine for radiological imaging studies. *Paediatr Anaesth.* 2010;20:265–272.

36. Campbell K, Torres L, Stayer S. Anesthesia and sedation outside the operating room. *Anesthesiology Clin.* 2014;32:25–43.

37. De Buck F, Deprest J, Van de Velde M. Anesthesia for fetal surgery. *Curr Opin Anaesthesiol.* 2008;21:293–297.

38. Lin EE, Tran KM. Anesthesia for fetal surgery. *Semin Pediatr Surg.* 2013;22:50–55.

39. Brusseau R, Mizrahi-Arnaud A. Fetal anesthesia and pain management for intrauterine therapy. *Clin Perinatol.* 2013;40:429–442.

40. Loepke AW, Soriano SG. An assessment of the effects of general anesthetics on developing brain structure and neurocognitive function. *Anesth Analg.* 2008;106:1681–1707.

41. Lin EP, Soriano SG, Loepke AW. Anesthetic neurotoxicity. *Anesthesiology Clin.* 2014;32:133–155.

IV

# 35 ELDERLY PATIENTS

Sheila R. Barnett

The change in demographics of the U.S. and world population has led to a significant shift in the age of the population and the absolute numbers of geriatric patients. Between 2005 and 2030, the percentage of individuals over 65 years of age is expected to increase from 12% to 20% of the U.S. population. This is an increase of almost 30 million: from 37 million to over 70 million individuals. The "oldest old" age group, over 80 years of age, represents the fastest growing segment of the population. At present there are approximately 11 million, and this number is expected to increase to over 20 million in the next 20 years. The increase in population is due to the combined effect of the aging baby boomers and the increase in longevity. The average life expectancy in the United States is now estimated at 78 years old.[1,2] The increase in population of older patients will place a burden on health care systems, and this will be reflected in an increase in the proportion of older patients with multiple comorbid conditions undergoing surgery and invasive procedures. Anesthesia providers must have a clear understanding of fundamental geriatric issues and the challenges inherent in caring for this segment of the population.[3-5]

## WHY GERIATRIC ANESTHESIOLOGY IS IMPORTANT

About one third of geriatric patients undergo at least one surgery with anesthesia prior to death, and this number is likely to increase given the frequent number of new procedures requiring anesthesia. In the United States, over 30% of inpatient surgeries are performed in patients older than 65 years of age, and when considering all procedures and surgeries, this increases to 50%. In addition, anesthetic and surgical morbidity and mortality rates in the elderly are also increased.[6,7]

Despite multiple population studies demonstrating that advanced age predicts adverse outcomes, prediction of how well a very elderly individual patient will tolerate a surgery can be challenging.[3,7] Numerous studies support surgery in the oldest old individuals, and advanced age by itself should not be considered a contraindication for surgery. A reduction in physiologic reserve associated with normal aging can be accelerated by certain disease conditions that may render older patients more vulnerable from complications and increase the risk of severe morbidity and death. Certain conditions are associated with increased risk from anesthesia and surgery and include emergency surgery, a high American Society of Anesthesiologists (ASA) physical status (classification greater than II), low functional capacity, intracavitary surgery, congestive heart failure, and trauma. Overall the presence of significant medical conditions indicated by a high ASA score is more important than chronologic age (Box 35.1) (Fig. 35.1).[5-9] More recently,

---

**Box 35.1** Challenges in Management of the Geriatric Patient

- Population is heterogeneous.
- Wide disparity between physiologic and chronologic age is common.
- Advancing age is associated with a steady decline in organ function.
- Preoperative reserve organ function is unknown.
- Multiple acute and chronic comorbid conditions are typical.
- Common conditions may have atypical clinical presentations.
- Emergency procedures are associated with increased mortality and morbidity rates.
- Patients often have complex medication regimens.
- Potential diminished mental capacity makes history taking difficult.

---

frailty has also been identified as an important predictor of postoperative outcomes. Frailty is a state of reduced physiologic reserve beyond what would be expected with normal aging, associated multisystem impairment, and subsequent diminished homeostatic reserve.[8,9] Diminished cognitive function in older patients can also be an important predictor of postoperative cognitive decline and morbidity.[10,11]

## MORBIDITY AND MORTALITY RATES

Morbidity and mortality rates in older patients range from 3% to 10% following noncardiac surgery. The higher mortality rate follows emergency surgery; the lower mortality rate accordingly reflects nonemergent, less invasive procedures. In a retrospective study using data from the American College of Surgeons National Surgical Quality Improvement Program database, authors found that postoperative fatality, overall morbidity, and postoperative complications all increased with age.[12] In individuals older than 80 years of age who developed cardiovascular, pulmonary, or renal complications, mortality rate was especially high—43% in patients developing renal insufficiency, 36% with a stroke, and 36% following a myocardial infarction. These results are similar to earlier studies by Hamel and associates,[13] who found that for elective noninvasive surgeries such as transurethral resection of the prostate (TURP), hernia repair, knee replacement, and carotid endarterectomy, the mortality rate in older patients was less than 2%. However, in patients over 80

IV

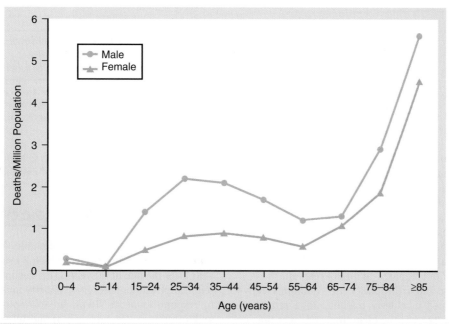

**Fig. 35.1** Mortality rates. (Redrawn from Li G, Warner M, Lang BH, et al. Epidemiology of anesthesia-related mortality in the United States, 1999-2005. *Anesthesiology.* 2009;110:759-765.)

| Table 35.1 | Age-Related Changes in Selected Organ Systems | |
|---|---|---|
| **Organ System** | **Structural Changes** | **Functional Changes** |
| Body composition | Decreased skeletal muscle mass<br>Increased percentage of body fat<br>Decreased total body water | Increased storage size for lipid-soluble drugs<br>Decreased $O_2$ consumption and heat production |
| Central nervous system | Loss of neural tissue<br>Decreased number of serotonin, acetylcholine, and dopamine receptors | Reduction in cerebral blood flow<br>Decline in memory, reasoning, perception<br>Disturbed sleep/wake cycle |
| Cardiovascular system | LV hypertrophy and decreased compliance<br>Increase in vascular rigidity<br>Decreased compliance of venous vessels | Decreased parasympathetic nervous system tone<br>Increased sympathetic neuronal activity<br>Desensitization of β-adrenergic receptors<br>Increase in SVR and SBP<br>Decrease in stroke volume and cardiac output<br>Diastolic LV dysfunction<br>Decreased maximally attainable HR |
| Pulmonary system | Increase in central airway size<br>Decrease in small airway diameter<br>Decrease in elastic tissue, reorientation of elastic fibers, increased amount of collagen<br>Decrease in respiratory muscle strength<br>Increased chest wall stiffness<br>Decrease in chest wall height and increase in AP diameter | Decreased respiratory center sensitivity<br>Decreased effectiveness of coughing and swallowing<br>Increase in lung compliance and decrease in chest wall compliance<br>Decreased functional alveolar surface area<br>Decrease in $D_{LCO}$<br>Decrease in $PI_{max}$ and $PE_{max}$<br>Decrease in ERV and VC<br>Increase in RV and FRC with no change in TLC<br>Increase in RV/TLC and FRC/TLC ratios<br>Increase in closing volume and closing capacity<br>Decrease in FVC, $FEV_1$, $FEV_1$/VC, and FEF at low lung volumes<br>Increased A-a gradient and decrease in $Pao_2$ |
| Renal system | Loss of tissue mass<br>Decreased perfusion | Decreased GFR<br>Reduced ability to dilute and concentrate urine and conserve sodium<br>Decreased drug clearance |
| Hepatic system | Decrease in tissue mass<br>Decrease in blood flow | Possible decrease in affinity for substrate<br>Possible decrease in intrinsic activity<br>Decreased first-pass metabolism of some drugs |

*A-a*, Alveolar-arterial; *AP*, anteroposterior; *$D_{LCO2}$*, single-breath carbon monoxide diffusion capacity; *ERV*, expiratory reserve volume; *FEF*, peak expiratory flow rate—the peak flow rate during expiration; *$FEV_1$*, the amount that can be forcefully exhaled in the first second from a full inspiration; *FRC*, functional residual capacity; *FVC*, forced vital capacity; *GFR*, glomerular filtration rate; *HR*, heart rate; *LV*, left ventricle; *RV*, residual volume; *SBP*, systolic blood pressure; *SVR*, systemic vascular resistance; *TLC*, total lung capacity; *VC*, vital capacity.

years of age who developed one or more complications, the 30-day mortality rate was 26% versus 4% in patients without a complication. Death occurred most frequently following a cardiac arrest (88%), acute renal failure (52%), and myocardial infarction (48%). In an analysis of surgical outcomes for patients 80 years of age and older, for every year above 80 years there is an associated 5% increase in mortality rate; thus, a 90-year-old had a 50% higher risk of death compared to an 80-year-old.[14]

Total knee and hip arthroplasty are common elective surgeries performed in elderly patients. In a retrospective study of 46,322 patients, including 12% over the age of 80 years, overall cardiac complications were relatively uncommon (<1%), but significant risk factors for a cardiac event included age over 80 years, hypertension treated with medication, and a history of cardiac disease.[15]

## AGE-RELATED PHYSIOLOGIC CHANGES

Aging is associated with predictable decline in organ function in all body systems, which is estimated at 1% per year after the age of 40 years. This decline leads to overall reduced physiologic reserve capacity and a limited ability to respond to acute stress, for example, during surgery and anesthesia. The addition of multiple comorbid conditions further reduces reserve capacity, increasing the risks from anesthesia and surgery (Table 35.1).[1,16,17]

2

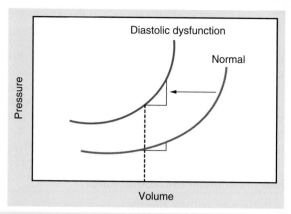

**Fig. 35.2** Depiction of the diastolic function.

## Cardiovascular Changes

Cardiovascular functional capacity is one of the most significant factors influencing perioperative outcome in elderly patients. Aging leads to progressive stiffening and loss of compliance in the vasculature and the myocardium. This results from the collective effects of a gradual loss of elastin, increases in collagen, and damage to collagen through glycosylation and the deposition of free radicals in connective tissue. Systolic arterial blood pressure and pulse wave velocity increase, and the left ventricle faces greater impedance to outflow and subsequent myocardial hypertrophy, further reducing ventricular compliance. Diastolic dysfunction refers to the reduction of left ventricular relaxation during diastole. The impaired relaxation of the ventricle leads to a decrease in early diastolic filling. In the elderly this may be reduced as much as 50% compared to younger patients. These alterations render the older patient very dependent on adequate atrial pressures and active atrial contraction to complete diastolic filling. Preoperatively diastolic dysfunction may be underestimated because patients frequently have vague symptoms, and studies suggest that one third or more of patients with normal preoperative left ventricular function may also have diastolic dysfunction. Older patients with diastolic dysfunction may not tolerate even brief periods of atrial fibrillation and readily develop congestive heart failure in the setting of intravascular volume overload (Fig. 35.2).[18,19]

Aging also alters cardiovascular autonomic function. Vagal or parasympathetic tone is decreased, and at the same time there is an increase in sympathetic nerve activity and plasma levels of noradrenaline. β-Adrenergic receptors are less responsive to stimulation with a lesser increase in heart rate and less arterial and venous relaxation with direct stimulation. α-Adrenergic receptor activity appears largely preserved. The reduction in baroreflex function and overall vascular stiffening leads to more labile arterial blood pressure and predisposes elderly patients to orthostatic hypotension. This condition may be exaggerated during anesthesia, especially in intravascularly volume-depleted patients. The impaired β-adrenergic receptor responsiveness reduces an older patient's ability to respond to an increase in demand through increased heart rate alone, and the elderly patient becomes very reliant on vascular tone and preload.

Myocardial fibrosis and fatty infiltration of pacemaker cells lead to conduction abnormalities such as sick sinus syndrome, atrial fibrillation, and frequent premature atrial contractions. The changes in the conduction system may lead to exaggerated bradycardia following the administration of opioids, such as remifentanil.

Cardiac function in the older patient is frequently compromised further by the development of cardiac disease. Cardiovascular disease occurs in over 75% of the U.S. population over the age of 75 years. The incidence of hypertension increases dramatically in older individuals and is a leading cause of congestive heart failure. Congestive heart failure is one of the most significant risk factors for death following anesthesia and surgery.

## Pulmonary Changes

In the perioperative period, 40% of deaths in patients older than 65 years are due to postoperative pulmonary complications. Postoperative pneumonia can be slow to evolve but is associated with increased 30-day mortality rate as well as increased length of hospital stay. The increased susceptibility reflects both loss of physiologic reserve and a diminished immune capacity. In addition, there is often increased colonization of the upper respiratory tract with gram-negative organisms.[20,21]

As with other organ systems, there are certain predictable changes that occur during aging, including a reduction in respiratory muscle strength, a decrease in chest wall compliance, and a decrease in the elastic recoil.

With aging the chest wall becomes stiffer, and at the same time muscle strength is diminished, leading to an increase in the work of breathing. The aging chest is more barrel-shaped, and the diaphragm can become flattened, negatively impacting chest wall dynamics. The combined impact of these changes can lead to diaphragmatic fatigue and a predisposition to respiratory failure in the postoperative period and difficulty weaning from a ventilator, especially in frail older patients. Pulmonary changes with aging are similar to those that occur with smoking-induced emphysema. They both have increased size of central airways and anatomic-physiologic dead space. The lack of elastic recoil in smaller airways can result in air-trapping with positive-pressure ventilation. Closing capacity is increased, and by the age of 65 years it exceeds functional residual capacity (FRC), leading to closure of small airways and increase in shunt fraction, predisposing older patients to hypoxemia.

In addition to structural changes with the lungs, alveolar gas exchange is also impacted by an age-related increase in ventilation-perfusion mismatch, decreased diffusing capacity, and an increase in dead space. There is a gradual decrease in resting arterial oxygen tension, leaving the older patient vulnerable to the development of significant hypoxemia with even minimal residual weakness or sedation.

Respiratory-related central nervous system changes also occur, leading to a decrease in hypoxemic and hypercapnic ventilatory drive by 50% or more. The elderly patient has an increased susceptibility to narcotic-induced apnea, potentially leading to hypoxemia and hypercapnia.

## Metabolic and Renal Changes

Metabolic and renal changes lead to significant changes in pharmacokinetics of anesthetic and analgesic drugs. Overall there is a decrease in the total body water and an increase in percentage of body fat, accompanied by a reduction of protein and muscle mass. Both plasma volume and intracellular water decline by 20% to 30% by the age of 75 years. Then the initial volume of distribution and plasma concentration of an anesthetic drug increase. This can have important hemodynamic consequences. For example, following the administration of propofol, older patients have an exaggerated and prolonged hypotensive reaction. This is due to the combined effect of a higher initial plasma concentration and probably to an age-related delay in the redistribution of propofol from the central compartment. These and other age-related changes have led to the broad recommendation to reduce the initial drug dose and increase the intervals between boluses in elderly patients. As total body water declines, the percentage of fat increases, which can lead to increases in drug deposition of lipid-soluble drugs and delayed elimination.

Renal changes include a 20% to 25% decrease in renal cortical mass by the age of 80 years that may be exacerbated by comorbid conditions such as hypertension and diabetes mellitus. Other renal changes include a decrease in renal blood flow with the number of functioning glomeruli and remaining glomeruli exhibiting an increase in sclerosis. There is a progressive reduction in glomerular filtration rate (GFR), from an average of 125 mL/min in a young adult to only 60 mL/min by age 80 years. As aging leads to significant reduction in muscle mass, the serum creatinine in the older patient will not accurately reflect the degree of renal insufficiency in the geriatric patient.

Several changes predispose the older patient to fluid and electrolyte abnormalities. These changes include a reduction in tubular function and limited ability to concentrate urine appropriately and a reduction in the renin-angiotensin system and the secretion of antidiuretic hormone (ADH). As a result, older patients are more likely to develop hyponatremia (e.g., in combination with diuretics) and hypernatremia (e.g., with reduced thirst perception). Renal failure accounts for 20% of all perioperative deaths, and acute renal failure in elderly patients in the postoperative period has a significant mortality rate.

Hepatic blood flow decreases and the sizes of the liver and enzyme systems decrease in elderly patients. Both qualitative and quantitative reductions in protein binding occur, potentially leading to an increase in free fraction of protein-bound drugs. Owing to the significant hepatic reserve, the impact on metabolism is less than on other systems, and hepatic aging has less clinical impact compared to age-related changes in renal function (Fig. 35.3).[22]

## Changes in Basal Metabolic Rate

Metabolic rate and the effectiveness of peripheral vasoconstriction decrease in the elderly, making it more difficult for them to maintain body temperature during surgery and anesthesia. Hypothermia can lead to significant negative effects such as slowed metabolism of medications, shivering with subsequent increased oxygen demand, and potential myocardial ischemia, as well as impaired coagulation. Active warming is an important component for most patients, especially for geriatric patients undergoing procedures.[23]

## Central Nervous System Changes

A gradual decrease in brain size occurs in aging, most likely secondary to a decrease in neuronal size. The loss in brain size is associated with an increase in ventricular volume and widening of sulci. The number of neuroreceptors and neurotransmitters decreases even in the absence of dementia or recognized neurodegenerative diseases. The most significant declines are observed in acetylcholine and serotonin receptors in the cortex, dopamine receptors in the neostriata, and dopamine levels in the substantia nigra and neostriata. Normal aging can be accompanied by cognitive changes such as memory difficulty and a decrease in speed of processing; however, the extent of these changes among individuals is widely variable.[24] Alzheimer disease is the most common dementia, accounting for 60% to 80% of cases, followed by vascular dementia, dementia associated with Parkinson disease, dementia with Lewy bodies, and frontotemporal dementia. The incidence of Alzheimer dementia increases significantly in aging patients and is estimated to affect 45% of people over 85 years of age. Mild cognitive impairment (MCI) may represent a precursor of Alzheimer disease. Cognitive impairment (with or without a formal dementia diagnosis) is a major risk factor for postoperative cognitive complications.[11,25]

## PERIOPERATIVE CARE IN THE ELDERLY

The preoperative evaluation (also see Chapter 13) in the older patient is challenging but remains an important aspect of the anesthetic.[16,17,26] In addition to certain

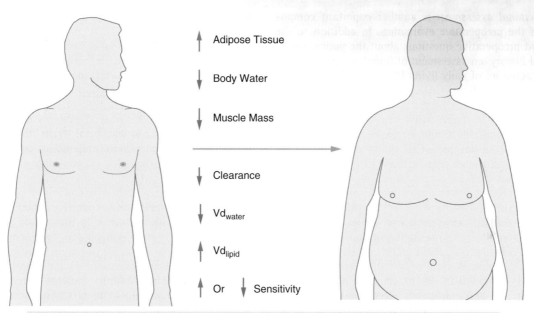

**Fig. 35.3** Changes in body composition in elderly patients. *Vd*, Volume of distribution. (From Rivera R, Antognini JF. Perioperative drug therapy in elderly patients. *Anesthesiology.* 2009;110(5):1176-1181.)

geriatric-specific elements described later, older patients should undergo standard risk stratification for cardiopulmonary risk prior to surgery. The 2014 American College of Cardiology/American Heart Association (ACC/AHA) Guideline on Perioperative Cardiovascular Evaluation and Management of Patients Undergoing Noncardiac Surgery provides an algorithmic approach for further cardiac testing and evaluation.[27] Laboratory testing[16,26,28] in older patients should be performed if clinically indicated, acknowledging that as a result of the increased number of comorbid conditions, older patients will often need more testing for surgeries and procedures in general. For the elderly patient the functional assessment is one of the most important aspects of the preoperative evaluation. Excellent medical fitness, as described by activity level, is associated with a reduction in postoperative complications.[29] In addition, the identification of significant geriatric syndromes, such as frailty and cognitive impairment, can identify "at risk" patients and potentially direct risk-reduction strategies as well as prepare patients and caregivers more realistically about the postoperative course. As stated, routine laboratory testing should not be performed based on advanced age alone. All laboratory testing should be based on the patient's medical history and the invasiveness of the anticipated surgery. Age-based criteria for electrocardiograms (ECGs) and other testing are no longer recommended. Instead, elderly patients with a cardiac history, hypertension, or a history of active cardiac disease may need a preoperative ECG if the surgery is more than a minimal risk and no recent ECG is available. The preoperative ECG may reveal significant abnormalities and confirm the presence of preexisting cardiac disease such as left ventricular hypertrophy and prior myocardial infarction. Comparison with a prior ECG is recommended to establish the timing of a possible cardiac event, yet preoperative abnormalities on ECGs have a low specificity for predicting postoperative complications. Furthermore, an older patient may have a normal ECG and still have significant occult cardiac dysfunction. A routine chest radiograph is not indicated preoperatively in the absence of pulmonary symptoms or abnormalities on physical examination. A chest radiograph may be indicated to assess cardiopulmonary status such as pulmonary congestion or the presence of pneumonia.

The preoperative evaluation of an elderly patient who resides in a skilled nursing facility ("nursing home") or rehabilitation facility can be especially challenging. These patients often have significant comorbid conditions that may make the preoperative interview challenging. In addition, a separate trip to a hospital for a preoperative evaluation may not be feasible. In these patients a history and list of medications may be reviewed prior to the day of surgery and anesthesia. This approach may also be useful for patients who have cataracts and carry an intense burden of disease but are undergoing a very low risk, noninvasive procedure. For all patients with cognitive dysfunction from dementia or neurologic disease, it is important to identify the person who can provide consent for the patient as well as how that person can be reached. Although sometimes uncomfortable, a discussion of advanced health care directives can be initiated during the preoperative assessment of these patients.

IV

*Functional assessment* is another important component of the preoperative evaluation. In addition to the standard preoperative questions about the patient's past medical history, an assessment of function using activity scores, activities of daily living (ADLs), and instrumental activities of daily living (IADLs) is recommended for frail older patients (Box 35.2).[16,26]

*Malnutrition* in elderly patients occurs in 13% of community dwelling elders, and increases to 39% and 50% for elders in the hospital or rehabilitation facility. Poor nutrition is associated with an increased risk of wound complications such as wound infection or anastomotic leak that increase postoperative length of stay. Recommended nutritional assessments include calculating body mass index (BMI), measuring baseline serum albumin and prealbumin levels, and inquiring about unintended weight loss in the prior 12 months. A BMI of less than 18.5 kg/m$^2$, serum albumin of less than 3.0 g/dL, and a weight loss of more than 10% in 6 months indicate severe nutritional risk, and appropriate referral for supplemental nutrition may be indicated, especially for elective surgeries that can be delayed or postponed. In addition, malnutrition is a frequent indicator of overall frailty.[17,26]

*Frailty* is characterized by a decrease in physiologic reserve across multiple systems in excess of normal age-related decline in function. The underlying cause of frailty is not totally understood, but frailty appears to be related to an inflammatory state and autonomic and immune dysregulation. Frailty impacts 7% to 10% of community dwelling elders, increasing with age to 25% in individuals over age 85 years. It appears to be particularly high in patients undergoing surgery—estimated between 25% and 56%.[8,30,31] Frailty is independently associated with increased postoperative mortality rate, morbidity, and delirium, and all contribute to an increased length of stay, readmission, and discharge to an institution as opposed to home.

Several tools and approaches can be employed to identify frailty preoperatively.[8,32,33] The clinical phenotype model, first described in 2001, identifies five observable conditions[9,33]: unintended weight loss (>10 lb in the past year), weakness (assessed by grip strength), self-reported exhaustion, slow walking speed, and low physical activity. Robinson identified additional "traits" to characterize susceptible frail individuals undergoing colorectal surgery.[34] These traits included (1) measures of daily function such as ADL or IADL (see Box 35.2), (2) a Timed Up and Go (TUG) test greater or equal to 15 seconds (Box 35.3),[35] (3) an assessment of cognitive function (e.g., the Mini-Cog test with a score < 3) (Box 35.4), (4) a measure of comorbid condition burden, (5) anemia defined as hematocrit less than 35%, (6) poor nutrition assessed as an albumin level less than 3.4 g/dL, and (7) a history of falls within 6 months. Patients were considered as frail if they had four or more traits, nonfrail if they had none or one trait, and intermediate with two to three traits. Researchers found that frailty was associated with increased complications and length of stay postoperatively.[30,36] In general, higher frailty scores defined using the phenotype model and adaptations are associated with poor outcomes following surgery, and frailty assessment is becoming a more accepted risk assessment tool. This is particularly valuable for older patients in whom the benefits of surgery need to be balanced with realistic expectations about postoperative complications and outcomes (Fig. 35.4).[17]

Although the phenotype frailty score provides an excellent assessment of an individual patient, such assessment is not always practical in the preoperative clinic or surgeon's office.[37] An alternative approach to identify frailty is to calculate a Frailty Index,[9,33] a multidimensional score that measures the number of deficits an individual has accumulated divided by the total number of preidentified deficits. The higher the score, the more frail

---

**Box 35.2** Activities of Daily Living and Instrumental Activities of Daily Living[a]

**Activities of Daily Living**
Bathing
Dressing
Toileting
Transferring
Eating

**Instrumental Activities of Daily Living**
Use of telephone
Use of public transportation
Shopping
Preparation of meals
Housekeeping
Taking medications properly
Managing personal finances

[a]The ability of the patient to perform the listed tasks independently, partially independently, or with complete assistance required is recorded.

---

**Box 35.3** Assessment of Gait and Mobility Limitations With the Timed Up and Go (TUG) Test

Patients should sit in a standard armchair with a line 10 feet in length in front of the chair. They should use standard footwear and walking aids and should not receive any assistance. Have the patient perform the following commands:
1. Rise from the chair (if possible, without using the armrests)
2. Walk to the line on the floor (10 feet)
3. Turn
4. Return to the chair
5. Sit down again

From Centers for Disease Control and Prevention. The Timed Up and Go (TUG) Test. http://www.cdc.gov/steadi/pdf/tug_test-a.pdf/. Accessed June 1, 2016.

the individual is considered to be. The number of deficits identified ranges from 10 (the modified Frailty Index) to 30 or 70 and includes multiple variables: comorbid

---

**Box 35.4** Cognitive Assessment With the Mini-Cog Test: Three-Item Recall and Clock Draw

1. Get the patient's attention, then say:
   "I am going to say three words that I want you to remember now and later. The words are: *banana, sunrise, chair*. Please say them for me now."
   Give the patient three tries to repeat the words. If unable after three tries, go to the next item.
2. Say all the following phrases in the order indicated:
   "Please draw a clock in the space below. Start by drawing a large circle. Put all the numbers in the circle and set the hands to show 11:10 (10 past 11)."
   If the subject has not finished clock drawing in 3 minutes, discontinue and ask for recall items.
3. Say:
   "What were the three words I asked you to remember?"

**Scoring**
Three-item recall (0 to 3 points); Clock draw (0 or 2 points)
- 1 point for each correct word; 0 points for abnormal clock; 2 points for normal clock
- A normal clock has all of the following elements:
  - All numbers 1 to 12, each only once, are present in the correct order and direction (clockwise) inside the circle.
  - Two hands are present, one pointing to 11 and one pointing to 2.
  - Any clock missing any of these elements is scored abnormal. Refusal to draw a clock is scored abnormal.
- Total score of 0, 1, or 2 suggests possible impairment.
- Total score of 3, 4, or 5 suggests no impairment.

From Mini-Cog.com. Copyright S. Borson (soob@uw.edu), used with permission.

---

conditions, laboratory values, assessment of function (e.g., ADLs), and other physical traits such as weakness and cognitive function. These indices may provide better discrimination of outcome compared to the phenotype classification.

The Comprehensive Geriatric Assessment (CGA) is a systematic multidimensional assessment that includes a medical evaluation (usually by a geriatrician), an assessment of the patient's cognitive and functional status, social support, and disability. Most CGAs include a screen for frailty. The CGA generally includes multidisciplinary recommendations for preoperative optimization of comorbid conditions and also postoperative recommendations, for example, to prevent and manage postoperative delirium. The CGA has been shown to provide a valuable predictive assessment of the risk of surgery for older patients.[38,39]

Cognitive assessment is an important aspect of the preoperative assessment in elderly patients. Patients with preexisting preoperative cognitive difficulties carry an increased risk of postoperative morbidity and complications such as delirium and postoperative cognitive dysfunction (POCD).[10,40,41] In addition, older patients with multiple comorbid conditions including cognitive disorders and disability may have limited decision-making ability, impacting their ability to appropriately participate in a discussion regarding recommendations for treatment. A review of decision-making capacity in elders found that 2.8% of healthy older patients lacked decision-making capacity. In comparison, 20% of these patients had MCI and 54% had Alzheimer disease. The American College of Surgeons and the American Geriatrics Society (ACS/AGS) preoperative guidelines recommend a simple cognitive assessment tool such as the

IV

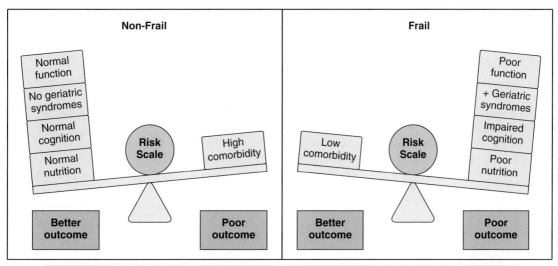

**Fig. 35.4** Frailty score as a predictor of complications after surgery in elderly patients. Simple frailty score predicts postoperative complications across surgical specialties. (From Robinson TN, Wu DS, Pointer L, et al. Simple frailty score predicts postoperative complications across surgical specialties. *Am J Surg.* 2013;206(4):544-550.)

Mini-Cog test (see Box 35.4). This simple test assesses several cognitive domains including memory, language, visual-motor skills, and executive function. Impaired cognitive function in surgical patients between age 60 and 90 years identified using the Mini-Cog test ranges from 17% to 100%, with an average of 44%.[11]

## Medications

The preoperative examination should include a complete history of all medications including over-the-counter drugs. More than 90% of persons older than 65 years of age use at least one drug, 40% take five or more drugs per week, and 12% use 10 or more drugs per week on average.[42]

These numbers increase in very old patients, especially those who are hospitalized. In general, most medications, especially cardiac and antihypertensive medications, should be continued through the morning of surgery, with the exception of angiotensin-converting enzyme (ACE) inhibitors and angiotensin II receptor blockers (ARBs). Continuation of ACE inhibitors has been associated with increased hypotension immediately following induction of anesthesia, which means that these drugs should not be taken for at least 12 hours prior to general anesthesia. Decisions regarding platelet antagonists and anticoagulants should be made with the patient's primary care doctor and the surgeon (Table 35.2).

## Intraoperative Monitoring

Standard ASA monitoring is required during the administration of any anesthetic. In the older patient additional hemodynamic monitoring is often required for invasive and prolonged surgeries and in patients with significant comorbid conditions (see Chapter 20).

## Choice of Anesthesia

As with all anesthetics, the choice of general versus regional anesthesia or sedation will depend on the surgical requirements, the patient's physical status, and the patient's preferences. In elderly patients, there is no evidence that one type of anesthesia is safer than another, although regional anesthesia may confer certain benefits such as improved postoperative pain control, decreased blood intraoperative loss during hip surgery, and decreased postoperative venous thrombosis.[43]

## General Anesthesia

Elderly patients are more likely to be edentulous compared with young patients. Thus, laryngoscopy may be easier, but difficulty during ventilation via a mask may necessitate the use of an oral or nasopharyngeal airway to maintain a patent airway (also see Chapter 16). Reduced extension of the neck secondary to advanced arthritis may limit head and neck manipulation during laryngoscopy, and vertebrobasilar disease may predispose older patients to cerebral ischemia with neck manipulation. Older patients present in more advanced stages of disease (for example, with end-stage rheumatoid arthritis), which may increase the frequency of a difficult airway. Elderly patients frequently exhibit exaggerated hemodynamic responses to laryngoscopy, which is an obvious concern in patients with underlying cardiac conditions. A small dose of lidocaine (e.g., 50 mg) intravenously or short-acting β-adrenergic blockade with induction of anesthesia can attenuate this response. An age-related decrease in pharyngeal reflexes predisposes older patients to pulmonary aspiration of gastric contents. Prolonged periods of intraoperative hypotension may lead to an increase in postoperative morbidity in older patients. Hypotension should be avoided in older patients, and arterial blood pressure probably should arbitrarily be maintained within 10% of starting levels.

| Table 35.2 | Drugs Often Taken by Elderly Patients That May Contribute to Adverse Effects or Drug Interactions |
|---|---|
| **Drug/Drug Class** | **Response** |
| Diuretics | Hypokalemia |
| | Hypovolemia |
| Centrally acting antihypertensives | Decreased autonomic nervous system activity |
| β-Adrenergic antagonists | Decreased autonomic nervous system activity |
| | Decreased anesthetic requirements |
| | Bronchospasm |
| | Bradycardia |
| Cardiac antidysrhythmics | Potentiation of neuromuscular blocking drugs |
| Digitalis | Cardiac dysrhythmias |
| | Cardiac conduction disturbances |
| Tricyclic antidepressants | Anticholinergic effects |
| Antibiotics | Potentiation of neuromuscular blocking drugs |
| Oral hypoglycemics | Hypoglycemia |
| Alcohol | Increased anesthetic requirements Delirium tremens |

## Anesthetic Drugs

Pharmacokinetic and pharmacodynamic changes with aging necessitate dosing adjustments for most anesthetic drugs.[22] In general, "start low, go slow" remains a valid axiom when taking care of elderly patients (Table 35.3).

### Intravenous Anesthetics (Also See Chapter 8)

Propofol is commonly used to induce general anesthesia. The mechanism of action appears to be mediated through the central γ-aminobutyric acid A (GABA$_A$) receptors. Propofol produces a rapid loss of consciousness, apnea in sufficient doses, and a dose-dependent reduction in vascular resistance and preload. The hemodynamic effects of propofol can be greatly exaggerated in older patients, especially if their intravascular volumes are depleted, possibly leading to significant cardiac or cerebral ischemia. The initial dose of propofol should be reduced and the time interval between repeated doses increased to prevent an exaggerated and potentially prolonged hypotension. Propofol does allow for rapid recovery with minimal delayed cognitive effects. Given in smaller total doses than in younger adults, propofol infusions probably provide a more stable hemodynamic course, but the dose required for sedation should be reduced.

Etomidate, a carboxylated imidazole ring, has the disadvantage of producing some disinhibitory effects leading to development of myoclonus, which has been observed in 30% to 60% of patients. Yet its minimal cardiovascular effects make it preferred in patients in whom a decrease in arterial blood pressure may not be tolerated. It is an excellent anesthetic for an emergency situation. The volume of distribution for etomidate is reduced with aging, and a 50% reduction in dose is recommended in patients 80 years of age or older.

The anxiolytic and sedative properties of midazolam make it an excellent premedication for anesthesia, and its short duration and absence of significant active metabolites or cardiovascular effects increase the utility in the elderly population. Although pharmacokinetic changes can prolong elimination, especially in obese elderly patients, the increase in sensitivity observed in geriatric patients appears to be due mainly to a pharmacodynamic change within the benzodiazepine GABA receptor unit.[43a] In general the dose of midazolam should be reduced by 50% and repeat doses administered in increments of 0.5 mg or less. Older patients are susceptible to midazolam-induced apnea, and when administered during spinal anesthesia there may be an increased risk of respiratory depression. Unwanted effects of midazolam can be reversed with flumazenil. Long-acting benzodiazepines have been associated with delirium in the elderly owing to prolonged clearance and active metabolites. For these reasons, diazepam and lorazepam are not recommended in elderly patients.

### Inhaled Anesthetics (Also See Chapter 7)

The minimum alveolar concentration (MAC) of inhaled anesthetics decreases predictably by 6% every decade after age 20 years. Thus, the MAC at age 90 years is reduced by 30% compared to the MAC for a 40-year-old. This change most likely reflects a combination of age-related cerebral atrophy and alterations in neurotransmitter balance.

### Muscle Relaxants (Also See Chapter 11)

Aging does not increase sensitivity to muscle relaxants at the neuromuscular junction. Of course, age-related diseases (e.g., kidney dysfunction) may increase sensitivity but more likely prolong the action of muscle relaxants. Furthermore, decreases in hepatic metabolism and renal clearance may lead to delayed elimination of nondepolarizing neuromuscular blocking drugs. This is most prominent for pancuronium, which is 85% eliminated through renal clearance, and the drug probably should be avoided in elderly patients. Vecuronium and rocuronium are less dependent on renal excretion, and their effects are less likely to be significantly prolonged. Cisatracurium and atracurium are dependent on Hoffman elimination that is not impacted by aging or renal or hepatic function. To ensure complete recovery from neuromuscular blockade, monitoring of neuromuscular blockade should be done to assure that successive doses are appropriate and complete

| Table 35.3 | Adjustments to Anesthetic and Adjuvant Drug Administration in Elderly Patients |
|---|---|
| **Drug/Drug Class** | **Adjustment** |
| Volatile anesthetics | Decrease inspired concentration |
| Intravenous induction drugs (thiopental, propofol) | Small to moderate decreases in initial dose<br>Decreased maintenance infusion |
| Opioids | Decrease initial dose[a]<br>Increased incidence of skeletal muscle rigidity<br>Increased duration of systemic and neuraxial effects<br>Increased incidence of depression of ventilation |
| Local anesthetics (spinal and epidural) | Small to moderate decrease in segmental dose requirements<br>Anticipate prolonged effects |
| Benzodiazepines | Modest decrease in initial dose<br>Anticipate marked increase in duration of action |
| Atropine | Increased dose needed for comparable heart rate response<br>Anticipate possible central anticholinergic syndrome |
| Isoproterenol | Increased dose needed for comparable heart rate response |

[a]Supportive data not available.

reversal from neostigmine or sugammadex has occurred prior to extubation of the trachea. Actually, monitoring of neuromuscular blockade is becoming a requirement in most or all patients, but especially with the elderly. In the older patient, even a small degree of weakness can result in a clinically significant respiratory incident during transport to and while in the postanesthesia care unit (PACU).

### Opioids (Also See Chapter 9)

Pharmacodynamic changes in elderly patients account for the increase in the sensitivity of the brain to opioids, and pharmacokinetic changes impacting elimination and distribution of opioids are less significant. Opioid doses should be reduced by 50% in older patients. Interindividual variability of opioid response is common among older patients, and it is important to titrate these drugs to desired effect. Fentanyl is a popular short-acting lipid-soluble opioid with a large volume of distribution. The dose should be reduced by 50%, largely as a result of pharmacodynamic changes. Remifentanil is an ultrashort-acting mu-receptor agonist that is metabolized by plasma esterases. The bolus dose and the infusion rates should be reduced in the elderly and titrated to effect. Morphine is one of the most popular postoperative analgesics administered. In elderly patients there is a reduction in the volume of distribution and a potential accumulation of active metabolites morphine 3-glucuronide and morphine 6-glucuronide that are eliminated via the kidneys.[9,37,38]

Meperidine has been a popular opioid for sedation and analgesia with nonanesthesia providers. In older patients, administration of meperidine causes delirium, possibly through anticholinergic mechanism and accumulation of active metabolite normeperidine. It is not recommended for elderly patients for sedation or analgesia.

## Monitored Anesthesia Care

Assistance from anesthesiology is more frequently requested for nonsurgical procedures such as endoscopic retrograde cholangiopancreatography (ERCP), advanced gastrointestinal procedures, bronchoscopy, and radiologic interventions (also see Chapters 14, 37, and 38). Elderly patients with complex medical conditions are frequent candidates for these noninvasive procedures, and administration of anesthesia can be especially challenging. In general, geriatric principles should be applied, and reduction of the dose, infusion, and an increase in bolus interval are recommended. Because of an age-related increase in sensitivity to narcotics and benzodiazepines, as well as pulmonary changes, older patients are particularly susceptible to developing hypoventilation and apnea during procedures. Supplemental oxygen and monitoring of ventilation through end-tidal $CO_2$ is recommended. Standard intravenously administered anesthetics that can be used for MAC include midazolam and the short-acting

opioids (e.g., fentanyl and remifentanil). In addition, small doses of ketamine, 10 mg to 30 mg intravenously, can be a valuable adjunct for procedures, especially if associated with painful stimuli. At these small doses the positive hemodynamic effects of ketamine are less pronounced and can be treated with small doses of labetalol. Dexmedetomidine has no adverse respiratory effects and can provide both analgesia and sedation. Side effects that may preclude its use are prolonged sedation, bradycardia, and hypotension.

## Neuraxial Anesthesia

Spinal and epidural anesthesia compared to general anesthesia do not alter the 30-day mortality rate in elderly patients (also see Chapter 17). However, these techniques may be particularly useful for a wide range of orthopedic procedures such as hip fracture repair, lower extremity joint replacement, TURP, and gynecologic and lower extremity vascular procedures.[43-45] Age-related changes including calcification of the interspinous ligaments and ligamentum flavum and narrowing of the intervertebral foramina, combined with a reduction in flexibility and difficulty positioning, may make the placement of the needle for a spinal or epidural block more challenging. Age-related changes can also lead to exaggerated spread of the local anesthetic within the epidural space and a higher than expected anesthetic level. Similarly for spinal anesthesia, the cephalad spread may be wider than expected and the dose of local anesthetic should be reduced in older patients. Hypotension is the most significant hemodynamic consequence of neuraxial anesthesia. Hypotension occurs when the sympathetic blockade leads to significant vasodilatation, causing a decrease in systemic vascular resistance and central venous pressure and a redistribution of blood volume to the extremities from central splanchnic and mesenteric vascular beds. Hypotension is of particular concern in very elderly patients with limited cardiac reserve and may be exaggerated in patients with baseline hypertension. Pretreatment with crystalloid does not consistently offset the hypotension following a spinal block. Treatment of hypotension with vasopressors, such as ephedrine and phenylephrine, is frequently required.

## POSTOPERATIVE CARE

### Pain

The treatment of intraoperative and postoperative pain in the elderly patient is an important part of the anesthetic plan.[46,47] Age-related reduction in nerve conductivity and receptors may lead older patients to experience less pain following surgery, but untreated pain can have significant adverse consequences. Postoperative pain is associated with increased length of stay, increased morbidity, pulmonary complications, and delirium. The longer a patient stays in the hospital, the greater the risk of complications. Generational and cultural issues may lead older patients to complain less about pain, and elderly patients frequently have lower expectations for successful treatment. For cognitively intact elders patient-controlled analgesia (PCA) is the preferred method for administering postoperative intravenous (IV) narcotics. Treatment of pain in patients with significant dementia or delirium is challenging both to assess and treat. If possible, pain should be assessed using a specially designed nonverbal pain scale such as the Pain Assessment IN Advanced Dementia (PAINAD), which is an observational scale of five items: breathing, vocalization, facial expression, body language, and consolability. For nonverbal elders and those with a diagnosis of dementia, pain medication should be offered on a regularly scheduled interval as opposed to an as-needed basis (also see Chapter 39).

Opioid use can be reduced by concomitant administration of acetaminophen. Nonsteroidal antiinflammatory drugs (NSAIDs) in older patients cause renal failure and gastrointestinal hemorrhage, and medications such as ibuprofen and ketorolac should be administered cautiously. When administered, the IV dose of ketorolac should be reduced to 15 mg IV every 6 hours, with a 60 mg 24-hour dose maximum.

Gabapentin, originally released for its antiepileptic properties, is another useful opioid adjunct for postoperative pain control. Although most commonly used to treat chronic neuropathic pain, it has been used preemptively before surgery as well as following surgery. It is an oral medication excreted via the kidneys, and in elderly patients a reduction in dose is recommended; larger doses are associated with sedation.

The role of nerve blocks for postoperative pain control in elderly patients is increasingly important (see Chapter 40). Adequate, but safe, postoperative analgesia is very important in the elderly. The total dose of local anesthetic should be reduced as the metabolism and clearance of local anesthetics are delayed in advanced age. Postoperative epidural analgesia with local anesthetics or opioids probably improves postoperative pulmonary outcomes including (1) improved postoperative pain control, (2) decline in atelectasis, (3) improved tracheal extubation variables, and (4) shorter intensive care unit stays.[43,44]

## Postoperative Neurologic Events

The most common postoperative neurologic events in the elderly are postoperative delirium and POCD.[40,48,49] Delirium refers to an acute state of confusion that generally occurs within 1 to 3 days following surgery. It can persist for weeks or months after surgery. Delirium is not unique to surgery patients; it also commonly develops in hospitalized elderly patients, especially those admitted to the intensive care unit. Delirium is a significant source of morbidity and occurs in 15% to 60% of elderly patients who have a hip fracture.[40,50]

POCD can increase length of hospital stay and require discharge to rehabilitation facilities as opposed to home and is associated with an increased mortality rate. There are multiple causes of delirium in the postoperative patient. The more common ones include acute metabolic derangements such as hypo- or hypernatremia, hypoxemia, anemia, uremia, sepsis, uncontrolled pain, disorientation, depression, residual effects of anticholinergic medications, and alcohol withdrawal. Treatment of delirium should start with a search for an underlying reversible condition such as hypoxemia or pain; unfortunately, often there is no single factor that is easily reversed. Agitated patients may benefit from intravenously administered small doses of haloperidol.[51]

POCD is a distinct cognitive disorder found in patients after anesthesia.[10,49,52] It is diagnosed through neuropsychological testing and results in subtle changes in mental ability. Unlike patients with delirium, POCD patients are not acutely confused or agitated. In some studies 10% of older patients developed POCD 3 months after major noncardiac surgery. In most cases it resolved by 6 to 12 months, although its occurrence has been associated with an increased mortality rate. The role of anesthetics in the development of POCD is a current focus of significant research.

Perioperative stroke is an uncommon event following general surgery; it occurs more frequently after head and neck, vascular, and cardiac surgery. Risk factors for a postoperative stroke include advanced age and predisposing comorbid conditions such as hypertension and reduced ejection fraction of less than 40%. The most frequent incidence of stroke occurs after cardiac and aortic surgery. Most perioperative strokes are embolic and ischemic. A perioperative stroke is associated with prolonged hospitalization, increased disability, and death following surgery.[50]

## REDUCTION OF PERIOPERATIVE RISK

Elderly patients have high mortality and morbidity rates after surgery, especially after major and emergent surgery. Reduction of risk should be aimed at avoiding complications and limiting risk. The patient should be in optimal condition preoperatively. Unfortunately it is not always possible to delay surgery, especially in emergent situations. Administration of perioperative β-adrenergic blockers may reduce postoperative cardiac events through a reduction in sympathetic tone, improved myocardial oxygen supply/demand, and reduction in ventricular arrhythmias as well as decreasing shear stress surrounding

---

**Box 35.5** Guidelines for Treating Geriatric Patients

1. Advanced chronologic age is not a contraindication to surgery.
2. Clinical presentation of disease may have been atypical, leading to delays and errors in diagnosis.
3. Assume interindividual variability and titrate medications to physiologic effect when possible.
4. Expect complexity: Multiple medications and illnesses are common, and persons older than 65 years of age have on average 3.5 medical diseases.
5. Diminished organ reserve can be unpredictable and difficult to measure preoperatively; limitations may become apparent only during stress.
6. A disproportionate increase in perioperative risk may occur without adequate preoperative optimization—for example, after emergent procedures.
7. Meticulous attention to detail can help avoid minor complications, which in elderly patients can rapidly escalate into major adverse events.
8. Impact of extrinsic factors, such as smoking or those related to the environment or socioeconomic status, is difficult to quantify.

---

atherosclerotic plaque. If a patient is already receiving chronic β-adrenergic blockade, it should be continued for the entire perioperative period; abrupt discontinuation can increase the incidence of adverse events. Patients with American Heart Association class I or IIa indications should receive β-adrenergic blockers (also see Chapter 13, Table 13.10). More data are still needed to establish the most effective use of perioperative β-adrenergic blockade for elderly patients.[27,53]

As mentioned previously, appropriate pain control is also important, and epidural analgesia may have a significant role in preventing pulmonary complications. Other measures that may be used to limit pulmonary complications include using positive end-expiratory pressure (5 to 10 cm $H_2O$) to maintain FRC above closing capacity. Maintaining a higher inspired oxygen concentration (60%-90%) during surgery has been evaluated for potential benefit in reducing surgical site infections and postoperative nausea and vomiting, but meta-analyses have not clearly demonstrated efficacy.[55,56]

## MEDICATIONS TO AVOID IN THE GERIATRIC POPULATION

An important aspect of risk reduction in geriatric patients is the avoidance of iatrogenic complications from medication side effects. Geriatric patients have decreased cholinergic reserve and are at risk from developing side effects from central anticholinergic medications.[10]

The most prominent side effects include cognitive decline and delirium, and patients with Alzheimer dementia or other types of dementia, such as multi-infarct and vascular dementia, are particularly sensitive. Perioperatively, antihistamines such as chlorpheniramine, promethazine, and the antiemetic scopolamine are the most commonly encountered anticholinergic medications to be avoided. Haloperidol also has anticholinergic properties but is well tolerated in the small doses typically prescribed for agitation or nausea. Tools available to screen patients for potentially inappropriate medications include both the 2012 AGS Beers Criteria for Potentially Inappropriate Medication Use in Older Adults and the Screening Tool of Older People's Prescriptions or STOPP criteria.[17,54]

## SUMMARY

In summary, aging is associated with significant physiologic changes and an increase in comorbid conditions that influence the administration and choice of anesthetics. In the future there will be even larger numbers of elderly patients undergoing surgical procedures. Anesthetic plans must be designed to reduce or minimize postoperative complications.

## QUESTIONS OF THE DAY

1. How does aging alter cardiovascular autonomic function? What are the implications for evaluation of intraoperative hypotension in an elderly patient?
2. What is frailty, and how can it be assessed using the clinical phenotype model? What measures of frailty can be used to predict postoperative complications after surgery?
3. What postoperative risks are increased in a patient with preoperative cognitive impairment? What are the elements included in the Mini-Cog test?
4. What are the expected changes in the minimum alveolar concentration (MAC) of inhaled anesthetics for each decade after 20 years of age?
5. What is the incidence of delirium in elderly postoperative patients? What factors can contribute to the development of delirium?
6. What medications should be avoided in the elderly patient undergoing surgery? What screening tools can be used to evaluate for potentially inappropriate medications?

# REFERENCES

1. Yang R, Wolfson M, Lewis MC. Unique aspects of the elderly surgical population: an anesthesiologist's perspective. *Geriatr Orthop Surg Rehabil.* 2011;2(2):56–64.

2. Arias E. United States life tables, 2010. National Center for Health Statistics. *Natl Vital Stat Rep.* 2014;63(7):1–63.

3. Peden CJ, Grocott MPW. National research strategies: what outcomes are important in peri-operative elderly care? *Anaesthesia.* 2013;69(Suppl 1):61–69.

4. Strøm C, Rasmussen LS. Challenges in anaesthesia for elderly. *Singapore Dent J.* 2014;35(C):23–29.

5. Griffiths R, Beech F, Brown A, et al. Peri-operative care of the elderly 2014: Association of Anaesthetists of Great Britain and Ireland. *Anaesthesia.* 2014;69(Suppl 1):81–98.

6. Kheterpal S, O'Reilly M, Englesbe MJ, et al. Preoperative and intraoperative predictors of cardiac adverse events after general, vascular, and urological surgery. *Anesthesiology.* 2009;110(1):58–66.

7. Turrentine FE, Wang H, Simpson VB, Jones RS. Surgical risk factors, morbidity, and mortality in elderly patients. *J Am Coll Surg.* 2006;203(6):865–877.

8. Partridge JSL, Harari D, Dhesi JK. Frailty in the older surgical patient: a review. *Age Ageing.* 2012;41(2):142–147.

9. Joseph B, Pandit V, Sadoun M, et al. Frailty in surgery. *J Trauma Acute Care Surg.* 2014;76(4):1151–1156.

10. Ramaiah R, Lam AM. Postoperative cognitive dysfunction in the elderly. *Anesthesiol Clin.* 2009;27(3):485–496.

11. Robinson TN, Wu DS, Pointer LF, et al. Preoperative cognitive dysfunction is related to adverse postoperative outcomes in the elderly. *J Am Coll Surg.* 2012;215(1):12–17.

12. Gajdos C, Kile D, Hawn MT, et al. Advancing age and 30-day adverse outcomes after nonemergent general surgeries. *J Am Geriatr Soc.* 2013;61(9):1608–1614.

13. Hamel MB, Henderson WG, Khuri SF, Daley J. Surgical outcomes for patients aged 80 and older: morbidity and mortality from major noncardiac surgery. *J Am Geriatr Soc.* 2005;53(3):424–429.

14. Pallati PK, Gupta PK, Bichala S, et al. Short-term outcomes of inguinal hernia repair in octogenarians and nonagenarians. *Hernia.* 2013;17(6):723–727.

15. Belmont PJ, Goodman GP, Kusnezov NA, et al. Postoperative myocardial infarction and cardiac arrest following primary total knee and hip arthroplasty: rates, risk factors, and time of occurrence. *J Bone Joint Surg.* 2014;96(24):2025–2031.

16. Kim S, Brooks A, Groban L. Preoperative assessment of the older surgical patient: honing in on geriatric syndromes. *Clin Interv Aging.* 2014;10:13–27.

17. Oresanya LB, Lyons WL, Finlayson E. Preoperative assessment of the older patient. *JAMA.* 2014;311(20):2110–2111.

18. Martin RS, Farrah JP, Chang MC. Effect of aging on cardiac function plus monitoring and support. *Surg Clin North Am.* 2015;95(1):23–35.

19. Sanders D, Dudley M, Groban L. Diastolic dysfunction, cardiovascular aging, and the anesthesiologist. *Anesthesiol Clin.* 2009;27(3):497–517.

20. Ramly E, Kaafarani HM, Velmahos GC. The effect of aging on pulmonary function: implications for monitoring and support of the surgical trauma patient. *Surg Clin North Am.* 2015;95(1):53–69.

21. Gupta H, Gupta PK, Schuller D, et al. Development and validation of a risk calculator for predicting postoperative pneumonia. *Mayo Clin Proc.* 2013;88(11):1241–1249.

22. Rivera R, Antognini JF. Perioperative drug therapy in elderly patients. *Anesthesiology.* 2009;110(5):1176–1181.

23. Kenney WL, Munce TA. Invited review: aging and human temperature regulation. *J Appl Physiol.* 2003;95:2598–2603.

24. World Health Organization. Health Topics, Dementia. http://www.who.int/topics/dementia/en/. Accessed June 1, 2016.

25. Seitz DP, Gill SS, Bell CM, et al. Postoperative medical complications associated with anesthesia in older adults with dementia. *J Am Geriatr Soc.* 2014;62(11):2102–2109.

26. Chow WB, Rosenthal RA, Merkow RP, et al. Optimal preoperative assessment of the geriatric surgical patient: a best practices guideline from the American College of Surgeons National Surgical Quality Improvement Program and the American Geriatrics Society. *J Am Coll Surg.* 2012;215(4):453–466.

27. Fleisher LA, Fleischmann KE, Auerbach AD, et al. 2014 ACC/AHA guideline on perioperative cardiovascular evaluation and management of patients undergoing noncardiac surgery: a report of the American College of Cardiology/American Heart Association Task Force on Practice Guidelines. *J Am Coll Cardiol.* 2014;64(22):e77–e137.

28. Kirkman KR, Wijeysundera DN, Pendrith C, et al. Preoperative testing before low-risk surgical procedures. *CMAJ.* 2015;187(11):E349–E358.

29. Wilson RJT, Davies S, Yates D, et al. Impaired functional capacity is associated with all-cause mortality after major elective intra-abdominal surgery. *Br J Anaesth.* 2010;105(3):297–303.

30. Makary MA, Segev DL, Pronovost PJ, et al. Frailty as a predictor of surgical outcomes in older patients. *J Am Coll Surg.* 2010;210(6):901–908.

31. Amrock LG, Deiner S. The implication of frailty on preoperative risk assessment. *Curr Opin Anaesthesiol.* 2014;27(3):330–335.

32. Rockwood K, Andrew M, Mitnitski A. A comparison of two approaches to measuring frailty in elderly people. *J Gerontol A Biol Sci Med Sci.* 2007;62(7):738–743.

33. Blodgett J, Theou O, Kirkland S, et al. Frailty in NHANES: comparing the frailty index and phenotype. *Arch Gerontol Geriatr.* 2015;60(3):464–470.

34. Robinson TN, Wu DS, Pointer L, et al. Simple frailty score predicts postoperative complications across surgical specialties. *Am J Surg.* 2013;206(4):544–550.

35. Centers for Disease Control and Prevention. The Timed Up and Go (TUG) Test. http://www.cdc.gov/steadi/pdf/tug_test-a.pdf. Accessed June 1, 2016.

36. Revenig LM, Canter DJ, Taylor MD, et al. Too frail for surgery? Initial results of a large multidisciplinary prospective study examining preoperative variables predictive of poor surgical outcomes. *J Am Coll Surg.* 2013;217(4):665–670.e1.

37. Sternberg SA, Schwartz AW, Karunananthan S, et al. The identification of frailty: a systematic literature review. *J Am Geriatr Soc.* 2011;59(11):2129–2138.

38. Kim SW, Han HS, Jung HW, et al. Multidimensional frailty score for the prediction of postoperative mortality risk. *JAMA Surg.* 2014;149(7):633–640.

39. Stotter A, Reed MW, Gray LJ, et al. Comprehensive geriatric assessment and predicted 3-year survival in treatment planning for frail patients with early breast cancer. *Br J Surg.* 2015;102(5):525–533.

40. The American Geriatrics Society Expert Panel on Postoperative Delirium in Older Adults. Postoperative delirium in older adults: best practice statement from the American Geriatrics Society. *J Am Coll Surg.* 2014;220(2):136–148.e1.

IV

41. van Meenen LCC, van Meenen DMP, de Rooij SE, ter Riet G. Risk prediction models for postoperative delirium: a systematic review and meta-analysis. *J Am Geriatr Soc.* 2014;62(12):2383–2390.

42. Barnett SR. Polypharmacy and perioperative medications in the elderly. *Anesthesiol Clin.* 2009;27(3):377–389.

43. Nordquist D, Halaszynski TM. Perioperative multimodal anesthesia using regional techniques in the aging surgical patient. *Pain Res Treat.* 2014; 2014(9):902174.

43a. Jacobs JR, Reves JG, Marty J, et al. Aging increases pharmacodynamic sensitivity to the hypnotic effects of midazolam. *Anesth Analg.* 1995;80(1): 143–148.

44. Mason SE, Noel-Storr A, Ritchie CW. The impact of general and regional anesthesia on the incidence of postoperative cognitive dysfunction and post-operative delirium: a systematic review with meta-analysis. *J Alzheimers Dis.* 2010;22(Suppl 3):67–79.

45. Aw D, Sahota O. Orthogeriatrics moving forward. *Age Aging.* 2014;43(3):301–305.

46. Schofield PA. The assessment and management of peri-operative pain in older adults. *Anaesthesia.* 2013;69(Suppl 1):54–60.

47. Sieber FE, Barnett SR. Preventing postoperative complications in the elderly. *Anesthesiol Clin.* 2011;29(1):83–97.

48. Lee HB, Mears SC, Rosenberg PB, et al. Predisposing factors for postoperative delirium after hip fracture repair in individuals with and without dementia. *J Am Geriatr Soc.* 2011;59(12):2306–2313.

49. Sieber FE. Postoperative delirium in the elderly surgical patient. *Anesthesiol Clin.* 2009;27(3):451–464.

50. Mashour GA, Woodrum DT, Avidan MS. Neurological complications of surgery and anaesthesia. *Br J Anaesth.* 2015;114(2):194–203.

51. Mu JL, Lee A, Joynt GM. Pharmacologic agents for the prevention and treatment of delirium in patients undergoing cardiac surgery. *Crit Care Med.* 2015;43(1):194–204.

52. Monk TG, Price CC. Postoperative cognitive disorders. *Curr Opin Crit Care.* 2011;17(4):376–381.

53. Wijeysundera DN, Duncan D, Nkonde-Price C, et al. Perioperative beta blockade in noncardiac surgery: a systematic review for the 2014 ACC/AHA guideline on perioperative cardiovascular evaluation and management of patients undergoing noncardiac surgery: a report of the American College of Cardiology/American Heart Association Task Force on practice guidelines. *J Am Coll Cardiol.* 2014;64(22):2406–2425.

54. Blanco-Reina E, Ariza-Zafra G, Ocaña-Riola R, León-Ortiz M. 2012 American Geriatrics Society Beers criteria: enhanced applicability for detecting potentially inappropriate medications in European older adults? A comparison with the screening tool of older person's potentially inappropriate prescriptions. *J Am Geriatr Soc.* 2014;62(7):1217–1223.

55. Wetterslev J, Meyhoff CS, Jørgensen LN, et al. The effects of high perioperative inspiratory oxygen fraction for adult surgical patients. *Cochrane Database Syst Rev.* 2015;6,CD008884.

56. Orhan-Sungur M, Kranke P, Sessler D, Apfel CC. Does supplemental oxygen reduce postoperative nausea and vomiting? A meta-analysis of randomized controlled trials. *Anesth Analg.* 2008;106(6):1733–1738.

# 36 ORGAN TRANSPLANTATION

## Randolph H. Steadman and Victor W. Xia

Patients waiting for a transplantable organ share a hope for the future that is predicated on the availability of an organ donor. Donor death must be declared prior to organ procurement. Donation after brain death (DBD) is the most common setting in which donation occurs.[1] Organ shortages have led to donation after cardiac death (DCD).[2] The ethical considerations related to DCD donation are challenging, yet DCD donation is increasing in response to the national organ shortage.[3,4]

## CONSIDERATIONS FOR ORGAN TRANSPLANTATION

Because of the shortage of available organs not all potential recipients on the waiting list survive long enough to undergo a transplant procedure. Those who do typically wait a year or more. Prelisting assessments may be outdated by the time an organ is identified, and supplemental testing may be indicated. This testing may necessitate a deferral of the scheduled transplant, which must be weighed against the risk of further deterioration that can preclude transplantation. Untreated systemic infection, incurable malignancy, untreated substance abuse, and the lack of sufficient social support to comply with posttransplant care can preclude transplantation.

Once the decision is made to proceed with transplantation, coordination between the donor procedure and multiple recipient hospitals may be involved. Because not all donor organs are suitable for transplantation, the recipient operation should not begin until visual or biopsy-based confirmation of organ suitability has been made. During the time between the identification of the donor and the procurement surgery, the recipient's latest laboratory values should be ascertained. If necessary, dialysis can be performed. The anesthetic plan should be reviewed with the patient and the family, questions and concerns are addressed, and the patient's consent is obtained.

---

**Box 36.1** Kidney Transplantation Facts

- The kidney is the most frequently transplanted solid organ.
- More than 10,000 deceased donor and 6000 live donor kidney transplant procedures are performed annually in the United States.
- Five-year posttransplantation survival rates are 91% for recipients of live donor grafts, 83% for standard (non-ECD) deceased donor recipients, and 70% for recipients of grafts from ECDs.
- Transplantation improves survival rate over that achieved with dialysis, which carries a 20% annual mortality risk.

*ECD*, Extended criteria donor.
From Annual Report of the U.S. Organ Procurement and Transplantation Network and the Scientific Registry of Transplant Recipients: Transplant Data 1998-2007. Rockville, MD: U.S. Department of Health and Human Services, Health Resources and Services Administration, Healthcare Systems Bureau, Division of Transplantation; 2008.

## KIDNEY TRANSPLANTATION

Kidney transplantation confers a survival advantage over dialysis for the management of renal failure.[5] The best organ survival occurs from transplantation with grafts (kidney) from living donors, but even kidneys from marginal deceased donors confer a survival advantage over continued dialysis (Box 36.1). Marginal or extended criteria donor (ECD) grafts have lower graft survival rates than standard grafts. The recently implemented kidney donor risk index (KDRI) provides a more detailed assessment of risk associated with donor kidneys than the non-ECD/ECD classification.[6] Donor factors in the KDRI include older, hypertensive, and diabetic donors, and grafts with a prolonged duration of cold or warm ischemia, as seen with long preservation times and DCD donors, respectively.

### Preoperative Assessment

Because of the shortage of deceased donor grafts, the number of candidates on the waiting list continues to increase (also see Chapter 13). The median time on the waiting list in the United States is longer than 5 years for recipients of deceased donor grafts.[7] This makes it challenging to maintain an up-to-date pretransplant assessment. Currently one third of kidney transplants are living-related, which facilitates scheduling preoperative evaluation and significantly shortens waiting time. Almost all living donations are performed laparoscopically; few are converted to open procedures.[7]

Diabetes is the most common cause of end-stage renal disease, followed by hypertension, and glomerulonephritis (Box 36.2). These three causes account for over two thirds of the cases of renal failure. Patients with these conditions should be medically managed to achieve treatment goals while on the waiting list.

**Box 36.2** Kidney Transplant Recipient: Preoperative Assessment

**Cardiovascular**
  Ischemic heart disease
  Congestive heart failure
  Hypertension
**Diabetes**
  Hyperkalemia
  Acidosis
  Anemia
  Dialysis history

Although cardiovascular disease is the leading cause of death in patients receiving dialysis, cardiovascular risk factors are often undertreated.[8] After transplant, the cardiovascular risk diminishes from a tenfold to a twofold increase compared to that of normal patients. Accordingly, the preoperative assessment should focus on screening for ischemic heart disease and management of hypertension, diabetes, and dyslipidemia. Ischemic heart disease may be silent, particularly in diabetic patients. As a result of preexisting vasodilatation stress, echocardiography is probably superior to thallium imaging in predicting postoperative cardiac events, although false positive and false negative findings occur with both techniques.[9] Coronary angiography, accompanied by therapeutic intervention for significant lesions, should be considered in patients with reversible cardiac ischemia or in those with significant risk.

Congestive heart failure is prevalent in dialysis patients but, in the absence of ischemic heart disease, does not preclude safe transplantation. Ejection fraction typically improves after transplantation. The preoperative focus is on optimal medical management of heart failure and maintenance of intravascular fluid balance.

Anemia may increase cardiovascular risk, particularly in patients with ischemic heart disease. A hemoglobin level of 12 g/dL is sufficient; higher hemoglobin concentrations may increase the risk of thrombotic events. Erythropoietin, when used to correct anemia to levels of 12 g/dL or less, lessens the risk of blood transfusion (see Chapter 24).

Hyperkalemia is common in patients with renal insufficiency and may be associated with increased risks during transplant surgery, particularly during reperfusion. However, mild increases in potassium may reflect normal homeostasis for renal failure, and potassium levels of 5.0 to 5.5 mEq/L are acceptable in this population. Dialysis-dependent patients may benefit from dialysis immediately prior to transplantation; however, a reduced intravascular central volume may offset the benefits of reduced potassium levels.

### Intraoperative Management

Donor kidneys are usually implanted in the iliac fossa. Vascular anastomoses are most frequently to the external iliac artery and vein, and the ureter is anastomosed

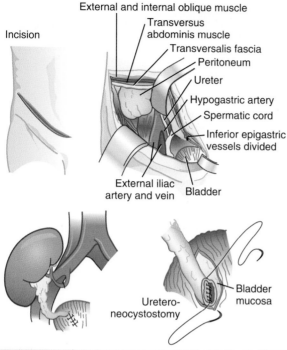

Incision

External and internal oblique muscle
Transversus abdominis muscle
Transversalis fascia
Peritoneum
Ureter
Hypogastric artery
Spermatic cord
Inferior epigastric vessels divided
External iliac artery and vein   Bladder

Uretero-neocystostomy
Bladder mucosa

**Fig. 36.1** Kidney recipient operation. (From Townsend CM Jr, Beauchamp RD, Evers BM, Mattox KL, eds. *Sabiston Textbook of Surgery.* 18th ed. Philadelphia: Saunders Elsevier; 2007, used with permission.)

directly to the bladder (Fig. 36.1). Chronic renal disease can affect drug excretion via the kidney but also through changes in plasma protein binding or hepatic metabolism. When the protein binding is diminished the free fraction of the drug is increased. This results in an increase in the volume of distribution and the clearance. The net effect for the unbound fraction is similar to that in normal patients.

Some drugs require particular caution when administered in patients with renal failure.[1] They include neuromuscular blocking (NMB) drugs (also see Chapter 11) and certain opioids (also see Chapter 9). Long-acting NMB drugs, which are excreted via the kidneys (e.g., pancuronium), are best avoided. Vecuronium and rocuronium may have a prolonged action in patients with renal failure. Cisatracurium's duration of action is more predictable because of spontaneous breakdown (also see Chapter 11). Although atracurium undergoes similar elimination, it is less potent than cisatracurium, so its breakdown product, laudanosine, is found in higher concentrations. Laudanosine's theoretical potential to cause seizures has never been clinically important.

The 6-glucuronide metabolite of morphine has clinical activity that can result in a prolonged duration of action. Meperidine should be avoided because of the seizure-inducing potential of its metabolite, normeperidine.

Inhaled anesthetics can be used in renal failure patients. Although sevoflurane's metabolite, compound A, is nephrotoxic in rats, similar effects have not been seen in humans. Serum fluoride concentrations of 30 μmol occur in humans after sevoflurane, but do not produce renal damage. Isoflurane is metabolized to fluoride, but the extent of metabolism is so small that fluoride levels are negligible. Desflurane is not contraindicated in renal failure; but like the other volatile anesthetics, it produces a decrease in renal blood flow and glomerular filtration rate in a dose-dependent manner.

Intravascular fluid balance should be maintained in patients undergoing kidney transplantation. Typically crystalloid is used for this purpose with colloids preferred by some centers. In an intensive care unit (ICU) population (also see Chapter 41), balanced salt solutions (e.g., lactated Ringer solution, Plasma-Lyte) are preferred over hyperchloremic crystalloids such as normal saline. These balanced salt solutions are associated with a lower incidence of acute kidney injury and a reduced need for renal replacement.[10] Paradoxically, their effect on serum potassium levels is less than that of potassium-free hyperchloremic solutions, which are more likely to increase serum blood potassium concentrations by generating a hyperchloremic acidosis. Albumin is the typical colloid of choice; hydroxyethyl starch solution is associated with a more frequent risk of acute kidney injury.[11]

Monitoring arterial blood pressure via an arterial catheter is avoided in some centers in order to preserve arterial access for dialysis, whereas other centers use arterial monitoring regularly in an aging recipient population with increasingly common comorbid conditions. Central venous pressure (CVP) monitoring is now recognized as a poor monitoring method of preload and fluid responsiveness.[12] Placement of a central intravenous line should be reserved for medications that require administration into a high flow vein such as rabbit antithymocyte globulin, an immunosuppression induction drug. Induction of immunosuppression is increasingly common as efforts to increase the living donor pool include use of unrelated living donors, nondirected donors, and donor exchange programs.

Delayed graft function and acute tubular necrosis can lead to renal replacement therapy after transplantation. The factors responsible include donor hemodynamics, graft warm ischemia, and recipient hemodynamics. Adequate hydration reduces the incidence of acute tubular necrosis. There are few data to support the intraoperative use of diuretics, and there is considerable variability between surgeons regarding the intraoperative use of diuretics.[13] Although of unproven benefit in preventing acute kidney injury in a general perioperative population, administration of osmotic diuretics, such as mannitol, during transplantation may be helpful.[14]

IV

## Postoperative Management

Maintaining renal perfusion is an important consideration and is best accomplished by maintaining an adequate intravascular volume. Dopamine, large-dose diuretics, and osmotic diuretics are of no proven benefit in the postoperative period. Postoperative analgesia can be achieved by epidural infusion, although many health care facilities prefer intravenously administered patient-controlled analgesia with fentanyl or morphine (also see Chapter 40). Nonsteroidal antiinflammatory drugs should be avoided.

## LIVER TRANSPLANTATION

The liver is second to the kidney as the most frequently transplanted solid organ. Patients with liver failure have no alternatives to liver transplantation.[1] The median time to transplant for waiting list candidates decreased significantly, from 14 months in 2012 to just over a month in 2013, owing to within-region sharing of liver grafts for the highest acuity recipients (those with model for end-stage liver disease [MELD] scores of 35 or more). The MELD score is used to allocate grafts based upon the recipient's 90-day mortality risk in the absence of transplantation. International normalized ratio (INR) of prothrombin time, creatinine, and bilirubin are used to derive the MELD score. The most common indication for liver transplantation in the United States is hepatitis C virus, followed by alcoholic liver disease, cholestatic disease, and malignancy. Combined, these diagnoses account for 70% of candidates who are on the waiting list. New antiviral agents for hepatitis C, introduced in 2013, are expected to reduce, if not eliminate, transplants for this diagnosis in the future. Nonalcoholic steatohepatitis (NASH), a diagnosis associated with metabolic syndrome and obesity, is expected to become an increasingly prevalent cause leading to transplantation in the coming years.

An ongoing shortage of donors has lead to the increased use of marginally viable grafts, defined as organs from elderly donors; DCD donors; donors with steatotic livers, obesity, malignancy, prolonged ICU stays, bacterial infection, or high-risk lifestyle; donors on multiple vasopressor infusions; or those who had suffered cardiac arrest.[15]

### Preoperative Assessment

Over 75% of transplant recipients are older than 50 years, compared to 63% 10 years ago (also see Chapter 13). A higher percentage are hospitalized and have comorbid conditions. Liver transplant candidates have many symptoms ranging from fatigue to multiple organ failure (Box 36.3). Encephalopathy, common in end-stage liver disease (ESLD), can lead to sensitivity to sedative and analgesic medications, increased risk of aspiration of gastric contents, and the need for endotracheal intubation to protect the airway.

---

**Box 36.3** Liver Transplant Recipient: Preoperative Assessment

Neurologic
    Encephalopathy
    Cerebral edema (acute liver failure)
Cardiovascular
    Hyperdynamic circulation
    Cirrhotic cardiomyopathy
    Portopulmonary hypertension
Pulmonary
    Restrictive lung disease
    Ventilation-perfusion mismatch
    Intrapulmonary shunts
    Hepatopulmonary syndrome
Gastrointestinal
    Portal hypertension
    Variceal bleeding
    Ascites
Renal/metabolic
    Hepatorenal syndrome
Acid-base abnormalities
    Hematologic
    Coagulopathy
    Anemia
Musculoskeletal
    Muscle atrophy

---

The pretransplant cardiac evaluation includes an assessment for ischemic heart disease and screening for portopulmonary hypertension (PPHTN). Dobutamine stress echocardiography and nuclear scans are common screening tests to rule out coronary artery disease; however, they are associated with both false positive and false negative results.[9] In older patients with diabetes, multiple risk factors, or a history of coronary disease, left-sided heart catheterization may be indicated (also see Chapters 25 and 35). More than two thirds of ESLD patients have a hyperdynamic circulation characterized by a high cardiac output and low systemic vascular resistance (SVR), most likely because of circulating vasoactive substances not cleared by the liver. This hyperdynamic state can be confused with sepsis and is exacerbated by graft reperfusion.

Resting echocardiography is the test of choice in screening for PPHTN. An estimated right ventricular systolic pressure less than 50 mm Hg by echocardiography rules out significant PPHTN. Right-sided heart catheterization is indicated if estimated right ventricular pressure exceeds 50 mm Hg. The definitive diagnosis of PPHTN is made when the mean pulmonary artery (PA) pressure is more than 25 mm Hg in the presence of an increased transpulmonary gradient (mean PA minus PA occlusion pressure > 12) and an increased pulmonary vascular resistance (>3 Wood units, or >240 dynes/s/cm$^5$). Mean PA pressures higher than 35 mm Hg are associated with a perioperative mortality rate of 50%, and treatment prior to transplant should be considered.

Hepatopulmonary syndrome (resting and breathing room air $Po_2 < 70$ mm Hg in the presence of an intrapulmonary shunt on bubble echocardiography) resolves after transplantation; however, $Pao_2$ levels less than 50 mm Hg while breathing room air are associated with increased acuity, longer postoperative hospital stays, and, in some studies, a higher postoperative mortality rate.

Renal disease is common in patients who present for liver transplantation. If not long-standing, hepatorenal syndrome may resolve after transplantation. Prior to transplantation, excessive intravascular volume, acidosis, or hyperkalemia may necessitate renal replacement therapy. The coagulopathy of ESLD is multifactorial and requires correction in the presence of active bleeding.

Acute liver failure (ALF) accounts for approximately 5% of liver transplants. ALF is distinct from chronic liver disease because of the potential for cerebral edema, which is the most common cause of death in ALF.[16] Cerebral edema is managed similarly to other causes of increased intracranial pressure (also see Chapter 30). The cause of ALF often predicts whether spontaneous recovery without transplant is likely. Approximately 25% of ALF patients undergo liver transplantation; survival rate in those receiving transplants is similar to posttransplant survival rate in patients with chronic liver disease.

## Intraoperative Management

Intraoperative management requires a consideration of the effects of liver failure on drug metabolism. Preoperative anxiolytic medication should be used sparingly in patients with a history of encephalopathy. The chosen anesthetic should maintain SVR. The intermediate duration NMB drugs metabolized by the liver can have a prolonged duration of action; however, after reperfusion, evidence of liver function typically occurs and metabolism of these drugs improves. Alternatively cisatracurium, which undergoes Hofmann elimination, can be selected to avoid these concerns. Seizures can also be caused by an accumulation of normeperidine, so meperidine should be avoided. The metabolite of morphine, 6-glucuronide morphine, can accumulate and cause a prolonged effect. Fentanyl and the other synthetic opioids are safe choices. Volatile anesthetics have similar, mild effects on hepatic blood flow. Sevoflurane undergoes metabolism by the liver, but the metabolite, compound A, is not toxic to the liver or kidneys in humans.

Intraoperative monitoring varies among medical centers (Box 36.4). An arterial line is placed, followed by a central venous catheter (CVC) and pulmonary artery catheter (PAC), or CVC alone. Continuous cardiac output measurement from arterial waveform analysis may not accurately reflect cardiac output in liver recipients as a result of low SVR, high cardiac output, and vasopressor administration. Stroke volume and pulse pressure variation, although more accurate than CVP monitoring for predicting

---

> **Box 36.4** Liver Transplantation: Unique Aspects of Case Preparation
>
> **Transfusion**
> Red blood cells: 6-10 units for adults
> Fresh frozen plasma: 6-10 units for adults
> Rapid infusion device
>
> **Medication**
> Vasopressors: phenylephrine, epinephrine (10 and 100 μg/mL), vasopressin
> Calcium chloride: for infusion and bolus
> Insulin: for infusion (poststeroid immunosuppression and/or hyperkalemia unresponsive to diuretics)
>
> **Monitors**
> Arterial line
> Central venous pressure catheter
> Pulmonary artery catheter
> Transesophageal echocardiography

---

fluid responsiveness, are less accurate during mechanical ventilation with smaller tidal volumes (<8 mL/kg) and in the presence of cardiac arrhythmias.[17] Transesophageal echocardiography (TEE) is often used, which may obviate the need for PAC monitoring in the operating room. TEE represents the gold standard for cardiac preload monitoring; however, interpretation is operator dependent and monitoring into the postoperative period is not feasible.

Venovenous bypass is used in some medical facilities to attenuate the effects of inferior vena cava (IVC) clamping on intravascular volume; however, it has risks and adds to the length of the procedure.

The operation is divided into three phases: preanhepatic, anhepatic, and neohepatic. In the preanhepatic phase dissection and preparation for the native hepatectomy occur. This phase is associated with blood loss, particularly in the presence of varices and prior abdominal surgery. Vascular isolation of the native liver (cross-clamping of the IVC, portal vein, and hepatic artery) begins the anhepatic phase. Excision of the native liver occurs next and is followed by implantation of the donor graft. The implantation involves anastomoses of the suprahepatic IVC, the infrahepatic IVC, and the portal vein (Fig. 36.2). An alternative "piggyback" technique involves anastomosis of the donor hepatic veins to the recipient vena cava, followed by portal anastomosis. The anhepatic period is typically quiescent from a hemodynamic perspective. Reperfusion follows portal anastomoses and begins the neohepatic period. Reperfusion is the most precarious event during the procedure because of the release of cold, acidotic effluent from the graft and lower extremities (Box 36.5). *Reperfusion syndrome* is characterized by a decrease in systemic blood pressure and SVR.[18] The portal effluent contains vasoactive peptides that reduce SVR and can increase pulmonary resistance. Hyperkalemia can be life threatening. If

**IV**

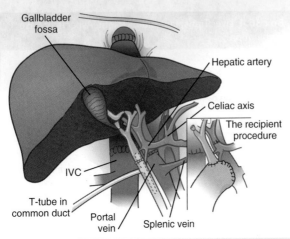

**Fig. 36.2** Liver recipient operation. *IVC,* Inferior vena cava. Illustrated are the anastomoses of the donor and recipient suprahepatic IVC, infrahepatic IVC, portal vein, hepatic artery, and duct-to-duct biliary anastomosis, which can be performed with or without T-tube placement. Alternatively *(inset),* in the presence of disease of the bile duct biliary drainage is via a choledochojejunostomy. (From Townsend CM Jr, Beauchamp RD, Evers BM, Mattox KL, eds. *Sabiston Textbook of Surgery.* 18th ed. Philadelphia: Saunders Elsevier; 2007, used with permission.)

---

**Box 36.5** Liver Transplantation: Treatment for the Physiologic Changes of Reperfusion

- *Hyperkalemia:* calcium, bicarbonate, insulin, and glucose
- *Acidosis:* bicarbonate, other buffers such as tris (hydroxymethyl) aminomethane
- *Decreased SVR:* α-agonists
- *Hypothermia:* warm saline peritoneal lavage

*SVR,* Systemic vascular resistance.

---

hyperkalemia is a concern, dialysis is helpful if started early in the preanhepatic period. Insulin is effective if given at least 10 to 15 minutes prior to reperfusion; infusions are preferred to repeated bolus dosing. Calcium given immediately prior to reperfusion blunts the effect of hyperkalemia on the myocardium. α-Adrenergic agonists and alkalizing drugs may be required to maintain SVR and pH, respectively.

During the neohepatic phase, fibrinolysis can occur resulting in ongoing oozing due to microvascular bleeding. If fibrinolysis is not self-limited, antifibrinolytic drugs can be administered. Metabolic acidosis, which worsens during the anhepatic phase and peaks after reperfusion, should improve when the liver starts functioning. Additional signs of liver function include increased core temperature and decreasing calcium requirement (indicating citrate metabolism by the liver). On occasion oliguric patients with hepatorenal syndrome may show an increase in urine output in the operating room.

## Postoperative Management

Posttransplant patient survival rates are 85% to 90% at 1 year and 72% to 78% after 5 years. Recipients of grafts from living donors have the most success with 1- and 5-year posttransplant survival rates. Thrombosis of the hepatic artery in the early postoperative period usually necessitates retransplantation. Infection is a major threat to survival in the initial months after transplant.

## HEART TRANSPLANTATION

Heart transplantation is the definitive treatment for patients with end-stage heart disease. Currently, the three most common indications for heart transplantation are idiopathic dilated cardiomyopathy, ischemic heart disease, and congenital heart disease, which account for more than 90% of the transplants.[19]

### Preoperative Evaluation

Although patients undergo extensive multidisciplinary evaluation before being listed, a detailed preanesthetic evaluation is often challenging owing to the urgent nature of the surgery, the complex clinical presentation, and multiple comorbid conditions.[20] Many patients require inotropic drugs or mechanical support at the time of heart transplantation. Preoperative evaluation should focus on current cardiac status, medications (particularly the need for inotropic and anticoagulant drugs), and mechanical support such as intra-aortic balloon pump or ventricular assist device. The patients should not have severe, irreversible pulmonary hypertension or an active infectious disease. For patients with multiple organ failure, combined heart transplantation with other organs (e.g., lung, kidney, liver) may be considered (also see Chapter 13).

### Intraoperative Management

In addition to standard monitors, invasive hemodynamic monitors (arterial lines, CVCs, and PACs) are routinely inserted for heart transplantation.[21] The right internal jugular vein remains a preferred site despite a concern that it may jeopardize postoperative biopsies. The PAC needs to be withdrawn to the jugular vein before the native heart is excised. Alternatively, the PAC is inserted at the central venous position and is advanced after the donor heart is implanted. In some institutions, a PAC with capability of continuous monitoring of mixed venous $O_2$ saturation and cardiac output is also used. TEE plays an important role in assessing intravascular volume status, contractility, and valvular function, while monitoring for thromboembolism (also see Chapter 25).

---

**Box 36.6** Heart Transplantation: Perioperative Goals

- Maintain systemic blood pressure to maintain coronary filling
- Optimize preload
- Reduce afterload to improve ejection fraction
- Avoid pulmonary vasoconstriction
  - Maintain oxygenation
  - Avoid hypercapnia
  - Avoid high tidal volumes
  - Correct acid-base abnormalities
- Support contractility
  - Pharmacologic drugs
  - Intra-aortic balloon pump
  - Assist devices

---

Patients who are having a heart transplant often have a full stomach due to the urgency of the procedure; therefore, a rapid sequence induction of anesthesia is needed. The choice of anesthetic is dictated by the patient's cardiac status. A failing heart is dependent on preload and sensitive to afterload. Even small changes in venous return, vascular resistance, rhythm, heart rate, and contractility can lead to hemodynamic collapse. Anesthetics with minimal hemodynamic impact are often chosen to induce anesthesia. Etomidate is a reasonable selection. Maintenance of anesthesia is often achieved by administration of a combination of a volatile anesthetic and an opioid. A large-dose opioid technique can be used as well. Nitrous oxide is usually avoided as cardiac suppression can be seen in heart transplant patients and is presumably due to catecholamine store depletion and β-adrenergic receptor downregulation.

Management goals during heart transplantation are dictated by the underlying congestive heart failure and the need to avoid conditions that increase PA pressure (Box 36.6). Weaning from cardiopulmonary bypass is similar to any other cardiac case. Patients are rewarmed. Acid-base and electrolytes should be in the normal range, the lungs are ventilated with 100% oxygen, and the cardiac chambers are free of air.

Several intraoperative issues are unique to heart transplantation. First, the transplanted heart is denervated and bradycardia can occur following reperfusion. The heart rate response to hemodynamic changes is absent and drugs acting indirectly on the heart are ineffective. Bradycardia can be treated by pacing (usually 90 to 110 beats/min) or chronotropic drugs such as isoproterenol. Second, failure to wean from cardiopulmonary bypass is often caused by right-sided heart failure. Several possible mechanisms are related to right-sided heart failure during heart transplantation: preexisting pulmonary hypertension can be worsened during reperfusion of the donor heart, and the right ventricle is particularly prone to ischemia/reperfusion injury. The

primary treatment goals for right-sided heart failure during heart transplantation are to increase contractility of the right ventricle and decrease PA resistance. Failure to respond may necessitate mechanical right ventricular support. Worsening pulmonary hypertension during heart transplantation is multifactorial. An increase in cardiac output, pulmonary vessel spasm, and blood or air embolism are all possible causes. Adequate ventilation and oxygenation, with avoidance of hypoxia and hypercarbia, can prevent an increase in pulmonary vasculature resistance. Treatment of pulmonary hypertension with nonselective vasodilators such as nitroglycerin and sodium nitroprusside can decrease SVR and result in systemic hypotension. Selective drugs such as inhaled nitric oxide, aerosolized iloprost (a carbacyclin analog of prostaglandin $I_2$), and sildenafil (inhaled or infused) may be helpful.

## Postoperative Management

Postoperative management targets adequate oxygenation, ventilation, intravascular volume, pulmonary and systemic pressures, coagulation, and body temperature. Extubation of the trachea is considered when stable hemodynamics and adequate spontaneous ventilation have been achieved. Some patients require permanent pacemaker implantation because of the loss of sinus node function.[21] Most patients require inotropic and chronotropic support in the first few days following heart transplant. Posttransplant bleeding and a nonfunctional graft are life threatening and need to be diagnosed and managed emergently.

## LUNG TRANSPLANTATION

Chronic obstructive lung disease and interstitial lung disease are two common indications for adult lung transplantation.[22] In children, cystic fibrosis is the most common indication for lung transplantation. The choice of transplant type (single, sequential, double lung) is dependent on the surgeon's preference and the nature and severity of disease. Each operative type requires slightly different anesthetic setup and intraoperative management.

## Preoperative Evaluation

Preoperative evaluation should focus on the severity of lung disease, the baseline function of other vital organs, the airway, and interval changes since the last examination (also see Chapter 13).[23] The preoperative administration of anxiolytic drugs should be performed with caution, as too much sedation or uncontrolled anxiety can worsen pulmonary hypertension. Supplemental administration of oxygen is carefully given because most lung transplant

**IV**

patients depend on their hypoxic drive. Epidural analgesia should be considered in lung transplant patients for postoperative pain control (also see Chapter 40).

## Intraoperative Management

In addition to standard monitors, arterial catheters, CVCs, and PACs are usually placed. In some institutions, a PAC with continuous mixed venous $O_2$ saturation and cardiac output monitoring is used. Endobronchoscopy is necessary during lung transplantation. In addition to assessing the position of the double-lumen endotracheal tube, endobronchoscopy can examine the airway anastomoses for stenosis, bleeding, and obstruction secondary to blood or sputum. TEE is often used during lung transplantation.

Induction of anesthesia needs to balance the risk of aspiration of gastric contents with hypoxia and hemodynamic instability. Positive-pressure ventilation can cause a decreased venous blood return. Patients with severe pulmonary hypertension are at risk of cardiac arrest during induction of anesthesia. Emergent cardiopulmonary bypass is established in this situation. Positive-pressure ventilation can cause further damage to diseased lungs and worsen hypoxia and hypercarbia. Air-trapping and barotrauma should be avoided. Protective ventilation strategies, including small tidal volumes, should be considered.[24]

The most challenging intraoperative issues associated with lung transplant involve ventilation-reperfusion mismatch and PA hypertension. Strategies to treat hypoxemia during lung transplant are similar to those seen in thoracic surgery (also see Chapter 27). At the time of PA clamping, increased PA pressure is often encountered. Methods to reduce PA pressure include intravascular fluid restriction and nonselective and selective pulmonary vasodilators in both intravenous and inhaled forms. Excessive intravascular fluid administration should be avoided because noncardiogenic pulmonary edema is a frequent development in lung transplant patients.

## Postoperative Management

Special care for lung transplant patients in the postoperative period is provided to avoid barotrauma, volutrauma, and anastomotic dehiscence during positive-pressure mechanical ventilation.

## PANCREAS TRANSPLANTATION

The most common indication for pancreas transplantation is type 1 diabetes. However, more transplants have been performed in patients with type 2 diabetes in recent years.[25] The transplanted pancreas can provide endogenous insulin and restore normoglycemia and the glucagon response. Diabetes mellitus affects cardiovascular, autonomic, nervous, renal, gastrointestinal, and metabolic systems. Preoperative evaluation should focus on functional status of the vital organs. Ischemic heart disease is a primary cause of perioperative death. Diagnosis of coronary artery disease in this patient population is difficult in the presence of neuropathy and silent ischemia. If coronary artery disease is suspected, a preoperative stress test or coronary artery angiogram should be performed. Preoperative evaluation should also include examination of renal function, acid-base status electrolytes, and hemoglobin. Most pancreas transplants are performed simultaneously with kidney transplantation. Compared with pancreas alone or pancreas after kidney transplant, simultaneous pancreas and kidney transplants experience the best graft survival rates.[25]

Pancreas transplantation can be performed under general or regional anesthesia. Invasive monitors should be considered if there is cardiovascular disease. The choice of anesthetic drugs should take into account the possibility of severe postinduction hypotension due to diabetic autonomic nervous system dysfunction. Administration of NMB drugs not dependent on renal excretion for their elimination is preferred if renal function is impaired (also see Chapter 11). Severe intraoperative hyperglycemia should be avoided because it may adversely affect islet function and promote posttransplant infection.

## CONCLUSIONS

Patients presenting for organ transplantation have end-stage disease of one or more organs, and many are critically ill. Anesthetic management tailored to the patient's comorbid conditions is vital for successful transplant. Vigilant anesthetic care, both before and after the transplant, can have a profound impact on minimizing these complications and improving posttransplant outcomes. Successful transplantation reverses organ failure and promotes the recovery of organ systems beyond the transplanted organ.

## QUESTIONS OF THE DAY

1. How should the risk of cardiovascular disease be evaluated in a patient who requires kidney transplantation?
2. What are the most common indications for liver transplantation in the United States? How is the model for end-stage liver disease (MELD) score used in the allocation of liver grafts?
3. What are the three phases of the liver transplant procedure? What are the manifestations of reperfusion syndrome?
4. A patient develops bradycardia immediately after heart transplantation. What are the unique aspects of managing the patient's hemodynamics in this setting?

# REFERENCES

1. Steadman H, Wray CL. Anesthesia for abdominal organ transplantation. In: Miller RD, Cohen NH, Eriksson LI, et al, eds. *Miller's Anesthesia*. 8th ed. Philadelphia: Saunders Elsevier; 2015:2262–2291. Chap. 74.

2. Centers for Medicare and Medicaid Services. Department of Health and Human Services. Medicare and Medicaid programs, conditions for coverage for organ procurement organizations (OPOs), final rule. *Fed Regist*. 2006;71:30981–31054. http://www.ustransplant.org/annual_reports/current/. Accessed March 7, 2010.

3. Bernat JL, D'Alessandro AM, Port FK, et al. Report of a National Conference on Donation after cardiac death. *Am J Transplant*. 2006;6(2):281–291.

4. Verheijde JL, Rady MY, McGregor JL. The United States Revised Uniform Anatomical Gift Act (2006): new challenges to balancing patient rights and physician responsibilities. *Philos Ethics Humanit Med*. 2007;2:19.

5. Reese PP, Shults J, Bloom RD, et al. Functional status, time to transplantation, and survival benefit of kidney transplantation among wait-listed candidates. *Am J Kidney Dis*. 2015;66(5):837–845.

6. Rao PS, Schaubel DE, Guidinger MK, et al. A comprehensive risk quantification score for deceased donor kidneys: the kidney donor risk index. *Transplantation*. 2009;88:231–236.

7. Matas AJ, Smith JM, Skeans MA, et al. OPTN/SRTR 2013 Annual Data Report: kidney. *Am J Transpl*. 2015;15(suppl 2):1–34.

8. Delville M, Sabbah L, Girard D, et al. Prevalence and predictors of early cardiovascular events after kidney transplantation: evaluation of pre-transplant cardiovascular work-up. *PLoS One*. 2015;10(6):e0131237.

9. Lentine KL, Costa SP, Weir MR, et al. Cardiac disease evaluation and management among kidney and liver transplantation candidates. *Circulation*. 2012;126:617–663.

10. Yunos NM, Bellomo R, Hegarty C, et al. Association between a chloride-liberal vs chloride-restrictive intravenous fluid administration strategy and kidney injury in critically ill adults. *JAMA*. 2012;308(15):1566–1572.

11. Mutter TC, Ruth CA, Dart AB, et al. Hydroxyethyl starch (HES) versus other fluid therapies: effects on kidney function. *Cochrane Database Syst Rev*. 2013;(7):CD007594.

12. Marik PE, Baram M, Vahid B. Does central venous pressure predict fluid responsiveness? *Chest*. 2008;134:172–178.

13. Hanif F, Macrae AN, Littlejohn MG, et al. Outcome of renal transplantation with and without intra-operative diuretics. *Int J Surg*. 2011;9(6):460–463.

14. Yang B, Xu J, Xu F, et al. Intravascular administration of mannitol for acute kidney injury prevention: a systematic review and meta-analysis. *PLoS One*. 2014;9(1):e85029.

15. Attia M, Silva MA, Mirza DF. The marginal liver donor—an update. *Transpl Int*. 2008;21:713–724.

16. Stravitz RT, Kramer AH, Davern T, et al. Intensive care of patients with acute liver failure: recommendations of the U.S. Acute Liver Failure Study Group. *Crit Care Med*. 2007;35:2498–2508.

17. Rudnick MR, de Marchi L, Plotkin JS. Hemodynamic monitoring during liver transplantation: a state of the art review. *World J Hepatol*. 2015;7(10):1302.

18. Paugam-Burtz C, Kavafyan J, Merckx P, et al. Postreperfusion syndrome during liver transplantation for cirrhosis: outcome and predictors. *Liver Transpl*. 2009;15:522–529.

19. Colvin-Adams M. OPTN/SRTR 2012 Annual Data Report: heart. *Am J Transpl*. 2014;14(suppl 1):97–111.

20. Ramakrishna H, Jaroszewski DE, Arabia FA. Adult cardiac transplantation: a review of perioperative management. Part I. *Ann Card Anaesth*. 2009;12:71–78.

21. Fischer S. A review of cardiac transplantation. *Anesth Clin*. 2013;31:383–403.

22. Yusen R. The registry of International Society for Heart and Lung Transplantation—2014. *J Heart Lung Transpl*. 2014;3:1009.

23. Castillo M. Anesthetic management for lung transplantation. *Curr Opin Anesth*. 2011;24(1):32–36.

24. Verbeek GL. Intraoperative protective ventilation strategies in lung transplantation. *Transpl Rev*. 2013;27:30–35.

25. Kandaswamy R, Skeans MA, Gustafson SK, et al. OPTN/SRTR 2013 Annual Data Report: pancreas. *Am J Transpl*. 2015;15(suppl 2):1–20.

IV

# 37 OUTPATIENT ANESTHESIA

## David M. Dickerson and Jeffrey L. Apfelbaum

## INTRODUCTION

Outpatient anesthesia embodies many of the technologic and pharmacologic perioperative advances of the past 200 years. Currently, most surgery is conducted on an outpatient basis; patients arrive from home at a surgical facility, have an interventional procedure or surgery, and return home with their friends and families to heal. The outpatient surgical and anesthetic experience, however, begins well before, and extends well beyond, the day of surgery and anesthesia.

The vision for outpatient anesthesia began 100 years ago when Dr. Ralph Waters opened the first modern ambulatory surgery center (ASC) in downtown Sioux City, Iowa, "the Downtown Anesthesia Clinic."[1] In the late 1950s and early 1960s, outpatient surgery facilities were opened in Canada and the United Kingdom to relieve waitlists for elective surgery in hospitals. In 1962, Dr. David Cohen and Dr. John Dillon opened an outpatient surgery clinic, which would be a precursor to the modern "surgicenter." They proposed attention to quality measures, patient evaluation and selection, and availability of equipment with an emphasis on standardizing the patient pathway and flow. They demonstrated significant savings to patients and insurance companies with good outcomes.[2] In 1970 when inpatient surgery became more expensive, Drs. Wallace Reed and John Ford opened the first modern American ASC, the Phoenix Surgicenter, with the primary goal of decreasing the cost of surgery for patients while maintaining quality and safety. These sites embodied the value that surgery centers and office-based surgical practices still provide today: high quality, convenience, and cost savings to patients, their families, and the surgical team. Timeliness, effective operations, and excellent clinical outcomes regarding the patient experience are fundamental to that convenience.

The editors and publisher would like to thank Dr. Douglas G. Merrill for contributing to this chapter in the previous edition of this work. It has served as the foundation for the current chapter.

This chapter serves as a primer on the unique aspects of modern outpatient anesthesia practice with an emphasis on optimizing outcomes and the patient experience while modulating costs.

## OUTPATIENT ANESTHESIA IS DIFFERENT

In 1985, when it was founded, the Society for Ambulatory Anesthesia (SAMBA) sought to define the field of outpatient anesthesia. Through promulgating standards of care and a myriad of guidelines, SAMBA shaped clinical care, research, and education.[2] With technologic advances in surgery and pharmacologic advances in anesthesiology, many surgeries performed nationally shifted to the ambulatory setting and with the shift, the practice patterns of the ambulatory anesthesia provider soon evolved. Although not all anesthesia providers are expected to provide anesthesia for complicated cardiac valve replacement surgery, they may be expected to administer a successful ambulatory anesthetic. An ambulatory or outpatient anesthetic is not simply an anesthetic that is followed by a patient discharge home. An outpatient anesthetic procedure respects the patient's and surgeon's time as valuable resources and maximizes predictability through preparation and prevention of even the most minor morbidities in the hours to days that follow the procedure. Outpatient anesthesia is multidisciplinary, readily accessible, cost-effective, patient-centered, and at its penultimate, a model for the "Surgical Home" (also see Chapter 51).

## OUTPATIENT ANESTHESIA IS PATIENT-CENTERED

Ambulatory surgery requires a minimally invasive anesthetic with maximal emphasis on patient safety, comfort, and recovery. The challenges inherent to this requirement have led to innovative and highly patient-centered methods by ambulatory groups. To provide the best service, the expectations of the patient and his or her family should be understood.[3-5] Box 37.1 outlines these expectations. Patient expectations and familial support should be assessed and addressed before performing outpatient anesthesia and surgery to ensure that the facility and its personnel can meet the patient's expectations. To achieve

**Table 37.1** Various Venues for Outpatient Surgery

| Facility | Potential Ownership Structure |
|---|---|
| Hospital outpatient department | Hospital or investment group, cannot be physician owned as of 2010, PPACA mandate |
| Ambulatory surgery center | Hospital, physician group, non-physician investors, ownership may preclude referring providers such as primary care physicians to preserve compliance with the Stark antikickback legislation |
| Surgeon, dentist, or proceduralist's office | Hospital, physician group, nonphysician investors |

*PPACA,* Patient protection and affordable care act.

the goals desired by patients, families, and the medical team, the anesthesia providers and the facility's leadership should subscribe to specific aims. Key aims for an outpatient care facility are described in Box 37.2.

## DEFINING THE VALUE OF AMBULATORY CARE

Outpatient surgery can be performed in various settings, and is typically defined by a same-day "come and go" experience for patients. The procedures can take place near or far from a hospital, in an office, freestanding ASC, freestanding hospital outpatient department, or a hospital-based outpatient department. The facility ownership can be equally diverse (Table 37.1). In both Canada and the United States, ambulatory surgical facilities have an established safety record.[6,7] Through accreditation and multidisciplinary oversight, well-established patient safety-related standards of care, careful patient and procedure selection, and a specialized workforce, favorable outcomes in a large volume of procedures are accomplished with a modicum of complications and an extremely small or even rare mortality rate.

Ambulatory surgical care has several economic and social benefits for patients, surgeons, and insurance payers. The outpatient surgical setting offers significant cost reduction with excellent outcomes in patient safety and satisfaction. From 1981 to 2011, outpatient procedures grew almost 10-fold and accounted for 19% to more than 60% of all surgeries performed in the United States.[8] Surgeries take less time at ASCs than at an inpatient facility.[9,10] From 2008 to 2010, new freestanding ASCs opened primarily in economically advantageous markets with the least amount of competition.[11] Commercial payer rates, case volume, cost control, and specialized billing practices influence ASC profitability.

## SELECTION

### Patient

Enabling successful outcomes requires the careful selection, evaluation, and preparation of patients with regard to comorbid conditions and social structure. Selectivity enables providers to anticipate the likely duration of the intake and preparation process, anesthesia evaluation, surgical period, and recovery. The ideal surgical candidate may differ depending on the practitioners involved, scheduled procedure, and the practice setting. Patient and procedure selection aimed at avoiding unexpected events is undoubtedly the reason that ASCs are historically safe venues.[12] Yet, more must be known about the patient characteristics (e.g., comorbid conditions and baseline pathophysiologic derangements) that occasionally can lead to quality and safety failures.[13]

Many comorbid conditions require intraoperative and postoperative consideration. Failure to recognize comorbid conditions may result in increased cost and, more importantly, perioperative morbidity. Facilities typically implement care pathways to ensure consistent, evidence-based care. No single list of acceptable patients or case types will work for all venues. These conditions should be approached in an organized and meticulous fashion, incorporating the existing guidelines from professional societies to create a personalized patient plan while seeking to minimize complexity and maximize predictability.

### Practitioner

Ambulatory anesthesia providers embody a distinct set of skills that, like all subspecialists, set them apart from their peers. An ambulatory anesthesia provider appreciates the value of standardized work, effectively communicates with the team, values the patient's and surgeon's time, employs broad but cost-effective multimodal analgesia, and administers minimally invasive short-acting, fast emergence anesthesia for a rapid and safe recovery. The specialization of the team that works in an operating

suite is a primary determinant of the duration and predictability of operative room time and postanesthesia care unit (PACU) stay.[14-16]

### Medical Direction

Leadership is critical to the well-being of outpatient care facilities. Differences exist between the specific practices of the various outpatient anesthesia venues, yet standardized monitoring of patient safety, crisis preparedness, personnel education, and cost control are required regardless of site and depend on the direction provided by the facility's leadership team.

ASC and office anesthesia providers typically find their responsibilities expanded to fulfill the role of medical director, helping the site maintain compliance with regulatory and legislative directives. Continued compliance requires awareness of state, payer, and federal regulations for a multitude of issues including, but not limited to, keeping medication records, restrictions on facility size, maintenance of emergency equipment, sterilizing systems, personnel-to-patient ratio, and availability of recovery beds. Because anesthesia providers are often present for the longest periods at ASCs and offices, they typically become advisors to the administrative teams who manage the facility and frequently become the de facto medical director. There are no courses or curricula for becoming a medical director of an ambulatory surgery facility. The ambulatory track at the annual meetings of the American Society of Anesthesiologists (ASA) and the SAMBA offer a modicum of continuing education in medical direction and a network for guidance and mentorship. A highly functioning medical director is essential to the success of the daily workflow of the facility as well as to the patient experience and safety. Maintenance of accreditation is a shared responsibility of the facility spearheaded by the medical director.

### Multidisciplinary Leadership and Standardized Care

Unnecessary variation and a hierarchical culture that fosters a lack of transparency and teamwork are often the sources of unsafe, inefficient, and high-cost practices in the delivery of health care.[17] One effective response is for health care delivery teams to integrate published studies and guidelines with analysis of local outcomes. The data should then be developed. Algorithm-driven policies to modulate or eliminate unnecessary variation should be used.[18-20] The ASC or office is a uniquely suitable location for this work. It is a homogeneous environment in which fewer providers perform a smaller set of procedures when compared to the inpatient operating suite.[21] Patient-care decisions in the most stable clinical environments achieve the best outcomes and best practice.[22]

To achieve maximal predictability, consistent guidelines and directives for management of specific patient comorbid conditions should be agreed upon by surgeons, facility leadership, and anesthesia providers and written into durable policies and procedures for reference. The most effective means to develop standard care plans use multidisciplinary teams of physicians and nurses to assay the literature, visit model peer sites, create protocols with specific exclusion criteria, measure the clinical outcomes of practitioners who do and do not adopt the protocols, and report those outcomes to the entire team. Guidelines of this sort vary by venue and should be reevaluated frequently to keep up with the dynamic landscape of patient care. The expectation should be that providers follow set practice guidelines or care pathways, unless an alternative method induces equal or better results than the published "best practice." At that time leadership should reassess the currently existing practice guidelines.

### Ancillary Personnel

The ancillary care staff in the outpatient setting is a specialized workforce that contributes substantively to the achievement of the facility's goals.[14] Specialized nursing and anesthesia personnel typically are trained and rehearsed in emergency care in the freestanding or office setting because of the facility's relative isolation. ASC operating room providers are often required by accrediting bodies to complete Advanced Cardiac Life Support (ACLS) and Pediatric Advanced Life Support (PALS) training because these individuals are primary caregivers in an emergency situation, usually for a longer period than is a nurse in the operating room of a tertiary care facility.

### Procedure

Much like patient selection, procedure selection seeks to minimize complexity to ensure a predictable operative course and recovery. A facility's resources, personnel, and patient population may make complex procedures possible. Among the majority of ambulatory surgical procedures are lens and cataract operations, orthopedic procedures, and laparoscopic cholecystectomy[23] (also see Chapters 29, 31, and 32). Increased complexity should be weighed against the potential for case delays, delayed discharge, unanticipated admission, and their impact on patient satisfaction and facility efficiency. Patients who have surgeries with a duration more than 1 hour and who are ASA physical status III or IV, of advanced age (also see Chapter 35), and have a large body mass index (BMI) have an increased risk of unanticipated admission.[24]

Some combinations of elective outpatient procedures increase the risk of venous thromboembolism.[25] Outpatient cholecystectomy has specifically been reported safe and, as a consequence, is frequently performed as an ambulatory procedure.[26] Yet, same-day discharge after appendectomy may be a challenge. Emergency laparoscopic appendectomy may be feasible in an ASC when a predictive scoring system is utilized to select candidates who need less than 12 hours of postoperative observation.[27] However, many patients need their appendectomy performed at hours when the ambulatory center is not open.[27] Hospital admission or observation times can be reduced when patients meet the validated criteria for a truncated observation.

Postoperative complication rates resulting in revisits may also determine procedure selection. Same-day thyroidectomy and parathyroidectomy have good postoperative morbidity and mortality profiles but may require revisits within the first postoperative week for hypocalcemia, bleeding, seroma, or hematoma.[28] Such complications can result in acute postoperative airway compromise, which strongly suggests that these cases be performed in locations where inpatient care can be obtained expeditiously.

## Place (Surgical Facility)

Maximizing predictability also influences the site selected for surgery. Location and resources typically foster or preclude procedures of significant complexity. Access to hospital-based care must be considered when nonhospital facilities are selected for the care of sicker patients or more complex procedures. If 98% of patients who have a specific surgery can be discharged home the same day, but 2% require overnight observation, that specific surgery should take place where 23-hour postoperative observation is possible. A hospital transfer, which is a rare event, serves as a quality metric for outpatient surgery.[29,30] The rate of hospital-based acute care encounters via the emergency department in one series was nearly 30-fold more frequent than hospital transfer.[31] The modern challenge for outpatient anesthesia is to safely incorporate more complex cases into the ambulatory setting.

### Office-Based Anesthesia

Historically, ASCs were thought to be a safer location to perform surgery than an office.[32] The reasons given for the supposed discrepancy were the careful attention to case and patient selection as well as the on-site preparation practiced by freestanding ASCs.[33] A 2014 study indicates that office-based anesthesia can be as safe as hospital- and ASC-based procedures.[34] Office accreditation, proper procedure and patient selection, provider credentialing, facility accreditation, patient safety checklists, and implementing professional society guidelines improve safety in office-based surgery.

Dental surgery, plastic surgery, and an ever-widening variety of surgical procedures are now being performed in offices rather than ambulatory surgery facilities or hospitals. The office setting is convenient, private, and cost-efficient. The facility requirements, case selection, and anesthesia techniques for office locations have been well defined.[35-37] The outcomes of office-based procedures have generally been excellent. A few notably high-profile

IV

tragedies after procedures in offices highlight the need for vigilant anesthesia care and oversight, regardless of the site of service.[38] A comparison of risk for anesthesia and surgery in an office setting, ASCs, or hospitals is difficult because reporting mechanisms for all are insufficient.[39] The Institute for Safety in Office-Based Surgery has developed a safety checklist to improve preparedness for office-based procedures.[40] Most remote-site injuries related to anesthesia occur as a result of inadequate monitoring, not errors in patient selection.[41] Factors associated with increased risk in the office setting include the use of unqualified surgical or anesthesia staff, a lack of proper equipment and training for resuscitation and other emergencies, and a lack of access to hospitals for the occasional life-threatening emergency.[42] If these factors are eliminated, office-based anesthesia administered by qualified providers in an accredited facility appears to be equally safe.[7]

### Simulation and Drills: Site Preparedness

Site preparation for unanticipated emergency situations must be meticulous. ASC and office personnel should simulate common emergencies to enhance system and provider readiness for such events. A SAMBA-endorsed publication provides in-depth drill scenarios with educational material for outpatient practices to assess and improve on preparedness and responsiveness for common emergencies.[43] Like their real counterparts, simulations and drills can be stressful and should be followed by debriefings that emphasize the potential improvements in system design and teamwork rather than individual failings.[44,45] Simulations may also afford insight into needed changes in patient and procedure selection and the policies and guidelines that shape them.

## THE PERIOPERATIVE JOURNEY OF AN AMBULATORY SURGICAL PATIENT

### An Itinerary for Success

In the ambulatory setting, the patient experience begins well before arrival at an ASC and lasts long after discharge from the recovery room. The need for predictability in ambulatory surgery necessitates a formalized discrete itinerary. The patient flow schematic depicted in Fig. 37.1 illustrates the patient's journey from selection through postsurgical follow-up and beyond. The ambulatory schematic may differ from site to site but in general several phases exist. Understanding the phases of care and the goals and challenges associated with each one is essential to delivering high value ambulatory care.

### Preoperative Phase: Days to Weeks Before Surgery

Patient, procedure, and site selection take place preliminarily in the surgeon's office and are congruent with the

guidelines, policies, and procedures developed by the medical site's leadership. The preoperative screening of candidates identifies patient characteristics that jeopardize predictability or create complexity or risk in the intraoperative, postoperative, or postdischarge phases of care (also see Chapter 13).

### Assessing for Adequate Social Support

The patient screening queries about social support, which includes an escort on the day of surgery, a driver to take the patient home, and a caregiver for postsurgical care and assistance with activities of daily living.[46] On the day of surgery, every patient should have an escort on site or immediately available. A driver to take the patient home also should be immediately available. Some centers require a signed statement by the patient that he or she will have a caregiver for the first night after surgery. The escort is present during patient admission and preparation for surgery. If the patient is not able to obtain an escort, driver, or caregiver the night after surgery, the procedure is not scheduled. These requirements are not popular with a few patients, but early identification of patients who lack these resources reduces patient risk and the potential for case cancellation of surgery on the day of surgery. The only patients who might be released alone are those who received only a small dose of local anesthesia and no other anesthesia-related drugs.[46-49]

### Evaluation and Testing: Before the Day of Surgery

Outpatient centers develop workflows for patient screening to avoid cancellations on the day of surgery and to ensure selection of the optimal care setting. Patients are deemed outpatient surgical candidates by their surgeon, but medical issues relevant to intraoperative care and recovery may preclude this outpatient status. The preliminary clinical history submitted at the time of surgical evaluation drives the initial preoperative evaluation and can be augmented by health assessment forms completed by the patient. Relevant health status can be assessed with a form completed on site for preoperative surgical evaluation. The completed form provides a review of systems, medical history, and identification of social support. The form is then transmitted to the surgery facility's anesthesia group with the booking for the case. A licensed practitioner from the group (physician, advanced practice nurse, certified registered nurse anesthetist [CRNA], or anesthesiology assistant) reviews the forms and determines whether a follow-up phone call is needed based on surgery type and patient comorbid condition. The status of medical conditions is reviewed and a preliminary anesthesia evaluation is then conducted. The need for further testing or evaluation is decided based on medical society guidelines, facility policies, and the anesthesia provider's judgment.

Testing should be cost-effective and evidence-based. Preoperative testing is overused in patients undergoing low-risk, ambulatory surgery despite a lack of influence on postoperative outcomes.[50] A systematic review has corroborated these findings in elective, noncardiac surgery as well.[51] Although practice in ASCs and office settings has reduced the cost of care delivery, routine preoperative evaluation for low-risk outpatient surgery remains costly. In 2011, 53% of Medicare beneficiaries undergoing cataract surgery had a preoperative evaluation. The health care costs for this cohort in the month preceding the cataract surgery were $12.4 million more than in the preceding 11 months.[52] A subsequent Cochrane Review found that routine testing beforehand did not increase safety for cataract surgery.[53] Yet not all ambulatory procedures have the favorable risk profile of cataract surgery and its minor anesthetic exposure. Preoperative screening should determine a patient's eligibility for specific outpatient procedures and the setting in which they are performed.

According to published guidelines there is a shift from routine testing to risk stratification-driven specific testing to modify risk and stabilize an existing medical condition. A 2014 review offers current evidence regarding central topics in risk assessment and management for the ambulatory surgical patient.[54] Successful ambulatory anesthesia groups use screening paradigms according to guidelines and communication with patients before the day of surgery to minimize last-minute cancellations, delayed discharge, unanticipated admission, and patient dissatisfaction. Several important clinical issues that should trigger further discussion before the day of surgery are reviewed here.

### Cardiovascular Risk Assessment (Also See Chapter 13)

The 2014 American College of Cardiology/American Heart Association (ACC/AHA) guidelines offer an

# The Journey of an Ambulatory Surgical Patient

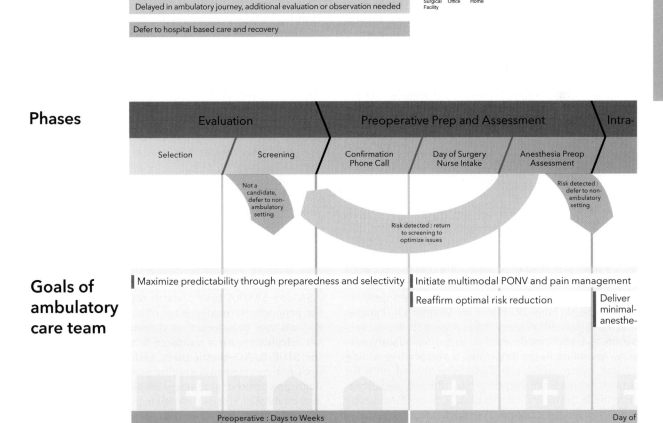

**Fig. 37.1** The journey of an ambulatory surgical patient. (Drawn by design researcher Amanda Rosenberg.)

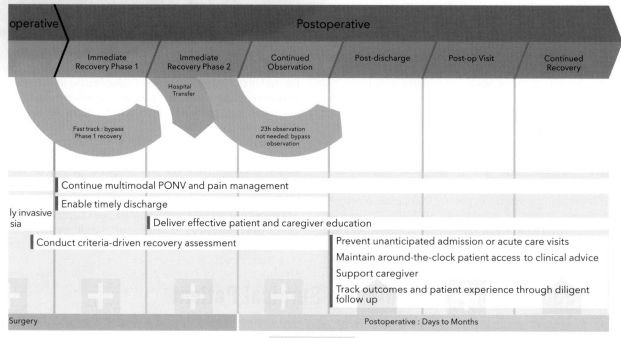

**Fig. 37.1, cont'd**

algorithm for the perioperative cardiovascular evaluation and care of patients with coronary artery disease who are having noncardiac surgery.[55] Because most ambulatory surgery procedures have infrequent perioperative cardiac complications, the guidelines recommend that a patient demonstrate a functional capacity of at least four metabolic equivalent (MET) values for activities; for example, the ability to asymptomatically ascend two flights of stairs. The risk of major adverse cardiac events depends on the surgical procedure and patient characteristics. The guidelines recommend utilizing one of two risk-calculating methods to determine combined risk before surgery. The surgical risk calculator of the National Surgical Quality Improvement Program or the revised cardiac risk index identifies high-risk patients.[56-58]

After detailed assessment and risk stratification, ambulatory procedures may be attempted in patients with a risky profile once medical status issues have been properly analyzed and addressed. Several key characteristics are associated with increased risk of perioperative complications (Table 37.2) (also see Chapter 13). Patients with the associated characteristics require in-depth evaluation and may not be candidates for ambulatory surgery. According to the guidelines, a preoperative resting 12-lead electrocardiogram (ECG) is performed only for patients with known coronary heart disease, significant arrhythmia, peripheral arterial disease, or cerebrovascular disease having intermediate- or high-risk procedures.[55] Such risk assessment is best performed well before the day of surgery (also see Chapter 13).

**Obstructive Sleep Apnea (Also See Chapters 27 and 50)**

Obstructive sleep apnea (OSA) influences patient physiology and intraoperative and postoperative care.[59] OSA activates sympathetic neurons and leads to hypertension and cardiovascular abnormalities that can cause morbidity or even death perioperatively.[60] OSA, which is undiagnosed in most patients,[61] increases the potential for cerebrovascular events, myocardial infarction, bleeding, perioperative respiratory events, difficult intubation, and death.[62,63] This diagnosis is critical to establish before ambulatory surgery.

In an ambulatory surgical cohort, patients with established OSA, regardless of severity or compliance with continuous positive airway pressure (CPAP) therapy, had no unanticipated admissions or delayed discharges, suggesting good patient selection and monitoring.[64] The ability to identify patients with OSA preoperatively may improve outcomes through risk stratification and preparation or through referral to a hospital setting. The ASA and SAMBA have updated separate guidelines on the perioperative management of patients with OSA.[65,66] Patients can be screened at the surgical evaluation or via telephone with a validated screening tool such as the STOP-BANG questionnaire (Table 37.3).[67] The ASA does not recommend a specific screening tool. A thorough preoperative assessment identifies patients at risk and establishes whether associated comorbid conditions are well managed. A licensed practitioner (physician, registered nurse [RN], CRNA, anesthesiology assistant) should screen patients with known or suspected OSA in a

| Table 37.2 | Clinical Factors That Increase Risk of Perioperative Complications |
|---|---|

| Organ System | Symptom or Medical Concern |
|---|---|
| Cardiovascular | New-onset or unstable angina<br>Hypertensive emergency<br>Myocardial infarction within 6 months<br>Newly diagnosed cardiac dysrhythmia<br>Decompensated heart failure<br>Severe valvular disease<br>Drug-eluting stent within 12 months<br>Bare metal stent within 4 weeks |
| Pulmonary | Symptomatic bronchospasm<br>Productive cough<br>Increased work of breathing<br>Severe obstructive sleep apnea<br>Hypoxia (decreased oxygen saturation) |
| Renal | Unknown or insufficient recent dialysis therapy |
| Endocrine | Symptomatic hypoglycemia<br>Symptomatic hyperglycemia |
| Neurologic | Recent cerebrovascular accident or unmanaged transient ischemic attack<br>Dementia or delirium |
| Hematologic | Insufficient cessation of anticoagulants |

| Table 37.3 | Components of the STOP-BANG Questionnaire and Score Interpretation |
|---|---|

| Components (each worth 1 point) | Interpretation of Scores |
|---|---|
| **S**noring<br>**T**iredness during the day<br>**O**bserved apnea<br>**P**ressure: increased blood pressure<br>**B**ody mass index (BMI) > 35 kg/m²<br>**A**ge > 50 years<br>**N**eck circumference > 40 cm<br>**G**ender = male | <3 points: Low likelihood of OSA<br>3 to 6 points: Adequate positive screen, further testing needed<br>≥5 points: High likelihood of OSA |

OSA, Obstructive sleep apnea.

systematic fashion before surgery via telephone at a minimum. The assessment confirms the presence or absence of an OSA diagnosis, compliance with CPAP therapy, the presence of a CPAP machine and well-fitting mask, and control of associated comorbid conditions. The type of surgery, the ability to minimize opioid exposure via local or regional anesthetic techniques, and the facility's ability to treat the complications associated with undiagnosed or uncontrolled OSA and its comorbid conditions may determine suitability. An inability to provide this heightened level of care should defer management to a hospital setting. Table 37.4 lists the comorbid conditions and perioperative concerns associated with OSA and patient characteristics associated with sleep-disordered breathing.

### Diabetes Mellitus (Also See Chapter 29)
There is no hemoglobin $A_{1c}$ ($HbA_{1c}$) value that precludes a patient from having outpatient surgery; however, adverse perioperative outcomes are associated with an $HbA_{1c}$ that is more than 7%. Poor glucose control may indicate the presence of other organ system dysfunction including cardiovascular and renal comorbid conditions, making the specific ambulatory procedure relevant. The underlying principle on the day of surgery is to prevent hypoglycemia while perioperatively maintaining basal physiologic insulin levels. The preoperative degree of baseline blood glucose control, end-organ dysfunction from hyperglycemia, and the current therapy must be known. Such information is obtained before the day of surgery. A SAMBA consensus statement provides practical expertise in perioperative management of the diabetic patient in the ambulatory setting.[68]

### Chronic Pain (Also See Chapter 44)
Patients with chronic pain, opioid dependence, or history of severe uncontrolled postsurgical pain or who are receiving buprenorphine or methadone therapy are best identified well in advance of the day of surgery for proper treatment planning. With pain and nausea as common causes of delayed discharge and unanticipated admission, a formal plan for postoperative pain control and follow-up should be established for patients with potential tolerance or intolerance to pain therapy, or for those patients who are currently under the care of a pain physician[29,69,70] (also see Chapters 40 and 44).

In the absence of neural blockade, opioid-dependent patients may require a 100% to 200% dose increase in baseline opioids postoperatively. Such "uptitration" may not be within the scope of practice of some surgeons or surgical facilities. For some surgeries or patients, regional anesthesia may not be indicated. Preoperative screening and planning may reduce pain-related unanticipated admission, discharge delays, or emergency department visits. Patients with chronic pain may have little faith preoperatively in their ability to go home immediately after surgery. Such fear or expectation should be identified preoperatively and addressed through treatment planning, patient education, and possible hospital-based care.

**Table 37.4** Comorbid Conditions and Periprocedural Complications Associated With Obstructive Sleep Apnea (OSA)

| Comorbid Conditions | Disease-Related Potential Complications | Characteristics That May Increase OSA |
|---|---|---|
| Hypertension | Difficult mask ventilation | Down syndrome |
| Arrhythmias | Difficult intubation | Neuromuscular disease |
| Cor pulmonale | Oxygen desaturation and hypoxemia | Cerebral palsy |
| Ischemic heart disease | Exacerbation of cardiac comorbid | History of difficult intubation |
| Diabetes | conditions | Enlarged tongue or tonsil size |
| Stroke | Delayed extubation | |
| Daytime sleepiness | Risk of reintubation | |
| Depression | Prolonged recovery room stay | |
| Decreased vitality and social functioning on SF-36 (reduced quality of life) | Hypoxic brain injury | |
| | Death | |

*SF-36,* Short form (36) health survey.

## Preoperative Phase: Day(s) Before Surgery

Once preoperative assessment, evaluation, and preparation are completed and the results reviewed, the patient's appointment with the facility is confirmed (also see Chapter 13). At that time, information regarding an escort and ride is also verified. A preoperative phone call several days before surgery confirms arrival time, reiterates medication and oral intake instructions, answers patient questions, and reconfirms the availability of the escort, ride, and postoperative caregiver. Within 24 hours of surgery a designated facility employee confirms the information about arrival time and need for an escort and ride. These measures reduce case delay and cancellation as well as the consumption of resources required for caring for an abandoned patient.

The days or weeks preceding the surgery are ample time for preliminary assessment of the patient's candidacy by the anesthesia group. The anesthesia provider may not be assigned to the case until the day before. Upon assignment, the final preparations commence. Health assessment forms are available the day before surgery for review by the anesthesia provider who will be caring for the patient. Timely review detects omissions or oversights in treatment planning so that additional directives or treatment can be added. Although such last-minute preparation is not ideal, even that is not possible if the chart review is delayed until the following morning.

## Preoperative Phase: Day of Surgery

### The Anesthesia Preoperative Assessment (Also See Chapter 13)

The ASA and Center for Medicaid Services (CMS) have determined that a preoperative review of the patient's medical and social history and a physical examination by an anesthesia provider are necessary.[71] As more complicated procedures and patients are accepted in the outpatient setting, the act of conducting a detailed history cannot be abbreviated. Anesthesia providers frequently uncover significant changes in patient health that can affect postoperative and long-term health.[72,73] Because physical status correlates with unanticipated admission and delayed discharge, a thorough assessment of the medical status of a patient may affect outcome. A brief motivational interview and counseling by anesthesia providers on preventive health issues, such as smoking cessation, can also be effective with minor time commitment.[74]

When patients present for day surgery not in their usual state of health, the anesthesia provider is faced with the challenging question: should we proceed with surgery for this patient today? The essence of this question is whether a patient's risk is increased. If not, does the added complexity jeopardize the predictability of the procedure and the anesthetic effects? The anesthesia provider asks this untimely question when patients become acutely ill, when the preoperative preadmission evaluation is incomplete, or when patients are noncompliant with previous recommendations for essential consultation, testing, or therapy. Several clinical conditions significantly impact outcome and are described in Table 37.2. The decision to proceed with surgery is always an individualized assessment best decided in an evidence-based, multidisciplinary manner.

### Acute Pulmonary Conditions

If a patient has been given therapy sufficient to achieve optimal medical condition (e.g., medications have been reviewed by the primary physician and no other therapy is believed to be needed) but is still symptomatic (e.g., wheezing at rest, a bedside forced expiratory time of less than 6 seconds, unable to climb a flight of stairs because of dyspnea) or has pulmonary hypertension, surgery should be performed in the hospital environment where respiratory therapy services are ideal.[75-78] Complicated pediatric airway surgery is not scheduled for a freestanding center but may be performed in a hospital-based center if pediatric intensivists and respiratory therapists with pediatric expertise are readily accessible (also see Chapter 34).

Present or recent acute upper respiratory infection (URI) is, in some instances, sufficient reason for postponing a case because of the potential for respiratory complications perioperatively. Supraglottic edema, stridor, laryngospasm, desaturation, and coughing can occur during general anesthesia in patients with URI, particularly when endotracheal intubation has been performed.[79] Although the use of supraglottic airway devices may be associated with fewer problems in these patients, there is still an opportunity for severely negative outcomes, such as laryngeal edema after use of a supraglottic airway device in a patient with a recent URI.[80] The choice of a particular type of anesthetic or technique, the value of an antisialagogue, or the decision to extubate the trachea while the patient is deeply or lightly anesthetized is not clear.[81,82]

Elective surgery can proceed in patients with a current or recent mild URI if the procedure can be performed safely without endotracheal intubation, the patient has no other cardiac or pulmonary problems (i.e., congenital heart disease, asthma, or chronic obstructive pulmonary disease [COPD]), and the surgical procedure will not impact the airway.[83] Severe, functionally compromising active, or recent pulmonary symptoms necessitate scrutiny and possible delay in elective surgery if more than a local anesthetic is required. Even then, the patient may best initially seek primary care rather than a procedure that could further limit function or activities of daily living during recovery.

### Hypertension (Also See Chapters 13 and 25)

Patients with hypertension requiring medication who undergo surgery have as much as a 50% more frequent risk of adverse cardiovascular problems in the first 30 days after a procedure.[84,85] Although angiotensin-converting enzyme (ACE) inhibitors improve hypertension, they may be associated with profound hypotension after induction of general anesthesia.[86,87] Others have questioned this conclusion.[88] For patients who experience postinduction of anesthesia hypotension, postoperative morbidity and mortality rates increase.[85] The decision to omit antihypertensive drugs preoperatively may increase arterial blood pressure even in a short 24-hour period. Although sedation and general anesthesia can decrease arterial blood pressure, the neurohumoral response to surgical stimuli can be profound, resulting in postoperative lability and difficult-to-treat hypertension in an at-risk population.

If new-onset angina, chronic unstable angina, new cardiac arrhythmia, signs of decompensated congestive heart failure, or recent angioplasty or percutaneous coronary stenting are identified, elective ambulatory surgery is best deferred.[55,89,90] No set arterial blood pressure reading calls for cancellation of surgery, but severe preoperative hypertension should trigger a multidisciplinary discussion. The patient's baseline arterial blood pressure range is a helpful reference for intraoperative management and

for deciding whether a surgery should be delayed. If there are symptoms of hypertensive emergency, the ambulatory procedure is rescheduled, and the patient is transferred to acute care.

### The Difficult Airway (Also See Chapter 16)

The "difficult" airway presents a serious challenge in the ambulatory setting. A history of difficult airway should be identified well before the day of surgery through preoperative communication with the patient or review of the health questionnaire. On the day of surgery, a preoperative airway assessment is requisite for reduction of risk.[91,92] A facility should be prepared for comprehensive airway management for every case. The occult lingual tonsil is defined by its unanticipated nature.[93] For this reason and many others, the equipment required for fully employing the ASA's difficult airway algorithm should be immediately available and regularly checked for functionality.[94-96] If regional or neuraxial anesthesia is selected for the patient with a known difficult airway, the contingency for inadequate anesthesia should be discussed preoperatively with the patient and surgeon to ensure all parties appreciate the risks "a touch of sedation" could carry. Endotracheal intubation with the patient awake (i.e., may include a small dose of preoperative medication) may be the safest option despite its perceived delay in workflow.

### Pregnancy Testing (Also See Chapters 33 and 34)

Some facilities require pregnancy tests for all women of childbearing age, and others offer it only to those women who say they may be pregnant. In one study, mandating that all women undergo pregnancy testing resulted in a cost of over $3000 per positive test, a particularly troubling price in view of an unknown level of benefit.[97] A separate study found that the cost per positive result was $1,005.32 with an unknown benefit of not performing elective surgery on a pregnant woman.[98] Some providers screen patients during preoperative evaluation: "Is there any chance you could be pregnant today?" A "yes" response triggers a test, and a "no" response triggers a statement of confirmation and further counseling: "If there is any chance, we should confirm to make sure we do not unknowingly expose a developing fetus to anesthesia."

### Preoperative Medications (Also See Chapter 13)

Anxious patients may benefit from a variety of nonpharmacologic techniques for anxiolysis including aromatherapy or listening to music of their choice.[99-101] Administration of short-acting benzodiazepines or 1200 mg of gabapentin may also improve the anxious or catastrophizing patient's perioperative experience.[102] Administration of acetaminophen, gabapentin, or pregabalin, and nonsteroidal antiinflammatory drugs (NSAIDs) during the preoperative period initiates preventive analgesia

IV

**Table 37.5** Benefits and Adverse Effects of Anesthesia Techniques

| Anesthesia Type | Benefits | Adverse Effects |
|---|---|---|
| General inhalational | Neuromuscular blockade and intraperitoneal procedures<br>Maximal intraoperative airway control when performed with intubation | PONV, PDNV<br>Airway injury<br>Cognitive dysfunction<br>Delayed discharge<br>Hyperalgesia<br>Succinylcholine-induced myalgia<br>Residual neuromuscular blockade |
| General intravenous | Less PONV with propofol<br>Neuromuscular blockade and intraperitoneal procedures<br>Maximal intraoperative airway control with intubation | Airway injury<br>Cognitive dysfunction<br>Delayed discharge<br>Hyperalgesia (remifentanil)<br>Succinylcholine-induced myalgia<br>Residual neuromuscular blockade |
| Regional | Prolonged postoperative analgesia<br>Less PONV<br>Less risk of airway injury<br>Rapid recovery<br>Reduced exposure to anesthesia | Local anesthetic systemic toxicity<br>Peripheral nerve injury<br>Spinal headache with neuraxial blockade<br>Equipment costs<br>Specialized training<br>Recall of operation and the associated stress |
| Monitored anesthesia care (MAC) | Less exposure to anesthetic doses<br>Rapid recovery<br>Less PONV/PDNV<br>Low incidence of sore throat | Minimal airway control<br>Patient dissatisfaction from unexpected recall<br>Oversedation<br>Operating room fires with an open system<br>Hypercarbia, hypoxemia<br>Patient discomfort |

*PONV*, Postoperative nausea and vomiting; *PDNV*, postdischarge nausea and vomiting.

so that serum concentrations are therapeutic before surgical stimuli, potentially reducing secondary hyperalgesia, postoperative opioid requirements, and opioid-related side effects.[103-105] Preoperative administration of dexamethasone also may improve the patient's emotional state, physical state, and pain dimensions postoperatively.[106] Postoperative nausea and vomiting (PONV) in the high-risk patient can be mitigated preoperatively with transdermal scopolamine (also see Chapter 39). A scopolamine patch applied before transfer to the operating room can be as effective as droperidol or ondansetron in prevention of PONV in adults.[107]

## Intraoperative Phase: Anesthesia Techniques

The overall goals of outpatient anesthesia today are unchanged from those espoused many decades ago by Drs. Ralph Waters, Wallace Reed, and John Ford: convenience, small cost, patient safety and care in alignment with the patient's and surgeon's goals. Accordingly, the techniques of anesthesia should be chosen for safety and to diminish or eliminate pain, nausea and vomiting, and prolonged cognitive impairment postoperatively. Anesthetic techniques are selected to enable timely recovery. Efficiency, however, should not put patients at risk or

jeopardize their comfort or satisfaction. For example, with remifentanil recovery is reliable and rapid, but the risk of hyperalgesia makes it unsuitable for patients having painful surgery or a history of chronic pain.[108] Table 37.5 lists the benefits and adverse effects of various anesthesia types.

The anesthetic selection of sedation, general anesthesia, or regional anesthesia depends on several factors: patient characteristics, expectations and positioning, surgical anatomy and technique, surgeon preference, anesthesia provider preference, and risk-reducing or efficiency-driven policies or facility guidelines (also see Chapter 14). Although no anesthetic technique is best for all patients, standardizing care may improve outcomes. Treatment pathways require patient education, patient selection, and potentially, various detours in the pathway for individualized care within the standardization. Presence of psychological concerns, need for a language translator, or other patient comorbid conditions may exclude a patient from the typically selected pathway.[22] Ethically, a fine line exists between preserving outpatient center efficiency and impeding access to care. Such deviation from the "typical" pathway should be identified in advance and accounted for in the day's schedule or the overall planned utilization of personnel and operating rooms.

## Sedation

Monitored anesthesia care (MAC), a term of anesthesia billing, describes sedation by an anesthesia provider. Titrated sedation and continuous monitoring often transition the patient in and out of general anesthesia, as required by changes in patient or surgical conditions. Only providers with anesthesia privileges should administer this technique. Thus sedation/general anesthesia by an anesthesia provider or MAC differs from other light sedation techniques used by nonanesthesia personnel.

Deep sedation (i.e., in between light sedation and general anesthesia) is chosen when general or regional anesthesia is considered too invasive or prolonged for the procedure or patient. The potential for catastrophic outcomes with deep sedation may be equal to or more than that associated with general anesthesia, with particular risks for oversedation and operating room fires.[109] Vigilance and monitoring are critical during deep sedation because of the possibility of hypoventilation and hypoxemia.[41] When choosing deep sedation or general anesthesia, the possible need for oxygen supplementation has to be considered. If the procedure will be so uncomfortable that the patient must be predominantly unresponsive, increased levels of supplemental oxygen may be required. When combined with electrocautery and surgery proximate to the airway, deep sedation without a secured airway may carry the risk of combustion from accumulated oxygen under the surgical drapes. General anesthesia in a closed system allows for safer supplemental oxygen delivery. A history of OSA, uncontrolled gastroesophageal reflux disease, or difficult endotracheal intubation or ventilation may create challenges or conflicts in patient safety if deeper planes of anesthesia are anticipated during deep sedation.

## Regional Anesthesia (Also See Chapters 17 and 18)

Regional anesthesia—alone or in conjunction with general anesthesia or sedation—may benefit patients and the facility.[110-112] The modern ambulatory anesthesia provider is an expert in regional anesthesia who modifies tried and true techniques while learning and applying new techniques as they are discovered. Performing regional nerve blocks in a preoperative area for patients undergoing orthopedic procedures decreases overall anesthesia time without increasing turnover time, when compared to general anesthesia.[113] PACU discharge time can be shortened and the immediate postoperative period made more pleasant for the patient.[114,115] Between 1994 and 2006 the use of peripheral nerve blocks during ambulatory ankle arthroscopy procedures increased from 6% to 26%, reflecting increased utilization by practitioners.[116] The use of regional catheters, in the presence of safe postdischarge conditions, can reduce pain for days after surgery while improving rehabilitation.[117-119]

Regional anesthesia techniques have revolutionized hernia and breast surgery. Paravertebral regional block decreases opioid exposure, PONV, urinary retention, and pain scores as compared to general or neuraxial anesthetics.[120-123] Multilevel paravertebral blocks combined with total intravenous anesthesia for breast tumor resection were reliable and improved postoperative analgesia, enhanced quality of recovery, and expedited PACU discharge compared with inhaled anesthetics or opioid-based general anesthesia.[124] Paravertebral block for patients undergoing mastectomy may decrease the incidence of chronic postsurgical chest wall pain and tumor recurrence or metastasis.[124-126] The serratus anterior plane block and pectoral nerve blocks (pecs I and II) are novel interfascial plane blocks for breast surgery analgesia.[127,128]

## Central Neuraxial Anesthesia (Also See Chapter 17)

Neuraxial blockade, with or without sedation, has been reported to reduce the incidence of PONV and pain after lower extremity, gynecologic, and abdominal surgery and for patients with chronic respiratory disease.[129,130] A short-duration "speed spinal" provides substantial value in the ambulatory setting.[131] Spinal doses of lidocaine, mepivacaine, and 2-chloroprocaine provide superb anesthesia for shorter procedures such as knee arthroscopy and inguinal hernia repair.[132-135] Low-dose spinal bupivacaine (e.g., 4 mg with 20 μg fentanyl) is effective, quick-acting, and rapidly resolving for transurethral procedures in elderly males, without delaying discharge.[136] For outpatient knee arthroscopy, 7.5 mg of 0.5% hyperbaric ropivacaine provides sufficient anesthesia, but with a duration of up to 2.5 hours and a time to discharge of up to 3.5 hours, much longer than with 2-chloroprocaine.[137,138]

## General Anesthesia

The natural airway creates a potential for risk for some patient-procedure combinations, especially those involving surgery in the airway. The decision to provide general anesthesia with or without endotracheal intubation should be determined by patient and procedure-related risk factors.[92] General anesthesia carries the potential for increased risk of PONV, postdischarge nausea and vomiting (PDNV), airway injury, postoperative hypothermia, postoperative cognitive dysfunction, and delayed discharge when compared to deep sedation or regional anesthesia. General anesthesia may be necessary, however, for procedures that require neuromuscular blockade or peritoneal insufflation. Some patients may refuse regional anesthesia or have conditions that contraindicate it, thus necessitating a general anesthetic.

General anesthesia can be accomplished through total intravenous techniques, combined maintenance with volatile anesthesia and intravenous drugs, or solely with volatile anesthetics. Nitrous oxide may be an adjunct to general anesthesia. Limiting duration of nitrous oxide exposure has been shown to reduce the risk of PONV.[139]

**IV**

---

**Box 37.3** Five General Principles for Improving Patient Outcomes and Experience

1. Thorough preoperative evaluation, patient and case selection, anesthesia delivery decisions, and postoperative recovery room care are required to provide optimal patient outcomes.[29,69,70]
2. Without opioids and with multimodal analgesia, postoperative pain and nausea decrease, cognitive function is preserved, and patient satisfaction is high.[142,143]
3. When possible choose only regional anesthesia (peripheral nerve block) or a combined regional-general anesthesia technique to improve patient satisfaction.[111]
4. Use evidence-based, preemptive antiemetic therapy for most patients given a general anesthetic.[144-146]
5. Favor total intravenous anesthesia over inhaled anesthetics for general anesthesia to improve patient outcomes.[147]

---

Infrequent perioperative morbidity is possible with total intravenous anesthesia or volatile anesthesia. Low-dose propofol infusions, multimodal analgesia, and antiemetic methods further reduce the postoperative risk for nausea and vomiting after general anesthesia.[140,141] The literature supports several principles for anesthetic selection described in Box 37.3.[111,142-147]

## Postoperative Phase: Beginning of Recovery

As patients emerge from anesthesia, they are transferred to the recovery phase of care (also see Chapter 39). A standard workflow for signout should be defined for communication from the operating room to the recovery room prior to patient transfer. Anesthetic type, patient comorbid conditions, procedure type, and the availability of recovery room personnel may dictate timing for patient transfer from operating room to recovery. For example, an experienced pediatric nurse may routinely be able to adequately monitor a still deeply anesthetized (but otherwise healthy) pediatric patient (also see Chapter 34). However, a less specialized postanesthetic nurse may provide better care if pediatric (or less than healthy) patients are fully awake and maintaining an airway before leaving the operating suite.

There are three phases of recovery: early, intermediate, and late. The early recovery (phase I) occurs until anesthesia or surgically induced derangements in protective reflexes and motor function resolve. Patients matriculate to phase II recovery when they meet these criteria and have well-controlled nausea and pain. Some patients meet these criteria prior to leaving the operating room and can be admitted directly to phase II. The modified Aldrete criteria and White criteria provide scoring systems for evaluating phase II readiness and are described in Table 37.6.[148,149] Phase II persists until discharge criteria are met, and phase III occurs at home as the patient returns to his or her preoperative physiologic state.

Upon arrival in the appropriate recovery setting, the anesthesia provider verbally relays the operative and anesthetic course, patient history and condition, and any other key clinical data for the responsible recovery nurse. Handoff forms or checklists can improve retention of important patient and perioperative information as communication failures contribute to preventable medical errors and resultant adverse events.[150,151]

### Fast-Tracking: Phase I Bypass

Some patients are transferred from the operating room directly to phase II of recovery, bypassing the first stage and potentially the PACU. Fast-tracking is suitable for patients who do not require airway support and have stable cardiopulmonary indices and adequate analgesia. Fast-tracking rapidly reunites patients with their loved ones, for a better experience for the patient and family, and may decrease cost in the outpatient facility, depending upon personnel management practices.[152] The use of multimodal analgesia and preemptive interventions to reduce PONV enable fast-tracking even with general anesthesia. The success of fast-tracking may be predicted by key preoperative patient characteristics such as age older than 60 years, ASA physical status score less than 3, and nongeneral surgery.[153] Immediate postoperative complications do not increase in frequency when fast-track anesthetic techniques and well-defined phase II criteria are utilized.[154,155] If patient selection is inaccurate, nursing workload reductions and potential cost saving may be marginal because workload is shifted from the PACU to the phase II recovery area.[156]

### Multimodal Analgesia and Systematic Pain Management (Also See Chapter 40)

Pain is a highly individualized, unpleasant sensory and emotional experience. For this reason, assessment of pain should be multidimensional. Surgical pain should be distinguished from potential chronic pain or even anxiety or emotional distress. A systematic approach to pain care seeks to adequately manage pain, minimize side effects, and prevent postoperative and postdischarge patient discomfort through risk stratification and treatment planning. Some practitioners advocate the three Is: identify, implement, and intervene.[157] *Identifying* at-risk patients requires an appreciation of the factors that contribute to the pain experience: mechanism of surgical injury, patient characteristics, and bandwidth of multimodal pain therapy.[158-160] The ASA practice guidelines on acute pain management recommend individualized care that prioritizes efficacy with minimal adverse events.[161] Counseling patients before surgery on the potential for pain after surgery and the methods that will be taken to ease it may influence patient satisfaction.[162]

*Implementing* an opioid-sparing, multimodal pain plan that incorporates regional anesthesia enables effective analgesia and minimizes side effects. Intradermal

| Table 37.6 | Scoring Systems for Determining PACU Discharge Readiness or PACU Bypass[148,149] | | | |
|---|---|---|---|---|
| **Modified Aldrete: Score ≥9 Required for PACU Discharge** | | | **White Scoring System: Score of 12 With No Category Being <1 Required for Fast-Track to Phase 1 Unit** | |
| *Clinical Finding* | *Score* | | *Clinical Finding* | *Score* |
| **Level of Consciousness** | | | | |
| Fully awake | 2 | | Awake and oriented | 2 |
| Arousable with verbal cue | 1 | | Arousable with minimal stimulation | 1 |
| Nonresponsive | 0 | | Responsive only to tactile stimuli | 0 |
| **Physical Activity (Voluntary Movement or on Command)** | | | | |
| Moves four extremities | 2 | | Able to move all extremities | 2 |
| Moves two extremities | 1 | | Some weakness in movement of extremities | 1 |
| Moves no extremities | 0 | | Unable to move extremities | 0 |
| **Circulation/Hemodynamic Stability** | | | | |
| Blood pressure within 20 mm Hg of preoperative level | 2 | | Blood pressure <15% of baseline MAP | 2 |
| Blood pressure within 20 mm Hg to 50 mm Hg of preoperative level | 1 | | Blood pressure 15%-30% of baseline MAP | 1 |
| Blood pressure greater than 50 mm Hg of preoperative level | 0 | | Blood pressure >30% of baseline MAP | 0 |
| **Respiration/Respiratory Stability** | | | | |
| Able to breathe deeply and cough freely | 2 | | Able to breathe deeply | 2 |
| Shortness of breath, shallow or limited breathing | 1 | | Tachypnea with good cough | 1 |
| Apneic | 0 | | Dyspneic with weak cough | 0 |
| **Oxygen Saturation Status** | | | | |
| $Sao_2$ maintained above 92% on room air | 2 | | Maintains $Sao_2$ > 90% on room air | 2 |
| Needs supplemental $O_2$ to maintain $Sao_2$ > 90% | 1 | | Requires supplemental $O_2$ | 1 |
| $Sao_2$ < 90% even with $O_2$ supplementation | 0 | | $Sao_2$ < 90% on room supplemental $O_2$ | 0 |
| **Postoperative Pain Assessment** | | | | |
| Not included in modified Aldrete | | | None, or mild discomfort | 2 |
| | | | Moderate to severe pain controlled with IV analgesics | 1 |
| | | | Persistent severe pain despite IV analgesics | 0 |
| **Postoperative Emetic Symptoms** | | | | |
| Not included in modified Aldrete | | | None, or mild nausea with no active emesis | 2 |
| | | | Intermittent emesis or retching | 1 |
| | | | Persistent moderate to severe nausea and emesis | 0 |
| Total Score Possible | 10 | | Total Score Possible | 14 |

*IV*, Intravenous; *MAP*, mean arterial pressure; *$O_2$*, oxygen; *PACU*, postanesthesia care unit; *$Sao_2$*, oxygen saturation.

local anesthesia reduces opioid exposure during preoperative regional anesthesia techniques. Not administering opioids before the postoperative period may lessen PONV. Increased postoperative sedation and opioid requirements are associated with preoperative and intraoperative opioid use.[163-165] Continuous peripheral neural blockade and single-shot peripheral nerve blocks reduced opioid exposure, improved patient comfort, reduced recovery time, increased patient satisfaction, and resulted in lower rates of adverse events.[166-168] Multimodal analgesia decreases pain for patients and contributes to high patient satisfaction and rapid throughput, or fast-tracking.[70,169,170] Multiple studies support preoperative administration of pregabalin and gabapentin,[104,171] COX-2 inhibitors,[105,172,173] intraoperative β-adrenergic blockers,[174-176] ketorolac,[177,178] subanesthetic-dose ketamine,[179-181] magnesium,[182,183] dexamethasone,[106,184,185] methylprednisolone,[186] dexmedetomidine,[187] and intravenous lidocaine infusion[179,188] to diminish the need for postoperative opioids, alleviate acute postoperative pain, and reduce PONV and time to discharge. With countless nonopioid analgesics available, at least one of these drugs is suitable for ambulatory surgical patients with risk of procedural pain. Pain scores in recovery can predict the length of stay in the PACU and are decreased by the use of nonopioids in the operating room.[189]

When multimodal analgesia falls short, the ambulatory anesthesia provider must *intervene* in a timely and potent fashion. After a multidimensional assessment of pain, additional nonopioids are administered during assessment for potential neural blockade. Opioids may be warranted for severe uncontrolled postoperative pain, but the potential for delayed discharge because of PONV and other opioid-related adverse events must be considered.[190] Nonpharmacologic techniques for pain management also should be incorporated.[102,191]

### Postoperative Nausea and Vomiting (Also See Chapter 39)

A definite link exists with pain, opioid-based pain medication, and nausea and vomiting. Patients place a high value on the prevention of PONV, ranking it equivalent to prevention and treatment of pain.[5,192] PONV and PDNV interfere with recovery of daily function after surgery and are therefore incompatible with the goals of ambulatory anesthesia care and perioperative medicine.[193,194] PONV frequently impairs quality of recovery, delays discharge, and may cause unanticipated admission.[70,195,196]

Apfel's scoring system is used to direct prophylaxis against PONV.[144] It is predictive of PONV in the PACU and the first 24 hours after discharge, but the scoring system is a poor predictor of nausea and vomiting 24 to 72 hours after discharge (PDNV).[197] PONV occurs in up to 74% of untreated at-risk outpatients, and PDNV in up to 33%.[198,199] The treatment of PONV begins preoperatively when baseline risk is assessed and multimodal analgesia and PONV prophylaxis are planned and implemented. For most patients, guideline-driven multimodal management reduces the incidence of PONV early in the discharge period.[47,146,200] A regimen of both intravenous dexamethasone 8 mg and ondansetron 4 mg intraoperatively, followed by oral tablets of 8 mg ondansetron at discharge and on postoperative days 1 and 2, virtually eliminates early and late PONV/PDNV in many patients including those in the highest risk categories.[201] Recent meta-analysis and guidelines, however, support an equivalent reduction in the incidence of PONV with a 4-mg to 5-mg dose of dexamethasone.[146,202] Despite triple prophylaxis

with dexamethasone, ondansetron, and scopolamine, and omitting anesthetic triggers, a small residual group of patients still experiences significant PONV.[203]

In some instances, intravenous hydration can reduce the incidence of both PONV and pain.[204] Most otherwise healthy pediatric patients (also see Chapter 34) can be aggressively hydrated and given dual prophylaxis (dexamethasone and ondansetron) to decrease the risk of PONV by as much as 80%.[205] Repeated use of ondansetron in adults for nausea and vomiting in the PACU, despite intraoperative administration, is less effective than a small intravenous dose of promethazine, 6.25 mg.[206]

## Postoperative Phase: Discharging Patients Home

### Patient Assessment

Recovery may continue for days after discharge, and most patients will recover at home. Before discharge there is a home readiness assessment of the patient by a physician or delegated health care professional.[49] One validated scoring system using standardized criteria is the post-anesthesia discharge scoring system (PADSS).[207] The use of such criteria has been associated with reduced length of stay in the PACU when compared to arbitrary PACU time requirements. When the criteria in the pediatric PADSS are applied, most children are safely discharged from the PACU 1 hour after surgery.[208] Practice guidelines further delineate necessary and unnecessary criteria for discharge.[47]

### Patient Instructions

Patient education and preparation are critical to excellent ambulatory surgical outcomes. The preparation of the patient and friends and family who will act as primary caregivers begins well before the procedure. Adverse events after discharge from ambulatory anesthesia may present a risk for legal action.[209] For patients receiving regional anesthesia, clear and effective instructions may prevent a patient from incurring additional injury or requiring acute care for pain or nausea. Instructions describe the care of the insensate limb, the use of crutches or immobilization devices, and the timing of analgesic and antiemetic therapy. Such instruction and education begin during the preoperative phase and may improve patient preparedness and reduce resource-consuming misunderstandings in the recovery room. Other instructions remind the patient not to make major life or financial decisions, consume alcohol, drive, or operate heavy machinery after any level of anesthesia or sedation.[210] The caregiver or escort must have the physical and mental ability to assist the patient, recognize when help is needed, facilitate communication with health care providers, or obtain acute care if needed. Criteria and adherence to discharge criteria should be routinely reviewed and modified.

| Table 37.7 | Themes in Patient and Caregiver Experience and Burden After Ambulatory Surgery[215] | |
|---|---|---|
| **Physical and Emotional Health** | **Hospital Experience** | **Caregiving** |
| Inadequate pain control<br>Analgesic-related side effects<br>Constipation<br>Inadequate guidance in wound care resulting in caregiver stress<br>Loss of function and independence<br>Physically challenging to help with necessities, washroom, eating, getting to bed<br>Caregiver maintenance of personal and professional relationships | Sense of inadequate preparation for the perioperative experience despite preoperative assessment and phone reminder the night before surgery<br><br>Written discharge instructions were unclear or contradictory<br><br>In attempts to solve the patient's concerns, institutional or physician's office support was lacking after hours | Burden of all tasks for the household and providing care<br><br>Caregiver concerns about mobility of the patient despite physician's encouragement of mobility |

### PACU Management (Also See Chapter 39)

In the absence of advanced planning, availability of anesthesia personnel to manage airway or cardiopulmonary emergencies can be limited in a fast-paced ambulatory surgery unit or office. An anesthesia provider should remain immediately available if a patient is unable to maintain an airway or is medically unstable.

The PACU is often the final opportunity for patient education and review of postdischarge care. Caregivers should be given specific instructions for communicating questions or concerns to the ambulatory care team. An ambulatory center may elect to have an answering service or hotline for 24-hour response for continued patient and caregiver reassurance and instruction.

### Patient Transfer or 23-Hour Observation

In the event a patient's condition has not met discharge criteria, the patient is transferred to a hospital facility or short-stay unit for continued observation or treatment. Admission to observation units typically costs less than emergency room visits or hospital admission.[211] Procedural sites should have a well-defined management plan for patient transfer. The ASC provides a detailed physician-to-physician hand-off detailing patient history, operative course, current status, concerns, and patient needs on transfer. For anticipated or unanticipated 23-hour observation, clinical status should dictate the appropriate level of care. If the monitoring and care capabilities of the observation unit are insufficient, the patient should be transferred to a hospital-based facility. The prompt identification of a need for transfer or admission may minimize delay in obtaining patient access to a bed at a busy health care facility. Delays in transfer can result in increased morbidity and additional cost through continued consumption of recovery resources.

## Postoperative Phase: Postdischarge Issues

The postdischarge phase (phase III) creates challenges for the patient and ambulatory clinicians.[29] After discharge many patients suffer moderate to severe pain, cognitive impairment, and PDNV. They may take several days to return to normal activity.[212]

The convenience of going home after a procedure can be quickly overshadowed by the needs of the recovering patient and the burden on the caregivers. Patients may require a longer recovery period than previously recognized. Increased pain and prolonged recovery contribute to increased caregiver burden. Informal caregiving can result in emotional and physical disturbances in the daily lives of patients and caregivers. Such findings can be comparable to those from studies of caregiver burden in chronic disease states.[213,214]

Several major themes have been identified concerning the patient's physical and emotional health, hospital experience, and caregiving after outpatient surgery.[215] These themes are described in Table 37.7. A 2012 study found a 25% accuracy rate for information retention and interpretation of information presented in a preoperative educational session in healthy volunteers, suggesting that patients should have longitudinal access to reeducation and redirection.[216] For this reason a hotline or answering service continues the multidisciplinary team approach; surgeons typically are not able to troubleshoot peripheral nerve catheters and anesthetists should not triage surgical wound drainage.

Quality of recovery in the first postoperative week has been assessed in several studies.[217,218] Despite early discharge from short-stay surgery (<24 hours), 33% of patients had suboptimal recovery 2 months after abdominal surgery. Patients who were older, suffered a complication, or had a low baseline health-related quality of life or a high baseline level of physical activity were less likely to recover to preoperative levels at 3 weeks after surgery.

### Postdischarge Nausea and Vomiting (Also See Chapter 39)

A validated prediction model for PDNV up to 48 hours after ambulatory surgery uses several components: operating room time, PONV history, use of ondansetron, and pain during days 3 to 7 to predict PDNV 3 to 7 days after discharge.[219,220] Patients at risk should receive triple therapy (dexamethasone, ondansetron, scopolamine), continuous regional anesthesia when appropriate, robust nonopioid analgesic treatment, and additional rescue drugs in the event triple therapy is insufficient.[201] Although newer, long-acting drugs have entered clinical practice, traditional and less expensive options appear equally efficacious.[221]

### Postdischarge Pain

As pain is one determinant of PDNV, effective multimodal pain management can ameliorate two primary postdischarge concerns. The use of continuous peripheral neural blockade offers continuous analgesia and reduces the need for opioids.[222,223] Patients given continuous blocks are contacted daily, and around-the-clock clinical access should be available. Patients should be advised of the painful area that is treated by the peripheral nerve catheter. In the example of ankle surgery, a sciatic nerve catheter's pump reservoir can be quickly emptied if the patient self-administers a bolus every hour for a saphenous-mediated, medial ankle pain. For this reason, visual reference materials are given. The materials illustrate the areas of the operated extremity that are treated by a dose of oral analgesic and those best treated with a patient-administered demand dose of local anesthesia. We recommend avoiding combination tablets (e.g., acetaminophen-hydrocodone, acetaminophen-codeine). Tramadol or small-dose oxycodone allows for "uptitration" or discontinuation of opioid via telephone directive without excessive or subtherapeutic exposure to acetaminophen. If necessary, acetaminophen can be administered around the clock acknowledging the FDA recommended daily limit of 3 g.

### Nerve Injury or Motor Deficits

As a part of routine follow-up, communication from the anesthesia group or a delegate from the ASC should verify that neural blockade has fully resolved in the days following surgery. In the event of persistent sensory or motor deficits, the surgeon and anesthesia provider involved in the patient's care are notified for assessment and management.[224,225] Iatrogenic injuries after orthopedic surgery may sometimes confound physician assessment of the cause of the injury.[226-228]

## Outcomes

The ambulatory anesthesia provider may or may not be aware of a patient's readmission after surgery for severe, uncontrolled, postoperative pain and nausea and vomiting. Without follow-up the anesthesia provider may be unaware of that patient's continued acute pain in the days to weeks that followed her discharge or the continued presence of severe pain 6 months thereafter. With awareness of this outcome, would the anesthesia provider be more likely to utilize alternative techniques for future such cases?[126]

Outcomes in ambulatory surgery include the events after discharge from the care facility and potentially weeks to months after the surgical experience. Evaluation of the recovery process is requisite for potential improvement in postoperative and postdischarge care as well as in preoperative and intraoperative management. An ambulatory anesthesia group should routinely track events such as PDNV, persistent moderate to severe pain, regional anesthetic failure or complication, emergency department visits, cognitive dysfunction, and service dissatisfaction.

The use of outcome measurement data to standardize care has successfully improved safety and service delivery in a variety of industries, including health care.[229-232] A recognized tenet of evidence-based medicine is to reference past patient outcomes when selecting therapies.[233] Data should be collected on the day of surgery through anesthesia information systems, combined with follow-up data from postdischarge phone calls and benchmarked across individual practitioners, peer institutions, and diverse practice settings through the multitude of outcomes databases.

## CONCLUSION

The future of outpatient anesthesia is clear. The number of patients will increase, the venues will grow more experientially distant from medical center operating rooms, and the technology of surgical intervention will increase the invasiveness of the procedures on the daily list. Advances in telemedicine and information technology will optimize preoperative and postdischarge interaction for better patient care and communication before and after surgery. As capitation seeks to reduce health care expense, the 23-hour ambulatory perioperative experience will increasingly become the norm for most surgeries. The ambulatory surgical home will enable patients to be remotely monitored and in continuous contact with health care providers with the expectation of safe and timely recovery and return of function. Through preparedness, selectivity, and enhanced communication, excellent ambulatory anesthesia outcomes will reflect the investment of the practitioners who choose this labor-intensive practice.

## QUESTIONS OF THE DAY

1. What patient factors increase the risk of perioperative complications after ambulatory surgery?
2. What social support must be ensured to facilitate safe ambulatory surgery?
3. How should the anesthesia provider decide whether a patient with recent upper respiratory infection (URI) should proceed with ambulatory surgery?
4. What are the phases of recovery after surgery (prior to discharge home)? Which patients are eligible for "fast-tracking" after surgery?

5. What medications can be administered as part of an opioid-sparing multimodal postoperative analgesia regimen?

6. What factors predict development of postdischarge nausea and vomiting (PDNV) after ambulatory surgery? What steps can be taken to prevent PDNV in the at-risk patient?

## Special Mention

The authors would like to acknowledge Sally Kozlik for her assistance in reference management and manuscript editing and design researcher Amanda Rosenberg for her designing with the authors' input Fig. 37.1, depicting the perioperative journey of an ambulatory surgical patient.

## REFERENCES

1. Waters RM. The downtown anesthesia clinic. *Am J Surg.* 1919;33(7):71–77.
2. Urman RD, Desai S. History of ambulatory anesthesia. *Curr Opin Anaesthesiol.* 2012;25(6):641–647.
3. Macario A, Weinger M, Carney S, Kim A. Which clinical anesthesia outcomes are important to avoid? The perspective of patients. *Anesth Analg.* 1999;89(3):652–658.
4. Macario A, Weinger M, Truong P, Lee M. Which clinical anesthesia outcomes are both common and important to avoid? The perspective of a panel of expert anesthesiologists. *Anesth Analg.* 1999;88(5):1085–1091.
5. Gan J, Sloan F, Dear G, et al. How much are patients willing to pay to avoid postoperative nausea and vomiting? *Anesth Analg.* 2001;92:393–400.
6. Ahmad J, Ho OA, Carman WW, et al. Assessing patient safety in Canadian ambulatory surgery facilities: a national survey. *Plast Surg.* 2014;22(1):34–38.
7. Keyes GR, Singer R, Iverson RE, et al. Mortality in outpatient surgery. *Plast Reconstr Surg.* 2008;122:245–250.
8. American Hospital Association. Chartbook: trends affecting hospitals and health systems. http://www.aha.org/research/reports/tw/chartbook/index.shtml Accessed August 15, 2015.
9. Khadim M, Gans I, Baldwin K, et al. Do surgical times and efficiency differ between inpatient and ambulatory surgery centers that are both hospital owned? *J Pediatr Orthop.* 2016;36(4):423–428.
10. Munnich EL, Parente ST. Procedures take less time at ambulatory surgery centers, keeping costs down and ability to keep demand up. *Health Aff.* 2014;33(5):764–769.
11. Suskind AM, Zhang Y, Dunn RL, et al. Understanding the diffusion of ambulatory surgery centers. *Surg Innov.* 2015;22(3):257–265.
12. Fleisher LA, Pasternak LR, Lyles A. A novel index of elevated risk of inpatient hospital admission immediately following outpatient surgery. *Arch Surg.* 2007;142(3):263–268.
13. Menachemi N, Chukmaitov A, Brown LS, et al. Quality of care differs by patient characteristics: outcome disparities after ambulatory surgical procedures. *Am J Med Qual.* 2007;22(6):395–401.
14. Sarin P, Philip BK, Mitani A, et al. Specialized ambulatory anesthesia teams contribute to decreased ambulatory surgery recovery room length of stay. *Ochsner J.* 2012;12(2):94–100.
15. Urman RD, Sarin P, Mitani A, et al. Presence of anesthesia resident trainees in day surgery unit has mixed effects on operating room efficiency measures. *Ochsner J.* 2012;12(1):25–29.
16. Eijkemans MJ, van Houdenhoven M, Nguyen T, et al. Predicting the unpredictable: a new prediction model for operating room times using individual characteristics and the surgeon's estimate. *Anesthesiology.* 2010;112:41–49.
17. Leape L, Berwick D, Clancy C. Transforming healthcare: a safety imperative. *Qual Saf Health Care.* 2009;18:424–428.
18. Berwick DM. The clinical process and the quality process. *Qual Manag Health Care.* 1992;1:1–8.
19. Brown EC, Kros J. Reducing room turnaround time at a regional hospital. *Qual Manag Health Care.* 2010;19(1):90–100.
20. Carlhed R, Bojestig M. Improved clinical outcome after acute myocardial infarction in hospitals participating in a Swedish quality improvement initiative. *Circ Card Qual Outcomes.* 2009;2(3):458–464.
21. Macario A. Truth in scheduling: is it possible to accurately predict how long a surgical case will last? *Anesth Analg.* 2009;108(3):681–685.
22. Merrill D. Management of outcomes in the ambulatory surgery center: the role of standard work and evidence-based medicine. *Curr Opin Anaesthesiol.* 2008;21:743–747.
23. Wier LM, Steiner CA, Owens PL. Surgeries in hospital-owned outpatient facilities. https://www.hcup-us.ahrq.gov/reports/statbriefs/sb188-Surgeries-Hospital-Outpatient-Facilities-2012.jsp Accessed August 15, 2015.
24. Whippey A, Kostandoff G, Paul J, et al. Predictors of unanticipated admission following ambulatory surgery: a retrospective case-control study. *Can J Anaesth.* 2013;60(7):675–683.
25. Saad AN, Parina R, Chang D, et al. Risk of adverse outcomes when plastic surgery procedures are combined. *Plast Reconstr Surg.* 2014;134(6):1415–1422.
26. Gurusamy K, Junnarkar S, Farouk M, et al. Meta-analysis of randomized controlled trials on the safety and effectiveness of day laparoscopic cholecystectomy. *Br J Surg.* 2008;95(2):161–168.
27. Lefrancois M, Lefevre JH, Chafai N, et al. Management of acute appendicitis in ambulatory surgery: is it possible? How to select patients? *Ann Surg.* 2015;261(6):1167–1172.
28. Orosco RK, Lin HW, Bhattacharyya N, et al. Ambulatory thyroidectomy: a multistate study of revisits and complications. *Otolaryngol Head Neck Surg.* 2015;152(6):1017–1023.
29. Coley KC, Williams BA, DaPos SV, et al. Retrospective evaluation of unanticipated admissions and readmissions after same day surgery and associated costs. *J Clin Anesth.* 2002;14(5):349–353.
30. Outpatient quality reporting slated. *OR Manager.* 2007;23(9):5.
31. Fox JP, Vashi AA, Ross JS, et al. Hospital-based, acute care after ambulatory surgery center discharge. *Surgery.* 2014;155(5):743–753.
32. Fleisher LA, Pasternak LR, Herbert R, Anderson GF. Inpatient hospital admission and death after outpatient surgery in elderly patients: importance of patient and system characteristics and location of care. *Arch Surg.* 2004;139(1):67–72.
33. Grisel J, Arjmand E. Comparing quality at an ambulatory surgery center and a hospital-based facility: preliminary findings. *Otolaryngol Head Neck Surg.* 2009;141(6):701–709.
34. Shapiro FE, Punwani N, Rosenberg NM, et al. Office-based anesthesia: safety and outcomes. *Anesth Analg.* 2014;119(2):276–285.

IV

35. Qualifications of anesthesia providers in the office-based setting. http://www.asahq.org/For-Healthcare-Professionals/Standards-Guidelines-and-Statements.aspx Accessed August 30, 2015.

36. Evron S, Ezri T. Organizational prerequisites for anesthesia outside the operating room. *Curr Opin Anaesthesiol.* 2009;22:514–518.

37. American Society of Anesthesiologists guidelines for office-based anesthesia. https://www.asahq.org/quality-and-practice-management/standards-and-guidelines Accessed September 4, 2015.

38. Vila H Jr, Soto R, Cantor AB, Mackey D. Comparative outcomes analysis of procedures performed in physicians' offices and ambulatory surgery centers. *Arch Surg.* 2003;138(9):991–995.

39. Li G, Warner M, Lang BH, et al. Epidemiology of anesthesia-related mortality in the United States, 1999-2005. *Anesthesiology.* 2009;110(4):759–765.

40. Institute for Safety in Office-based Surgery. SOBS safety checklist for office-based surgery. http://isobsurgery.org/wp-content/uploads/2012/03/safety-checklist.jpg Accessed August 15, 2015.

41. Metzner J, Posner KL, Domino KB. The risk and safety of anesthesia at remote locations: the US closed claims analysis. *Curr Opin Anaesthesiol.* 2009;22:502–508.

42. Vila H Jr, Desai MS, Miguel RV. Office-based anesthesia. In: Twersky RS, Philip BK, eds. *Handbook of Ambulatory Anesthesia.* New York: Springer Science & Business Media; 2008:283–324.

43. Butz S, ed. *Perioperative Drill-Based Crisis Management.* Cambridge, England: Cambridge University Press; 2015.

44. Salas E, Wilson KA, Burke CS, et al. Using simulation-based training to improve patient safety: what does it take? *Jt Comm J Qual Patient Saf.* 2005;31(7):363–371.

45. Rosen MA, Salas E, Wilson KA, et al. Measuring team performance in simulation-based training: adopting best practices for healthcare. *Simul Healthcare.* 2008;3(1):33–41.

46. Ip HY, Chung F. Escort accompanying discharge after ambulatory surgery: a necessity or a luxury? *Curr Opin Anaesthesiol.* 2009;22:748–754.

47. Apfelbaum J, Silverstein J, Chung F, et al. Practice guidelines for postanesthetic care: an updated report by the American Society of Anesthesiologists Task Force on Postanesthetic Care. *Anesthesiology.* 2013;118:291–307.

48. American Association for Accreditation of Ambulatory Facilities. Medicare Standards and Checklist for Accreditation of Ambulatory Surgery Facilities, version 6.5, 2014. http://www.aaaasf.org/standards.html Accessed September 4, 2015.

49. Whitaker DK, Booth H, Clyburn P, et al. Guidelines: immediate post anaesthesia recovery. *Anaesthesia.* 2013;68:288–297.

50. Bennarroch-Gampel J, Sheffield KM, Duncan CB, et al. Preoperative laboratory testing in patients undergoing elective, low-risk ambulatory surgery. *Ann Surg.* 2012;256(3):518–528.

51. Johansson T, Fritsch G, Flamm M, et al. Effectiveness of non-cardiac preoperative testing in non-cardiac elective surgery: a systematic review. *Br J Anaesth.* 2013;110(6):926–939.

52. Chen CL, Lin GA, Bardach NS, et al. Preoperative medical testing in Medicare patients undergoing cataract surgery. *N Engl J Med.* 2015;372(16):1530–1538.

53. Keay L, Lindsley K, Tielsch J, et al. Routine preoperative medical testing for cataract surgery. *Cochrane Database Syst Rev.* 2012;14:3.

54. Fong R, Sweitzer BJ. Preopeartive optimization of patients undergoing ambulatory surgery. *Curr Anesthesiol Rep.* 2014;4:303–315.

55. Fleisher LA, Fleischmann KE, Auerbach AD, et al. 2014 ACC/AHA guideline on perioperative cardiovascular evaluation and management of patients undergoing noncardiac surgery: a report of the American College of Cardiology/American Heart Association Task Force on Practice Guidelines. *Circulation.* 2014;130(24):e278–e333.

56. Bilimoria KY, Liu Y, Paruch JL, et al. Development and evaluation of the universal ACS NSQIP surgical risk calculator: a decision aid and informed consent tool for patients and surgeons. *J Am Coll Surg.* 2013;217(5):833–842.

57. Ford MK, Beattie WS, Wijeysundera DN. Prediction of perioperative cardiac complications and mortality by the Revised Cardiac Risk Index: a systematic review. *Ann Intern Med.* 2010;152:26–35.

58. Lee TH, Marcantonio ER, Mangione CM, et al. Derivation and prospective validation of a simple index for prediction of cardiac risk of major noncardiac surgery. *Circulation.* 1999;100:1043–1049.

59. Memtsoudis S, Liu SS, Ma Y, et al. Perioperative pulmonary outcomes in patients with sleep apnea after noncardiac surgery. *Anesth Analg.* 2011;112(1):113–121.

60. Dincer HE, O'Neill W. Deleterious effects of sleep-disordered breathing on the heart and vascular system. *Respiration.* 2006;73:124–130.

61. Singh M, Liao P, Kobah S, et al. Proportion of surgical patients with undiagnosed obstructive sleep apnoea. *Br J Anaesth.* 2013;110:629–636.

62. Siyam MA, Benhamou D. Difficult endotracheal intubation in patients with sleep apnea syndrome. *Anesth Analg.* 2002;95:1098–1102.

63. Chung S, Yuan H, Chung F. A systematic review of obstructive sleep apnea and its implications for anesthesiologists. *Anesth Analg.* 2008;107:1543–1563.

64. Bryson GL, Gomez CP, Jee RM, et al. Unplanned admission after day surgery: a historical cohort study in patients with obstructive sleep apnea. *Can J Anaesth.* 2012;59(9):842–851.

65. Joshi GP, Ankichetty SP, Gan TJ, et al. Society for Ambulatory Anesthesia Consensus statement on preoperative selection of adult patients with obstructive sleep apnea scheduled for ambulatory surgery. *Anesth Analg.* 2012;115:1060–1068.

66. American Society of Anesthesiologists Task Force on Perioperative Management of patients with obstructive sleep apnea. Practice guidelines for the perioperative management of patients with obstructive sleep apnea: an updated report by the American Society of Anesthesiologists Task Force on Perioperative Management of patients with obstructive sleep apnea. *Anesthesiology.* 2014;120(2):268–286.

67. Chung F, Subramanyam R, Liao P, et al. High STOP-Bang score indicates a high probability of obstructive sleep apnoea. *Br J Anaesth.* 2012;108:768–775.

68. Joshi GP, Chung F, Vann MA, et al. Society for Ambulatory Anesthesia consensus statement on perioperative blood glucose management in diabetic patients undergoing ambulatory surgery. *Anesth Analg.* 2010;111:1378–1387.

69. Pavlin DJ, Rapp SE, Polissar NL, et al. Factors affecting discharge time in adult outpatients. *Anesth Analg.* 1998;87:816–826.

70. Chung F, Mezei G. Factors contributing to a prolonged stay after ambulatory surgery. *Anesth Analg.* 1999;89:1352–1359.

71. Committee on Standards and Practice Parameters, Apfelbaum JL, Connis RT, Nickinovich DG. American Society of Anesthesiologists Task Force on Preanesthesia Evaluation, Pasternak LR, Arens JF, Caplan RA, et al. Practice advisory for preanesthesia evaluation: an updated report by the American Society of Anesthesiologists Task Force on Preanesthesia Evaluation. *Anesthesiology.* 2012;116(3):522–538.

72. Chung F, Yegneswaran B, Herrera F, et al. Patients with difficult intubation may need referral to sleep clinics. *Anesth Analg.* 2008;107:915–920.

73. Van Klei WA, Moons KG, Rutten CL, et al. The effect of outpatient preoperative evaluation of hospital inpatients on cancellation of surgery and length of hospital stay. *Anesth Analg.* 2002;94:644–649.

74. Warner DO. American Society of Anesthesiologists Smoking Cessation Initiative Task Force. Feasibility of tobacco interventions in anesthesiology practices: a pilot study. *Anesthesiology.* 2009;110(6):1223–1228.

75. Woods BD, Sladen RN. Perioperative considerations for the patient with asthma and bronchospasm. *Br J Anaesth.* 2009;103(suppl 1):i57–i65.

76. Licker M, Schweizer A, Ellenberger C. Perioperative medical management of patients with COPD. *Int J Chron Obstruct Pulmon Dis.* 2007;2(4):493–515.

77. Carmosino MJ, Friesen RH, Doran A. Perioperative complications in children with pulmonary hypertension undergoing noncardiac surgery or cardiac catheterization. *Anesth Analg.* 2007;104:521–527.

78. Lai HC, Lai HC, Wang KY, et al. Severe pulmonary hypertension complicates postoperative outcome of noncardiac surgery. *Br J Anaesth.* 2007;99:184–190.

79. Tait AR, Pandit UA, Voepel-Lewis T, et al. Use of the laryngeal mask airway in children with upper respiratory tract infections: a comparison with endotracheal intubation. *Anesth Analg.* 1998;86:706–711.

80. Chin KJ, Chee VW. Laryngeal edema associated with the ProSeal laryngeal mask airway in upper respiratory tract infections. *Can J Anaesth.* 2006;53(4):389–392.

81. Tait AR, Burke C, Voepel-Lewis T, et al. Glycopyrrolate does not reduce the incidence of perioperative adverse events in children with upper respiratory tract infections. *Anesth Analg.* 2007;104:265–270.

82. Tait AR, Malviya S, Voepel-Lewis T, et al. Risk factors for perioperative adverse respiratory events in children with upper respiratory tract infections. *Anesthesiology.* 2001;95:299–306.

83. Tait AR, Malviya S. Anesthesia for the child with an upper respiratory tract infection: still a dilemma? *Anesth Analg.* 2005;100:59–65.

84. Wax DB, Porter SB, Lin HM, et al. Association of preanesthesia hypertension with adverse outcomes. *J Cardiothorac Vasc Anesth.* 2010;24:927–930.

85. Kheterpal S, O'Reilly M, Englesbe MJ, et al. Preoperative and intraoperative predictors of cardiac adverse events after general, vascular and urological surgery. *Anesthesiology.* 2009;110:58–66.

86. Coriat P, Richer C, Douraki T, et al. Influence of chronic angiotensin-converting enzyme inhibition on anesthetic induction. *Anesthesiology.* 1994;81:299–307.

87. Colson P, Saussine M, Seguin JR, et al. Hemodynamic effects of anesthesia in patients chronically treated with angiotensin-converting enzyme inhibitors. *Anesth Analg.* 1992;74:805–808.

88. Reich DL, Hossain S, Krol M, et al. Predictors of hypotension after induction of general anesthesia. *Anesth Analg.* 2005;101:622–628.

89. Hernandez AF, Whellan DJ, Stroud S, et al. Outcomes in heart failure patients after major noncardiac surgery. *J Am Coll Cardiol.* 2004;44:1446–1453.

90. Brotman DJ, Bakhru M, Saber W, et al. Discontinuation of antiplatelet therapy prior to low-risk noncardiac surgery in patients with drug-eluting stents: a retrospective cohort study. *J Hosp Med.* 2007;2:378–384.

91. el-Ganzouri AR, McCarthy RJ, Tuman KJ, et al. Preoperative airway assessment: predictive value of a multivariate risk index. *Anesth Analg.* 1996;82:1197–1204.

92. Cook TM, Woodall N, Frerk C. Major complications of airway management in the UK: results of the Fourth National Audit Project of the Royal College of Anaesthetists and the Difficult Airway Society. Part 1: anaesthesia. *Br J Anaesth.* 2011;106(5):617–631.

93. Ovassapian A, Glassenberg R, Randel GI, et al. The unexpected difficult airway and lingual tonsil hyperplasia: a case series and a review of the literature. *Anesthesiology.* 2002;97(1):124–132.

94. Apfelbaum JL, Hagberg CA, Caplan RA, et al. Practice guidelines for management of the difficult airway: an updated report by the American Society of Anesthesiologists Task Force on Management of the Difficult Airway. *Anesthesiology.* 2013;118(2):251–270.

95. Greenland KB. Difficult airway management in an ambulatory surgical center? *Curr Opin Anaesthesiol.* 2012;25(6):659–664.

96. Berkow LC, Greenberg RS, Kan KH, et al. Need for emergency surgical airway reduced by a comprehensive difficult airway program. *Anesth Analg.* 2009;109(6):1860–1869.

97. Kahn RL, Stanton MA, Tong-Ngork S, et al. One-year experience with day-of-surgery pregnancy testing before elective orthopedic procedures. *Anesth Analg.* 2008;106:1127–1131.

98. Hutzler L, Kraemer K, Palmer N, et al. Cost benefit analysis of same day pregnancy tests in elective orthopaedic surgery. *Bull Hosp Jt Dis.* 2014;72(2):164–166.

99. Ni CH, Hou WH, Kao CC, et al. The anxiolytic effect of aromatherapy on patients awaiting ambulatory surgery: a randomized controlled trial. *Evid Based Complement Alternat Med.* 2013;2013:927419.

100. Angioli R, De Cicco Nardone C, Plotti F, et al. Use of music to reduce anxiety during office hysteroscopy: prospective randomized trial. *J Minim Invasive Gynecol.* 2014;21(3):454–459.

101. Hole J, Hirsch M, Ball E, Meads C. Music as an aid for postoperative recovery in adults: a systematic review and meta-analysis. *Lancet.* 2015;386(10004):1659–1671.

102. Clarke H, Kirkham KR, Orser BA, et al. Gabapentin reduces preoperative anxiety and pain catastrophizing in highly anxious patients prior to major surgery: a blinded randomized placebo-controlled trial. *Can J Anaesth.* 2013;60(5):432–442.

103. Ong CK, Seymour RA, Lirk P, et al. Combining paracetamol (acetaminophen) with nonsteroidal anti-inflammatory drugs: a qualitative systematic review of analgesic efficacy for acute postoperative pain. *Anesth Analg.* 2010;110(4):1170–1179.

104. Kim SY, Song JW, Park B, et al. Pregabalin reduces post-operative pain after mastectomy: a double-blind randomized, placebo-controlled study. *Acta Anaesthesiol Scand.* 2011;55(3):290–296.

105. White PF, Tang J, Wender RH, et al. The effects of oral ibuprofen and celecoxib in preventing pain, improving recovery outcomes and patient satisfaction after ambulatory surgery. *Anesth Analg.* 2011;112(2):323–329.

106. Murphy GS, Szokol JW, Greenberg SB, et al. Preoperative dexamethasone enhances quality of recovery after laparoscopic cholecystectomy: effect on in-hospital and postdischarge recovery outcomes. *Anesthesiology.* 2011;114(4):882–890.

107. White PF, Tang J, Song D. Transdermal scopolamine: an alternative to ondansetron and droperidol for the prevention of postoperative and post-discharge emetic symptoms. *Anesth Analg.* 2007;104:92–96.

108. Kim SH, Stoicea N, Soghomonyan S, Bergese SD. Intraoperative use of remifentanil and opioid induced hyperalgesia/acute opioid tolerance: systematic review. *Front Pharmacol.* 2014;5:108.

IV

109. Bhananker SM, Posner KL, Cheney FW, et al. Injury and liability associated with monitored anesthesia care: a closed claims analysis. *Anesthesiology.* 2006;104:228–234.

110. Kessler J, Marhofer P, Hopkins PM, Hollmann MW. Peripheral regional anaesthesia and outcome: lessons learned from the last 10 years. *Br J Anaesth.* 2015;114(5):728–745.

111. Liu SS, Strodtbeck WM, Richman J, et al. A comparison of regional versus general anesthesia for ambulatory anesthesia: a meta-analysis of randomized controlled trials. *Anesth Analg.* 2005;101(6):1634–1642.

112. O'Donnell BD, Iohom G. Regional anesthesia techniques for ambulatory orthopedic surgery. *Curr Opin Anaesthesiol.* 2008;21(6):723–728.

113. Mariano ER, Chu LF, Peinado CF, et al. Anesthesia-controlled time and turnover time for ambulatory upper extremity surgery performed with regional versus general anesthesia. *J Clin Anesth.* 2009;21:253–257.

114. Hadzic A, Williams BA, Karaca PE, et al. For outpatient rotator cuff surgery, nerve block anesthesia provides superior same-day recovery over general anesthesia. *Anesthesiology.* 2005;102:1001–1007.

115. Hadzic A, Alris J, Kerimoglu B, et al. A comparison of infraclavicular nerve block versus general anesthesia for hand and wrist day-case surgeries. *Anesthesiology.* 2004;101:127–132.

116. Best MJ, Buller LT, Miranda A. United States trends in ankle arthroscopy: analysis of the national survey of ambulatory surgery and national hospital discharge survey. *Foot Ankle Spec.* 2015;8(4):266–272.

117. Klein SM, Pietrobon R, Nielsen KC, et al. Peripheral nerve blockade with long-acting local anesthetics: a survey of the Society for Ambulatory Anesthesia. *Anesth Analg.* 2002;94:71–76.

118. Ilfeld BM, Morey TE, Enneking FK. Continuous infraclavicular brachial plexus block for post-operative pain control at home: a randomized, double-blinded, placebo-controlled study. *Anesthesiology.* 2002;96:1297–1304.

119. Swenson JD, Bay N, Loose E, et al. Outpatient management of continuous peripheral nerve catheters placed using ultrasound guidance: an experience in 620 patients. *Anesth Analg.* 2002;103:1436–1443.

120. Hadzic A, Kerimoglu B, Loreio D, et al. Paravertebral blocks provide superior same-day recovery over general anesthesia for patients undergoing inguinal hernia repair. *Anesth Analg.* 2006;102:1076–1081.

121. Iohom G, Abdalla H, O'Brien J, et al. The associations between severity of early post-operative pain, chronic post-surgical pain and plasma concentration of stable nitric oxide products after breast surgery. *Anesth Analg.* 2006;103:995–1000.

122. Naja Z, Lonnqvist PA. Somatic paravertebral nerve blockade. Incidence of failed block and complications. *Anaesthesia.* 2001;56:1181–1201.

123. Eid H. Paravertebral block: an overview. *Curr Anaesth Crit Care.* 2009;20:65–70.

124. Abdallah FW, Morgan PJ, Cil T, et al. Ultrasound-guided multilevel paravertebral blocks and total intravenous anesthesia improve the quality of recovery after ambulatory breast tumor resection. *Anesthesiology.* 2014;120(3): 703–713.

125. Exadaktylos AK, Buggy DJ, Moriarty DC, et al. Can anesthetic technique for primary breast cancer surgery affect recurrence or metastasis? *Anesthesiology.* 2006;105:660–664.

126. Andreae MH, Andreae DA. Local anaesthetics and regional anaesthesia for preventing chronic pain after surgery. *Cochrane Database Syst Rev.* 2012;(10). CD007105.

127. Bashandy GM, Abbas DN. Pectoral nerves I and II blocks in multimodal analgesia for breast cancer surgery: a randomized clinical trial. *Reg Anesth Pain Med.* 2015;40(1):68–74.

128. Bouzinac A, Brenier G, Dao M, Delbas A. Bilateral association of pecs I block and serratus plane block for postoperative analgesia after double modified radical mastectomy. *Minerva Anestesiol.* 2015;81(5):589–590.

129. Korhonen AM, Valanne JV, Jokela RM, et al. A comparison of selective spinal anesthesia with hyperbaric bupivacaine and general anesthesia with desflurane for outpatient knee arthroscopy. *Anesth Analg.* 2004;99:1668–1673.

130. Kodeih MG, Al-Alami AA, Atiyeh BS, Kanazi GE. Combined spinal epidural anesthesia in an asthmatic patient undergoing abdominoplasty. *Plast Reconstr Surg.* 2009;123(3):e118–e120.

131. Wulf H, Hampl K, Steinfeldt T. Speed spinal anesthesia revisited: new drugs and their clinical effects. *Curr Opin Anaesthesiol.* 2013;26(5):613–620.

132. Lacasse MA, Roy JD, Forget J, et al. Comparison of bupivacaine and 2-chloroprocaine for spinal anesthesia for outpatient surgery: a double-blind randomized trial. *Can J Anaesth.* 2011;58:384–391.

133. Yoos JR, Kopacz DJ. Spinal 2-chloroprocaine for surgery: an initial 10-month experience. *Anesth Analg.* 2005;100:553–558.

134. Casati A, Danelli G, Berti M, et al. Intrathecal 2-chloroprocaine for lower limb outpatient surgery: a prospective, randomized, double-blind, clinical evaluation. *Anesth Analg.* 2006;103: 234–238.

135. Pawlowski J, Orr K, Kim KM, et al. Anesthetic and recovery profiles of lidocaine versus mepivacaine for spinal anesthesia in patients undergoing outpatient orthopedic arthroscopic procedures. *J Clin Anesth.* 2012;24(2): 109–115.

136. Zohar E, Noga Y, Rislick U, et al. Intrathecal anesthesia for elderly patients undergoing short transurethral procedures: a dose-finding study. *Anesth Analg.* 2007;104(3):552–554.

137. Cappelleri G, Aldegheri G, Danelli G, et al. Spinal anesthesia with hyperbaric levobupivacaine and ropivacaine for outpatient knee arthroscopy: a prospective, randomized, double-blind study. *Anesth Analg.* 2005;101:77–82.

138. Smith KN, Kopacz DJ. Spinal 2-chloroprocaine: a dose-ranging study and the effect of added epinephrine. *Anesth Analg.* 2004;98:81–88.

139. Peyton PJ, Wu CY. Nitrous oxide-related postoperative nausea and vomiting depends on duration of exposure. *Anesthesiology.* 2014;120: 1137–1145.

140. Fredman B, Nathanson MH, Smith I, et al. Sevoflurane for outpatient anesthesia: a comparison with propofol. *Anesth Analg.* 1995;81: 823–828.

141. Gupta A, Stierer T, Zuckerman R, et al. Comparison of recovery profile after ambulatory anesthesia with propofol, isoflurane, sevoflurane and desflurane: a systematic review. *Anesth Analg.* 2004;98(3):632–641.

142. Pavlin JD, Horvarth KD, Pavlin EG, et al. Preincisional treatment to prevent pain after ambulatory hernia surgery. *Anesth Analg.* 2003;97: 1627–1632.

143. White PF. The changing role of nonopioid analgesic techniques in the management of postoperative pain. *Anesth Analg.* 2005;101(suppl 5): S5–S22.

144. Apfel CC, Laara E, Koivuranta M, et al. A simplified risk score for predicting postoperative nausea and vomiting: conclusions from cross-validations between two centers. *Anesthesiology.* 1999;91:693–700.

145. Kolodzi K, Apfel CC. Nausea and vomiting after office-based anesthesia. *Curr Opin Anaesthesiol.* 2009;22:532–538.

146. Gan TJ, Diemunsch P, Habib AS, et al. Consensus guidelines for management of postoperative nausea and vomiting. *Anesth Analg.* 2014;118(1): 85–113.

147. Visser K, Hassingk EA, Bonsel GJ, et al. Randomized controlled trial of total intravenous anesthesia with propofol versus inhalation anesthesia with isoflurane-nitrous oxide: postoperative nausea with vomiting and economic analysis. *Anesthesiology.* 2001;95:616–626.

148. Aldrete JA. The post-anesthetic recovery score revisited. *J Clin Anesth.* 1995;7:89–91.

149. White PF, Song D. New criteria for fast-tracking after outpatient anesthesia: a comparison with the modified Aldrete's scoring system. *Anesth Analg.* 1999;88(5):1069–1072.

150. Milby A, Bohmer A, Gerbershagen MU, et al. Quality of post-operative patient handover in the post-anesthesia care unit: a prospective analysis. *Acta Anaesthesiol Scand.* 2014;58(2):192–197.

151. Agarwala AV, Firth PG, Albrecht MA, et al. An electronic checklist improves transfer and retention of critical information at intraoperative handoff of care. *Anesth Analg.* 2015;120(1):96–104.

152. Lubarsky DA. Fast-track in the postanesthesia care unit: unlimited possibilities. *J Clin Anesth.* 1996;8:70–72.

153. Twersky RS, Sapozhnikova S, Toure B. Risk factors associated with fast track ineligibility after monitored anesthesia care in ambulatory surgery patients. *Anesth Analg.* 2008;106:1421–1426.

154. Apfelbaum JL, Lichtor JL, Lane BS, et al. Awakening, clinical recovery, and psychomotor effects after desflurane and propofol anesthesia. *Anesth Analg.* 1996;83:721–725.

155. White PF, Eng M. Fast-track anesthetic techniques for ambulatory surgery. *Curr Opin Anaesthesiol.* 2007;20:545–557.

156. Song D, Chung F, Ronayne M, et al. Fast tracking (bypassing the PACU) does not reduce nursing workload after ambulatory surgery. *Br J Anaesth.* 2004;93:768–774.

157. Dickerson DM. Acute pain management. *Anesthesiol Clin.* 2014;32(2):495–504.

158. Ip HY, Abrishami A, Peng PW, et al. Predictors of postoperative pain and analgesic consumption: a qualitative systematic review. *Anesthesiology.* 2009;111:657–677.

159. Gerbershagen HJ, Aduckathil S, van Wijck AJ, et al. Pain intensity on the first day after surgery: a prospective cohort study comparing 179 surgical procedures. *Anesthesiology.* 2013;118(4):934–944.

160. Schwenkglenks M, Gerbershagen HJ, Taylor RS, et al. Correlates of satisfaction with pain treatment in the acute postoperative period: results from the international PAIN OUT registry. *Pain.* 2014;155:1401–1411.

161. American Society of Anesthesiologists Task Force on Acute Pain Management. Practice guidelines for acute pain management in the perioperative setting: an updated report by the American Society of Anesthesiologists Task Force on Acute Pain Management. *Anesthesiology.* 2012;116(2):248–273.

162. Hanna MN. Does patient perception of pain control affect patient satisfaction across surgical units? *J Med Qual.* 2012;27:411–416.

163. Lentschener C, Tostivint P, White PF, et al. Opioid-induced sedation in the postanesthesia care unit does not insure adequate pain relief: a case-control study. *Anesth Analg.* 2007;105:1143–1147.

164. Angst MS, Clark JC. Opioid-induced hyperalgesia: a qualitative systematic review. *Anesthesiology.* 2006;104:570–587.

165. White PF. Prevention of postoperative nausea and vomiting: a multimodal solution to a persistent problem. *N Engl J Med.* 2004;350:2511–2512.

166. Carli F, Kehlet H, Baldini G, et al. Evidence basis for regional anesthesia in multidisciplinary fast-track surgical care pathways. *Reg Anesth Pain Med.* 2011;36:63–72.

167. Lenart MJ, Wong K, Gupta RK, et al. The impact of peripheral nerve techniques on hospital stay following major orthopedic surgery. *Pain Med.* 2012;13(6):828–834.

168. Ilfeld BM. Continuous peripheral nerve blocks: a review of the published evidence. *Anesth Analg.* 2011;113(4):904–925.

169. White PF, Kehlet H, Neal JM, et al. The role of the anesthesiologist in fast-track surgery: from multimodal analgesia to perioperative medical care. *Anesth Analg.* 2007;104:1380–1396.

170. Fung D, Cohen MM, Stewart S, et al. What determines patient satisfaction with cataract care under topical local anesthesia and monitored sedation in a community hospital setting? *Anesth Analg.* 2005;100:1644–1650.

171. Turan A, White PF, Karamanlioglu B, et al. Premedication with gabapentin: the effect on tourniquet pain and quality of intravenous regional anesthesia. *Anesth Analg.* 2007;104(1):97–101.

172. White PF. Changing role of COX-2 inhibitors in the perioperative period. Is parecoxib really the answer? *Anesth Analg.* 2005;100:1306–1308.

173. Kaye AD, Baluch A, Kaye AJ, et al. Pharmacology of cyclooxygenase-2 inhibitors and preemptive analgesia in acute pain management. *Curr Opin Anaesthesiol.* 2008;21:439–445.

174. Coloma M, Chiu JW, White PF. The use of esmolol as an alternative to remifentanil during desflurane anesthesia for fast-track outpatient gynecologic laparoscopic surgery. *Anesth Analg.* 2001;92:352–357.

175. Collard V, Mistraletti G, Taqi A, et al. Intraoperative esmolol infusion in the absence of opioids spares postoperative fentanyl in patients undergoing ambulatory laparoscopic cholecystectomy. *Anesth Analg.* 2007;105(5):1255–1262.

176. White PF, Wang B, Tang J, et al. The effect of intraoperative use of esmolol and nicardipine on recovery after ambulatory surgery. *Anesth Analg.* 2003;97:1633–1638.

177. De Oliveira GS, Agarwal D, Benzon HT. Perioperative single dose ketorolac to prevent postoperative pain: a meta-analysis of randomized trials. *Anesth Analg.* 2012;114:424–433.

178. Norman PH, Daley MD, Lindsey RW. Preemptive analgesic effects of ketorolac in ankle fracture surgery. *Anesthesiology.* 2001;94(4):599–603.

179. Viscomi CM, Friend A, Parker C, et al. Ketamine as an adjuvant in lidocaine intravenous regional anesthesia: a randomized, double-blind, systematic control trial. *Reg Anesth Pain Med.* 2009;34:130–133.

180. Suzuki M. Role of N-methyl-D-aspartate receptor antagonists in postoperative pain management. *Curr Opin Anaesthesiol.* 2009;22(5):618–622.

181. Laskowski K, Stirling A, McKay WP, et al. A systematic review of intravenous ketamine for postoperative analgesia. *Can J Anaesth.* 2011;58:911–923.

182. Ryu JH, Kang MH, Park KS, et al. Effects of magnesium sulphate on intraoperative anaesthetic requirements and postoperative analgesia in gynaecology patients receiving total intravenous anaesthesia. *Br J Anaesth.* 2008;100(3):397–403.

183. Hwang JY, Na HS, Jeon YT, et al. I.V. infusion of magnesium sulphate during spinal anaesthesia improves postoperative analgesia. *Br J Anaesth.* 2010;104(1):89–93.

184. Mattila K, Kontinen VK, Kalso E, et al. Dexamethasone decreases oxycodone consumption following osteotomy of the first metatarsal bone: a randomized controlled trial in day surgery. *Acta Anaesthesiol Scand.* 2010;54:268–276.

185. De Oliveira GS, Almeida MD, Benzon HT, et al. Perioperative single dose systemic dexamethasone for postoperative pain. *Anesthesiology.* 2011;115:575–588.

IV

186. Romundstad L, Breivik H, Roald H, et al. Methylprednisolone reduces pain, emesis, and fatigue after breast augmentation surgery: a single-dose, randomized, parallel-group study with methylprednisolone 125 mg, parecoxib 40 mg and placebo. *Anesth Analg.* 2006;102(2):418–425.

187. Salman N, Uzun S, Coskun F, et al. Dexmedetomidine as a substitute for remifentanil in ambulatory gynecologic laparoscopic surgery. *Saudi Med J.* 2009;102:117–122.

188. De Oliveira GS, Fitzgerald P, Streicher LF, et al. Systemic lidocaine to improve postoperative quality of recovery after ambulatory laparoscopic surgery. *Anesth Analg.* 2012;115(2):262–267.

189. Pavlin DJ, Chen C, Penaloza DA, et al. Pain as a factor complicating recovery and discharge after ambulatory surgery. *Anesth Analg.* 2002;95(3):627–634.

190. Zhao J, Chung F, Hanna DB, et al. Dose-response relationship between opioid use and adverse effect after ambulatory surgery related events. *Pain Symptom Manage.* 2004;28(1):35–46.

191. Chen L, Tang J, White PF, et al. The effect of location of transcutaneous electrical nerve stimulation on postoperative opioid analgesic requirement: acupoint versus nonacupoint stimulation. *Anesth Analg.* 1998;87:1129–1134.

192. Lee A, Gin T, Lau AS, et al. A comparison of patients' and health care professionals' preferences for symptoms during immediate postoperative recovery and the management of postoperative nausea and vomiting. *Anesth Analg.* 2005;100:87–93.

193. White PF, O'Hara JF, Roberson CR, et al. The impact of current antiemetic practices on patient outcomes: a prospective study on high-risk patients. *Anesth Analg.* 2008;107:452–458.

194. Lichtor JL, Glass PS. We're tired of waiting. *Anesth Analg.* 2008;107(2):353–355.

195. Roh YH, Gong HS, Kim JH, et al. Factors associated with postoperative nausea and vomiting in patients undergoing an ambulatory hand surgery. *Clin Orthop Surg.* 2014;6(3):273–278.

196. Dzwonczyk R, Weaver TE, Puente EG, Bergese SD. Postoperative nausea and vomiting prophylaxis from an economic point of view. *Am J Ther.* 2012;19(1):11–15.

197. White PF, Sacan O, Nuangchamnong N, et al. The relationship between patient risk factors and early versus late postoperative emetic symptoms. *Anesth Analg.* 2008;107:459–463.

198. Candiotti KA, Kovac AL, Melson TI, et al. A randomized, double-blind study to evaluate the efficacy and safety of three different doses of palonosetron versus placebo in preventing postoperative nausea and vomiting. *Anesth Analg.* 2008;107:445–451.

199. Gupta A, Wu CL, Elkassabany N, et al. Does the routine prophylactic use of antiemetics affect the incidence of post-discharge nausea and vomiting following ambulatory surgery? A systematic review of randomized controlled trials. *Anesthesiology.* 2003;99:488–495.

200. Scuderi PE, James RL, Harris L, et al. Multimodal antiemetic management prevents early postoperative vomiting after outpatient laparoscopy. *Anesth Analg.* 2000;91:1408–1414.

201. Pan PH, Lee SC, Harris LC. Antiemetic prophylaxis for post-discharge nausea and vomiting and impact on functional quality of living during recovery in patients with high emetic risks: a prospective, randomized, double-blind comparison of two prophylactic antiemetic regimens. *Anesth Analg.* 2008;107:429–438.

202. De Oliveira GS, Castro-Alves LJ, Ahmad S, et al. Dexamethasone to prevent postoperative nausea and vomiting: an updated meta-analysis of randomized controlled trials. *Anesth Analg.* 2013;116(1):58–74.

203. Apfel CC, Korttila K, Abdalla M, et al. A factorial trial of six interventions for the prevention of postoperative nausea and vomiting. *N Engl J Med.* 2004;350(24):2441–2451.

204. Maharaj CH, Kallam SR, Malik A. Preoperative intravenous fluid therapy decreases postoperative nausea and pain in high risk patients. *Anesth Analg.* 2005;100:675–682.

205. Engelman E, Salengros J, Barvais L. How much does pharmacologic prophylaxis reduce postoperative vomiting in children? *Anesthesiology.* 2008;109:1023–1035.

206. Habib AS, Reuveni J, Taguchi A, et al. A comparison of ondansetron with promethazine for treating postoperative nausea and vomiting in patients who received prophylaxis with ondansetron: a retrospective database analysis. *Anesth Analg.* 2007;104:548–551.

207. Chung F. Recovery pattern and home-readiness after ambulatory surgery. *Anesth Analg.* 1995;80(5):896–902.

208. Moncel JB, Nardi N, Wodey E, et al. Evaluation of the pediatric post anesthesia discharge scoring system in an ambulatory surgery unit. *Paediatr Anaesth.* 2015;25(6):636–641.

209. Metzner J, Kent CD. Ambulatory surgery: is the liability risk lower? *Curr Opin Anaesthesiol.* 2012;25:654–658.

210. Chung F, Kayumov L, Sinclair DR, et al. What is the driving performance of ambulatory surgical patients after general anesthesia? *Anesthesiology.* 2005;103(5):951–956.

211. Abbass IM, Krause TM, Virani SS, et al. Revisiting the economic efficiencies of observation units. *Manag Care.* 2015;24(3):46–52.

212. Wu CL, Berenholtz SM, Provonost PJ. Systematic review and analysis of post-discharge symptoms after outpatient surgery. *Anesthesiology.* 2002;96:994–1003.

213. Manohar A, Cheung K, Wu CL, et al. Burden incurred by patients and their caregivers after outpatient surgery: a prospective observational study. *Clin Orthop Relat Res.* 2014;473(5):1416–1426.

214. Yabroff KR, Kim Y. Time costs associated with informal caregiving for cancer survivors. *Cancer.* 2009;115(suppl 18):4362–4373.

215. Bryson GL, Mercer C, Varpio L. Patient and caregiver experience following ambulatory surgery: qualitative analysis in a cohort of patients 65 yr and older. *Can J Anaesth.* 2014;61(11):986–994.

216. Sandberg EH, Sharma R, Sandberg WS. Deficits in retention for verbally presented medical information. *Anesthesiology.* 2012;117:772–779.

217. Chanthong P, Abrishami A, Wong J, et al. Systematic review of questionnaires of measuring patient satisfaction in ambulatory anesthesia. *Anesthesiology.* 2009;110(5):1061–1067.

218. Idvall E, Berg K, Unosson M, et al. Assessment of recovery after day surgery using a modified version of quality of recovery-40. *Acta Anaesthesiol Scand.* 2009;53(5):673–677.

219. Odom-Forren J, Jalota L, Moser DK, et al. Incidence and predictors of postdischarge nausea and vomiting in a 7-day population. *J Clin Anesth.* 2013;25(7):551–559.

220. Apfel CC. Who is at risk for postdischarge nausea and vomiting after ambulatory surgery? *Anesthesiology.* 2012;117:475–486.

221. Meltron M, Nielsen K, Tucker M, et al. Long-acting serotonin antagonist (palonosetron) and the NK-1 receptor antagonists. *Anesthesiol Clin.* 2014;32(2):505–516.

222. Bingham AE, Fur R, Horn JL, et al. Continuous peripheral nerve block compared with single-injection peripheral nerve block: a systematic review and meta-analysis of randomized controlled trials. *Reg Anesth Pain Med.* 2012;37(6):583–594.

223. Ilfeld BM. Continuous peripheral nerve blocks in the hospital and at home. *Anesthesiol Clin.* 2011;29(2):193–211.

224. Neal JM, Barrington MJ, Brull R, et al. The second ASRA practice advisory on neurologic complications associated with regional anesthesia and pain medicine: executive summary. *Reg Anesth Pain Med.* 2015;40(5):401–430.

225. Watson JC, Huntoon MA. Neurologic evaluation and management of perioperative nerve injury. *Reg Anesth Pain Med.* 2015;40(5):491–501.

226. Veljkovic A, Dwyer T, Lau JT, et al. Neurological complications related to elective orthopedic surgery: part 3: common foot and ankle procedures. *Reg Anesth Pain Med.* 2015;40(5):431–432.

227. Dwyer T, Drexler M, Chan VW, et al. Neurological complications related to elective orthopedic surgery: part 2: common hip and knee procedures. *Reg Anesth Pain Med.* 2015;40(5):443–454.

228. Dwyer T, Henry PD, Cholvisudhi P, et al. Neurological complications related to elective orthopedic surgery: part 1: common shoulder and elbow procedures. *Reg Anesth Pain Med.* 2015;40(5):455–466.

229. Laffel G, Blumenthal D. The case for using industrial quality management science in health care organizations. *JAMA.* 1989;262(20):2869–2873.

230. Spear S. Learning to lead at Toyota. *Harv Bus Rev.* 2004;82(5):78–86.

231. Spencer FC. Human error in hospitals and industrial accidents: current concepts. *J Am Coll Surg.* 2000;191(4):410–418.

232. Uhlig P. Interview with a quality leader: Paul Uhlig on transforming healthcare. Interviewed by Jason Trevor Fogg. *J Health Care Qual.* 2009;31(3):5–9.

233. Jamtvedt G, Young JM, Kristoffersen DT, et al. Audit and feedback: effects on professional practice and health care outcomes. *Cochrane Database Syst Rev.* 2006;(2). CD:000259.

IV

# 38 ANESTHESIA FOR PROCEDURES IN NON-OPERATING ROOM LOCATIONS

## Wilson Cui and Chanhung Z. Lee

**CHARACTERISTICS OF NORA LOCATIONS**
Importance of Communication
Standard of Care and Equipment

**SAFETY AND CONCERNS IN RADIOLOGY SUITES**
Radiation Safety Practices
Monitoring the Radiation Dose
Adverse Reactions to Contrast Materials

**MAGNETIC RESONANCE IMAGING**
MRI Safety Considerations
Monitoring Issues in MRI Suites
Compatible Equipment

**ANESTHESIA FOR NONINVASIVE IMAGING PROCEDURES**
Physiologic Monitoring
Oxygen Administration
Pharmacologically Induced Sedation
Management of Anesthesia for Computed Tomography
Management of Anesthesia for MRI

**INTERVENTIONAL RADIOLOGY**
Interventional Neuroradiology
Body Interventional Radiology

**ENDOSCOPY AND ENDOSCOPIC RETROGRADE CHOLANGIOPANCREATOGRAPHY**
Anesthesia Evaluation and Management
Challenges and Complications

**CATHETER-BASED CARDIOLOGY PROCEDURES**
Adult Cardiac Catheterization
Electrophysiology Studies
Structural Heart Disease Intervention
Pediatric Studies
Challenges and Complications

**ELECTROCONVULSIVE THERAPY**
Electrically Induced Seizures
Anesthesia Evaluation
Psychotropic Medications
Induction of Anesthesia and Seizure
Physiologic Responses to Seizure and Treatment

**QUESTIONS OF THE DAY**

Procedures performed outside the operating room fall under the term non–operating room anesthesia (NORA), which refers to providing anesthesia care at any location away from traditional operating room suites (Box 38.1). In response to the need for minimally invasive interventions as well as the rapid advancement in imaging and other technologies, the number of NORA procedures has markedly increased in many medical and surgical specialties. Even as more hybrid operating rooms are being built inside or close to the main operating rooms, NORA is increasingly becoming a significant part of anesthesia care.

Many patients treated in NORA locations are deemed "too sick" to undergo traditional surgical interventions. As with most anesthetics, both patient and procedure factors must be considered (Table 38.1). Anesthesia-related concerns include (1) maintenance of patient immobility and physiologic stability, (2) perioperative management of anticoagulation, (3) readiness for sudden unexpected complications during the procedure, (4) provision of smooth and rapid emergence from

The editors and publisher would like to thank Drs. Lawrence Litt and William L. Young for contributing to this chapter in the previous edition of this work. It has served as the foundation for the current chapter.
This chapter is dedicated to the memory of our esteemed colleague and mentor, Dr. William L. Young.

---

**Box 38.1** NORA Locations That Commonly Require Anesthesia Services

**Radiology and Nuclear Medicine**
Diagnostic radiology and nuclear medicine
  Computed tomography
  Fluoroscopy
Therapeutic radiology
  Interventional body angiography (can involve embolization or stent placement)
  Interventional neuroangiography (can involve embolization or stent placement)
Magnetic resonance imaging
Positron emission tomography (PET) scan
Ultrasound imaging

**Radiation Therapy**
Standard x-ray therapy with collimated beams
Gamma Knife x-ray surgery for brain tumors and arteriovenous malformations
CyberKnife x-ray surgery for central nervous system, body tumors, and arteriovenous malformations
Electron beam radiation therapy (usually intraoperative)

**Cardiology**
Cardiac catheterization with or without electrophysiologic studies
Cardioversion
Structural cardiac intervention

**Gastroenterology**
Upper gastrointestinal endoscopy
Colonoscopy
Endoscopic retrograde cholangiopancreatography

**Pulmonary Medicine**
Tracheal and bronchial stent placement
Bronchoscopy
Pulmonary lavage

**Psychiatry**
Electroconvulsive therapy

**Urology**
Extracorporeal shock wave lithotripsy
Nephrostomy tube placement

**General Dentistry and Oral and Maxillofacial Surgery**
Dental surgery

**Reproductive Health**
In vitro fertilization procedures

*NORA*, Non-operating room anesthesia.

---

**Table 38.1**   Factors Considered for the Involvement of Anesthesia Services

| Patient | Procedure |
|---|---|
| History of anxiety | Duration |
| Chronic opiate dependency | Nonsupine position |
| High oxygen requirement | Breath holding |
| Sleep apnea | Immobilization |
| Altered mental status | Degree of invasiveness |
| Inability to follow command | |
| Comorbid conditions | |

anesthesia and sedation at appropriate times (which may even be required during the procedure), and (5) appropriate postprocedure monitoring and management during transport. A study of the National Anesthesia Clinical Outcomes Registry (NACOR) database has revealed that patients receiving NORA were older, and monitored anesthesia care was more commonly performed as compared to anesthesia given in the main operating room.[1] NACOR's report of complications in NORA locations also indicated that the most common major complications were serious hemodynamic instability and increased rates of death in cardiology and radiology locations. This chapter emphasizes the unique aspects of working in some of the common NORA locations, which often include special medical and procedure concerns and approaches.

## CHARACTERISTICS OF NORA LOCATIONS

### Importance of Communication

Remote locations are structured differently from the typical operating room, but clear communication is prudent for efficient and safe practice in either site. With clear communication, the actions of anesthesia personnel can be integrated with those of the procedural team involved in the NORA intervention. The anesthesia provider should have a detailed plan for communicating with more centrally located anesthesia colleagues and technicians, especially when help is required urgently. For instance, an unexpected difficult airway can be especially challenging because of the remote nature of many NORA locations. Additional anesthesia personnel and resources should be immediately available if needed. Sometimes the anesthesia providers in NORA locations feel isolated from the facilities available to operating room personnel. The lack of mutual experience and vocabulary presents challenges for anesthesia providers and other staff working in NORA locations. Anesthesia providers and proceduralists should have a mutual understanding of the specifics and challenges in the procedures as well as in medical care. Anesthesia providers working in an unfamiliar remote location must keep track of the identity and role of personnel participating in the interventional procedure or patient care. During times when the anesthesia provider may need experienced medical assistance (e.g., tracheal intubation, placement of an invasive monitor, or intravenous access), the availability of qualified staff members must be identified. Readily available

IV

preoperative documents for all patients in remote locations must include the attending proceduralist's patient history and physical examination. Patient arrival and check-in arrangements should be similar to those for patients undergoing procedures in a traditional operating room setting.

## Standard of Care and Equipment

Anesthesia care provided in remote locations must adhere to the same standards as the operating room. The American Society of Anesthesiologists (ASA) has issued a Statement on Nonoperating Room Anesthetizing Locations that posts minimal guidelines for NORA procedures. In summary, these guidelines recommend adequate monitoring capabilities, the means to deliver supplemental oxygen via a face mask with positive-pressure ventilation, the availability of suction, the equipment for providing controlled mechanical ventilation, an adequate supply of anesthetic drugs and ancillary equipment, and supplemental lighting for procedures that involve darkness. Although portable anesthesia machines should be placed in close proximity to the patient to facilitate breathing circuit connections, this is not always possible owing to the presence of equipment such as fluoroscopy "C-arms."

If anesthetic gases are to be used, scavenging must be sufficient to ensure that trace amounts are below the upper limits set by the Occupational Safety and Health Administration (OSHA). Remote locations frequently involve additional hazards, such as exposure to radiation, loud sound levels, and heavy mechanical equipment. Advance preparation should be made to have all needed equipment available, such as lead aprons, portable lead-glass shields, and earplugs. At the end of the procedure one may often travel distances longer than the usual distance to the postanesthesia care unit or other patient units. So that patients can be safely and expeditiously transported to a recovery area, remote locations should always have available sufficient supplies of supplemental oxygen, transport monitors, and elevator and passageway keys. The anesthesia provider should always know the location of the nearest defibrillator, fire extinguisher, gas shutoff valves, and exits.

## SAFETY AND CONCERNS IN RADIOLOGY SUITES

Imaging-related procedures for both diagnostic and interventional purposes have been presented as a major component in current NORA operations.

## Radiation Safety Practices

Ionizing radiation and radiation safety issues are often encountered in these locations.[2] Radiation intensity and exposure decrease with the inverse square of the distance from the emitting source. Frequently, the anesthesia provider can be located immediately behind a movable lead-glass screen. Regardless of whether this is possible or not, the anesthesia provider should wear a lead apron and a lead thyroid shield and remain at least 1 to 2 m from the radiation source. A 2011 study also highlighted the importance of eye protection for anesthesia providers working for a significant time in the radiology suite.[3] Clear communication between the radiology and anesthesia teams is crucial for limiting radiation exposure.

## Monitoring the Radiation Dose

Anesthesia providers, like all other health care workers who are at risk for radiation exposure, can monitor their monthly dosage by wearing radiation exposure badges. The physics unit of measurement for a biologic radiation dose is the sievert (Sv): 100 rem = 1 Sv. Because some types of ionizing radiation are more injurious than others, the biologic radiation dose is a product of the type-specific radiation weighting factor (or "quality factor") and the ionizing energy absorbed per gram of tissue. Radiation exposure can be monitored with one or more film badges. In the United States, the average annual dose from cosmic rays and naturally occurring radioactive materials is about 3 mSv (300 mrem). Patients undergoing a chest radiograph receive a dose of 0.04 mSv, whereas those undergoing a computed tomography (CT) scan of the head receive 2 mSv. Federal guidelines set a limit of 50 mSv for the maximum annual occupational dose.

## Adverse Reactions to Contrast Materials

Contrast materials are used in more than 10 million diagnostic radiology procedures performed each year. In 1990, fatal adverse reactions after the intravenous administration of contrast media were estimated to occur approximately once every 100,000 procedures, whereas serious adverse reactions were estimated to occur 0.2% of the time with ionic materials and 0.4% of the time with low osmolarity materials. Radiocontrast materials can produce anaphylactoid reactions in sensitive patients, and such reactions necessitate aggressive intervention, including the administration of oxygen, intravenous fluids, and epinephrine, with epinephrine being the essential component of therapy (also see Chapter 45).

Adverse drug reactions are more common after the injection of iodinated contrast agents (used for x-ray examinations such as CT) than after gadolinium contrast agents (used for magnetic resonance imaging [MRI]). The signs and symptoms of anaphylactoid reactions can be mild (nausea, pruritus, diaphoresis), moderate (faintness, emesis, urticaria, laryngeal edema, bronchospasm), or severe (seizures, hypotensive shock, laryngeal edema, respiratory distress, cardiac arrest) (also see Chapter 45). Prophylaxis against anaphylactoid reactions is directed against the massive vasodilation that results from mast cell and basophil release of inflammatory cytokines such as histamine, serotonin, and bradykinin. The main approach to prophylaxis is steroid and antihistamine administration on the night before and the morning of the procedure. A typical regimen for a 70-kg adult is 40 mg prednisone, 20 mg famotidine, and 50 mg diphenhydramine.[4] Patients undergoing contrast procedures usually have induced diuresis from the intravenous osmotic load presented by the contrast agent. In this regard, adequate hydration of these patients is important to prevent aggravation of coexisting hypovolemia or azotemia. Chemotoxic reactions to contrast media are typically dose-dependent (unlike anaphylactoid and anaphylactic reactions) and related to osmolarity and ionic strength of the contrast agent.

Intravenous contrast material is often administered for radiologic imaging. A serious adverse reaction called nephrogenic systemic fibrosis (NSF) can occur after exposure to gadolinium-based MRI contrast agents.[5] In NSF there is fibrosis of the skin, connective tissue, and sometimes internal organs. The severity of NSF can range from mild to severe and it can also be fatal. However, NSF apparently occurs only when severe renal impairment (e.g., dialysis-dependent renal failure) also exists. Anesthesia providers should not casually administer gadolinium-containing MRI contrast agent to patients with renal disease.

## MAGNETIC RESONANCE IMAGING

MRI is a standard diagnostic tool and is likely to supplant or replace conventional x-ray techniques. However, MRI image quality is degraded significantly with patient movement, and scanning sequences can take an hour or more. The MRI "bore" where the patient is positioned is a tube with diameter of only 60 cm to 70 cm and length of approximately 120 cm. Thus, patient immobility is the primary indication for sedation or general anesthesia. Patients who routinely require anesthesia services for MRI include children, adults who are claustrophobic or in pain, and critical care patients.

### MRI Safety Considerations

Although ionizing radiation is not a safety issue because no x-rays or radioactive substances are involved, other safety issues are prominent in the magnet suite. Hearing loss may occur from high sound levels during the scan. Electrical burns can occur if incompatible monitoring equipment is attached to the patient. Similarly, patients with incompatible implanted devices or ferromagnetic material should never be placed inside a large magnetic

field as device heating and malfunction can result in patient injury. Finally, missile injury can occur if ferromagnetic objects are brought within the vicinity of the magnetic field.

Objects in the magnet room need to be both MRI safe and MRI compatible. The term "MR conditional" was defined by the American Society for Testing and Materials to describe an item that poses no known hazards in a specified MRI environment (with specifications that include the static magnetic field strength and spatial gradient field generated by a particular MRI model). Before an MRI scan is started, the anesthesia provider should ensure the patient has been screened and cleared by MRI technicians responsible for knowing that the patient's body does not contain susceptible metal objects such as incompatible orthopedic hardware, cardiac implantable electronic devices (CIEDs), wire-reinforced epidural catheters, or a pulmonary artery catheter with a temperature wire. Pulse oximetry is essential during MRI scans, and only an MRI-compatible fiberoptic pulse oximeter should be used. Patient burns can result at the point of attachment if one uses a standard pulse oximeter. Similar concerns pertain to any other monitoring or management devices that make actual or potential patient contact.

Missile injury in an MRI suite is a serious and life-threatening risk. The superconducting electrical currents that generate an MRI scanner's large magnetic field are always "on." Therefore, MRI scanners are always surrounded by large magnetic field gradients (up to 6 m away). Magnetic field gradients can pull metallic objects into the magnet with alarming speed and force. Certain metals such as nickel and cobalt are dangerous because they are magnetic, whereas other metals such as aluminum, titanium, copper, and silver do not pose a missile danger. These metals are used to make MRI-compatible intravenous poles, fixation devices, and nonmagnetic anesthesia machines. MRI-compatible intravenous infusion pumps are clinically available. If one must bring susceptible metal items such as infusion pumps into the MRI magnet room, they should be safely located and fixed, preferably bolted to a wall or floor. The additional equipment should be placed and verified as secure before the patient enters the MRI scanner. In the event that an object is pulled into the magnet causing patient injury and equipment damage, the superconducting magnet can be turned off immediately. This process, called *quenching*, should only be performed by MRI technicians. The superconducting magnet of an MRI operates at cryogenic temperatures near absolute zero and requires coolant (cryogen) such as liquid helium to maintain the low temperature. The quenching process involves a rise in temperature of the superconducting magnet with escape of cryogen into a venting system outside the MRI room. However, cryogen can escape into the MRI room and displace oxygen, which can cause cold injury and asphyxiation.

IV

## Monitoring Issues in MRI Suites

Many anesthesia providers prefer to be outside the magnet room during the scan. This practice is acceptable as long as the provider (1) has access to all vital sign monitor displays and (2) can view the patient through a window or video camera. Critically ill patients undergoing MRI may require an arterial line for blood pressure monitoring. If the pressure transducer is classified as "MR conditional" for the particular MRI scanner, then it may be used during the procedure along with an MRI-compatible pressure cable and monitoring system. Otherwise, long lengths of pressure tubing must be added so that pressure transducers and their electrical cables can be located far from the magnet, preferably outside the magnet room. The radiofrequency pulse from an MRI can cause a pressure transducer to generate artifactual spikes. This can lead to erroneously high arterial blood pressure readings that could mislead the anesthesia provider. Visual inspection of the waveform allows rapid detection of this artifact. All arterial and venous line stopcocks should be capped so that hemorrhage will not occur if the stopcock is inadvertently manipulated.

## Compatible Equipment

The MRI-compatible equipment that goes into the magnet room functions as a second anesthesia workstation. Although suction, physiologic monitoring, and mechanical ventilation must be possible inside the magnet room, a primary anesthesia workstation must be located just outside the magnet room. If a potentially life-threatening problem arises, the patient must be promptly transferred from the scanner room to the primary anesthesia workstation so that optimal care and additional help can be provided.

## ANESTHESIA FOR NONINVASIVE IMAGING PROCEDURES

Because noninvasive imaging procedures do not cause pain, most adult patients do not need sedation or general anesthesia. The ASA has described a continuum of depth of sedation that includes progressive levels of sedation, including minimal sedation (anxiolysis), moderate sedation (so-called "conscious sedation"), deep sedation, and general anesthesia (also see Chapter 14, Table 14.1). For those adult patients who require sedation, anxiolysis (pharmacologic or nonpharmacologic) may be all that is required. In many medical centers, minimal sedation and moderate sedation can be provided by appropriately trained nonanesthesia personnel, whereas deep sedation and general anesthesia must be administered by anesthesia providers. For pediatric patients, deep sedation or general anesthesia is often required to facilitate the imaging procedure. In addition to the requirements for sedation, patient comorbid conditions such as airway compromise, severe cardiac or respiratory disease, or morbid obesity may require an anesthesia provider to assure patient immobility, maintenance of adequate oxygenation, hemodynamic stability, and minimization of pain and anxiety during the radiology procedure.

## Physiologic Monitoring

The ASA Standards of Basic Anesthetic Monitoring (also see Chapter 20) are applicable to all noninvasive imaging procedures. Anesthesia providers commonly use specially constructed nasal cannulas that have an integrated $CO_2$ sampling line. Capnography can provide the respiratory rate and pattern, as well as the end-tidal $CO_2$ concentration, although readings are more prone to artifacts in a nonintubated patient. If capnography is not possible, ventilation must be assessed by continuous visual inspection, auscultation, or both.

## Oxygen Administration

Supplemental oxygen via a nasal cannula should come from a dedicated flowmeter instead of the anesthesia machine common gas outlet. This approach permits more rapid deployment of the anesthesia machine breathing circuit for delivering face mask oxygen or positive-pressure ventilation if the patient develops hypoventilation, hypoxemia, or apnea. For procedures of long duration, humidified oxygen should be given via nasal cannula to promote patient comfort by minimizing drying of the nasal and pharyngeal passages. Certain patients, including infants and small children, will not tolerate a nasal cannula but can receive oxygen with a "blow-by" technique.

## Pharmacologically Induced Sedation

Many medications can be used to provide sedation for imaging procedures (also see Chapters 8, 9, and 14). For example, sedation can usually be managed successfully with a continuous propofol infusion, with or without supplemental intravenous opioids or benzodiazepines (or both). For brief procedures, a small dose of a rapid-onset, short-acting opioid such as remifentanil or alfentanil is often an appropriate selection. Dexmedetomidine is another useful drug, primarily in procedures lasting more than an hour. Because dexmedetomidine has less frequent risk of respiratory depression compared to propofol, it is especially useful for patients with severe pulmonary hypertension, or those who require frequent assessment of mental status. Because dexmedetomidine tends to decrease systemic arterial blood pressure and has relatively long lasting duration, its use might require intravenous vasopressor support. Dexmedetomidine should be used cautiously in patients undergoing procedures that require arterial blood pressure to remain at baseline values or that require induced hypertension. Patients with atherosclerotic lesions in cerebral, cardiac, or renal arteries, as well as patients with brain or spinal cord compression from tumors, are particularly vulnerable.

## Management of Anesthesia for Computed Tomography

CT is often used for intracranial imaging and for studies of the thorax and abdomen. Because CT is painless, noninvasive, and generally of short duration, adult patients undergoing elective diagnostic scans rarely require more than emotional support. In addition, the bore of the CT scan is much more open than an MRI, so claustrophobia is rarely an issue. CT scanning is a crucial diagnostic tool in several acute settings, including traumatic injury (head and abdominal), acute stroke, and acute altered mental status of unknown cause. CT scanning is also used for urgent assessments of gastrointestinal integrity in critically ill patients in the intensive care unit (ICU), who may require complex care during ICU transport. Sedation or general anesthesia is often essential for such patients, as well as for children and adults who have difficulty remaining motionless.

Unlike MRI, the concerns about magnetic fields are not present for CT scanning; however, the anesthesia provider is at risk for exposure to ionizing radiation. During the CT scan, the anesthesia provider should remain behind radiation shielding while the mechanized table moves the patient through the scanner. In addition to patient medical issues, complications during a CT scan could include disconnection of oxygen tubing or breathing circuits, inadvertent removal of intravenous catheters, and disconnection of monitors.

## Management of Anesthesia for MRI

For pediatric patients (also see Chapter 34), a common technique consists of (1) inhaled induction of anesthesia with sevoflurane, (2) placement of intravenous catheter, (3) intravenous infusion of propofol, and (4) either nasal cannula, laryngeal mask airway, or endotracheal tube for airway management, based on patient comorbid conditions. For adults who require general anesthesia for MRI, the location of planned imaging may influence airway management choice. For example, a patient with a laryngeal mask airway may still have slight airway obstruction resulting in unacceptable motion artifact during brain MRI scan, which would not occur with an endotracheal tube.

Certain MRI image sequences (e.g., fluid-attenuated inversion recovery [FLAIR]) are influenced by the patient's oxygenation, which is managed by the anesthesia provider. Hyperoxia can increase signal intensity in brain cerebrospinal fluid, so the radiologist may request a decrease in the inspired oxygen concentration and must interpret the MRI scan accordingly.[6]

## INTERVENTIONAL RADIOLOGY

Interventional radiology (IR) is a rapidly changing field as a result of continuing improvement in imaging quality and technological advances. The ability to combine real-time, noninvasive imaging with minimally invasive, often catheter-based, interventions offers great benefits to patients who otherwise have to experience the stress of an open surgery and possibly lengthier recovery. Interventional neuroradiology (INR), also called endovascular neurosurgery, mixes traditional neurosurgery with neuroradiology while also including certain aspects of head and neck surgery. Body IR mixes general surgery with general radiology. In angiographic procedures, the relevant blood vessel trees are imaged, after which a decision is made to advance to one or more therapeutic interventions via drugs, devices, or both. The list of IR procedures is extensive and continues to grow.

### Interventional Neuroradiology

#### Anesthesia Choice
Most medical centers routinely use general endotracheal anesthesia for complex procedures or those of long duration, but there is no clearly superior anesthetic technique.[7] The specific choice of anesthesia may be guided primarily by the procedure needs as well as cardiovascular and cerebrovascular considerations.[8] Advantages of general anesthesia include control of ventilation and immobility, which improves image quality. Intermittent apnea may be requested by the interventional team to even further reduce motion artifact during digital subtraction angiography. Mechanical ventilation goals include maintenance of normocapnia or slight hypocapnia as long as intracranial pressure is normal. A patient with increased intracranial pressure may benefit from mild hyperventilation prior to anesthesia induction as well as during maintenance of anesthesia, in order to counteract inhaled anesthetic-induced cerebral vasodilation (also see Chapter 30). As an alternative to general anesthesia, minimal or moderate sedation has the advantage of allowing assessment of neurologic function during the procedure. A variety of medications can be used for sedation based on the experience of the provider and the goals of anesthetic management.

#### Access and Monitoring
The INR suite requires multiple imaging screens and a large fluoroscopy C-arm device that is capable of extensive movement around the patient. As a result, the distance from the intravenous catheter to the intravenous fluid bag can be twice as long as normal. The tubing extensions must be securely connected and of sufficient length to prevent accidental dislodgement. Infusions of intravenous anesthetics or vasoactive drugs should be connected as close to the intravenous catheter as possible

**IV**

to minimize tubing dead space. For procedures involving the blood supply to the central nervous system (CNS), arterial line placement for continuous blood pressure monitoring is prudent. A significant volume of fluid (e.g., heparinized flush solution and radiographic contrast agent) can be administered through catheters placed by the interventional team, in addition to the fluid administered by the anesthesia provider. Foley catheter placement will facilitate assessment of urine output and assist in fluid management decisions, and will promote patient comfort by avoiding bladder distention.

### Arterial Blood Pressure Management

Baseline arterial blood pressure and cardiovascular reserve should be assessed carefully because blood pressure manipulation is commonly required during INR procedures and treatment-related perturbations regularly occur. Maintenance of arterial blood pressure within a predetermined range is particularly important in patients with cerebrovascular disease. Arterial blood pressure targets should always be discussed preoperatively with the interventional team. Deliberate hypertension, that is, maintaining a higher than normal arterial blood pressure, is used in INR patients with occlusive cerebrovascular disease to promote collateral cerebral blood flow. Such cases include patients undergoing emergency thrombolysis[9,10] and patients with aneurysmal subarachnoid hemorrhage in whom vasospasm has developed. Maintaining normal or supranormal arterial pressure is also important in patients with tumors that compromise blood flow to the spinal cord, kidneys, and other organs. Conversely, prevention of arterial hypertension may be critical in certain patients, including those with recently ruptured intracranial aneurysms or recently obliterated intracranial arteriovenous malformation. Patients who have undergone cerebrovascular angioplasty and stent placement in extracranial conductance vessels such as the carotid artery are susceptible to posttreatment cerebral hyperperfusion injury and require careful control of systemic blood pressure after the procedure[11] (also see Chapter 30).

### Management of Neurologic and Procedural Crises

Crisis management during an INR procedure requires a well-thought-out plan coupled with rapid and effective communication between the anesthesia and radiology teams. The initial responsibility of the anesthesia provider is to assure that airway patency, gas exchange, and hemodynamic status remain intact. Then the anesthesia provider should communicate with the procedural team and determine whether the INR problem is hemorrhagic or occlusive.

In the setting of vascular occlusion, the goal is to increase distal perfusion by augmentation of arterial blood pressure with or without direct thrombolysis. This may require preparation and administration of a vasopressor infusion.

If the problem is hemorrhage, the anesthesia provider should discuss with the interventional team whether to immediately cease heparin administration and administer reversal with protamine. Complications of protamine administration include hypotension, anaphylaxis, and pulmonary hypertension. Most cases of vascular rupture can be managed in the angiography suite. The INR team can attempt to seal the rupture site via endovascular approach and may abort the originally planned procedure. In addition, a ventriculostomy catheter may be placed emergently in the angiography suite if elevated intracranial pressure is suspected. Patients with suspected rupture will require emergent head CT scan, but emergent craniotomy may not be needed.

## Body Interventional Radiology

Interventional radiologists use x-rays, CT, ultrasound, MRI, and other imaging modalities to perform image-guided procedures throughout the body. These procedures are usually performed using needles and catheters, which are regarded as minimally invasive compared to traditional surgery. This section highlights the general approaches and challenges of anesthesia management for the most common image-guided procedures, such as diagnostic procedures, catheter drainage, stent placement, tumor ablation, vascular angioplasty and embolization treatment, and site-specific delivery of therapeutic agents (Table 38.2). Transjugular intrahepatic portosystemic shunt (TIPS) procedure deserves special recognition because of the severity of illness in its patient population.[12]

### Anesthesia Evaluation and Management

The anesthesia requirements of patients undergoing IR procedures can vary greatly. Because of the minimally invasive nature, many procedures in the IR suites are performed with minimal sedation without an anesthesia provider present. However, a number of factors can prompt the involvement of the anesthesia provider (see Table 38.1). The presence of an anesthesia provider allows the proceduralists to focus their complete attention on the intervention at hand. A clear and detailed discussion should take place among the team members, so the proceduralists can specify their intraprocedural needs and the anesthesia provider can express any anesthetic concerns.

The preprocedure evaluation by the anesthesia provider follows the same approach as with any other anesthetic (also see Chapter 13). The choice of anesthetic technique follows the same principles outlined earlier in this chapter (also see Chapter 14). Patients who have altered mental status, or cognitive dysfunction—dementia, delirium, encephalopathy, or developmental delay—may not be candidates for sedation if they will be expected to cooperate and breath-hold during the procedure. The

| Table 38.2 | List of Common Interventional Radiology Procedures | | |
|------------|--------------------|------------|------------------|
| **Vascular** | **Liver/Biliary** | **Cancer** | **Miscellaneous** |
| Angiography | Biliary drainage and stenting | Percutaneous (needle) biopsy | Abscess drainage |
| Balloon angioplasty | Transjugular liver biopsy | Chemoembolization | Chest tube |
| Embolization | Transjugular intrahepatic portosystemic shunt | Radiofrequency ablation | Percutaneous nephrostomy tube |
| Central venous/hemodialysis access | | | Gastrostomy tube |
| Thrombolysis | | | |
| Vena cava filter | | | |

medication list should be reviewed. Special concerns for body interventional procedures include therapy with the oral antihyperglycemic metformin, which may cause lactic acidosis if administered with intravenous contrast agent in the setting of renal failure. Lactic acidosis is extremely rare when a patient with normal renal function receives both metformin and intravenous contrast agent. ASA Practice Guidelines for Preoperative Fasting should be followed as with any other elective procedure.

If general anesthesia is not the initial anesthetic choice, the anesthesia provider should be prepared to escalate the level of sedation as needed, up to and including general anesthesia. Therefore, all necessary equipment, monitors, and medications should be available.

### Transjugular Intrahepatic Portosystemic Shunt

Patients who are scheduled to undergo the TIPS procedure have significant liver disease and complications of portal hypertension, which can include variceal bleeding, ascites, and hepatorenal syndrome. The Model for End-Stage Liver Disease (MELD) score serves as a marker of liver disease severity and is a predictor of short-term mortality risk in these patients, some of whom may be candidates for liver transplantation. Anesthetic evaluation should focus on the multisystem effects of liver failure, including cardiovascular, pulmonary, neurologic, renal, and hematologic manifestations (also see Chapter 28). Hepatic encephalopathy is a common finding in this patient population and is a contraindication for TIPS. Coagulopathy and thrombocytopenia may increase bleeding risk and require correction prior to the procedure.

The anesthetic management of a patient undergoing TIPS procedure can be quite challenging. Because of the presence of cardiopulmonary comorbid conditions, coagulopathy, and the unpredictable length of the procedure, most proceduralists prefer general anesthesia. Medications that have significant liver metabolism and biliary clearance should be avoided or minimized. The presence of tense ascites and gastroesophageal reflux are obvious risk factors for pulmonary aspiration of gastric contents.

An endotracheal tube is preferred for airway management (as opposed to a laryngeal mask airway) because the neck must be rotated to provide internal jugular venous access. Lastly, the anesthesia provider must be aware of several important post-TIPS complications: altered mental status because of post-TIPS encephalopathy, massive hemorrhage from intrahepatic bleeding or vascular injury, and worsening liver failure from decreased portal vein blood flow.

### Challenges: Hemostasis and Anticoagulation

Many IR procedures involve access of the arterial tree with large-diameter catheters. To minimize the risk of thromboembolic complication, the anesthesia provider is often asked to maintain intraprocedural anticoagulation. This is usually achieved with intravenous heparin, and monitored with whole blood activated clotting time (ACT). Heparin has the advantage of a short half-life and reliable reversal with protamine. For patients with heparin or protamine allergy or heparin-induced thrombocytopenia, direct thrombin inhibitors are alternatives. However, there is no reliable reversal for these drugs.

On the other hand, IR embolization is frequently performed as urgent therapy for acute hemorrhage. Common applications include gastrointestinal or uterine bleeding. Diagnostic angiography is performed to identify the site and mechanism of bleeding. Often, coils and thrombotic agents can be injected to stop the bleeding. To safely induce anesthesia and to rapidly secure the airway in a bleeding patient can be challenging. In addition, the patient's vital signs may further deteriorate after induction of anesthesia and require resuscitation with fluids and blood transfusion (also see Chapters 23 and 24). In addition to acute anemia, coagulopathy and thrombocytopenia are common, either as the cause of the initial hemorrhage or as the result of dilution from fluid replacement or factor consumption. The correction of coagulopathy should ideally be guided by laboratory data and a treatment algorithm. Because data may not be available during an emergency, the decision whether to transfuse

**IV**

will need to rely on the patient's medical history (e.g., presence of hematologic and hepatic diseases), medications (e.g., anticoagulant or antiplatelet therapy), physical findings (e.g., of disseminated intravascular coagulopathy), and the clinician's judgment. In addition to platelets, plasma, and cryoprecipitate, recombinant factors and factor concentrates may offer similar benefit of correcting factor deficiency without the risk of transfusion-related complications (see Chapters 22 and 24).

# ENDOSCOPY AND ENDOSCOPIC RETROGRADE CHOLANGIOPANCREATOGRAPHY

Endoscopy is frequently performed for the diagnosis and screening of gastrointestinal conditions. Indications for upper endoscopy (esophagogastroduodenoscopy, EGD) include gastroesophageal reflux, bleeding, dysphagia, protracted pain or nausea, accidental ingestion, and abnormal imaging. Additionally, therapeutic interventions such as treatment of bleeding source, ablation of Barrett esophagus, biopsy and removal of abnormal growth, dilation and stenting of stricture, and feeding tube placement can be performed. The development of high-frequency endoscopic ultrasound (EUS) using a small-caliber catheter through the biopsy channel of the endoscope can provide high-resolution images of benign and neoplastic lesions in the gastrointestinal tract.

For EGD, the patient is typically placed in a left lateral position with the neck flexed. The usual sequence of events includes (1) application of topical anesthesia to the patient's pharynx with either lidocaine or benzocaine, (2) placement of a plastic mouth guard to minimize risk of damage to teeth or endoscope, (3) administration of medications to achieve minimal to moderate sedation, (4) insertion of endoscope through mouth into esophagus, (5) examination of esophagus, gastroesophageal junction, stomach, pylorus, and duodenum as required, and (5) performance of therapeutic maneuvers when necessary.

Endoscopic retrograde cholangiopancreatography (ERCP) is often performed for the diagnosis and possible treatment of bile duct and pancreatic duct diseases. ERCP requires specialized equipment including a dedicated fluoroscopy machine. Common indications include jaundice, acute biliary pancreatitis, chronic pancreatitis of unknown cause, pancreatic pseudocyst, suspected biliary or pancreatic malignancy, sphincter of Oddi disorders, duct stricture, and postoperative bile leak. Often, intervention such as sphincterotomy, dilation and stenting of biliary duct, stenting of fistulas, stricture or postoperative bile leak, drain placement, and tissue biopsy is also performed. The patient is typically placed in a left lateral or prone position with the head turned toward the endoscopist. The first portion of the procedure is similar to EGD whereby the endoscope is advanced past the pharynx and is inserted into the esophagus. Once the endoscope is in the duodenum, it is rotated to face the papilla. A cannula is inserted into the papilla, contrast agent is injected, and the duct is visualized under fluoroscopy. Excessive intestinal motility can impede endoscopic examination and can be inhibited by the administration of either anticholinergic drugs or glucagon.

## Anesthesia Evaluation and Management

Anesthesia providers are often asked to care for patients requiring procedures in the gastrointestinal endoscopy suites. The standard approach to preprocedure evaluation (also see Chapter 13) and anesthetic choice (also see Chapter 14) applies in this setting. Simple EGD and ERCP in otherwise healthy patients can be performed with minimal or moderate sedation administered by a trained nonanesthesia provider. However, anesthesia service (whether monitored anesthesia care or general anesthesia) may be requested if the procedure is expected to be challenging or prolonged, patient immobility is desired, or the patient's history suggests airway difficulty or other comorbid conditions. Hepatobiliary dysfunction is common in patients who require ERCP. These patients may have coagulopathy because of decreased synthesis of coagulation factors and thrombocytopenia (also see Chapter 28). Blood product transfusion may be necessary prior to the endoscopy, especially for the more invasive ERCP.[13]

The choice of anesthetic techniques requires clear communication between the patient, endoscopist, and the anesthesia provider. Although minimal or moderate sedation is the most common technique for uncomplicated EGD, deep sedation or general anesthesia may be necessary for EGD based on patient comorbid conditions or severity of clinical status (e.g., critically ill patient with massive hematemesis).

ERCP is considered to be a riskier procedure compared to EGD, based on the nature of the procedure and the typical patient population. The patient is most often in the prone position and the anesthesia provider has limited access to the patient's airway because the endoscopist stands next to the patient's head. Finally, the room is darkened to allow better viewing of the fluoroscopy screen, and the provider must wear protective lead shields to minimize exposure to ionizing radiation. Many patients undergo repeat ERCP and have developed a preference for monitored anesthesia care versus general anesthesia based on their experience.

## Challenges and Complications

Complications of EGD or ERCP can generally be grouped by sedation and airway, procedure, and patient-related factors (Table 38.3). Topical benzocaine administration can lead to methemoglobinemia (also see Chapter 10). Procedure-related

| Table 38.3 | Complications of Esophagogastroduodenoscopy or Endoscopic Retrograde Cholangiopancreatography | | |
|---|---|---|---|
| **Sedation and Airway** | **Procedure** | **Patient-Related** | |
| Hypoxemia | Bleeding | Bleeding | |
| Excessive secretion | Perforation | Coagulopathy | |
| Aspiration | Pancreatitis (ERCP) | Thrombocytopenia | |
| Laryngospasm | Air embolism (insufflation) | Cardiac arrhythmia | |
| Bronchospasm | Hypercarbia ($CO_2$ insufflation) | | |
| Methemoglobinemia | Contrast agent allergy | | |

*ERCP*, endoscopic retrograde cholangiopancreatography.

complications, such as esophageal perforation, are rare but can be life threatening.[14] Esophageal perforation is more likely to occur in someone who has a history of stricture, previous perforation, previous surgery, or other anatomic abnormalities. Symptoms may include neck, chest, or abdominal pain. Clinical signs are often nonspecific (i.e., tachycardia, tachypnea, hypotension, abdominal distention, and even sepsis). Clinical suspicion should be intense especially if the symptoms do not resolve or are self-limited. The diagnosis of perforation is usually made radiographically, often with the use of water-soluble contrast material. Depending on the lesion, some perforations can be managed medically whereas others constitute surgical emergencies.

The anesthetic management of a patient with upper gastrointestinal bleeding can be especially challenging. Tracheal intubation may be complicated by ongoing hematemesis. Large-bore, possibly central, venous access is required to continue resuscitation with fluid, blood, and vasopressors. Often the patient may have an underlying cause of coagulopathy, or the hemorrhage can cause a coagulopathy. A typical example is a patient who has end-stage liver disease with deficiency in coagulation factors, thrombocytopenia, portal hypertension, and variceal bleeding. For anesthesia providers caring for such critically ill patients, anesthesia management is further complicated by the location outside the operating room, where resources and help are often far way.

## CATHETER-BASED CARDIOLOGY PROCEDURES

### Adult Cardiac Catheterization

Patients needing coronary artery or peripheral artery angiography usually show evidence of coronary ischemia on noninvasive cardiac stress tests, or other clinical evidence of atherosclerosis. Preprocedural assessment and preparation should be focused on their cardiopulmonary functional status, airway, relevant medications, and other common comorbid conditions such as diabetes mellitus and renal insufficiency.

The procedure usually involves the cannulation of one or more peripheral arteries, such as the radial, brachial, or femoral. A noninvasive arterial blood pressure monitor should be placed on an extremity that is not involved with the procedure. The cardiologist will inject local anesthetic at the site of cannulation in addition to sedation using intravenous midazolam and fentanyl. The procedure itself is usually well tolerated by the patient. Anesthesia care is requested when the patient has a history of severe anxiety, because sedation by an anesthesia provider may be safer. Sometimes, high-risk coronary angioplasty is planned and may require mechanical extracorporeal circulatory life support (ECLS), in which case the anesthesia provider should be readily available so that if hemodynamic instability occurs the airway can be secured rapidly. General anesthesia is rarely indicated unless a surgical exposure for ECLS cannulation is planned. The risk of hemodynamic instability during general anesthesia is clearly high. Because the procedure is usually short, an opiate-dominated induction of anesthesia is not desirable. Small-dose propofol, etomidate, ketamine, or an inhaled induction of anesthesia may be appropriate. Either a small concentration of inhaled anesthetic or small dose of propofol via an infusion is usually sufficient to maintain anesthesia. The use of vasoconstrictors may be needed to maintain systemic vascular resistance, and inotropic drugs such as dobutamine, epinephrine, or dopamine can be given to those patients with severely depressed left ventricular ejection fraction. Finally, as with any non–operating room location, the anesthesia provider may be called to the catheterization suite emergently to help resuscitate a patient including securing a patent airway, and possibly organizing the transport to the ICU or operating room.

### Electrophysiology Studies

Catheter-Based Ablation
Electrophysiology (EP) covers the diagnosis of cardiac dysrhythmias, detailed mapping of their circuitry, and treatment with catheter-based ablation.[15] With rapid advancements in cardiac monitors, computer tomography,

**IV**

MRI, and catheter technologies, a wide variety of dysrhythmia—atrial fibrillation, supraventricular tachyarrhythmias (SVTs), and ventricular tachycardia—are amendable to EP study and treatment. Patients undergoing EP studies and ablation can vary greatly, ranging from healthy young adults with isolated dysrhythmia to patients with end-stage heart failure with left ventricular assist devices. Preprocedural evaluation of these patients should focus on their cardiopulmonary reserve (particularly signs and symptoms when arrhythmias occur), airway, comorbid conditions, and relevant medications, especially anticoagulants such as heparin, warfarin and the newer direct factor Xa inhibitors, and direct thrombin inhibitors.

The intracardiac catheters are usually placed via the femoral and internal jugular veins, unless a retrograde approach to the left side of the heart via the femoral artery is planned. Endocardial mapping studies are performed with stimulation and recording from the internal and external electrodes, followed by catheter ablation of the endocardium (usually with radiofrequency energy) to produce a scar that disrupts dysrhythmia generation or propagation. Generous subcutaneous injection of local anesthetics and intravenous sedation administered drugs (also see Chapters 8, 9, and 10) during cannulation is sufficient for most patients. In fact, many electrophysiologists believe that excessive sedation or general anesthesia during the study can suppress dysrhythmia and negatively affect the success of mapping. The anesthetic plan and monitoring should be determined by the patient's overall clinical picture.[16] A history of syncope or angina during a tachycardic episode may suggest depressed cardiac output and significant hypotension, and an invasive arterial pressure monitor may be warranted as the study can induce or elicit periods of rapid heart rates. The anesthetic plan usually involves more profound sedation (often deep sedation) and analgesia during the initial cannulation and catheter insertion, and minimal sedation thereafter. One exception is atrial fibrillation ablation, which involves endocardial ablation that isolates pulmonary vein ostia from the rest of the left atrium. General anesthesia with endotracheal intubation may be helpful for this procedure. It allows predictable respiratory movement during ablation, monitoring of esophageal temperature to avoid left atrial perforation, and detection of any phrenic nerve stimulation. For procedures involving catheters in the left side of the heart, anticoagulation is usually achieved with intravenous heparin to avoid thromboembolic complications.[17] Finally, EP catheters are irrigated with fluid, and because the amount can be substantial over a long procedure, patients with a history of congestive heart failure may require a diuretic to avoid excessive intravascular volume.

### Cardiac Implantable Electronic Devices

Another common group of procedures performed in the EP suite is the placement of CIEDs, such as implantable cardioverter-defibrillators (ICDs) and pacemakers (PMs).

The anesthesia provider should understand the indication of the device, whether it is heart block, primary prevention for sudden cardiac death in cardiomyopathy, secondary prevention for a history of ventricular tachycardia, or biventricular pacing for cardiac resynchronization therapy. Transcutaneous pacing and defibrillator devices should be attached to the patient, and the anesthesia provider should understand how to operate these devices to institute emergency pacing or defibrillation. Again, the procedure can be performed successfully with subcutaneous local anesthetic injection and intravenous sedation and analgesia medications. However, the anesthesia provider may decide that general anesthesia may be safer, for example, in someone with altered mental status. The cardiologist may choose to perform a defibrillation threshold test, in which fibrillation is intentionally induced and the device's ability to sense and terminate fibrillation is confirmed. In some patients such as those with severe systolic left ventricular dysfunction (e.g., ischemic cardiomyopathy), the brief loss of cardiac output and perfusion, even for seconds, may be poorly tolerated. Invasive pressure monitoring is advisable to facilitate timely treatment of hypotension. Prior to the test, administration of oxygen and a small intravenous dose of a short-acting anesthetic to produce amnesia is appropriate.

### Cardioversion

The anesthesia provider is frequently involved in caring for patients who are undergoing cardioversion for atrial fibrillation or atrial flutter. Because of the risk of thromboembolic disease in these patients, cardioversion is often immediately preceded by a transesophageal echocardiogram (TEE) to examine the left atrium for thrombus. TEE may be bypassed if the patient has been on therapeutic anticoagulation. The echocardiographer may choose to topicalize the upper airway with local anesthetics to suppress gag reflex during probe insertion. The drawback with topicalization is that the loss of airway reflex may linger beyond the procedure and have a potentially negative effect on the patient's ability to handle excessive secretions. A good choice is the use of a short-acting sedative such as propofol. Before TEE probe insertion, the patient should have standard monitors attached and have been breathing supplemental oxygen. Sedation with propofol is then titrated to accommodate the passage of the probe and should be maintained during the examination. Maneuvers such as jaw thrust, chin lift, or pharyngeal suctioning may be necessary to avoid obstruction or clear secretions. For cardioversion without TEE, small doses of propofol after preoxygenation to render the patient amnestic should be sufficient. After cardioversion, the anesthesia provider should continue to monitor the patient, relieve any airway obstruction, and provide additional oxygen until recovery of mentation and airway reflex is satisfactory before transferring patient care to the recovery room.

## Structural Heart Disease Intervention

Similar to EP, catheter-based intervention for the treatment of structural heart diseases is a rapidly evolving field. Balloon valvuloplasty or even valve replacement can be performed on all of the intracardiac valves. Atrial septal defect (ASD), patent foramen ovale (PFO), ventricular septal defect (VSD), and coronary fistula can be closed with expandable devices. These procedures are performed using fluoroscopy with additional guidance from echocardiography. Because a large portion of this patient population has had previous sternotomy for cardiac intervention, the transcatheter approach avoids the morbidity and risk of repeat sternotomy and inadvertent cardiac injury. General anesthesia has a number of advantages: an immobile patient, controlled ventilatory movement, ease of continuous TEE examination, and a secured airway in the case of hemodynamic instability or when open surgery is needed. The induction of anesthesia may be challenging, however, given the existent severe cardiac defect. Pediatric patients with cyanotic heart lesions or adult patients with palliative treatment of congenital heart diseases may be especially challenging. A thorough preprocedural discussion between the anesthesia provider, congenital cardiologist, interventional cardiologist, and cardiac surgeon regarding the cardiac anatomy and surgical history and its implication is invaluable.

## Pediatric Studies

Caring for neonates, infants, and children who are undergoing invasive cardiac studies and procedures is one of the most challenging tasks faced by the anesthesia provider (also see Chapters 26 and 34). To safely anesthetize these patients requires a mastery of the neonatal cardiopulmonary physiology, complex anatomy of cardiac lesions, pharmacology, pediatric airway, and other coexisting congenital diseases. Because of their age and cognitive development, most pediatric patients require either general anesthesia or deep sedation for these procedures. Special attention must be paid to the possibility of a difficult airway, the rapidity of ventilation problems adversely affecting cardiovascular stability, the pharmacodynamic and pharmacokinetic properties of anesthetic drugs, and the avoidance of hypothermia in the smaller patient. The onset of intravenous and inhaled anesthetics will be significantly altered owing to the presence of intra- or extracardiac shunts. Similarly, the onset of medication effect can be delayed as a result of congestive heart failure and low cardiac output. Hypoxia, hypercapnia, excessive positive airway pressure, metabolic acidosis, hypothermia, and painful stimulation can lead to increases in pulmonary vascular resistance and right-sided heart failure and should be avoided. However, in patients with intracardiac shunts, hyperoxia and resulting pulmonary vasodilation may promote excessive left-to-right shunt and cause systemic hypotension. Also, cyanotic patients become polycythemic to compensate for chronic oxygen deprivation. This places them at a higher risk of thrombotic complications during the procedures. The rule of thumb is to have the cyanotic patient remain at preanesthetic hemodynamic and oxygenation baseline, which can be a considerable challenge during anesthesia.

## Challenges and Complications

Providing anesthetic care in interventional cardiology locations can be challenging. The typical arrangement of a room designed for the interventional cardiologist frequently places the anesthesia provider far away from the patient, with other equipment serving as obstacles. Despite the infrequent use of general anesthesia in many cases, the anesthesia provider should always be prepared to escalate the depth of anesthesia, secure the airway, and provide resuscitation in case of emergency. The most common complications with interventional cardiology procedures are related to vascular access and include bleeding, hematoma, pneumothorax, and vascular injury. In addition, intracardiac catheters can trigger arrhythmia and heart blocks, which may cause significant cardiovascular changes.

Rarely, cardiac perforation can occur, resulting in pericardial effusion and tamponade. Clinical signs include persistent hemodynamic instability unrelated to the induced arrhythmia and refractory to routine administration of vasoconstrictors and intravenous fluids. The procedural team should be informed if perforation is suspected. The diagnosis can be confirmed with echocardiography. Blood products should be ordered immediately. Perhaps anticoagulation should be reversed after a consultation with the proceduralist. One or more of the venous sheaths can be used for intravascular volume resuscitation. The options for managing a new pericardial effusion in this setting could include the following: (1) "wait-and-watch" approach if the effusion is small and self-limiting; (2) emergent pericardial drain placement; or (3) rapid mobilization for surgical decompression of tamponade. Thus, communication and understanding of the procedural plan between the anesthesia provider and the cardiologist are crucial. The cardiologist's specialty expertise can be an asset during a cardiovascular emergency. In addition, vascular access placed by the cardiologist can be used for invasive monitoring (arterial line) and fluid resuscitation (central venous line).

## ELECTROCONVULSIVE THERAPY

Electroconvulsive therapy (ECT) is an effective treatment for patients suffering from severe depression (both unipolar and bipolar types), psychotic depression, and schizophrenia.[18] For severe depression, ECT, compared with antidepressants, produces faster remission, reduces

IV

acute suicidal risk, and lowers relapse rate. Most guidelines recommend ECT as a treatment reserved for those who have failed medical therapy with antidepressants, or those with severe psychotic features (catatonia) or at risk of suicide in need of rapid, definitive response. The American Psychiatric Association (APA) also recommends its use as maintenance therapy. ECT exerts its therapeutic effect by inducing generalized seizures, and its efficacy on depression is affected by techniques, such as electrode placement and length of convulsion, and by the length of ECT treatment. It is thought that grand mal seizure changes the neurobiology of depression by increasing CNS γ-aminobutyric acid (GABA) concentration, normalizing serotonin function, and suppressing hypothalamic-pituitary-adrenal axis hyperactivity.[19]

## Electrically Induced Seizures

A trained ECT physician produces generalized seizure by placing two electrodes in bifrontotemporal (bilateral), right unilateral, or bifrontal positions on the patient's head. Right unilateral or bifrontal position is chosen in order to minimize the side effects of ECT, especially short-term cognitive dysfunction. On the other hand, bilateral position has the advantages of ease of use, lower energy, and higher efficacy for remission. A brief (0.5-2 ms) or an ultra-brief (<0.5 ms) pulse of electrical charge, usually 100 to 600 μC (microcoulombs) is applied with the goal to trigger a seizure of sufficient duration (>15 seconds). Seizure threshold can either be determined empirically during the initial ECT treatment or based on the patient's age (for bilateral position). Threshold can be affected by a number of factors, including medication and blood pH, and may also increase over the course of the treatment series. The duration of seizure is monitored with single-channel electroencephalography (EEG). Motor seizure activity can also be followed; however, motor activity typically stops before the electrical activity. Seizures shorter than 15 seconds or a complete lack of seizure may be subtherapeutic, whereas prolonged seizures (>120 seconds) may be harmful to the patient. Adjustment by the ECT physician and possible intervention by the anesthesia provider may be necessary. A typical course may involve 3 treatments per week and a total of 6 to 20 treatments.

## Anesthesia Evaluation

Before starting ECT, a patient should undergo a full medical evaluation by the ECT physician and the anesthesia provider (also see Chapter 13). Any interval change in health and side effects from previous treatments should be elicited during subsequent visits. Special attention should be given to any cardiopulmonary comorbid conditions, CNS disease, surgical (e.g., orthopedic) history, and relevant medications. Patients are often older and common concerns include cardiovascular diseases (e.g.,

hypertension, coronary artery disease, valvulopathy, cardiomyopathy, arrhythmia, or aortic aneurysm) and CNS diseases (e.g., cerebrovascular diseases and intracranial hypertension). Patients who are symptomatic or have unstable cardiac disease, such as malignant hypertension, decompensated heart failure, or hemodynamic significant arrhythmia, should be evaluated and optimized by a cardiologist. Those with CIEDs and pregnant women can undergo ECT safely. Patients with unstable fractures may be at risk owing to motor seizure. Standard nil per os or nothing by mouth (NPO) guidelines should be followed. Chronic medication for cardiovascular or pulmonary diseases usually should be continued. One exception is the bronchodilator drug theophylline, which can increase the risk of status epilepticus. Chronic anticoagulation (e.g., warfarin) should be continued as the risk of bleeding is minimal. Chronic medication for treatment of gastro-esophageal reflux disease should be taken, but there is no evidence for routine prophylactic use of antacid, $H_2$ antagonist, or proton-pump inhibitor in an asymptomatic patient.

## Psychotropic Medications

Many ECT patients are receiving psychotropic medications. Lithium, anticonvulsants, and benzodiazepines, which may shorten seizure duration, may be tapered under the direction of the ECT physician. However, many psychotropic medications (e.g., monoamine oxidase inhibitors, serotonin reuptake inhibitors, tricyclic antidepressants, lithium, and benzodiazepines) have sympathomimetic, anticholinergic, and CNS effects and can cause serious drug-drug interactions with commonly used perioperative medications.

## Induction of Anesthesia and Seizure

Preparation for ECT treatment is similar to that of induction for general anesthesia.[20] Standard monitors are applied and vital signs are continually checked. Invasive pressure monitoring is rarely necessary, but may be useful for someone with unstable or severe cardiovascular disease. Oxygen should be given via face mask, and the patient is encouraged to breathe deeply to maximize oxygen content of the functional residual capacity (FRC) before induction of anesthesia. A second blood pressure cuff is placed on a distal limb. A peripheral nerve stimulator placed distal to the cuff is useful to determine the onset of neuromuscular paralysis by succinylcholine or any evidence of prolonged blockade likely because of pseudocholinesterase deficiency. If the patient has an ICD, the defibrillation function should be temporarily deactivated so that the device does not misinterpret the ECT electrical stimulus as an arrhythmia. Depending on the ICD programming, a magnet placed over the ICD can deactivate the defibrillator function. Similarly, for a patient with a PM who is PM-dependent, a magnet placed over the PM should convert it to an asynchronous mode. Otherwise, the electrical artifact from the ECT stimulus and resulting motor movement can cause PM inhibition leading to severe bradycardia. An external defibrillator machine with PM capabilities should be immediately available for those patients with CIEDs.

The most common induction drug is intravenous methohexital (0.5 to 1 mg/kg), a short-acting barbiturate that is superior to propofol, a potent anticonvulsant that may increase seizure threshold and shorten seizure duration. An alternative is intravenous etomidate (0.2 to 0.3 mg/kg),[21] which has the advantage of maintaining hemodynamic stability and can decrease seizure threshold and augment seizure duration in some patients; however, it can induce nonepileptic myoclonic activity and can cause adrenal insufficiency with just a single dose. Ketamine is another alternative, but its use is controversial as it may cause posttreatment confusion. If a patient has undergone prior ECT, the anesthesia provider should determine what induction drug and dose were administered, the resulting seizure duration, and the presence of any adverse effects. Subtherapeutic seizure may prompt a dose adjustment or a change of drug to induce anesthesia. In consultation with the ECT physician, an appropriate drug and dose can be selected.

Once the patient loses consciousness, the cuff on the distal limb is inflated. A fast-acting neuromuscular blocker, usually succinylcholine (0.5 to 1 mg/kg), is then injected to produce paralysis. For those patients with contraindications for succinylcholine, rocuronium can be substituted, which can be rapidly reversed with sugammadex (see Chapter 11). The distal tourniquet allows the monitoring of isolated motor activity. A bite guard is placed in the patient's mouth. The anesthesia provider continues to support the patient's breathing with bag-mask ventilation and may be asked to provide hyperventilation, as hypocarbia can decrease the seizure threshold. Once fasciculation stops, electrodes are applied and the electrical stimulus is delivered. The seizure activity can be followed on EEG with visual confirmation of the motor activity of the injured limb. A prolonged seizure (>2 minutes) can be terminated by a small propofol bolus. As the neuromuscular paralysis subsides, maneuvers to relieve airway obstruction such as jaw thrust or chin lift may be necessary. Endotracheal intubation is rarely necessary. Laryngeal mask airway may be useful for airway management in patients with risk factors for difficult face mask ventilation or history of obstructive sleep apnea.

## Physiologic Responses to Seizure and Treatment

The electrically induced seizure can have profound effects on the patient's vital signs. The first (tonic) phase is characterized by profound parasympathetic discharge that can lead to bradycardia, atrioventricular block, atrial arrhythmia, premature atrial or ventricular contraction, or even asystole. Hypotension may occur. Intervention with atropine or glycopyrrolate may be necessary. This is rapidly followed by the second (clonic) phase of sympathetic overstimulation characterized by tachycardia and hypertension, which can also be profound. This may be exacerbated by hypoventilation and the resultant hypercarbia. Although the hemodynamic response usually subsides quickly after seizure termination, persistent hypertension and tachycardia, especially in those with significant cardiovascular diseases at risk for ischemia, may require treatment such as β-adrenergic antagonists (e.g., esmolol or labetalol) and other antihypertensives (e.g., hydralazine).

As discussed, these patients undergo a series of ECT treatments over time. The anesthesia provider should review the prior anesthesia record to determine the intraoperative hemodynamic response as well as post-ECT experience of the patient. If the patient had an excessive sympathetic response during past treatments, the anesthesia provider may choose to administer prophylactic β-adrenergic antagonists before seizure induction. Severe post-ECT complaints such as headache, muscle pain, or nausea suggest that small doses of opiates, acetaminophen, nonsteroidal antiinflammatory drugs, or antiemetics should be considered in future treatments.

## QUESTIONS OF THE DAY

1. How can the anesthesia provider minimize exposure to ionizing radiation from C-arm fluoroscopy?

2. What is meant by the term *MR conditional* in the context of magnetic resonance imaging (MRI) and the safety of monitoring equipment?

3. A patient requires anesthesia for ablation of a renal mass in the CT scanner. What are the specific anesthetic considerations for this procedure?

4. A patient with an intracranial aneurysm is receiving general anesthesia for interventional neuroradiology coil embolization. The radiologist announces that the aneurysm suddenly ruptured during manipulation. What are the most important next steps in the management of this patient?

5. A patient with hepatic cirrhosis and upper gastrointestinal bleeding is scheduled for urgent esophagogastroduodenoscopy (EGD). What are the anesthetic priorities in caring for a patient in this situation?

6. A patient with history of ventricular fibrillation requires placement of an implantable cardioverter-defibrillator (ICD). What intraoperative complications related to this procedure should be anticipated?

7. A patient is about to undergo electroconvulsive therapy (ECT) for severe depression. What are the expected cardiovascular responses to the induced seizure? How can these responses be attenuated?

IV

## REFERENCES

1. Chang B, Kaye AD, Diaz JH, et al. Complications of non-operating room procedures: outcomes from the National Anesthesia Clinical Outcomes Registry. *J Patient Saf.* Epub 2015 Apr 7.
2. Orme NM, Rihal CS, Gulati R, et al. Occupational health hazards of working in the interventional laboratory: a multisite case control study of physicians and allied staff. *J Am Coll Cardiol.* 2015;65:820–826.
3. Anastasian ZH, Strozyk D, Meyers PM, et al. Radiation exposure of the anesthesiologist in the neurointerventional suite. *Anesthesiology.* 2011;114:512–520.
4. Robertson PS, Rhoney DH. Prophylaxis for anaphylactoid reactions in high risk patients receiving radiopaque contrast media. *Surg Neurol.* 1997;48:292–293.
5. Marckmann P, Skov L. Nephrogenic systemic fibrosis: clinical picture and treatment. *Radiol Clin North Am.* 2009;47:833–840.
6. Mehemed TM, Fushimi Y, Okada T, et al. Dynamic oxygen-enhanced MRI of cerebrospinal fluid. *PloS One.* 2014;9:e100723.
7. McDonagh DL, Olson DM, Kalia JS, et al. Anesthesia and sedation practices among neurointerventionalists during acute ischemic stroke endovascular therapy. *Front Neurol.* 2010;1:118.

8. Lee CZ, Young WL. Anesthesia for endovascular neurosurgery and interventional neurology. *Anesthesiol Clin.* 2012;30:127–147.
9. Lee CZ, Litt L, Hashimoto T, et al. Physiologic monitoring and anesthesia considerations in acute ischemic stroke. *J Vasc Interv Radiol.* 2004;15:S13–S19.
10. Davis MJ, Menon BK, Baghirzada LB, et al. Anesthetic management and outcome in patients during endovascular therapy for acute stroke. *Anesthesiology.* 2012;116:396–405.
11. Abou-Chebl A, Reginelli J, Bajzer CT, Yadav JS. Intensive treatment of hypertension decreases the risk of hyperperfusion and intracerebral hemorrhage following carotid artery stenting. *Catheter Cardiovasc Interv.* 2007;69(5):690–696.
12. Scher C. Anesthesia for transjugular intrahepatic portosystemic shunt. *Int Anesthesiol Clin.* 2009;47:21–28.
13. Kapoor H. Anaesthesia for endoscopic retrograde cholangiopancreatography. *Acta Anaesthesiol Scand.* 2011;55:918–926.
14. Garmon EH, Contreras E, Conley J. Tension pneumothorax and widespread pneumatosis after endoscopic retrograde cholangiopancreatography. *Anesthesiology.* 2013;119:699.

15. Patel KD, Crowley R, Mahajan A. Cardiac electrophysiology procedures in clinical practice. *Int Anesthesiol Clin.* 2012;50:90–110.
16. Malladi V, Naeini PS, Razavi M, et al. Endovascular ablation of atrial fibrillation. *Anesthesiology.* 2014;120:1513–1519.
17. Mittnacht AJ, Dukkipati S, Mahajan A. Ventricular tachycardia ablation: a comprehensive review for anesthesiologists. *Anesth Analg.* 2015;120:737–748.
18. Fink M. What was learned: studies by the consortium for research in ECT (CORE) 1997-2011. *Acta Psychiatr Scand.* 2014;129:417–426.
19. Lisanby SH. Electroconvulsive therapy for depression. *N Engl J Med.* 2007;357:1939–1945.
20. Saito S. Anesthesia management for electroconvulsive therapy: hemodynamic and respiratory management. *J Anesth.* 2005;19:142–149.
21. Singh PM, Arora S, Borle A, et al. Evaluation of etomidate for seizure duration in electroconvulsive therapy: a systematic review and meta-analysis. *J ECT.* 2015;31(4):213–225.

# THE RECOVERY PERIOD

# 39 POSTANESTHESIA RECOVERY

## Dorre Nicholau and Melissa Haehn

The postanesthesia care unit (PACU), sometimes referred to as the recovery room, is designed and staffed to monitor and care for patients who are recovering from the immediate physiologic effects of anesthesia and surgery. PACU care spans the transition from delivery of anesthesia in the operating room to the less acute monitoring on the hospital ward and, in some cases, independent function of the patient at home. Also, PACUs provide critical care to patients for whom there is no intensive care unit bed in busy medical centers. To serve this unique transition period, the PACU must be equipped to monitor and resuscitate unstable patients while simultaneously providing a tranquil environment for the "recovery" and comfort of stable patients. The proximity of the unit to the operating room facilitates rapid access to postoperative patients by anesthesia providers and surgical caregivers.

## ADMISSION TO THE POSTANESTHESIA CARE UNIT

Upon arrival in the unit, the anesthesia provider should inform the PACU nurse of pertinent details on the patient's history, medical condition, anesthesia, and surgery. Particular attention is directed to monitoring oxygenation (pulse oximetry), ventilation (breathing frequency, airway patency, capnography), and circulation (systemic arterial blood pressure, heart rate, electrocardiogram [ECG]).

Vital signs are recorded as often as necessary but at least every 15 minutes while the patient is in the unit. The American Society of Anesthesiologists (ASA) has adopted Standards for Postanesthesia Care that delineate the minimal requirements for PACU monitoring and care.[1] More specific recommendations addressing clinical evaluation and therapeutic intervention can be found in the ASA Practice Guidelines for Postanesthesia Care.[2]

## EARLY POSTOPERATIVE PHYSIOLOGIC DISORDERS

A variety of physiologic disorders affecting multiple organ systems must be diagnosed and treated in the PACU during emergence from anesthesia and surgery (Box 39.1). Nausea and vomiting, the need for upper airway support, and systemic hypotension are among the most frequently encountered complications.[3] Not surprisingly, serious outcomes may result from airway, respiratory, or cardiovascular compromise.[4] Airway problems and cardiovascular events accounted for the majority (67%) of 419 recovery room incidents reported to the 2002 Australian Incident Monitoring Study (AIMS).[5] In addition, transport of the patient from the operating room to the PACU is also a time when patients are especially vulnerable to airway obstruction, as discussed next.

---

**Box 39.1** Physiologic Disorders Manifested in the Postanesthesia Care Unit

Upper airway obstruction
Arterial hypoxemia
Hypoventilation
Hypotension
Hypertension
Cardiac dysrhythmias
Oliguria
Bleeding
Decreased body temperature
Delirium (emergence agitation)
Delayed awakening
Nausea and vomiting
Pain

---

## UPPER AIRWAY OBSTRUCTION

### Loss of Pharyngeal Muscle Tone

Airway obstruction is a common and potentially devastating complication in the postoperative period (also see Chapter 16). The most frequent cause of airway obstruction in the PACU is the loss of pharyngeal tone in a sedated or obtunded patient. The residual depressant effects of inhaled and intravenous anesthetics and the persistent effects of neuromuscular blocking drugs (also see Chapter 11) contribute to the loss of pharyngeal tone in the immediate postoperative period.

In an awake, unanesthetized patient, the pharyngeal muscles contract synchronously with the diaphragm to pull the tongue forward and tent the airway open against the negative inspiratory pressure generated by the diaphragm. This pharyngeal muscle activity is depressed during sleep, and the resulting decrease in tone promotes airway obstruction. With the collapse of compliant pharyngeal tissue during inspiration, a vicious circle may ensue in which a reflex compensatory increase in respiratory effort and negative inspiratory pressure promotes further airway obstruction. This effort to breathe against an obstructed airway is characterized by a paradoxic breathing pattern consisting of retraction of the sternal notch and exaggerated abdominal muscle activity. Collapse of the chest wall plus protrusion of the abdomen with inspiratory effort produces a rocking motion that becomes more prominent with increasing airway obstruction.

Obstruction secondary to loss of pharyngeal tone can be relieved by simply opening the airway with the "jaw thrust maneuver" or continuous positive airway pressure (CPAP) applied via a face mask (or use of both). Support of the airway is needed until the patient has adequately recovered from the effects of drugs administered during anesthesia. In selected patients, placement of an oral or nasal airway, laryngeal mask airway, or endotracheal tube may be required (also see Chapter 16).

### Residual Neuromuscular Blockade

When evaluating upper airway obstruction in the PACU, the possibility of residual neuromuscular blockade must be considered in any patient who received neuromuscular blocking drugs during anesthesia (also see Chapter 11). Residual neuromuscular blockade may not be evident on arrival in the PACU because the diaphragm recovers from neuromuscular blockade before the pharyngeal muscles do. With an endotracheal tube in place, end-tidal carbon dioxide concentrations and tidal volumes may indicate adequate ventilation while the ability to maintain a patent upper airway and clear upper airway secretions remain compromised. The stimulation associated with tracheal extubation, followed by the activity of patient transfer to the gurney and subsequent mask airway support, may keep the airway open during transport. Only after the patient is calmly resting in the PACU does upper airway obstruction become evident. Even patients treated with intermediate- and short-acting neuromuscular blocking drugs may manifest residual paralysis in the PACU despite what was deemed clinically adequate pharmacologic reversal in the operating room (OR).

The association between intermediate-acting neuromuscular blocking drugs and postoperative respiratory complications is dose dependent.[6] Also, inappropriate dosing of the reversal drug neostigmine can cause postoperative respiratory complications. A large prospective study of over 3000 PACU patients showed the unwarranted use or inappropriate dosing of neostigmine to be an independent risk factor for reintubation of the trachea.[7,8] Therefore, determining the appropriate dose of neostigmine, and specifically avoiding inappropriate dosing or overdosage, is essential to assure full recovery of neuromuscular function in the PACU. Over the years qualitative measurement of the train-of-four (TOF) ratio by tactile response or visualization was the most commonly used method to assess the degree of reversal of neuromuscular blockade at the end of surgery. However, more recent evidence suggests that the qualitative measurement of the TOF ratio may not accurately reflect recovery of neuromuscular function. Instead, the use of quantitative TOF measurement using acceleromyography provides a more objective and accurate method of monitoring neuromuscular function.[9] It is hoped that use of a newly approved reversal drug, sugammadex, will decrease the frequency of inadequate reversal of neuromuscular blockade.

When patients with residual neuromuscular blockade are awake in the PACU, their struggle to breathe may manifest as agitation. In an awake patient, clinical assessment of reversal of neuromuscular blockade is preferred to the application of painful TOF or tetanic stimulation. Clinical evaluation includes grip strength, tongue protrusion, the ability to lift the legs off the bed, and the ability to lift the head off the bed for a full 5 seconds. Of these maneuvers, the 5-second sustained head lift is considered the gold standard because it reflects not only generalized motor strength but, more important, the patient's ability to maintain and protect the airway. In patients whose tracheas have been extubated, the ability to strongly oppose the incisor teeth against a tongue depressor is another reliable indicator of pharyngeal muscle tone in the awake patient. This maneuver correlates with an average TOF ratio of 0.85. Inadequate ventilation or airway obstruction is less likely if the neuromuscular blockade has been reversed with neostigmine or sugammadex (also see Chapter 11).

If persistence or return of neuromuscular weakness in the PACU is suspected, prompt review of possible etiologic factors is indicated (Box 39.2). Common factors include respiratory acidosis and hypothermia, alone or in combination. Residual depressant effects of volatile anesthetics or opioids (or both) may result in progressive respiratory acidosis only after the patient is admitted to the PACU and external stimulation is minimized. Similarly, a patient who becomes hypothermic during anesthesia and surgery may show signs of weakness in the PACU that were not noted following extubation in the operating room. Simple measures such as warming the patient, airway support, and correction of electrolyte abnormalities can facilitate recovery from neuromuscular blockade.

## Laryngospasm

Laryngospasm refers to a sudden spasm of the vocal cords that completely occludes the laryngeal opening. It typically occurs in the transitional period when the patient whose trachea has been extubated is emerging

---

**Box 39.2** Causes of Prolonged Neuromuscular Blockade

**Factors Contributing to Prolonged Nondepolarizing Neuromuscular Blockade**
Drugs
　Inhaled anesthetic drugs
　Local anesthetics (lidocaine)
　Cardiac antidysrhythmics (procainamide)
　Antibiotics (polymyxins, aminoglycosides, lincosamines [clindamycin], metronidazole [Flagyl], tetracyclines)
　Corticosteroids
　Calcium channel blockers
　Dantrolene
　Furosemide
Metabolic and physiologic states
　Hypermagnesemia
　Hypocalcemia
　Hypothermia
　Respiratory acidosis
　Hepatic/renal failure
　Myasthenia syndromes

**Factors Contributing to Prolonged Depolarizing Neuromuscular Blockade**
Excessive dose of succinylcholine
Reduced plasma cholinesterase activity
　Decreased levels
　Extremes of age (newborn, old age)
　Disease states (hepatic disease, uremia, malnutrition, plasmapheresis)
　Hormonal changes
　Pregnancy
　Contraceptives
　Glucocorticoids
Inhibited activity
　Irreversible (echothiophate)
　Reversible (edrophonium, neostigmine, pyridostigmine)
Genetic variant (atypical plasma cholinesterase)

V

from general anesthesia. Although it is most likely to occur in the operating room at the time of tracheal extubation, patients who arrive in the PACU asleep after general anesthesia are also at risk for laryngospasm when awakening.

Jaw thrust with CPAP (up to 40 cm $H_2O$) is often sufficient stimulation to "break" the laryngospasm. If jaw thrust and CPAP maneuvers fail, immediate skeletal muscle relaxation can be achieved with intravenously (IV) or intramuscularly (IM) administered succinylcholine (0.1 to 1.0 mg/kg IV or 4 mg/kg IM). A tracheal tube should not be passed forcibly through a glottis that is closed because of laryngospasm.

## Airway Edema

Airway edema is a possible postoperative complication in patients undergoing prolonged procedures in the prone or Trendelenburg position and in procedures with large amounts of blood loss requiring aggressive intravascular fluid resuscitation. Surgical procedures on the tongue, pharynx, and neck, including thyroidectomy, carotid endarterectomy, and cervical spinal procedures, can result in upper airway obstruction because of tissue edema or hematoma, or both. Although facial and scleral edema are important physical signs that can alert the clinician to the presence of airway edema, significant edema of pharyngeal tissue is often not accompanied by visible external signs. If tracheal extubation is attempted in these patients in the PACU, evaluation of airway patency must precede removal of the endotracheal tube (ETT). The patient's ability to breathe around the ETT can be evaluated by suctioning the oral pharynx and deflating the ETT cuff. With occlusion of the proximal end of the ETT, the patient is then asked to breathe around the tube. This qualitative assessment of adequate air movement suggests that the patient's airway will remain patent after tracheal extubation. More quantitative methods include (1) measuring the intrathoracic pressure required to produce an audible leak around the ETT when the cuff is deflated and (2) measuring the exhaled tidal volume before and after ETT cuff deflation in a patient receiving volume control ventilation. Though helpful, none of these cuff leak "tests" takes the place of sound clinical judgment when deciding when to safely extubate the patient.[10] If concern for airway compromise is significant, a tracheal tube exchange catheter can be used.

## Obstructive Sleep Apnea

Special consideration must be given to patients with obstructive sleep apnea (OSA) in the PACU (also see Chapters 27 and 50).[11] Patients with OSA have a more frequent risk for postoperative desaturation, respiratory failure, postoperative cardiac events, and the need for intensive care unit transfer.[12] As such, it is important to recognize and diagnose OSA in the preoperative setting and be mindful of its implications in the intraoperative and postoperative settings. Many screening tools such as the STOP-BANG questionnaire are effective in predicting OSA.[13] Because patients with OSA are particularly prone to airway obstruction, their tracheas should not be extubated until they are fully awake and following commands. Any redundant compliant pharyngeal tissue in these patients not only increases the incidence of airway obstruction but also makes mask ventilation and intubation by direct laryngoscopy difficult or at times impossible. Once in the PACU, a patient with OSA whose trachea has been extubated is exquisitely sensitive to opioids, and, when possible, regional anesthesia and multimodal analgesia techniques should be used to provide postoperative analgesia and minimize opioid consumption. The combination of benzodiazepines and opioids can cause significant episodes of hypoxemia and apnea in patients with OSA.[14]

For patients with OSA, plans should be made preoperatively to provide CPAP in the immediate postoperative period. Patients are often asked to bring their CPAP machines with them on the day of surgery so that the equipment can be set up before the patient's arrival in the PACU. Patients who do not routinely use CPAP at home or who do not have their machines with them may require additional attention from the respiratory therapist to ensure proper fit of the CPAP delivery device (mask or nasal airways) and to determine the amount of positive pressure needed to prevent upper airway obstruction. For patients with known or suspected OSA, consideration should also be given to postoperative continuous pulse oximetry monitoring.

## Management of Airway Obstruction

A patient who has an obstructed upper airway requires immediate attention. Efforts to open the airway by noninvasive measures should be attempted before reintubation of the trachea. Jaw thrust with CPAP (5 to 15 cm $H_2O$) is often enough to tent the upper airway open in patients with decreased pharyngeal muscle tone. If CPAP is not effective, an oral, nasal, or laryngeal mask airway can be inserted rapidly. After successfully opening the upper airway and ensuring adequate ventilation, the cause of the upper airway obstruction should be identified and treated. The sedating effects of opioids and benzodiazepines can be reversed with persistent stimulation or small, titrated doses of naloxone or flumazenil, respectively (see Chapter 8). Residual effects of neuromuscular blocking drugs can be reversed pharmacologically or by correcting contributing factors such as hypothermia (see Chapter 11).

Ventilating the lungs of a patient with severe upper airway obstruction as a result of edema or hematoma may not be possible via a mask. In the case of hematoma after thyroid or carotid surgery, an attempt can be made to decompress the airway by releasing the clips or sutures on the wound and evacuating the hematoma. This maneuver is recommended as a temporizing measure, but it will not effectively decompress the airway if a significant amount of fluid or blood (or both) has infiltrated the tissue planes of the pharyngeal wall. If emergency tracheal intubation is required, ready access to difficult airway equipment should be arranged and, if possible, surgical backup for performance of an emergency tracheostomy. If the patient is able to move air by spontaneous ventilation, an awake endotracheal intubation technique is preferred because visualization of the cords by direct laryngoscopy may not be possible.

### Monitoring Airway Patency During Transport

Upper airway patency and the effectiveness of the patient's respiratory efforts must be monitored during transportation from the operating room to the PACU. Hypoventilation in a patient receiving supplemental oxygen will not be reliably detected by monitoring with pulse oximetry during transport.[15] Adequate ventilation must be confirmed by watching for the appropriate rise and fall of the chest wall with inspiration, listening for breath sounds, or simply feeling for exhaled breath with the palm of one's hand over the patient's nose and mouth. As indicated previously, this can be a critically dangerous time in the immediate postoperative period.

## HYPOXEMIA IN THE POSTANESTHESIA CARE UNIT

Atelectasis and alveolar hypoventilation are the most common causes of transient postoperative arterial hypoxemia in the immediate postoperative period. Filling the patient's lungs with oxygen at the conclusion of anesthesia, as well as the administration of supplemental oxygen, should blunt any effect of diffusion hypoxia as a contributor to arterial hypoxemia. Review of the patient's history, operative course, and clinical signs and symptoms will direct the workup to determine possible causes of persistent hypoxia (Box 39.3) (also see Chapter 5).

### Alveolar Hypoventilation

Postoperative ventilatory failure can result from a depressed drive to breathe or generalized weakness from either residual neuromuscular blockade or underlying neuromuscular disease. Restrictive pulmonary conditions such as preexisting chest wall deformity, postoperative abdominal binding, or abdominal distention can also contribute to inadequate ventilation (Box 39.4).

Review of the alveolar gas equation demonstrates that hypoventilation alone is sufficient to cause arterial hypoxemia in a patient breathing room air (Fig. 39.1). At sea level, a normocapnic patient breathing room air will have an alveolar oxygen partial pressure of 100 mm Hg.

---

**Box 39.3** Causes of Postoperative Hypoxemia

Right-to-left shunt
    Pulmonary: atelectasis
    Intracardiac: congenital heart disease
Mismatching of ventilation to perfusion
Congestive heart failure
Pulmonary edema—fluid overload, postobstructive
Alveolar hypoventilation—residual effects of anesthetics and neuromuscular blocking drugs
Diffusion hypoxia—unlikely if patient is receiving supplemental oxygen
Aspiration of gastric contents
Pulmonary embolus
Pneumothorax
Posthyperventilation hypoxia
Increased oxygen consumption (e.g., shivering)
Acute respiratory distress syndrome (ARDS)
Sepsis
Transfusion-related acute lung injury
Advanced age
Obesity

---

**Box 39.4** Factors Leading to Postoperative Hypoventilation

Drug-induced central nervous system depression (volatile anesthetics, opioids)
Residual effects of neuromuscular blocking drugs
Suboptimal ventilatory muscle mechanics
Increased production of carbon dioxide
Coexisting chronic obstructive pulmonary disease

---

$$PAO_2 = FIO_2(PB - PH_2O) - \frac{PaCO_2}{RQ}$$

**$PaCO_2$ = 40 mm Hg**
$$PAO_2 = 0.21(760 - 47) - \frac{40}{0.8} = 150 - 50 = 100 \text{ mm Hg}$$

**$PaCO_2$ = 80 mm Hg**
$$PAO_2 = 0.21(760 - 47) - \frac{80}{0.8} = 150 - 100 = 50 \text{ mm Hg}$$

$PAO_2$ = alveolar oxygen pressure
$FIO_2$ = fraction of inspired oxygen concentration
PB   = barometric pressure
$PH_2O$ = vapor pressure of water
RQ   = respiratory quotient

**Fig. 39.1** Hypoventilation as a cause of arterial hypoxemia.

---

Thus, a healthy patient without a significant alveolar-arterial (A-a) gradient will have a $PaO_2$ near 100 mm Hg. In the same patient, an increase in $PaCO_2$ from 40 to 80 mm Hg (alveolar hypoventilation) results in an alveolar oxygen partial pressure ($PAO_2$) of 50 mm Hg. This exercise

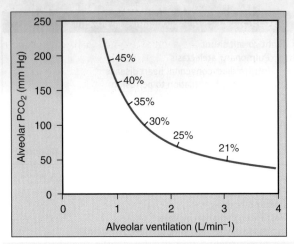

**Fig. 39.2** Alveolar $P_{CO_2}$ as a function of alveolar ventilation at rest. The percentages indicate the inspired oxygen concentration required to restore alveolar $P_{O_2}$ to normal. (Adapted from Lumb AB, ed. *Nunn's Applied Respiratory Physiology*. 6th ed. Philadelphia: Elsevier/Butterworth-Heinemann; 2005, used with permission.)

demonstrates that even a patient with normal lungs will become hypoxic if allowed to significantly hypoventilate while breathing room air.

Normally, minute ventilation increases by approximately 2 L/min for every 1 mm Hg increase in arterial $P_{CO_2}$. This linear ventilatory response to carbon dioxide can be significantly depressed in the immediate postoperative period by the residual effects of drugs (e.g., inhaled anesthetics, opioids, sedative-hypnotics) administered during anesthesia.

Arterial hypoxemia secondary to hypercapnia alone can be reversed by the administration of supplemental oxygen or by restoring the $Pa_{CO_2}$ to normal, or both (Fig. 39.2).[16] In the PACU, $Pa_{CO_2}$ can be returned to normal by external stimulation of the patient to wakefulness, pharmacologic reversal of opioid or benzodiazepine effect, or controlled mechanical ventilation. Fig. 39.2 demonstrates why pulse oximetry is an unreliable marker of hypoventilation in a patient receiving supplemental oxygen.

### Decreased Alveolar Partial Pressure of Oxygen

Diffusion hypoxia refers to the rapid diffusion of nitrous oxide into alveoli at the end of a nitrous oxide anesthetic. Nitrous oxide dilutes the alveolar gas and produces a transient decrease in $Pa_{O_2}$ and $Pa_{CO_2}$. In a patient breathing room air, the resulting decrease in $Pa_{O_2}$ can produce arterial hypoxemia. In the absence of supplemental oxygen administration, diffusion hypoxia can persist for 5 to 10 minutes after a nitrous oxide anesthetic and thus contribute to arterial hypoxemia in the initial moments as the patient is admitted to the PACU.

When providing supplemental oxygen to a patient during transport to the PACU, care should be taken to avoid the relative decrease in the fraction of inspired oxygen ($F_{IO_2}$) that can result from an unrecognized disconnection of the oxygen source or from an empty oxygen tank.

### Ventilation-to-Perfusion Mismatch and Shunt

Hypoxic pulmonary vasoconstriction (HPV) is an attempt of normal lungs to optimally match ventilation and perfusion. This response constricts vessels in poorly ventilated regions of the lung and directs pulmonary blood flow to well-ventilated alveoli. The HPV response is inhibited by many conditions and medications, including pneumonia, sepsis, and vasodilators. In the PACU, the residual effects of inhaled anesthetics and vasodilators such as nitroprusside and dobutamine will blunt HPV and contribute to arterial hypoxemia.

Unlike a ventilation-to-perfusion mismatch, a true shunt will not respond to supplemental oxygen. Causes of postoperative pulmonary shunt include atelectasis, pulmonary edema, gastric aspiration, pulmonary emboli, and pneumonia. Of these, atelectasis is probably the most common cause of pulmonary shunting in the immediate postoperative period. Mobilization of the patient to the sitting position, incentive spirometry, and positive airway pressure via a face mask can be effective in treating atelectasis.

### Increased Venous Admixture

Increased venous admixture typically refers to low cardiac output states. It is due to mixing of desaturated venous blood with oxygenated arterial blood. Normally, only 2% to 5% of cardiac output is shunted through the lungs, and this small amount of shunted blood with a normal mixed venous saturation has a minimal effect on $Pa_{O_2}$. In low cardiac output states, blood returns to the heart severely desaturated. Additionally, the shunt fraction increases significantly in conditions that impede alveolar oxygenation, such as pulmonary edema and atelectasis. Under these conditions, mixing of desaturated shunted blood with saturated arterialized blood decreases $Pa_{O_2}$.

### Decreased Diffusion Capacity

A decreased diffusion capacity is caused by underlying lung disease such as emphysema, interstitial lung disease, pulmonary fibrosis, or primary pulmonary hypertension. The differential diagnosis of arterial hypoxemia in the PACU must include the contribution of any preexisting pulmonary condition.

### PULMONARY EDEMA IN THE POSTANESTHESIA CARE UNIT

Pulmonary edema in the immediate postoperative period is often cardiogenic in nature, the result of increased intravascular volume or cardiac dysfunction. Noncardiogenic edema may occur in the PACU as a result of pulmonary aspiration of gastric contents or sepsis. Rarely, postoperative pulmonary edema is the result of airway obstruction (postobstructive pulmonary edema) or transfusion of blood products (transfusion-related acute lung injury) (also see Chapter 24).

## Postobstructive Pulmonary Edema

Postobstructive pulmonary edema (POPE), also referred to as negative-pressure pulmonary edema, and the resulting arterial hypoxemia are rare but significant consequences of upper airway obstruction and may follow tracheal extubation at the conclusion of anesthesia and surgery. POPE is characterized by a transudative edema produced by one of two mechanisms: the exaggerated negative pressure generated by inspiration against acute airway obstruction (type I) or following relief of a chronic partial airway obstruction (type II).[17] The pathophysiology of type I POPE involves exaggerated negative intrathoracic pressure, which increases venous return, afterload, and pulmonary venous pressures, and promotes the transudation of fluid. Muscular healthy patients are at increased risk because of their ability to generate significant inspiratory force.

Laryngospasm is the most common cause of upper airway obstruction leading to type I POPE, but it may result from any condition that occludes the upper airway including epiglottitis, bilateral vocal cord paralysis, goiter, and occlusion of the ETT. Arterial hypoxemia with respiratory distress is usually manifested within 90 minutes after relief of airway obstruction and is frequently accompanied by tachypnea, tachycardia, rales, rhonchi, and evidence of bilateral pulmonary edema on the chest radiograph. The diagnosis depends on clinical suspicion once other causes of pulmonary edema are ruled out. Treatment is supportive and includes supplemental oxygen, diuresis, and, in severe cases, positive-pressure ventilation utilizing CPAP or mechanical ventilation.

## Transfusion-Related Acute Lung Injury

The differential diagnosis of pulmonary edema in the PACU should include transfusion-related acute lung injury (TRALI) in any patient who received blood, coagulation factor, or platelet transfusions intraoperatively and is described in Chapter 24. Treatment is generally supportive and includes supplemental oxygen and diuresis. Rarely, TRALI results in a prolonged course of acute respiratory distress syndrome (ARDS). Historically, the lack of specific diagnostic criteria has led to the underdiagnosis and underreporting of TRALI. In a 2007-2008 study, implementation of TRALI risk mitigation policies that utilized a predominantly male plasma supply indicated a significant reduction in the incidence of TRALI[18] (see Chapter 24 for more details).

## OXYGEN SUPPLEMENTATION

The delivery of supplemental oxygen in the immediate postoperative period is usually routine for the prevention of possible hypoxemia. Still, the "optimal" perioperative oxygenation procedure remains controversial. Whether increased oxygenation delivery results in a reduction in the incidence of postoperative nausea and vomiting (PONV) and promotion of surgical wound healing is not clear.[19]

### Oxygen Delivery

The choice of oxygen delivery systems in the PACU is determined by the degree of hypoxemia, the surgical procedure, and patient compliance. Patients who have undergone head and neck surgery may not be candidates for administration of oxygen via a face mask owing to the risk of pressure necrosis of incision sites and microvascular flaps, whereas nasal packing prohibits the use of nasal cannulas in others.

Delivery of oxygen by traditional nasal cannula should be limited to 6 L/min flow to minimize discomfort and complications that result from inadequate humidification. As a general rule each 1 L/min of oxygen flow through nasal cannula increases $F_{IO_2}$ by 0.04, with 6 L/min resulting in approximately 0.44 $F_{IO_2}$.

Until recently maximum oxygen delivery to patients whose tracheas have been extubated required a nonrebreather mask or high-flow nebulizer. Delivery of oxygen via mask can be inefficient when mask fit is inadequate or large minute ventilation is required, which results in significant entrainment of room air. Alternatively, oxygen can be delivered up to 40 L/min by high-flow nasal cannulas. These high-flow nasal cannula delivery systems humidify and warm the gas to 99.9% relative humidity and 37° C. Unlike nonrebreather masks, these devices deliver oxygen directly to the nasopharynx throughout the respiratory cycle. The efficacy of these systems may be enhanced by a CPAP effect produced by the high gas flow.

### Continuous Positive Airway Pressure and Noninvasive Positive-Pressure Ventilation

Approximately 8% to 10% of patients who undergo abdominal surgery require endotracheal intubation and mechanical ventilation for hypoxemia postoperatively. Application of CPAP in the PACU reduces the incidence of reintubation of the trachea, pneumonia, infection, and sepsis.[18-21] Even with the application of CPAP in the PACU, many patients will require additional ventilatory support. Ventilatory failure in the immediate postoperative period may result from many conditions including excessive intravascular volume, splinting due to pain,

V

diaphragmatic dysfunction, muscular weakness, and pharmacologically depressed respiratory drive.

Although the use of noninvasive positive-pressure ventilation (NPPV) in both chronic and acute respiratory failure is well established, there is limited experience with its application in the PACU. NPPV can be used in the PACU for patients with increased risk for pulmonary complications and as a rescue technique for patients in postoperative respiratory distress. NPPV is often avoided in the immediate postoperative period because of the potential for gastric distention, aspiration of gastric contents, and wound dehiscence, especially in patients who have undergone gastric or esophageal surgery. Thus, the decision to use noninvasive modes of ventilation in the PACU must be guided by careful consideration of both patient and surgical factors. Contraindications include hemodynamic instability or life-threatening arrhythmias, altered mental status, increased risk of aspiration of gastric contents, inability to use a nasal or face mask (head and neck procedures), and refractory hypoxemia. In the appropriate patient population, particularly for prophylactic use in patients following bariatric surgery and for patients in postoperative respiratory distress, NPPV is effective in avoiding endotracheal intubation in the PACU.[22]

## HEMODYNAMIC INSTABILITY

Hemodynamic instability in the immediate postoperative period can have a negative impact on outcome. Surprisingly, postoperative systemic hypertension and tachycardia are more predictive of unplanned admission to the critical care unit and mortality rate than are hypotension and bradycardia.[23]

### Systemic Hypertension

Patients with a history of essential hypertension are at greatest risk for significant systemic hypertension in the PACU. Additional factors include pain, hypoventilation and associated hypercapnia and hypoxia, emergence excitement, advanced age, a history of cigarette smoking, and preexisting renal disease (Box 39.5). Complications that may arise as a result of postoperative hypertension include myocardial ischemia, cardiac arrhythmia, congestive heart failure with pulmonary edema, stroke, and encephalopathy.[24] Acute postoperative hypertension increases the risk for intracranial hemorrhage following craniotomy and postoperative bleeding at the surgical site, and may compromise vascular anastomoses.[25] Surgical procedures that predispose the patient to postoperative hypertension include craniotomy, carotid endarterectomy, cardiothoracic procedures, and head and neck procedures.[24]

---

**Box 39.5** Factors Leading to Postoperative Hypertension

Arterial hypoxemia
Preoperative essential hypertension
Enhanced sympathetic nervous system activity—hypercapnia from hypoventilation, pain, gastric distention, bladder distention
Hypervolemia
Emergence agitation
Shivering
Drug or alcohol withdrawal—clonidine, β-blockers, narcotics
Increased intracranial pressure

---

**Box 39.6** Causes of Hypotension in the Postanesthesia Care Unit

Intravascular fluid volume depletion
    Ongoing fluid losses—bowel preparation, gastrointestinal losses, surgical bleeding
    Increased capillary permeability—sepsis, burns, transfusion-related lung injury
Decreased cardiac output
    Myocardial ischemia/infarction
    Cardiomyopathy
    Valvular disease
    Pericardial disease
    Cardiac tamponade
    Cardiac dysrhythmias
    Pulmonary embolus
    Tension pneumothorax
    Drug-induced—β-blockers, calcium channel blockers
Decreased vascular tone
    Sepsis
    Allergic reactions—anaphylactic, anaphylactoid
    Spinal shock—cord injury, iatrogenic: spinal or epidural anesthesia
Adrenal insufficiency

---

### Systemic Hypotension

Postoperative hypotension may be characterized as (1) hypovolemic, (2) cardiogenic, or (3) distributive (Box 39.6). Regardless of the cause, postoperative hypotension can lead to decreased tissue perfusion and impaired end organ function and requires immediate attention (also see Chapter 5).

#### Hypovolemia (Decreased Preload)

Systemic hypotension in the PACU is usually due to decreased intravascular fluid volume and preload and, as such, responds favorably to intravenous fluid administration. The most common causes of decreased intravascular volume in the immediate postoperative period include ongoing third-space translocation of fluid, inadequate intraoperative fluid replacement (especially in patients who undergo major intra-abdominal procedures or preoperative bowel preparation), and loss of sympathetic nervous system tone as a result of neuraxial (spinal or epidural) blockade (also see Chapter 23).

Persistent bleeding should be ruled out in hypotensive patients who have undergone a surgical procedure in which significant blood loss is possible. This is true regardless of the estimated intraoperative blood loss. If the patient is unstable, hemoglobin can be measured at the bedside to eliminate laboratory turnover time. It is also important to remember that tachycardia may not be a reliable indicator of hypovolemia or anemia (or both) if the patient is taking β-adrenergic or calcium channel blockers.

### Cardiogenic Hypotension (Intrinsic Pump Failure)

Significant cardiogenic causes of postoperative systemic hypotension include myocardial ischemia and infarction, cardiomyopathy, and cardiac dysrhythmias. The differential diagnosis depends on the surgical procedure, intraoperative course, and the patient's preoperative medical condition.

### Distributive Hypotension (Decreased Afterload)

#### Iatrogenic Sympathectomy

Iatrogenic sympathectomy secondary to regional anesthetic techniques is an important cause of hypotension in the PACU. An extensive sympathetic block (to T4) will decrease vascular tone and block the cardioaccelerator fibers. If not treated promptly, the resulting bradycardia in the presence of severe hypotension can lead to cardiac arrest, even in young healthy patients. Vasopressors, including phenylephrine and ephedrine, are pharmacologic treatments of hypotension caused by residual sympathetic nervous system blockade.

#### Critically Ill Patients

Critically ill patients may rely on exaggerated sympathetic nervous system tone to maintain systemic blood pressure and heart rate. In these patients even minimal doses of inhaled anesthetics, opioids, or sedative-hypnotics can decrease sympathetic nervous system tone and produce marked systemic hypotension.

#### Allergic Reactions

Allergic (anaphylactic or anaphylactoid) reactions may be the cause of hypotension in the PACU. These reactions are likely underreported and have an estimated incidence of 100 per 1 million procedures.[26] Anaphylaxis should be considered in all cases of sudden refractory extreme hypotension, even when not accompanied by the classic sequelae of bronchospasm and rash. Increased serum tryptase concentrations confirm the occurrence of an allergic reaction, but this change does not differentiate anaphylactic from anaphylactoid reactions. The blood specimen for tryptase determination must be obtained within 30 to 120 minutes after the allergic reaction, but the results may not be available for several days. Neuromuscular blocking drugs (also see Chapter 11) are the most common cause of anaphylactic reactions in the operative setting, followed by latex and antibiotics. Treatment begins with withdrawal of the triggering agent, and epinephrine is the drug of choice for severe reactions. Patients should receive counseling after a suspected anaphylactic reaction, and allergy testing is recommended 4 to 6 weeks after the initial reaction.[27]

#### Sepsis

If sepsis is suspected as the cause of hypotension in the PACU, blood should be obtained for culture, after which empiric antibiotic therapy should be initiated before transfer of the patient to the ward (also see Chapter 41). Urinary tract manipulations and biliary tract procedures are examples of interventions that can result in a sudden onset of severe systemic hypotension in the PACU. In these cases hypotension is often accompanied by fever and rigor.

## Myocardial Ischemia

Detection of myocardial ischemia in the PACU can be challenging because of the patient's inability to identify or communicate symptoms related to cardiac ischemia. In one study, only approximately 35% of postoperative patients with myocardial infarction complained of typical chest pain.[28] The ASA Practice Guidelines for Postanesthesia Care recommend routine pulse, blood pressure, and ECG monitoring to detect cardiovascular complications such as myocardial ischemia.[2]

### Low-Risk Patients

Interpretation of ST-segment changes on the ECG in the PACU should be interpreted in light of the patient's cardiac history and risk index. In low-risk patients (<45 years of age, no known cardiac disease, only one risk factor), postoperative ST-segment changes on the ECG do not usually indicate myocardial ischemia. Relatively benign causes of ST-segment changes in these low-risk patients include anxiety, esophageal reflux, hyperventilation, and hypokalemia. In general, low-risk patients require only routine PACU observation unless associated signs and symptoms warrant further clinical evaluation. A more aggressive evaluation is indicated if the changes are accompanied by cardiac rhythm disturbances, hemodynamic instability, angina, or associated symptoms.

### High-Risk Patients

In contrast to low-risk patients, ST-segment and T-wave changes on the ECG in high-risk patients can be significant even in the absence of typical signs or symptoms of myocardial ischemia. In this patient population, any ST-segment, T-wave, or rhythm changes that are compatible with myocardial ischemia should prompt further

V

**Box 39.7** Factors Leading to Postoperative Cardiac Dysrhythmias

Hypoxemia
Hypercarbia
Intravascular volume shifts
Pain, agitation
Hypothermia
Hyperthermia
Anticholinesterases
Anticholinergics
Myocardial ischemia
Electrolyte abnormalities
Respiratory acidosis
Hypertension
Digitalis intoxication
Preoperative cardiac dysrhythmias

evaluation to rule out myocardial ischemia. Determination of serum troponin levels is indicated when myocardial ischemia or infarction is suspected in the PACU. Once blood samples for measurement of troponin and a 12-lead ECG are completed, arrangements must be made for the appropriate cardiology follow-up.

### Routine Postoperative 12-Lead Electrocardiogram and Troponin Measurement

Even small increases of troponin in the postoperative period are associated with an increased 30-day mortality rate, and there is currently no defined management strategy for these patients.[27-30] As a result, current American Heart Association/American College of Cardiology (AHA/ACC) guidelines cite insufficient evidence regarding routine postoperative 12-lead ECG or troponin measurements in patients at high risk for perioperative myocardial ischemia but without ongoing signs or symptoms of myocardial ischemia. These guidelines recommend against routine screening of an unselected patient population using troponin measurements.[31]

## Cardiac Dysrhythmias

Perioperative cardiac dysrhythmias are frequently transient and multifactorial in cause (Box 39.7). Reversible causes of cardiac dysrhythmias in the perioperative period include hypoxemia, hypoventilation and associated hypercapnia, endogenous or exogenous catecholamines, electrolyte abnormalities, acidemia, excessive intravascular fluid, anemia, and substance withdrawal.

### Tachydysrhythmias

Common causes of sinus tachycardia in the PACU include postoperative pain, agitation (rule out arterial hypoxemia), hypoventilation with associated hypercapnia, hypovolemia (continued postoperative bleeding), shivering, and the presence of a tracheal tube. Additional causes

include cardiogenic or septic shock, pulmonary embolism, thyroid storm, and malignant hyperthermia.

### Atrial Dysrhythmias

The incidence of new postoperative atrial dysrhythmias may be as high as 10% after major noncardiothoracic surgery. The incidence is even higher after cardiac and thoracic procedures when the cardiac dysrhythmia is often attributed to atrial irritation. These new-onset atrial dysrhythmias are not benign because they are associated with a longer hospital stay and increased mortality rate.[32]

### Atrial Fibrillation

Control of the ventricular response rate is the immediate goal in the treatment of new-onset atrial fibrillation. Hemodynamically unstable patients may require prompt electrical cardioversion, but most patients can be treated pharmacologically with intravenous β-blocker or calcium channel blocker. Diltiazem is the calcium channel blocker of choice for patients in whom β-blockers are contraindicated. Ventricular rate control with these drugs is often enough to chemically cardiovert the postoperative patient whose arrhythmia may be catecholamine driven. If the goal of therapy is chemical cardioversion, an amiodarone infusion can be initiated in the PACU.

### Ventricular Dysrhythmias

Ventricular tachycardia is uncommon, whereas premature ventricular contractions (PVCs) and ventricular bigeminy are common. PVCs often reflect increased sympathetic nervous system stimulation, as may accompany tracheal intubation and transient hypercapnia. True ventricular tachycardia is indicative of underlying cardiac disease, and in the case of torsades de pointes, QT-interval prolongation on the ECG may be intrinsic or drug related (amiodarone, procainamide, haloperidol [Haldol], or droperidol).

### Bradydysrhythmias

Bradycardia in the PACU is often iatrogenic. Drug-related causes include β-adrenergic blocker therapy, neostigmine reversal of neuromuscular blockade, opioid administration, and treatment with dexmedetomidine. Procedure- and patient-related causes include bowel distention, increased intracranial or intraocular pressure, and spinal anesthesia. A high spinal block of cardioaccelerator fibers originating from T1 through T4 can produce severe bradycardia. The resulting sympathectomy, and possible intravascular volume depletion and associated decreased venous return can result in sudden cardiac arrest, even in young healthy patients.

### Treatment

The urgency of treatment of a cardiac dysrhythmia depends on the physiologic consequences (principally systemic hypotension and myocardial ischemia) of the dysrhythmia. Tachydysrhythmia decreases diastolic and coronary perfusion time and increases myocardial oxygen consumption. Its impact depends on the patient's underlying cardiac function, and it is most harmful in patients with coronary artery disease. Bradycardia has a more deleterious effect in patients with a fixed stroke volume, such as infants and patients with restrictive pericardial disease or cardiac tamponade.

## DELIRIUM

Delirium is a transient disturbance in attention, awareness, and cognition that is not otherwise explained by another disorder or process (also see Chapter 35). The estimated incidence of postoperative delirium ranges from 4% to 75% of patients, depending on patient characteristics and type of surgery. The incidence is much higher for certain procedures, such as repair of a hip fracture, cardiac surgery, abdominal aneurysm repair, and bilateral knee replacement, as opposed to outpatient cataract surgery. Early recognition and treatment of postoperative delirium are important because it is associated with increased morbidity and mortality rates, length of stay, and cost.[33,34] Additionally, delirium following cardiac surgery was associated with prolonged cognitive impairment at 1 year follow-up, indicating that postoperative delirium is not just a short-term disorder.[35]

### Risk Factors

Persistent postoperative delirium is generally a condition of elderly patients. In adults, patients should be screened in the preoperative setting to identify those at risk for postoperative delirium. Risk factors for postoperative delirium can be divided between predisposing factors, such as advanced age, and precipitating factors, such as medication administration or withdrawal (Box 39.8). Other intraoperative and postoperative factors that increase the likelihood of postoperative delirium include larger surgical blood loss and intraoperative blood transfusions, anemia, and use of a urinary bladder catheter.[34] Intraoperative hemodynamic derangements and the anesthetic technique do not seem to be predictors of postoperative delirium. Patients with an increased risk for postoperative delirium should be identified in the preoperative period using patient history, physical examination, and a cognitive screening tool such as the Mini-Cog.[36] Early identification of patients at risk for delirium can help guide management in the preoperative, intraoperative, and postoperative settings.

In addition, the workup of postoperative delirium must include evaluation to exclude arterial hypoxemia, hypercapnia, pain, sepsis, and electrolyte abnormalities (Box 39.9). Clinical evaluation of a delirious patient in the PACU includes a thorough evaluation of any underlying disease and metabolic derangements, such as hepatic- and renal-related encephalopathy.

---

**Box 39.8**  Risk Factors for Delirium

**Predisposing**
Reduced cognitive reserve: dementia, depression, advanced age
Reduced physical reserve: atherosclerotic disease, renal impairment, pulmonary disease, advanced age, preoperative β-blockade
Sensory impairment (vision, hearing)
Alcohol abuse
Malnutrition
Dehydration

**Precipitating**
Medications or medication withdrawal: anticholinergics, muscle relaxants, antihistamines, GI antispasmodics, opioid analgesics, antiarrhythmics, corticosteroids, more than six total medications, more than three new inpatient medications
Pain
Hypoxemia
Electrolyte abnormalities
Malnutrition
Dehydration
Environmental change (e.g., ICU admission)
Sleep-wake cycle disturbances
Urinary catheter use
Restraint use
Infection
Psychotropic medications: antidepressants, antiepileptics, antipsychotics, benzodiazepines

*GI*, Gastrointestinal; *ICU*, intensive care unit.

---

**Box 39.9**  Differential Diagnosis of Postoperative Delirium in the Postanesthesia Care Unit

Arterial hypoxemia
Preexisting cognitive disorder—Parkinson disease, baseline dementia
Hypoventilation with hypercapnia
Metabolic derangements—renal, hepatic, endocrine
Drugs—anticholinergics, benzodiazepines, opioids, β-blockers
Drug or ETOH withdrawal
Electrolyte abnormalities
Incomplete muscle relaxant reversal
Acute CNS event—hemorrhage, ischemic stroke
Infection
Seizures

*CNS*, Central nervous system; *ETOH*, ethanol.

---

### Management

Management of postoperative delirium begins with nonpharmacologic treatments including withdrawal of any inciting stimulus and environmental modifications such as frequent reorientation. Pharmacologic treatment may be necessary for severely agitated patients, and the typical antipsychotic haloperidol (0.5 to mg IV) is considered first-line therapy if

V

no contraindications exist. Severely agitated patients may require restraints and additional personnel to control their behavior and avoid self-inflicted injury or dislodgement of intravascular catheters and the endotracheal tube.

Because the elderly population (also see Chapter 35) may become delirious from both pain and sedating drugs such as opioids, a multimodal pain relief strategy utilizing nonopioid medications may be beneficial in reducing the likelihood of postoperative delirium in this population. On the contrary, patients with tolerance to opioids may require increased opioid doses to treat pain and anxiety and avoid the onset of withdrawal.

## Emergence Agitation

Emergence agitation is a transient period of excitation characterized by inconsolable crying, agitation, and delirium that is associated with emergence from general anesthesia. Emergence agitation is common in children, with more than 30% experiencing agitation or delirium at some period during their PACU stay (also see Chapter 34). The peak age of emergence agitation in children is between 2 and 4 years.

Unlike delirium, emergence agitation typically resolves quickly and is followed by uneventful recovery. Emergence excitement is more frequent with rapid "waking up" from inhaled anesthetics. In children, preoperative medication with midazolam may increase the incidence and duration of postoperative delirium, but whether midazolam is an independent factor or merely a reflection of other preoperative variables remains unclear.

## RENAL DYSFUNCTION

The risk of postoperative acute kidney injury (AKI) ranges from 5% to 10%.[37] The differential diagnosis of postoperative renal dysfunction includes preoperative, intraoperative, and postoperative causes (Box 39.10) (also see Chapter 28). Frequently, the cause is multifactorial, with a preexisting renal insufficiency that is exacerbated by an intraoperative insult. For example, preoperative or intraoperative angiography can result in ischemic injury secondary to renal vasoconstriction and direct renal tubular injury. Intravascular volume depletion can exacerbate hepatorenal syndrome or acute tubular necrosis caused by sepsis. In the PACU, diagnostic efforts should focus on identification and treatment of the readily reversible causes of oliguria (urine output < 0.5 mL/kg/h). For example, urinary catheter obstruction or dislodgement is easily remedied and often overlooked.

## Oliguria

### Postoperative Urinary Retention

The reported incidence of urinary retention in the PACU is between 5% and 70%. Clinical postoperative urinary retention is defined as the inability to void despite a

---

> **Box 39.10** Causes of Postoperative Renal Dysfunction
>
> **Prerenal**
> Hypovolemia (bleeding, sepsis, third-space fluid loss, inadequate volume resuscitation)
> Hepatorenal syndrome
> Low cardiac output
> Renal vascular obstruction or disruption
> Intra-abdominal hypertension
>
> **Renal**
> Ischemia (acute tubular necrosis)
> Radiographic contrast dyes
> Rhabdomyolysis
> Tumor lysis
> Hemolysis
>
> **Postrenal**
> Surgical injury to the ureters
> Obstruction of the ureters with clots or stones
>
> **Other**
> Mechanical (urinary catheter obstruction or malposition)

---

bladder volume of more than 500 to 600 mL. Risk factors include age older than 50 years, male gender, volume of intraoperative intravascular fluid infusion, duration of surgery, and bladder volume on admission. Type of surgery is also predictive, with urinary retention occurring most commonly in anorectal and joint replacement surgery. Commonly used perioperative medications such as anticholinergics, β-blockers, and narcotics also contribute to urinary retention. Diagnosis can be made by clinical examination, bladder catheterization, or ultrasound assessment. Bladder volumes measured by ultrasound imaging correlate well with volumes obtained by urinary catheterization, an uncomfortable procedure that can be complicated by catheter-related infections and urethral trauma. Bladder ultrasound is an efficient and accurate method to evaluate patients at risk for oliguria.[38]

### Decreased Intravascular Volume

The most common cause of oliguria in the immediate postoperative period is a decrease of intravascular volume. An intravascular fluid challenge (500 to 1000 mL of crystalloid) is usually effective in restoring urine output. The hematocrit should be measured when surgical blood loss is suspected and repeated intravascular boluses of fluid are required to maintain urine output. Resuscitation by intravenous administration of fluids to maximize renal perfusion is particularly important in order to prevent ongoing ischemic injury and the development of acute tubular necrosis.

If an intravascular fluid challenge is contraindicated or oliguria persists, assessment of intravascular volume or cardiac function is indicated to differentiate hypovolemia from sepsis and low cardiac output states. Fractional excretion of sodium can be useful in determining the adequacy of renal perfusion (assuming that diuretics have not been given), but the diagnosis of prerenal azotemia will not differentiate between hypovolemia, congestive heart failure, or hepatorenal syndrome. In these cases evaluation with central venous monitoring or echocardiography may facilitate the diagnosis.

## Intra-Abdominal Hypertension

Intra-abdominal hypertension (IAH) is a sustained measured intra-abdominal pressure higher than 12 mm Hg and should be considered as a cause of oliguria in patients following abdominal surgery, major trauma, or burns, and in those who are critically ill. Abdominal compartment syndrome is defined as sustained intra-abdominal pressure higher than 20 mm Hg that is associated with new organ dysfunction or failure.[39] In addition to cardiovascular effects, IAH may impede renal perfusion and lead to renal ischemia and postoperative renal dysfunction. Intra-abdominal pressure should be measured (via bladder pressure) in patients in whom intra-abdominal hypertension is suspected so that prompt intervention can be initiated to relieve intra-abdominal pressure and restore renal perfusion.

## Rhabdomyolysis

Rhabdomyolysis is a possible cause of postoperative renal insufficiency in patients who have suffered major crush or thermal injury as well as with patients undergoing elective surgery. The incidence is increased in morbidly obese patients, particularly those having bariatric surgery. Risk factors include increased body mass index (BMI), prolonged duration of surgery, male gender, and patient positioning (lithotomy and lateral decubitus).[40] Patient history and the operative course should guide the decision to measure creatinine phosphokinase in the PACU. Severe postoperative pain is characteristic of myonecrosis and rhabdomyolysis, often in the areas of contact with the operating room table such as the gluteal, lumbar, and shoulder muscles. Volume loading, mannitol, and alkalinization of urine may help prevent rhabdomyolysis from progressing to AKI. Loop diuretics can be used to maintain urine output and avoid fluid overload.

## Contrast Nephropathy

Angiography with intravascular stent placement is replacing open procedures to treat carotid stenosis, aortic aneurysms, and peripheral vascular disease. Patients undergoing these procedures often have chronic renal insufficiency and are at risk for developing renal failure secondary to intravenous contrast infusion. Management of these patients in the PACU includes particular attention to intravascular volume status in order to prevent AKI. Although aggressive hydration with normal saline provides the single most effective protection against contrast nephropathy, alkalinization with bicarbonate has been shown to provide additional protection. If bicarbonate is used for renal protection in this setting, 154 mEq/L should be infused at a rate of 1 mL/kg/h for 6 hours after the procedure. Mucomyst can be given and is a relatively inexpensive and easily administered medication (single oral dose before and after procedure) that may also provide renal protection.[27]

## BODY TEMPERATURE AND SHIVERING

Postoperative shivering is a dramatic consequence of general and epidural anesthesia. The incidence of postoperative shivering may be as high as 65% (range 5% to 65%) after general anesthesia and 33% after epidural anesthesia. Identified risk factors include male gender and the choice of drug for induction of anesthesia (i.e., more likely with propofol than thiopental).

## Mechanism

Postoperative shivering is usually associated with a decrease in the patient's body temperature. Although thermoregulatory mechanisms can explain shivering in a hypothermic patient, a separate mechanism has been proposed to explain shivering in normothermic patients. The proposed mechanism is based on the observation that the brain and spinal cord do not recover simultaneously from general anesthesia. The more rapid recovery of spinal cord function results in uninhibited spinal reflexes manifested as clonic activity. This theory is supported by the fact that doxapram, a central nervous system stimulant, is somewhat effective in abolishing postoperative shivering.

## Treatment

Intervention includes the identification and treatment of hypothermia if present. In addition to shivering, mild to moderate hypothermia (33° to 35° C) inhibits platelet function, coagulation factor activity, and drug metabolism. It exacerbates postoperative bleeding, prolongs neuromuscular blockade, and may delay awakening. Shivering also increases oxygen consumption and is potentially detrimental in the postoperative patient with history of cardiac disease or limited reserve. Accurate core body temperatures can be most quickly and easily obtained using a temporal artery thermometer.[41] Forced air warmers can be used preoperatively to prevent hypothermia as well as to actively warm the hypothermic patient in the PACU.[42] A number of opioids and $\alpha_2$-agonists are effective in abolishing shivering once it starts, but meperidine (12.5 to 25 mg IV) is the most effective treatment.

## POSTOPERATIVE NAUSEA AND VOMITING

The consequences of PONV in the PACU include delayed discharge from the PACU, unanticipated hospital admission, increased incidence of pulmonary aspiration, and significant postoperative discomfort and patient dissatisfaction. Therefore, the ability to identify high-risk patients for prophylactic intervention can significantly improve the quality of patient care and satisfaction in the PACU (also see Chapter 37).

## High-Risk Patients

Risk factors for PONV can be grouped into three categories: patient, anesthetic, and surgery-related factors. A subset of factors has been established for each. The most significant patient-related factors include female gender (postpuberty), nonsmoking status, age less than 50 years, and history of motion sickness or PONV. Anesthesia-related factors include the use of volatile anesthetics or nitrous oxide and the administration of large doses of neostigmine and perioperative opioids. The most significant surgical risk factor is duration of surgery (Box 39.11).

---

**Box 39.11** Factors Associated With Increased Incidence of Postoperative Nausea and Vomiting (PONV)

History of PONV or motion sickness
Female gender
Age less than 50 years
Postoperative opioids
Nonsmoking status
Type of surgery—eye muscle surgery, middle ear surgery, cholecystectomy, gynecologic surgery—laparoscopic approach
Duration of surgery
Anesthetic drugs—opioids, nitrous oxide, volatile anesthetics
Gastric distention—swallowed blood

---

High-risk patients can be identified by a simplified risk score consisting of four mostly patient-related factors: (1) female gender, (2) history of motion sickness or PONV, (3) nonsmoking, and (4) the use of postoperative opioids. The incidence of PONV correlates with the number of these factors present: zero, one, two, three, and four factors correspond to an incidence of 10%, 21%, 39%, 61%, and 79%, respectively.

Cost-effective management of PONV takes into consideration the patient's underlying risk. A single intervention in a patient with four risk factors will result in an absolute risk reduction of 21% compared with a 3% risk reduction in a patient with an initial risk of only 10%. These numbers correlate to a number of 5 and 40, respectively, needed to treat.[43]

## Prevention and Treatment

Prophylactic measures against PONV include modification of the anesthetic technique and pharmacologic intervention. Strategies to reduce baseline risk include avoidance of general anesthesia by the use of regional anesthesia, preferential use of propofol infusions, avoidance of nitrous oxide and volatile anesthetics, minimization of giving postoperative opioids, and adequate hydration.[44] Although prophylactic measures to prevent PONV are clearly more effective than rescue, a subset of patients will require treatment in the PACU even after receiving appropriate prophylactic treatment. When choosing an antiemetic for these patients, both the class of drug and the timing of administration are important factors (Box 39.12). For instance, dexamethasone is effective when given prophylactically at

---

**Box 39.12** Commonly Used Antiemetics, With Adult Doses

**Anticholinergics**
Scopolamine: transdermal patch, 1.5 cm$^2$
    Apply to a hairless area behind the ear before surgery; remove 24 hours postoperatively

**Antihistamines**
Hydroxyzine: 12.5-25 mg IM

**Phenothiazines**
Promethazine: 12.5-25 mg IV/IM
Prochlorperazine: 2.5-10 mg IV/IM

**Butyrophenones**
Droperidol: 0.625-1.25 mg IV
    See black box warning regarding torsades de pointes: monitor the ECG for prolongation of the QT interval for 2-3 hours after administration—preoperative 12-lead ECG recommended

**Nk-1 Receptor Antagonists**
Aprepitant: 40 mg PO prior to induction of anesthesia

**Prokinetic**
Metoclopramide: 10-20 mg IV
    Minimal antiemetic properties, avoid in patients with any possibility of gastrointestinal obstruction

**Serotonin Receptor Antagonists**
Ondansetron: 4 mg IV 30 minutes before conclusion of surgery
Granisetron: 0.35-3 mg IV near the conclusion of surgery
Tropisetron: 2 mg IV near the conclusion of surgery
Palonosetron: 0.075 mg IV with induction of anesthesia
Dolasetron: 12.5 mg IV 15-30 minutes before conclusion of surgery (no longer marketed in the United States due to risk of QTc prolongation and torsades de pointes)

**Corticosteroids**
Dexamethasone: 4-8 mg IV with induction of anesthesia
Methylprednisolone: 40 mg IV with induction of anesthesia

**Other Antiemetics**
Propofol: subhypnotic doses such as 20 µg/kg/min IV infusion intraoperatively

---

*ECG*, Electrocardiogram; *IM*, intramuscularly; *IV*, intravenously; *PO*, by mouth.

the start of surgery, whereas serotonin receptor antagonists are effective when given near the end of anesthesia administration.

Upon admission to the PACU, the patient's risk profile and anesthetic technique should be noted, along with whether a prophylactic antiemetic was administered intraoperatively. If an adequate dose of antiemetic given at the appropriate time proves ineffective, simply giving more of the same class of drug in the PACU is unlikely to be of significant benefit. If no prophylactic drug was given, the recommended treatment is a low dose 5-$HT_3$ antagonist.

## DELAYED AWAKENING

Even after prolonged surgery and anesthesia, a response to stimulation in 60 to 90 minutes should be expected. When delayed awakening occurs, the vital signs (systemic blood pressure, arterial oxygenation, ECG, body temperature) should be evaluated and a neurologic examination performed. Monitoring with pulse oximetry and analysis of arterial blood gases should be used to rule out hypoxemia and hypoventilation. Additional studies may be indicated to evaluate possible electrolyte derangements, metabolic disturbances, and hypoglycemia. Rarely, computed tomographic imaging is indicated to rule out an acute intracerebral event.

### Treatment

Residual sedation from drugs used during anesthesia is the most frequent cause of delayed awakening in the PACU. If residual effects of opioids are a possible cause of delayed awakening, carefully titrated doses of naloxone (20- to 40-µg IV increments in adults) should be given, while keeping in mind that this treatment will also antagonize opioid-induced analgesia. Physostigmine may be effective in reversing the central nervous system sedative effects of anticholinergic drugs (especially scopolamine). Flumazenil is a specific antagonist for the residual depressant effects of benzodiazepines. In the absence of pharmacologic effects to explain delayed awakening, other causes, such as hypothermia (especially <33° C) and hypoglycemia, should be considered.

## DISCHARGE CRITERIA

Specific PACU discharge criteria may vary, but certain general principles are universally applicable (Box 39.13) (also see Chapter 37). For example, a mandatory minimum stay in the PACU is not required. Patients must be observed until they are no longer at risk for ventilatory depression and their mental status is clear or has returned to baseline. Hemodynamic criteria are based on the patient's baseline hemodynamics without specific systemic blood pressure and heart rate requirements (Table 39.1).[2]

---

**Box 39.13**  General Principles for Discharge From the Postanesthesia Care Unit

Patients should be routinely required to have a responsible person accompany them home.

Requiring patients to urinate before discharge should not be part of a routine discharge protocol and may be necessary only in selected patients.

The demonstrated ability to drink and retain clear fluids should not be part of a routine discharge protocol but may be appropriate for selected patients.

A minimum mandatory stay in the unit should not be required.

Patients should be observed until they are no longer at increased risk for cardiorespiratory depression.

---

**Table 39.1**  Criteria for Determination of Discharge Score for Release From the Postanesthesia Care Unit

| Variable Evaluated | Score |
| --- | --- |
| **Activity** | |
| Able to move four extremities on command | 2 |
| Able to move two extremities on command | 1 |
| Able to move no extremities on command | 0 |
| **Breathing** | |
| Able to breathe deeply and cough freely | 2 |
| Dyspnea | 1 |
| Apnea | 0 |
| **Circulation (systemic blood pressure)** | |
| Within 20% of the preanesthetic level | 2 |
| 20% to 49% of the preanesthetic level | 1 |
| ≥50% of the preanesthetic level | 0 |
| **Consciousness** | |
| Fully awake | 2 |
| Arousable | 1 |
| Not responding | 0 |
| **Oxygen Saturation (pulse oximetry)** | |
| >92% while breathing room air | 2 |
| Needs supplemental oxygen to maintain saturation >90% | 1 |
| <90% even with supplemental oxygen | 0 |

Adapted from Aldrete JA. The post anaesthesia recovery score revisited. *J Clin Anesth*. 1995;7:89-91.

V

| Table 39.2 | Criteria for Determination of Discharge Score for Release Home to a Responsible Adult |
| --- | --- |

| Variable Evaluated | Score[a] |
| --- | --- |
| **Vital signs** (stable and consistent with age and preanesthetic baseline) | |
| Systemic blood pressure and heart rate within 20% of the preanesthetic level | 2 |
| Systemic blood pressure and heart rate 20% to 40% of the preanesthetic level | 1 |
| Systemic blood pressure and heart rate >40% of the preanesthetic level | 0 |
| **Activity level** | |
| Steady gait without dizziness or meets the preanesthetic level | 2 |
| Requires assistance | 1 |
| Unable to ambulate | 0 |
| **Nausea and vomiting** | |
| None to minimal | 2 |
| Moderate | 1 |
| Severe (continues after repeated treatment) | 0 |
| **Pain** (minimal to no pain, controllable with oral analgesics) | |
| Yes | 2 |
| No | 1 |
| **Surgical bleeding** (consistent with that expected for the surgical procedure) | |
| Minimal (does not require dressing change) | 2 |
| Moderate (up to two dressing changes required) | 1 |
| Severe (more than three dressing changes required) | 0 |

[a]Patients achieving a score of at least 9 are ready for discharge.
Modified from Marshall SI, Chung F. Discharge criteria and complications after ambulatory surgery. *Anesth Analg.* 1999;88:508-517.

To facilitate PACU discharge, discharge scoring systems have been developed and modified over time to reflect current technology and anesthesia practice (Tables 39-1 and 39-2).[45] The ASA Standards of Care require that a physician accept responsibility for discharge of patients from the unit (Standard V). This is the case even when the decision to discharge the patient is made by the bedside nurse in accordance with the hospital-sanctioned discharge criteria or scoring system. If discharge scoring systems are to be used in this way, they must first be approved by the department of anesthesia and the hospital medical staff. A responsible physician's name must be noted on the record.

## QUESTIONS OF THE DAY

1. What are the most likely causes of upper airway obstruction for a patient in the postanesthesia care unit (PACU)? What steps can be taken to differentiate the causes?
2. What are the potential manifestations of residual neuromuscular blockade for a patient who has just arrived in the PACU?
3. A patient who had prolonged surgery in the prone position arrives to the PACU with the trachea intubated. What steps can be taken to determine the presence of significant upper airway edema prior to extubation?
4. A patient with coronary artery disease is recovering in the PACU after noncardiac surgery. What monitoring should be done to evaluate for postoperative myocardial ischemia or infarction?
5. What factors can predict the risk of postoperative nausea and vomiting (PONV)? How does the degree of risk affect the approach to preventing and treating PONV?
6. What criteria can be used to determine whether a patient is ready for discharge from the PACU? What is the utility of scoring systems in making a discharge decision?

## REFERENCES

1. American Society of Anesthesiologists. Standards for Postanesthesia Care. Last amended on October 15, 2014. http://www.asahq.org/quality-and-practice-management/standards-and-guidelines/ accessed March 24, 2017.
2. Apfelbaum JL, Silverstein JH, Chung FF, et al. Practice guidelines for postanesthetic care: an updated report by the American Society of Anesthesiologists Task Force on Postanesthetic Care. *Anesthesiology.* 2013;118(2):291–307.
3. Hines R, Barash PG, Watrous G, O'Connor T. Complications occurring in the postanesthesia care unit: a survey. *Anesth Analg.* 1992;74(4):503–509.
4. Ellis SJ, Newland MC, Simonson JA, et al. Anesthesia-related cardiac arrest. *Anesthesiology.* 2014;120(4):829–838.
5. Kluger MT, Bullock MF. Recovery room incidents: a review of 419 reports from the anaesthetic incident monitoring study (AIMS). *Anaesthesia.* 2002;57(11):1060–1066.
6. Grosse-Sundrup M, Henneman JP, Sandberg WS, et al. Intermediate acting non-depolarizing neuromuscular blocking agents and risk of postoperative respiratory complications: prospective propensity score matched cohort study. *BMJ.* 2012;345:e6329.
7. McLean DJ, Diaz-Gil D, Farhan HN, et al. Dose-dependent association between intermediate-acting neuromuscular-blocking agents and postoperative respiratory complications. *Anesthesiology.* 2015;122(6):1201–1213.

8. Sasaki N, Meyer MJ, Malviya SA, et al. Effects of neostigmine reversal of non-depolarizing neuromuscular blocking agents on postoperative respiratory outcomes: a prospective study. *Anesthesiology*. 2014;121(5):959–968.

9. Murphy GS, Szokol JW, Marymont JH, et al. Intraoperative acceleromyographic monitoring reduces the risk of residual neuromuscular blockade and adverse respiratory events in the postanesthesia care unit. *Anesthesiology*. 2008;109(3):389–398.

10. Zhou T, Zhang HP, Chen WW, et al. Cuff-leak test for predicting postextubation airway complications: a systematic review. *J Evid Based Med*. 2011;4(4):242–254.

11. American Society of Anesthesiologists Task Force on Perioperative Management of patients with obstructive sleep apnea. Practice guidelines for the perioperative management of patients with obstructive sleep apnea: an updated report by the American Society of Anesthesiologists Task Force on Perioperative Management of patients with obstructive sleep apnea. *Anesthesiology*. 2014;120(2):268–286.

12. Kaw R, Chung F, Pasupuleti V, et al. Meta-analysis of the association between obstructive sleep apnoea and postoperative outcome. *Br J Anaesth*. 2012;109(6):897–906.

13. Chung F, Subramanyam R, Liao P, et al. High STOP-BANG score indicates a high probability of obstructive sleep apnoea. *Br J Anaesth*. 2012;108(5):768–775.

14. Vasu TS, Grewal R, Doghramji K. Obstructive sleep apnea syndrome and perioperative complications: a systematic review of the literature. *J Clin Sleep Med*. 2012;8(2):199–207.

15. Fu ES, Downs JB, Schweiger JW, et al. Supplemental oxygen impairs detection of hypoventilation by pulse oximetry. *Chest*. 2004;126(5):1552–1558.

16. Lumb A. *Nunn's Applied Respiratory Physiology*. 6th ed. Philadelphia: Butterworth-Heinemann; 2005.

17. Udeshi A, Cantie SM, Pierre E. Postobstructive pulmonary edema. *J Crit Care*. 2010;25(3):508.e1–508.e5.

18. Toy P, Gajic O, Bacchetti P, et al. Transfusion-related acute lung injury: incidence and risk factors. *Blood*. 2012;119(7):1757–1767.

19. Meyhoff CS, Staehr AK, Rasmussen LS. Rational use of oxygen in medical disease and anesthesia. *Curr Opin Anaesthesiol*. 2012;25(3):363–370.

20. Squadrone V, Coha M, Cerutti E, et al. Continuous positive airway pressure for treatment of postoperative hypoxemia: a randomized controlled trial. *JAMA*. 2005;293(5):589–595.

21. Ireland CJ, Chapman TM, Mathew SF, et al. Continuous positive airway pressure (CPAP) during the postoperative period for prevention of postoperative morbidity and mortality following major abdominal surgery. *Cochrane Database Syst Rev*. 2014;8:CD008930.

22. Neligan PJ. Postoperative noninvasive ventilation. *Anesthesiol Clin*. 2012;30(3):495–511.

23. Rose DK, Cohen MM, DeBoer DP. Cardiovascular events in the postanesthesia care unit: contribution of risk factors. *Anesthesiology*. 1996;84(4):772–781.

24. Marik PE, Varon J. Perioperative hypertension: a review of current and emerging therapeutic agents. *J Clin Anesth*. 2009;21(3):220–229.

25. Basali A, Mascha EJ, Kalfas I, Schubert A. Relation between perioperative hypertension and intracranial hemorrhage after craniotomy. *Anesthesiology*. 2000;93(1):48–54.

26. Mertes PM, Alla F, Trechot P, et al. Groupe d'Etudes des Reactions Anaphylactoides Peranesthesiques. Anaphylaxis during anesthesia in France: an 8-year national survey. *J Allergy Clin Immunol*. 2011;128(2):366–373.

27. Dewachter P, Mouton-Faivre C, Emala CW. Anaphylaxis and anesthesia: controversies and new insights. *Anesthesiology*. 2009;111(5):1141–1150.

28. Devereaux PJ, Xavier D, Pogue J, et al. Characteristics and short-term prognosis of perioperative myocardial infarction in patients undergoing noncardiac surgery: a cohort study. *Ann Intern Med*. 2011;154(8):523–528.

29. Vascular Events In Noncardiac Surgery Patients Cohort Evaluation (VISION) Study Investigators, Devereaux PJ, Chan MT, Alonso-Coelho P, et al. Association between postoperative troponin levels and 30-day mortality among patients undergoing noncardiac surgery. *JAMA*. 2012;307(21):2295–2304.

30. Botto F, Alonso-Coello P, Chan MT, et al. Myocardial injury after noncardiac surgery: a large, international, prospective cohort study establishing diagnostic criteria, characteristics, predictors, and 30-day outcomes. *Anesthesiology*. 2014;120(3):564–578.

31. Fleisher LA, Fleischmann KE, Auerbach AD, et al. 2014 ACC/AHA guideline on perioperative cardiovascular evaluation and management of patients undergoing noncardiac surgery: executive summary: a report of the American College of Cardiology/American Heart Association Task Force on practice guidelines. *Circulation*. 2014;130(24):2215–2245.

32. Bhave PD, Goldman LE, Vittinghoff E, et al. Incidence, predictors, and outcomes associated with postoperative atrial fibrillation after major noncardiac surgery. *Am Heart J*. 2012;164(6):918–924.

33. Rudolph JL, Marcantonio ER. Review articles: postoperative delirium: acute change with long-term implications. *Anesth Analg*. 2011;112(5):1202–1211.

34. Whitlock EL, Vannucci A, Avidan MS. Postoperative delirium. *Minerva Anestesiol*. 2011;77(4):448–456.

35. Saczynski JS, Marcantonio ER, Quach L, et al. Cognitive trajectories after postoperative delirium. *N Engl J Med*. 2012;367(1):30–39.

36. Long LS, Shapiro WA, Leung JM. A brief review of practical preoperative cognitive screening tools. *Can J Anaesth*. 2012;59(8):798–804.

37. Chenitz KB, Lane-Fall MB. Decreased urine output and acute kidney injury in the postanesthesia care unit. *Anesthesiol Clin*. 2012;30(3):513–526.

38. Baldini G, Bagry H, Aprikian A, Carli F. Postoperative urinary retention: anesthetic and perioperative considerations. *Anesthesiology*. 2009;110(5):1139–1157.

39. Kirkpatrick AW, Roberts DJ, De Waele J, et al. Intra-abdominal hypertension and the abdominal compartment syndrome: updated consensus definitions and clinical practice guidelines from the World Society of the abdominal compartment syndrome. *Intensive Care Med*. 2013;39(7):1190–1206.

40. Chakravartty S, Sarma DR, Patel AG. Rhabdomyolysis in bariatric surgery: a systematic review. *Obes Surg*. 2013;23(8):1333–1340.

41. Calonder EM, Sendelbach S, Hodges JS, et al. Temperature measurement in patients undergoing colorectal surgery and gynecology surgery: a comparison of esophageal core, temporal artery, and oral methods. *J Perianesth Nurs*. 2010;25(2):71–78.

42. Horn E, Bein B, Böhm R, et al. The effect of short time periods of pre-operative warming in the prevention of perioperative hypothermia. *Anaesthesia*. 2012;67(6):612–617.

43. Apfel CC, Korttila K, Abdalla M, et al. A factorial trial of six interventions for the prevention of postoperative nausea and vomiting. *N Engl J Med*. 2004;350(24):2441–2451.

44. Gan TJ, Diemunsch P, Habib AS, et al. Consensus guidelines for the management of postoperative nausea and vomiting. *Anesth Analg*. 2014;118(1):85–113.

45. Abdullah HR, Chung F. Postoperative issues: discharge criteria. *Anesthesiol Clin*. 2014;32(2):487–493.

**V**

**691**

# 40 PERIOPERATIVE PAIN MANAGEMENT

## Meredith C.B. Adams and Robert W. Hurley

Postoperative pain is a complex physiologic reaction to tissue injury. Commonly, patients' primary concern about surgery is how much pain they will experience following the procedure. Postoperative pain produces acute adverse physiologic effects with manifestations on multiple organ systems that can lead to significant morbidity (Box 40.1). For example, pain after upper abdominal or thoracic surgery often leads to hypoventilation from splinting. This promotes atelectasis, which impairs ventilation-to-perfusion relationships, and increases the likelihood of arterial hypoxemia and pneumonia. Pain that limits postoperative ambulation, combined with a stress-induced hypercoagulable state, may contribute to an increased incidence of deep vein thrombosis. Catecholamines released in response to pain may result in tachycardia and systemic hypertension, which may induce myocardial ischemia in susceptible patients. In a 2015 observational study, 54% of patients experienced moderate to extreme acute postoperative pain at the time of their discharge from the hospital.[1] This represents an insignificant or slight improvement in postoperative pain management as compared to an earlier (2003) study in which 64% of patients had the same level of pain at hospital discharge.[2] However, it is concerning that in the more recent study[1] 46% of the patients had moderate to extreme level of postoperative pain 2 weeks following discharge.

Factors that positively correlate with severity of postoperative pain include preoperative opioid intake, increased body mass index, anxiety, depression, pain intensity level, characteristics of fibromyalgia, and the duration of surgical operation. Factors that are negatively correlated include the patient's age and the level of the surgeon's operative experience. Although these findings have been replicated in numerous studies, the immediate postoperative pain assessment may suffer from significant observer bias. Besides the postoperative pain-related factors, the accepting postanesthesia care unit (PACU) nurse had a greater impact on the initial postoperative pain score than the anesthesiologist's intraoperative care.[3]

| Box 40.1 Adverse Physiologic Effects of Postoperative Pain |
|---|

**Pulmonary System (decreased lung volumes)**
Atelectasis
Ventilation-to-perfusion mismatching
Arterial hypoxemia
Hypercapnia
Pneumonia

**Cardiovascular System (sympathetic nervous system stimulation)**
Systemic hypertension
Tachycardia
Myocardial ischemia
Cardiac dysrhythmias

**Endocrine System**
Hyperglycemia
Sodium and water retention
Protein catabolism

**Immune System**
Decreased immune function

**Coagulation System**
Increased platelet adhesiveness
Decreased fibrinolysis
Hypercoagulation
Deep vein thrombosis

**Gastrointestinal System**
Ileus

**Genitourinary System**
Urinary retention

A perioperative plan should be developed that encompasses these factors in order to lessen the severity of the patient's postoperative pain. Despite having a lower predictive risk for postoperative pain, elderly patients can represent significant management challenges (also see Chapter 35). Elderly patients are at a greater risk than younger patients for cognitive dysfunction in the perioperative period because of various factors, including increased sensitivity to drugs and other medical comorbid conditions. Patients taking opioids for chronic pain relief preoperatively have higher pain scores, more opioid consumption, and lower pain thresholds in the immediate postoperative period. Perioperative management plans that incorporate these variables may favor the use of regional anesthesia because of the decreased mortality rate and infrequent incidence of postoperative cognitive dysfunction and pain (also see Chapters 17 and 18). Preemptive regional analgesia may enhance pain control, decrease adverse cognitive effects, and improve postoperative recovery overall. Well-controlled pain postoperatively will enhance postoperative rehabilitation, which may improve short- and long-term recovery as well as the quality of life after surgery.

Postoperative pain also may have long-term consequences as well. Poorly controlled postoperative pain may be an important predictive factor for the development of chronic postsurgical pain (CPSP),[4] defined as pain after a surgery lasting longer than the normal recuperative healing time. CPSP is a largely unrecognized problem that may occur in 10% to 65% of postoperative patients, with 2% to 10% of these patients experiencing severe CPSP.[5] Transition from acute to chronic pain occurs very quickly, and long-term behavioral and neurobiologic changes occur much earlier than previously anticipated.[6] CPSP is relatively common after surgical procedures, such as limb amputation (30% to 83%), thoracotomy (22% to 67%), sternotomy (27%), breast surgery (11% to 57%), and gallbladder surgery (up to 56%).[7]

Improved understanding of the epidemiology and pathophysiology of postoperative pain has increased the use of multimodal management of pain in an effort to improve patient comfort, decrease perioperative morbidity, and reduce cost by shortening the time spent in PACUs, intensive care units, and hospitals. Multimodal approaches involve the use of multiple, mechanistically distinct medications with the application of peripheral nerve or neuraxial analgesia. The added complexity of a true multimodal approach to perioperative pain requires the formation of perioperative pain management services, most often directed by an anesthesiologist or pain medicine physician.

## COMMON TERMINOLOGY

- *Pain (nociception):* Pain is described as an unpleasant sensory and emotional experience caused by actual or potential tissue damage, or described in terms of such damage.[8]
- *Acute pain:* Acute pain follows injury to the body, and generally disappears when the bodily injury heals. For instance, acute pain occurs during the time needed for inflammation to subside or for acute injuries, such as lacerations or incisions, to repair with the union of separated tissues. Acute pain is commonly thought to last up to 7 days, but prolongation up to 30 days is common. Acute pain is often, but not always, associated with objective physical signs of autonomic nervous system activity (e.g., increased heart rate).
- *Chronic (persistent) pain:* Chronic pain is pain that persists beyond the time of healing.[8] The length of time is determined by the nature of the injury or surgical operation, but the pain is considered to be chronic (persistent) when it exceeds 3 months in duration.
- *Pain management:* Pain management is the clinical practice of relieving acute, subacute, and chronic (persistent) pain through the implementation of psychological, physical therapeutic, pharmacologic, and interventional methods. Physicians and pain psychologists practice pain management in a team model with the assistance of advanced practice providers and physical therapists in the inpatient and outpatient settings (also see Chapter 44).

V

## Pain Services

- *Perioperative (acute) pain medicine service:* The perioperative pain medicine service is a team of highly specialized members who practice acute pain medicine and regional analgesic interventions for the patient who is about to have surgery, undergoing surgery, and in the process of recovery from surgery, and for trauma-induced pain. The role of the perioperative pain physician is to reduce the pain resulting from surgery and minimize the period of recuperation, and to inhibit the development of chronic (persistent) pain through early intervention. This service is most commonly found in the inpatient setting but crossover to the outpatient setting is expected for continuity of care.

- *Chronic (persistent) pain medicine service:* The chronic pain medicine service is a multidisciplinary team of providers who treat chronic (persistent) pain and cancer pain using diverse treatment modalities including psychological interventions, analgesic medications, and regional analgesic and chronic pain procedural interventions. The patient population served includes the perioperative patient with preoperative chronic/persistent pain issues, the inoperable patient with chronic/persistent pain issues, and patients who have not undergone surgery but have comorbid persistent pain. The role of the inpatient chronic pain physician is to attenuate the patient's pain, provide rationalized pain medication care, and transition the patient to outpatient pain care. The diagnosis and treatment of chronic pain is most commonly and most successfully performed in the outpatient setting, not in the acute care inpatient setting (also see Chapter 44).

## NEUROBIOLOGY OF PAIN

### Nociception

Nociception involves the recognition and transmission of painful stimuli. Stimuli generated from thermal, mechanical, or chemical tissue damage may activate nociceptors, which are free afferent nerve endings of myelinated Aδ and unmyelinated C fibers. These peripheral afferent nerve endings send axonal projections into the dorsal horn of the spinal cord, where they synapse with second-order afferent neurons. Axonal projections of second-order neurons cross to the contralateral side of the spinal cord, and ascend as afferent sensory pathways (e.g., spinothalamic tract) to the level of the thalamus.[9] Along the way, these neurons divide and send axonal projections to the reticular formation and periaqueductal gray matter. In the thalamus, second-order neurons synapse with third-order neurons, which send axonal projections into the sensory cortex.

### Modulation of Nociception

Surgical incision produces tissue injury, with consequent release of histamine and inflammatory mediators, such as peptides (e.g., bradykinin), lipids (e.g., prostaglandins), neurotransmitters (e.g., serotonin), and neurotrophins (e.g., nerve growth factor).[10] The release of inflammatory mediators activates peripheral nociceptors, which initiate transduction and transmission of nociceptive information to the central nervous system (CNS). Noxious stimuli are transduced by peripheral nociceptors and transmitted by Aδ and C nerve fibers from peripheral visceral and somatic sites to the dorsal horn of the spinal cord, where integration of peripheral nociceptive and descending inhibitory modulatory input (i.e., serotonin, norepinephrine, γ-aminobutyric acid [GABA], and enkephalin) or descending facilitatory input (i.e., cholecystokinin, excitatory amino acids, dynorphin) occurs. Further transmission of nociceptive information is determined by complex modulating influences in the spinal cord. Some impulses pass to the ventral and ventrolateral horns to initiate spinal reflex responses. These segmental responses may include increased skeletal muscle tone, inhibition of phrenic nerve function, or even decreased gastrointestinal motility. Other signals are transmitted to higher centers through the spinothalamic and spinoreticular tracts, where they produce cortical responses to ultimately generate the perception of pain.

The question of how the disease of chronic pain develops from the symptom of acute pain remains unanswered. The traditional dichotomy between acute and chronic pain is somewhat arbitrary, as animal and clinical studies demonstrate that acute pain may become chronic pain. The duration of painful or noxious stimuli, type of stimuli, genetic or phenotypic makeup, or other possible factors that lead to the transition from the symptom of acute pain to the disease of chronic pain remain unclear.

Noxious stimuli can produce expression of new genes (the basis for neuronal sensitization) in the dorsal horn of the spinal cord within 1 hour, and these changes are sufficient to alter behavior within the same time frame.[11,12] Also, the intensity of acute postoperative pain is a significant predictor of chronic postoperative pain.[7] Continuous release of inflammatory mediators in the periphery sensitizes functional nociceptors and activates dormant nociceptors (Box 40.2).[6] Sensitization of peripheral nociceptors results in a decreased threshold for activation, increased discharge rate with activation, and increased rate of spontaneous discharge. Intense noxious input from the periphery may also produce central sensitization and hyperexcitability. Central sensitization is the development of "persistent post-injury changes in the CNS that result in pain hypersensitivity."[13] Hyperexcitability is the "exaggerated and prolonged responsiveness of neurons to normal afferent input after tissue damage."[13]

**Box 40.2** Endogenous Mediators of Inflammation

Prostaglandins (PGE$_1$ > PGE$_2$)
Histamine
Bradykinin
Serotonin
Acetylcholine
Lactic acid
Hydrogen ions
Potassium ions

*PGE$_1$, PGE$_2$*, Prostaglandins E$_1$ and E$_2$.

**Box 40.3** Examples of Pain-Modulating Neurotransmitters

**Excitatory**
Glutamate
Aspartate
Vasoactive intestinal polypeptide
Cholecystokinin
Gastrin-releasing peptide
Angiotensin
Substance P

**Inhibitory**
Enkephalins
Endorphins
Somatostatin

Noxious input can trigger the cascade that leads to functional changes in the dorsal horn of the spinal cord and other sequelae. Ultimately, these changes may later cause postoperative pain to be perceived as more painful than would otherwise have been experienced. The neural circuitry in the dorsal horn is extremely complex, and we are just at the beginning of understanding the specific role of the various neurotransmitters and receptors in the process of nociception.[10,12]

Key receptors (e.g., *N*-methyl-D-aspartate [NMDA]) may play a significant role in the development of chronic pain after an acute injury. Neurotransmitters or second messenger effectors (e.g., substance P, protein kinase C-γ) may also play important roles in spinal cord sensitization and chronic pain (Box 40.3).[11] Our understanding of the neurobiology of nociception includes the dynamic integration and modulation of nociceptive transmission at several levels. Still, the specific roles of various receptors, neurotransmitters, and molecular structures in the process of nociception are not fully understood.

## Preemptive and Preventive Analgesia

The development of central or peripheral sensitization after traumatic injury or surgical incision can result in amplification of postoperative pain. Therefore, preventing the establishment of altered central processing by analgesic treatment may, in the short term, reduce post-procedural or traumatic pain and accelerate recovery. In the long term, the benefits may include a reduction in chronic pain and improvement in the patient's quality of recovery and life satisfaction. Although the concept of preemptive analgesia in decreasing postinjury pain is valid, clinical trials are difficult to objectively conduct, which partly accounts for inconsistent conclusions.[14-16]

The precise definition of preemptive analgesia is one of the major controversies in perioperative pain medicine, and this lack of precision contributes to the confusion regarding its clinical relevance. Preemptive analgesia can be defined as an analgesic intervention initiated before the noxious stimulus develops in order to block peripheral and central pain transmission. Preventive analgesia can be functionally defined as an attempt to block pain transmission prior to the injury (incision), during the noxious insult (surgery itself), *and* after the injury and throughout the recovery period. Unfortunately, the concept of preventive analgesia has not been examined in a rigorous fashion. Confining the definition of preemptive analgesia to only the immediate preoperative or early intraoperative (incisional) period may not be clinically relevant or appropriate because the inflammatory response may last well into the postoperative period and continue to maintain peripheral sensitization. However, preventive analgesia is a clinically relevant phenomenon. Katz and McCartney[4] described an analgesic benefit of preventive analgesia but no such benefit with the preemptive strategy. Maximal clinical benefit is observed when there is complete blockade of noxious stimuli, with extension of this blockade into the postoperative period. Central sensitization and persistent pain after surgical incision are predominantly maintained by the incoming barrage of sensitized peripheral pain fibers throughout the perioperative period,[17] extending into the postsurgical recovery period. By avoiding central sensitization and its prolongation by peripheral input, preventive analgesia along with intensive multimodal analgesic interventions could, theoretically, reduce acute postprocedure pain/hyperalgesia and, therefore, chronic pain after surgery.[7]

## Opioid-Induced Hyperalgesia

Short-term administration of opioids in the perioperative setting may unfortunately lead to opioid-induced hyperalgesia (OIH), a paradoxical increase in the patient's pain severity and decrease in pain tolerance. This has been demonstrated in humans who received intraoperative opioid infusion for operative analgesia as well as in human and animal experimental models.[18] Although the clinical impact of OIH has not been fully elucidated, the possibility of it contributing to acute postoperative pain should be considered. OIH has also

V

been implicated as a risk for the development of CPSP and the pronociceptive process involves the activation of the NMDA receptor.[18]

## Multimodal Approach to Perioperative Recovery

A multimodal approach to analgesia is a broad definition that may include a combination of interventional analgesic techniques (epidural catheter or peripheral nerve catheter analgesia) and a combination of systemic pharmacologic therapies (nonsteroidal antiinflammatory drugs [NSAIDs], α-adrenergic agonists, NMDA receptor antagonists, membrane stabilizers, and opioid administration) (also see Chapters 9 and 17). Postprocedural or posttraumatic pain is best managed through this multimodal approach.[19] For instance, basic perioperative therapy, such as including a single dose of the membrane stabilizer, gabapentin, can attenuate postoperative pain and decrease opioid dosage with minimal side effects in various types of surgeries.[20]

The principles of a multimodal strategy include a sufficient improvement of the patient's pain to instill a sense of control over the pain, enable early mobilization, allow early enteral nutrition, and attenuate the perioperative stress response. The secondary goal of this approach is to maximize the benefit (analgesia) while minimizing the risk (i.e., side effects of the medication being used). These goals are often achieved through regional anesthetic techniques (also see Chapters 17 and 18) and a combination of analgesic drugs (also see Chapters 9 and 10). Epidural anesthesia and analgesia form an integral part of the multimodal strategy because of the superior analgesia and physiologic benefits conferred by epidural analgesia.[21] A multimodal approach involving a combination of neuraxial analgesia and systemic analgesics during recovery from radical prostatectomy resulted in a reduction of opioid use, lower pain scores, and decreased length of hospital stay.[22] Patients undergoing major abdominal or thoracic procedures and managed with a multimodal strategy have a reduction in hormonal and metabolic stress, preservation of total-body protein, shorter times to tracheal extubation, lower pain scores, earlier return of bowel function, and earlier attainment of criteria for discharge from the intensive care unit.[23] Integrating the most recent data and techniques for surgery, anesthesiology, and pain treatment, the multimodal approach is an extension of clinical pathways or fast track protocols by revamping traditional care programs into effective postoperative rehabilitation pathways.[23] This approach may potentially decrease perioperative morbidity, decrease the length of hospital stay, and improve patient satisfaction without compromising safety. However, the widespread implementation of these programs requires multidisciplinary collaboration, changes in the traditional principles of postoperative care, additional resources, and expansion of the traditional acute pain service, all of which may be challenging in the current medical economic climate.

## ANALGESIC DELIVERY SYSTEMS

The traditional delivery systems for the management of perioperative pain have oral and parenteral on-demand administration of analgesics. More efficacious mechanisms, such as patient-controlled analgesia (PCA), are increasingly being used. A PCA mechanism can refer to oral, parenteral, neuraxial, or peripheral administration of an analgesic (Tables 40.1 to 40.3). This medication delivery technique is based on improved understanding of the neurobiology of pain and the potential deleterious effects of postoperative pain. The formation of perioperative pain management services, directed by anesthesiologists with expertise in the pharmacology of analgesics and regional analgesia, has facilitated the widespread application of these techniques and improved the care of the postoperative patient.

### Patient-Controlled Analgesia

PCA can be delivered via oral, intravenous, subcutaneous, epidural, and intrathecal routes, as well as by peripheral nerve catheter. Upon activation of the delivery system, limits are placed on the number of doses per unit of time that will be administered to the patient. There is also a minimum time interval that must elapse between dose administrations (lockout interval). Also, a continuous background infusion superimposed on patient-controlled boluses can be implemented. Most patients determine a level of pain that is acceptable and taper their dosage requirements as they recover. Patients usually accept PCA because it restores their feeling of having control of their therapy. When compared with traditional methods of intermittent intramuscular or intravenous injections of opioids to manage perioperative pain, PCA provides better analgesia with more safety, less total drug use, less sedation, fewer nocturnal sleep disturbances, and more rapid return to physical activity.[24] Some institutions employ pulse oximetry monitoring to assess the respiratory depression associated with opioid administration. Although pulse oximetry is better than having no specific monitor at all, it may not capture the relationship between respiratory depression and opioid administration. The addition of supplemental oxygen lowers the detection sensitivity of pulse oximetry as a monitor for respiratory depression and renders this monitor ineffective. Capnography and respiratory rate are more specific monitors of respiratory depression. However, capnography is not readily available in all institutions and is not needed universally for patients receiving opioid therapy. Capnography is best reserved for patients with substantial

| Table 40.1 | Oral and Parenteral Analgesics for Treatment of Perioperative Pain | | | | | |
|---|---|---|---|---|---|---|
| Agent | Route of Administration | Dose (mg) | Half-Life (h) | Onset (h) | Analgesic Action (h) | Peak Duration (h) |
| **Opioids and Opioid Derivatives** | | | | | | |
| Morphine | Intravenous | 2.5-15 | 2-3.5 | 0.25 | 0.125 | 2-3 |
| | Intramuscular | 10-15 | 3 | 0.3 | 0.5-1.5 | 3-4 |
| | Oral | 30-60 | 3 | 0.5-1 | 1-2 | 4 |
| Codeine[a] | Oral | 15-60 | 4 | 0.25-1 | 0.5-2 | 3-4 |
| Hydromorphone | Intravenous | 0.2-1.0 | 2-3 | 0.2-0.25 | 0.25 | 2-3 |
| | Intramuscular | 1-4 | 2-3 | 0.3-0.5 | 1 | 2-3 |
| | Oral | 1-4 | 2-3 | 0.5-1 | 1 | 3-4 |
| Fentanyl | Intravenous | 20-50 µg | 0.5-1 | 5-10 min | 5 min | 1-1.5 |
| | Transmucosal[b] | 200-1600 µg | 2-12 | 0.1-0.25 | 0.5-1 | 0.25-0.5 |
| | Transdermal | 12.5-100 µg | 20-27 | 12-24 | 20-72 | 72 |
| Oxymorphone | Oral | 5-10 | 3.3-4.5 | 0.5 | 1 | 2-6 |
| | Intravenous | 0.5-1 | 3-5 | 0.15 | 0.25 | 3-6 |
| | Subcutaneous | 1-1.5 | 3-5 | 0.15 | 0.25 | 3-6 |
| | Intramuscular | 1-1.5 | 3-5 | 0.15 | 0.25 | 3-6 |
| Hydrocodone | Oral | 5-7.5 | 2-3 | 30 | 90 | 3-4 |
| Oxycodone | Oral | 5 | 3-5 | 0.5 | 1-2 | 4-6 |
| Methadone | Oral | 2.5-10 | 3-4 | 0.5-1 | 1.5-2 | 4-8 |
| Propoxyphene | Oral | 32-65 | 12-16 | 0.25-1 | 1-2 | 3-6 |
| **Other** | | | | | | |
| Tramadol[c] | Oral | 50-100 | 5-6 | 0.5-1 | 1-2 | 4-6 |

[a]Not recommended for postoperative analgesia due to genetic variable metabolism.
[b]Transmucosal fentanyl is most appropriately reserved for breakthrough malignant (cancer) pain.
[c]Not classified by the U.S. Food and Drug Administration (FDA) as an opioid; however, tramadol possesses naloxone partial-reversal analgesia.

comorbid conditions that increase the risks associated with opioid therapy. Perhaps monitors that directly display respiratory rate with sufficient sensitivity and specificity will soon be available.

## SYSTEMIC THERAPY

### Oral Administration

Oral administration of analgesics is not optimal for the management of moderate to severe perioperative pain, primarily because of the nil per os (NPO, nothing by mouth) status of patients in the immediate postoperative period. Traditionally, postoperative patients are switched to oral analgesics (aspirin, acetaminophen, cyclooxygenase [COX-1/COX-2] inhibitors, opioids) when pain has diminished enough to eliminate the need for rapid adjustments of analgesia level.

Perioperative administration of opioid and nonopioid analgesic medications is an integral component of multimodal analgesic treatment plans. The increased complexity of outpatient surgical procedures has introduced the need for perioperative analgesia plans that enable moderate to severe postoperative pain to be effectively treated in the outpatient setting. Membrane stabilizers (gabapentin and pregabalin) used in the pre- and postoperative settings decrease postoperative pain and opioid consumption.[20,25] The optimal dose of gabapentin is 900 mg or more preoperatively followed by 400 to 600 mg three times a day postoperatively for 14 days; 300 mg of pregabalin followed by 150 mg two times a day should be given for maximal benefit. These drugs may provide postoperative pain relief but also may reduce CPSP.[26] NSAIDs including COX-2 predominant medications are effective when given intraoperatively and postoperatively but have not been found to have significant impact when given

V

**Table 40.2**  Guidelines for Delivery Systems Used in Intravenous Patient-Controlled Analgesia

| Drug Concentration | Size of Bolus[a] | Lockout Interval (min) | Continuous Infusion |
|---|---|---|---|
| **Agonists** | | | |
| Morphine (1 mg/mL) | 0.5-2.5 mg | 6-10 | 1-2 mg/h |
| Fentanyl (0.01 mg/mL) | 20-50 μg | 5-10 | 10-100 μg/h |
| Hydromorphone (0.2 mg/mL) | 0.05-0.25 mg | 10-20 | 0.2-0.4 mg/h |
| Alfentanil (0.1 mg/mL) | 0.1-0.2 mg | 5-10 | — |
| Methadone (1 mg/mL) | 0.5-1.5 mg | 10-30 | — |
| Oxymorphone (0.25 mg/mL) | 0.2-0.4 mg | 8-10 | — |
| Sufentanil (0.002 mg/mL) | 2-5 μg | 4-10 | 2-8 μg/h |
| **Agonists-Antagonists** | | | |
| Buprenorphine (0.03 mg/mL) | 0.03-0.1 mg | 8-20 | — |
| Nalbuphine (1 mg/mL) | 1-5 mg | 5-15 | — |
| Pentazocine (10 mg/mL) | 5-30 mg | 5-15 | — |

[a]All doses are for a 70-kg adult patient. The anesthesia provider should proceed with titrated intravenous loading doses if necessary to establish initial analgesia. Individual patient's requirements vary widely, with smaller doses typically given for elderly or compromised patients. Continuous infusions are not recommended for opioid-naïve adult patients. Continuous opioid infusion doses often are considerably higher in the cancer pain population.
Modified from Hurley RW, Murphy JD, Wu CL. Acute postoperative pain. In Miller RD, Cohen NH, Eriksson LI, et al, eds. *Miller's Anesthesia*. 8th ed. Philadelphia: Elsevier Saunders; 2015:2974-2998.

**Table 40.3**  Neuraxial Analgesics

| Drug | Intrathecal or Subarachnoid Single Dose | Epidural Single Dose | Epidural Continuous Infusion |
|---|---|---|---|
| **Opioid[a]** | | | |
| Fentanyl | 5-25 μg | 50-100 μg | 25-100 μg/h |
| Sufentanil | 2-10 μg | 10-50 μg | 10-20 μg/h |
| Alfentanil | — | 0.5-1 mg | 0.2 mg/h |
| Morphine | 0.1-0.3 mg | 1-5 mg | 0.1-1 mg/h |
| Hydromorphone | — | 0.5-1 mg | 0.1-0.2 mg/h |
| Extended-release morphine[†] | Not recommended | 5-15 mg | Not recommended |
| **Local Anesthetic[b]** | | | |
| Bupivacaine | 5-15 mg | 25-150 mg | 1-25 mg/h |
| Ropivacaine | Not recommended | 25-200 mg | 6-20 mg/h |
| **Adjuvant Medications** | | | |
| Clonidine | Not recommended | 100-900 μg | 10-50 μg/h |

[a]Doses are based on use of a neuraxial opioid alone. No continuous intrathecal or subarachnoid infusions are provided. Smaller doses may be effective when administered to the elderly or when injected in the cervical or thoracic region. Units vary across drugs for single dose (mg versus μg) and continuous infusion (mg/h versus μg/h).
[b]Most commonly used in combination with an opioid, in which case the total dose of local anesthetic is reduced.
Modified from Hurley RW, Murphy JD, Wu CL. Acute postoperative pain. In Miller RD, Cohen NH, Eriksson LI, et al, eds. *Miller's Anesthesia*. 8th ed. Philadelphia: Elsevier Saunders; 2015:2974-2998.

alone and preoperatively. However, they are effective for acute postsurgical pain and CPSP when given as part of a preoperative polypharmacologic regimen including gabapentinoids. Preoperative administration of acetaminophen may improve acute postoperative pain but has not been shown to reduce CPSP. Amine reuptake inhibitors such as tricyclic antidepressants and serotonin-norepinephrine reuptake inhibitors have not received sufficient investigation to draw conclusions about their efficacy in acute postoperative pain or the prevention of CPSP. Preoperative doses of vitamin C may reduce the incidence of complex regional pain syndrome following orthopedic extremity surgery although the quality of evidence is not strong.[27]

## Intravenous Administration

Intermittent intravenous (IV) administration of small doses of opioids (see Tables 40.1 and 40.2) is commonly used to treat acute and severe pain in the PACU or intensive care unit, where continuous nursing surveillance and monitoring are available. With a small intravenous dose of an opioid, the time delay for analgesia and the variability in plasma concentrations characteristic of intramuscular injections are minimized. Rapid redistribution of the opioid produces a shorter duration of analgesia after a single intravenous administration than after an intramuscular injection.

Ketamine is traditionally recognized as an intraoperative anesthetic; however, it is also effective in small dose (subanesthetic or analgesic dose, up to 15 µg/kg/min) infusions for postoperative analgesia partly because of its direct analgesic properties through antagonism of the NMDA receptor. It has also been shown to reduce the OIH associated with intraoperative opioid infusion.[18] Patients receiving large doses of opioids may experience hyperalgesia, resulting in increased excitatory amino acid release in the spinal cord. Ketamine directly inhibits the actions of the excitatory amino acids and reverses OIH, leading to improved postoperative pain outcome. Microdosing of ketamine (2 µg/kg/min) was ineffective for either postoperative pain or CPSP. Preoperative intravenous ketamine bolus dose of 0.5 mg/kg followed by an intraoperative infusion of a subanesthetic dose (4 to 5 µg/kg/min) of ketamine reduces postoperative pain and CPSP. This indirect antihyperalgesic effect may occur through suppression of central sensitization.[28] The benefit of subanesthetic dosing of ketamine also includes a decrease in postoperative nausea and vomiting, with minimal adverse effects. Subanesthetic ketamine infusions do not cause hallucinations or cognitive impairment. The incidence of side effects, such as dizziness, itching, nausea, or vomiting, is comparable to that seen with opioids. Therefore, the use of perioperative ketamine in patients at high risk for the development of CPSP is warranted.

Acetaminophen can be given intravenously in addition to orally and rectally. This has increased the ability to provide additional nonopioid analgesia to patients who are NPO but refuse rectal administration. Despite patient, and often provider, assumptions that intravenous preparations are more potent or effective, no clinical trial has demonstrated a difference in efficacy between oral and intravenous formulations.[29] Although the formulations differ in bioavailability and time to onset of analgesia, intravenous dosing has not been associated with improved efficacy.

Preoperative administration of dexamethasone decreases acute postoperative pain scores and decreases opioid consumption on a dose-dependent basis when more than 10 mg are given.[30] Intraoperative administration of clonidine decreases postoperative pain, but bradycardia and hypotension limit the benefits of its modest analgesic properties. Intraoperative magnesium administration reduces postoperative pain and opioid requirements.[31] The mechanism of action is likely the increased blockade of the NMDA receptor.

## Subcutaneous Administration

Subcutaneous administration of select medications (hydromorphone) is highly efficacious and is a very practical approach for providing analgesia in patients without intravenous access or those in need of long-term, home-based analgesic care. The administration of hydromorphone exerts basically the same pharmacokinetics whether it is administered subcutaneously or intravenously. This modality is primarily used in palliative care populations.

## Transdermal/Iontophoretic Administration

The development of iontophoretic fentanyl and the validation of its efficacy in postoperative patients may expand the possibilities of parenteral administration. However, because the intramuscular or subcutaneous route possesses a rapid onset time, it may be the best alternative for patients who are without immediate intravenous access.

## Transmucosal Administration

Transmucosal delivery of analgesics, such as fentanyl, may serve as an alternative to the oral administration of NSAIDs and opioids, especially when a rapid onset of drug effect is desirable. However, these medications rarely have a role in the management of postoperative pain because intravenous, intramuscular, subcutaneous, and oral delivery routes are usually sufficient for the delivery of analgesic medications.

## NEURAXIAL ANALGESIA

A variety of neuraxial (intrathecal and epidural) and peripheral regional analgesic techniques are employed for postoperative pain. In general, when compared to

V

systemic opioids, epidural and peripheral techniques can provide superior analgesia, especially when local anesthetics are applied; furthermore, these techniques may decrease morbidity and mortality rates.[32] Clinical judgment is important with regard to the concerns regarding the use of these techniques in the presence of various anticoagulants (see later discussion; also see Chapter 17).

## Intrathecal Administration

Intrathecal administration of an opioid can provide short-term to intermediate length postoperative analgesia after a single injection. The intrathecal route offers the advantage of precise and reliable placement of small concentrations of the drug near its site of action. The onset of analgesic effects after intrathecal administration of an opioid is directly proportional to the lipid solubility of the drug. Duration of effect is longer with more hydrophilic compounds. Morphine produces peak analgesic effects in 20 to 60 minutes and postoperative analgesia for 12 to 36 hours. Adding a small dose of fentanyl to the morphine-containing opioid solution may speed the onset of analgesic effect. For lower abdominal surgical procedures performed with spinal anesthesia (cesarean section, transurethral resection of the prostate), morphine may be added to the local anesthetic solution to increase the duration of analgesia.

The primary disadvantage of an intrathecal opioid injection is the lack of flexibility inherent to a single-shot modality. Clinicians must either repeat the injection or consider other options when the analgesic effect of the initial dose diminishes. The practical aspects of leaving a catheter in the intrathecal space for either continuous or repeated intermittent opioid injections is controversial, especially in view of reports of cauda equina syndrome after continuous spinal anesthesia with hyperbaric local anesthetic solutions injected through a small-diameter catheter.

## Epidural Administration

Epidural administration of a local anesthetic as a continuous infusion through an epidural catheter is a common method of providing perioperative analgesia (also see Chapter 17). Epidural infusions of local anesthetic alone may be used for postoperative analgesia but usually are not as effective in controlling pain as local anesthetic-opioid epidural analgesic combinations. This is due to the significant failure rate (from regression of sensory block and inadequate analgesia) and relatively high incidence of motor block and hypotension. Epidural infusions of local anesthetic alone may be warranted for postoperative analgesia, with the goal of avoiding opioid-related side effects.

The benefit of opioid monotherapy in epidural infusions is that they generally do not cause motor block or hypotension from sympathetic blockade. There are mechanistic differences between continuous epidural infusions of lipophilic (e.g., fentanyl, sufentanil) and hydrophilic (e.g., morphine, hydromorphone) opioids. The analgesic site of action (spinal versus systemic) for continuous epidural infusions of lipophilic opioids is not clear, although several randomized clinical trials suggest that it is systemic[33] because there were no differences in plasma concentrations, side effects, or pain scores between those who received intravenous and those who received epidural infusions of fentanyl. A continuous infusion, rather than an intermittent bolus of epidural opioids, may provide superior analgesia with fewer side effects. Hydrophilic opioid epidural infusions have a spinal mechanism of action. The impact of epidural analgesia is dependent upon the total dose administered rather than the volume or concentration; therefore, a larger concentration of local anesthetic delivered in a small volume is functionally equivalent to that of a small concentration in a larger volume.

Epidural analgesia (local anesthetic with and without opioids) for abdominal surgeries provides superior pain relief in the initial postoperative period, with fewer gastrointestinal-related side effects compared to systemic opioid therapy; however, pruritus often occurs. Epidural analgesia is beneficial for major joint surgery of the lower extremity but has the associated disadvantages of neuraxial analgesia. Thoracic epidural analgesia has been the mainstay of analgesia for thoracotomy, but paravertebral blockades may be just as effective with a more favorable side effect profile.[34] One of the primary benefits of epidural analgesia for traumatic rib fractures is the decreased duration of mechanical ventilation required when compared to using a local anesthetic alone.

## Side Effects of Neuraxial Analgesic Drugs

Many medication-related (opioid and local anesthetic) side effects can occur with postoperative epidural analgesia. When side effects are suspected, the patient's overall clinical status should be evaluated so that serious comorbid conditions are not inappropriately attributed to epidural analgesia. The differential diagnosis for a patient with neuraxial analgesia and hypotension should also include hypovolemia, bleeding, and a decreased cardiac output. Patients with respiratory depression should also be evaluated for cerebrovascular accident, pulmonary edema, and evolving sepsis. Standing orders and nursing protocols for analgesic regimens, neurologic monitoring, treatment of side effects, and physician notification about critical variables should be standard for all patients receiving neuraxial and other types of postoperative analgesia.

## Most Common Side Effects

The most frequent side effects of neuraxial analgesia include the following:

- *Hypotension* (0.3% to 7%)—Local anesthetics used in an epidural analgesic regimen may block sympathetic fibers and contribute to postoperative hypotension.
- *Motor block* (2% to 3%)—In most cases, motor block resolves within 2 hours after discontinuing the epidural infusion. Persistent or increasing motor block should be promptly evaluated, and spinal hematoma, spinal abscess, and intrathecal catheter migration should be considered as part of the differential diagnosis.
- *Nausea, vomiting, and pruritus* (15% to 18%)—Pruritus is one of the most common side effects of epidural or intrathecal administration of opioids, with an incidence of approximately 60% compared with about 15% to 18% for local epidural anesthetic administration or systemic opioids.
- *Respiratory depression* (0.1% to 0.9%)—Neuraxial opioids administered in appropriate doses are not associated with a higher incidence of respiratory depression than that seen with systemic administration of opioids. Risk factors for respiratory depression with neuraxial opioids include larger dose, geriatric age group, concomitant administration of systemic opioids or sedatives, the possibility of prolonged or extensive surgery, the presence of comorbid conditions, and thoracic surgery.
- *Urinary retention* (10% to 30%)—Epidural administration of local anesthetics and opioids is associated with urinary retention.

## Anticoagulation

The concurrent use of anticoagulants with neuraxial anesthesia and analgesia has always been a relatively controversial issue. However, the introduction of low-molecular-weight heparin in North America in 1993 increased the incidence of spinal hematomas. Traditionally, the incidence of spinal hematoma is estimated at approximately 1 in 150,000 for epidural block, with a lower incidence of 1 in 220,000 for spinal blocks.[35] Before its introduction in North America, low-molecular-weight heparin was used in Europe without significant problems. However, the incidence of spinal hematoma increased to as high as 1 in 40,800 for spinal anesthetics and 1 in 6600 for epidural anesthetics (1 in 3100 for postoperative epidural analgesia) in the United States between 1993 and 1998. The estimate of the higher incidence of spinal hematomas after epidural catheter removal is based in part on the Food and Drug Administration MedWatch data, which suggest that epidural catheter removal may be a traumatic event, although this is still a relatively controversial issue.

Different types and classes of anticoagulants vary in pharmacokinetic properties that affect the timing of neuraxial catheter or needle insertion and catheter removal. Despite a number of observational and retrospective studies investigating the incidence of spinal hematoma in the setting of various anticoagulants and neuraxial techniques, there is no definitive conclusion regarding the absolute safety of neuraxial anesthesia and anticoagulation. The American Society of Regional Anesthesia and Pain Medicine (ASRA) lists a series of consensus statements, based on the available literature, for the administration (insertion and removal) of neuraxial techniques in the presence of various anticoagulants, including oral anticoagulants (warfarin), antiplatelet agents, fibrinolytics-thrombolytics, standard unfractionated heparin, and low-molecular-weight heparin. The ASRA consensus statements include the concepts that (1) the timing of neuraxial needle or catheter insertion or removal should reflect the pharmacokinetic properties of the specific anticoagulant; (2) frequent neurologic monitoring is essential; (3) concurrent administration of multiple anticoagulants may increase the risk of bleeding; and (4) the analgesic regimen should be tailored to facilitate neurologic monitoring, which may be continued in some cases for 24 hours after epidural catheter removal. An updated version of the ASRA consensus statements on neuraxial anesthesia and anticoagulation[36] can be found on their website,[36] with some of these statements addressing the newer anticoagulants (also see Chapter 13).

## Infection

Infection associated with postoperative epidural analgesia may result from exogenous or endogenous sources. Serious infections (e.g., meningitis, spinal abscess) associated with epidural analgesia are rare (<1 in 10,000), although some researchers report a higher incidence (approximately 1 in 1000 to 1 in 2000).[37] Closer examination of the studies that report a higher incidence of epidural abscesses reveal that the patients had a relatively longer duration of epidural analgesia or the presence of coexisting immunocompromising or complicating diseases (e.g., malignancy, trauma). Use of epidural analgesia in the general surgical population, with a typical duration of postoperative catheterization of approximately 2 to 4 days, is generally not associated with epidural abscess formation. A trial of postoperative epidural analgesia (mean catheterization of 6.3 days) in more than 4000 surgical cancer patients did not reveal any abscesses.

## SURGICAL SITE (INCISION) INFILTRATION

Surgical site infiltration with local anesthetic prior to incision and prior to tissue closure is recommended for the reduction of postoperative pain.[38] Liposomal bupivacaine (EXPAREL, Pacira Pharmaceuticals) was approved in 2011 for surgical site administration following bunionectomy and hemorrhoidectomy. Although this extended release

V

formulation is designed to slowly release bupivacaine to surrounding tissues over 96 hours, it was superior to placebo only for the first 24 hours after administration.[39]

## INTRA-ARTICULAR ADMINISTRATION

Intra-articular injection of opioids may provide analgesia for up to 24 hours postoperatively and prevent the development of chronic postsurgical pain. Opioid receptors are found in the peripheral terminals of primary afferent nerves, which may explain this improved analgesia, despite the lack of response with the addition of opioids to perineural anesthetic injections. The analgesic benefit of intra-articular opioids over systemic administration has not been demonstrated, and the systemic analgesic effect of these injections has not been excluded. Extended-release bupivacaine was found to be less effective than traditional local anesthetic and opioid infiltration in one study and no different from traditional bupivacaine alone in another.[39] Glenohumeral intra-articular continuous catheters have been associated with chondrolysis when bupivacaine is used and therefore should be avoided.[40]

## INTRAPLEURAL ANALGESIA

Intrapleural regional analgesia is produced by the injection of a local anesthetic solution through a catheter inserted percutaneously into the intrapleural space. The local anesthetic diffuses across the parietal pleura to the intercostal neurovascular bundle and produces a unilateral intercostal nerve block at multiple levels. Effective postoperative pain relief requires intermittent intrapleural injections approximately every 6 hours of large volumes of local anesthetic (20 mL of 0.25% to 0.5% bupivacaine). This large bolus of local anesthetic introduced into the intrapleural space produces significant side effects while providing minimal analgesia. Pleural drainage tubes placed after a thoracotomy will result in a large loss of the local anesthetic solution and, consequently, poor analgesia. This technique is recommended only if all other options have been exhausted.

## PERIPHERAL NERVE BLOCK

Peripheral nerve blockade can provide analgesia as part of an autonomous or multimodal pain regimen. Single-shot injections can provide coverage for intraoperative pain control. However, many providers feel that the risk of the intervention warrants the prolonged benefit, which includes postoperative pain control, and have driven the need for flexible duration of action. Intermediate-term pain relief (<24 hours) can be achieved with a combination of a local anesthetic and adjuvant drugs in a single injection. Longer-acting pain control may be indicated by the surgical technique, rehabilitation needs, and patient comorbid conditions and can be achieved by utilizing perineural catheters for continuous local anesthetic infusions.

### Techniques

Nerve blocks can be inserted using anatomic landmarks, nerve stimulation, and ultrasound guidance. The efficacy between ultrasound-guided techniques and nerve stimulation varies, depending on the skill of the provider, primarily resulting in differences in comfort during placement and procedural time of the blockade. Nonetheless, these techniques provide a comparable quality of analgesia and similar complication profile.[43]

### Adjuvant Drugs

Commonly used adjuvant drugs include epinephrine, clonidine, and opioids. Epinephrine for peripheral nerve blockade significantly increases the duration of the blockade, with minimal side effects. Epinephrine can also increase the sensitivity of intravascular injection; concentrations of 2.5 to 5 µg/mL are generally used. The mechanism of this effect is primarily through vasoconstriction. Opioids probably should not be added to a peripheral nerve blockade. Clonidine is beneficial in extending the duration of preoperative blockade but has less value with perineural catheters. The mechanism is most likely peripheral $\alpha_2$-adrenergic receptor–mediated and dose-dependent. Clonidine is a better preemptive analgesic when added to a local anesthetic block than when used as a single drug. Side effects, including hypotension, bradycardia, and sedation, are less likely to occur with doses less than 1.5 µg/kg.[44] The use of clonidine increases the duration of analgesia and motor blockade by approximately 2 hours. More recently, the addition of dexmedetomidine to peripheral nerve blocks has been shown to improve analgesia duration and opioid reduction.[45]

## REGIONAL ANALGESIA

Efficacy and safety are primary limiting factors in the implementation of any therapeutic measure. Regional analgesia is becoming an increasingly popular technique for perioperative pain control and has several specific advantages and disadvantages. The technical details of these blocks are covered in the regional anesthesia chapter; this section focuses on the utility and comparative efficacy of these blocks (also see Chapter 18).

### Catheter Versus Single-Shot Techniques

#### Upper Extremity

Continuous interscalene blockade allows for longer duration of action compared with single-shot techniques.

This technique has increased utility with the posterior interscalene approach for moderate to severely painful shoulder surgeries. The continuous administration allows for increased pain relief, with minimal opioid supplementation and increased patient satisfaction and sleep quality.[46]

### Lower Extremity

Lower extremity orthopedic surgeries resulting in moderate to severe perioperative pain also benefit from long-acting regional techniques. Lower extremity perineural catheters are utilized for major joint surgery of the hip, knee, ankle, and foot. This type of catheter may decrease clinical signs of inflammation for some lower extremity procedures, although inflammation is not decreased at the cellular level. Epidural catheters are utilized to provide good analgesia for major joint surgeries of the lower extremities, but expose patients to neuraxial analgesia risks, and generally have bilateral effects. Lumbar plexus catheters have been utilized as part of a multimodal regimen, with better pain scores at rest and with physical therapy than multimodal regimens that include PCA with or without femoral catheters for unilateral hip repairs.[47] Patients undergoing major foot and ankle surgeries under continuous perineural blockade are not only potentially able to obtain pain relief comparable to single-shot and systemic analgesia but also are discharged from PACUs in a shorter period of time.[48]

## PARAVERTEBRAL BLOCKS

The increased utilization of paravertebral blockade can be directly correlated with the beneficial effects for patients undergoing breast surgery. This block provides an effective mechanism for controlling acute pain associated with this procedure, but has also demonstrated benefit in decreasing the development of chronic postsurgical pain over other analgesic regimens.[41] This technique can be performed as a single-shot technique or as a continuous catheter infusion to provide ongoing perioperative analgesia. This use of the technique has expanded to thoracic, cardiac, and pediatric applications.[42]

## TRANSVERSUS ABDOMINIS PLANE BLOCK

Neuraxial analgesia techniques are starting to face competition from the transversus abdominis plane (TAP) block for many abdominal procedures. Theoretical advantages of this technique over other modalities include avoidance of both neuraxial involvement and lower extremity blockade, decreased urinary retention, and decreased systemic side effects. Compared with placebo blocks, TAP block provides increased analgesia and decreased systemic medication requirements as part of a multimodal analgesic regimen for total abdominal hysterectomy, cesarean section, and laparoscopic cholecystectomy. Moreover, guidance by ultrasound has made this a more reliably efficacious treatment modality.[49]

## QUESTIONS OF THE DAY

1. How many organ systems are affected by acute postoperative pain? What are the adverse physiologic effects in each system?

2. What is the rationale for a multimodal approach to perioperative pain management? What medications and routes of delivery can be used as part of a multimodal analgesic plan?

3. What are the typical parameters that should be ordered for patient-controlled analgesia (PCA) with hydromorphone in an opioid-naïve patient?

4. A patient is receiving postoperative epidural analgesia with an infusion of ropivacaine and fentanyl. What side effects are most likely to occur? What are the risk factors for respiratory depression with neuraxial opioids?

5. What surgical procedures are most suitable for postoperative analgesia with a transversus abdominis plane (TAP) block?

V

## REFERENCES

1. Buvanendran A, Fiala J, Patel KA, et al. The incidence and severity of postoperative pain following inpatient surgery. *Pain Med.* 2015;16:2277–2283.

2. Apfelbaum JL, Chen C, Mehta SS, et al. Postoperative pain experience: results from a national survey suggest postoperative pain continues to be undermanaged. *Anesth Analg.* 2003;97(2):534–540.

3. Wanderer JP, Shi Y, Schildcrout JS, et al. Supervising anesthesiologists cannot be effectively compared according to their patients' postanesthesia care unit admission pain scores. *Anesth Analg.* 2015; 120(4):923–932.

4. Katz J, McCartney CJ. Current status of preemptive analgesia. *Curr Opin Anaesthesiol.* 2002;15(4):435–441.

5. Kehlet H, Jensen TS, Woolf CJ. Persistent postsurgical pain: risk factors and prevention. *Lancet.* 2006;367(9522): 1618–1625.

6. Carr DB, Goudas LC. Acute pain. *Lancet.* 1999;353(9169):2051–2058.

7. Perkins FM, Kehlet H. Chronic pain as an outcome of surgery. A review of predictive factors. *Anesthesiology.* 2000;93(4):1123–1133.

8. Merskey H. Pain and psychological medicine. In: Wall PD, Melzack R, eds. *Textbook of Pain.* 3rd ed. New York: Churchill Livingstone; 1994:903–920.

9. Basbaum AI, Fields HL. Endogenous pain control systems: brainstem spinal pathways and endorphin circuitry. *Annu Rev Neurosci.* 1984;7:309–338.

10. Julius D, Basbaum AI. Molecular mechanisms of nociception. *Nature.* 2001;413(6852):203–210.

11. Basbaum AI. Spinal mechanisms of acute and persistent pain. *Reg Anesth Pain Med.* 1999;24(1):59–67.

12. Besson JM. The neurobiology of pain. *Lancet.* 1999;353(9164):1610–1615.

13. Kissin I. Preemptive analgesia. *Anesthesiology.* 2000;93(4):1138–1143.

14. Moiniche S, Kehlet H, Dahl JB. A qualitative and quantitative systematic review of preemptive analgesia for postoperative pain relief: the role of timing of analgesia. *Anesthesiology.* 2002;96(3):725–741.

15. Dahl JB, Moiniche S. Pre-emptive analgesia. *Br Med Bull.* 2004;71:13–27.

16. Ong CK, Lirk P, Seymour RA, et al. The efficacy of preemptive analgesia for acute postoperative pain management: a meta-analysis. *Anesth Analg.* 2005;100(3):757–773.

17. Pogatzki-Zahn EM, Zahn PK. From preemptive to preventive analgesia. *Curr Opin Anaesthesiol.* 2006;19(5):551–555.

18. Joly V, Richebe P, Guignard B, et al. Remifentanil-induced postoperative hyperalgesia and its prevention with small-dose ketamine. *Anesthesiology.* 2005;103(1):147–155.

19. Kehlet H. Multimodal approach to control postoperative pathophysiology and rehabilitation. *Br J Anaesth.* 1997;78(5):606–617.

20. Hurley RW, Cohen SP, Williams KA, et al. The analgesic effects of perioperative gabapentin on postoperative pain: a meta-analysis. *Reg Anesth Pain Med.* 2006;31(3):237–247.

21. Block BM, Liu SS, Rowlingson AJ, et al. Efficacy of postoperative epidural analgesia: a meta-analysis. *JAMA.* 2003;290(18):2455–2463.

22. Ben-David B, Swanson J, Nelson JB, et al. Multimodal analgesia for radical prostatectomy provides better analgesia and shortens hospital stay. *J Clin Anesth.* 2007;19(4):264–268.

23. Kehlet H, Wilmore DW. Multimodal strategies to improve surgical outcome. *Am J Surg.* 2002;183(6):630–641.

24. Egbert AM, Parks LH, Short LM, et al. Randomized trial of postoperative patient-controlled analgesia vs intramuscular narcotics in frail elderly men. *Arch Intern Med.* 1990;150(9):1897–1903.

25. Elia N, Lysakowski C, Tramer MR. Does multimodal analgesia with acetaminophen, nonsteroidal antiinflammatory drugs, or selective cyclooxygenase-2 inhibitors and patient-controlled analgesia morphine offer advantages over morphine alone? Meta-analyses of randomized trials. *Anesthesiology.* 2005;103(6):1296–1304.

26. Buvanendran A, Kroin JS, Della Valle CJ, et al. Perioperative oral pregabalin reduces chronic pain after total knee arthroplasty: a prospective, randomized, controlled trial. *Anesth Analg.* 2010;110(1):199–207.

27. Evaniew N, McCarthy C, Kleinlugtenbelt YV, et al. Vitamin C to prevent complex regional pain syndrome in patients with distal radius fractures: a meta-analysis of randomized controlled trials. *J Orthop Trauma.* 2015;29(8):e235–e241.

28. De Kock M, Lavand'homme P, Waterloos H. 'Balanced analgesia' in the perioperative period: is there a place for ketamine? *Pain.* 2001;92(3):373–380.

29. Jibril F, Sharaby S, Mohamed A, et al. Intravenous versus oral acetaminophen for pain: systematic review of current evidence to support clinical decision-making. *Can J Hosp Pharm.* 2015;68(3):238–247.

30. Nielsen RV, Siegel H, Fomsgaard J, et al. Preoperative dexamethasone reduces acute but not sustained pain after lumbar disc surgery: a randomized, blinded, placebo-controlled trial. *Pain.* 2015;156(12):2538–2544.

31. De Oliveira Jr GS, Castro-Alves LJ, Khan JH, et al. Perioperative systemic magnesium to minimize postoperative pain: a meta-analysis of randomized controlled trials. *Anesthesiology.* 2013;119(1):178–190.

32. Wu CL, Fleisher LA. Outcomes research in regional anesthesia and analgesia. *Anesth Analg.* 2000;91(5):1232–1242.

33. Loper KA, Ready LB, Downey M, et al. Epidural and intravenous fentanyl infusions are clinically equivalent after knee surgery. *Anesth Analg.* 1990;70(1):72–75.

34. Gulbahar G, Kocer B, Muratli SN, et al. A comparison of epidural and paravertebral catheterisation techniques in post-thoracotomy pain management. *Eur J Cardiothorac Surg.* 2010;37(2):467–472.

35. Tryba M. [Epidural regional anesthesia and low molecular heparin: Pro]. *Anasthesiol Intensivmed Notfallmed Schmerzther.* 1993;28(3):179–181.

36. Horlocker TT, Wedel DJ, Rowlingson JC, et al. Regional anesthesia in the patient receiving antithrombotic or thrombolytic therapy: American Society of Regional Anesthesia and Pain Medicine Evidence-Based Guidelines (Third Edition). *Reg Anesth Pain Med.* 2010;35(1):64–101. Also available at www.asra.com.

37. Horlocker TT, Wedel DJ. Neurologic complications of spinal and epidural anesthesia. *Reg Anesth Pain Med.* 2000;25(1):83–98.

38. Group TPW. PROSPECT (Procedure Specific Postoperative Pain Management). http://www.postoppain.org/; Accessed October, 1, 2015.

39. Uskova A, O'Connor JE. Liposomal bupivacaine for regional anesthesia. *Curr Opin Anaesthesiol.* 2015;28(5):593–597.

40. Busfield BT, Romero DM. Pain pump use after shoulder arthroscopy as a cause of glenohumeral chondrolysis. *Arthroscopy.* 2009;25(6):647–652.

41. Vila Jr H, Liu J, Kavasmaneck D. Paravertebral block: new benefits from an old procedure. *Curr Opin Anaesthesiol.* 2007;20(4):316–318.

42. Wardhan R. Update on paravertebral blocks. *Curr Opin Anaesthesiol.* 2015;28(5):588–592.

43. Fredrickson MJ, Ball CM, Dalgleish AJ, et al. A prospective randomized comparison of ultrasound and neurostimulation as needle end points for interscalene catheter placement. *Anesth Analg.* 2009;108(5):1695–1700.

44. Neal JM, Gerancher JC, Hebl JR, et al. Upper extremity regional anesthesia: essentials of our current understanding, 2008. *Reg Anesth Pain Med.* 2009;34(2):134–170.

45. Fritsch G, Danninger T, Allerberger K, et al. Dexmedetomidine added to ropivacaine extends the duration of interscalene brachial plexus blocks for elective shoulder surgery when compared with ropivacaine alone: a single-center, prospective, triple-blind, randomized controlled trial. *Reg Anesth Pain Med.* 2014;39(1):37–47.

46. Mariano ER, Afra R, Loland VJ, et al. Continuous interscalene brachial plexus block via an ultrasound-guided posterior approach: a randomized, triple-masked, placebo-controlled study. *Anesth Analg.* 2009;108(5):1688–1694.

47. Marino J, Russo J, Kenny M, et al. Continuous lumbar plexus block for postoperative pain control after total hip arthroplasty. A randomized controlled trial. *J Bone Joint Surg Am.* 2009;91(1):29–37.

48. Hunt KJ, Higgins TF, Carlston CV, et al. Continuous peripheral nerve blockade as postoperative analgesia for open treatment of calcaneal fractures. *J Orthop Trauma.* 2010;24(3):148–155.

49. El-Dawlatly A, Turkistani A, Kettner S, et al. Ultrasound-guided transversus abdominis plane block: description of a new technique and comparison with conventional systemic analgesia during laparoscopic cholecystectomy. *Br J Anaesth.* 2009;102(6):763–767.

# CONSULTANT ANESTHETIC PRACTICE

# 41 CRITICAL CARE MEDICINE

## John H. Turnbull and Linda L. Liu

**RESPIRATORY FAILURE**
Mechanical Ventilation
Noninvasive Positive-Pressure Ventilation
Weaning From Mechanical Ventilation and
    Tracheal Extubation
Acute Respiratory Distress Syndrome
Tracheostomies

**SHOCK**
Hypovolemic Shock
Cardiogenic Shock
Vasodilatory Shock
Hemodynamic Monitoring
Sepsis

**ACUTE RENAL FAILURE**
Epidemiology
Diagnosis
Treatment
Dialysis

**PAIN AND SEDATION**
Analgesia
Sedation
Sedation Interruption

**OTHER TOPICS IN CRITICAL CARE**
Delirium
Nutrition
Glucose Control
Prophylaxis
Hospital-Acquired Infections
ICU Staffing and Organization

**QUESTIONS OF THE DAY**

From the late 20th century to the present, critical care medicine has evolved as a dynamic, multidisciplinary field focused on the care of patients with life-threatening diseases. Anesthesia providers can play an important role in the care of the critically ill patient both in the operating room and intensive care unit (ICU). A few key topics in critical care with which the practicing anesthesia provider should be familiar include respiratory failure, shock, renal failure, and management of pain and sedation.

## RESPIRATORY FAILURE

Respiratory failure remains a primary indication for admission to an ICU. The type of respiratory failure can be categorized based on the acuity of the process (e.g., acute vs. chronic) and the physiologic perturbation present (e.g., hypercapnia vs. hypoxemia). Such distinctions help to direct decision making for various treatment options. However, multiple processes can occur simultaneously. For example, a patient may have an acute and chronic respiratory failure with the presence of both hypoxemia and hypercapnia.

Hypoxemic respiratory failure generally occurs because of ventilation/perfusion ($\dot{V}/\dot{Q}$) mismatch leading to a large alveolar-arterial (A-a) gradient. Causes include trauma, acute respiratory distress syndrome (ARDS), sepsis, pneumonia, pulmonary embolism, cardiogenic pulmonary edema, and obstructive lung disease. Other physiologic causes of hypoxemia include intrapulmonary shunt, hypoventilation, and increased $O_2$ extraction (also see Chapter 5).

Causes of hypercapnic respiratory failure include hypoventilation, as may occur from a drug intoxication or

The editors and publisher would like to thank Drs. Lundy Campbell and Michael Gropper for contributing to this chapter in the previous edition of this work. It has served as the foundation for the current chapter.

| Table 41.1 | Different Settings of Mechanical Ventilation | | |
|---|---|---|---|
| **Mode** | **Control** | **Limit** | **Cycle** |
| AC | Volume | Volume | Volume |
| | Pressure | Pressure | Time |
| SIMV | Volume | Volume | Volume |
| | Pressure | Pressure | Time |
| PS | | Pressure | Flow |

*AC,* Assist control; *PS,* pressure support; *SIMV,* synchronized intermittent mandatory ventilation.

neuromuscular weakness, or increased dead space, which occurs with chronic obstructive pulmonary disease (COPD) or asthma. Hypercapnia may also be present in severe forms of an infiltrative pulmonary process, such as ARDS. Both hypercapnic and hypoxemic respiratory failure may require initiation of mechanical ventilator support.

## Mechanical Ventilation

In modern ICUs, mechanical ventilation is performed entirely via positive-pressure ventilation. It may be accomplished through a noninvasive approach (via face mask or nasal mask) or an invasive approach (via endotracheal tube [ETT] or tracheostomy). The goals of mechanical ventilation include (1) decreasing the work of breathing; (2) improving oxygen delivery; (3) facilitating carbon dioxide removal; and (4) minimizing ventilator-associated lung injury. The settings for mechanical ventilation describe how the ventilator interacts with the patient (Table 41.1).

### Modes
#### Assist Control
In assist control (AC) mode, the ventilator is set to deliver a minimum number of breaths per minute, while allowing the patient to initiate breaths as well. All mandatory and spontaneous breaths are fully supported to the same degree. So, if tidal volume is set at 500 mL, then all breaths (i.e., mandatory and spontaneous) will receive a tidal volume of 500 mL.

#### Synchronized Intermittent Mandatory Ventilation
With synchronized intermittent mandatory ventilation (SIMV), the ventilator attempts to synchronize the mandatory mechanical breaths with the patient's spontaneous breaths in order to decrease ventilator dyssynchrony. If there are no spontaneous breaths within the preset time interval, then the ventilator will deliver the mandatory breath. The breaths in between the mandatory breaths are not fully supported, unlike the AC mode. For these non-mandatory breaths, the ventilator can be set to deliver pressure support (PS), as described next.

### Pressure Support
PS mode is used only with spontaneously breathing patients, as all breaths are triggered by patient effort. The driving pressure ($\Delta P$), positive end-expiratory pressure (PEEP), and fraction of inspired oxygen ($F_{IO_2}$) are the only variables set in this mode. Inspiratory flows are based on patient demand. The ventilator ends inspiration when the flow rate has decreased to a predetermined level (usually 25% of the peak flow rate). There is no backup respiratory rate in PS mode unless it is combined with SIMV.

### Other Modes
The sophisticated microprocessors in current ventilators enable novel modes such as adaptive support ventilation, airway pressure release ventilation, and proportional assist ventilation. These modes offer potential physiologic benefits but have not been subject to large clinical trials with enough power to demonstrate improved mortality rate.

### Limits
With AC or SIMV mode, the limit or control needs to be specified. With volume control (VC), a preset tidal volume is delivered during inspiration. With pressure control (PC), a preset inspiratory pressure is delivered by the ventilator.

### Volume Control
Sample mechanical ventilation orders for AC and SIMV with VC are listed in Table 41.2. The tidal volume, rate, PEEP, and $F_{IO_2}$ must be specified. The inspiratory flow rate is not typically part of a standard ventilator order set and is set by the respiratory therapist. A typical inspiratory flow rate is 60 L/min. By increasing inspiratory flow, the set tidal volume is delivered in a shorter time, which allows more time for exhalation. This strategy may be beneficial for an asthmatic patient in respiratory distress to increase expiratory time. The flow waveform in VC can be decelerating or constant (so-called square wave).

### Pressure Control
In AC or SIMV mode with PC, a driving pressure must be specified. Additionally, an inspiratory time or inspiratory-expiratory time (I:E) ratio is set. The peak flows in PC are variable and based on demand. By default, the flow waveform must be decelerating in order to maintain a constant peak inspiratory pressure. Tidal volumes are not guaranteed and if lung compliance changes quickly, vigilance is necessary to make sure minute ventilation does not drop rapidly.

### Dual Control
The choice between VC or PC is not supported by definitive evidence. Modern ventilators can combine the features of both, targeting specified tidal volumes, but delivering each breath in a PC mode with decelerating flows. If pulmonary compliance changes, then the ventilator automatically adjusts the pressure gradually over a few breaths to maintain the targeted tidal volumes. Many

| Table 41.2 | Sample Orders for Mechanical Ventilation | | |
|---|---|---|---|
| **Example** | **Ventilator Orders Written** | **Additional Settings That Can Be Ordered** | **Explanation** |
| Example 1: Assist control–volume control (AC-VC) | Mode AC/VC<br>Rate 10<br>$V_T$ 500 mL<br>PEEP 5 cm $H_2O$<br>$F_{IO_2}$ 1.0 | Flow rate: typically 60 L/min<br>Trigger: flow or pressure | Ventilator will deliver the preset tidal volume of 500 mL 10 times a minute; if the patient's respiratory rate is greater than 10, each breath will also be 500 mL |
| Example 2: Assist control–pressure control (AC-PC) | Mode AC/PC<br>Rate 10<br>PIP 20 cm $H_2O$<br>PEEP 5 cm $H_2O$<br>$F_{IO_2}$ 1.0 | I:E ratio: typically 1:2<br>Inspiratory time<br>Trigger: flow or pressure | Ventilator will deliver 10 breaths per minute; each breath will reach a peak pressure of 20 cm $H_2O$; if the patient's respiratory rate is greater than 10, each breath will also reach peak pressure of 20 cm $H_2O$ |
| Example 3: Synchronized intermittent mandatory ventilation–volume control (SIMV-VC) | Mode SIMV-VC<br>Rate 10<br>$V_T$ 500 mL<br>Pressure support 5 cm $H_2O$<br>PEEP 5 cm $H_2O$<br>$F_{IO_2}$ 0.5 | Flow rate: typically 60 L/min<br>Trigger: flow or pressure (this applies to all the breaths, SIMV, or pressure support) | Ventilator will deliver 10 breaths per minute with tidal volume 500 mL; if the patient's respiratory rate is greater than 10, those nonmandatory breaths will receive inspiratory pressure support to peak pressure 5 cm $H_2O$ above the PEEP of 5 cm $H_2O$ |
| Example 4: Pressure support ventilation (PSV) | Mode PSV<br>Driving pressure 8 cm $H_2O$<br>PEEP 5 cm $H_2O$<br>$F_{IO_2}$ 0.5 | Trigger: flow or pressure | Patient must be breathing spontaneously; each breath will receive inspiratory pressure support to peak pressure 8 cm $H_2O$ above the PEEP of 5 cm $H_2O$ |

$F_{IO_2}$, Fraction of inspired oxygen; *I:E*, inspiratory to expiratory ratio; *PEEP*, positive end-expiratory pressure; *PIP*, peak inspiratory pressure; *V_T*, tidal volume.

proprietary names exist, such as *pressure control ventilation-volume guaranteed, pressure-regulated volume control,* or *volume control plus.*

### Cycle

The cycle determines how the ventilator switches from inspiration to expiration. For AC-VC or SIMV-VC modes, volume determines the ventilator cycle. Inspiration is complete when the tidal volume is delivered (see Table 41.1). For AC-PC or SIMV-PC, inspiration is complete when the inspiratory time has ended. With PS mode, a decrease in the inspiratory flow rate determines the end of the inspiratory cycle. Knowledge of how the ventilator cycles can allow better understanding of patient/ventilator dyssynchrony. For example, a patient in respiratory distress receiving mechanical ventilation in the AC-VC mode may find the set tidal volume too small and "double stack" (i.e., take a second breath during the start of the ventilator's exhalation phase). Or, a patient receiving AC-PC ventilation may begin exhalation prior to the end of the set inspiratory time.

### Other Settings

#### Positive End-Expiratory Pressure

PEEP is constant positive airway pressure that is applied throughout the respiratory cycle. PEEP is generated by a pressure relief valve on the expiratory limb of the ventilator circuit. The use of PEEP leads to an increased mean airway pressure, which decreases atelectasis and improves oxygenation. PEEP also increases functional residual capacity and can improve pulmonary compliance.

If PEEP is too large, alveolar overdistention can occur, which may lead to barotrauma. Excessive PEEP can also reduce preload and cause hypotension. Auto-PEEP occurs when a buildup of end-expiratory pressure results from insufficient exhalation time. Emergent treatment of auto-PEEP entails disconnecting the patient from the ventilator to release the PEEP. Treatment of auto-PEEP requires increasing expiratory time (i.e., changing the ratio of the duration of inspiration to the duration of expiration, or I:E ratio).

### Trigger

The trigger refers to the manner by which the ventilator detects patient inspiration and delivers positive pressure in synchrony with the patient's efforts. The trigger variable, which can be based on flow or pressure, is not part of a typical ventilator order set and is often managed by respiratory therapists. Usual triggers are a change in flow of 2 L/min or a change in pressure of 2 cm $H_2O$. Smaller or larger triggers can be set based on the clinical situation.

VI

For example, patients with bronchopleural fistulas may constantly trigger mechanical ventilation breaths if the flow trigger is too sensitive.

## Noninvasive Positive-Pressure Ventilation

Noninvasive positive-pressure ventilation (NIPPV) delivers positive-pressure breaths via a face mask, nasal pillows, or helmet without an ETT present. For patients with COPD and acute hypercapnic respiratory failure (AHRF), appropriate use of NIPPV can reduce mortality rate, avoid endotracheal intubation, improve dyspnea, and reduce hospital length of stay. Other established indications for NIPPV include acute cardiogenic pulmonary edema, postoperative respiratory failure, and hypoxic respiratory failure in immunocompromised patients (e.g., organ and bone marrow transplant recipients).

The data for NIPPV are often impressive, but the patients chosen for these studies were judiciously selected in trials with close clinical observation. NIPPV is most beneficial in patients who have a potentially rapidly reversible pulmonary process that requires some ventilator support. Delays in endotracheal intubation can lead to an emergent event that is more prone to complications. Contraindications for using NIPPV are listed in Box 41.1. The most commonly used ventilator mode for NIPPV is PS.

### High-Flow Nasal Cannula

Use of high-flow nasal cannula (HFNC) has emerged as an alternative to NIPPV. HFNC uses heated and humidified oxygen that is delivered at high flow rates through nasal cannula. This delivery system provides a small amount of positive airway pressure and reduces dead space by flushing expired carbon dioxide from the upper airways. Most patients find HFNC to be more comfortable and easier to tolerate than NIPPV via a face mask. A 2015 multicenter trial in patients with acute hypoxemic, nonhypercarbic respiratory failure showed that high-flow oxygen therapy, as compared with standard oxygen therapy or noninvasive ventilation, resulted in reduced mortality rate in the ICU and at 90 days, although there was no difference in the rate of tracheal intubation.[1]

---

**Box 41.1** Contraindications for Noninvasive Positive-Pressure Ventilation

- Impaired neurologic state (coma, seizures, encephalopathy)
- Respiratory arrest or upper airway obstruction
- Shock or severe cardiovascular instability
- Severe upper gastrointestinal bleeding
- Recent gastroesophageal surgery
- Vomiting
- Excessive airway secretions
- Facial lesions that prevent proper fit of nasal or facial masks

---

## Weaning From Mechanical Ventilation and Tracheal Extubation

Weaning may account for more than 40% of the patient's time on mechanical ventilation depending on the definition of when weaning commences. To decrease the risk of ventilator-associated pneumonia (VAP), patients should be weaned from mechanical ventilation as soon as they have recovered from the process that originally required mechanical ventilator support.

The average rate of failed tracheal extubation (i.e., inadequate ventilation following extubation of the trachea) in surgical ICUs is 5% to 8%, whereas in medical and neurologic ICUs the rate is 17%. Although many criteria are listed in the following section, no one algorithm can accurately predict successful tracheal extubation. A cautiously applied aggressive approach to weaning from mechanical ventilation and tracheal extubation results in fewer ICU-related complications, although definitive data from randomized trials are lacking.

### Criteria for Weaning Trial

#### A-a Gradient

The patient should have adequate oxygenation, usually defined as $Pa_{O_2}/F_{I_{O_2}}$ more than 150 mm Hg with PEEP less than 8 cm $H_2O$. This amount of oxygen is chosen because this level can be reliably delivered via face mask or nasal cannula. An oxygen requirement greater than this denotes that the patient still has a large shunt fraction and the underlying pulmonary process may not have resolved adequately. In the end, these criteria are just guidelines. The final decision regarding what is an appropriate A-a gradient is often based on clinical judgment and experience.

### Respiratory Mechanics

#### Rapid Shallow Breathing Index

Rapid shallow breathing index (RSBI) is the ratio of respiratory rate (breaths/min) to tidal volume (in liters). This index is the most extensively studied and commonly used weaning predictor. A RSBI less than 105 breaths/min/L (i.e., positive RSBI) is associated with weaning success, but a negative RSBI (RSBI more than 105 breaths/min/L) is likely better at identifying patients who will fail than a positive RSBI is at identifying patients who can succeed.

#### Maximum Inspiratory Force

Patients must have the respiratory muscle strength to generate an adequate tidal volume. One attempt to measure this is via the maximum inspiratory force (MIF). For weaning, a MIF of at least −20 cm $H_2O$ is preferable. A normal MIF indicates little or no increase in the probability of weaning success, but a small MIF predicts a small increase in the probability of weaning failure. One reason for the poor predictive ability of the MIF is the challenge of obtaining an accurate measurement in a spontaneously breathing patient. In many ICUs, MIF is not routinely measured prior to weaning from ventilation. However, if a patient is not progressing in the weaning process, measurement of a MIF may suggest a cause such as muscle weakness or deconditioning.

### Other Criteria

Other respiratory criteria may impact success of weaning from ventilation, including the nature and amount of airway secretions and the ability to clear secretions, which involves the gag reflex and cough strength. The presence of upper airway edema may promote airway obstruction and hypoxemia after tracheal extubation. The cuff leak test is one method to assess for airway edema. The ETT cuff is deflated and positive pressure is delivered through the ETT until an air leak is heard. A leak pressure of less than 10 cm $H_2O$ suggests the absence of airway edema. In contrast, a leak pressure greater than 20 cm $H_2O$ may indicate significant airway edema and should be considered prior to the decision for tracheal extubation.

Other patient factors that impact weaning include mental status and hemodynamics. Patients should have an adequate level of consciousness to protect their airway from aspiration of gastric contents. In addition, patients should be hemodynamically stable, because discontinuation of positive-pressure ventilation can lead to increased work of breathing and alter left ventricular preload and afterload.

### Weaning Strategies

Regardless of the weaning strategy used in ICUs, early identification of patients who are able to breathe spontaneously results in better outcomes. A common strategy is for the mechanically ventilated patient to undergo a daily assessment of readiness.[2] If the patient is deemed ready, a spontaneous breathing trial (SBT) is performed. If the factors described previously (respiratory mechanics, mental status, hemodynamics) remain adequate throughout the SBT, a decision for tracheal extubation can be made. Protocol-based weaning by nurses and respiratory therapists allows more rapid tracheal extubation compared to physician-directed weaning.

The SBT can be conducted with different ventilation modes, including PS ventilation or T-piece trial. There is no definitive evidence of a superior mode associated with more frequent weaning success, less need for tracheal reintubation, or lower ICU fatality.[3] However, for an individual patient, a specific mode may have clinical advantages. For example, in patients with heart failure and reduced cardiac ejection fraction, the change from positive-pressure ventilation to negative-pressure ventilation can increase left ventricular afterload and worsen cardiovascular strain. This patient may benefit from T-piece trial for the SBT, because even low levels of positive pressure and PEEP may provide afterload reduction. If the patient does not develop signs of pulmonary edema during the T-piece trial, the decision for tracheal extubation can proceed.

The optimal duration of an SBT is unknown, but most range from 30 minutes to 2 hours. Longer periods may be required for patients with chronic respiratory failure whose tracheas have been intubated for an extended duration or for patients who fail their initial SBT. In select patients, weaning strategies that include NIPPV can reduce the rate of mortality, VAP, and weaning failure without increasing the risk of tracheal reintubation.[4] This approach may be considered in patients who do not have difficult to manage airways, excessive secretions, or an impaired mental status and should be coupled with an early decision regarding tracheal reintubation if the patient remains tachypneic or in distress. Tracheal reintubation, especially if delayed, is associated with increased mortality rate, longer hospital stay, and lower likelihood of returning home.

Automated closed-loop systems (e.g., SmartCare/PS, adaptive support ventilation, proportional assist ventilation, volume support ventilation) were developed to adapt ventilation in response to real-time changes with the patient's respiratory mechanics. A recent meta-analysis showed that closed-loop systems reduced the duration of ventilation and ICU length of stay in mixed (combined medical-surgical ICUs) or medical ICU patients; however, more randomized controlled trials are needed for surgical ICU patients and patients using other automated systems.[5] Currently, this area of research is in its infancy.

## Acute Respiratory Distress Syndrome

ARDS, characterized as a diffuse, inflammatory injury of the lung, results in the development of noncardiogenic pulmonary edema with resultant $\dot{V}/\dot{Q}$ mismatch, hypoxemia, and decreased pulmonary compliance. ARDS typically follows an inciting event that can lead to direct or indirect lung injury (Table 41.3). Although the underlying cause of lung injury may predict outcome, patient-specific factors such as age, immunocompromised status, and organ dysfunction are stronger predictors for survival. In

| Table 41.3 | Causes of Acute Respiratory Distress Syndrome |

| Causes of Direct Lung Injury | Causes of Indirect Lung Injury |
|---|---|
| Pneumonia | Sepsis |
| Aspiration of stomach contents | Severe trauma |
| Pulmonary contusion | Cardiopulmonary bypass |
| Reperfusion pulmonary edema | Drug overdose |
| Amniotic fluid embolus | Acute pancreatitis |
| Inhalational injury | Near-drowning, transfusion-related acute lung injury |

Data from Ware LB, Matthay MA. The acute respiratory distress syndrome. *N Engl J Med*. 2000;342:1334-1349.

VI

| Table 41.4 | Comparison of the American-European Consensus Conference and Berlin Definition of Adult Respiratory Distress Syndrome | |
|---|---|---|
| | **AECC Definition** | **Berlin Definition** |
| Timing | Acute onset | Within 1 week of a known clinical insult or new or worsening respiratory symptoms |
| Oxygenation | **ALI**: $PaO_2/FiO_2 \leq$ 300 mm Hg<br>**ARDS**: $PaO_2/FiO_2 \leq$ 200 mm Hg | **Mild**: 200 mm Hg $< PaO_2/FiO_2 \leq$ 300 mm Hg with PEEP or CPAP $\geq$ 5 $cmH_2O$<br>**Moderate**: 100 mm Hg $< PaO_2/FiO_2 \leq$ 200 mm Hg with PEEP $\geq$ 5 $cmH_2O$<br>**Severe**: $PaO_2/FiO_2 \leq$ 100 mm Hg with PEEP $\geq$ 5 $cmH_2O$ |
| Chest radiograph | Bilateral infiltrates | Bilateral opacities not fully explained by effusions, lobar/lung collapse, or nodules |
| Edema | PAWP $\leq$ 18 mm Hg when measured or no clinical evidence of left atrial hypertension | Respiratory failure not fully explained by cardiac failure or fluid overload |
| Risk factor | Not included in definition | If no risk factor for lung injury identified, then need objective assessment such as echocardiography to exclude hydrostatic edema |

AECC, American-European consensus Conference; ALI, acute lung injury; ARDS, acute respiratory distress syndrome; $FiO_2$, fraction of inspired oxygen; $PaO_2$, arterial partial pressure of oxygen; PAWP, pulmonary artery wedge pressure; PEEP, positive end-expiratory pressure.
From Liu LL, Gropper MA: Critical care anesthesiology. Ch 101. In Miller RD (ed): Miller's Anesthesia, 8e. Philadelphia: Elsevier, 2015.

such as echocardiography are required to rule out cardiogenic pulmonary edema as the cause of bilateral infiltrates.

### Management

Because many clinical trials of pharmacologic immune modulation have shown no benefit, treatment for ARDS remains largely supportive, with a focus on the prevention of further lung injury. The central tenet for ARDS care involves lung protective ventilation when mechanical ventilation is required. In the landmark ARDS Network (ARDSnet) trial, "lower tidal volume (6 mL/kg of ideal body weight)" ventilation reduced mortality rate (31% vs. 40%) as compared to standard ventilation practices (12 mL/kg).[7] The theory is that by accepting decreased $Po_2$ and increased $Pco_2$ values ("permissive" hypoxemia and hypercapnia), the avoidance of large tidal volumes and high airway pressures decreases the incidence of barotrauma and volutrauma, and mortality rate.

Physician-directed lung protective ventilation protocols allow respiratory therapists to proactively adjust ventilator settings to maintain lung protective criteria. A lower threshold should be used to initiate lung protective ventilation, as patients who are ventilated with lung protective protocols and who are later ruled out for ARDS suffer no worse clinical outcomes.[8] Furthermore, intraoperative lower tidal volume ventilation may reduce the risk for developing ARDS postoperatively.

Patients with moderate to severe ARDS may benefit from administration of neuromuscular blocking drugs (NMBDs) (also see Chapter 11). NMBDs often improve pulmonary compliance and oxygenation. A clinical trial of early cisatracurium infusion in ARDS patients demonstrated improved 90-day survival rate although the mechanism for the benefit is not clear.[9] The prone position may improve oxygenation and clinical outcomes and should be used in the management of severe ARDS. However, a medical facility's experience and comfort in caring for critically ill patients while prone should be considered prior to initiating this procedure. Finally, referral for extracorporeal life support (ECLS) may be indicated, although data for improved outcomes do not currently exist. Clinical trials are being conducted to explore this resource intensive therapy.

### Tracheostomies

A small, but significant portion of patients may require prolonged mechanical ventilation during their critical illness. Tracheostomies often facilitate rehabilitation and allow for weaning of sedation. However, the timing of tracheostomies remains a controversial topic. Early tracheostomies ($\leq$4 days) do not decrease 30-day mortality rate, 2-year mortality rate, or ICU length of stay in patients when compared to those who received late tracheostomies ($\geq$10 days).[10] Physicians are poor at predicting those patients requiring prolonged mechanical ventilation. Only 45% of the patients who were predicted to require more

some patients, ARDS resolves following an acute phase but others experience a chronic alveolitis leading to pulmonary fibrosis. Such patients often experience continued hypoxemia, increased physiologic dead space, and decreased compliance with chronic ventilator dependence.

Although classically defined by an increased A-a gradient in the setting of diffuse bilateral noncardiogenic pulmonary infiltrates, the clinical definition of ARDS continues to evolve—most recently with the Berlin criteria (Table 41.4).[6] In this new definition, the clinical distinction between ARDS and acute lung injury disappears and is replaced by categories of severity (i.e., mild, moderate, and severe). Additionally, the requirement for pulmonary artery occlusion pressure (PAOP) measurement no longer exists. In the absence of a known cardiac event, objective data

| Table 41.5 | Characteristics of Various Shock States | | | | |
|---|---|---|---|---|---|
| Shock Type | Cardiac Output | Systemic Vascular Resistance | Central Venous Pressure | Pulmonary Capillary Wedge Pressure | Mixed Venous Oxygen Saturation |
| Hypovolemic | ↓ | ↑ | ↓ | ↓ | ↓ |
| Cardiogenic | ↓ | ↑ | ↑ | ↑a | ↓ |
| Vasodilatory | ↑ or ↔ | ↓ | ↓ | ↓ | ↑ or ↔ |

aPulmonary capillary wedge pressure is normal to low in right ventricular failure.

than 7 days of mechanical ventilation actually required a tracheostomy. The remaining 55% were successfully extubated. Because of this, with the exception of certain clinical situations, tracheostomies are often deferred until 10 to 14 days after tracheal intubation. Placement of tracheostomies can lead to the loss of mean airway pressure and derecruitment of alveolar units, so tracheostomies should be deferred in unstable patients and those with high PEEP and oxygen requirements.

Inadvertent dislodgement of the tracheostomy tube during the first 7 days after placement is a potentially life-threatening problem. In this circumstance, blind tracheostomy tube advancement may result in tube passage through a false subcutaneous track rather than into the trachea. When feasible, orotracheal intubation should be the first maneuver to obtain a secure airway. Otherwise, a pediatric laryngoscope blade may be inserted into the stoma and a new tracheostomy tube or ETT can be inserted under direct visual identification of tracheal rings.

## SHOCK

Shock is a common clinical condition encountered in critically ill patients. Many clinical processes can cause shock that leads to inadequate perfusion to major organ systems, such as the brain, heart, kidney, liver, and abdominal viscera. This in turn leads to anaerobic metabolism, multiorgan failure, and death when adequate perfusion cannot be restored. Shock is categorized by the underlying physiologic process that induced the state of hypoperfusion. Major categories include hypovolemic, cardiogenic, and vasodilatory shock. Vasodilatory shock can be further categorized as septic, anaphylactic, and neurogenic shock. Characteristics of the major categories of shock are listed in Table 41.5.

### Hypovolemic Shock

Hypovolemic shock occurs following an acute, decompensated decrease in circulating blood volume (also see Chapters 42 and 45. Decreases in intravascular volume reduce cardiac preload (left ventricular end-diastolic volume), which is a major determinant of cardiac output. Hypovolemia most commonly occurs during massive blood loss from trauma, surgery, or gastrointestinal hemorrhage (also see Chapter 24). When compensatory mechanisms are unable to restore adequate perfusion of the vital organs, shock and hemodynamic collapse result.

### Clinical Manifestations

Acute blood loss initially results in the translocation of interstitial fluid into the circulating blood volume to transiently restore cardiac output. This response helps to explain some of the physical examination findings found in patients with hypovolemic shock, including dry mucous membranes and decreased skin turgor. Following this fluid shift, activation of the renin-angiotensin-aldosterone system results in sodium conservation by the kidneys and restoration of interstitial fluid loss.

If cardiac output continues to decrease from inadequate circulating blood volume (>15% reduction), the baroreceptor reflex triggers an increase in the heart rate to maintain cardiac output. Sympathetic stimulation through the release of endogenous catecholamines from the adrenal glands produces vasoconstriction of nonessential organs. Blood is redirected away from the skin, skeletal muscle, and the splanchnic circulation to maintain perfusion of vital organs. Patients may appear cold, clammy, and vasoconstricted. Mesenteric ischemia may result if the condition persists. If circulating volume loss continues (>40% reduction) in the absence of adequate resuscitation, compensatory mechanisms may no longer be able to maintain cardiac output and decompensated hypovolemic shock follows.

### Treatment

Adequate intravascular volume resuscitation and source control are key to the treatment of hypovolemic shock. First, adequate intravenous access must be obtained quickly. Ideal access involves short, large-bore intravenous peripheral catheters, preferably 16-gauge or greater. Central access should be reserved for patients for whom large-bore peripheral access cannot be obtained. If intravenous access cannot be readily obtained, an intraosseous (IO) catheter can be placed to allow for the initiation of resuscitation (also see Chapter 24). Fluids, blood products, and vasopressors may be administered through this line. IO access should be exchanged for intravenous access once the patient has been stabilized because of concerns about compartment syndrome from extravasation or osteomyelitis from prolonged needle placement.

VI

In patients with mild to moderate intravascular volume loss, cardiovascular resuscitation may begin with the intravenous administration of isotonic fluids. Balanced salt solutions, such as lactated Ringer solution or Plasma-Lyte, may be preferable, as their composition and osmolality more closely resemble that of human plasma. If vital signs improve in response to resuscitation, then laboratory measurements (especially hemoglobin values) may be obtained to guide the need for blood products (also see Chapter 24). In trauma patients (also see Chapter 42), permissive hypotension may need to be employed until bleeding is controlled in patients requiring emergent surgical intervention.

In the event of moderate to severe hypovolemic shock because of acute blood loss, the empiric administration of blood products may be necessary prior to obtaining laboratory measurements. Additionally, an initial hematocrit value may be misleading if compensatory mechanisms or crystalloid resuscitation has not led to the dilution of the remaining red blood cell mass. During massive transfusion, defined as the need for 10 units packed red blood cells in 24 hours or 4 units in 1 hour, fresh frozen plasma and platelets should be administered in a 1:1:1 ratio to packed red blood cells[11] (also see Chapter 24).

## Cardiogenic Shock

Cardiogenic shock results when either the left or right ventricle is unable to contract efficiently to generate an adequate stroke volume. Ventricular end-diastolic volume rises leading to distention of the ventricle and the development of pulmonary edema in left-sided failure or distended neck veins, peripheral edema, and hepatic congestion in right-sided failure. Biventricular failure can result when the pulmonary congestion from left ventricular failure leads to pulmonary artery hypertension and concomitant right ventricular failure.

### Clinical Manifestations

Causes of cardiogenic shock include acute myocardial infarction, severe cardiomyopathy, myocarditis, arrhythmia, valvular rupture, or ventricular septal defect. A decreased stroke volume reduces cardiac output and arterial blood pressure. To maintain systolic blood pressure, compensatory tachycardia occurs to offset the decreased stroke volume. This often worsens myocardial oxygen balance as the tachycardia increases oxygen consumption by allowing less time for diastolic subendocardial perfusion. Increasing end-diastolic pressure further reduces subendocardial blood flow, worsening oxygen delivery to the failing ventricle. As ventricular function continues to fail, the compensatory tachycardia is unable to maintain cardiac output and hypotension follows. Patients often develop poorly perfused extremities as sympathetic outflow leads to peripheral vasoconstriction.

### Treatment

Pharmacologic interventions aim to improve cardiac output, cardiac filling pressures, and myocardial oxygen balance. Invasive monitors, including arterial and central venous lines, help to guide therapy. PAOP measurements may be indicated, but the risks and benefits of pulmonary artery line placement must be carefully considered. In severe cardiogenic shock with hypotension, the administration of inotropic and vasopressor support helps to increase perfusion to the myocardium and other vital organs, but may increase myocardial oxygen demand. For severe hypotension, administration of norepinephrine as compared to dopamine improves outcomes with fewer arrhythmias.[12]

When hypotension is absent, dobutamine should be given to provide inotropic support. As an inodilator, dobutamine often decreases arterial blood pressure but improves forward flow and perfusion of vital organs. Often norepinephrine and dobutamine are administered in combination to improve cardiac output while maintaining adequate coronary artery filling pressures. Diuresis is key to improving cardiac filling pressures but should be undertaken judiciously if the hemodynamics are tenuous. In patients with evidence of cardiogenic shock accompanied by hypertension, vasodilators such as nitroprusside or nitroglycerin may help to decrease afterload and preload and improve forward flow.

Reversible causes of cardiogenic shock should be identified and addressed. For patients with cardiogenic shock complicating an acute myocardial infarction, early revascularization improves mortality rate.[13] Angiography with stenting is preferred when this procedure can be accomplished within 90 minutes. Otherwise, fibrinolytic therapy should be considered when not contraindicated. In the case of tachyarrhythmias precipitating cardiogenic shock, the preferred antiarrhythmic is amiodarone as it possesses less negative inotropic affects than β-adrenergic blockers or calcium channel blockers.

For selected patients with severe heart failure (i.e., left ventricular ejection fraction < 25% and hemodynamic compromise), mechanical support (i.e., intra-aortic balloon pump, extracorporeal membrane oxygenator, or left ventricular assist device) is a treatment option.

## Vasodilatory Shock

Vasodilatory shock encompasses an array of well-defined clinical entities that include septic, anaphylactic, and neurogenic shock. Vasodilatory shock results from profound dilation of the arterial vascular system leading to decreased systemic vascular resistance (SVR) and hypotension. Capillary leakage of intravascular volume into the extracellular space further worsens the hemodynamics and leads to tissue hypoperfusion, which results in anaerobic metabolism and lactic acidosis. Tachycardia and increased stroke volume attempt to compensate for the decrease in SVR to restore arterial blood pressure. If the underlying process continues to evolve, multiorgan ischemia and failure develop.

## Clinical Manifestations

Vasodilation occurs via different mechanisms in septic, anaphylactic, and neurogenic shock. Septic shock occurs because of release of cytokines and an inflammatory response. Anaphylaxis is due to release of mediators from white blood cells triggered by immunologic mechanisms. Neurogenic shock generally follows a traumatic injury to the brain or spinal cord in which sympathetic outflow to the periphery is interrupted. The pooling of blood in vascular beds from low SVR leads to hypotension and circulatory failure. In early vasodilatory shock, patients may present with warm extremities. However, with disease progression, the skin can become cool and cyanotic as a result of poor end-organ perfusion.

## Treatment

Treatment first involves replacement of the effective circulatory volume initially lost owing to pooling of venous blood or capillary leakage. When resuscitation of intravascular volume is unable to restore circulation, vasopressors should be given.

For septic shock, norepinephrine is considered the vasopressor of choice. Norepinephrine helps to restore SVR and arterial blood pressure through its $\alpha_1$-adrenergic effects, while also providing cardiac support through its $\beta_1$-adrenergic effects. When compared to dopamine, norepinephrine results in fewer arrhythmias. When norepinephrine alone is not adequate to restore arterial blood pressure, epinephrine or vasopressin can be added. Epinephrine can also substitute for norepinephrine, but vasopressin is not recommended as the single initial vasopressor, and doses larger than 0.03 to 0.04 units/min should be reserved for salvage therapy.

In neurogenic shock, adequate perfusion to the injured spinal cord must be maintained to limit secondary ischemic injury, so the goal is to institute early appropriate fluid resuscitation. If there is an inadequate response to intravascular fluid resuscitation, vasopressors with $\alpha$- and $\beta$-adrenergic activity should be initiated to counter the loss of sympathetic tone and provide chronotropic cardiac support if bradycardia is present.

Anaphylactic shock is treated initially with epinephrine as the vasopressor of choice. Epinephrine helps alleviate the bronchospasm that accompanies severe anaphylaxis, through its $\beta_2$-adrenergic effects, while also increasing SVR, stroke volume, and heart rate. Secondary treatments for anaphylaxis (i.e., histamine $H_1$ and $H_2$ blockers, bronchodilators, and glucocorticoids) do not prevent airway edema, hypotension, or shock and should not delay the administration of epinephrine.

## Hemodynamic Monitoring

Appropriate monitoring of patients with shock plays a key role in treatment. Intensive care settings not only allow for more frequent monitoring but also for the placement of continuous, invasive monitors (i.e., arterial, central, and pulmonary artery catheters [PACs]).

### Arterial Pressure

Arterial catheters are the most commonly inserted invasive monitors in the ICU. Besides obtaining minute-to-minute information regarding arterial blood pressure, arterial waveform analysis has gained acceptance as a tool to predict a patient's hemodynamic response to intravascular volume expansion. Chapter 20 describes variables derived from the arterial line, including systolic pressure variation (SPV) and pulse pressure variation (PPV). PPV is more accurate than cardiac filling pressures (central venous pressure [CVP], PAOP) to predict intravascular fluid responsiveness.

### Central Venous Pressure

CVP monitoring, generally recorded at the junction of the superior vena cava and the right atrium, traditionally guided fluid therapy. However, CVP is a poor predictor of fluid responsiveness[14] (also see Chapter 20). Given their risks, central venous catheters should rarely be placed solely for measurement of CVP.

### Pulmonary Artery Catheter

In the ICU, PAC use has associated insertion risks and lack of documented benefit. Randomized controlled trials in patients with ARDS were unable to demonstrate improved outcomes with the use of PACs as compared to CVP catheters. Clinical care has shifted more toward the use of noninvasive hemodynamic monitoring that offers dynamic measures of intravascular fluid responsiveness.

### Bedside Ultrasonography

The use of bedside ultrasonography (including echocardiography) has increased in the ICU because of its ability to provide rapid information to aid in clinical diagnosis and management. The goal is to perform a focused examination to answer a specific clinical question.

With training in focused point-of-care echocardiography, critical care physicians are able to correctly identify ventricular dysfunction more than 80% of the time. The limitation of echocardiography is that it cannot provide continuous monitoring, but it can offer additional information such as valvular or pericardial anatomy.

In terms of fluid management, ultrasonography evaluation of the inferior vena cava (IVC) offers a noninvasive method to assess fluid responsiveness in patients who are mechanically ventilated. IVC size alone can be an indicator of volume status but not volume responsiveness (improved cardiac output after fluid challenge). IVC diameter variation (>15%) with positive-pressure

**VI**

ventilation has correlated well with volume responsiveness. However, measurements should be taken during positive-pressure ventilation, the tidal volume should be at least 8 mL/kg, and the heart should be in sinus rhythm. Measurements taken during spontaneous respiration are less reliable because of variability in tidal volume and degree of IVC collapse.

Bedside ultrasonography can also provide procedural guidance for placement of peripheral intravenous catheters, arterial lines, and central venous catheters. Use of real-time ultrasound for internal jugular central line placement has been associated with fewer complications, fewer failed attempts, and shorter procedure times. There are fewer studies of ultrasound guidance for placement of arterial lines or subclavian central lines, but use of ultrasonography may improve the success rates of those procedures as well.

Ultrasonography can also help identify many pulmonary diseases in the ICU such as pleural effusion, pulmonary edema, pneumonia, and pneumothorax. For example, when alveoli are filled with fluid, reverberation artifacts can be seen on the pleural surface, which are called "B-lines" or "lung rockets." Identification of these B-lines indicates airspace disease, consistent with the diagnosis of ARDS, pulmonary edema, or pneumonia.

## Sepsis

Sepsis is the leading cause of death in the ICU and is the most common reason for admission to the ICU. Patients with septic shock suffer an overwhelming systemic inflammatory response, which often ends in multiple organ dysfunction syndrome (MODS) and death. Many approaches have been proposed and negated over the past 10 years (e.g., activated protein C, tight glucose control, and use of glucocorticoids). However, the fundamental approach of early recognition, rapid cardiorespiratory resuscitation, immediate antibiotic administration, and identification and treatment of the infectious source has withstood the test of time.

The 2001 clinical trial of early goal-directed therapy (EGDT) in sepsis was based on (1) intravascular fluid resuscitation, (2) vasopressors to achieve a mean arterial pressure goal, and (3) packed red blood cell transfusion or dobutamine infusion to improve central venous oxygen saturation. The entire protocol-based algorithm occurred in the emergency department for 6 hours prior to ICU transfer.[15] The trial was monumental because the protocol group had improved clinical outcomes (shorter length of hospitalization and lower mortality rate). Subsequently, the algorithm was integrated into many ICU sepsis treatment bundles. However, three multicenter randomized controlled trials were recently published comparing EGDT with usual care or protocol-based standard care.[16-18] All three trials showed no decrease in mortality rate from EGDT compared with usual care, which did not mandate the more controversial components of the 2001 protocol

---

> **Box 41.2** Updated Surviving Sepsis Campaign Bundle
>
> Complete within 3 hours of presentation
>     Measure lactate level
>     Obtain blood cultures prior to antibiotic administration
>     Administer antibiotics
>     Give 30 mL/kg crystalloid for hypotension or lactate
>       ≥ 4 mmol/L
> Complete within 6 hours of presentation
>     For hypotension unresponsive to fluid resuscitation, start
>       vasopressors for MAP ≥ 65 mm Hg
>     Assess volume status and tissue perfusion if persistent hypotension (MAP < 65 mm Hg) or initial lactate ≥ 4 mmol/L
>     Repeat lactate if initial value was elevated

MAP, Mean arterial pressure.

(i.e., central venous oxygen saturation monitoring, blood transfusions, and inotropes).

The Surviving Sepsis Campaign (SSC) Executive Committee recently revised their guidelines because of the new evidence presented[19] (Box 41.2). Based on the current data, sepsis care should involve early aggressive intravascular fluid resuscitation targeting end points such as fluid responsiveness and lactate clearance (as opposed to central venous oxygen saturation monitoring or CVP measurements). Early antibiotic administration and source control are important components to sepsis management. Vasopressors can be used to support organ perfusion after intravascular volume repletion, and central lines should not be inserted in all patients unless indicated clinically.

Finally, goal-directed, liberal fluid administration during the acute phase of sepsis offers important benefits, but excess fluid is not beneficial when it is not physiologically needed during the established phase of sepsis. In the Fluid and Catheter Treatment Trial (FACTT) of patients with acute lung injury (mostly owing to pneumonia or sepsis), patients in the "conservative fluid" (i.e., minimal use of fluids) management group had improved lung function, improved central nervous system (CNS) function, and a decreased need for sedation, mechanical ventilation, and intensive care when compared to a liberal fluid group.[20] In addition, the patients in the conservative fluid management group did not have an increased incidence of complications, such as organ failure or shock. Perhaps the final lesson from all these studies is that management should be based on clinical examination findings and patient requirements as opposed to absolute numbers obtained by invasive monitors.

## ACUTE RENAL FAILURE

### Epidemiology

The incidence of acute kidney injury (AKI) in the ICU is highly variable and can be as high as 35%. Despite improvements in renal replacement technology, mortality rate caused by AKI in the ICU has remained at more than 50%.

**Table 41.6**   The RIFLE Criteria

| RIFLE Category | GFR Criteria | UO Criteria | OR Hospital Mortality |
|---|---|---|---|
| Risk | Cr increased × 1.5 or GFR decreased >25% | UO <0.5 mL/kg/h × 6 h | 2.2 (95% CI 2.17-2.3) |
| Injury | Cr increased × 2 or GFR decreased >50% | UO <0.5 mL/kg/h × 12 h | 6.1 (95% CI 5.74-6.44) |
| Failure | Increased Cr × 3 or GFR decrease >75% or Cr > 4 mg/dL | UO <0.3 mL/kg/h × 24 h or Anuria × 12 h | 8.6 (95% CI 8.07-9.15) |
| Loss | Complete loss of renal function For > 4 wk | | |
| ESRD | End-stage disease | | |

*Cr*, Creatinine; *ESRD*, end-stage renal disease; *GFR*, glomerular filtration rate; *OR*, odds ratio; *UO*, urine output.
Data modified from Global KDI, Group OKAKIW. Kidney Disease Improving Global Outcomes (KDIGO) clinical practice guideline for acute kidney injury. *Kidney Int.* 2012;(suppl 2):1-138.

## Diagnosis

The definition of AKI has not been straightforward and multiple criteria are used in the literature. The Acute Dialysis Quality Initiative (ADQI) group, an alliance of experts consisting of nephrologists and intensivists, proposed the RIFLE criteria (Table 41.6), which stands for risk, injury, failure, and two outcome classes (loss and end-stage kidney disease).[21] For each increasing RIFLE class, there is a stepwise increase in mortality rate independent of a comorbid condition. Strategies to prevent even mild AKI may improve survival, and recovery of renal function in the ICU should be a specific therapeutic target.

Acute renal failure (ARF) is normally categorized by prerenal, renal, and postrenal causes (Box 41.3). The workup should include careful physical examination and assessment of intravascular volume status in order to differentiate hypovolemia leading to prerenal azotemia versus hypervolemia from oliguria. Laboratory evaluations should include serum and urine electrolytes, urinalysis, and examination of urinary sediment. Urine sodium concentration and fractional excretion of sodium can help identify prerenal azotemia. In patients who have received a diuretic, the fractional excretion of urea may be a more sensitive test than fractional excretion of sodium.

## Treatment

Supportive care should be focused on maintenance of euvolemia, avoidance of nephrotoxic drugs, medication

**Box 41.3**   Causes of Acute Renal Failure

**Prerenal**
Hypovolemia
Low effective circulating volume (decompensated heart failure or liver disease)
**Renal**
Glomerulonephritis
Toxins (NSAIDs, cisplatin, aminoglycosides, contrast agent, myoglobin, hemoglobin)
Vasculitis (TTP/HUS)
AIN (PCN, cephalosporins, cimetidine, SLE, sarcoidosis)
Tubular disease (ATN, tumor lysis syndrome)
**Postrenal**
Obstructive nephropathy

*AIN,* Acute interstitial nephritis; *ATN,* acute tubular necrosis; *NSAIDs,* nonsteroidal antiinflammatory drugs; *PCN,* penicillin; *SLE,* systemic lupus erythematosus; *TTP/HUS,* thrombotic thrombocytopenic purpura/hemolytic uremic syndrome.

dose adjustments for creatinine clearance, and electrolyte and acid-base monitoring. Platelet dysfunction may occur as a result of uremia and require desmopressin (DDAVP) for support if bleeding is problematic. Pharmacologic approaches to improve renal function such as low-dose dopamine, diuretics, and *N*-acetylcysteine have not shown benefit. Dialysis is often required in patients with advanced renal failure to help with excessive intravascular volume and electrolyte disturbances.

## Dialysis

Dialysis in the ICU patient is often accomplished by continuous renal replacement therapy (CRRT). Although CRRT has several theoretical advantages over intermittent hemodialysis (IHD), randomized trials have not supported its superiority.[22] The difference in efficacy lies not in the type of dialysis (IHD vs. CRRT), but in the dialysis dose. Inadequate dialysis appears to be harmful, but intensive dose dialysis is also not beneficial in terms of mortality rate, renal function recovery, or ICU length of stay.[23,24] The important factor seems to be achieving the prescribed dose.

## PAIN AND SEDATION

Pain and agitation are commonly underrecognized and undertreated in the ICU, yet there are important hemodynamic and psychological consequences associated with unrelieved pain and agitation, such as impaired wound healing, increased levels of catecholamines, and development of posttraumatic stress disorder (also see Chapter 40). Unfortunately, many patients in the ICU are unable to self-report pain and discomfort. Although vital signs may indicate the presence of pain and agitation, hypertension and tachycardia should not be used alone in the assessment.

VI

**Table 41.7** Commonly Used Sedatives and Analgesics

| Drug | Elimination Half-Time | Peak Effect[a] | Suggested Dose |
|------|----------------------|----------------|----------------|
| Morphine | 2 to 4 h | 30 min | 1 to 4 mg bolus 1 to 10 mg/h |
| Fentanyl | 2 to 5 h | 4 min | 25 to 100 μg bolus 25 to 200 μg/h |
| Hydromorphone | 2 to 4 h | 20 min | 0.2 to 1 mg bolus 0.2 to 5 mg/h |
| Ketamine | 2 to 3 h | 30 to 60 s | 1 to 5 ug/kg/min |
| Midazolam | 3 to 5 h | 2 to 5 min | 1 to 2 mg bolus 0.5 to 10 mg/h |
| Lorazepam | 10 to 20 h | 2 to 20 min | 1 to 2 mg bolus 0.5 to 10 mg/h |
| Propofol | 20 to 30 h | 90 s | 25 to 100 μg/kg/min |
| Dexmedetomidine | 2 h | 1 to 2 min | 0.2 to 0.7 μg/kg/h |

[a]With intravenous administration.

Commonly used sedatives and analgesics are listed in Table 41.7 (also see Chapters 8 and 9). The choice of which drug to use should depend on the effect that is desired. Pain control should be treated with analgesics, whereas anxiolysis should be accomplished with sedatives. Specific concerns related to the use of these medications in the ICU will be addressed in the next sections.

## Analgesia

Opioids are the first-line treatment for pain (also see Chapter 9). They can be administered by continuous infusion, as needed boluses, or patient-controlled methods if the patient is neurologically intact and not heavily sedated. Fentanyl is the most frequently used opioid in the ICU owing to its pharmacokinetics (e.g., relatively short duration of action) and lack of active metabolites. Methadone is a synthetic, long-acting opioid that has a unique place in the ICU. It is often administered to patients who have been receiving narcotic infusions for a prolonged time or who require large narcotic doses because of chronic pain. Because of its long half-life, methadone dose should be increased slowly to avoid oversedation. Methadone has been associated with QT-interval prolongation and torsades de pointes, so electrocardiogram (ECG) monitoring is essential for ICU patients.

Multimodal analgesia with nonopioid drugs may help limit the narcotic side effects and is encouraged in ICU patients. Adjuncts include acetaminophen, ketamine, antiepileptics (gabapentin and carbamazepine), $\alpha_2$-adrenergic agonists (clonidine and dexmedetomidine), tramadol, antidepressants, and topical lidocaine. In addition, for postoperative pain, regional anesthesia techniques may also limit total narcotic dose (also see Chapter 40).

## Sedation

Sedation is used in the ICU to provide anxiolysis, amnesia, and comfort and ensure the safety of life-sustaining interventions (e.g., inadvertent patient removal of central lines, ETTs, or drains). Sedatives can also assist with mechanical ventilator dyssynchrony, seizure control, intracranial pressure reduction, and alcohol withdrawal.

### Benzodiazepines

Benzodiazepines are commonly administered for ICU sedation because they provide anxiolysis and anterograde amnesia. In addition, they are often used to prevent or treat seizures and alcohol withdrawal symptoms. Midazolam causes less ventilatory and cardiovascular depression when compared with propofol. However, benzodiazepines may contribute to the development of ICU delirium, especially in elderly patients.

### Propofol

Propofol has pharmacologic properties such as rapid onset and relatively short duration of action, which are ideal for the mechanically ventilated ICU patient who requires frequent neurologic evaluation. It is also useful in treating seizures and decreasing intracranial pressure. Propofol has no analgesic effects, so an opioid may be necessary concurrently.

In addition, propofol decreases myocardial contractility and SVR, so it may not be the drug of choice in severely hypotensive patients. Because of its respiratory depressant effects, propofol should be used for sedation only in intubated patients or for procedural sedation in nonintubated patients with the presence of an anesthesia provider.

The propofol preparation contains lecithin and has a high fat content, so patients on prolonged infusions should be monitored for hypertriglyceridemia and the development of pancreatitis. For ICU patients on total parenteral nutrition, the propofol infusion needs to be accounted for when calculating caloric requirements.

Propofol infusion syndrome (PRIS) is a rare syndrome caused by mitochondrial dysfunction and characterized by metabolic acidosis, hyperkalemia, rhabdomyolysis, and fatty liver infiltration. Cardiac complications may include nonspecific symptoms such as acute refractory bradycardia and right bundle branch block. It is more common in children, but predisposing factors include infusion rates of more than 5 mg/kg/h for more than 48 hours in patients with critical illness receiving vasopressors or glucocorticoids. Early recognition of the syndrome and discontinuation of the propofol infusion reduce morbidity and mortality rates, which can be as high as 80%.

### $\alpha_2$-Receptor Agonists

The sedative effect from dexmedetomidine resembles more of a physiologic sleep state than the other sedatives. In the ICU, a dexmedetomidine infusion of 0.2 to 1.2 µg/kg/h can be started without an initial bolus dose. Dexmedetomidine use in critically ill adults reduced the duration of mechanical ventilation and ICU length of stay compared with traditional sedatives such as propofol, midazolam, and lorazepam.[25]

### N-Methyl-D-Aspartate Receptor Antagonist

A ketamine infusion (1 to 5 µg/kg/min) can be used in the ICU to limit opioid tolerance and provide analgesia without respiratory depression. Ketamine is also useful in small bolus doses (0.2 to 0.8 mg/kg IV) for patients who need to undergo brief, painful procedures (e.g., burn dressing changes). The sympathomimetic properties of ketamine are associated with better preservation of arterial blood pressure and heart rate, but ketamine is still a direct myocardial depressant and may lead to hypotension when given to patients in shock.

## Sedation Interruption

Meta-analyses have not shown strong evidence for protocol-directed sedation and daily sedation interruption because of the heterogeneity between trials. However, lighter levels of sedation or daily sedation interruption (also called "sedation wake-up") are the expected standard instead of deep, uninterrupted sedation.[26] In single center studies, daily sedation wake-up with retitration led to shorter durations of mechanical ventilation and ICU lengths of stay when compared with weaning based on the discretion of the intensivist.[27,28] Rapid weaning of sedation did not increase complications such as unplanned tracheal extubation, myocardial ischemia, or delirium. Combining sedation wake-up with protocol-driven ventilator weaning reduced duration of mechanical ventilation, mortality rate, and ICU length of stay.[29] This practice has become the preferred method and the standard of care in most ICUs.

## OTHER TOPICS IN CRITICAL CARE

## Delirium

Delirium, characterized as an acute onset of waxing and waning mental status, occurs frequently in critically ill

| Table 41.8 | Confusion Assessment Method for the Intensive Care Unit (CAM-ICU) Delirium Assessment |
|---|---|

**CAM-ICU Worksheet**

| | |
|---|---|
| Feature 1: Acute onset of mental status changes or a fluctuating course | |
| Feature 2: Inattention | Ask patient to squeeze your hand whenever he hears the letter "A." Read S...A...V...E...A...H...A...A...R...T. |
| | Points are given when patient squeezes on "A" and does not squeeze on other letters. |
| | This feature is positive if score is 8 or less |
| Feature 3: Disorganized thinking | Ask patient questions, 1 point for each correct answer. |
| | Will a stone float on water? Are there fish in the sea? Does one pound weigh more than two pounds? Can you use a hammer to pound a nail? |
| | Ask patient to hold up fingers on left hand and right hand: 1 point if able to successfully complete the entire command. |
| | This feature is positive if score is less than 4. |
| Feature 4: Altered level of consciousness | Considered positive if the RASS score is anything other than zero |

Overall CAM-ICU is positive if Features 1 and 2 and either Feature 3 or 4 are positive.
RASS, Richmond Agitation-Sedation Scale.
Modified from E. Wesley Ely, MD, MPH, and Vanderbilt University, all rights reserved. Copyright © 2002.

patients. Delirium can be divided into two subtypes, hyperactive and hypoactive. Hyperactive delirium is characterized by periods of agitation, restlessness, and emotional lability. This patient is often pulling out lines and catheters or hitting and biting. Hypoactive delirium is characterized by flat affect and apathy. Patients may seem calm and alert, but they suffer from the same cognitive changes as the hyperactive form. Both forms occur with equal frequency.

Delirium independently predicts ICU outcomes such as mortality rate, hospital length of stay, cost of care, and the development of post-ICU syndrome. All ICU patients should routinely be screened for delirium with tools such as the Confusion Assessment Method for the ICU (CAM-ICU) (Table 41.8).

The causes of delirium are numerous. Factors that can contribute to delirium in the ICU patient include

**VI**

preexisting cognitive impairment, advanced age, increasing severity of illness, multiorgan dysfunction, sepsis, immobilization, sleep deprivation, pain, mechanical ventilation, and the use of benzodiazepines. Nonpharmacologic prevention strategies, such as early mobilization, physical and occupational therapy visits, and reorientation help to reduce the incidence of delirium and improve other ICU outcomes. When these strategies are unsuccessful, antipsychotic medications, including haloperidol and atypical antipsychotics, may be administered, but their efficacy has yet to be adequately demonstrated in randomized controlled trials.[30]

## Nutrition

The goal of nutrition in the ICU is to preserve lean body mass and avoid malnourishment, which can lead to increased mortality rate, prolonged hospital stay, poor wound healing, and increased risk for infection. However, there are no reliable laboratory markers to determine the patients at risk, because of fluctuating volume status and impaired protein synthesis associated with critical illness and multiorgan failure.

Estimates of daily caloric requirements can be calculated from various equations. The Harris Benedict equation estimates basal energy expenditure based on weight, height, age, and gender, but then adjustments must be made for the underlying disease processes such as infections, multisystem organ dysfunction, trauma, and burns. A quick estimate of whether the patient is receiving enough calories can be based on weight and level of stress or illness (Table 41.9). Sometimes, a simple nutritional plan can be started based on these estimates, and then further tests (e.g., nitrogen balance study) can be obtained to assess the adequacy of the protein-based calories.

Enteral nutrition is always preferred to parenteral nutrition in order to maintain gut integrity, but achieving goal rate or goal calories is not urgent, at least for the first week.[31] Vomiting and aspiration of gastric contents have long been a concern for critically ill patients fed via a feeding tube. In the past, feedings were often reduced or held for minimal gastric residual volume (GRV), leading patients to receive only a small portion of their estimated caloric requirement over time. Current literature does not support this practice, so significantly larger GRVs are now accepted (500 mL or more in some institutions).

Patients undergoing frequent surgeries (like burn débridements) may end up malnourished from frequent nutritional holds that start at midnight or 8 hours prior to surgery. With increased emphasis on continuing enteral nutrition, there has been a shift toward decreasing nil per os or nothing by mouth (NPO) times for critically ill patients having surgical procedures. One approach is to continue enteral feeding until just prior to transport to the operating room for patients receiving postpyloric or jejunal feeding.[32] At some institutions, this "short duration NPO" approach is also used for ICU patients with gastric tubes (oral, nasal, or percutaneous gastrostomy), with the added step of aspiration of the gastric tube with a syringe to empty the stomach prior to transport. Standard NPO times may still be necessary prior to procedures involving the airway (tracheostomies or laryngectomies). No definitive data exist to guide practice and ultimately the decision is based on a hospital's practice and the clinical discretion of the anesthesia provider.

## Glucose Control

Based on a landmark 2001 study, intensive insulin therapy to achieve a blood glucose level between 80 and 110 mg/dL was thought to be essential for improving survival in the ICU.[33] However, more recent (2009, 2010) data have shown that intensive insulin therapy does not improve survival and actually increases the risks of hypoglycemia and mortality.[34,35] Currently, it appears that tight glycemic control, and even routine normalization of plasma glucose, may not be the right goal, and instead, moderate glucose levels (between 140 to 180 mg/dL) are more appropriate for the ICU patient. Using moderate glucose levels as a goal can minimize the risk of severe hypoglycemia (less than 40 mg/dL) and hyperglycemia (more than 200 mg/dL). The optimal glucose target is not known and will vary by patient, clinical scenario, and even rate of glucose change.

## Prophylaxis

### Venous Thromboembolism

Critically ill patients are at increased risk for venous thromboembolisms (VTEs), including deep vein thrombosis (DVT) and pulmonary embolism. Along with risk factors for the general population, independent risk factors specific to critically ill patients include mechanical ventilation, central venous catheterization, vasopressor administration, and platelet transfusion.

| Table 41.9 | Quick Estimate of Caloric Needs |
| --- | --- |

| Level of Illness/Stress | Estimated Caloric Need |
| --- | --- |
| Maintenance or minimal | 25-30 kcal/kg/day |
| Moderate | 30-35 kcal/kg/day |
| Severe | 35-40 kcal/kg/day |

The nutritional intake composition should be 1.2-2 g/kg/day protein, 15% to 30% of calories should be from lipids, and the remainder of the calories should be from carbohydrates (30% to 70%).

Randomized controlled trials reveal that chemoprophylaxis significantly reduces the occurrence of DVTs. Chemoprophylaxis may be achieved with unfractionated heparin (UFH) or low-molecular-weight heparin (LMWH).[36] The American College of Chest Physicians recommends either UFH or LMWH in patients with moderate risk for VTE, whereas high-risk patients, such as trauma and orthopedic patients, should receive LMWH. In patients at increased risk for bleeding complications, mechanical thromboprophylaxis (e.g., graduated compression stockings, intermittent pneumatic compression devices) provides some level of protection against VTE, but it is less effective than chemoprophylaxis.

### Gastrointestinal Prophylaxis

Gastrointestinal stress ulcers occur in critically ill patients owing to an increase in gastric acid production in conjunction with a functionally impaired mucosal barrier. Gastrointestinal bleeding occurs more frequently in patients who are mechanically ventilated for more than 48 hours and in those with a coagulopathy (Box 41.4). Patients in the ICU who are considered high risk for gastrointestinal hemorrhage should be started on prophylaxis. Either $H_2$ blockers or proton-pump inhibitors provide protection with the data somewhat favoring proton-pump inhibitors. Because of cost, an enteral route is preferred. The potential risks of developing hospital-associated pneumonia or *Clostridium difficile* infection because of an increased gastric pH should be weighed against the benefits in patients at risk for ICU-related gastrointestinal hemorrhage.

## Hospital-Acquired Infections

The most common hospital-acquired infections (HAIs) in ICUs are urinary tract infections (31%), followed by pneumonia (27%), and primary bloodstream infections (19%). By reducing HAIs, hospitals can improve mortality rate and reduce cost. The Centers for Medicare and Medicaid

---

> **Box 41.4** Indications for Gastrointestinal Prophylaxis
>
> History of GI bleed within last year
> Mechanical ventilation > 48 hours
> Coagulopathy not from pharmacologic anticoagulation (platelet count < $50 \times 10^9$/L, INR > 1.5, or PTT > 2 × control)
> Trauma
> Spinal cord injury
> Severe traumatic brain injury
> Extensive thermal injury or burns
> High-dose steroids in patients with severe sepsis or septic shock

*GI*, Gastrointestinal; *INR*, international normalized ratio; *PTT*, partial thromboplastin time.

---

Services no longer reimburse hospitals for additional costs associated with HAI.

### Catheter-Associated Urinary Tract Infections

No single strategy prevents catheter-associated urinary tract infections. The only recommendations have been to use aseptic techniques for placement and to limit the duration of indwelling urinary catheters by assessing for daily need.

### Ventilator-Associated Pneumonia

Positioning the head of the bed at 30 degrees is the most cost-effective intervention to prevent VAP. In patients anticipated to have a prolonged course of tracheal intubation with mechanical ventilation, the use of ETTs with subglottic suctioning appears effective for prevention. Excessive use of medications for stress ulcer prophylaxis increases gastric pH and increases the risk for VAP. Clinicians will need to balance the risks and benefits of using $H_2$-receptor antagonists or proton-pump inhibitors. The concept of preventing mechanical ventilation adverse events, including VAP, by use of a bundle (multiple single interventions implemented simultaneously) is common practice in many ICUs.[37]

### Catheter-Related Bloodstream Infections

The prevention of catheter-related bloodstream infections (CRBSIs) is achievable through large-scale quality improvement projects that involve a bundle of evidence-based interventions. Recommendations include the use of ultrasound guidance for line placement, skin preparation with chlorhexidine, chlorhexidine sponge for site dressing, antimicrobial impregnated central lines, and maximal sterile barrier use during line placement. Broad implementation of these interventions can substantially reduce the risk and morbidity of these infections.[38]

## ICU Staffing and Organization

Because of the increased complexity of care, ICUs have required more specialized staff, which can include physicians, nurses, nurse practitioners, physician assistants, respiratory therapists, physical therapists, pharmacists, nutritionists, and patient care assistants. The use of nonphysician providers, such as nurse practitioners and physician assistants under the supervision of attending critical care physicians, has become more prevalent with the institution of resident duty hour limitations in the United States. The presence of pharmacists reduces fatalities in patients with infections and sepsis, and the rate of adverse drug events. Respiratory therapist involvement improves compliance with weaning protocols and decreases duration of mechanical ventilation. The multidisciplinary team has been shown to improve mortality rate for critically ill patients.[39]

VI

## QUESTIONS OF THE DAY

1. A spontaneously breathing, mechanically ventilated patient is receiving pressure support ventilation. What determines the inspiratory flow rate and duration of each breath?

2. Which type of intensive care unit (ICU) patient is most likely to benefit from noninvasive positive-pressure ventilation (NPPV)? What are the most commonly encountered contraindications to NPPV?

3. What respiratory criteria predict successful weaning from mechanical ventilation? What nonrespiratory criteria can have an impact on the weaning process?

4. What mechanical ventilation strategy is most appropriate for a patient with acute respiratory distress syndrome (ARDS)?

5. What are the most common clinical conditions that can cause vasodilatory shock?

6. How can bedside ultrasonography be used to predict intravascular fluid responsiveness (improvement in blood pressure with intravenous fluid bolus) in a patient receiving positive-pressure ventilation?

7. In a patient who is mechanically ventilated, what is the impact of "sedation interruption" strategies on duration of ventilation and length of ICU stay?

8. What is the confusion assessment method for the intensive care unit (CAM-ICU) method of delirium assessment? What nonpharmacologic methods can help to prevent delirium in the ICU patient?

9. Which critically ill patients are most likely to develop gastrointestinal stress ulcers?

10. What are the most common hospital-acquired infections in the ICU?

## REFERENCES

1. Frat JP, Thille AW, Mercat A, et al. High-flow oxygen through nasal cannula in acute hypoxemic respiratory failure. *N Engl J Med.* 2015;372:2185–2196.

2. McConville JF, Kress JP. Weaning patients from the ventilator. *N Engl J Med.* 2012;367:2233–2239.

3. Ladeira MT, Vital FMR, Andriolo RB, et al. Pressure support versus T-tube for weaning from mechanical ventilation in adults. *Cochrane Database Syst Rev.* 2014;(5):CD006056.

4. Burns KEA, O'Meade M, Premji A, et al. Noninvasive positive-pressure ventilation as a weaning strategy for intubated adults with respiratory failure. *Cochrane Database Syst Rev.* 2013;(12):CD004127.

5. Rose L, Schultz MJ, Cardwell CR, et al. Automated versus non-automated weaning for reducing the duration of mechanical ventilation for critically ill adults and children. *Cochrane Database Syst Rev.* 2014;(6):CD009235.

6. The ARDS Definition Task Force, Ranieri VM, Rubenfeld GD, Thompson BT, et al. Acute respiratory distress syndrome: the Berlin definition. *JAMA.* 2012;307(23):2526–2533.

7. The Acute Respiratory Distress Syndrome Network. Ventilation with lower tidal volumes as compared with traditional tidal volumes for acute lung injury and the acute respiratory distress syndrome. *N Engl J Med.* 2000;342(18):1301–1308.

8. Serpa Neto A, Cardoso SO, Manetta JA, et al. Association between use of lung-protective ventilation with lower tidal volumes and clinical outcomes among patients without acute respiratory distress syndrome: a meta-analysis. *JAMA.* 2012;308:1651–1659.

9. Papazian L, Forel JM, Gacouin A, et al. Neuromuscular blockers in early acute respiratory distress syndrome. *N Engl J Med.* 2010;363:1107–1116.

10. Young D, Harrison DA, Cuthbertson BH, et al. Effect of early vs late tracheostomy placement on survival in patients receiving mechanical ventilation: the TracMan randomized trial. *JAMA.* 2013;309:2121–2129.

11. Holcomb JB, Tilley BC, Baranuik S, et al. Transfusion of plasma, platelets, and red blood cells in a 1:1:1 vs a 1:1:2 ratio and mortality in patients with severe trauma: the PROPPR randomized clinical trial. *JAMA.* 2015;313:471–482.

12. De Backer D, Biston P, Devriendt J, et al. Comparison of dopamine and norepinephrine in the treatment of shock. *N Engl J Med.* 2010;362:779–789.

13. Hochman JS, Sleeper LA, Webb JG, et al. Early revascularization in acute myocardial infarction complicated by cardiogenic shock. SHOCK Investigators. Should we emergently revascularize occluded coronaries for cardiogenic shock. *N Engl J Med.* 1999;341:625–634.

14. Marik P, Baram M, Vahid B. Does central venous pressure predict fluid responsiveness? A systemic review of the literature and the tale of seven mares. *Chest.* 2008;134:172–178.

15. Rivers E, Nguyen B, Havstad S, et al. Early goal-directed therapy in the treatment of severe sepsis and septic shock. *N Engl J Med.* 2001;345:1368–1377.

16. ProCESS Investigators, Yealy DM, Kellum JA, Huang DT, et al. Randomized trial of protocol-based care for early septic shock. *N Engl J Med.* 2014;370(18):1683–1693.

17. ARISE Investigators; ANZICS Clinical Trials Group, Peake SL, Delaney A, Bailey M, et al. Goal-directed resuscitation for patients with early septic shock. *N Engl J Med.* 2014;371(16):1496–1506.

18. Mouncey PR, Osborn TM, Power GS, et al. Trial of early, goal-directed resuscitation for septic shock. *N Engl J Med.* 2015;372:1301–1311.

19. Dellinger RP, Levy MM, Rhodes A, et al. Surviving Sepsis Campaign: international guidelines for management of severe sepsis and septic shock, 2012. *Intensive Care Med.* 2013;39(2):165–228.

20. The National Heart, Lung, and Blood Institute Acute Respiratory Distress Syndrome (ARDS) Clinical Trials Network, Wiedemann HP, Wheeler AP, Bernard GR, et al. Comparison of two fluid-management strategies in acute lung injury. *N Engl J Med.* 2006;354(24):2564–2575.

21. Bellomo R, Kellum J, Ronco C, et al. Defining and classifying acute renal failure: from advocacy to consensus and validation of the RIFLE criteria. *Intensive Care Med.* 2007;33:409–413.

22. Vinsonneau C, Camus C, Combes A, et al. Continuous venovenous haemodiafiltration versus intermittent haemodialysis for acute renal failure in patients with multiple-organ dysfunction syndrome. A multicentre randomised trial. *Lancet.* 2006;368:379–385.

23. Joannidis M. Acute kidney injury in septic shock—do not under-treat! *Intensive Care Med.* 2006;32:18–20.

24. Bellomo R, Cass A, Cole L, et al. Intensity of continuous renal-replacement therapy in critically ill patients. *N Engl J Med.* 2009;361:1627–1638.

25. Chen K, Lu Z, Xin YC, et al. Alpha-2 agonists for long-term sedation during mechanical ventilation in critically ill patients. *Cochrane Database Syst Rev.* 2015;(1):CD010269.

26. Aitken LM, Bucknall T, Kent B, et al. Protocol-directed sedation versus non-protocol directed sedation to reduce duration of mechanical ventilation in mechanically ventilated intensive care patients. *Cochrane Database Syst Rev.* 2015;(1):CD009771.

27. Kress JP, Pohlman AS, O'Connor MF, et al. Daily interruption of sedative infusions in critically ill patients undergoing mechanical ventilation. *N Engl J Med.* 2000;342:1471–1477.

28. Burry L, Rose L, McCullagh IJ, et al. Daily sedation interruption versus no daily sedation interruption for critically ill adult patients requiring invasive mechanical ventilation. *Cochrane Database Syst Rev.* 2014;(7):CD009176.

29. Girard TD, Kress JP, Fuchs BD, et al. Efficacy and safety of a paired sedation and ventilator weaning protocol for mechanically ventilated patients in intensive care (Awakening and Breathing Controlled trial): a randomised controlled trial. *Lancet.* 2008;371(9607):126–134.

30. Barr J, Fraser GL, Puntillo K, et al. Clinical practice guidelines for the management of pain, agitation, and delirium in adult patients in the intensive care unit. *Crit Care Med.* 2013;41(1):263–306.

31. National Heart, Lung, and Blood Institute Acute Respiratory Distress Syndrome (ARDS) Clinical Trials Network, Rice TW, Wheeler AP, Thompson BT, et al. Initial trophic vs full enteral feeding in patients with acute lung injury: the EDEN randomized trial. *JAMA.* 2012;307(8):795–803.

32. McElroy LM, Codner PA, Brasel KJ. A pilot study to explore the safety of perioperative postpyloric enteral nutrition. *Nutr Clin Pract.* 2012;27:777–780.

33. van den Berghe G, Wouters P, Weekers F, et al. Intensive insulin therapy in critically ill patients. *N Engl J Med.* 2001;345:1359–1367.

34. The COIITSS Study Investigators. Corticosteroid treatment and intensive insulin therapy for septic shock in adults. *JAMA.* 2010;303:341–348.

35. The NICE-SUGAR Study Investigators, Finfer S, Chittock DR, Su SY, et al. Intensive versus conventional glucose control in critically ill patients. *N Engl J Med.* 2009;360:1283–1297.

36. Minet C, Potton L, Bonadona A, et al. Venous thromboembolism in the ICU: main characteristics, diagnosis and thromboprophylaxis. *Crit Care.* 2015;19:287.

37. O'Grady NP, Murray PR, Ames N. Preventing ventilator-associated pneumonia: does the evidence support the practice? *JAMA.* 2012;307:2534–2539.

38. Pronovost PJ, Goeschel CA, Colantuoni E, et al. Sustaining reductions in catheter related bloodstream infections in Michigan intensive care units: observational study. *BMJ.* 2010;340:c309.

39. Costa DK, Wallace DJ, Kahn JM. The association between daytime intensivist physician staffing and mortality in the context of other ICU organizational practices: a multicenter cohort study. *Crit Care Med.* 2015;43:2275–2282.

**VI**

# ANESTHESIA FOR TRAUMA

Marc Steurer, Tony Chang, and Benn Lancman

## INTRODUCTION

### Background

Injury is the leading cause of fatality worldwide, causing more than 5 million deaths, or 9% of the world's deaths, each year.[1] According to the Centers for Disease Control and Prevention (CDC), trauma accounted for approximately 192,900 deaths in 2013, costing over $400 billion in health care cost and productivity loss in the United States. Trauma is the most frequent cause of fatality in those aged 1 to 44 years, accounting for 31.9% of deaths in age group 1 to 9 years, 40.5% in age group 10 to 24 years, and 27.1% in age group 25 to 44 years.[2] The relative burden of disease of trauma disproportionately affects younger age groups with trauma responsible for over 30% of years of potential life lost in people younger than the age of 65 years.[3]

During the past decades, mortality trends have continued to decrease as care for the severely injured patient has improved. Emergent care for the severely injured is aggregated at designated trauma centers, which are independently verified by a strict criteria stipulated by the American College of Surgeons. The most specialized trauma centers, designated as Level I, have the ability to deliver 24-hour specialized multidisciplinary care. Trauma care delivered at Level I trauma centers decreases overall mortality risk by 25% when compared to nontrauma centers.[4] Anesthesia providers, in particular, play a vital role in the acute resuscitation and management of severely injured patients. In this chapter, the basics of trauma care for anesthesia providers will be discussed.

The editors and publisher would like to thank Dr. Eric Y. Lin for contributing to this chapter in the previous edition of this work. It has provided the framework for much of this chapter.

| Table 42.1 | Classes of Hemorrhagic Shock in Adults | | | |
|---|---|---|---|---|
| | **Class I** | **Class II** | **Class III** | **Class IV** |
| Blood loss[a] (mL) | Up to 750 | 750-1500 | 1500-2000 | >2000 |
| Blood loss (% blood volume) | Up to 15% | 15%-30% | 30%-40% | >40% |
| Pulse rate (BPM) | <100 | 100-120 | 120-140 | >140 |
| Systolic BP | Normal | Normal | Decreased | Decreased |
| Pulse pressure | Normal or increased | Decreased | Decreased | Decreased |
| Respiratory rate | 14-20 | 20-30 | 30-40 | >35 |
| Urine output (mL/h) | >30 | 20-30 | 5-15 | Negligible |
| CNS/mental status | Slightly anxious | Mildly anxious | Anxious, confused | Confused, lethargic |

[a]For 70-kg adult.
*BP*, Blood pressure; *BPM*, beats per minute; *CNS*, central nervous system.
Modified from the Advanced Trauma Life Support (ATLS) program.

## Physiology in Trauma

Physiologic derangements in patients who have suffered trauma-induced injuries depend on the mechanism and severity of injury. Most commonly, hypotension in trauma is the result of severe blood loss or "hemorrhagic shock," which is the main cause of fatality in critically injured patients. After sources of hemorrhagic shock are investigated, other causes of shock must also be considered when encountering hypotension in the setting of trauma. Relative hypovolemia from obstructed venous return in cases of tension pneumothorax or cardiac tamponade, cardiogenic shock, and neurogenic shock must be considered.

The initial presenting arterial blood pressure values of a trauma patient may be misleading in early hemorrhage. The degree of hemorrhage can be masked by compensatory reflexes via sympathetics, carotid sinus and aortic arch baroreceptors, and other low-pressure receptors. The renin-angiotensin system and vasopressin secretion from the pituitary play a later compensatory role. These responses allow sympathetic vasoconstriction of the arterioles to increase total peripheral resistance, venoconstriction to increase venous return, and an increase in heart rate. With extreme hypoxia and acidosis, the central nervous system also provides additional sympathetic stimulation.

Hemorrhagic shock can generally be divided into a compensated and progressive phase. Each phase has different characteristics depending on the acuity and volume of blood lost (Table 42.1).

In compensated hemorrhage, physiologic compensatory mechanisms that are intact may be adequate to sustain systemic perfusion without clinical intervention. About 10% to 15% of blood loss may be adequately compensated by physiology alone. As blood loss continues, hemorrhagic shock progresses and ultimately leads to multiorgan failure if resuscitation has been inadequate. If inadequate perfusion persists, generalized tissue and cellular necrosis, cardiac dysfunction, and metabolic acidosis occur.

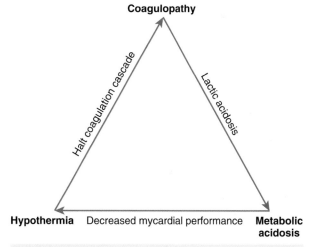

**Fig. 42.1** Lethal triad.

Hemorrhagic shock and tissue hypoperfusion subsequently lead to complex interactions between inflammatory factors, intrinsic anticoagulants, and other cellular dysfunctions that can cause an acute traumatic coagulopathy after injury. This coagulopathy is attributed to factor deficiency, hyperfibrinolysis, and platelet dysfunction. Iatrogenic factors of resuscitation can further disrupt the coagulation process. These factors include hemodilution, hypocalcemia, hypothermia, and acidosis. This is known as *trauma-induced coagulopathy*. All of these processes lead to a positive feedback loop that eventually ends in death. Hypothermia, coagulopathy, and acidosis are commonly termed the *triad of death* or *lethal triad* (Fig. 42.1). Hemorrhagic shock may cross a threshold at which it becomes irreparable despite blood transfusions and other therapies owing to severe, irreversible multiorgan failure.

VI

## INITIAL MANAGEMENT

Successfully managing a patient who has suffered a major trauma requires a coordinated systematic approach to history, examination, diagnosis, and treatment and these processes must run in parallel. Often initial management is commenced before a definitive diagnosis has been established.

Each patient has a unique constellation of injuries and mechanisms, and when combined with his or her premorbid status there are an immeasurable number of potential presentations. To prepare for the unpredictability of trauma, many of the initial assessment and management processes are standardized and clinicians must be familiar with their local institution's policies and guidelines.

This section will focus on the initial management of a major trauma patient, focusing primarily on the time in the emergency department. The initial management can significantly influence intraoperative care. The components of a mature trauma system can be divided into prearrival, the trauma bay, adjuncts, and definitive care.

### Prearrival Preparation

Preparation for the arrival of an intensely injured patient enables the trauma team to deliver rapid, effective care, which is essential for a positive outcome to occur. This involves more than just confirming that essential equipment is present and functioning. Although these checks are very important, there are also organizational and patient-specific preparations that need to be considered.

#### Universal/Organization Preparation
Caring for a major trauma patient requires the mobilization and deployment of a large and diverse range of health care resources to a single point. Preparations are not limited to, but should include the following considerations:

- Designated trauma bay in the emergency department
- Who attends trauma call? How are they notified?
- Policies and protocols regarding activation of
  - Emergency radiology
  - Emergency operating room (OR) use (also see Chapter 46)
  - Massive blood transfusion (also see Chapter 24)
  - Transport
  - Referral pathways to internal and external providers

Needless to say, these issues should be addressed before the arrival of a critically ill patient. Because of the unpredictable nature of trauma, it is reasonable to expect a novel set of circumstances that can overwhelm or bypass an organization's existing preparation. In this eventuality, it is the responsibility of the clinicians involved as members of a learning organization to alert those providing the required resources.

| Box 42.1 IMIST—Paramedic Handover Tool | |
|---|---|
| **I**dentification of the patient | Age |
| | Gender |
| | Name (if known) |
| **M**echanism/medical complaint | What happened? |
| **I**njuries/information relative to the complaint | Known/suspected injuries |
| **S**igns (vital signs and Glasgow Coma Scale score) | Presence of breath sounds |
| | Tracheal deviation |
| **T**reatment and trends/response to treatment | Vital signs |
| | Drugs |
| | Fluids |
| | Splints |

#### Patient-Specific Preparation
This should occur immediately before the arrival of a major trauma patient. Information regarding the patient's injury and status should be provided to emergency department staff by the ambulance service to facilitate resource mobilization.

Most ambulance services around the world use a standardized handover tool to provide essential information in a succinct and efficient manner. An example of this tool is IMIST, a mnemonic for *I*dentification of the patient, *M*echanism/medical complaint, *I*njuries/information relative to the complaint, *S*igns (including vital signs and Glasgow Coma Scale [GCS] score), *T*reatment and trends/response to treatment (Box 42.1).[5] With this information, the health care team can begin to anticipate what the patient's clinical needs may be and prepare accordingly.

#### Prearrival Briefing
The purpose of this briefing is to optimize team efficiency and performance. This enables all members of the team to introduce themselves, develop group situational awareness about the known condition of the patient, and to assign appropriate team roles.

### Trauma Bay

#### Primary Survey
Once the patient arrives the focus of the team shifts to rapid and simultaneous diagnosis and treatment of life-threatening conditions.

The Advanced Trauma Life Support (ATLS) approach has been widely adopted throughout the world. It is structured into primary, secondary, and tertiary surveys. This chapter will only address the primary survey.

The purpose of the primary survey is to identify and treat immediately life-threatening injuries. It is organized into the ABCDE mnemonic (*A*irway and cervical spine control, *B*reathing and oxygenation, *C*irculation and hemorrhage control, *D*isability, and *E*xposure; also see Box 42.2). The ATLS course is highly recommended as an

| Box 42.2 | Primary Survey |
|---|---|
| **A** | Airway and cervical spine control |
| **B** | Breathing and oxygenation |
| **C** | Circulation and hemorrhage control |
| **D** | Disability |
| **E** | Exposure |

Modified from the Advanced Trauma Life Support (ATLS) program.

| Box 42.3 | Patients Who May Require Endotracheal Intubation |
|---|---|

- Maxillofacial trauma
- Major hemodynamic instability
- Low $Sao_2$
- Burns
- Head injury
- Intoxicated/behavioral/safety issues
- Transport (radiology/OR/ICU/external)

*ICU*, Intensive care unit; *OR*, operating room.

introduction to trauma management. Most importantly it provides a common language and framework to organize thinking required for optimal individual and team performance.

### Airway and Oxygenation (Also See Chapter 16)

Establishment of a patent airway is of paramount importance to ensure a positive outcome for the patient. Rapid assessment is most easily achieved by asking the patient some simple questions. If the patient can speak, then the airway is usually patent. Intervention may still be required, but there is time to plan the safest treatment.

### Management of the Airway and Trauma

The need to provide a definitive patent airway for the patient (an endotracheal tube) can occur for many reasons (Box 42.3). First, the process of induction of anesthesia for the purpose of endotracheal intubation may be a high-risk and dangerous procedure. The top priority is always to maintain adequate tissue oxygenation. If a patent airway is maintained with simple airway maneuvers, then there is time to optimize the patient's physiology and properly prepare for attempting endotracheal intubation. Consideration should be given to performing a focused neurologic assessment preinduction, if the clinical situation allows. This can provide invaluable information that is very difficult to obtain in the sedated, endotracheally intubated patient.

There are several differences in the approach to intubating the trachea in a trauma patient in the emergency department as compared to an elective surgical patient in the OR.

### Preoxygenation (Administration of Oxygen Before Induction of Anesthesia)

Preoxygenation in the patient who has injuries from trauma can be challenging. The objective of preoxygenation is to "denitrogenate" the lung, thus providing a reservoir of oxygen in the patient's functional residual capacity (FRC) to prevent desaturation during the apneic phase of intubation of the trachea (also see Chapter 16). However, many of the injuries sustained by trauma patients prevent this process from being as effective as in a patient with less severe injuries. Specifically, any injury that reduces FRC or creates a shunt (lung units that are perfused but not ventilated) will increase the likelihood of desaturation despite technically adequate preoxygenation. Examples of such injuries include direct lung parenchymal injury, hemothorax or pneumothorax, tracheal aspiration of blood or gastric contents, intra-abdominal bleeding, diaphragmatic injury, and rib fractures. Addition of an alternate oxygen source to provide apneic oxygenation throughout the peri-intubation period has been discussed in the emergency department literature.[6] Despite a theoretical benefit, as a result of all the issues with preoxygenation in trauma patients, no benefit has been demonstrated in experienced laryngoscopists' hands.[7] The best defense against desaturation is reducing total apneic time.

### Fasting

All trauma patients should be assumed to have a "full stomach" even when many hours have elapsed since their last oral intake. As such, a rapid sequence induction (RSI) is considered standard practice. The use of cricoid pressure is common clinical practice but may worsen the view at laryngoscopy. A review of the evidence is presented in Chapter 16.

### Altered Physiology

Major trauma patients who require emergent tracheal intubation are often the most critically ill patients in the hospital. The justification for endotracheal intubation and the impact of that physiologic insult on their response to laryngoscopy must be clearly defined. For example, if the reason for endotracheal intubation is respiratory distress from a major lung injury, then optimal preoxygenation may still result in rapid desaturation after apnea has been instituted.

### Hemodynamic Status

The hemodynamic response to anesthetics given to induce anesthesia is often exaggerated for two main reasons. First, acute intravascular volume loss from bleeding results in an inability to maintain arterial blood pressure and cardiac output in the face of the vasodilatory effects of anesthetic drugs. Second, sympathetic overstimulation caused by pain and distress can mask the true intravascular volume state; if so, induction of anesthesia can cause marked hemodynamic instability. This can usually be

**VI**

anticipated by the appropriate intravascular administration of fluids (i.e., crystalloids, blood, colloids) and the availability of vasopressors.

## Anesthetic Drug Choices

The choice of drugs to induce anesthesia in the critically ill patient is an area of much controversy (also see Chapter 8). Propofol and, to a lesser extent, thiopental are often used. Ketamine and etomidate may be more hemodynamically stable when used to induce anesthesia. Most important is for the clinician to be very familiar and experienced with the anesthetic drugs they plan to use rather than using a new, unfamiliar drug. In general, the dose of anesthetic drug should be decreased because of a relatively reduced volume of distribution of drugs in a very ill or hypovolemic patient. Preferential perfusion to essential organs, such as the brain, heart, and kidneys, occurs in such patients. So, a vasopressor should be immediately available to manage any transient hypotension caused by the anesthetic drugs.

### Manual In-Line Stabilization

The process of laryngoscopy can produce an unacceptable amount of force through the cervical spine. Attempts should always be made to reduce this force. Any patient with a suspected spinal injury should be placed in a hard collar. The front of the collar should be loosened at the time of laryngoscopy and the head and neck stabilized by an additional clinician (also see Chapter 16). The objective is to minimize movement of the cervical spine during laryngoscopy. It is important to have a pragmatic approach though, because a failed endotracheal intubation attempt presents a much greater immediate risk (i.e., hypoxia) to the patient than small movements of the neck. In the event of poor visualization of the glottic structures, consideration should be given to relaxing manual in-line stabilization (MILS) to facilitate endotracheal intubation before replacing the hard cervical collar.

### Choice of Laryngoscope

Video laryngoscopy has transformed the manner in which airways are managed in the emergency department and OR. The advantages of video laryngoscopy are numerous:

- Gives adequate tracheal intubating view with reduced pressure and force
- Provides group situational awareness of progress of laryngoscopy
- Improves visualization of larynx in more difficult patients without the need to change equipment
- Allows supervisors and trainers to provide dynamic feedback throughout the laryngoscopy

As stated before, clinicians must be familiar with the equipment they expect to use in the trauma bay.

### Failed Endotracheal Intubation Drills

Failed endotracheal intubations are rare. Even so, it is important to prepare and be explicit about planning for the management of the unanticipated difficult airway (also see Chapter 16). Endotracheal intubation in traumatized patients is likely to be more difficult than with their elective counterparts. Factors contributing to the increased difficulty include spinal precautions, blood or foreign body in the airway, and the stress experienced by the person performing the intubation. Plans for failed intubation must be made explicit, such as what equipment will be needed, its location, and discussion on the immediate availability of staff who are assisting with intubation before induction of anesthesia. Staff who work outside the OR environment may not be familiar with equipment such as laryngeal masks or surgical airway kits and their comfort with using this type of equipment should be known in advance.

### Posttracheal Intubation Care

Endotracheal intubation is a mechanism for providing physiologic support—it is not therapeutic treatment itself. The focus of the emergency department team needs to remain on the patient's transition to definitive care. Several issues need to be managed immediately after intubation:

- Ongoing sedation—postintubation hypertension is common and should be avoided because of its effect on uncontrolled bleeding
- Ventilator and settings
- Disposition—where is the patient going next? To the computed tomography (CT) scanner, the OR, or intensive care unit (ICU)?
- Additional intravenous or arterial access, or both—these technical requirements should not delay movement to definitive care

### Special Groups

Several special circumstances need to be considered when making a decision on the management of the trauma patient's airway.

1. Airway burns: Patients with airway burns require expedited management of their airway. Within a very short time they can progress from minimal or no respiratory distress to a completely occluded airway due to edema. Warning signs of potential airway burns include facial burns, soot in mouth/nose, carbonaceous sputum, explosive injuries to upper body, and stridor.
2. Oral trauma: Blood is often in the upper airway in trauma patients. Bleeding can range from a minor nuisance to a life-threatening hemorrhage. It is important to recognize this situation (i.e., blood in the airway) because induction of anesthesia can result in the rapid

loss of a patent airway. Video laryngoscopes and fiberoptic scopes do not perform well when blood obscures the field of view. An additional suction source is mandatory and a surgical airway team should be immediately available.

3. Direct airway injury: Although uncommon, tracheal trauma should be suspected in any patient with direct penetrating or blunt trauma to the neck. Warning signs such as stridor and subcutaneous emphysema may be present. These airways should be managed only by experienced clinicians with early involvement of a head and neck surgeon (also see Chapter 31).

### Circulation and Hemorrhage Control

Adequate circulation and perfusion need to be reestablished to ensure sufficient oxygen delivery to essential organs. The priority is to stop any bleeding. This can be achieved through a combination of interventions performed in the emergency department (direct pressure, suturing wounds), surgical intervention, or angioembolization. Simultaneously, it is the role of the anesthesia provider to ensure adequate oxygen delivery to essential organs such as the brain and heart. Damage control resuscitation (DCR) is the term given to a resuscitative strategy that provides circulatory support sufficient to prevent permanent end-organ damage while avoiding the pitfalls of excessive resuscitation. The damage control approach is explained in more detail in Chapter 24. Hypothermia, acidosis, and calcium supplementation are additional considerations.

### Disability

The assessment of the neurologic system is important to identify potentially catastrophic injuries that require prompt management. This rapid assessment is based on the GCS score, pupillary response, and gross limb function. Intubation is usually required for patients with a GCS score less than 8 (Box 42.4).

### Exposure

To avoid missing major injuries that are not visible, the patient needs to be exposed and inspected on all sides, including the back, for other injuries. Simultaneously, attention is required to avoid hypothermia in the patient as this affects coagulation, oxygen consumption, and mortality risk.

## Adjuncts and Investigations

Any tests or investigations that are ordered should have an impact on diagnosis and management. Because clinical events can change rapidly and dramatically in trauma patients, timely access to information can be a considerable challenge. Results that are especially useful are ones that have a rapid turnaround time, are performed serially to follow trends, and that correlate with possible treatments that can improve outcome (Box 42.5).

---

**Box 42.4** The Glasgow Coma Scale (GCS) Score[a]

Eyes (E)
    4—Open spontaneously
    3—Open to voice
    2—Open to pain
    1—Do not open
Verbal (V)
    5—Oriented
    4—Confused
    3—Inappropriate words
    2—Incomprehensible sounds
    1—No sounds
Motor (M)
    6—Obeys commands
    5—Localizes to pain
    4—Withdraws to pain
    3—Abnormal flexion to pain
    2—Abnormal extension to pain
    1—No response
Total score = best responses for eyes, verbal, and motor
    E = 4
    V = 5
    M = 6
    Total GCS score = 15

[a]Best response used.
The Glasgow Coma Scale score is the sum of the best scores in each of the three categories, eye opening, verbal response, and motor response. The 15-point scale is the predominant one in use.

---

**Box 42.5** Initial Investigations

Minimum "standard" major trauma investigations
    Complete blood count
    Electrolytes/BUN
    Blood gas (preferably arterial)
    Chest radiograph
    Pelvis radiograph
    Coagulation testing—ideally viscoelastic testing (ROTEM/TEG)
    Blood group and antibody screen
Additional investigations to consider
    ECG
    CT scan
    General radiograph

*BUN*, Blood urea nitrogen; *CT*, computed tomography; *ECG*, electrocardiogram; *ROTEM*, rotational thromboelastometry; *TEG*, thromboelastography.

## Definitive Care and Transport

Definitive care is the process of fixing the underlying physiologic problem. Examples include stopping the bleeding, plating the fracture, or removing the spleen. Some components of definitive care should be performed emergently while others can wait for the patient's condition to improve. Depending on the patient's injuries and the capabilities of

VI

**Box 42.6** Questions to Ask Locally to Be an Effective Part of a Trauma Team

- How do we alert a major trauma?
- How do we define a major trauma?
- Who responds to trauma calls?
- What is our massive transfusion protocol?
- How do we get more help if we need it?
- What are the limits of what we can deal with locally?

**Box 42.7** Leadership

Qualities of a good leader
    Listens to the team
    Provides clear direction and expectations for patient care
    Shares uncertainty
    Delegates appropriately
    Stands back and maintains "big picture" situational awareness
Good leaders do NOT need to
    Know the most
    Be the most experienced clinician
    Always be right

**Box 42.8** Followership

Qualities of a good follower
    Uses closed-loop communication (e.g., clarify instructions, report back when task is complete)
    Offers suggestions (e.g., would you like me to…)
    Alerts the leader to changes in clinical status of patient (e.g., hypotension)
    Provides feedback on personal limitations, skills, experience
    Uses communication techniques such as graded assertiveness (see Box 42.9)

individual institutions, definitive care may require transfer to another health care facility. Either way the patient will need to move out of the emergency department.

Setting Priorities: What Is Next?

Conflict often arises when trying to decide the most appropriate location to treat the patient. Depending on the injuries sustained, there can be disagreement about the most clinically urgent injury, and thus most appropriate location for treatment; or the logistical barriers to treatment can be such that it is impossible to do everything the patient needs in a single location.

An example is major pelvic and neurosurgical trauma. The most appropriate place for management of neurosurgical trauma is the OR; however, current guidelines for pelvic trauma recommend angioembolization (also see Chapter 38). The decision about which injury to prioritize is a difficult one and should be made on the clinical nuances of that individual patient. Many Level 1 trauma centers now have hybrid ORs where both angiographic and operative interventions can be performed; thus, the treatment is coming to the patient rather than vice versa.

A reasonable alternative for many conditions is conservative management during the acute phase. This allows time for restoration of normal physiology, clarification of medical history, and a more complete assessment of the extent of injuries. Providing intensive care level observation and regular review of conditions is an extremely appropriate and responsible course of action.

Local Care Versus Transfer

Once a patient's clinical needs exceed the services provided by the institution, the process for timely transfer begins. A key aspect is to understand the local referral pathways and to seek help from the accepting hospital early. Moving a critically ill patient takes time, and timely communication with the accepting hospital enables the resources required to be mobilized and ready. Regardless of the ultimate destination, the patient's clinical status can be optimized by regular review of the ATLS primary survey. When transporting critically ill patients, the level of care received at the hospital should be continued during transfer to the new facility. Specific equipment, staff skill mix, routes, and oxygen supplies should all be considered before initiating a transfer (Box 42.6).

## Decision Making in Trauma

Mature and complex systems such as health care and trauma require multiple individuals with different and complementary skill sets to work together toward the common goal of achieving the best patient outcomes. Some simple strategies can be employed to optimize team performance and bring some order to the potential chaos of a major trauma.

Leadership and Followership

Traditional medical teaching reinforces the need for a clearly defined leader to ensure that any resuscitation runs smoothly. The role of the leader is to act as a central point for information and decision making (Box 42.7). Conversely, what makes a good follower is less often discussed. Although each team will have only one leader at any time, there will be several followers. The qualities of a good follower support the leader in the ability to make the right decisions at any given point in time (Box 42.8).

Graded Assertiveness

Graded assertiveness is one technique for communicating personal concerns about decision making or priorities to the team leader in a way that maintains constructive group performance. It is based on the assumption that poor decision making is based on incorrect or insufficient information. Followers are in

**Box 42.9** Graded Assertiveness—PACE (as defined in table)

**P**robe

"I thought our goal was to keep the arterial blood pressure higher than 90/-."

**A**lert

"Did you realize the arterial blood pressure is low? Would you like me to give some blood?"

**C**hallenge

"Is there a reason you are tolerating hypotension in this patient?"

**E**mergency action

"The arterial blood pressure is dangerously low. I am going to treat it now."

| Table 42.2 | Differential Diagnosis of Shock in the Trauma Patient |
| --- | --- |
| **Medical Condition** | **Investigation Modalities** |
| Massive hemorrhage | Clinical examination |
| | Bedside TTE—assess volume status |
| | FAST scan—abdominal source |
| Tension pneumothorax | Clinical examination (percussion/trachea) |
| | Lung ultrasound |
| Cardiac tamponade | TTE (subcostal view best) |
| Severe cardiac contusion | TTE |

*FAST*, Focused assessment with sonography for trauma; *TTE*, transthoracic echocardiogram.

a position to see the situation from a unique perspective and can communicate their concerns. They can then use the Probe, Alert, Challenge, Emergency action (PACE) technique (described in Box 42.9) to communicate their concerns in a constructive manner.[8] The team leader is very important and is usually aware of information that the follower may not be, and as such those concerns may not be the priority at that point in time.

## INTRAOPERATIVE MANAGEMENT

The spectrum of patients who need to go to the OR for surgical or interventional procedures as a result of trauma is vast. It encompasses injuries of all levels of magnitude in all organs and structures of the human body. Some are very minor and simple, and others involve specific organs with explicit implications and treatment. The latter group consists of life-threatening injury to one or multiple organs and is the main focus of this section. All current concepts that should be applied to the severely injured and bleeding patient can be applied to the lesser injured to varying degrees.

The severely injured and massively bleeding patient usually presents in hemodynamic shock and is in need of lifesaving interventions. The differential diagnosis of a trauma patient in shock consists of massive hemorrhage, tension pneumothorax, cardiac tamponade, and severe cardiac contusion. Underlying medical conditions can lead to exaggeration of the degree of shock (Table 42.2).

The management of severely injured patients with massive hemorrhage can be divided into three discrete phases. This distinction is based on different physiologic aspects, a varying approach, and management principles. Early, in the first phase, patients suffer from uncontrolled hemorrhage. The second phase begins when at least partial control of the hemorrhage has been achieved. The third and last phase is reached when the patient's physiology starts to achieve normal values (e.g., arterial blood pressure). The breakdown into these three phases takes into account the different treatment goals for each phase plus the varying speed and pragmatism of the approach. It allows the provider to appreciate the specific goals for the given phase. These three phases exist in a continuum and the borders are very fluid (Table 42.3).

### Phase 1: Uncontrolled Hemorrhage

The medical team has one goal only for trauma patients with massive hemorrhage that warrants emergent surgical procedures in the OR—to stop the bleeding as soon as possible. Everyone involved facilitates that aim by all means. There is no time to wait for study results, to order additional tests, or for consultation with other specialists. The anesthesia team's role is to facilitate achievement of hemostasis as quickly as possible. Massively bleeding patients who come to the OR for resuscitation and hemostasis present a challenge to the anesthesia providers, who are faced with a very hectic and dynamic situation. Additional personnel can be very helpful, but have to be managed, ideally in a standardized fashion. Having too many team members can be a hindrance and may prevent the team from functioning efficiently. The airway has to be secured and the patient should be ventilated with 100% oxygen. Details and consideration of airway management can be found in the section, Initial Management, earlier in this chapter, and in Chapter 16. The maximization of the fraction of inspired oxygen ($F_{IO_2}$) restores the oxygen delivery, to a certain extent, by compensating for lost hemoglobin via an increase of the dissolved oxygen fraction. Another important institutional protocol to have in place is the massive transfusion protocol

**Table 42.3** Phases of Major Traumatic Resuscitation

| | Phase 1 | Phase 2 | Phase 3 |
|---|---|---|---|
| Clinical status | Life-threatening uncontrolled hemorrhage | Ongoing hemorrhage—not immediately life threat-ening—partial surgical control | Hemorrhage controlled |
| Clinical priorities | • STOP THE BLEEDING<br>• Call for HELP<br>• Control airway, $F_{IO_2}$ 100%<br>• Damage control resuscitation (DCR)<br>  • SBP < 100 mm Hg<br>  • MAP 50-60 mm Hg<br>  • Consider modifications if TBI, carotid stenosis, CAD | • TAILORED RESUSCITATION<br>• Place supportive lines (arterial/CVC)<br>• Prevent hypothermia<br>  • Esophageal temperature probe<br>  • Warmed fluids<br>  • Warming blankets (upper and lower body)<br>  • Increase room temperature | • RESTORE PHYSIOLOGY<br>• Rapid intravascular filling<br>• Stepwise deepening of anesthesia<br>  • Fentanyl boluses<br>  • Increased volatile anesthetics<br>  • Additional lines (urinary catheter, nasogastric tube)<br>  • Communicate with all team members and ICU |
| Blood products | • Activate massive transfusion protocol (MTP)<br>• Consider emergency (unmatched) blood products<br>• Early use<br>• Empiric 1:1:1 | • TEG/ROTEM to guide coagulation products<br>• ABG to guide red blood cell transfusion | • Only as required on testing<br>• Deactivate MTP when appropriate |
| Crystalloids/ colloids | • Cautious use | • Use for hypovolemia with normal coagulation/Hb<br>• Use serial lactate/BE to guide fluid requirements | • Attempt to normalize BE/ lactate |
| Special points | • Consider $CaCl_2$ 1 g for every three blood products<br>• Large bore IV access (>16 G) or CVC<br>• Rapid infusing system (e.g., Belmont)<br>• Avoid vasoconstrictors | • Consider cell salvage<br>• Aim to repeat TEG/ROTEM/ABG every 30 min<br>• Consider TEE for difficult cases | • Consider vasoactive infusions if necessary |

*ABG*, Arterial blood gas; *BE*, base excess; *CAD*, coronary artery disease; *CVC*, central venous catheter; *ICU*, intensive care unit; *IV*, intravenous; *MAP*, mean arterial pressure; *MTP*, massive transfusion protocol; *ROTEM*, rotational thomboelastometry; *SBP*, systolic blood pressure; *TBI*, traumatic brain injury; *TEE*, transesophageal echocardiography; *TEG*, thromboelastography.

(MTP) (also see Chapter 24). The MTP facilitates communication, optimizes the response time of the blood bank, and minimizes errors. Although all of these procedures are essential to taking care of such patients, the absolute mainstay of this phase is the hemostatic resuscitation of the patient.

Historically, the anesthesia provider would deploy large volumes of crystalloids early in order to aggressively restore the circulating volume and restore normal arterial blood pressure values. This can lead to a direct escalation in the bleeding rate by increasing cardiac output as well as both the arterial and venous pressures. This abandoned practice would also lead to a dilution of coagulation factors and hypothermia, further increasing the bleeding. Over the past 10 to 15

---

**Box 42.10** Principles of Damage Control Resuscitation (DCR)

Permissive hypotension
Stop bleeding early—pressure, angiography, operating room
Early use of hemostatic products
Minimize crystalloid use

---

years, the initial resuscitation has been revolutionized and the concept entirely changed.[9] The main goal of the initial resuscitation is on bridging the patient for as long as possible until the bleeding can be stopped. DCR is the term used to describe the new concept[10] (Box 42.10).

## Damage Control Resuscitation (Also See Chapter 24)

Permissive hypotension, limited use of crystalloids and colloids, and the early use of blood products represent the cornerstones of DCR.[10]

Permissive hypotension aims to utilize the body's physiologic response to hemorrhage. The resulting low venous and arterial blood pressures and the decrease in cardiac output lead to a reduction in the driving force behind the bleeding. At the same time, the providers can take advantage of the normal response to blood loss: vasoconstriction in nonvital regions and redirection of the blood flow to the most important organs. The ultimate goal is to benefit from this compensatory mechanism for as long as possible. Unfortunately, there are no direct and accurate measures of when this mechanism is at its limits and the oxygenation of vital organs is starting to be impaired. Systolic blood pressure (SBP, invasive or noninvasive) continues to serve as a very basic surrogate variable, even though there is no reliable correlation between SBP and organ microcirculation. Animal models of shock demonstrate that resuscitation to 60% of the baseline mean arterial pressure (MAP) does not reduce the regional organ perfusion compared to normotensive resuscitation, but the less aggressive resuscitation does lead to a decreased blood loss. At the same time, brain perfusion was not different between the two groups. Consequently, there is some expert consensus to tolerate SBP around 80 to 90 mm Hg in actively hemorrhaging patients until hemostasis is achieved with adjustment to the patient's age, preexisting medical conditions, and injury pattern. For example, on one extreme, there is the young and healthy patient with a massive abdominal bleed. In that case, SBP in the 60 mm Hg range can be tolerated for a short duration. On the other end of the spectrum, keeping SBP well above 100 mm Hg for elderly patients with multiple medical conditions and multisystem trauma involving the brain should be considered. These measures are temporarily in place until hemostasis is achieved or the patient's condition further deteriorates. In the latter case, the intravascular volume has to be replenished.

At the point when the patient needs additional intravascular fluids, crystalloids and colloids should be limited in this early phase.[11] Otherwise, the cardiac output and intravascular pressures will increase, as will the rate of bleeding; coagulation factors will continually be consumed in an effort to clot the bleeding sites; and their plasma levels will rapidly decline. All of these conditions will negatively affect a patient's ability to survive a disastrous bleeding episode. Restoring vital signs to normal values will bring a short period of better physiology before the disastrous combination of an increased bleeding rate and rapid deterioration of the patient's coagulation capability significantly worsen the overall situation. In addition, large volumes of crystalloids will worsen reperfusion injury, and augment inflammatory response. Administration of synthetic colloids will even further increase coagulopathy by impairing both fibrinogen polymerization and platelet function.

As a result, the use of crystalloids and colloids has been reduced in the setting of severe hemorrhage. Instead blood products are the fluids of choice for the resuscitation of massively bleeding patients (also see Chapter 24). Packed red blood cells (PRBCs), fresh frozen plasma (FFP), and platelets are the mainstays for the initial resuscitation. Evidence is emerging that demonstrates the pragmatic and early use of these blood products in a fixed ratio (i.e., 1:1:1, PRBC:FFP:platelets).[12] The benefit of using this approach is that the oxygen-carrying capacity is maintained or restored with the PRBCs, and the patient's ability to form clots is supported with the plasma factors in the FFP and platelet infusions. When transfusing large amounts of this combination of blood products, one should consider the additional supplementation of fibrinogen in the form of cryoprecipitate because fibrinogen is one of the key components of hemostasis. Cryoprecipitate is expended much faster than can be resynthesized by the liver under such circumstances, and as a result, tranexamic acid, an antifibrinolytic, is given for preventing coagulopathy in severely injured hypotensive patients early in their course (Figs. 42.2 and 42.3).[13,14] The role of vasopressors for hemodynamic support in this phase remains largely controversial. They should generally be avoided, because in an already severely hypovolemic state, further vasoconstriction may compromise the blood flow to vital organs.

### Access for Intravascular Resuscitation

In order to deploy an adequate resuscitation in a severely bleeding patient, proper access to the patient's vascular system needs to be obtained. Every patient with significant trauma or mechanism of trauma should have two large-bore peripheral intravenous (PIV) lines placed. They should be 16 gauge or larger and preferably inserted in the upper extremities. The integrity and the time to meaningful venous access are of equal importance. It is better to quickly obtain a well-functioning 18-gauge PIV than to waste valuable time on obtaining an elusive 14-gauge PIV.

Prolonged or significant massive transfusions usually benefit from large-bore central access. Classically, a large-bore (e.g., 8.5F) catheter introducer sheath is placed in either the femoral, internal jugular, or subclavian vein. If the circumstances permit, this is performed with ultrasound guidance.

Intraosseous (IO) access is suitable as a first-line access if PIV access is poor or delayed. Although an IO line cannot be used for rapid volume resuscitation, it can serve as a line to administer medications. With better overall flow rates and the proximity to the heart, the humeral approach is the preferable location for an IO line in adults.

The use of a modern rapid infuser system is of paramount importance. The rapid infuser provides the

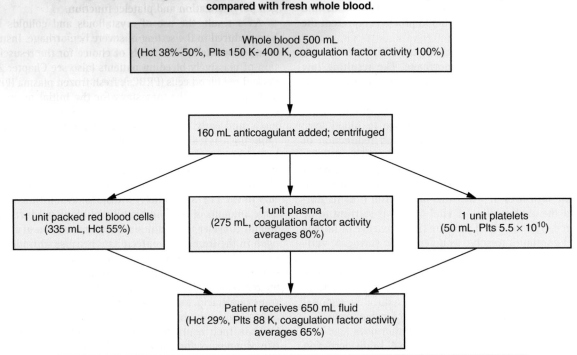

**Dilution and storage loss reduce the effectiveness of component blood product therapy compared with fresh whole blood.**

Whole blood 500 mL
(Hct 38%-50%, Plts 150 K- 400 K, coagulation factor activity 100%)

160 mL anticoagulant added; centrifuged

1 unit packed red blood cells
(335 mL, Hct 55%)

1 unit plasma
(275 mL, coagulation factor activity averages 80%)

1 unit platelets
(50 mL, Plts $5.5 \times 10^{10}$)

Patient receives 650 mL fluid
(Hct 29%, Plts 88 K, coagulation factor activity averages 65%)

**Fig. 42.2** Resultant blood component activity after transfusion compared with whole blood. (Redrawn from Dutton R. Haemostatic resuscitation. *Br J Anaesth.* 2012;109(suppl 1):i39-i46.)

| | |
|---|---|
| 1st Cooler | 4 units PRBC<br>4 units FFP |
| 2nd Cooler | 4 units PRBC<br>4 units FFP<br>6 units platelets (1 pooled) |
| 3rd Cooler | As 1st |
| 4th Cooler | As 2nd |
| Repeat | Consider adding cryoprecipitate after 4th cooler or if fibrinogen <1 |

**Fig. 42.3** Example of a massive transfusion protocol. *FFP,* Fresh frozen plasma; *PRBC,* packed red blood cells.

anesthesia team with the capability to deliver large amounts of warmed blood products very quickly and safely. Rapid infuser systems are very potent and the patient and the clinical situation should be closely monitored to avoid excessive resuscitation (Fig. 42.4).

When all the aforementioned measures and techniques are properly deployed, the anesthesia team can provide the patient and surgical team the valuable extra time

needed until hemostasis can be achieved. Once the bleeding is mostly under control, the priorities and speed of approach change and phase 2 of resuscitation begins.

### Phase 2: Controlled Hemorrhage

In phase 2, after the major aspects of the bleeding source have been controlled, the anesthesia team should focus on a more individualized, tailored approach. Depending on the dynamics of a given case and the number and experience of anesthesia providers available, phase 2 items can happen earlier and in parallel with phase 1.

Invasive monitoring should begin at this point. The insertion should never delay or distract from the massive transfusion, the placement of intravenous lines, and the surgical hemostasis. Additionally, it is technically much easier to place an arterial line in a properly resuscitated patient.

In phase 2 the dynamics of the case slow down, the process becomes less blind, and the patient's needs should be reanalyzed. A mainstay during phase 2 is the utilization of point-of-care testing (POCT) to guide the resuscitation.[15] In order to do so, one has to reflect on the main physiologic goals of resuscitation: guaranteeing adequate oxygen delivery and coagulation function. Oxygen delivery depends mostly on the oxygen-carrying capacity and normal intravascular filling. The first

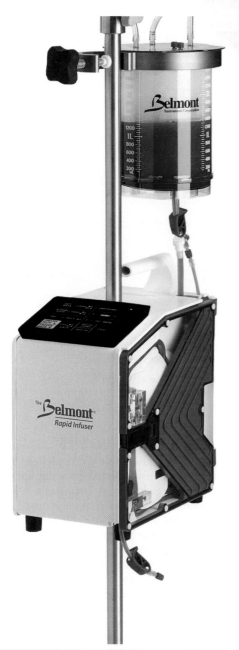

**Fig. 42.4** The Belmont rapid infuser. (Courtesy of Belmont Instrument Corporation, Billerica, MA.)

is measured via hemoglobin (Hb) concentration or the hematocrit (Hct) in the patient's blood. Depending on the patient's age, comorbid conditions, and injuries, Hct values between 18% and 28% are targeted. The intravascular volume status can be assessed by a combination of a multitude of clinical clues, such as vital signs, urine output, and, if applicable, direct observation of the patient's heart and major vessels. In more challenging cases (e.g., suspected cardiac comorbid conditions,

cardiac contusions, arrhythmias), a transesophageal echocardiogram (TEE) can further quantify the intravascular volume.

To best assess the coagulation status of a patient, the clinician has to collect information from the four main pillars of perioperative coagulation monitoring: the patient's medical history, clinical presentation, standard laboratory coagulation tests, and point-of-care coagulation tests. If obtainable, the patient's medical history can provide information on medications and medical conditions relevant to the coagulation system. The clinical presentation of the phenotype of bleeding is a simple but critical tool for the existence and differential diagnosis of coagulopathy. Any abnormal coagulation test needs to be correlated to the clinical presentation. Without any clinically relevant diffuse bleeding, no procoagulant therapy should be initiated, as it can increase the risk of thrombosis. The clinical picture can also help differentiate between a surgical versus nonsurgical origin of the bleeding. Nonsurgical bleeding presents itself with a diffuse and more widespread pattern and must be addressed by correcting the coagulation abnormalities. In contrast, surgical bleeding has to be controlled via mechanical hemostasis. The standard laboratory coagulation tests consist of prothrombin time and international normalized ratio (PT/INR), activated partial thromboplastin time (aPTT), platelet count, and fibrinogen concentration. These tests come with significant limitations such as sensitivity, specificity, validity, and timeliness that render them virtually useless early in dynamic massive transfusion scenarios (also see Chapter 24).

### Viscoelastic Testing

Over the past decade, viscoelastic point-of-care coagulation tests have become a mainstay for timely assessment of the situations previously described. The thromboelastograph (TEG) and rotational thromboelastometry (ROTEM) are standard tools to assess the magnitude and nature of the coagulation disturbance and help guide interventions (Fig. 42.5). Both devices provide the clinician with a graphical output that can guide the procoagulant interventions. The readout of TEG/ROTEM can be divided into parts: (1) preclot formation phase, (2) clot formation phase, and (3) clot stability phase (Fig. 42.6). The first phase, preclot formation, starts with the addition of reagents that trigger the plasma coagulation cascade and activate the platelets. This phase lasts less than 5 minutes and can inform the anesthesia provider about the coagulation cascade. If there are deficiencies in this phase, prothrombin complex concentrate (PCC) and FFP can be given. The second phase starts with the beginning of the clot formation and ends when the maximum clot firmness is reached. This phase reflects the functional platelet mass and the availability of fibrinogen. Any defects in the second phase can be corrected with the transfusion of

**VI**

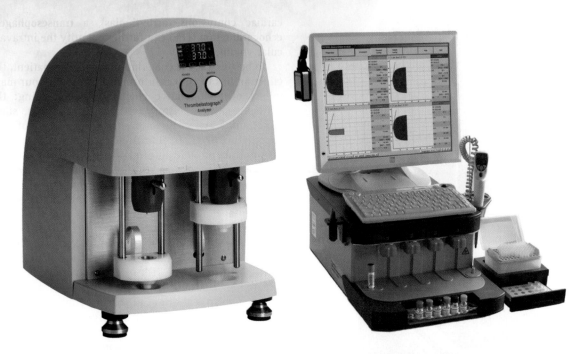

**TEG 5000, Haemoneics Corp.**    **ROTEM Delta, TEM Systems**

**Fig. 42.5** Tools for viscoelastic point-of-care coagulation testing. *Left,* Thromboelastograph (TEG). *Right,* Rotational thromboelastometry (ROTEM).

cryoprecipitate, fibrinogen concentrate, or platelet concentrates. The third and last phase reflects the stability of the clot, allowing fibrinolysis to be detected and quantified. When identified, it can be effectively treated with an antifibrinolytic product.

With the information from the four pillars of coagulation monitoring, the treatment can be tailored using a goal-directed approach and predefined algorithms. This approach also must take into account that any procoagulant therapy always has to be used with caution. A coagulopathy should never be excessively corrected; otherwise the risk for serious thromboembolic events can increase (Fig. 42.7).

After hemorrhage has been controlled, frequent analysis of arterial blood gases should be obtained because they help guide PRBC transfusions as well as adjustments in ventilation to the patient's needs. Additionally, electrolyte disturbances (e.g., hypocalcemia and hyperkalemia) frequently occur and warrant treatment.

During resuscitation, hypothermia should be prevented. This is achieved by only administering warmed fluids, increasing room temperature, and the use of forced air warmers. The insertion of an esophageal temperature probe helps the clinician to monitor the success of these interventions and serves as a reminder to try to achieve normothermia.

## Phase 3: Restoration of Physiology

The third and final resuscitation phase includes the fine-tuning and restoration of the patient's physiology. This should occur once the surgical hemostasis is complete and the dynamic of the resuscitation is under control. The DCR principles no longer apply as the potential for harm may outweigh the benefits. The intravascular volume is replenished during this phase. Additional cardiac output monitoring devices can help guide this process. If not already achieved, the anesthetic should be incrementally increased to a level near 1 minimum alveolar concentration (MAC) (see Chapter 7). At this point, low-dose vasoactive infusions can be considered to counteract anesthesia-induced vasodilation. They should not be used to compensate for inadequate intravascular volume resuscitation. Continued serial POCT is useful in determining the success of the resuscitation. Normal serum lactate and base deficit levels are excellent indicators for this achievement.

### Anesthetics

Except for the most uncontrolled hemorrhage, it is very important to use a stepwise approach to restoring adequate anesthetic levels using arterial blood pressure values as a guide. This concept goes hand in hand with the rapid filling of the intravascular space and allows for a restoration of a normal blood flow to all tissues.

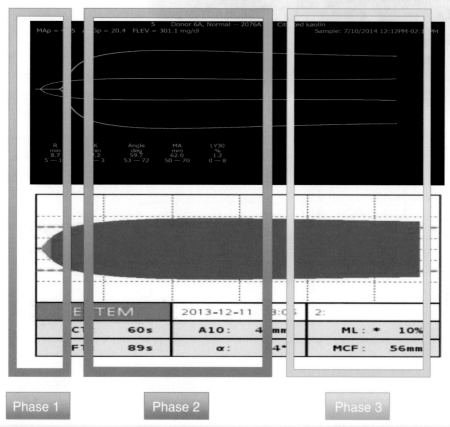

**Fig. 42.6** Three phases of viscoelastic tests: phase 1 (preclot), phase 2 (formation), and phase 3 (stability). TEG tracing in top panel and ROTEM tracing in bottom panel. *ROTEM,* Rotational thromboelastometry; *TEG,* thromboelastograph.

Slow administration of anesthetics should be started in phase 2. The stepwise deepening of the anesthetic can be achieved by either repeated boluses of opioids or increasing inhaled anesthetic concentrations in an incremental manner.[16]

## SPECIAL GROUPS

### Traumatic Brain Injury

Traumatic brain injury (TBI) is defined as injury to the head that disrupts normal brain function (also see Chapter 30). Over 15 million people are seen in emergency departments for TBI each year and it contributes to 30% of trauma deaths in the United States.[17] Long-term effects of TBI may lead to cognitive and functional impairment, disability, and an overall reduction in quality of life.

Primary neurologic injury is irreversible, occurring at the moment of injury and causing immediate neuronal damage. The magnitude of the primary injury is a significant prognostic factor of TBI. Secondary injury is the subsequent injury to the brain after the primary injury occurs. Common causes of secondary injury include intracranial hypertension, hypotension, hypoxia, hyperthermia, coagulopathy, hyperglycemia or hypoglycemia, and acidosis. The focus of TBI management for the anesthesia provider is to limit secondary injury in the perioperative period in order to improve neurologic outcomes.

Neurologic manifestations of TBI largely depend on the mechanism, severity, and type of injury that have occurred. Types of injuries include skull fractures; intracerebral, subdural, and epidural hematomas; hemorrhagic contusions; and diffuse axonal injuries. These injuries may be focal or diffuse. The GCS is commonly used to initially assess and classify TBI patients, though iatrogenic intoxication and other factors may sometimes lead to misclassification. GCS score should be reported for each of the three components (eye, verbal, motor) separately. Untestable components of GCS should be documented. Early CT scan is critical in delineating the type and extent of injury.

Like other trauma patients, the initial evaluation begins with ATLS. An early definitive airway should be established in a TBI patient who does not have the ability to maintain a patent airway owing to loss of reflexes and cannot adequately oxygenate or ventilate. These factors

VI

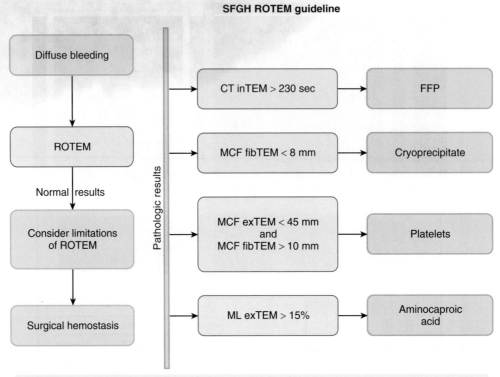

**SFGH ROTEM guideline**

**Fig. 42.7** An example of a rotational thromboelastometry (ROTEM) treatment algorithm for use in trauma. (Courtesy of San Francisco General Hospital and Trauma Center.)

are usually related to a deteriorating GCS score, usually 8 or less, or other concurrent injuries. Nasal airways (and nasogastric tubes) should be avoided if possible in TBI patients with facial or suspected skull base fractures because of the risk of intracranial insertion. Other indications for intubating the trachea of TBI patients include signs of intracranial hypertension or uncontrollable seizure activity. Securing the airway should always be considered prior to transport if the patient's mental status and GCS score are worsening.

Many of the same considerations must be taken when intubating the trachea of a TBI patient as for other trauma patients, such as inadequate fasting, hypoxia, uncertain intravascular volume status, and presumed cervical spine injury in blunt trauma. Approximately 4% to 8% of moderate to severe TBI patients have concurrent cervical spine injury, with greater risk for high cervical injuries and mechanically unstable injuries.[18] Of particular attention to the anesthesia provider should be the integrity of the cervical spine. Cervical collars should be opened and mechanical in-line stabilization should be held by experienced personnel during a rapid sequence induction of anesthesia and tracheal intubation. Additional factors such as increased intracranial pressure (ICP) or pending herniation, concurrent airway injuries, uncooperative patients, and combativeness should also be considered. It is not clear whether video

laryngoscopy (e.g., GlideScope) is superior to intubation compared to conventional laryngoscopy. Video laryngoscopy (GlideScope) may produce slightly less cervical spine motion and obtain better glottis visualization at the cost of a slightly longer time to endotracheal intubation in an experienced laryngoscopist's hands.[19,20] Selection of the intubation method should be based on speed of establishing a definitive airway and experience of the laryngoscopist.

The use of anesthetics should focus on hemodynamic stability to maintain cerebral perfusion pressure (CPP). Propofol and etomidate are commonly selected for their reduction in cerebral blood flow (CBF), which is coupled to a reduction in cerebral metabolic rate of oxygen ($CMRO_2$) requirement. Although traditionally controversial, use of ketamine in this population has not led to increases in ICP or worsened outcomes.[21] Nondepolarizing neuromuscular blocking drugs have no significant effect on cerebral hemodynamics. Succinylcholine may theoretically increase ICP, but this effect has not been demonstrated to be clinically significant and may be attenuated with a defasciculating dose of a nondepolarizing drug (also see Chapter 11).

Emergent surgical management may sometimes be indicated after imaging is performed. Volatile anesthetics may increase CBF while decreasing $CMRO_2$, known as "uncoupling." Increased CBF does not occur until after 0.5 MAC, and over 1 MAC for sevoflurane. If volatile anesthetics are used, less than 1 MAC should be used, with a preference for sevoflurane. Total intravenous anesthesia (TIVA) may be preferred because it decreases ICP but is generally less titratable during sudden, profound hypotension that may occur during dural decompression. Although data exist for the effects of volatile anesthetics and TIVA on cerebral hemodynamics, no definitive prospective outcome studies exist. A retrospective study in combat-related TBI did not show significant difference between neurologic outcomes at discharge when comparing the two anesthetic strategies.[22]

The patient is usually placed in reverse Trendelenburg position of approximately 30 degrees during the procedure to facilitate venous drainage. Large-bore intravenous access is necessary for intraoperative fluid administration. Blood should be checked for availability of transfusion. Surgery for compound depressed skull fractures near venous sinuses are at particularly intense risk for massive hemorrhage. Coagulopathy may be checked with a traditional laboratory coagulation panel or viscoelastometric testing. An arterial line should be inserted for continuous arterial blood pressure monitoring and withdrawal of blood for serial laboratory analysis. Brain Trauma Foundation guidelines should be followed throughout the perioperative period.[23] Hypotension should be promptly treated to maintain a CPP of 50 to 70 mm Hg. Intravascular fluid administration-resuscitation is usually required to achieve euvolemia, especially after administration of mannitol. Isotonic crystalloid is usually preferred. The use of albumin may increase mortality risk in the resuscitation of ICU brain-injured patients when compared to crystalloid.[24] Hypoxemia should be avoided. Attention should be paid to peak inspiratory pressure and positive end-expiratory pressure to avoid obstruction of cerebral venous drainage. Hyperventilation is not recommended within the first 24 hours of injury unless treating impending herniation. Prophylactic administration of mannitol and antiseizure administration is recommended. Glucose should be monitored regularly. Hyperglycemia and hypoglycemia should be treated to avoid exacerbation of secondary injury. General recommendations are to treat blood glucose levels above 180 mg/dL. Most importantly, close communication with the operative team must be maintained prior to decompression and dural opening.

Systemically, high ICP may trigger intense sympathetic activity to maintain CPP. This is known as Cushing reflex. The catecholamine release and increased systemic vascular resistance may mask intravascular volume depletion. Sudden, profound hypotension may sometimes occur after decompression and normalization of ICP, especially in those who are not adequately resuscitated. Anesthetic drugs should be gradually decreased and vasopressors and inotropes should be available for administration prior to major decompression. Blood should be immediately available for sudden, abrupt bleeding.

The decision to leave the trachea intubated or to extubate the trachea should be discussed with the surgeon. Many TBI patients remain tracheally intubated owing to the risks of postoperative hypoventilation, hypoxia, depressed level of consciousness, other concurrent injuries, and the need for further diagnostic studies or therapies. These patients should be transported with full monitoring. Sedation and a transport ventilator may be necessary if the patient remains intubated. For transporting TBI patients, small-dose muscle relaxant may be considered to reduce episodes of agitation, bucking, or coughing. The use of large-dose muscle relaxation at the end of the procedure or for transport may delay postoperative neurologic examination and is not recommended. TBI variables should continue throughout the immediate perioperative period.

## Spinal Cord Injury

Spinal cord injury (SCI) occurs when acute trauma disrupts normal sensory, motor, or autonomic function. It is estimated that there are 12,500 new cases per year in the United States with over 200,000 people currently living with SCI.[25] The most common causes of injury are motor vehicle accidents, falls, and assault.

The presentation of SCI depends largely on the level, extent, and severity at which injury occurs. An injury may be described as "complete" if the patient has no motor or sensory function below the level of injury. Incomplete SCIs describe partial injury to the cord that results in varying degrees of residual sensory and motor function. The American Spinal Injury Association (ASIA) classification is the preferred impairment scale to describe findings of neurologic examinations.

Spinal cord precautions should be immediately undertaken when suspecting an injury, including a cervical collar and strict roll precautions whenever transporting or moving patients. Adequacy of ventilation and oxygenation should be quickly evaluated. Cervical spine injuries, especially those with complete injuries, may result in diaphragmatic impairment and weakness. This leads to decreased vital capacity and the inability to cough and clear secretions. Concurrent lung injury associated with trauma or chronic lung disease may exacerbate the patient's ability to ventilate and oxygenate. Signs of inadequate ventilation may include rapid, shallow breathing, increased work of breathing, and paradoxic abdominal movement. These signs may appear with thoracic and high lumbar injuries affecting intercostal and abdominal muscles. The airway should be secured with an endotracheal tube in similar fashion as used with TBI patients. Up to 16% of patients admitted

VI

with SCI are diagnosed with concurrent TBI. In this population with concurrent diagnoses, the cervical spine was most frequently injured.[26] Succinylcholine may be used to safely provide neuromuscular blockade in an SCI patient within the first 24 hours of injury. However, it should be avoided after 48 hours of injury because of the risk of severe hyperkalemia that may result with administration. Exaggerated bradycardic response and hypotension have been reported with direct laryngoscopy and intubation of the trachea of patients with cervical or high thoracic injuries.

During the acute phase, high thoracic (usually T4 and above) and cervical SCIs may result in significant bradyarrhythmia and atrioventricular block (AV block) owing to disruption of sympathetic cardiac accelerator fibers leading to unopposed parasympathetic innervation. Sympathetic blockade may also lead to systemic vasodilation and result in severe hypotension. In addition to the motor and sensory findings below the level of injury, this physiologic constellation has been referred to as "spinal shock." Treatment is supportive and includes administration of isotonic fluid, vasopressors, and inotropes. Caution should be taken to not over-resuscitate the patient with fluids intravenously as this may lead to pulmonary edema after spinal shock has resolved.

MAP should be kept at 85 to 90 mm Hg for patients with SCI to maintain adequate spinal cord perfusion, unless otherwise contraindicated by concurrent injuries. Administration of methylprednisolone is no longer recommended by the American Association of Neurological Surgeons, as there is evidence that large-dose steroids are associated with mostly negative effects, including death.[27]

## Burns

Major burns can occur in isolation or in combination with other forms of traumatic injury. They can result in rapid deterioration. Organized and systematic advanced trauma management is paramount. In addition, there are some special considerations for patients with burns. This section will address some of the issues in the immediate management of a major acute burn patient. This section does not address issues that arise later in the management or intraoperative care.

### Burn Severity
Burns are categorized based on their severity as superficial, partial thickness, or full thickness burns:

Superficial—This burn affects the epidermis only (e.g., sunburn). It does not require any specific treatment other than first aid. Superficial burns are not included in the calculation of percentage body surface area (%BSA) affected.

Partial thickness—This burn involves all of the epidermis and part of the dermis. It can further be divided into superficial dermal, mid-dermal, and deep dermal. These burns change in appearance as the burn destroys more of the dermis and vasculature; the pain ranges from minimal to extreme; color can be red to pale/white; and exudates can be high fluid to relatively dry. Blisters are often present. They may require surgical management.

Full thickness—This burn involves complete destruction of all of the epidermis and dermis. It is white, insensate, and has a waxy or leathery appearance. This type of skin is called an *eschar*.

### Estimating Burn Surface Area
A patient's future management and need for transfer to tertiary centers is based on the percentage of body surface area that is affected by burns. The rule of nines is helpful for localized burns to a particular body part, although the patient's palmar surface is considered approximately 1% of total BSA; this method underestimates in the obese population (Fig. 42.8).

### Types of Burns: Chemical, Electrical, and Thermal
The first priority in managing the burn is to halt the burning process. The most appropriate method to do this depends on what caused the burn. Remove any clothing that can be removed easily. Irrigate the area thoroughly with running water. This can take several hours with some chemical burns.

#### Chemical Burns: Special Considerations
Try to prevent irrigation fluid running across unaffected skin. Continue irrigation until skin pH or fluid pH is neutral (use litmus paper). DO NOT use water for elemental metal burns (lithium, magnesium, potassium, sodium) as they react with water, worsening the burn; use mineral oil.

#### Electrical Burns: Special Considerations
Look for entry and exit points because injury has occurred along that trajectory. Beware of underlying muscle damage; there is the risk of compartment syndrome and rhabdomyolysis. There is a slightly increased fluid requirement.

#### Thermal Burns: Special Considerations
Remove source of heat as soon as possible (e.g., burning clothing). Continue prolonged irrigation with cold fluid but beware of hypothermia. Be suspicious for associated injuries (inhalational, other forms of trauma).

### Intravascular Fluid Management
Fluid management is an important cornerstone of modern burns management; however, controversy still exists about the correct amount of fluid to give and the appropriate end points to be monitoring. There is increasing recognition of the adverse effects of excessive intravenous fluid resuscitation and the increased risk of precipitating acute respiratory distress syndrome (ARDS) 3 to 5 days after injury.

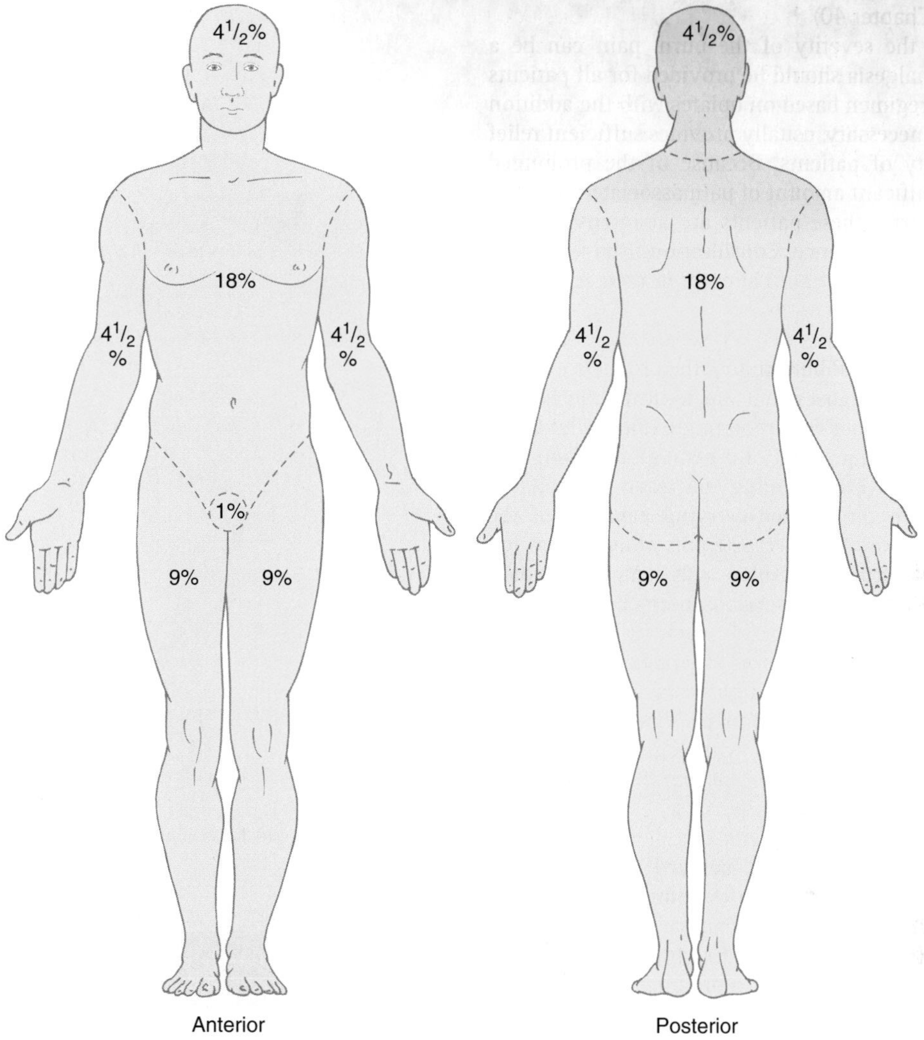

**Fig. 42.8** The rule of nines—used to calculate %BSA (body surface area) burns.

Multiple formulas are in use for estimating fluid resuscitation requirements (also see Chapter 23). Most were developed approximately 30 to 40 years ago. One of the most common is the modified Parkland formula: 4 mL/kg/% burn (adults) over first 24 hours after burn injury.

Only crystalloid fluid is used for the first 24 hours as the amount of protein leak into the interstitial space is thought to be greatest during this period, thus rendering colloids ineffective. The most commonly used fluid is a balanced salt solution such as lactated Ringer solution or Plasma-Lyte.

### Airway (Also See Chapter 16)

Burns are characterized by erythema and the rapid onset of edema in affected tissues. When this happens in the upper airway the swelling can result in total airway obstruction and death. As a consequence, it is

---

**Box 42.11** Signs of Potential Airway Burns

- Carbonaceous sputum
- Stridor
- Voice changes
- Facial burns
- Explosive injuries involving upper torso/head
- Prolonged entrapment in fire

---

important to maintain a high level of attentiveness for burns affecting the airway and to take steps to intubate early before swelling makes it impossible. Some warning signs are presented in Box 42.11. Consider inserting an endotracheal tube 0.5 to 1 mm internal diameter less than normally would be used to allow for the expected swelling.

VI

### Pain (Also See Chapter 40)

Depending on the severity of the burn, pain can be a major issue. Analgesia should be provided for all patients as required. A regimen based on opiates with the addition of ketamine, if necessary, usually provides sufficient relief for the majority of patients. Because of the prolonged nature and significant amount of pain associated with the treatment of burns, these patients are at intense risk of developing opiate tolerance. Consultation from a specialist pain service should be sought early in their recovery.

### Inhalation

In addition to the actual burn injury, the products of combustion can produce gases that are toxic to the human body. The most common is carbon monoxide (CO). CO has a much higher binding affinity for hemoglobin compared with oxygen. Thus, CO poisoning can result in a significant reduction in the oxygen-carrying capacity of the blood. The only way to detect CO poisoning is through CO-oximetry performed on a blood gas sample. Standard pulse oximetry monitors are unable to detect CO poisoning and will read a normal value even in the presence of profound tissue hypoxemia. The application of high concentration oxygen significantly reduces the half-life of CO in the blood and any patient with suspected CO inhalation should be provided with high concentration oxygen as an initial measure.

### Infection

Infection is a major cause of delayed morbidity and death. Although empiric antibiotics addressing skin flora are sufficient for the immediate management, coverage of the burn surface with sterile dressings is essential to reestablish the external barrier to organisms. Over-resuscitation with fluids is also associated with increased risk of infectious complications.

### Eshcarotomies

The eschar of full thickness burns significantly reduces the compliance of body tissues. If the eschars are circumferential around any part, it can result in a compartment-like syndrome. This is particularly concerning around the torso where ventilation can be impeded. In this eventuality, eshcarotomies may need to be performed. The preferred location for incisions is outlined in Fig. 42.9.

### Transfer of Burn Patients

In general, most locations have a burn center or unit that provides specialized treatment of burn victims. Such expert care improves outcomes for burn victims. When it comes to transferring the patient, consideration must be given as to any other associated injuries and where these can best be managed. Sometimes it may be appropriate to stabilize the major visceral injuries at the trauma center before transferring care to the burn unit at a later stage. Commonly used transfer criteria are listed in Box 42.12.

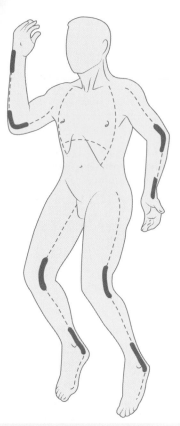

**Fig. 42.9** Locations for escharotomy incisions.

---

**Box 42.12** Criteria for Transfer of Patients to a Tertiary Burn Center (American Burn Association)

- >10% total BSA partial thickness burns
- Full thickness burns in any age group
- Burns involving sensitive areas (hands, feet, perineum, face, genitals, major joints)
- Inhalation injuries
- Electrical/lightning burns
- Circumferential burns to limbs or torso
- Significant chemical burn risking cosmetic or functional outcome
- Major preexisting comorbid conditions

*BSA*, Body surface area.

## Extremes of Age

### Pediatric Trauma (Also See Chapter 34)

Trauma is the most common cause of major morbidity and fatality in the pediatric population (Box 42.13). The presentation of an injured child to a hospital is usually a source of anxiety for most clinicians. By delivering high-quality, advanced trauma care the burden of the child's injury can be lessened and an improved outcome attained.

---

**Box 42.13** Common Injuries in Pediatrics

- Simple fractures—falls from height/play equipment, sports
- Pedestrian versus car—more chest/head injuries—especially with SUVs
- More major visceral injury without overlying fractures

*SUVs,* Sport-utility vehicles.

---

**Box 42.15** Blood Volume Estimations

- Preterm neonate—95 mL/kg
- Full-term neonate—85 mL/kg
- Infant—80 mL/kg
- Adult (male)—75 mL/kg
- Adult (female)—65 mL/kg

---

**Box 42.14** Key Points—Pediatric Trauma

- Late physiologic decompensation
- Potential for difficult intravenous access—consider intraosseous line
- Look out for nonaccidental injury
- Any blood loss is significant

---

**Box 42.16** Key Points—Geriatric Trauma

- Reduced physiologic reserve
- Consider preexisting conditions
- Check medications—beware the β-blocked bleeding patient
- Consider elder abuse
- Discuss end-of-life care if appropriate

---

This section will present a brief overview of some of the issues that are unique to trauma in the pediatric patient (Box 42.14). Fundamentally, the principles of ATLS form the basis of management of the pediatric patient.

Special Considerations

*Nonaccidental injury*
This differential diagnosis should always be considered in pediatric injury. The majority of jurisdictions have mandatory reporting for child abuse. Warning signs include the following:

- Injury pattern inconsistent with developmental milestones (e.g., a 2-month-old rolling off the diaper changing table)
- Multiple injuries (especially if these appear to have been inflicted over a period of time)
- Frequent presentations
- Inconsistent history of incident

*Pediatric physiology*
Children are able to mask significant hemodynamic compromise because of their robust physiology. There are also confounders for signs such as tachycardia, pain, and a fear or stress response. Beware of rapid deterioration once compensatory threshold is reached.

*Vascular access*
Pediatric venous cannulation can present a challenge even in a well-hydrated patient. In the presence of hemorrhagic shock it can be almost impossible. The priority should be restoring a circulating volume, and early IO access is advocated. A rule of thumb used by some institutions is two attempts in two locations before you use the IO approach.

*Drug dosing*
Because the majority of drug doses and fluids are weight based, it is essential to get an accurate estimation of the child's weight. The clinician's choices are to ask a caregiver or parent, or to use a tool such as the Broselow Pediatric Emergency Tape to get an estimate.

The considerations for dose reduction of some drugs in the trauma patient still apply to pediatrics.

*Behavior*
It is often difficult to get children to be compliant with treatment depending on their age. There should be consideration for the appropriateness of diagnostic tests such as CT and the requirement for the child to be still. Intubation may be required to facilitate the process.

*Blood dosing* (Box 42.15)
Small children have a substantially reduced circulating blood volume, and a small amount of blood loss can be significant. In a 20-kg 4-year-old child, the estimated circulating blood volume is only 1600 mL. Loss of 375 mL (equivalent to a 12-oz can of soft drink) is over 20% of the total circulating volume. It is important to be vigilant for occult sources of bleeding and intervene early. Transfusing red blood cells will increase hemoglobin by 2 to 2.5 g/dL for every 10 mL/kg administered.

Geriatric Trauma (Also See Chapter 35)
As with pediatrics, the elderly trauma patient also requires some unique considerations for management. Although trauma is not a major contributor to morbidity and fatality in the geriatric population, their physiologic age, coexisting diseases, and medications make this group much more susceptible to poor outcomes if their care is not of the highest standards. Once again, the principles of advanced trauma management are paramount and the basis of all interventions (Box 42.16). This section will briefly outline some of the unique considerations for the trauma patient of advanced age.

Special Considerations

*Preexisting illness and physiologic reserve*
With advancing age comes the potential for a variety of medical conditions that may affect a patient's ability to survive a major trauma. This combines with the decline in

VI

physiologic reserve that occurs with healthy aging, placing these patients at serious risk of major morbidity or fatality.

### Medications

Medications, such as antihypertensives, for relatively minor and well-controlled conditions can exacerbate hemodynamic instability following a trauma. β-Adrenergic blocking drugs can mask the tachycardia associated with blood loss.

### Minimal impact trauma

Relatively minor mechanisms can result in significant injuries. Geriatric patients are more prone to fractures and head injuries. Subdural hematomas are particularly common.

### Elder abuse (also see Chapter 35)

An increasingly recognized cause of injury to the geriatric population in long-term care facilities is abuse. This should be considered and explored especially in patients who are in care facilities and have reduced mobility or cognitive function.

### End-of-life care

It is important to consider what is appropriate when providing an intervention to a patient. When possible, determine the patient's wishes and any preexisting limitation of treatment orders. Remain focused on interventions that can return the patient to a level of function that she or he would find fulfilling. This can be very difficult in the chaos of a major trauma, but when there is an opportunity, discuss this with the patient, or the family, or both.

## Trauma in Pregnancy

Fundamentally, the management of a pregnant patient is the same as that for any other trauma victim (also see Chapter 33). A focus on delivering advanced trauma management will optimize the outcomes for both the mother and the fetus. Still, some specific issues need to be considered when managing a pregnant trauma patient (Box 42.17). This section will present a brief outline of some of the considerations and differences when managing a pregnant trauma patient.

### Causes of Trauma

Pregnant women suffer the same types of trauma as nonpregnant women, yet they can be more vulnerable to injury. There are a few special situations worth considering. For example, intimate partner violence increases during pregnancy and should always be actively considered. In addition, pregnant women are at risk of improper seatbelt use, which can significantly reduce the effectiveness of this countermeasure and result in a different injury pattern.

### Anatomy of Injury

As the fetus develops during the pregnancy, the nature of maternal and fetal injury changes.

---

| **Box 42.17** Key Points—Trauma in Pregnancy |
| --- |
| • Normal signs of blood loss are late—look to urine output or fetal distress |
| • Fetal distress is first sign of maternal compromise |
| • Don't forget left tilt—uterine displacement to reduce aortocaval compression |
| • Reduced FRC—rapid desaturation |

*FRC,* Functional residual capacity.

*First trimester*: 0 to 13 weeks' gestational age
The uterus remains an intrapelvic organ; thus, it is well protected from blunt force trauma. There are the "usual" adult injuries to abdominal viscera. The embryo is nonviable; vaginal bleeding is a poor prognostic sign.

*Second trimester*: 14 to 26 weeks' gestational age
The uterus moves into an extrapelvic position. There is a progressive, increased risk of direct fetal injury. The maternal organs gradually become more shielded.

*Third trimester*: 27 to 40 weeks' gestational age
The maternal organs are relatively protected from injury by the uterus and fetus. Exception—the bladder is at increased risk. There is an increased likelihood of precipitating early labor.

### Special Considerations

#### Maternal Physiology

Maternal physiology undergoes significant change to accommodate the growing fetus (also see Chapter 33). Health care providers should be aware of specific changes that have a significant impact on treatment:

- Increased circulating blood volume that can mask significant blood loss
- Compensated respiratory alkalosis with the normal carbon dioxide partial pressure ($P_{CO_2}$) of about 30 mm Hg
- Increased clotting factors or hypercoagulable state toward the end of pregnancy; at term, a fibrinogen of 300 mg/dL would be abnormally low

#### Aortocaval Compression

This is a phenomenon in which the mass of the uterus and fetus can apply compression to the inferior vena cava and abdominal aorta, causing a drop in cardiac output of up to 30%. The risk of aortocaval compression becomes clinically significant from approximately 20 weeks. To prevent this phenomenon, a wedge is placed under the right hip (left tilt) of approximately 15 to 30 degrees or the use of a spine board to rotate the patient is appropriate. An alternative approach during a resuscitation is to have an assistant manually displace the uterus to the patient's left (Fig. 42.10).

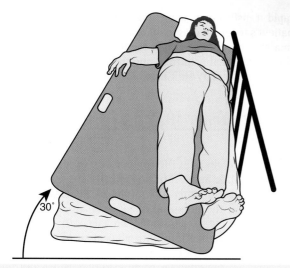

**Fig. 42.10** Left tilt of pregnant patient on spine board.

## Maternal Airway

There is a higher likelihood of difficulty intubating a pregnant patient. This is due to several changes in anatomy and biomechanics:

- Increased generalized soft tissue edema that affects pharyngeal/laryngeal structures
- Increased breast size affecting chest compliance and positioning in the supine position
- Reduced FRC resulting in relatively rapid desaturation
- Lower esophageal sphincter incompetence resulting in higher risk of aspiration

The approach to the maternal airway requires meticulous attention to detail to ensure there are no preventable adverse events. As with nonpregnant patients, consideration to spinal immobilization and adjuncts such as video laryngoscopy should be considered.

## Anti-D Immunoglobulin

For women with Rh (rhesus)-negative blood type, there is a risk of isoimmunization with fetal Rh-positive antigen. Pregnant patients of major trauma, and particularly any with injuries that involve the abdomen, should be considered at risk of contact between maternal and fetal circulations. To prevent longer-term impact on future pregnancies, an Rh-negative mother should be given anti-D immunoglobulin. This can be given any time after maternal blood group is determined but should be less than 72 hours after the trauma.

## Radiation Exposure

Understandably, great effort is made to reduce radiation exposure to pregnant women. In the context of a major trauma, the insult most likely to cause morbidity or fatality to the patient and her fetus is delayed diagnosis of major life-threatening conditions. If there is a diagnostic modality that is immediately available that uses less radiation (e.g., ultrasound), then it is appropriate to use it. The objective is to minimize the use of ionizing radiation but ensure the diagnosis is not delayed.

## Fetal Monitoring

Fetal monitoring should not be commenced until maternal stability has been achieved. Monitoring should be performed by those with appropriate skills and training to interpret the information. Continuous fetal monitoring is not recommended for a fetus younger than 24 weeks unless there are plans to offer full resuscitation and neonatal intensive care support. The duration of monitoring is controversial, but most authorities recommend an initial 2 to 4 hours. The perfusion to the uteroplacental unit is not autoregulated. As such, any reduction in maternal cardiac output, even if asymptomatic, can demonstrate a significant reduction in perfusion to the fetus. Any deterioration in fetal condition should prompt reassessment of maternal hemodynamics.

## Delivery

It may be necessary to expedite delivery of the fetus to optimize maternal or fetal survival. Delivery of the fetus may be the only way to control massive uterine or placental bleeding and ensure a successful resuscitation. Consultation with obstetric and pediatric colleagues should be sought before undertaking any operative delivery. In the event of sustained cardiac arrest, a perimortem cesarean section should be considered if 5 minutes have elapsed without return of spontaneous circulation.[28]

## Specific Differential Diagnoses

The following diagnoses are unique to the pregnant patient and should always be considered in addition to standard differential diagnoses.

- Amniotic fluid embolus can cause potentially life-threatening hemodynamic collapse (see Chapter 33).
- Placental abruption is the process of inappropriate separation of the placenta from the uterine wall. The effect on the mother and fetus depends on the size and location of the disruption. Large disruptions can result in massive hemorrhage and fetal hypoxia.
- Uterine rupture: A major trauma can result in loss of containment of the fetus in the uterine cavity. This results in fetal parts being in the mother's abdominal cavity. It is a life-threatening obstetric emergency for both mother and fetus. Women who have had previous cesarean sections are at higher risk.
- Eclampsia: Although rare, eclampsia should be considered in any pregnant woman with an altered conscious state. It is usually associated with hypertension (i.e., arterial blood pressure more than 140/90 mm Hg) and proteinuria.

VI

## Care for Trauma Patients in Non-OR Settings

Many procedures that are performed on trauma patients outside the ORs require anesthesia providers (also see Chapter 38). These procedures occur at varying stages of resuscitation. Care in these environments can present unique challenges because of the unfamiliarity with surroundings, equipment, and staff. Patients are often evaluated in the CT scanner prior to further triage. Other locations may include radiologic suites, such as magnetic resonance imaging (MRI) or interventional radiology (IR), or the ICU. Importantly, a full accounting of the mechanism of trauma as well as known information of past medical history, injuries, laboratory values, interventions already performed, and the planned procedure should be gathered as time allows. The focus of the anesthesia provider should remain on airway patency and the hemodynamic stability of the patient. Adequate patient monitoring throughout the transport and procedure must be maintained. Trauma surgeons should be notified immediately of any acute or unexpected changes in the patient's status. If the patient requires any additional airway interventions or has a preexisting airway in place, respiratory therapists may be available for additional support. Emergency airway equipment should always be readily available along with medications for anesthetic induction and hemodynamic support. Suction should also be available in each location, particularly if thoracostomy tubes have been placed. Interventions performed in IR that require the presence of an anesthesia provider should have an anesthesia machine available, as well as a standard OR cart with basic equipment and medications. If the patient is still in the acute phase of care while undergoing a procedure outside the OR, the anesthesia provider must be ready for active cardiopulmonary resuscitation, which may require the availability of blood, fluid warmers, large-bore intravenous access, rapid transfusion machines, and invasive monitoring. The patient's temperature should be monitored and normothermia maintained. Because of the remoteness of some locations, additional help from anesthesia technicians, nurses, and other ancillary staff may be critical.

## QUESTIONS OF THE DAY

1. What are the ABCDE components of the Advanced Trauma Life Support (ATLS) primary survey?
2. For patients with airway burns or oral trauma, what are the potential hazards of airway management? What steps should be taken to reduce the risk of complications with placement of a definitive airway?
3. What are the qualities of an effective leader and follower in a trauma team? How can followers communicate their concerns in a constructive manner?
4. What is the rationale for damage control resuscitation (DCR) compared to traditional approaches to fluid management in trauma care? What are the key components of DCR?
5. How should anesthetics be administered in a stepwise fashion in a patient undergoing exploratory laparotomy for acute hemorrhage after major trauma?
6. After traumatic brain injury (TBI), what is the difference between primary neurologic injury and secondary injury?
7. In a patient with traumatic spinal cord injury (SCI), what are the physiologic manifestations of spinal shock?
8. What criteria should be used to decide whether an acute burn patient should be transferred to a dedicated burn center?

## REFERENCES

1. World Health Organization. *Injuries and Violence: The Facts 2014.* Geneva: World Health Organization; 2014.
2. Heron M. Deaths: leading causes for 2011. *Natl Vital Stat Rep.* 2015;64(7):1–96.
3. Centers for Disease Control and Prevention. *Injury Prevention & Control: Data & Statistics (WISQARS).* Atlanta, GA: Centers for Disease Control and Prevention; 2015.
4. MacKenzie E, Rivara F, Jurkovich G. A national evaluation of the effect of trauma-center care on mortality. *N Engl J Med.* 2006;354:366–378.
5. Dawson S, King L, Grantham H. Improving the hospital clinical handover between paramedics and emergency department staff in the deteriorating patient. *Emerg Med Aust.* 2013;(25):393–405.
6. Weingart S, Levitan R. Preoxygenation and prevention of desaturation during emergency airway management. *Ann Emerg Med.* 2012;59(3):165–175.
7. Vourch M, Asfar P, Volteau C. High-flow nasal cannula oxygen during endotracheal intubation in hypoxemic patients: a randomized controlled clinical trial. *Intensive Care Med.* 2015;41(9):1538–1548.
8. Lancman B, Jorm C. Taking the heat in critical situations: being aware, assertive and heard. In: Iedema R, Piper D, Manidis M, eds. *Communicating Quality and Safety in Healthcare.* Cambridge, England: Cambridge University Press; 2015.
9. Spahn D. Management of bleeding and coagulopathy following major trauma: an updated European guideline. *Crit Care.* 2013;17(2):R76.
10. Duchesne JC, McSwain Jr NE, Cotton BA, et al. Damage control resuscitation: the new face of damage control. *J Trauma.* 2010;69(4):976–990.
11. Feinman M, Cotton B, Haut E. Optimal fluid resuscitation in trauma: type, timing, and total. *Curr Opin Crit Care.* 2014;20(4):366–372.
12. Study Group PROPPR, Holcomb JB, Tilley BC, Baraniuk S, et al. Transfusion of plasma, platelets, and red blood cells in a 1:1:1 vs a 1:1:2 ratio and mortality in patients with severe trauma: the PROPPR randomized clinical trial. *JAMA.* 2015;313(5):471–482.
13. Roberts I, Shakur H, Coats T, et al. The CRASH-2 trial: a randomised controlled trial and economic evaluation of the effects of tranexamic acid on death, vascular occlusive events and transfusion requirement in bleeding trauma patients. *Health Technol Assess.* 2013;17(10):1–79.

14. Morrison J, Dubose JJ, Rasmussen TE, et al. Military Application of Tranexamic Acid in Trauma Emergency Resuscitation (MATTERs) Study. *Arch Surg.* 2012;147(2):113–119.

15. Steurer M, Ganter M. Trauma and massive blood transfusions. *Curr Anesthesiol Rep.* 2014;4:200–208.

16. Dutton R. Haemostatic resuscitation. *Br J Anaesth.* 2012;109(suppl 1):i39–i46.

17. Frieden T, Houry D, Baldwin G. *Report to Congress on traumatic brain injury in the United States: epidemiology and rehabilitation.* Atlanta, GA: National Center for Injury Prevention and Control, Division of Unintentional Injury Prevention; 2014.

18. Holly LT, Kelly DF, Counelis GJ, et al. Cervical spine trauma associated with moderate and severe head injury: incidence, risk factors, and injury characteristics. *J Neurosurg.* 2002;96(3 suppl):285–291.

19. Robitaille A, Williams SR, Tremblay MH, et al. Cervical spine motion during tracheal intubation with manual in-line stabilization: direct laryngoscopy versus GlideScope videolaryngoscopy. *Anesth Analg.* 2008;106(3):935–941.

20. Turkstra T, Craen RA, Pelz DM, Gelb AW. Cervical spine motion: a fluoroscopic comparison during intubation with lighted stylet, GlideScope, and Macintosh laryngoscope. *Anesth Analg.* 2005;101(3):910–915.

21. Zeiler F, Teitelbaum J, West M, Gillman LM. The ketamine effect on ICP in traumatic brain injury. *Neurocrit Care.* 2014;21(1):163–173.

22. Grathwohl K, Black I, Spinella P. Total intravenous anesthesia including ketamine versus volatile gas anesthesia for combat-related operative traumatic brain injury. *Anesthesiology.* 2008;109:44.

23. Brain Trauma Foundation; American Association of Neurological Surgeons; Congress of Neurological Surgeons. Guidelines for the management of severe traumatic brain injury. *J Neurotrauma.* 2007;24(suppl 1):S1–106.

24. The SAFE Study Investigators; Australian and New Zealand Intensive Care Society Clinical Trials Group; Australian Red Cross Blood Service; George Institute for International Health; Myburgh J, Cooper DJ, Finfer S, et al. Saline or albumin for fluid resuscitation in patients with traumatic brain injury. *N Engl J Med.* 2007;357(9):874–884.

25. National Spinal Cord Injury Statistical Center. *Facts and Figures at a Glance.* Birmingham, AL: University of Alabama; 2013.

26. Ghobrial G, Amenta P, Maltenfort M. Longitudinal incidence and concurrence rates for traumatic brain injury and spine injury—a twenty year analysis. *Clin Neurol Neurosurg.* 2014;123:174–180.

27. Walters B, Hadley M, Hurlbert R. Guidelines for the management of acute cervical spine and spinal cord injuries: 2013 update. *Neurosurgery.* 2013;60(suppl 1):82–91.

28. Enlav S, Sela H, Weiniger C. Management and outcomes of trauma during pregnancy. *Anesthesiol Clin.* 2013;31(1):141–156.

VI

# 43 HUMAN-INDUCED AND NATURAL DISASTERS

## Catherine Kuza and Joseph H. McIsaac, III

Disasters can be broadly characterized into two categories: those that happen to someone else and those that happen to you. We typically define a disaster as an event that overwhelms the usual capacity of the facility or geographic area, often requiring outside resources in management. Disasters come in many different forms. They include human-driven intentional acts of violence (e.g., terrorism, riots, and war) and natural phenomena (e.g., severe weather, seismic events, or epidemics). The range of a disaster may vary from a localized event to one covering entire regions or continents. It can result from a single event in time, like an earthquake, or be extended over months to years (i.e., droughts, pandemics). Disasters universally create a mismatch between need and available resources including medical supplies, pharmaceuticals, food and water, shelter, and skilled responders such as police officers, firefighters, and health care professionals. In recent years, an increasing number of casualties have been caused by disasters such as earthquakes (e.g., Haiti in 2010 and Japan in 2011), shootings (e.g., Paris in 2015, San Bernardino in 2015, and Orlando in 2016), and other terrorist attacks (e.g., New York City World Trade Center attacks in 2001, London bombings in 2005, and Boston bombing in 2013). Thus, it is important for anesthesia providers to be educated and trained on disaster management to help save lives. It takes disciplined individuals to sustain their education and training because traumatic events of this nature rarely happen (outside a busy urban trauma center or war zone).

## DISASTER TYPES AND NOMENCLATURE

Communities often require outside help and international assistance, depending on the severity of the disaster.[1] Various disasters can result in mass casualty events (MCEs)

The editors and publisher would like to thank Dr. Eric Y. Lin for contributing to this chapter in the previous edition of this work. It has provided the framework for much of this chapter.

| Table 43.1 | Types of Disasters Resulting in Mass Casualty Events |
|---|---|
| **Category** | **Examples** |
| Natural | Hurricane, tornado, flood, earthquake, fire, volcano, tsunami, drought, avalanche, extreme heat or cold, rain, ice, snow, bacterial/viral pandemics |
| Unintentional | Public transportation accident, boat accident, nuclear accident, industrial accident, building collapse |
| Intentional | Bombing, nuclear/biologic/chemical attack, environmental interference |
| Human-induced | Oil spill, fire, chemical/nuclear plant explosion, terror attack, war |

Aitken P, Leggat P. Considerations in mass casualty and disaster management. In Blaivas M, ed. *Emergency Medicine—An International Perspective*. Rijeka, Croatia: InTech; 2012:143-182. Also available from http://www.intechopen.com/books/emergency-medicine-an-international-perspective/considerations-in-mass-casualty-and-disaster-management/; TFQCDM/WADEM (Task Force on Quality Control of Disaster Management/World Association for Disaster and Emergency Medicine). Health disaster management: guidelines for evaluation and research in the "utstein style." Chapter 3: overview and concepts. *Prehosp Disaster Med*. 2002;17(suppl 3):31-55; Dudaryk R, Pretto EA. Resuscitation in a multiple casualty event. *Anesthesiol Clin*. 2013;31:85-106.

(Table 43.1), in which the number of victims surpasses the treatment ability and resources provided by a medical center.[2] Even at Level I trauma centers with an activated disaster plan, it is difficult to provide care to more than seven casualties per hour.[3,4]

A health disaster constitutes decreased quality of public health and medical care to victims and an overall decline in the health status of a community, which is unable to adequately recover. Syria is an extreme example of such a continuous disaster. Conversely, a medical disaster refers to the suspension of providing health care to individuals because of a disaster event. Hazards are any conditions that may pose a threat to safety, well-being, or environment and can be natural, human-induced, or mixed.[5,6] The probability of a negative event occurring is defined as a risk. A schematic representation of these definitions is provided in Fig. 43.1.[5]

## EPIDEMIOLOGY

Various types of disasters occur frequently around the world leading to environmental and resource destruction, injury, and death of large populations. Disasters can be natural, human-induced, or mixed with contributions from nature and people. Table 43.2 shows the incidence of various disaster subgroups that occurred over the past 5 years globally and the number of people who were injured, affected, and died.[7] Table 43.3 shows the frequency of disaster types by continents.[1]

There has been an increased frequency of disastrous events over the past century (Fig. 43.2). Improved technology, database development, and increased reporting of these casualties may contribute to the rising number of disasters, but there are additional contributing factors. The advances in technology, chemicals, weapons, and increasing use of transportation vehicles contribute to the increasing number of human-induced disasters. Additionally, the world population has significantly increased, with an increase in the number of inhabitants of desolate regions, where disaster planning, preparedness, resource availability, and response may not be as well established as in larger cities.[1] In less developed countries, the access to resources and emergency preparedness plans may not be well established, resulting in higher death tolls compared to developed countries. International organizations such as the World Health Organization (WHO) and Pan American Health Organization (PAHO) work to help such countries implement cost-effective emergency preparedness plans to mitigate the effects of disasters.[1,8] Yet, mortality statistics do not reflect the severity of the disaster. Communities can be affected by interrupting employment, education, transportation, food resources, and security. The vast damage created by disasters may also affect health care workers by preventing them from safely reporting to work. In addition, power failures or floods can damage hospital equipment and cause secondary health hazards.

## DISASTER PREPARATION AND RESPONSE

### Phases of a Disaster

The goals of disaster management are to reduce or prevent the potential losses from hazards, provide prompt and appropriate assistance to victims, and achieve rapid and effective recovery. Disaster responsiveness requires the coordination among responders, civilians, and government agencies to plan for and reduce the impact of disasters. Disaster management also incorporates developing public policies and plans that prevent or minimize the harmful effects of disasters on people, structures, and communities. There are four phases of a disaster, and they are described in Table 43.4. The phases can sometimes overlap and do not necessarily proceed in order.[9-12]

Disaster Preparedness and Mitigation
Disaster preparedness consists of actions taken to prevent or minimize the negative impacts of disasters. Previous experiences with natural disasters and mass casualties have led to the development of preparedness plans and protocols to be implemented for future events. Preparedness also entails public education, simulation drills and training, hospital and national organization coordination, and expectant management. Not all disasters can be prevented, but proper planning, education, evacuation, and

VI

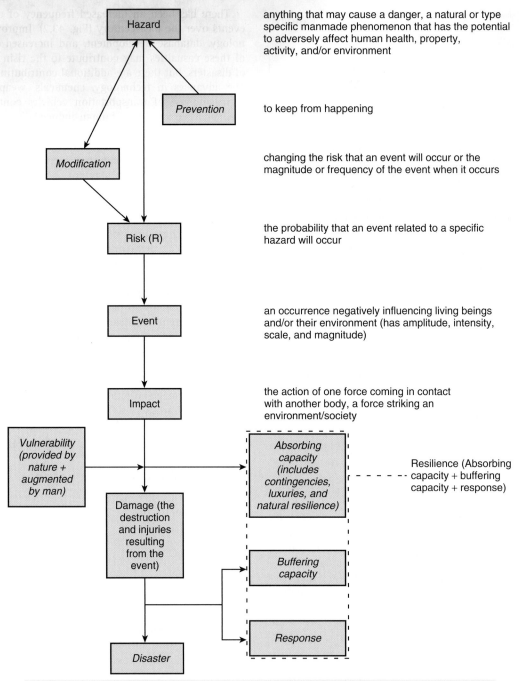

**Fig. 43.1** Schematic illustration of definitions. (From TFQCDM/WADEM [Task Force on Quality Control of Disaster Management/World Association for Disaster and Emergency Medicine]. Health disaster management: guidelines for evaluation and research in the "utstein style." Chapter 3: overview and concepts. *Prehosp Disaster Med.* 2002;17(suppl 3):31-55.)

preparation of necessary resources can help mitigate the consequent effects.[1]

A community's socioeconomic status, quality of structures (bridges, roads, buildings), hospital systems, and emergency medical services are important factors in disaster preparedness. Those communities with poor predisaster resources may not be equipped to deal with the repercussions of such disasters. This can result in increased injuries, fatality, destruction of infrastructures, and quickly exhausting resources. Such communities

| Table 43.2 | International Disaster Subgroups and Mortality Data from 2011 to 2016 | | | | |
|---|---|---|---|---|---|
| **Year** | **Disaster Subgroup** | **Occurrence** | **Total Deaths** | **Injured** | **Affected** |
| 2011 | Biologic | 27 | 3,174 | 420 | 1,156,317 |
| 2011 | Climatologic | 23 | 10 | 5 | 30,423,594 |
| 2011 | Geophysical | 34 | 20,767 | 11,663 | 1,274,378 |
| 2011 | Hydrologic | 172 | 6,472 | 2,403 | 135,241,070 |
| 2011 | Meteorologic | 94 | 3,537 | 34,778 | 42,341,557 |
| 2011 | Technologic | 241 | 6,588 | 5,640 | 10,156 |
| 2012 | Biologic | 25 | 1,887 | 149 | 156,302 |
| 2012 | Climatologic | 25 | 21 | 422 | 23,554,769 |
| 2012 | Complex disasters | 2 | | | 1,482,214 |
| 2012 | Geophysical | 29 | 727 | 41,776 | 2,799,144 |
| 2012 | Hydrologic | 142 | 3,961 | 9,144 | 63,490,304 |
| 2012 | Meteorologic | 137 | 4,922 | 12,419 | 20,147,336 |
| 2012 | Technologic | 185 | 5,720 | 10,090 | 13,504 |
| 2013 | Biologic | 22 | 526 | 2,509 | 306,851 |
| 2013 | Climatologic | 15 | 32 | 17 | 7,949,631 |
| 2013 | Extraterrestrial | 1 | | 1,491 | 300,000 |
| 2013 | Geophysical | 31 | 1,156 | 21,566 | 7,158,348 |
| 2013 | Hydrologic | 158 | 10,071 | 6,701 | 31,777,995 |
| 2013 | Meteorologic | 116 | 10,418 | 92,133 | 48,878,386 |
| 2013 | Technologic | 191 | 6,701 | 5,032 | 10,016 |
| 2014 | Biologic | 22 | 12,923 | 69,276 | 122,941 |
| 2014 | Climatologic | 20 | 14 | 500 | 68,821,066 |
| 2014 | Geophysical | 31 | 876 | 5,973 | 3,317,439 |
| 2014 | Hydrologic | 146 | 4,428 | 5,022 | 40,237,519 |
| 2014 | Meteorologic | 111 | 2,440 | 26,493 | 26,828,377 |
| 2014 | Technologic | 205 | 6,389 | 4,233 | 284,893 |
| 2015 | Biologic | 16 | 1,089 | 44,108 | 26,952 |
| 2015 | Climatologic | 30 | 76 | 1,017 | 46,938,206 |
| 2015 | Geophysical | 30 | 9,563 | 81,865 | 7,907,683 |
| 2015 | Hydrologic | 176 | 4,455 | 23,343 | 34,685,784 |
| 2015 | Meteorologic | 118 | 8,662 | 22,072 | 11,151,582 |
| 2015 | Technologic | 202 | 9,726 | 8,643 | 71,600 |
| 2016 | Biologic | 5 | 40 | 2,160 | |
| 2016 | Climatologic | 10 | 4 | | 335,107,656 |
| 2016 | Geophysical | 13 | 1,185 | 234,952 | 1,172,679 |

VI

**Table 43.2** International Disaster Subgroups and Mortality Data from 2011 to 2016—cont'd

| Year | Disaster Subgroup | Occurrence | Total Deaths | Injured | Affected |
|------|-------------------|------------|--------------|---------|----------|
| 2016 | Hydrologic | 116 | 3,655 | 8,190 | 9,068,011 |
| 2016 | Meteorologic | 50 | 1,953 | 3,062 | 5,665,433 |
| 2016 | Technologic | 118 | 3,406 | 2,855 | 12,202 |

From Centre for Research on the Epidemiology of Disasters (CRED). Emergency Events Database (EM-DAT). http://www.emdat.be. Accessed on: December 1, 2016.

**Table 43.3** Frequency of Disaster Types by Continent

| Disaster Type | Asia | Americas | Africa | Europe | Oceania | Total |
|---------------|------|----------|--------|--------|---------|-------|
| Transport | 668 | 233 | 437 | 186 | 11 | 1535 |
| Floods | 362 | 216 | 207 | 153 | 25 | 963 |
| Windstorms | 322 | 283 | 49 | 71 | 58 | 783 |
| Industrial | 225 | 55 | 37 | 67 | 2 | 386 |
| Misc. accidents | 178 | 45 | 57 | 53 | 5 | 338 |
| Droughts/ famines | 77 | 39 | 113 | 13 | 11 | 253 |
| Earthquakes | 112 | 48 | 10 | 37 | 8 | 215 |
| Avalanches/ landslides | 101 | 40 | 12 | 25 | 5 | 183 |
| Forest fires | 18 | 55 | 11 | 39 | 9 | 132 |
| Extreme temperatures | 35 | 30 | 6 | 51 | 4 | 126 |
| Volcanic eruptions | 16 | 23 | 3 | 2 | 6 | 50 |

From Aitken P, Leggat P. Considerations in mass casualty and disaster management. In Blaivas M, ed. *Emergency Medicine—An International Perspective*. Rijeka, Croatia: InTech; 2012:143-182.

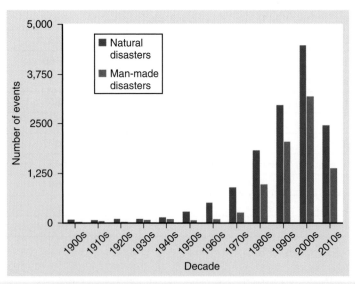

**Fig. 43.2** Graphic depiction of the frequency of disasters each decade. (From Centre for Research on the Epidemiology of Disasters [CRED]. Emergency Events Database [EM-DAT]. http://www.emdat.be. Accessed on December 1, 2016.)

| Table 43.4 | Four Phases of Disaster | |
|---|---|---|
| **Phase** | **Action** | **Example** |
| Mitigation | Predisaster; preventing or minimizing the effects of the disaster | Public education, building codes and zoning |
| Preparedness | Planning how to respond | Preparedness plans, emergency drills, warning systems |
| Response | Efforts to minimize the hazards created by a disaster | Search and rescue, emergency relief |
| Recovery | Returning the community to normal, rebuilding, data collection of lessons learned | Temporary housing, medical care |

Baird ME. The phases of emergency management. 2010. Prepared for the Intermodal Freight Transportation Institute (ITFI). http://www.vanderbilt.edu/vector/research/emmgtphases.pdf. Accessed December 1, 2016; Wisner B, Adams J. Environmental health in emergencies and disasters: a practical guide. World Health Organization, 2002. http://www.who.int/water_sanitation_health/hygiene/emergencies/em2002intro.pdf. Accessed December 1, 2016; Federal Emergency Management Agency (FEMA). Principles of emergency management: independent study. 2006. https://training.fema.gov/emiweb/downloads/is230.pdf. Accessed December 1, 2016; American Society of Anesthesiologists Committee on Trauma and Emergency Preparedness (ASA COTEP). Emergence Preparedness Resources. https://www.asahq.org/resources/resources-from-asa-committees/committee-on-trauma-and-emergency-preparedness/emergency-preparedness. Accessed December 1, 2016.

become reliant on assistance from other towns or countries (e.g., Haiti after the 2010 earthquake).[6]

### Personal Preparedness

A personal and family emergency preparedness plan should be in place and routinely updated. Families should also perform drills to prepare for unanticipated emergencies. There are numerous online websites of organizations such as the Federal Emergency Management Agency (FEMA), which have family plans, materials geared toward kids, communication resources, and updated information on what to do in the event of certain disasters. The American Society of Anesthesiologists Committee on Trauma and Emergency Preparedness (ASA COTEP) has also provided a document on necessary supplies, first aid and disaster kits, clothing, utilities, and items needed to pack in the event of an emergency or evacuation (Box 43.1).[12,13] Families should expect that telephones or electricity may not work in certain situations and devise alternative methods of communication.[14] Additionally, resources should be shared with neighbors, and one should provide assistance and help to neighbors and other community members.

### Government Plans

If a disaster or critical event has extensive impact requiring more assistance and resources than can be offered locally, national agencies often intervene. These various disaster management agencies have specific responsibilities in response to the type of crisis event as given in Table 43.5.[15]

In the United States, agencies such as the Centers for Disease Control and Prevention (CDC) prepare for disasters related to public health threats and have resources to

provide equipment, specially trained medical personnel, and medications within 6 hours of notification. There are also national pharmaceutical stores that can be rapidly dispensed to regions affected by disasters when needed. In certain situations, such as terrorist threats or attacks and biochemical exposure, military services may be called upon to create field hospitals, isolate exposures, and provide public safety.[15]

The National Disaster Medical System (NDMS) is a partnership between the Departments of Health and Human Services (HHS), Defense (DOD), Homeland Security (DHS), and Veterans Affairs (VA). NDMS provides medical response to a disaster area, moves patients from a disaster site to unaffected areas, and delivers medical care at participating hospitals. NDMS has formed specific disaster response teams such as the International Medical Surgical Response Team (IMSuRT), Disaster Medical Assistance Team (DMAT), Disaster Mortuary Operational Response Team (DMORT), National Veterinary Response Team (NVRT), and, most recently, Medical Specialty Enhancement Teams (MSETs). The response team descriptions and responsibilities are provided in Table 43.6. Despite the presence of these governmental response teams, the number of teams is small and the activation and deployment of resources to a specific location can take up to 2 hours.[14]

### Risk Assessment and Management

The components of risk assessment and management include predicting the probability of adverse outcomes, identifying and monitoring risks associated with the disaster event, and implementing policies and practices aimed at mitigating these risks.[1,16-18] Risks must be prioritized to identify those most likely to occur and have the most severe impact. There are several

**VI**

**Box 43.1** Family Emergency Preparedness Checklist[a] by ASA COTEP

**Shelter**
Supplies (at least 3 days)
- Medications
- Food and water (1 gallon per person per day)
- Pet care
- Batteries
First aid and disaster kit
Communications (battery-powered radio)
Security plan
Sanitation/hygiene plan
Cash
Utilities
- Ability to safely shut off
- Establish alternative power and lighting

**Evacuate**
Supplies (72 hours or more)
- Medications
- Food and water (1 gallon per person per day)
- Pet care
- Batteries
Communications (battery-powered radio)
Clothing (weather/climate appropriate)
Transportation and fuel
- Preplanned routes and alternatives
- Utilities
- Shut off water and electricity if instructed
- "Go bags"
- Documents/supplies
- Maps/compass
- Flashlight
- First aid and disaster kit
- Cash
Meeting place
- Right outside home
- Outside neighborhood
Critical documents (in waterproof container)
- Identity (passport, driver's license)
- Marriage license, divorce decree
- Birth certificates
- Medical license
- Insurance documents
- Financial records and deeds
- Irreplaceable photos

[a]Make sure every member of the family knows the plan, that you post in it an accessible place, and that you practice yearly. For more details see www.ready.gov.
*ASA COTEP*, American Society of Anesthesiologists Committee on Trauma and Emergency Preparedness.
From American Society of Anesthesiologists Committee on Trauma and Emergency Preparedness (ASA COTEP). Emergence Preparedness Resources. https://www.asahq.org/resources/resources-from-asa-committees/committee-on-trauma-and-emergency-preparedness/emergency-preparedness. Accessed December 1, 2016.

risk assessment scores and matrices (Fig. 43.3) that help distinguish such risks, allowing organizations to focus planning and interventions in these areas.

**Table 43.5** U.S. Government Agencies and Responsibilities in Mass Casualty Events

| Agency | Responsibility |
|---|---|
| Federal Bureau of Investigation (FBI) | Domestic terrorism and crisis management |
| Federal Emergency Management Agency (FEMA) | Coordinates national emergency response and provides assistance to local and state governments, emergency relief to affected persons and businesses, and support for public safety |
| Department of Health and Human Services (HHS) | Provides health-related and medical services |
| Department of Defense (DOD) | Assists with biologic or chemical terrorism, bomb disposal, and decontamination |
| Centers for Disease Control and Prevention (CDC) | Coordinates response to public health threats and provides resources to local and state organizations |

From Lin EY. Trauma, bioterrorism, and natural disasters. In Miller RD, ed. *Basics of Anesthesia*. 6th ed. Philadelphia: Elsevier Saunders; 2011:681-697.

Risk modification or prevention strategies should be reviewed regularly so that implementation plans can be adapted accordingly.[1]

### Response Systems
#### Hospital Incident Command System
In the United States and internationally, the Hospital Incident Command System (HICS) can be used during emergencies, planned events, or in managing threats. HICS is based on the Incident Command System (ICS), a management system that was developed after analysis of catastrophic wildfires in the state of California in the 1970s. The elements of ICS include command, operations, planning, logistics, and finance/administration. HICS, like ICS, is an adaptable system that can be employed at any hospital. The principles presented in HICS apply to the mission areas of prevention, protection, mitigation, response, and recovery. Although HICS is most often considered for hazardous events, it can also be used for nonemergent purposes such as hosting large hospital events and administering annual influenza vaccinations.

HICS utilizes a standard format for responses that is both effective and recognized by other responding agencies, thus facilitating coordination among various organizations during a disaster. The principles of HICS include facilitating smooth transitions of care between hospitals and outside responding providers, assigning

| Table 43.6 | U.S. Government Medical Response Teams: Description and Responsibilities |
|---|---|

| Response Team | Description and Responsibilities |
|---|---|
| International Medical Surgical Response Team (IMSuRT) | Three teams that provide care to U.S. citizens injured in areas of conflict. |
| Disaster Medical Assistance Team (DMAT) | Rapidly mobilizes and sets up staff with physicians, nurses, and other support personnel, emergency facilities, and pharmaceutical dispensaries near the disaster site. Response personnel must complete 1 weekend of training each month. |
| Disaster Mortuary Operational Response Team (DMORT) | Manages mass deaths; handles bodies and performs forensic examinations. |
| National Veterinary Response Team (NVRT) | Provides veterinary services and zoonotic disease surveillance. |
| Medical Specialty Enhancement Teams (MSETs) | Team composed of 30 surgeons, 30 anesthesiologists, and pediatricians who are federally employed during deployments of at least 2 weeks. They respond to domestic/international crises and deploy either to the disaster site or specified facility. |

From Murray MJ. Emergency preparedness for and disaster management of casualties from natural disasters and chemical, biologic, radiologic, nuclear, and high-yield explosive (CBRNE) events. In Barash PG, ed. *Clinical Anesthesia*. 7th ed. Philadelphia: Lippincott Williams & Wilkins; 2013:1535-1549.

| | | Potential Severity Rating | | | |
|---|---|---|---|---|---|
| | | Minor | Moderate | Significant | Catastrophic |
| Likelihood Severity Occurs | Very Likely | Moderate | High | Extreme | Extreme |
| | Likely | Low | Moderate | High | Extreme |
| | Unlikely | Very Low | Low | Moderate | High |
| | Rare | Very Low | Very Low | Low | Moderate |

**Fig. 43.3** Risk management using risk matrix. (From Risk Assessment. http://www.arriscar.com.au/services/risk-assessment/. Accessed December 1, 2016.)

responsibilities to personnel and designated teams, planning and coordinating support requirements, emphasizing efficient communication, and obtaining necessary equipment or supplies from outside sources. HICS provides job action sheets that define responder roles and list the tasks to be performed.[19-23] The implementation of HICS in individual hospitals requires education and training in order to provide a structured system that results in successful management of any pertinent event or disaster.[24]

### Hospital Emergency Management Plans

Hospitals should have emergency management plans in order to provide prompt medical care, justly allocate resources, and minimize deaths from disasters or MCEs. Emergency management plans should address situations in which large numbers of victims require treatment. Examples include MCEs due to terror attacks as well as incidents that affect the hospital itself, such as earthquakes and other natural disasters. The plans should educate and prepare the staff on disaster management, with the goal of appropriately allocating and using hospital resources to provide the best care possible. The main principles of hospital disaster plans are provided in Box 43.2.

Emergency management plans are developed by a hospital disaster/emergency management committee. This committee should have multidisciplinary membership of clinical and nonclinical staff from key departments and units in the hospital. In a large hospital, the committee may include the following groups: hospital administration, clinical division chiefs (e.g., surgery, orthopedics, anesthesiology, emergency medicine, pathology, blood bank, radiology, nutrition, nursing), clinical support services (e.g., radiology, laboratory, blood bank, pathology, social services), and hospital operations (e.g., engineering, materials management, security, sanitation/environmental services). Emergency plans should utilize HICS principles to assign roles and organize response efforts. Specific details of these plans include approaches to increase bed capacity, distribute information to the public regarding the disaster, ensure hospital security and safety during the disaster, communicate with other first responders (e.g., police officers), coordinate care with other health care facilities, allocate and obtain necessary supplies and equipment, and prepare for hospital evacuations in the event of natural disasters.

Finally, the hospital emergency management plan should specify when to implement disaster deactivation. A postdisaster debriefing should occur among disaster committee members to evaluate the hospital's performance and identify areas of strength and weakness and accordingly modify the plan in order to improve future performance.[25-27]

### Training, Education, and Planning

Planning is extremely important in emergency preparedness. It involves the coordinated efforts of several

**Box 43.2** Principles of Hospital Disaster Plans

Predictable chain of management
Simple
Flexible with organizational charts and applicable to various disasters
Clearly define authority, roles, and responsibilities
Comprehensive (must be compatible with other hospitals and facilitate interhospital transfer)
Adaptable
Anticipatory
Part of regional health plan in disasters

organizations to develop an agreed-upon emergency protocol based on current evidence and experiences. The planning process involves conducting risk analysis, creating a planning committee, assigning responsibilities, analyzing resources, developing emergency management systems, and testing the emergency preparedness plan. Periodically, these plans need to be reassessed and revised as part of a quality improvement process.[1]

Additionally, education and training for emergency disaster events are recommended. This applies to both civilians as well as medical professionals. Most training hospitals do not adequately prepare health care professionals to deal with disasters. Disaster events present a challenging environment because of the large number of patients and the limited resources. If hospitals do provide staff with training, responsiveness is often plagued with lag times and the inability to apply what was learned to all situations. Providers who have participated in an emergency response rarely have this experience again in the future, and thus most responders are novices. There is an increasing need for personnel who are trained to deal with disasters and who have good communication, teamwork, and decision-making skills.[1] The Hospital Preparedness Exercises Guidebook, which was prepared by the Agency for Healthcare Research and Quality (AHRQ), is a resource that gives hospitals a guide for developing and assessing hospital preparedness exercises.[28,29]

Because of the lack of hospital emergency drills, several programs and curricula have been developed to provide training and improve disaster management education. These include educational materials designed by the World Association for Disaster and Emergency Management (WADEM) and the International Society for Disaster Medicine (ISDM).[1] Additionally, there are courses such as Advanced Trauma Life Support (ATLS), Emergency and Trauma Care Training courses through the WHO, Primary Trauma Care courses, and the Disaster Management and Emergency Preparedness (DMEP) course offered through the American College of Surgeons Committee on Trauma (ACS COT), which are available to anesthesia providers. The teaching methods employed include self-study aids,

problem-based learning and case discussions, disaster drills, simulation exercises testing specific functions of plans (e.g., calling staff to the hospital), and mock field exercises using real resources, vehicles, staff, and equipment. There are also courses that focus on specific areas of emergency preparedness, such as decontamination, active shooter, and MCEs. Although some of these exercises may be expensive, be time consuming, and require significant resources,[1] it is important for providers to have training in order to develop the knowledge and skills required for disaster management.

## MASS CASUALTY EVENTS

Natural disasters, disease epidemics (e.g., severe acute respiratory syndrome [SARS], Ebola), transportation accidents, biochemical and radioactive disasters, and the increasing number of terrorist acts can occur at any time, and anesthesia providers should be trained and prepared to provide care. The mechanisms of injury include blunt and penetrating trauma, burns, and chemical and radiation injuries. MCEs occur when the number of victims surpasses the treatment ability and resources provided by a medical center. An MCE is a dynamic situation that requires the coordination and organization of many personnel through various phases of care in an attempt to decrease the strain put on health care personnel and systems. By their very nature, MCEs create overwhelming demand for medical attention in the setting of seemingly less available resources, equipment, and providers.[2] Even at Level I trauma centers with an activated disaster plan, providing care to more than seven casualties per hour is difficult.[3,4] Medical services and anesthesia skills are needed during an MCE. The centralized point for managing response is the Hospital Emergency Operations Center (HEOC). HEOC may assign anesthesia providers to provide care at the prehospital disaster site, emergency department, decontamination areas, operating room (OR), recovery area, or intensive care unit (ICU). The advent of the Perioperative Surgical Home and the expanding role of anesthesiologists outside the OR (also see Chapters 38 and 51) position them to be among those responders.

### Role of the Anesthesia Provider

Anesthesia providers have a broad knowledge base ranging from physiology to pharmacology. They are familiar with surgical injuries and procedures; capable of managing critically ill, surgically complex, and trauma patients; and possess valuable skills such as airway management, intravenous catheter insertion, and resuscitation, which makes them a valuable member of the disaster/MCE response team. Their training teaches them to be adaptable and provide care for patients in different hospital settings. Other countries have already expanded the role of anesthesiologists to prehospital, emergency department, and postoperative care phases in traumas and disasters.[30]

## Triage of Victims

There are several MCE triage systems: SALT (*s*ort, *a*ssess, *l*ifesaving interventions, *t*reatment/transport) (Fig. 43.4); START (*s*imple *t*riage *a*nd *r*apid *t*reatment for mass casualties) (Fig. 43.5); and MASS (*m*ove, *a*ssess, *s*ort, and *s*end), which may be used in a particular institution. All of these triage systems share the common goals of prioritizing care to the most severely injured and distributing the limited resources to those patients who are likely to survive and receive the greatest benefit.[15,31-33] Anesthesia providers may need to triage patients and assign them into one of four groups: immediate care, delayed care, first aid, and expectant.[14,34] The expectant group includes patients unlikely to survive, and efforts should focus on likely survivors. Anesthesia providers may help decide which patients require ICU or OR care.[2,14] Resources (e.g., imaging) should be allocated to those who are in critical condition but likely to survive. Triage decisions should be based on the available treatment capability and the patient's anatomic/physiologic status rather than the mechanism of injury. Only those with potentially reversible injuries should receive immediate interventions.[2] Those who are unlikely to survive may require medications to provide comfort, and anesthesia providers may be involved in minimizing their suffering.[14] It is also important to remember that in addition to dealing with MCE victims, hospitals are also required to provide routine medical care to patients unaffected by the disaster, such as patients with septic shock, acute appendicitis, stroke, and acute coronary syndrome. These patients cannot be ignored, and the role of triage is important in allocation of resources and prioritizing care, or redirecting care to less burdened facilities. Special patient populations such as pediatric or obstetric patients, may be victims of disasters, and specialized protocols must be in place to aid in the specific management of these patients.

## Prehospital Care

During an MCE, anesthesia providers may be required to provide care outside the hospital. Military anesthesia experiences have demonstrated that anesthesia providers are well equipped to provide care in the early management of trauma and possess skills for providing life support, resuscitation, and an understanding of shock and dysfunction of multiple organ systems.[30] Anesthesia providers can deliver a wide range of disaster scene care including airway management, intravenous line placement, resuscitation, and medication management. Sometimes, they may even provide anesthesia for field surgeries near disaster

sites.[15,23,30,35] Skills learned from programs such as ATLS, Basic Life Support (BLS), and Advanced Cardiac Life Support (ACLS) are important and often used. Early interventions such as chest tube placement may need to be performed. Actively bleeding patients may require splinting, the use of tourniquets, hemostatic bandages, direct pressure, or pelvic binder application. Surgeons may have to perform "damage control surgery" (rapid control of bleeding followed by abdominal packing) on-site, especially in combat situations, to stabilize and save the patient's life. "Field block anesthesia" or nearly "on-site" anesthesia is often required in these situations.[15] For over 30 years in France, anesthesiologists have been an integral part of the prehospital care team. There is a continuum of care provided to these patients by the same anesthesiologists upon arrival to the hospital.[23,30] During the London subway bombings, anesthesiologists were dispatched to the disaster site to help stabilize patients and provide anesthesia and analgesia to those who were trapped under the rubble.[30] Additionally, in cases of biochemical exposure, anesthesiologists aided in patient decontamination at the scene.[15,36] The role of anesthesiologists in the prehospital setting reduces 30-day mortality rate.[37]

### Airway Management in Mass Casualty Events

Anesthesia providers are often responsible for airway management (also see Chapter 16) in MCEs. Under these circumstances, airway management can be particularly challenging because of the emergent nature, risk of aspiration, presence of injuries affecting the airway, hemodynamic instability, and possible exposure to infectious biochemical pathogens. Establishing a secure airway early is preferred over an extended period of bag-mask ventilation. With known biochemical toxicity, providers may need to secure the airway wearing a hazardous material (HAZMAT) suit, which encumbers manual dexterity, impairs visualization of the airway, and requires more time. Endotracheal intubation is considered to be the gold standard and safest method of securing the airway in MCEs. Supraglottic devices such as laryngeal mask airways may be used during difficult intubations; however, they should be replaced by an endotracheal tube as soon as possible.[38] Usually, a rapid sequence intubation is recommended.[39-42] Manual in-line neck stabilization should be provided when applicable[43]; cricoid pressure is considered optional.[44] In nerve agent poisoning, neuromuscular blockers should be used with caution, and an awake intubation should be considered.[39,45] Confirmation of endotracheal tube placement is achieved with capnometry and auscultation.[38]

## Hospital Care

### Emergency Department Care
Although some Level I trauma hospitals have a strong anesthesia presence in the emergency department, this is

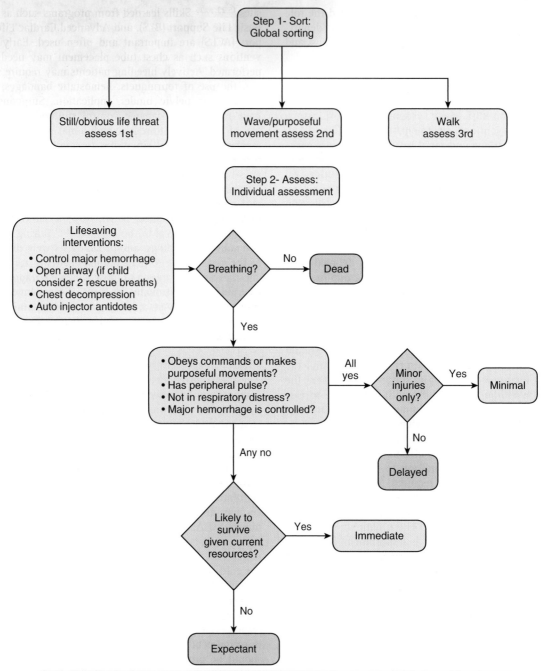

**Fig. 43.4** SALT triage algorithm. (From https://chemm.nlm.nih.gov/salttriage.htm. Accessed December 1, 2016.)

not typical of many centers. In MCEs, anesthesia providers may be required to assist in the emergency department with patient care activities including airway management, vascular access placement, cardiopulmonary resuscitation, and treatment of chemical or biologic toxicity.[14] Hospitals should have equipment needed to perform decontamination in the event of biochemical or radiologic disasters.[15]

Anesthesia providers may also be responsible for ensuring availability of appropriate equipment and supplies.[46] Although having staff who typically do not work in the emergency department participate in MCE care may be counterproductive, anesthesia providers who often assist with airway management or patient care in the emergency department may be extremely effective in this role.[47]

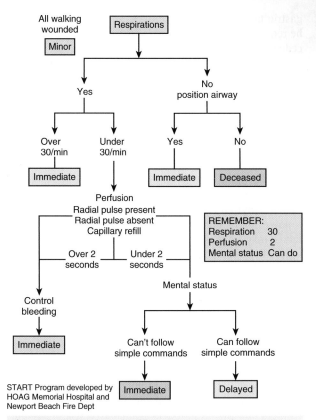

All walking wounded
**Minor**

Respirations

Yes — No position airway

**Over 30/min** → **Immediate**
**Under 30/min**

Yes → **Immediate**
No → **Deceased**

Perfusion
Radial pulse present
Radial pulse absent
Capillary refill

Over 2 seconds — Under 2 seconds

Control bleeding → **Immediate**

REMEMBER:
Respiration       30
Perfusion          2
Mental status  Can do

Mental status

Can't follow simple commands → **Immediate**
Can follow simple commands → **Delayed**

START Program developed by HOAG Memorial Hospital and Newport Beach Fire Dept

**Fig. 43.5** START triage algorithm. (From http://citmt.org/Start/flowchart.htm#Simplified. Accessed December 1, 2016.)

## Operating Room

The OR should be reserved for immediate life-threatening injuries such as a compromised airway, hemorrhagic shock, hollow viscus injuries, penetrating wounds, and persistent active bleeding. Less urgent surgeries should be deferred.[34] The surgeon should perform a damage control operation, in which the life-threatening injury is rapidly addressed and the patient is stabilized. Definitive management should be delayed so other patients requiring surgery can be treated in a timely fashion.[2] Anesthesia providers play a crucial role in the OR by providing airway management, resuscitation, and analgesia/anesthesia and employing massive transfusion protocols. Anesthesia providers should anticipate that patients are often hypovolemic, malnourished, and hemodynamically unstable. Anesthesia providers should practice balanced resuscitation, when a lower than normal arterial blood pressure (systolic pressures of 80 to 100 mm Hg) is tolerated to balance organ perfusion with rebleeding risk, as a bridge to definitive surgical bleeding control.[15,48] The administration of large volumes of blood products (also see Chapters 24 and 42) and crystalloids (also see Chapter 23) to achieve a normal arterial blood pressure is unacceptable in the absence of definitive control of hemorrhage. Administration of large

volumes of fluids can result in acidosis, hypothermia, activation of the inflammatory cascade, and coagulopathy. In hemorrhagic shock, blood products are favored over colloids and crystalloids and should be given in a packed red blood cell (PRBC) to fresh frozen plasma (FFP) to platelet ratio of 1:1:1, as it improves survival (also see Chapters 24 and 42).[15,48,49] Vasopressors impair tissue perfusion and should be avoided if possible.[48] Antifibrinolytics, such as tranexamic acid, may be given in bleeding trauma patients within 3 hours of injury to reduce the risk of death from bleeding; administration after 3 hours is harmful and increases the mortality rate.[50]

Communication with the surgeon and OR staff is of utmost importance.[4] The ASA COTEP released two checklists, one for mass casualty OR management (Box 43.3) and another for trauma anesthesia (Box 43.4),[51] to help organize tasks, promote teamwork, and ensure equipment and blood product availability.[13] It is likely that complex and numerous surgeries may last for many hours and this may emotionally and physically wear on the anesthesia team. Appropriate staff should be recruited to provide help with challenging OR cases, give breaks, provide relief after 24 hours of work, and help restock drugs and equipment.[46]

### Postoperative Care

Anesthesiologists may also need to provide postoperative care to mechanically ventilated patients in the recovery area or ICU because of personnel and bed shortages (also see Chapter 42).[52] Additonally, they may need to help manage complications experienced by these patients including but not limited to infections, gangrene, acute respiratory distress syndrome (ARDS), compartment syndrome, rhabdomyolysis, acute renal failure, disseminated intravascular coagulation, arrhythmias, and electrolyte abnormalities, as well as complications from excessive administration of fluids.[35]

## NUCLEAR EXPOSURE

Exposure to ionizing radiation is likely to occur from terrorist attacks, nuclear bomb detonation, and nuclear power plant accidents. Radiation exposure may result from external sources (i.e., beta particles, gamma rays), contaminated debris, or inhaled gases and particulates. Predictable injuries include radiation burns, bone marrow suppression, destruction of the gastrointestinal tract mucosa and bleeding with translocation of bacteria, and septic shock.[15] Patients may require care in burn centers for appropriate resuscitation, wound care, and surgeries.

Patients exposed to radiation are often decontaminated at the exposure site by removing all clothing and washing the skin with warm soapy water. Any wounds should be irrigated. Providers should wear protective gear while stabilizing patients as well as dosimeters to gauge the level of nuclear exposure. Internal decontamination with

VI

---

**Box 43.3** ASA Committee on Trauma and Emergency Preparedness Operating Room Procedures for Mass Casualty: Management Step by Step

**Objective:** To be able to manage the flow of patient care in the ORs during a mass casualty situation.

**Steps:** Indicate date and time for each item

- Refer to facility's operations manual
  Open up appropriate annex.
- Activate call-in tree
  Assign an individual to activate. Use clerical personnel or automatic paging system, if available.
- Assess status of operating rooms
  Determine staffing of ORs 0-2, 2-12, and 12-24 hours. Hold elective cases.
- Alert current ORs
  Finish current surgical procedures as soon as possible and prepare to receive trauma.
- Assign staff
  Set up for trauma/emergency cases.
- Anesthesia Coordinator should become OR Medical Director
  Work with OR Nursing Manager to facilitate communication and coordination of staff and facilities.
- Report OR status to Hospital Command Center (HCC)
  Enter telephone, email address of HCC.
- Ensure adequate supplies
  Coordinate with anesthesia techs/supply personnel to ensure adequate supplies of fluids, medications, disposables, other.
- Contact PACU
  Accelerate transfer of patients to floors/ICUs in preparation for high volume of cases.
- Anesthesiologist should act as liaison in Emergency Department (ED)
  Send an experienced practitioner to the ED to act as a liaison (your eyes and ears) and keep communications open to Anesthesia Coordinator.
- Consider assembly of Stat Teams
  Combination of anesthesia, surgical, nursing, respiratory personnel to triage, as needed.
- HAZMAT/WMD event
  Review special personal protective procedures, such as DECON and isolation techniques. Consider if part of the OR or hallways should be considered "hot" or should have ventilation altered. Good resources include CHEMM/REMM websites.
- Coordinate with blood bank
  Verify blood availability.
- Coordinate with other patient care areas
  ICUs, OB, Peds, etc., to ensure continuity of care for new and existing patients.

*DECON,* Decontamination; *HAZMAT,* hazardous materials; *ICU,* intensive care unit; *OB,* obstetrics; *OR,* operating room; *PACU,* postanesthesia care unit; *Peds,* pediatrics; *WMD,* weapons of mass destruction. From American Society of Anesthesiologists Committee on Trauma and Emergency Preparedness (ASA COTEP). Emergence Preparedness Resources. https://www.asahq.org/resources/resources-from-asa-committees/committee-on-trauma-and-emergency-preparedness/emergency-preparedness. Accessed December 1, 2016.

gastric lavage, emetics, laxatives, and diuretics may also be required. Life-threatening injury treatment should precede the treatment of radiologic injuries.[15]

Once patients are stabilized, they should be monitored in the ICU for signs of acute radiation syndrome (e.g., thrombocytopenia, granulocytopenia, nausea, vomiting, and diarrhea).[15] If internal contamination is suspected, all body orifices (nostrils, ears, mouth, rectum) should be swabbed and 24-hour stool and urine collections should be performed. The white blood cell count should be monitored, and neutropenic precautions should be exercised when appropriate. Potassium iodide must be given within 24 hours to be effective against preventing radiation-induced thyroid cancer from iodine-131 ($^{131}$I) release after a power plant incident. Granulocyte colony-stimulating factor may be helpful in the treatment of postirradiation sepsis. Certain medications may be administered to facilitate renal excretion (ammonium chloride, calcium gluconate, diuretics) and minimize gastrointestinal absorption of radionuclides (calcium and zinc diethylenetriamine penta-acetic acid chelating agents).[15]

## CHEMICAL AND BIOLOGIC TERRORISM

Biochemical weapons can rapidly cause morbidity and death. They also induce panic and place health care workers and first-responders at increased risk of secondary exposure. These agents include toxins, bacteria and viruses, neuropeptides, nerve agents, vesicants, cyanogens, and others that cause pulmonary damage. Large groups of patients with similar symptoms and exposure should alert providers to a possible biochemical exposure/attack. It is crucial to demarcate a contamination zone; ensure protective gear is worn (including respirators); notify hospitals, public health and government officials; and decontaminate victims.[36] Antidotes to specific agents should be administered as soon as they are identified in order to be effective. Protective equipment and respirators should continue to be worn by providers, even after on-site decontamination of patients, to prevent cutaneous absorption. The most common biochemical agents will be discussed here; more in-depth information on the most recent agents of bioterrorism can be found on the CDC, DOD, and federal and state public health organization websites.[15,35]

### Decontamination

During chemical disasters, patients must be decontaminated by emergency personnel. Health care providers should perform decontamination by wearing proper protective attire and in a designated decontamination area with its own water outlet to prevent environmental pollution. In an MCE, decontamination triage algorithms are used to prioritize patient decontamination. A crucial step in the management of chemical disasters is removing hazardous material; removed materials and clothing should be stored in a double polyvinyl chloride (PVC) bag. Decontamination may be delayed in order to first address life-threatening injuries or administer antidotes or medical treatments. Decontamination is performed with warm or cold water (although there is a risk for hypothermia with cold water); hot water is contraindicated because it increases absorption of chemicals. A soft brush or sponge and mild soap should be used on the skin, and then the whole body should be flushed with running water for 1 minute.[53]

## Personal Protective Equipment

Anesthesia providers should have education and training on self-protection because they have a key role in the management of trauma and MCE victims. Victims could have easily transmissible infections (such as tuberculosis) or be contaminated with chemicals (e.g., nerve agents) that can spread to providers not wearing proper protective gear.

Anesthesia providers need to know the location of decontamination areas in their hospital and basic decontamination techniques, which includes the proper use of protective gear such as suits and respirators. When the hazardous agent is known, proper protective equipment can be prepared in advance. However, it is difficult to determine what protective gear should be worn when the hazardous agent is unknown, or when victims bypass prehospital responders. This occurred in the 1995 Tokyo sarin incident when victims presented directly to the hospital without being decontaminated, thus transmitting the agent to unsuspecting health care providers.[54] There are four levels of protective equipment, as described in Table 43.7.[55] In most cases of toxin poisoning, level C equipment is adequate and allows for tactile dexterity to provide care.[35] Level A protection is required when the greatest potential for exposure to hazards exists.[55]

### Bioterrorism Agents

Biologic weapons are divided into three categories, A through C, based on their potential to cause widespread harm (Table 43.8).[15] Category A poses the greatest threat to public health and will be discussed in greater detail. Health care providers should recognize symptom patterns and diagnostic clues that are suggestive of a bioterrorist attack (Box 43.5).[15]

### Anthrax

*Bacillus anthracis* is a gram-positive, spore-forming bacillus transmitted to humans from contaminated animals or their by-products. The three primary types of anthrax are cutaneous, inhalational, and gastrointestinal.

---

**Box 43.4** Trauma Anesthesia Checklist

**Before Patient Arrival**
- Room temperature 25° C or higher
- Warm IV line
- Machine check
- Airway equipment
- Emergency medications
- *BLOOD BANK: "6 units O Neg PRBC, 6 units AB FFP, 5-6 units of random donor platelets (1 standard adult dose) available"*

**Patient Arrival**
- Patient identified for trauma/emergency surgery?
- *BLOOD BANK: "Send blood for T&C and initiate MTP now!"*
- IV access
- Monitors (Sao$_2$, BP, ECG)
- *SURGEON: "Prep and drape!"*
- Preoxygenation

**Induction**
- Sedative hypnotic (ketamine vs. propofol vs. etomidate)
- Neuromuscular blockade (succ vs. roc)

**Intubation**
- (+) ETCO$_2$ → SURGEON: "Go!"
- Place orogastric tube

**Anesthetic**
- (Volatile anesthetic and/or benzodiazepine) + narcotic
- Consider TIVA
- Insert additional IV access if needed and an arterial line

**Resuscitation**
- Send baseline labs
- Follow MAP trend
- Goal FFP:PRBC controversial, but consider early FFP
- Goal urine output 0.5-1 mL/kg/h
- Consider tranexamic acid if <3 h after injury; 1 g over 10 min × 1, then 1 g over 8 h
- Consider calcium chloride 1 g
- Consider hydrocortisone 100 mg
- Consider vasopressin 5-10 IU
- Administer appropriate antibiotics
- Special considerations for TBI (SBP >90-100 mm Hg, Sao$_2$ >90%, Pco$_2$ 35-45 mm Hg)

**Closing/Postoperative**
- ICU: "Do you have a bed?"
- Initiate low lung volume ventilation (TV = 6 mL/kg ideal body weight)

*BP*, Blood pressure; *ECG*, electrocardiogram; *ETCO$_2$*, end-tidal carbon dioxide; *FFP*, fresh frozen plasma; *IU*, international unit; *IV*, intravenous; *MAP*, mean arterial pressure; *PRBC*, packed red blood cell; *roc*, rocuronium; *SBP*, systolic blood pressure; *succ*, succinylcholine; *TBI*, traumatic brain injury; *T&C*, typing and crossmatch; *TIVA*, total intravenous anesthesia; *TV*, tidal volume.
From Tobin JM, Grabinsky A, McCunn M, et al. A checklist for trauma and emergency anesthesia. *Anesth Analg.* 2013;117(5):1178-1184.

VI

Weaponized anthrax causes infection via inhalation and presents with flu-like symptoms. There is a symptom-free period that is followed by chest pain, cyanosis, hemoptysis, and respiratory failure. A widened mediastinum secondary to central lymphadenopathy is often seen on chest radiographs. When profound dyspnea develops, death ensues within 1 to 2 days. Weaponized anthrax can be treated with ciprofloxacin or doxycycline as it is often engineered to have penicillin G resistance.[15]

## Smallpox

The WHO announced in 1980 that the world was free of the *variola* virus, or smallpox. Smallpox vaccination was stopped in 1972 in the United States. The disease is highly infective with only 10 to 100 organisms required to infect an individual. Transmission occurs through inhaled aerosolized droplets and materials that have been in direct contact with pustules. The disease course begins with fatigue, headache, and high fevers. Over the next 3 to 4 days the fever resolves and then a rash with same-stage lesions appears. Immediate isolation is of utmost importance and exposed contacts should be vaccinated within the first 3 to 7 days after exposure to be effective.[15]

## Plague

*Yersinia pestis* is a gram-positive bacillus that is carried by rodents and fleas and transmitted to humans via flea bites. Bubonic and pneumonic plagues are the two types of diseases caused by *Y. pestis*. In patients with pneumonic plague, human-to-human transmission occurs through aerosolized *Y. pestis*, which is highly contagious. Aerosolized *Y. pestis* has been studied as a biologic weapon; however, it is only viable for 1 hour after being dispersed. This limits its infectivity to only 10 km from the site of dispersion if it were released by an airplane.[14] Bubonic plague is primarily spread by an infected flea bite. After a 2- to 6-day incubation period, the patient develops sudden fevers, chills, headache, and weakness. Painful and tender lymph node enlargement or bubo (up to 10 cm in diameter) occurs, often surrounded by skin lesions such as pustules. In untreated individuals, this is followed by gangrene and septic shock. The infection can be seeded

| Table 43.7 | Description of Levels of Personal Protective Equipment |
|---|---|
| **Level** | **Personal Protective Equipment** |
| A | Positive pressure self-contained breathing apparatus (SCBA) <br> Fully encapsulating chemical-resistant suit <br> Double layer of chemical-resistant gloves <br> Chemical-resistant boots <br> Airtight seal between suit and gloves and boots |
| B | Positive-pressure SCBA <br> Chemical-resistant long-sleeved suit <br> Double layer of chemical-resistant gloves <br> Chemical-resistant boots |
| C | Full face air purification device (respirator) <br> Chemical-resistant suit <br> Chemical-resistant outer gloves <br> Chemical-resistant boots |
| D | Equipment does not provide specific respiratory or skin protection but may include gloves, gowns, or safety glasses or face shield |

Baker DJ. The role of the anesthesia provider in natural and human-induced disasters. In Miller RD, ed. *Miller's Anesthesia*. 8th ed. Philadelphia: Elsevier Saunders; 2015:2479-2511; Personal Protective Equipment. U.S. Environmental Protection Agency (EPA). https://www.epa.gov/emergency-response/personal-protective-equipment. Accessed December 1, 2016.

| Table 43.8 | Bioterrorism Agents and Diseases | | |
|---|---|---|---|
| | **Category A** | **Category B** | **Category C** |
| Definition | Highest priority; easily disseminated or transmitted, high mortality rate, public panic | Second highest priority; moderate dissemination and morbidity rates, low mortality rates | Third-highest priority; emerging pathogens, not yet mass-engineered |
| Examples | *Bacillus anthracis* (anthrax) | *Coxiella burnetii* (Q fever) | Various equine encephalitic viruses |
| | *Variola major* (smallpox) | *Brucella species* (brucellosis) | |
| | *Yersinia pestis* (plague) | *Burkholderia mallei* (glanders) | |
| | *Clostridium botulinum* (botulism) | Enteric pathogens (*Escherichia coli, Salmonella, Shigella*) | |
| | *Francisella tularensis* (tularemia) | Pathogens associated with water safety threats (*Vibrio cholerae, Cryptosporidium*) | |
| | Hemorrhagic fever viruses (Ebola, Lassa, Marburg) | Various encephalitic viruses and various biologic toxins (e.g., ricin) | |

From Lin EY. Trauma, bioterrorism, and natural disasters. In Miller RD, ed. *Basics of Anesthesia*. 6th ed. Philadelphia: Elsevier Saunders; 2011:681-697.

into the lungs causing pneumonic plague, which manifests as cough, pneumonia, and rapidly developing respiratory failure. Both forms of the disease have a mortality rate of over 50%. The disease may be diagnosed by Gram stains of blood, sputum, and bubo cultures. Streptomycin is the treatment of choice, but gentamicin, tetracycline, and chloramphenicol are effective alternatives that can also be used as prophylaxis for those directly exposed.[15]

### Tularemia

*Francisella tularensis* is a gram-negative coccobacillus, carried by several animal hosts, most notably the cottontailed rabbit. Transmission can occur through several routes, including direct contact with an infected animal, ingestion of infected food, infected tick or deerfly bite, or aerosolization of the bacteria. Acute respiratory symptoms, fevers, pleuritic pain, hilar lymphadenopathy, and pneumonia develop 3 to 5 days after exposure. Isolation is not required as there are no documented cases of person-to-person transmission. The treatment of choice is streptomycin. In exposed individuals, streptomycin, doxycycline, or ciprofloxacin can be used as prophylactic treatment.[15]

### Botulism

*Clostridium botulinum* toxin is the most potent known poison and causes a neuroparalytic disease. The disease is caused by the toxin; thus, the live organism is not contagious. *C. botulinum* is an anaerobic gram-positive spore found in marine and agriculture products and soil. When ingested or inhaled, the effects do not manifest until the organism releases the toxin. The toxin reaches cholinergic receptors and inhibits intracellular fusion of acetylcholine vesicles to nerve-terminal membranes, thus preventing acetylcholine release. Symptoms usually develop between 12 and 36 hours after toxin exposure and include diplopia, dysphagia, dysarthria, dyspnea,

---

**Box 43.5** Epidemiologic Features Suggesting Exposure or Infection With Biologic Weapons

| Unusually high incidence or mortality rate from a disease cluster |
| --- |
| Single case of an unusual pathogen (inhaled anthrax, smallpox) |
| Cluster of patients with a suspicious clinical illness (i.e., flu-like illness leading to ARDS, shock, meningitis with anthrax; acute febrile illness with pustular lesions with smallpox) |
| Occurrence of a disease outside its natural geographic boundary (hemorrhagic fever, tularemia, plague) |
| Cluster of patients with acute flaccid paralysis (botulism) Clustering of diseases that affect animals as well as humans |

*ARDS,* Acute respiratory distress syndrome.
From Lin EY. Trauma, bioterrorism, and natural disasters. In Miller RD, ed. *Basics of Anesthesia.* 6th ed. Philadelphia: Elsevier Saunders; 2011:681-697.

---

and, finally, paralysis. The muscarinic effects include ileus, urinary retention, and decreased salivation. Treatment requires trivalent antitoxin, possible intubation and mechanical ventilation, and toxin removal through cathartics, enemas, and gastric lavage.[15]

### Ricin

Ricin is a naturally occurring polypeptide that poses a serious terrorist threat because it can be easily extracted from seeds of the castor bean plant and because exposure to it has a high mortality rate. The mechanism of ricin's toxicity is profound inhibition of protein synthesis. After exposure there is a latent period followed by fevers, diarrhea, weakness, seizures, respiratory failure, cardiovascular collapse, and multiple organ failure culminating in death within 36 to 72 hours. Patients require supportive care in the ICU (also see Chapter 41). Although there is no specific treatment for ricin, an antitoxin has been developed for use in animals.[35]

### Viral Hemorrhagic Fevers

There are numerous viruses carried by arthropod and rodent vectors causing viral hemorrhagic fever syndromes. Incubation periods range from 2 to 18 days. Presenting symptoms can include fever, myalgia, malaise evolving into shock, generalized mucus membrane hemorrhage, edema, and death.[36] Some of these viruses have been weaponized because they are highly infectious, requiring only a few organisms to cause disease. Mortality rates can be as high as 60%, depending on the virus. An intense index of suspicion, early isolation, and reporting to hospital and public health departments are required to prevent disease spread.[15] Initial treatment is supportive. Ribavirin, interferon-α, and hyperimmune globulin have been used in some cases, but most viruses do not have specific therapies.[14,15] There are no vaccines against these infectious agents except for yellow fever, which has a live attenuated vaccine.[14] There is ongoing vaccine development research for the most life-threatening viruses, such as ebola.[14,56]

### Chemical Terrorism Agents and Toxic Industrial Chemicals

A toxic industrial chemical (TIC) or HAZMAT[35] is defined as a substance used for industrial purposes, which has potentially harmful effects owing to the nature of its biochemical properties. When improperly stored or accidentally released, a TIC may cause damage to the environment, community, and animals and cause significant injuries or death in humans. The toxicity of TICs is significantly less than that of traditional chemical warfare agents, but the release of large quantities of TICs can result in significant damage and destruction. TICs may be released as a result of natural disasters, terrorist attacks (toxic war or infiltrating chemical plants), and accidental release during transportation or industrial site accidents. As a result of previous TIC disasters, the United States

**VI**

| Table 43.9 | Toxic Industrial Chemicals That Can Be Used as Weapons | | |
|---|---|---|---|
| **High Hazard TICs** | **Medium Hazard TICs** | **Low Hazard TICs** | |
| *Tissue Irritants:* | Acrolein | Arsenic | |
| Ammonia | Nitrogen dioxide | Trichloride | |
| Fluoride | Phosphine | Bromine | |
| Formaldehyde | Carbon monoxide | Nitric oxide | |
| Phosgene | Methyl bromide | Parathion | |
| Hydrogen chloride | Stibine | Tetraethyl lead | |
| Nitric acid | | Toluene 2,4- | |
| Sulfur dioxide | | diisocyanate | |
| *Systemic Poisons:* | | | |
| Arsine | | | |
| Diborane | | | |
| Hydrogen fluoride | | | |
| Cyanide | | | |
| Tungsten hexafluoride | | | |

TICs, Toxic industrial chemicals.
Modified from Hincal F, Erkekoglu P. Toxic industrial chemicals (TICs)—chemical warfare without chemical weapons. *FABAD J Pharm Sci.* 2006;31:220-229.

passed the Emergency Planning and Community Right-to-Know Act (EPCRA), which requires industries to disclose security and storage reports on hazardous TICs, provide chemical release inventories, and have in place emergency release notifications and response plans. Chemical agents appeal to terrorist organizations because they are readily available, less securely protected, easy to access or disperse, and cheaper. They may be used as poisons, incendiaries, and in the construction of explosive devices. There are about 70 known chemical warfare agents and 70,000 TICs produced, stored, and transported through countries. A list of the TICs that could be used as weapons was identified by the North Atlantic Treaty Organization (NATO) International Task Force-25, and several examples are provided in Table 43.9.[57]

Chemical weapons used in terrorist attacks and warfare create panic and place overwhelming strain on health care systems.[15,36] Examples of the most commonly seen chemical weapons, including nerve, pulmonary, and blood agents and vesicants, will be discussed.[15,35]

### Nerve Agents

Nerve agents, which were originally used as pesticides, were developed after World War II for military purposes. These chemical agents have a similar structure to organophosphates. They are known by their chemical name and a two-letter military designation. Examples include soman (GD), *N,N*-diethyl-2(methyl-(2-methylpropoxy)phosphoryl) sulfanylethanamide (VR), 22-(diisopropylamino)ethyl-*O*-ethyl methylphosphonothioate (VX), cyclosarin (GF), tabun (GA), and sarin (GB). The agent most commonly used by terrorists has been sarin.[35] Most nerve agents are lipophilic, clear liquids that vaporize at room temperature and are absorbed through lungs, mucus membranes, skin, and the gastrointestinal tract. They can also penetrate through clothing and leather with VX as the most potent agent (as little as one drop can be fatal).[15,36] Nerve agents can be classified as "persistent" or "nonpersistent" based on their volatility. Tabun, VX, and VR are persistent and are absorbed through the skin, whereas sarin, soman, and cyclosarin are nonpersistent and pose a respiratory threat. The gases inhibit acetylcholinesterase, resulting in the accumulation of acetylcholine at nerve terminals. Patients will present with increased salivation and airway secretions, rhinorrhea, bronchoconstriction, miosis, sweating, nausea, diarrhea, altered mental status, bradycardia (muscarinic effects), muscle cramping and weakness, fasciculations, hyperthermia, and, most importantly, respiratory failure (nicotinic effects). Early recognition of this toxidrome is important to prevent delaying antidote administration. Atropine minimizes the nicotinic symptoms and can be given at a dose of 2 to 6 mg administered intravenously or intramuscularly every 5 to 10 minutes until secretions decrease and ventilation improves. Diazepam is an anxiolytic and prevents seizures. 2-Pralidoxime is a longer-acting anticholinergic drug that unbinds the nerve agents from acetylcholinesterase and reactivates the enzyme. Pyridostigmine reversibly binds to acetylcholinesterase and can provide protection from nerve agents if administered 30 minutes before exposure.[15] Most patients exposed to nerve agents will require tracheal intubation for airway protection. Patients exposed to G-series agents should undergo decontamination with alkaline solutions; however, decontamination with alkaline solutions is not recommended in V-series agent exposures as it produces toxic by-products.[35] The V-series agents permeate through clothing and leather, so providers should wear personal protective equipment made of rubber or synthetic materials resistant to the nerve agents. These patients require supportive ICU care, and anesthesia providers can play a vital role in their management[58] (also see Chapter 41).

### Pulmonary Agents

Phosgene and chlorine are the two most likely pulmonary agents to be used by terrorists.[14] Phosgene is the deadliest pulmonary agent. It smells of freshly cut hay, is colorless, and accumulates in low-lying areas. Phosgene is extremely lipid soluble and easily infiltrates the pulmonary epithelium and alveoli. It reacts with water to form carbon dioxide and hydrochloric acid, which irritate soft tissues, and causes pulmonary edema and acute lung injury (ALI). Both chlorine and phosgene gases, when released in sufficient quantities, cause death by displacing oxygen, resulting in asphyxia.[14] After exposure, there may be a symptom-free period of 1 to 24 hours, but during this time lung injury is occurring and pulmonary edema will eventually follow. There is no antidote and the treatment is supportive, with endotracheal intubation and lung protective mechanical ventilation protocols similar to those used for ARDS.[15]

### Blood Toxins

These agents are typically cyanogens, such as hydrogen cyanide and cyanogen chloride. Cyanogen chloride is a highly volatile toxin that is difficult to use as a biologic weapon. Hydrogen cyanide is more likely to be used by terrorists as an aerosol.[14] When inhaled, the cyanide disrupts the electron transport chain in the mitochondria by binding to cytochrome c oxidase, thus preventing electron transfer to oxygen and hindering adenosine triphosphate (ATP) production.[14,35] This results in cellular hypoxia and metabolic acidosis leading to death. Patients present with dyspnea and restlessness and may develop seizures, coma, and cardiac arrest.[15] Exposure to high concentrations can produce death within minutes.[35] The treatment is supportive with intubation, mechanical ventilation with 100% oxygen, and cardiovascular support with vasopressors and/or inotropes. Similar to nitroprusside toxicity, thiosulfate or hydroxocobalamin is administered intravenously to promote conversion of cyanide to thiocyanate, which is considerably less toxic.[14,15]

### Vesicants

These chemicals are also known as "blister agents," producing burns and blisters on contact. The best known vesicants include sulfur mustard, nitrogen mustard, lewisite, and phosgene oxime. On inhalation, they cause pulmonary damage and a multiorgan failure syndrome. Lewisite and phosgene oxime exposure result in immediate symptoms, whereas mustard exposure may not cause symptoms for 2 to 24 hours. Exposed individuals should be decontaminated, and a protective suit and gas mask should be worn by health care providers. Mild symptoms including erythema, tearing, hoarseness, and cough do not require treatment beyond supportive care. Severe poisoning can result in blindness, erythematous and bullous skin lesions, leukopenia, central nervous system effects, respiratory failure, and permanent respiratory damage. Supportive treatment includes endotracheal intubation and mechanical ventilation. There is no specific antidote for sulfur mustard, but combination treatment with thiosulfate, vitamin E, and dexamethasone may improve outcomes. Lewisite may be treated with its antidote, dimercaprol.[15,36]

## INFECTIOUS DISEASE DISASTERS AND PANDEMICS

Anesthesia providers should be familiar with contagious diseases such as influenza, SARS, Zika virus, and West Nile virus (WNV). Avian viruses can mutate, infect humans, and result in pandemics after human-to-human transmission resulting in high death tolls. In 2009, the H1N1 strain of influenza A resulted in almost 600,000 deaths internationally. There are few antiviral treatments with the exception of oseltamivir, zanamivir, and peramivir for influenza.[59] Supportive care and intubation and mechanical ventilation are often crucial in the treatment of these patients. Health care providers have several important responsibilities in infectious disease disasters. They must have an intense level of suspicion of these infections, wear proper protective gear, employ appropriate contact and isolation precautions, and notify the pertinent public health organizations to assist in diagnosis, treatment, and prevention of the spread of infection.[15] Pandemics occur on a semiregular basis, pose a significant strain on health care resources and costs, and result in significant morbidity and mortality rates. Although pandemics typically have a gradual onset, the 2009 influenza A pandemic demonstrated that they can also occur abruptly and without warning.[60] The CDC, infectious disease experts, and epidemiologists help develop vaccines, determine treatments, and provide educational materials and resources for hospitals, communities, and health care providers on disease transmission and prevention strategies to prepare for and mitigate infectious disease disasters.[60] The CDC website also provides a list of infectious organisms, modes of transmission, and the type of precautions that need to be implemented when patients are infected.[61] Table 43.10 gives a summary of antidotes and treatment options for biochemical agents.

## CYBER ATTACKS AND HIGH ALTITUDE ELECTROMAGNETIC PULSE EVENTS

Cyber attacks can compromise computer infrastructures of governmental and local agencies. Disruption of these computer systems can interfere with coordination, operational decision making, and allocation of resources. Communication between fire, law enforcement, hospitals, and public heath agencies can also be disrupted. Cyber attacks can compromise economic and national security, and the ensuing chaos can impede the efforts of response teams during disaster management, resulting in deaths.[62,63] Preventive measures that can be taken to protect against cyber attacks include using strong security protocols, locking down hospital operating systems, backing up and protecting hardware, and storing backups in secure locations.

High altitude electromagnetic pulse (HEMP) events result from nuclear weapon detonation above the earth's surface, which produces gamma radiation that interacts with the atmosphere creating an electromagnetic energy field that is harmless to people but disrupts the earth's magnetic field. The resulting current and voltage surges can melt circuitry and cause damage to computers and other electronic devices; equipment may fail immediately, or over a period of days to weeks. HEMP events can affect

VI

**Table 43.10**  Summary of Antidotes and Treatment Options for Biochemical Agents

| Offending Agent | Antidote | Treatment |
|---|---|---|
| *Bacillus anthracis* | | Streptomycin, ciprofloxacin, doxycycline |
| *Yersinia pestis* | | Streptomycin, doxycycline, chloramphenicol |
| Viral hemorrhagic fevers | | Ribavirin, immunoglobulin |
| *Francisella tularensis* | | Streptomycin, gentamicin |
| Variola | | Cidofovir |
| *Burkholderia mallei* | | Co-amoxiclav |
| *Coxiella burnetii* | | Doxycycline |
| *Brucella* | | Doxycycline |
| *Escherichia* | | No antibiotics |
| Cyanide; HCN | Sodium thiosulfate, amyl and sodium nitrite, dicobalt edatate, 4-DMAP, hydroxycobalamin | |
| Nerve agents/organophosphates | 2-Pralidoxime | Atropine, benzodiazepines |
| Sulfur mustard | | Thiosulfate, vitamin E, dexamethasone |
| Lewisite | Dimercaprol | |
| Influenza A virus | | Oseltamivir, zanamivir, penamivir |

Table derived from Lin EY. Trauma, Bioterrorism, and Natural Disasters. In Miller RD, ed. Basics of Anesthesia, 6th ed. Philadelphia: Elsevier Saunders: 2011:681-697, and references 24, 36, 59, and the CDC website: https://emergency.cdc.gov/agent/agentlist.asp.

many square miles of area, causing widespread power surges and disruption of equipment connected to power grids, telecommunication infrastructures, and communication systems. The effects are less severe over greater distances, and electronic equipment that is powered off at the time of the incident is less likely to be affected.[64] The effects can be severe enough to cause a blackout lasting months to years. It can also destroy transformers and generators in critical electrical grid infrastructures that may take years to replace.[65] These attacks can affect hospital equipment and computer systems. Actions that can be taken to protect against such events include shielding and filtering of a few key devices such as monitors and pulse oximetry, unplugging and turning off unused electronic equipment, rotating backup equipment to keep batteries charged, and having backup power systems, batteries, and solar-powered equipment. Storing small items like pulse oximeters in bubble wrap surrounded by aluminum foil may also protect it from most HEMP events.

## POSTDISASTER SYNDROMES SURVEILLANCE

A variety of postdisaster disease patterns emerge after severe natural disasters because of the destruction of homes and disruption of health care systems and available resources. The disease patterns seen may reflect a variety of factors including specifics of the affected region, type of natural disaster, lack of medical care and pharmaceutical resources, and living conditions (e.g., crowded shelters). A surveillance tool called the Surveillance for Post Extreme Emergencies and Disasters (SPEED) was developed to monitor and detect postdisaster disease trends that occurred after three natural disasters in the Philippines. After all three types of natural disasters (flood, earthquake, and typhoon), communicable disease was the most predominant syndrome. Other syndromes included acute respiratory infections, open wounds, bruises and burns, hypertension, skin disease, fever, and acute watery diarrhea (leptospirosis). Similarly, after the 2010 earthquake in Haiti, the National Sentinel Site Surveillance (NSSS) system was created to monitor disease trends and detect outbreaks. Respiratory infections, injuries, suspected malaria, and fever of unknown origin were the most commonly reported conditions. Monitoring postdisaster disease trends reflected the degree to which the health care system was disrupted as a result of the disaster. The decrease in the incidence of disease signals the beginning of the recovery phase. By using disease surveillance tools, data can be obtained that can help identify health needs that may differ in the recovery phase and may be specific to a certain region or type of disaster.

The data obtained from these tools can help identify necessary public health interventions, suggest resource allocation, and guide decision making. Efforts aimed at providing clean water, shelter, hygiene, and routine health care services may prevent a majority of the post-disaster diseases that have been observed.[66,67]

## RECOVERY

The recovery phase can last much longer than the response phase depending on the severity of destruction by the disaster. The recovery phase includes providing support services (medical and psychological) to victims, cleaning and reconstruction of damaged structures, and rebuilding the economy. It is important to begin planning the recovery phase during the response phase. Communicating that a disaster has happened to governmental agencies and the media attracts attention to the disaster, helps provide resources, and helps raise financial support for victims. Resources needed to rebuild a community after a disaster should be identified early in order to determine what future recovery resources will be needed. The involvement of community members in this process is crucial to ensure their concerns are being heard and that they are involved in recovery planning. The financial resources needed to rebuild a community are the major limiting factor of how quickly a region can recover from a disaster, especially in underdeveloped countries where insurance plans may not be available.[1] Support from other nations may be required during this time. Disasters put enormous strains on resources, communities, and victims, and recovery from them may take years.

## QUESTIONS OF THE DAY

1. What types of events can result in disasters? What are the common features of any type of disaster?
2. What are the four phases of a disaster? What are the components of a family preparedness checklist?
3. What is the role of personal protective equipment during a biologic or chemical disaster event? How do the different levels of protection impact the ability to care for a patient?
4. What are the goals of triage systems during a mass casualty event (MCE)?
5. What are the most important aspects of managing a patient who has been exposed to nerve agents?
6. What types of disease patterns can emerge after a natural disaster has occurred?

## REFERENCES

1. Aitken P, Leggat P. Considerations in mass casualty and disaster management. In: Blaivas M, ed. *Emergency Medicine–An International Perspective*. Rijeka, Croatia: InTech; 2012:143–182. Also available from http://www.intechopen.com/books/emergency-medicine-an-international-perspective/considerations-in-mass-casualty-and-disaster-management.
2. Bar-Joseph G, Michaelson M, Halberthal M. Managing mass casualties. *Curr Opin Anaesthesiol*. 2003;16:193–199.
3. Hirshberg A, Holcomb JB, Mattox KL. Hospital trauma care in multiple-casualty incidents: a critical view. *Ann Emerg Med*. 2001;37:647–652.
4. Murray MJ. Communicating during a disaster. *Anesth Analg*. 2010;110(3):657–658.
5. TFQCDM/WADEM (Task Force on Quality Control of Disaster Management/World Association for Disaster and Emergency Medicine). Health disaster management: guidelines for evaluation and research in the "utstein style." Chapter 3: overview and concepts. *Prehosp Disaster Med*. 2002;17(suppl 3):31–55.
6. Dudaryk R, Pretto EA. Resuscitation in a multiple casualty event. *Anesthesiol Clin*. 2013;31:85–106.
7. Centre for Research on the Epidemiology of Disasters (CRED). Emergency Events Database (EM-DAT). http://www.emdat.be. Accessed on December 1, 2016.
8. Iwan WD, Cluff LS, Kimpel JF, et al. Mitigation emerges as major strategy for reducing losses caused by natural disasters. *Science*. 1999;284(5422):1943–1947.
9. Lindsay BR. Federal emergency management: a brief introduction. *Congressional Research Service*. 2012. https://www.fas.org/sgp/crs/homesec/R42845.pdf. Accessed December 1, 2016.
10. Baird ME. The phases of emergency management. 2010. Prepared for the Intermodal Freight Transportation Institute (ITFI). http://www.vanderbilt.edu/vector/research/emmgtphases.pdf. Accessed December 1, 2016.
11. Wisner B, Adams J. Environmental health in emergencies and disasters: a practical guide. World Health Organization, 2002. http://www.who.int/water_sanitation_health/hygiene/emergencies/em2002intro.pdf. Accessed December 1, 2016.
12. Federal Emergency Management Agency (FEMA). Principles of emergency management: independent study. https://training.fema.gov/emiweb/downloads/is230.pdf; 2006. Accessed December 1, 2016.
13. American Society of Anesthesiologists Committee on Trauma and Emergency Preparedness (ASA COTEP). Emergence Preparedness Resources. https://www.asahq.org/resources/resources-from-asa-committees/committee-on-trauma-and-emergency-preparedness/emergency-preparedness. Accessed December 1, 2016.
14. Murray MJ. Emergency preparedness for and disaster management of casualties from natural disasters and chemical, biologic, radiologic, nuclear, and high-yield explosive (CBRNE) events. In: Barash PG, ed. *Clinical Anesthesia*. 7th ed. Philadelphia: Lippincott Williams & Wilkins; 2013:1535–1549.
15. Lin EY. Trauma, bioterrorism, and natural disasters. In: Miller RD, ed. *Basics of Anesthesia*. 6th ed. Philadelphia: Elsevier Saunders; 2011:681–697.
16. Carey R, ed. *Australian Emergency Management Handbook. Handbook 1*. Canberra: Australian Emergency Management Institute (AEMI), Commonwealth Attorney General's Department; 2011:1–112.
17. Arriscar. Risk Assessment. http://www.arriscar.com.au/services/risk-assessment/. Accessed December 1, 2016.

VI

18. City Redland. Disaster Risk Management. http://www.redlandsdisasterplan.com.au/disaster-risk-management/. Accessed December 1, 2016.

19. Yarmohammadian MH, Atighechian G, Haghshenas A, Shams L. Establishment of hospital emergency incident command system in Iranian hospitals: a necessity for better response to disasters. *Iran Red Crescent Med J.* 2013;15(12):e3371–e3373.

20. Djalali A, Castren M, Hosseinijenab V, et al. Hospital incident command system (HICS) performance in Iran; decision making during disasters. *Scand J Trauma Resusc Emerg Med.* 2012;20:14–21.

21. Zane RD, Prestipino AL. Implementing the hospital emergency incident command system: an integrated delivery system's experience. *Prehosp Disaster Med.* 2004;19(4):311–317.

22. Hospital Incident Command System. California Emergency Medical Services Authority. http://www.emsa.ca.gov/disaster_medical_services_division_hospital_incident_command_system_resources; 2014. Accessed November 13, 2016.

23. Katoh K, Marukawa S. The anesthesiologist's role in the French emergency medical system. *Masui.* 1990;39(11):1547–1553.

24. Backer H. *California Emergency Medical Services Authority (EMSA). HICS Guidebook.* 5th ed. 2014. http://www.emsa.ca.gov/media/default/HICS/HICS_Guidebook_2014_10.pdf. Accessed December 1, 2016.

25 Gupta A. Guidelines for Hospital Emergency Preparedness Planning. Assam State Disaster Management Authority. http://asdma.gov.in/pdf/publication/undp/guidelines_hospital_emergency.pdf. Accessed December 1, 2016.

26. World Health Organization. Mass casualty management systems: Strategies and guidelines for building health sector capacity. http://www.who.int/hac/techguidance/tools/mcm_guidelines_en.pdf. 2007. Accessed December 1, 2016.

27. Barbera JA, Macintyre AG. *Medical Surge Capacity and Capability: A Management System for Integrating Medical and Health Resources During Large-Scale Emergencies.* 2nd ed. Washington, DC: U.S. Department of Health and Human Services; 2007:1–274. http://www.phe.gov/preparedness/planning/mscc/handbook/documents/mscc080626.pdf. Accessed December 1, 2016.

28. Cheung M, Vu AT, Varlese D, et al. *Hospital Preparedness Exercises Guidebook.* Rockville, MD: Agency for Healthcare Research and Quality (AHRQ); 2010: 1–104.

29 Healthcare Security Services. Hospital preparedness exercises. http://hss-us.com/emergency-management/preparedness-exercises/. Accessed December 1, 2016.

30. Baker DJ, Telion C, Carli P. Multiple casualty incidents: the prehospital role of the anesthesiologist in Europe. *Anesthesiol Clin.* 2007;25:179–188.

31. SALT triage algorithm. SALT mass casualty triage: concept endorsed by the American College of Emergency Physicians, American College of Surgeons Committee on Trauma, American Trauma Society, National Association of EMS Physicians, National Disaster Life Support Education Consortium, and State and Territorial Injury Prevention Directors Association. *Disaster Med Public Health Prep.* 2008;2(4):245–246. https://chemm.nlm.nih.gov/salttriage.htm. Accessed December 1, 2016.

32 START triage flowchart. http://citmt.org/Start/flowchart.htm#Simplified. Accessed December 1, 2016.

33. Lerner EB, Schwartz RB, Coule PL, et al. Mass casualty triage: an evaluation of the data and development of a proposed national guideline. *Disaster Med Public Health Prep.* 2008;2:S25–S34.

34. Frykberg R. Triage: principles and practice. *Scand J Surg.* 2005;94:272–278.

35. Baker DJ. The role of the anesthesia provider in natural and human-induced disasters. In: Miller RD, Cohen NH, Eriksson LI, eds. *Miller's Anesthesia.* 8th ed. Philadelphia: Elsevier Saunders; 2015:2479–2511.

36. Murray MJ. Chemical weapons compromise provider safety. *Anesth Patient Safety Found Newsletter (Spring).* 2002:12–14. http://www.apsf.org.

37. Yeguiayan JM, Garrigue D, Binquet C, et al. Medical pre-hospital management reduces mortality in severe blunt trauma: a prospective epidemiological study. *Crit Care.* 2011;15: R34–R45.

38. Talmor D. Airway management during a mass casualty event. *Respir Care.* 2008;53(2):226–231.

39. Weinbroum AA, Rudick V, Paret G, et al. Anaesthesia and critical care considerations in nerve agent warfare trauma casualties. *Resuscitation.* 2000;47: 113–123.

40. Sansom GW. Emergency department personal protective equipment requirements following out-of-hospital chemical biological or radiological events in Australasia. *Emerg Med Australas.* 2007;19(2):86–95.

41. Morrison JJ, Oh J, DuBose JJ, et al. En-route care capability from point of injury impacts mortality after severe wartime injury. *Ann Surg.* 2013;257: 330–334.

42. Alfici R, Ashkenazi I, Kessel B. Management of victims in a mass casualty incident caused by a terrorist bombing: treatment algorithms for stable, unstable, and in extremis victims. *Milit Med.* 2006;171(12):1155–1162.

43. Como JJ, Smith CE, Grabinsky A. Trauma epidemiology, mechanisms of injury, and pre-hospital care. In: Varon AJ, ed. *Essentials of Trauma Anesthesia.* New York: Cambridge University Press; 2012:1–15.

44. Grissom TE, Varon AJ. Airway management controversies. *ASA Monitor.* 2013;77(4):12–14.

45. Ben-Abraham R, Rudick V, Weinbroum AA. Practical guidelines for acute care of victims of bioterrorism: conventional injuries and concomitant nerve agent intoxication. *Anesthesiology.* 2002;87:989–1004.

46. Shamir MY, Weiss YG, Willner D, et al. Multiple casualty terror events: the anesthesiologist's perspective. *Anesth Analg.* 2004;98:1746–1752.

47. Lavery GG, Horan E. Clinical review: communication and logistics in the response to the 1998 terrorist bombing in Omagh, Northern Ireland. *Crit Care.* 2005;9:401–408.

48. American College of Surgeons. *Advanced Trauma Life Support (ATLS) Student Course Manual.* 9th ed. Chicago: American College of Surgeons; 2012:63–75.

49. Holcomb JB, Tilley BC, Baraniuk S, et al. PROPPR Study Group. Transfusion of plasma, platelets, and red blood cells in a 1:1:1 vs a 1:1:2 ratio and mortality in patients with severe trauma: the PROPPR randomized clinical trial. *JAMA.* 2015;313(5):471–482.

50. CRASH-2 Collaborators, Roberts I, Shakur H, Afolabi A, et al. The importance of early treatment with tranexamic acid in bleeding trauma patients: an exploratory analysis of the CRASH-2 randomised controlled trial. *Lancet.* 2011;377(9771):1096–1101.

51. Tobin JM, Grabinsky A, McCunn M, et al. A checklist for trauma and emergency anesthesia. *Anesth Analg.* 2013;117(5):1178–1184.

52. Dara SI, Ashton RW, Farmer JC. Engendering enthusiasm for sustainable disaster critical care response: why this is of consequence to critical care professionals? *Crit Care.* 2005;9:125–127.

53. Sarc L. Incident caused by hazardous material. In: Lennquist S, ed. *Medical Response to Major Incident and Disasters: A Practical Guide for all Medical Staff.* New York: Springer; 2012:229–274.

54. Candiotti KA, Kamat A, Barach P, et al. Emergency preparedness for biological and chemical incidents: a survey of anesthesiology residency programs in the United States. *Anesth Analg.* 2005;101:1135–1140.

55 Personal Protective Equipment. U.S. Environmental Protection Agency (EPA). https://www.epa.gov/emergency-response/personal-protective-equipment. Accessed December 1, 2016.

56. Centers for Disease Control and Prevention. Sierra Leone Trial to Introduce a Vaccine against Ebola (STRIVE) Q&A. http://www.cdc.gov/vhf/ebola/strive/qa .html. April 20, 2016. Accessed on December 1, 2016.

57. Hincal F, Erkekoglu P. Toxic industrial chemicals (TICs)—chemical warfare without chemical weapons. *FABAD J Pharm Sci.* 2006;31:220–229.

58. Talmor D. Nonconventional terror—the anesthesiologist's role in a nerve agent event. *Anesthesiol Clin.* 2007;25:189–199.

59. Centers for Disease Control and Prevention. Treating Flu. https://www.cdc.gov/ flu/pdf/freeresources/updated/treating-in fluenza.pdf. Accessed February 24, 2017.

60. Rebman T. Infectious disease disasters: bioterrorism, emerging infections, and pandemics. In: Grota P, ed. *APIC Text of Infection Control and Epidemiology.* 4th ed. Arlington, VA: APIC Text Online; 2014:1201–1202.

61. Centers for Disease Control and Prevention. Isolation Precautions. Updated 2007. http://www.cdc.gov/hicpac/pdf/is olation/Isolation2007.pdf. Accessed December 1, 2016.

62 Federal Emergency Management Agency (FEMA). Cyber Security Guidance. https://www.fema.gov/pdf/governme nt/grant/hsgp/fy09_hsgp_cyber.pdf. Accessed December 1, 2016.

63 Lesperance A, Stein S. Cybersecurity as an Emergency Management Function. Domestic Preparedness. Updated: January 21, 2015. https:// www.domesticpreparedness.com/res ilience/cybersecurity-as-an-emergen cy-management-function/. Accessed December 1, 2016.

64. Wilson C. *High Altitude Electromagnetic Pulse (HEMP) and High Power Microwave (HPM) Devices: Threat Assessments.* CRS Reports for Congress; 2008:1–22. https://www.fas.org/sgp/cr s/natsec/RL32544.pdf.

65. Schnurr A. *The Catastrophic Effect of an EMP Attack or Severe Solar Storm: Our alarming and needless vulnerability to subcontinent-scale disaster.* A publication of the EIS council; 2013. https://www. centerforsecuritypolicy.org/wp-content/ uploads/2013/08/Catastrophic-Effect-of- an-EMP-Attack-or-Severe-Solar-Storm- 5-13.pdf. Accessed December 1, 2016.

66. Salazar MA, Pesigan A, Law R, Winkler V. Post-disaster health impact of natural hazards in the Philippines in 2013. *Glob Health Action.* 2016;9:31320– 31327.

67. Maglorie R, et al. Launching a national surveillance system after an earthquake— Haiti. *MMWR.* 2010;2010(59):933–938.

VI

# 44 CHRONIC PAIN MANAGEMENT

## Omar Hyder and James P. Rathmell

Anesthesia providers first ventured into the treatment of patients with chronic pain as an extension of their use of regional anesthesia in the operating room setting. Pain medicine is now a well-established subspecialty of anesthesiology, with many practitioners dedicating their entire clinical practice to caring for patients with chronic pain and employing a wide range of diagnostic and therapeutic modalities that now extend far beyond the scope of regional anesthesia. The International Association for the Study of Pain (IASP) defines pain as "an unpleasant sensory and emotional experience associated with actual or potential tissue damage, or described in terms of such damage" and chronic pain as "pain without apparent biological value that has persisted beyond the normal tissue healing time usually taken to be 3 months." Chronic pain leads to enormous personal and societal costs in lost productivity and prolonged, often seemingly futile, medical treatment.

## CLASSIFICATION OF CHRONIC PAIN

Chronic pain can be classified as cancer-related pain or noncancer pain, to distinguish the former, which is often associated with the issues that arise near the end of life. However, as more effective treatments for some cancers have emerged, more patients are surviving for prolonged periods of time on treatment or emerging as long-term survivors, and some of these patients suffer from persistent pain. Chronic pain is often divided into nociceptive pain in which activity in peripheral pain neurons is due to ongoing tissue injury, such as the pain of osteoarthritis, and neuropathic pain in which abnormal function of the nervous system causes ongoing pain, such as the pain associated with postherpetic neuralgia (PHN) or painful diabetic peripheral neuropathy (DPN).

The editors and publisher would like to thank Dr. Pankaj Mehta for contributing to this chapter in the previous edition of this work. It has served as the foundation for the current chapter.

## MULTIDISCIPLINARY PAIN MANAGEMENT

Chronic pain is a complex disorder and patients suffering with chronic pain often have biologic disease that is inextricably intertwined with cognitive, affective, behavioral, and social factors. Thus, managing patients with chronic pain necessitates employing the expertise of practitioners from a range of medical disciplines to properly address all the physical and psychological aspects of their illness to allow them to regain control over their lives and optimize their overall level of function. Such a multidisciplinary team approach is the most effective and cost-efficient means for the treatment of chronic pain. The core of the multidisciplinary pain team consists of a physician, a psychologist, and a physical therapist often working in conjunction with an occupational therapist and nurse specialists. The physician coordinates diagnosis and medical treatment, including drug therapy and appropriate pain-relieving interventions; the psychologist typically incorporates patient education, cognitive behavioral therapy (CBT), and relaxation training; and the physical therapist plans various exercise regimens, including muscle conditioning and aerobics, aimed at optimizing the patient's overall function.

## COMMON PAIN SYNDROMES

### Low Back Pain

#### Definitions

Low back pain, a nonspecific term, refers to pain centered over the lumbosacral junction. The diagnosis and treatment must be as precise as possible. Low back pain can be differentiated as pain that is centered primarily over the axis of the spinal column from pain that refers primarily to the leg (Fig. 44.1).[1] Lumbar spinal pain is pain inferior to the tip of the twelfth thoracic spinous process and superior to the tip of the first sacral spinous process. Sacral spinal pain is inferior to the first sacral spinous process and superior to the sacrococcygeal joint. Lumbosacral spinal pain is in either or both regions and constitutes "low back pain." Other patients present with "sciatica," or pain predominantly localized in the leg. The proper term is radicular pain because stimulation of the spinal nerve or the dorsal root ganglion of a spinal nerve evokes the pain.

Pain is a normal physiologic process and serves as a signal of actual or impending tissue injury. Pain from tissue injury is usually well localized and associated with sensitivity in the region. Pain signals are carried toward the central nervous system (CNS) via the peripheral sensory nerves. This type of pain is termed *nociceptive pain,* or physiologic pain. In contrast, persistent pain following injury to the nervous system is termed *neuropathic pain.*

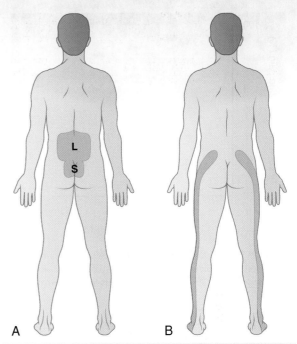

**Fig. 44.1** The definition of low back pain. (A) "Low back pain" is more precisely termed lumbosacral spinal pain, which encompasses both lumbar spinal pain (L) and sacral spinal pain (S). (B) Radicular pain describes pain that is referred to the lower extremity and is caused by stimulation of a spinal nerve.

#### Epidemiology

Low back pain is among the most common problems leading patients to seek medical attention. In a nationwide health survey, 28% of U.S. adults reported low back pain in the 3 months preceding the survey.[2] The majority of episodes of acute low back pain, with or without radicular pain, resolve without treatment. Overall, 60% to 70% of those affected recover by 6 weeks, and 80% to 90% recover by 12 weeks (Fig. 44.2).[3] However, recovery after 12 weeks is slow and uncertain. Fewer than half of patients disabled for longer than 6 months will return to work. The return-to-work rate for those out of work for 2 years is near zero. Low back pain is frequently recurrent; the vast majority of patients with a single episode experience another episode at some later time. Risk factors for developing chronic low back pain include age, gender, socioeconomic status, education level, body mass index, tobacco use, perceived general health status, physical activity (e.g., bending, lifting, twisting), repetitive tasks, job dissatisfaction, depression, spinal anatomic variations, and imaging abnormalities.[4]

#### Pathophysiology

The basic functional unit of the spine is composed of two adjacent vertebral bodies with two posterior facet joints,

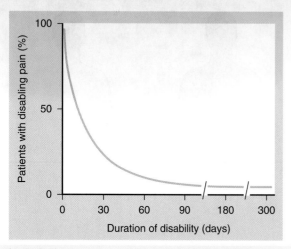

**Fig. 44.2** The time course of acute low back pain. (Redrawn from Andersson GB. Epidemiological features of chronic low-back pain. *Lancet.* 1999;354(9178):581-585, used with permission.)

an intervertebral disk, and the surrounding ligamentous structures. The intervertebral disk absorbs energy and distributes weight evenly from one spinal segment to the next while allowing movement of the protective bony elements. Lifting, bending, twisting, or whole body vibration can damage elements of the spine. With injury and aging, progressive degenerative changes appear in each element of the functional spinal unit, along with the onset of characteristic symptoms (Fig. 44.3). The earliest change in the lumbar facet joints is synovitis, which progresses to degradation of the articular surfaces, capsular laxity and subluxation, and finally enlargement of the articular processes (facet hypertrophy). Progressive degeneration also occurs within the intervertebral disks, starting with loss of hydration of the nucleus pulposus followed by the appearance of circumferential or radial tears within the annulus fibrosis (internal disk disruption). Lumbosacral pain can arise from the facet joints or the annulus fibrosis.[5] With internal disruption of the annulus, some of the gelatinous central nucleus pulposus can extend beyond the disk margin as a disk herniation (herniated nucleus pulposus, or HNP). When an HNP extends to the region adjacent to the spinal nerve, it incites an intense inflammatory reaction. Patients with HNP typically present with acute radicular pain. Hypertrophy of the facet joints and calcification of the ligamentous structures can reduce the size of the intervertebral foramina and central spinal canal (spinal stenosis), with onset of radicular pain and neurogenic claudication.

Patients with prior lumbar surgery and either recurrent or persistent low back pain, often termed *failed back surgery syndrome*, may require a more complex evaluation. Knowing the type of surgery performed, the indications for and results of the surgery, and the

time course and characteristics of any changes in the pattern and severity of postoperative pain is essential. Recurrent pain or progressive symptoms signal the need for further diagnostic evaluation.

### Initial Evaluation and Treatment

When first evaluating a patient with low back pain, several features termed *red flag* conditions require prompt investigation, including new-onset or worsening back pain after trauma, infection, or previous cancer. Patients with progressive neurologic deficits (i.e., typically worsening numbness or weakness) or bowel or bladder dysfunction also warrant immediate radiologic imaging to rule out a compressive lesion.[5] Diagnosis and treatment usually rely on location and duration of symptoms, and determining if the pain is acute or chronic and primarily radicular or lumbosacral in nature. Acute low back pain is pain that is present for less than 3 months, and chronic low back pain is defined as being present for a longer period of time.

### Acute Radicular Pain

HNP typically causes acute radicular pain, with or without radiculopathy (signs of dysfunction including numbness, weakness, or loss of deep tendon reflexes referable to a specific spinal nerve). In elderly patients and those with extensive lumbar spondylosis, acute radicular symptoms caused by narrowing of one or more intervertebral foramina can occur. Initial treatment is symptomatic, and following HNP, symptoms resolve without specific treatment in about 90% of patients.[6] Epidural steroid injections have shown efficacy for symptom control in acute radicular pain from HNP.[7] For those with more than 6 weeks of persistent pain after HNP, lumbar diskectomy may be indicated. A controlled trial of surgical versus nonoperative treatment in selected patients showed significant improvement in pain alleviation, quality of life, and physical functioning among both groups over short- and long-term follow-up but remained inconclusive about the superiority of either approach.[8]

### Chronic Radicular Pain

Persistent leg pain in the distribution of a spinal nerve may occur in patients with a disk herniation with or without subsequent surgery. In those with persistent pain, a search for a reversible cause of nerve root compression is warranted. In many individuals, scarring around the spinal nerve at the operative site on magnetic resonance imaging and abnormalities on electrodiagnostic studies can suggest chronic radiculopathy. There is a lack of consensus in the field of pain management on how to approach the workup and treatment of chronic radicular pain. As this patient group has characteristics similar to those suffering from other nerve injuries who respond to specific drugs, it is reasonable that initial management

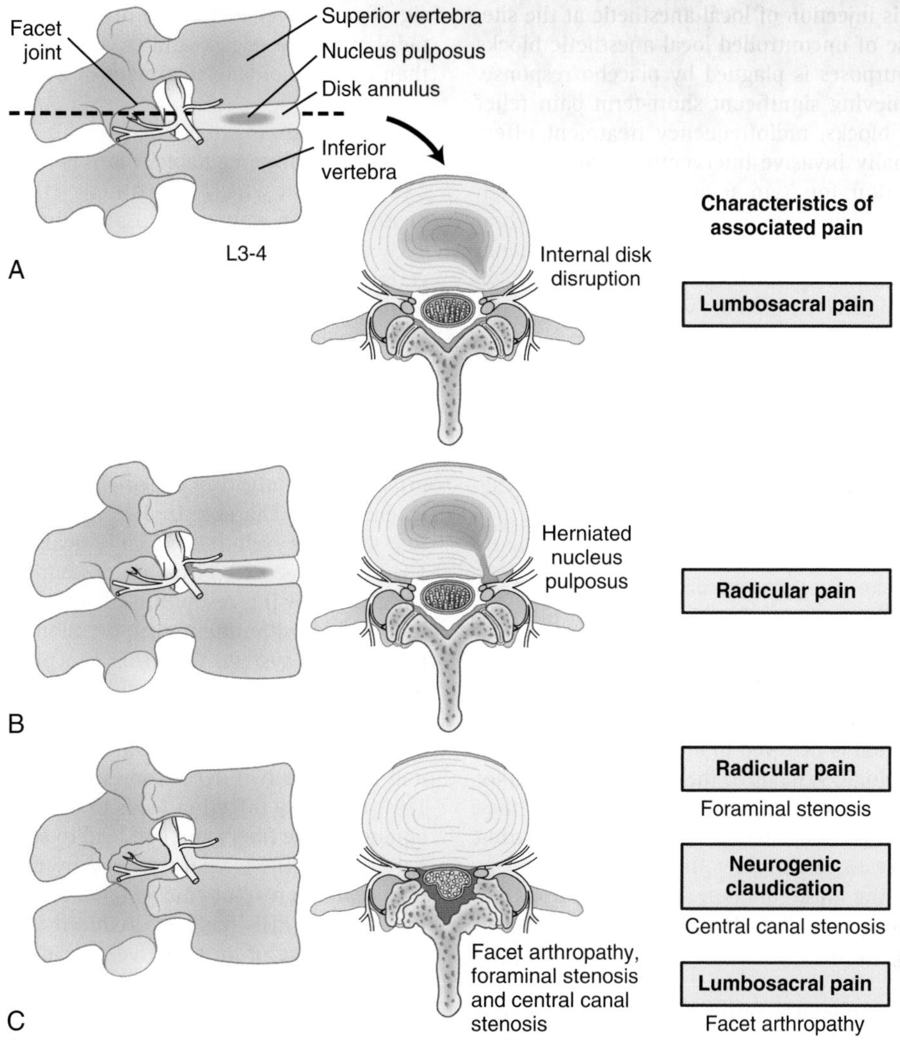

**Fig. 44.3** The functional spinal unit and the degenerative changes that lead to lumbosacral and radicular pain. (A) The normal functional spinal unit. (B) The degenerative changes leading to lumbosacral pain (disk disruption, facet joint arthropathy) and radicular pain (herniated nucleus pulposus). (C) The degenerative changes of lumbar spondylosis leading to lumbosacral (facet joint) pain, radicular (foraminal stenosis) pain, and neurogenic claudication (central canal stenosis).

consist of pharmacologic treatment for neuropathic pain using gabapentin, pregabalin, tricyclic antidepressants (TCAs), or serotonin-norepinephrine reuptake inhibitors (SNRIs).[9]

### Acute Lumbosacral Pain

Most patients presenting with acute onset of lumbosacral pain without radicular symptoms have no obvious abnormal physical findings, and radiologic imaging is unlikely to be helpful.[10,11] Traumatic sprain of the muscles and ligaments of the lumbar spine or the zygapophyseal joints, and early internal disk disruption, are significant causes of acute lumbosacral pain. As with patients with acute radicular pain, this group is best managed symptomatically.

### Chronic Lumbosacral Pain

There are many causes of chronic lumbosacral pain, and identification of the anatomic cause cannot be done with certainty in many cases. The structures most commonly implicated include the sacroiliac joint, lumbar facets, and lumbar intervertebral disks.[12] In chronic low back pain, the incidence of internal disk disruption has been estimated to be 39% (range 29% to 49%), facet joint pain 15% (10% to 20%), and sacroiliac joint pain 15% (7% to 23%). The gold standard for diagnosing sacroiliac and facet joint pain is injection of local anesthetic at the site. However, the use of uncontrolled local anesthetic blocks for diagnostic purposes is plagued by placebo response. For patients achieving significant short-term pain relief with diagnostic blocks, radiofrequency treatment offers a simple, minimally invasive intervention that can provide pain reduction for 3 to 6 months in those with facet-related pain. Pain from degenerating intervertebral disks is also a source of chronic axial back pain. Spinal cord stimulators with implanted epidural electrodes have shown efficacy in selected patients who fail medical and surgical therapy for chronic axial low back pain.[13]

## Neuropathic Pain

Persistent pain following injury to the nervous system is termed *neuropathic pain* and has unique characteristics:

- Spontaneous pain—pain that occurs with no stimulus (e.g., sudden lancinating pain described with PHN)
- Hyperalgesia—an exaggerated painful response to a normally mildly noxious stimulus (e.g., light pinprick leading to extreme, prolonged pain)
- Allodynia—a painful response to a normally non-noxious stimulus (e.g., light touch causing pain)

Neuropathic pain is believed to arise when the normal protective physiologic systems of the nervous system that produce sensitization of the peripheral and central nervous systems (sensitization that affords protection during the healing process) persist after the injured tissue has healed. Three of the most common forms of neuropathic pain include PHN, painful DPN, and complex regional pain syndrome (CRPS).

### Painful Diabetic Peripheral Neuropathy

Diabetes mellitus is the most common cause of neuropathic pain, and DPN is caused by damage to small unmyelinated nerve fibers. DPN can result in painless sensory loss or painful neuropathy. DPN typically begins with symmetric numbness in the toes associated with paresthesias, dysesthesias, and pain. The pain is often described as burning but equally common is a simple deep aching pain in the area affected. The neuropathy progresses slowly over many years. As the sensory changes reach the proximal portion of the feet, the same symptoms often appear in the hands. The incidence of painful DPN is directly related to glycemic control, with marked reduction in the incidence, severity, and rate of progression of the neuropathy in those with the tightest control of blood glucose levels. The strongest evidence for efficacy in pharmacologic management of pain-related symptoms exists for TCAs (amitriptyline, desipramine, and imipramine), SNRIs (duloxetine, venlafaxine), and anticonvulsants (gabapentin, pregabalin, carbamazepine, oxcarbezapine). Use of opioids is controversial because of potential for long-term dependence, abuse, and their significant adverse effects profile. In clinical trials, tepentadol extended release and oxycodone are more effective than other opioids in treatment of DPN.[14]

### Sympathetically Maintained Pain

Sympathetically mediated pain is a subset of neuropathic pain in which sympathetic efferent activity augments chronic pain and loss of function. As a result, early blockade of sympathetic neurotransmission during certain acute pain conditions may reduce the development of chronic pain. Typical examples of sympathetically mediated pain are PHN, CRPS, and stump neuroma in amputees.

### Postherpetic Neuralgia

The varicella-zoster virus produces a highly contagious primary viral infection called *chickenpox* that is common in childhood, characterized by the appearance of a diffuse vesicular rash that typically heals without scarring.[13] The varicella-zoster virus lies dormant in the dorsal root ganglia following resolution of the primary infection. In individuals with immunosuppression or with aging of the immune system, the virus can produce a secondary infection called *shingles* in which the virus replicates and travels from the ganglia along one or more spinal nerves erupting in an acute vesicular rash that is typically limited to one or two dermatomes on one side of the body. This secondary infection leads to damage to small unmyelinated nerve fibers and can lead to severe and persistent pain, PHN. PHN is characterized by episodic lancinating pain and severe allodynia in the affected dermatome. The incidence of PHN has been reduced in recent years with the emergence of an effective vaccine. Antiviral therapy with acyclovir, famcyclovir, or valacyclovir started within the first few days after eruption of vesicles also appears to reduce the incidence of PHN. The incidence rate of herpes zoster ranges from 1.2 to 3.4 per 1000 person-years among healthy individuals, increasing to 3.9 to 11.8 per 1000 person-years among those older than 65 years. Sympathetic blockade during acute herpes zoster can produce excellent analgesia, but is ineffective in treating established PHN.[14] Treatment of established PHN is difficult. Topical lidocaine can reduce pain in those with marked allodynia. TCAs and anticonvulsants remain the primary treatment for PHN.

### Complex Regional Pain Syndrome

CRPS develops as a localized pain disorder within 4 to 6 weeks following a trauma to an extremity (Box 44.1).[15] The incidence of CRPS is between 5.5 to 26.2 per 100,000 per year. Women are twice as frequently affected. Typically, symptoms are preceded by trauma. As the traumatized area heals, patients who develop CRPS are left with persistent pain that has the characteristics of neuropathic pain associated with signs and symptoms of dysfunction of the sympathetic nervous system (swelling, edema,

---

**Box 44.1** Budapest Clinical Diagnostic Criteria for Complex Regional Pain Syndrome

1. Continuing pain, which is disproportionate to any inciting event
2. Must report at least one symptom in *three of the four* following categories:
   - *Sensory:* reports of hyperesthesia or allodynia
   - *Vasomotor:* reports of temperature asymmetry or skin color changes or skin color asymmetry
   - *Sudomotor/edema:* reports of edema or sweating changes or sweating asymmetry
   - *Motor/trophic:* reports of decreased range of motion or motor dysfunction (weakness, tremor, dystonia) or trophic changes (hair, nail, skin)
3. Must display at least one sign at time of evaluation in *two or more* of the following categories:
   - *Sensory:* evidence of hyperalgesia (to pinprick) or allodynia (to light touch or deep somatic pressure or joint movement)
   - *Vasomotor:* evidence of temperature asymmetry or skin color changes or asymmetry
   - *Sudomotor/edema:* evidence of edema or sweating changes or sweating asymmetry
   - *Motor/trophic:* evidence of decreased range of motion or motor dysfunction (weakness, tremor, dystonia) or trophic changes (hair, nail, skin)
4. No other diagnosis better explains the signs and symptoms

---

erythema or bluish discoloration, temperature asymmetry when compared with the contralateral limb). CRPS can be divided into two subgroups based on absence (CRPS type 1) or presence (CRPS type 2) of distinct nerve lesions.

CRPS can lead to long-term, severe, persistent pain, and loss of function related to loss of use of the painful extremity. There is consensus that early therapeutic intervention is desirable and may prevent the transition to chronic CRPS. The central tenet of managing patients with CRPS is to focus on maintenance and restoration of function through aggressive physical and occupational rehabilitative therapy. Patients often fear the transient increase in pain and exacerbation of visible symptoms with use of the affected extremity. Reassurance and pain reduction can facilitate functional restoration. Pain is decreased with bisphosphonates administered both in early (first 6 to 9 months) and established CRPS. Although medications are widely prescribed in CRPS, clinical trial evidence for improvement in long-term pain is either negative (gabapetin) or is lacking (TCAs, carbamazepine). These medications may address the neuropathic components of CRPS. Sympathetic nerve blocks have been used for many years in managing patients with CRPS; they can produce dramatic pain reduction that facilitates physical therapy, but they are rarely useful in the long-term management of these patients.[16] Spinal cord stimulation (SCS) has emerged in recent years as a more effective long-term means to produce pain reduction and facilitate functional

restoration in patients with CRPS. Multidisciplinary treatment teams that include a provider that oversees medical management working in close coordination with a physical therapist and a psychologist appear to be the most effective means to help this group of patients.

## Musculoskeletal Pain

Two of the most common syndromes involving myofascial or widespread musculoskeletal pain are myofascial pain syndrome (MPS) and fibromyalgia. MPS is typically characterized by regional pain, fibromyalgia by generalized pain. In spite of distinct diagnostic criteria and clinical features in typical cases, they frequently coexist in the same patient and may be pathophysiologically interconnected.

### Myofascial Pain Syndrome

Although MPS lacks a consensus on definition and diagnostic criteria, it is characterized by the regional presence of spots of exquisite tenderness and hyperirritability in muscles or fascia, termed *myofascial trigger points.* Over 30% to 50% of middle-aged men and women, respectively, may complain of acute, recurrent, or chronic forms of regional musculoskeletal pain that may be MPS.[17] Trigger point injections are frequently employed in the treatment of MPS in addition to physical therapy. Although effective in relieving symptoms in a significant proportion of these patients, the pain relief mechanism of trigger point injections is poorly understood.

### Fibromyalgia

Fibromyalgia is a condition defined by widespread, chronic musculoskeletal pain, present for more than 3 months, and accompanied by other somatic symptoms such as fatigue, waking unrefreshed, and cognitive dysfunction. Two thirds of the symptom burden is due to pain.[18] It affects over 2% of the U.S. population, predominantly women (3.4% of women vs. 0.5% of men). In 25% to 65% of cases, fibromyalgia co-occurs with other rheumatic conditions such as rheumatoid arthritis, systemic lupus erythmatosus, and ankylosing spondylitis. Prevalence of fibromyalgia increases with aging. Although precise causation of fibromyalgia remains mostly speculative, dysregulation of pain-processing mechanisms and central pain sensitization have been postulated as major mechanisms underlying its clinical manifestations. Nonpharmacologic treatments (primarily promoting increased physical activity) are the cornerstone of therapy. TCAs, typically in doses smaller than those used to treat depression, are the traditional drug treatment. SNRIs, such as duloxetine and milnacipran, consistently augment pain alleviation and function in fibromyalgia. Although widely prescribed, opioids, with the exception of tramadol, have not been formally studied in fibromyalgia. Tramadol has effects on serotonin and norepinephrine uptake, which

**VI**

---

**Box 44.2** World Health Organization (WHO) Analgesic Ladder for the Treatment of Cancer Pain

**Step 1: Mild Pain**
Nonopioid analgesics (acetaminophen, NSAIDs)
± adjuvant analgesics (TCAs, anticonvulsants) for neuropathic pain

**Step 2: Moderate Pain**
Use of short-acting opioids (e.g., hydrocodone, oxycodone) in starting doses
± nonopioid analgesics (acetaminophen, NSAIDs)
± adjuvant analgesics (TCAs, anticonvulsants) for neuropathic pain

**Step 3: Severe Pain**
Use of potent opioids (e.g., morphine, hydromorphone) in higher doses
± nonopioid analgesics (acetaminophen, NSAIDs)
± adjuvant analgesics (TCAs, anticonvulsants) for neuropathic pain

---

*NSAIDs,* Nonsteroidal antiinflammatory drugs; *TCAs,* tricyclic antidepressants.

may explain its positive effects on pain and quality of life in fibromyalgia.[19]

## Cancer-Related Pain

Pain related to cancer and its treatment is common; indeed, pain is the most common presenting symptom of undiagnosed malignancy. The pain may be due to direct invasion of the malignancy or result from cancer treatment; chronic pain of various types often coexists with cancer-related pain. The primary focus of pain reduction in cancer patients is direct treatment of the malignancy, because successful treatment often leads to complete pain resolution. Nonetheless, ongoing pain during the course of treatment or as the disease progresses is all too common. More than 3 decades ago, the World Health Organization (WHO) revolutionized the treatment of cancer pain by introducing a simple, three-step analgesic ladder (Box 44.2). This approach has been adopted worldwide and promotes the aggressive treatment of cancer-related pain by tailoring the analgesic used to the severity of the pain, starting with oral non-opioids and moving toward more potent oral and parenteral nonopioid and opioid analgesics as necessary to control pain.[20,21] Anesthesia providers are often called upon to apply their knowledge of regional anesthesia and neuraxial drug delivery in caring for a small group of patients whose pain cannot be controlled with the more conservative approaches specified in the WHO approach. One of the more common nerve blocks used to successfully treat patients with pain associated with abdominal malignancy is the neurolytic celiac plexus block (described later). With the advent of implantable intrathecal drug delivery systems, long-term treatment of patients with intractable cancer-related pain using intrathecal opioids and other drugs (local anesthetics, clonidine, ziconotide) has become routine.

## PHARMACOLOGIC MANAGEMENT OF CHRONIC PAIN

### Acetaminophen and Nonsteroidal Antiinflammatory Drugs

Acetaminophen and the nonsteroidal antiinflammatory drugs (NSAIDs) are among the most common medications used to treat mild to moderate pain, ranging from headache to acute muscle sprain and strain. The NSAIDs reduce the long-term pain and stiffness associated with osteoarthritis. Acetaminophen is a novel nonopioid analgesic with a poorly understood mechanism of action; aspirin and the NSAIDs produce potent inhibition of the enzyme cyclooxygenase, resulting in decreased levels of prostaglandins. The long-term use of NSAIDs and acetaminophen in other chronic painful conditions such as low back pain is common but poorly supported by scientific evidence, which shows little utility in the use of these drugs.[22,23] These two groups of analgesics also represent the first step in the WHO analgesic ladder and are recommended as the initial drugs to treat mild to moderate cancer-related pain.

### Antidepressants

TCAs (e.g., amitriptyline, nortriptyline, desipramine) and newer selective SNRIs (e.g., venlafaxine, duloxetine) have a long history of use as first-line drugs in the treatment of neuropathic pain, including PHN and painful DPN. In this setting, TCAs are usually prescribed in doses smaller than those indicated for treatment of depression. Side effects can be problematic in maintaining long-term therapy. Common side effects of the TCAs include dry mouth and urinary retention; TCAs can also worsen preexisting heart block. The SNRIs have a more favorable side-effect profile at the cost of lesser efficacy when compared with the TCAs.[24] Milnacipran is a recently introduced SNRI that has shown modest benefit for fibromyalgia pain relief. Although clinical experience with milnacipran for chronic neuropathic pain has been positive, strong research evidence to support its use for this indication is awaited.[25]

### Anticonvulsants

Antiepileptic drugs (e.g., gabapentin, pregabalin) are effective as first-line treatment for neuropathic pain. These drugs are generally well tolerated; the most common side effects are dizziness, somnolence, and peripheral edema. Decisions regarding pharmacologic treatment of neuropathic pain (Box 44.3) may be based on an analysis of the number needed to treat (NNT); the NNT (with 95%

**Box 44.3** Stepwise Pharmacologic Management of Neuropathic Pain

**Step 1**

Assessment and diagnosis of the neuropathic pain syndrome followed by detailed explanation of the pain management plan setting realistic goals

**Step 2**

Initial pharmacologic therapy including one of the following agents:

*First-Line Medications*

- TCAs (nortriptyline, desipramine) or SNRIs (duloxetine, venlafaxine)
- Anticonvulsants, either gabapentin or pregabalin
- Topical lidocaine

*Second-Line Medications*

- Opioid analgesics and tramadol, which can be used alone or in combination for acute exacerbations, neuropathic cancer pain, or when prompt relief is required

**Step 3**

If follow-up evaluation demonstrates substantial pain relief with tolerable side effects (pain <3/10), treatment is continued. If the relief is partial after an adequate trial (pain >4/10), another first-line drug is added. If pain relief is inadequate at the target dosage (<30% reduction), an alternative first-line medication is started.

**Step 4**

If the initial trial fails, a second-line or third-line medication is considered.

*Third-Line Medications*

- Certain other antiepileptic agents (carbamazepine, oxcarbazepine) and antidepressants (citalopram, paroxetine), NMDA receptor antagonists, topical capsaicin

*NMDA,* N-methyl-ᴅ-aspartate; *SNRIs,* serotonin-norepinephrine reuptake inhibitors; *TCAs,* tricyclic antidepressants.

Modified from Dworkin RH, O'Connor AB, Backonja M, et al. Pharmacologic management of neuropathic pain: evidence-based recommendations. *Pain.* 2007;32:237-251, used with permission.

confidence interval [CI]) are TCA 3.6 (3.0 to 4.4), SNRI 6.4 (5.2 to 8.4), gabapentin 7.2 (5.9 to 9.1), and pregabalin 7.7 (6.5 to 9.4).[24]

## Opioids

### Chronic Opioid Therapy

Opioids have established efficacy for treatment of acute pain and are also routinely administered for moderate to severe cancer pain. Chronic opioid therapy in the long-term management of noncancer pain remains controversial. Advocates point to long-term efficacy and improvement in function in patients with chronic painful conditions, including low back pain. Opponents cite difficulties in prescribing these drugs over the long term. Assessment of maximum efficacy based on high-quality randomized controlled trials (RCTs) has shown no significant difference between opioids and other pharmacologic and nonpharmacologic treatments for chronic pain. Although opioids inhibit nociception, it is highly contentious whether opioids improve or deteriorate other factors inciting and sustaining chronic noncancer pain, such as psychological, cognitive, social, and financial aspects of health care. Treating acute pain in the opioid tolerant patient is difficult, and it is becoming evident that chronic opioid use can worsen pain by inducing hyperalgesia.[26-28] Although opioids are the most commonly prescribed class of drugs for back pain, there are no high-quality RCTs with long-term follow-up to guide the use of opioids in treating this set of conditions. Studies comparing opioids with placebo show short-term improvement in pain with unclear long-term benefits. There are no high-quality studies comparing opioids with nonopioid pain medications for chronic back pain. Despite the absence of conclusive evidence for long-term benefit, chronic opioid use is widely prevalent both for back pain and other chronic painful conditions. When treating a patient with long-term opioids, many drugs are available. The traditional paradigm for opioid treatment is based on cancer pain management. In this approach, patients with significant chronic pain are given a long-acting opioid for continuous analgesia; short-acting opioids may cause fluctuations in pain control. A small dose of a short-acting drug is also available for intermittent pain that occurs with activity and "breaks through" the control provided by the long-acting drug alone. Nearly every available opioid has been used successfully in treating chronic low back pain, including short-acting analgesics (e.g., hydrocodone, oxycodone) alone or in combination with ibuprofen or acetaminophen, and long-acting drugs (e.g., methadone, controlled-release morphine, transdermal fentanyl, controlled-release oxycodone). "Ultrafast onset" opioids (e.g., oral transmucosal fentanyl citrate, fentanyl buccal tablet) can also be used for the rapid treatment of breakthrough pain. As with the patient selection process, choosing the opioid drug and the appropriate dose remains empiric. The decision to use short- or long-acting drugs alone or in combination should be tailored to the individual patient's pattern of pain.

### Chronic Pain and the Opioid Epidemic

Tens of millions of Americans suffer from chronic persistent pain. In the United States, managing chronic pain costs over $500 billion every year.[29] In the last 2 decades, opioid use for noncancer pain—albeit controversial—has skyrocketed and so have deaths from prescription opioid overdoses.[30] Americans consume 84% of the world's entire supply of oxycodone and 99% of hydrocodone.[31] Although aberrant drug-related behavior (e.g., losing prescriptions, escalating drug use) is relatively common in patients receiving opioids for chronic pain, overt addiction is unusual. The risk of overdose

VI

and death increases significantly with increasing daily doses and use of extended release/long-acting formulations. Patients with chronic pain are not the only ones susceptible to harm from abuse and overdose; opioid diversions constitute a significant problem. The National Survey on Drug Use and Health has showed that nearly one third of people aged 12 years or older who used drugs for the first time began by using a prescription drug nonmedically. Seventy percent got prescription opioids from friends or relatives, whereas only 5% got them from drug dealers or from the Internet.[32] The opioid epidemic has been sustained and exacerbated largely by physician prescription practices. Although prescription opioids may be effective for short-term pain relief, there is limited evidence of improvement in pain alleviation and improvement in physical functioning with long-term opioid use.[33] Important aspects in preventing opioid abuse among patients already on chronic prescription opioids include frequent monitoring, periodic urine screens, opioid therapy agreements, opioid checklists, motivational counseling, and the active use of state-sponsored prescription drug monitoring programs by all prescribers of opioids, as well as sustained opioid tapering. It is important for prescribing physicians to strongly consider nonopioid analgesic options for opioid naïve patients presenting to them with painful conditions, thus preventing chronic opioid dependence.[26]

### Tapering Opioids

Increasing concern about the risks and limited evidence supporting the therapeutic benefit of long-term opioid therapy for chronic noncancer pain is leading prescribers to consider discontinuing the use of opioids. Criteria have been proposed to identify patients who will benefit from tapering long-term opioid therapy (Table 44.1). Central issues during tapering of long-term opioid treatment are many and can be divided into short-term and long-term risks. Among short-term risks, opioid withdrawal syndrome, fear of increasing pain, refusal to taper opioids or resumption of long-term opioid treatment with a new prescriber, or aggressive behavior toward the prescriber create concern for many clinicians. Long-term issues of relapse, interventions to improve or maintain function, treatment of psychiatric comorbid conditions, and medicolegal issues surrounding deaths by unintentional overdose or suicide represent serious concerns.

Depression, high pain scores, high opioid doses, and the absence of provision for taper failure are key predictors of opioid-tapering dropout or relapse. There is an absence of validated protocols on tapering opioids. A typical approach involves an initial reduction of the opioid dose to the smallest commonly available unit dosage followed by an increase in the amount of time between doses. For example, in a patient prescribed 60 mg of extended-release morphine every 8 hours, the dose would first be reduced to 15 mg, then the time interval between

| Table 44.1 | Criteria Identifying Patients in Whom Discontinuation of Long-Term Opioid Therapy Should Be Considered |
|---|---|

1. Inability to achieve or maintain anticipated pain relief or functional improvement despite reasonable dose escalation
2. Intolerable adverse effects at the minimum dose that produces effective analgesia, with reasonable attempts at opioid rotation unsuccessful
3. Persistent nonadherence with patient treatment agreement, including inappropriate use, failure to comply with monitoring (after excluding this failure is due to personal cost burden), selling prescription drugs, forging prescriptions, stealing or borrowing drugs, aggressive demand for opioids, injecting oral or topical opioids, unsanctioned use of opioids, unsanctioned dose escalation, concurrent use of illicit drugs, obtaining opioids from multiple prescribers or multiple pharmacies, recurring emergency department visits for chronic pain management
4. Deterioration in physical, emotional, or social functioning attributed to opioid therapy
5. Resolution or healing of the painful condition

doses would be increased to 12 hours, then 24 hours. It may be preferable to taper using the patient's long-term opioid treatment medications as opposed to switching to methadone or buprenorphine, which does not have strong evidence in support. Continued pain management, including optimized nonopioid regimens and interventional approaches, should be offered. The use of $\alpha_2$-agonists such as clonidine, lofexidine, guanfacine, and tizanidine for symptomatic treatment of increased sympathetic activity and NSAIDs or acetaminophen for muscle aches and pains are often part of tapering protocols. Considering the risk factors for dropout and adverse functional outcomes in these patients, as reviewed earlier, psychological support with interventions such as CBT may be needed to address anxiety related to the taper, underlying depression, and deficient pain and stress coping strategies.[33]

## INTERVENTIONAL PAIN THERAPIES

Interventional pain therapy refers to a group of targeted treatments used for specific spine disorders, ranging from epidural injection of steroids to percutaneous intradiskal techniques. Some have been rigorously tested in RCTs, and others are in widespread use without critical evaluation. When these treatment techniques are used for the disorders they are most likely to benefit (Table 44.2), they can be highly effective; however, when used haphazardly, they are unlikely to be helpful, are expensive, and may cause harm.

**Table 44.2**   Application of Medical Therapies in Treating Low Back Pain

| Type of Pain | Initial Therapy | Therapy for Persistent Pain |
|---|---|---|
| Acute radicular pain | • A 7- to 10-day course of an oral analgesic (NSAID or acetaminophen, ± opioid analgesic) with a relaxant drug, for those with superimposed muscle spasm. (LEVEL I) | • Between 2 and 6 weeks after onset of acute radicular pain, consider lumbar epidural steroid injection for attenuation of radicular symptoms. (LEVEL II) |
| Chronic radicular pain | • Initial treatment of chronic radicular pain is similar to treatment of other types of neuropathic pain and should begin with a trial of a tricyclic antidepressant, SNRI, or anticonvulsant. (LEVEL 1)<br>• Chronic radicular pain may respond to treatment with chronic opioids, but neuropathic pain is less responsive to opioids than nociceptive pain. (LEVEL II) | • Consider evaluation for a trial of spinal cord stimulation. (LEVEL II) |
| Acute lumbosacral pain | • A 7- to 10-day course of an oral analgesic (NSAID or acetaminophen, ± opioid analgesic) with a relaxant drug, for those with superimposed muscle spasm. (LEVEL I) | • Between 2 and 6 weeks after onset of chronic radicular pain, consider referral for physical therapy for stretching, strengthening, and aerobic exercise in conjunction with patient education. (LEVEL I) |
| Chronic lumbosacral pain | • Diagnostic medial branch blocks of the nerves to the facet joints. If >50% pain relief is obtained with the diagnostic blocks, radiofrequency treatment may be effective. (LEVEL II) | • Consider enrollment in a formal pain program that incorporates medical management, behavioral therapy, and physical therapy. (LEVEL I)<br>• Consider cognitive-behavioral therapy. (LEVEL I)<br>• If no response is obtained with diagnostic facet blocks and MRI shows evidence of early degenerative disk disease affecting fewer than two intervertebral disks, consider diagnostic provocative diskography. (LEVEL III) If diskography is concordant (pain is reproduced at anatomically abnormal level[s] and no pain is present at an adjacent anatomically normal level), consider treatment with intradiskal electrothermal therapy (IDET) at the symptomatic level(s). (LEVEL II) |

**Note:** Level of evidence is based on the Oxford Evidence-Based Medicine Levels for Treatment: LEVEL I, high-quality RCTs or systematic reviews of RCTs; LEVEL II, low-quality RCTs, cohort studies, or systematic reviews of cohort studies; LEVEL III, case-control studies or systematic reviews of case-control studies; LEVEL IV, case-series; LEVEL V, expert opinion.
*MRI,* Magnetic resonance imaging; *NSAID,* nonsteroidal antiinflammatory drug; *RCTs,* randomized controlled trials; *SNRI,* serotonin-norepinephrine reuptake inhibitor.
Modified with permission from Rathmell JP. A 50-year-old man with chronic low back pain. *JAMA.* 2008;299:2066-2077.

## Epidural Injection of Steroids

Numerous RCTs have examined the efficacy of epidural corticosteroid injection for acute radicular pain.[22] Such injections into the epidural space may combat the inflammatory response that is associated with acute disk herniation. In acute radicular pain with HNP, epidural steroids reduce the severity and duration of leg pain if given between 3 and 6 weeks after onset. Adverse effects, such as injection site pain and transient worsening of radicular pain, occur in less than 1% of treated subjects. Beyond 3 months from treatment, there are no long-term reductions in pain or improvements in function. This therapy has never proved helpful for lumbosacral pain without radicular symptoms. Epidural injection of steroids can be accomplished by the interlaminar route (Fig. 44.4) or the transforaminal route (Fig. 44.5). The rationale for use of the transforaminal route is to place the steroid in high concentration directly adjacent to the spinal nerve close to the site of inflammation. The transforaminal approach may be more effective than the interlaminar approach, but additional studies are needed.

## Facet Blocks and Radiofrequency Treatment

Pain from the lumbar facet joints affects up to 15% of chronic low back pain patients.[12] Patients are identified based on typical patterns of referred pain, with maximal pain located directly over the facet joints and their reports of pain on palpation over the facets; radiographic findings are variable, but some degree of facet arthropathy

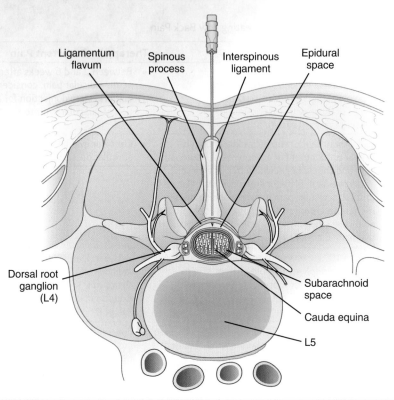

**Fig. 44.4** Axial diagram of interlaminar lumbar epidural injection. The epidural needle is advanced in the midline between adjacent spinous processes to traverse the ligamentum flavum and enter the dorsal epidural space in the midline. The normal epidural space is approximately 4 to 6 mm wide (from the ligamentum flavum to the dura mater in the axial plane). Note the proximity of the underlying cauda equina during lumbar epidural injection. (Redrawn from Rathmell JP. Atlas of image-guided intervention in regional anesthesia and pain medicine. Philadelphia: Lippincott Williams & Wilkins; 2006:47, used with permission.)

is typically present. The intra-articular injection of anesthetics and corticosteroids may lead to intermediate-term (1 to 3 months) pain relief in patients with an active inflammatory process. Radiofrequency denervation delivers energy through an insulated, small-diameter needle positioned adjacent to the sensory nerve to the facet joint (Fig. 44.6), creating a small area of tissue coagulation that denervates the facet joint. Radiofrequency denervation probably provides better pain relief than sham intervention for facet-related pain.[23] Approximately 50% of patients treated report at least 50% pain reduction. Pain typically returns 6 to 12 months after treatment, and denervation can be repeated without lessening of efficacy. Adverse events are uncommon; in 1% of treated patients, pain at the treatment site lasted 2 weeks or less.

## Sympathetic Blocks

Blockade of sympathetic nerve fibers can produce pain relief in specific pain syndromes, including CRPS and ischemic pain produced by vascular insufficiency. There is little scientific evidence to support long-term reductions in pain or improvements in physical function associated with the use of sympathetic blocks; nonetheless, they are still widely used to produce short-term pain reduction in order to facilitate active involvement in physical therapy.[16] One exception to this rule is the use of neurolytic celiac plexus block for the treatment of pain associated with abdominal malignancies, for which significant pain reduction can extend over weeks to months after treatment.[28]

### Stellate Ganglion Block

Stellate ganglion block is an established method for the diagnosis and treatment of sympathetically maintained pain of the head, neck, and upper extremity. Sympathetic fibers to and from the head, neck, and upper extremities pass through the stellate ganglion. In most individuals, the stellate ganglion is formed by fusion of the inferior cervical and first thoracic sympathetic ganglia. The ganglion is commonly found just lateral to the lateral border of the longus colli muscle, anterior to the neck of the first rib and the transverse process of the seventh cervical

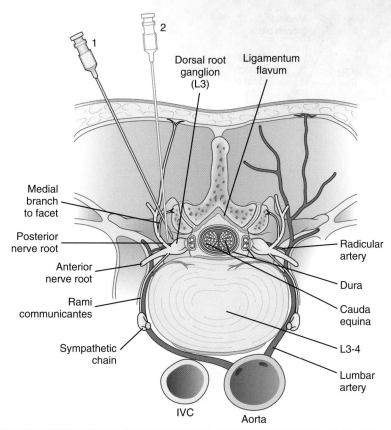

**Fig. 44.5** Axial view of lumbar transforaminal and selective nerve root injection. The anatomy and proper needle position (axial view) for right (1) L3-L4 transforaminal injection and (2) L3 selective nerve root injection. *IVC*, Inferior vena cava. (Redrawn from Rathmell JP. Atlas of image-guided intervention in regional anesthesia and pain medicine. Philadelphia: Lippincott Williams & Wilkins; 2006:58, used with permission.)

vertebra (Fig. 44.7). In this position, the ganglion lies posterior to the superior border of the first part of the subclavian artery and the origin of the vertebral artery posterior to the dome of the lung. Although several approaches to stellate ganglion block have been described, the most common is the anterior paratracheal approach at C6 using surface landmarks. Performing the block at C6 reduces the likelihood of pneumothorax, which is more likely when the block is performed close to the dome of the lung at C7. The anterior tubercle of the transverse process of C6 (Chassaignac tubercle) is readily palpable in most individuals. To perform the block without radiographic guidance, the operator palpates the cricoid cartilage, and then slides a finger laterally into the groove between the trachea and the sternocleidomastoid muscle, retracting the muscle and adjacent carotid and jugular vessels laterally. Chassaignac tubercle is typically palpable in this groove at the C6 level. Once the tubercle has been identified, a needle is advanced through the skin and seated on the tubercle, where local anesthetic is injected. The local anesthetic spreads along the prevertebral fascia in a caudal direction to anesthetize the stellate ganglion, which lies just inferior to the point of injection in the same plane. In practice, the marked variation in the size and shape of Chassaignac tubercle reduces the rate of successful block. Signs of successful stellate ganglion block include the appearance of Horner syndrome (miosis [pupillary constriction]); ptosis (drooping of the upper eyelid); and enophthalmos (recession of the globe within the orbit). Other signs of successful block include anhidrosis (lack of sweating), nasal congestion, venodilation in the hand and forearm, and increase in temperature of the blocked limb by at least 1° C. The adjacent vertebral artery and C6 nerve root must be avoided to safely conduct this block. A simple modification of technique in which the needle is directed medially toward the base of the transverse process using radiographic guidance is a safe and simple means of improving the reliability of stellate ganglion block (see Fig. 44.7).

Stellate ganglion block has long been the standard approach to diagnosis and treatment of sympathetically maintained pain syndromes involving the upper extremity,

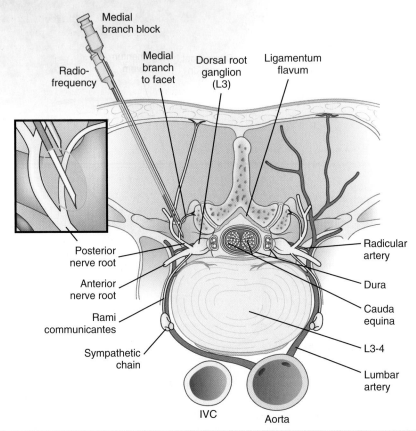

**Fig. 44.6** Axial diagram of lumbar medial branch nerve blocks and radiofrequency treatment. A 22-gauge, 3½-inch spinal needle (or 22-gauge, 10-cm radiofrequency cannula with a 5-mm active tip) is advanced toward the base of the transverse process, where it joins with the superior articular process. Cannula placement for conventional radiofrequency treatment should be carried out with 25 to 30 degrees of caudal angulation of the C-arm to bring the axis of the active tip parallel to the course of the medial branch nerve in the groove between the transverse process and the superior articular process. *IVC*, Inferior vena cava. (Redrawn from Rathmell JP. Atlas of image-guided intervention in regional anesthesia and pain medicine. Philadelphia: Lippincott Williams & Wilkins; 2006:89, used with permission.)

such as CRPS. Other neuropathic pain syndromes, including ischemic neuropathies, herpes zoster (shingles), early PHN, and postradiation neuritis may also respond to stellate ganglion block. Blockade of the stellate ganglion has also proved successful in reducing pain and improving blood flow in vascular insufficiency conditions such as intractable angina pectoris, Raynaud disease, frostbite, vasospasm, and occlusive and embolic vascular disease. Finally, the sympathetic fibers control sweating; thus, stellate ganglion block can be quite effective in controlling hyperhidrosis (recurrent and uncontrollable sweating of the hands). There are many structures within the immediate vicinity of the needle's tip once it is properly positioned for stellate ganglion block (see Fig. 44.7). Diffusion of local anesthetic can block the adjacent recurrent laryngeal nerve. This often leads to hoarseness, a feeling of having a lump in the throat, and a subjective feeling of shortness of breath and difficulty swallowing. Bilateral

stellate ganglion block should not be performed because bilateral recurrent laryngeal nerve blocks may well lead to loss of laryngeal reflexes and respiratory compromise. The phrenic nerve is also commonly blocked by direct spread of local anesthetic, which can lead to unilateral diaphragmatic paresis. Diffusion of local anesthetic as well as direct placement of local anesthetic adjacent to the posterior tubercle will result in somatic block of the upper extremity. This may take the form of a small area of sensory loss due to diffusion of local anesthetic or a complete brachial plexus block when the local anesthetic is placed within the nerve sheath. Patients with significant somatic block to the upper extremity should be sent home with a sling in place and counseled to guard their limb, just as one would instruct a patient who had received a brachial plexus block.

Major complications associated with stellate ganglion block include neuraxial block (spinal or epidural) and

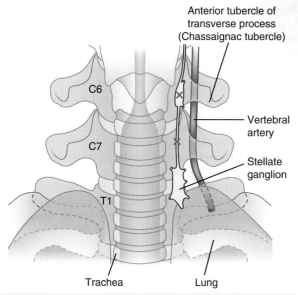

Anterior tubercle of transverse process (Chassaignac tubercle)

Vertebral artery

Stellate ganglion

C6

C7

T1

Trachea

Lung

**Fig. 44.7** Anatomy of the stellate ganglion. The stellate ganglion conveys sympathetic fibers to and from the upper extremities and the head and neck. The ganglion comprises the fused superior thoracic ganglion and the inferior cervical ganglion and is named for its fusiform shape (in many individuals, the two ganglia remain separate). The stellate ganglia lies over the head of the first rib at the junction of the transverse process and uncinate process of T1. The ganglion is just posteromedial to the cupola of the lung and medial to the vertebral artery. Stellate ganglion block is typically carried out at the C6 or C7 level to avoid pneumothorax, and a volume of solution that will spread along the prevertebral fascia inferiorly to the stellate ganglion is employed (usually 10 mL). When radiographic guidance is not used, the operator palpates the anterior tubercle of the transverse process of C6 (Chassaignac tubercle), and a needle is seated in the location. With radiographic guidance it is simpler and safer to place a needle over the vertebral body just inferior the uncinate process of C6 or C7. Particular care should be taken when performing the block at the C7 level to assure that the needle does not stray lateral to the uncinate process, as the vertebral artery courses anterior to transverse process at this level and is often not protected within a bony foramen transversarium. (Redrawn from Rathmell JP. Atlas of image-guided intervention in regional anesthesia and pain medicine. Philadelphia: Lippincott Williams & Wilkins; 2006:116, used with permission.)

seizures. Extreme medial angulation of the needle from a relatively lateral skin entry point may lead to needle placement into the spinal canal through the anterolaterally oriented intervertebral foramen. In this manner, local anesthetic can be deposited in the epidural space, or if the needle is advanced far enough, it may penetrate the dural cuff surrounding the exiting nerve root and lie within the intrathecal space. More likely is placement of the needle tip on the posterior tubercle and spread of local anesthetic proximally along the nerve root to enter the epidural space. In this case, partial or profound neuraxial

block, including high spinal or epidural block with loss of consciousness and apnea, may ensue. Airway protection, ventilation, and intravenous sedation should be promptly administered and continued until the patient regains airway reflexes and consciousness. Because the maximal effects of epidural local anesthetic may require 15 to 20 minutes to develop when using longer acting local-anesthetics, it is imperative that patients are monitored for at least 30 minutes after stellate ganglion block. Intravascular injection during stellate ganglion block will likely result in immediate onset of generalized seizures. The carotid artery lies just anteromedial to the Chassaignac tubercle, and the vertebral artery lies within the bony transverse foramen just posteromedial to the tubercle.

If injection occurs into either structure, the local anesthetic injected enters the arterial supply traveling directly to the brain, and generalized seizures typically begin rapidly and after only small amounts of local anesthetic (as little as 0.2 mL of 0.25% bupivacaine have led to seizure). However, because the local anesthetic rapidly redistributes, the seizures are typically brief and do not require treatment. In the event of seizure, halt the injection, remove the needle, and begin supportive care.

### Celiac Plexus Block

Neurolytic celiac plexus block (NCPB) is among the most widely applicable of all neurolytic blocks. NCPB has a long-lasting benefit for 70% to 90% of patients with pancreatic and other intra-abdominal malignancies.[29] Several techniques have been described for localizing the celiac plexus. The classic technique employs a percutaneous posterior approach using surface and bony landmarks to position needles in the vicinity of the plexus. Numerous reports have described new approaches for celiac plexus block using guidance from plain radiographs, fluoroscopy, computed tomography (CT), and ultrasound (an endoscopic transgastric technique).

No single methodology has proved clearly superior in either its safety or success rate. In recent years, general agreement has arisen that radiographic guidance is necessary to perform celiac plexus block. Some practitioners have turned to routine use of CT, taking advantage of the ability to visualize adjacent structures when performing this technique. The celiac plexus comprises a diffuse network of nerve fibers and individual ganglia that lie over the anterolateral surface of the aorta at the T12-L1 vertebral level. Sympathetic innervation to the abdominal viscera arises from the anterolateral horn of the spinal cord between the T5 and T12 levels. Nociceptive information from the abdominal viscera is carried by afferents that accompany the sympathetic nerves. Presynaptic sympathetic fibers travel from the thoracic sympathetic chain toward the ganglion, traversing over the anterolateral aspect of the inferior thoracic vertebrae as the greater (T5 to T9), lesser (T10 to T11), and least (T12) splanchnic nerves (Fig. 44.8). Presynaptic fibers

VI

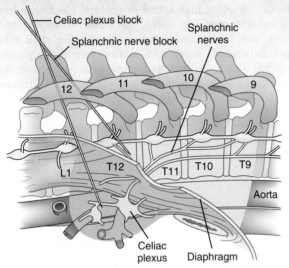

**Fig. 44.8** Anatomy of the celiac plexus and splanchnic nerves. The celiac plexus comprises a diffuse network of nerve fibers and individual ganglia that lie over the anterolateral surface of the aorta at the T12-L1 vertebral level. Presynaptic sympathetic fibers travel from the thoracic sympathetic chain toward the ganglion, traversing over the anterolateral aspect of the inferior thoracic vertebrae as the greater (T5-T9), lesser (T10-T11), and least (T12) splanchnic nerves. Celiac plexus block using a transcrural approach places the local anesthetic or neurolytic solution directly on the celiac ganglion anterolateral to the aorta. The needles pass directly through the crura of the diaphragm to the celiac plexus. In contrast, for splanchnic nerve block the needles remain posterior to the diaphragmatic crura in close apposition to the T12 vertebral body. Shading indicates the pattern of solution spread for each technique. (Redrawn from Rathmell JP. Atlas of image-guided intervention in regional anesthesia and pain medicine. Philadelphia: Lippincott Williams & Wilkins; 2006:124, used with permission.)

traveling via the splanchnic nerves synapse within the celiac ganglia, over the anterolateral surface of the aorta surrounding the origin of the celiac and superior mesenteric arteries at approximately the L1 vertebral level. Postsynaptic fibers from the celiac ganglia innervate all of the abdominal viscera with the exception of the descending colon, sigmoid colon, rectum, and pelvic viscera. Celiac plexus block using a transcrural approach places the local anesthetic or neurolytic solution directly on the celiac ganglion anterolateral to the aorta (see Fig. 44.8). The needles pass directly through the crura of the diaphragm en route to the celiac plexus. Spread of the solution toward the posterior surface of the aorta may thus be limited, perhaps reducing the chance of nerve root or spinal segmental artery involvement. In contrast, splanchnic nerve block (see Fig. 44.8) avoids the risk of penetrating the aorta, uses smaller volumes of solution, and the success is unlikely to be affected by anatomic distortion caused by extensive tumor or adenopathy within the pancreas. Because the needles remain posterior to the

diaphragmatic crura in close apposition to the T12 vertebral body, this has been termed the *retrocrural technique*. Splanchnic nerve block is a minor modification of the classic retrocrural celiac plexus block, the only difference being that for splanchnic block, the needles are placed over the midportion of the T12 vertebral body rather than the cephalad portion of L1. Retrocrural celiac plexus block at the superior aspect of the L1 vertebral body and splanchnic nerve block at the mid T12 vertebral body have both been described, and they are essentially the same technique relying on cephalad spread of solution to block the splanchnic nerves in a retrocrural location. In most cases, celiac plexus (transcrural or retrocrural) and splanchnic nerve block can be used interchangeably to effect the same results. Even though there are those who strongly advocate one approach or the other, there is no evidence that either approach results in superior clinical outcomes. Celiac plexus and splanchnic nerve block are used to control pain arising from intra-abdominal structures. These structures include the pancreas, liver, gallbladder, omentum, mesentery, and alimentary tract from the stomach to the transverse colon. The most common application of NCPB is to treat pain associated with intra-abdominal malignancy, particularly pain associated with pancreatic cancer. Neurolysis of the splanchnic nerves or celiac plexus can produce dramatic pain relief, reduce or eliminate the need for supplemental analgesics, and improve quality of life in patients with pancreatic cancer and other intra-abdominal malignancies.

The long-term benefit of NCPB in those with chronic nonmalignant pain, particularly those with chronic pancreatitis, is debatable. Many patients with pancreatic cancer have a short remaining life span. Analgesia sometimes lasts the rest of their lives.

Several physiologic side effects are expected following celiac plexus block and include diarrhea and orthostatic hypotension. Blockade of the sympathetic innervations to the abdominal viscera results in unopposed parasympathetic innervation of the alimentary tract and may produce abdominal cramping and sudden diarrhea. Likewise, the vasodilation that ensues often results in orthostatic hypotension. These effects are invariably transient, but may persist for several days after neurolytic block. The hypotension seldom requires treatment other than intravenous hydration.

Complications of celiac plexus and splanchnic nerve block include hematuria, intravascular injection, and pneumothorax. The kidneys extend from between T12 and L3 with the left kidney slightly more cephalad than the right. The aorta lies over the left anterolateral border of the vertebral column. The celiac arterial trunk arises from the anterior surface of the aorta at the T12 level and divides into the hepatic, left gastric, and splenic arteries. Using the transaortic technique, caution must be used to avoid needle placement directly through the axis of the celiac trunk as it exits anteriorly. The inferior vena cava lies just to the right of the aorta over the anterolateral surface of the vertebral column. The medial pleural reflection extends inferomedially as low as the T12-L1 level. NCPB carries small but significant additional risk. Intravascular injection of 30 mL of 100% ethanol will result in a blood ethanol level well above the legal limit for intoxication but below danger of severe alcohol toxicity. Intravascular injection of phenol is associated with clinical manifestations similar to those of local anesthetic toxicity: CNS excitation, followed by seizures and, in extreme toxicity, cardiovascular collapse.

The most devastating complication associated with NCPB using either alcohol or phenol is paraplegia. The theoretical mechanism is spread of the neurolytic solution toward the posterior surface of the aorta to surround the spinal segmental arteries. At the level of T12 or L1, it is common to have a single, dominant spinal segmental artery, the artery of Adamkiewicz. In some individuals, this artery is the dominant arterial supply to the anterior two thirds of the spinal cord in the low thoracic region. Neurolytic solution may cause spasm or even necrosis and occlusion of the artery of Adamkiewicz leading to paralysis. The actual incidence of this complication is unknown, but appears to be less than 1:1000.

### Lumbar Sympathetic Block

The sympathetic nervous system is involved in the pathophysiology that leads to a number of different chronic pain conditions, including CRPS and ischemic pain. The lumbar sympathetic chain consists of four to five paired ganglia that lie over the anterolateral surface of the L2 through L4 vertebrae (Fig. 44.9). The cell bodies that travel to the lumbar sympathetic ganglia lie in the anterolateral region of the spinal cord from T11 to L2, with variable contributions from T10 and L3. The preganglionic fibers leave the spinal canal with the corresponding spinal nerve root, join the sympathetic chain as white communicating rami, and then synapse within the appropriate ganglion. Postganglionic fibers exit the chain to join either the diffuse perivascular plexus around the iliac and femoral arteries or via the gray communicating rami to join the nerve roots that form the lumbar and lumbosacral plexuses. Sympathetic fibers accompany all of the major nerves to the lower extremities. The majority of the sympathetic innervation to the lower extremities passes through the L2 and L3 lumbar sympathetic ganglia, and blockade of these ganglia results in near complete sympathetic denervation of the lower extremities. Lumbar sympathetic blockade has been used extensively in the treatment of sympathetically maintained pain syndromes involving the lower extremities. The most common of these are the CRPS type 1 (reflex sympathetic dystrophy) and type 2 (causalgia). The local anesthetic block can produce marked pain relief of long duration, and

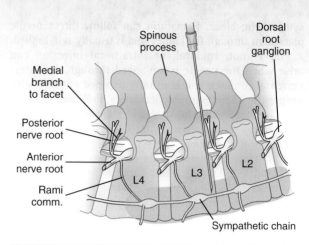

**Fig. 44.9** Anatomy of the lumbar sympathetic chain. The lumbar sympathetic ganglia are variable in number and location from one individual to another. Most commonly, the ganglia lie over the anteromedial surface of the vertebral bodies between L2 and L4. Temporary lumbar sympathetic block using local anesthetic is best performed by advancing a single needle cephalad to the transverse process of L3 in order to avoid the exiting nerve root. The needle tip is placed adjacent to the superior portion of the anteromedial surface of the L3 vertebral body. Use of 15 to 20 mL of local anesthetic solution will spread to cover multiple vertebral levels (shaded region). (Redrawn from Rathmell JP. Atlas of image-guided intervention in regional anesthesia and pain medicine. Philadelphia: Lippincott Williams & Wilkins; 2006:136, used with permission.)

this block is used as part of a comprehensive treatment plan to provide analgesia and facilitate functional restoration. Patients with peripheral vascular insufficiency due to small vessel occlusion may also be treated effectively with lumbar sympathetic blockade. Proximal fixed lesions are best treated with surgical intervention using bypass grafting or intra-arterial stent placement to restore blood flow. In those patients with diffuse, small vessel occlusion, lumbar sympathetic block can improve microvascular circulation and reduce ischemic pain. If local anesthetic block improves blood flow and reduces pain, these patients will often benefit from surgical or chemical sympathectomy.

Other patients with neuropathic pain involving the lower extremities have shown variable response to lumbar sympathetic block. In those with acute herpes zoster and early PHN, sympathetic block may reduce pain. However, once PHN is well established (beyond 3 to 6 months from onset), sympathetic blockade is rarely helpful. Likewise, deafferentation syndromes such as phantom limb pain and neuropathic lower extremity pain following spinal cord injury have shown variable and largely disappointing responses to sympathetic blockade.

Significant and potentially toxic levels of local anesthetic can result from direct needle placement into a blood vessel and intravascular injection during lumbar sympathetic block. Hematuria can follow direct needle placement through the kidney and is usually self-limited.

Nerve root, epidural, or intrathecal injection can arise when the needle is advanced through the intervertebral foramen and is usually avoided entirely with proper use of radiographic guidance. Following neurolytic lumbar sympathetic block, significant postsympathectomy pain arises in the L1 and L2 nerve root distribution over the anterior thigh in as many as 10% of treated patients. This observation stems from the results following open surgical sympathectomy, but such postsympathectomy neuralgia has also been reported after both chemical and radiofrequency sympathectomy. Postsympathectomy neuralgic pain in the anterior thigh has been postulated to result from partial neurolysis of adjacent sensory fibers, most often the genitofemoral nerve.

## Spinal Cord Stimulation

Based on the theory that nonnoxious sensory input interferes with the perception of pain, direct activation of the ascending fibers within the dorsal columns of the spinal cord that transmit nonpainful stimuli is used to treat chronic back pain. Modern systems make use of pacemaker-like, implanted pulse generators connected to a small electrode array positioned within the dorsal epidural space of the spinal column. These systems are implanted in a simple, brief surgical procedure. Spinal cord stimulation (SCS) is safe and effective in management of CRPS, unilateral radicular pain, and failed back surgery syndrome. Typically, patients undergo an initial externalized lead trial lasting approximately 1 week. Those with successful trials can receive surgical implantation of the spinal cord stimulator. This can be done with a percutaneous approach or with surgical paddle lead placement.[34] Pain scores and analgesic use are decreased in cancer pain patients implanted with spinal cord stimulators.[35] Adverse effects are declining and complications are less frequent with the advent of newer devices and improved surgical techniques. Common complications and their frequency are as follows: cerebrospinal fluid leakage (0.3% to 7%), pain or discomfort over the implanted pulse generator site (1% to 12%), and subcutaneous hematoma or seroma (0% to 9%).[36]

## Intrathecal Drug Delivery

Evidence that direct application of morphine to the spinal cord produces spinally mediated analgesia first appeared in the mid-1970s. The advent of small, programmable pumps that can be implanted in the abdominal wall, and deliver precise, continuous drug infusions into the thecal space via a catheter, has allowed application of this technology to patients with chronic noncancer-related pain. Intrathecal drug delivery is usually reserved for patients

with either severe pain that does not respond to conservative management or oral analgesic dose escalations over many years to the point that intolerable side effects or ineffective pain control obviate oral therapy.[37] A comparison of maximal medical therapy (oral or parenteral opioids) with intrathecal drug delivery for cancer-related pain showed similar improvement in analgesia and reduction in opioid-related side effects (less somnolence and fatigue) in those who received intrathecal therapy. Morphine is currently the only opioid that is approved for intrathecal use by the Food and Drug Administration, but other drugs singly and in combination are also used. Ziconotide delivered intrathecally provides significant analgesia in patients with severe chronic pain, but side effects are common, the most common being CNS side effects. Intrathecal drug delivery in noncancer-related pain has not been subject to controlled trials and remains controversial, but numerous observational studies suggest it provides significant pain reduction in some patients whose chronic low back pain fails to respond to more conservative management.

## SUMMARY

A brief overview of the most common chronic pain problems and treatments used in the modern practice of pain medicine is presented. Our understanding of chronic pain as a discrete disease of the nervous system continues to evolve, as does our understanding of the link between acute and chronic pain. The anesthesia provider is well poised in the perioperative arena to help with gaining a better understanding of how new approaches to the treatment of acute pain following surgery can be used to effectively reduce the incidence and severity of chronic pain and to provide precise delivery of new therapeutics to the neuraxis.

## QUESTIONS OF THE DAY

1. What is the typical clinical course of a patient with acute lower back pain? What are the risk factors for chronic low back pain?
2. What are the clinical characteristics of neuropathic pain? What are the most common presentations of diabetic peripheral neuropathy (DPN) and postherpetic neuralgia (PHN)?
3. What are the diagnostic criteria for complex regional pain syndrome (CRPS)? What are the most important aspects of CRPS management?
4. For a patient with cancer-related pain, what is the approach to providing analgesia?
5. What is the efficacy of opioid therapy for the following types of pain: acute postoperative pain, moderate to severe cancer pain, chronic noncancer pain?

6. What is the magnitude of the opioid epidemic in the United States? What approaches can be used to prevent opioid abuse for patients undergoing chronic opioid therapy?

7. What are the anatomic landmarks relevant to performance of stellate ganglion block via the anterior paratracheal approach?

## REFERENCES

1. International Association for the Study of Pain Task Force on Taxonomy. In: Merskey NB, ed. *Classification of Chronic Pain*. 2nd ed. Seattle: IASP Press; 1994:209–214.
2. Blackwell DL, Lucas JW, Clarke TC. Summary health statistics for U.S. adults: National Health Interview Survey, 2012. National Center for Health Statistics. *Vital Health Stat*. 2014;10(260):1–171.
3. Andersson GB. Epidemiological features of chronic low-back pain. *Lancet*. 1999;354(9178):581–585.
4. Rubin DI. Epidemiology and risk factors for spine pain. *Neurol Clin*. 2007; 25(2):353–371.
5. Koes BW, van Tulder MW, Thomas S. Diagnosis and treatment of low back pain. *Br Med J*. 2006;332(7555):1430–1434.
6. Saal JA, Saal JS. Nonoperative treatment of herniated lumbar intervertebral disc with radiculopathy. An outcome study. *Spine (Phila PA 1976)*. 1989;14(4): 431–437.
7. Cohen SP, Bicket MC, Jamison D, et al. Epidural steroids: a comprehensive, evidence-based review. *Reg Anesth Pain Med*. 2013;38(3):175–200.
8. Lurie JD, Tosteson TD, Tosteson AN, et al. Surgical versus nonoperative treatment for lumbar disc herniation: eight-year results for the spine patient outcomes research trial. *Spine (Phila PA 1976)*. 2014;39(1):3–16.
9. Yildirim K, Deniz O, Gureser G, et al. Gabapentin monotherapy in patients with chronic radiculopathy: the efficacy and impact on life quality. *J Back Musculoskelet Rehabil*. 2009;22(1):17–20.
10. Deyo RA, Weinstein JN. Low back pain. *N Engl J Med*. 2001;344(5):363–370.
11. Jarvik JG, Deyo RA. Diagnostic evaluation of low back pain with emphasis on imaging. *Ann Intern Med*. 2002;137(7): 586–597.
12. Bogduk N, McGuirk B. Causes and sources of chronic low back pain. In: Bogduk N, McGuirk B, eds. *Medical Management of Acute and Chronic Low Back Pain. An Evidence Based Approach: Pain Research and Clinical Management*. Amsterdam: Elsevier Science; 2002:115–126.
13. Stidd DA, Rivero S, Weinand ME. Spinal cord stimulation with implanted epidural paddle lead relieves chronic axial low back pain. *J Pain Res*. 2014;7:465–470.
14. Javed S, Petropoulos IN, Alam U, Malik RA. Treatment of painful diabetic neuropathy. *Ther Adv Chronic Dis*. 2015;6(1):15–28.
15. Birklein F, O'Neill D, Schlereth T. Complex regional pain syndrome: an optimistic perspective. *Neurology*. 2015;84(1):89–96.
16. Cossins L, Okell RW, Cameron H, et al. Treatment of complex regional pain syndrome in adults: a systematic review of randomized controlled trials published from June 2000 to February 2012. *Eur J Pain*. 2013;17(2):158–173.
17. Giamberardino MA, Affaitati G, Fabrizio A, Costantini R. Effects of treatment of myofascial trigger points on the pain of fibromyalgia. *Curr Pain Headache Rep*. 2011;15(5):393–399.
18. Wolfe F, Clauw DJ, Fitzcharles MA, et al. The American College of Rheumatology preliminary diagnostic criteria for fibromyalgia and measurement of symptom severity. *Arthritis Care Res (Hoboken)*. 2010;62(5):600–610.
19. Fitzcharles MA, Ste-Marie PA, Shir Y, Lussier D. Management of fibromyalgia in older adults. *Drugs Aging*. 2014;31(10):711–719.
20. Vardy J, Agar M. Nonopioid drugs in the treatment of cancer pain. *J Clin Oncol*. 2014;32(16):1677–1690.
21. Auret K, Schug SA. Pain management for the cancer patient—current practice and future developments. *Best Pract Res Clin Anaesthesiol*. 2013;27(4):545–561.
22. Machado LA, Kamper SJ, Herbert RD, et al. Analgesic effects of treatments for non-specific low back pain: a meta-analysis of placebo-controlled randomized trials. *Rheumatology (Oxford)*. 2009;48(5):520–527.
23. Machado GC, Maher CG, Ferreira PH, et al. Efficacy and safety of paracetamol for spinal pain and osteoarthritis: systematic review and meta-analysis of randomised placebo controlled trials. *BMJ*. 2015;350:h1225.
24. Finnerup NB, Attal N, Haroutounian S, et al. Pharmacotherapy for neuropathic pain in adults: a systematic review and meta-analysis. *Lancet Neurol*. 2015;14(2):162–173.
25. Derry S, Gill D, Phillips T, Moore RA. Milnacipran for neuropathic pain and fibromyalgia in adults. *Cochrane Database Syst Rev*. 2012;(3):CD008244.
26. Jamison RN, Mao J. Opioid analgesics. *Mayo Clin Proc*. 2015;90(7):957–968.
27. Cheung CW, Qiu Q, Choi SW, et al. Chronic opioid therapy for chronic non-cancer pain: a review and comparison of treatment guidelines. *Pain Physician*. 2014;17(5):401–414.
28. Reinecke H, Weber C, Lange K, et al. Analgesic efficacy of opioids in chronic pain: recent meta-analyses. *Br J Pharmacol*. 2015;172(2):324–333.
29. Gaskin DJ, Richard P. The economic costs of pain in the United States. *J Pain*. 2012;13(8):715–724.
30. Franklin GM. Opioids for chronic noncancer pain: a position paper of the American Academy of Neurology. *Neurology*. 2014;83(14):1277–1284.
31. Manchikanti L, Helm S 2nd, Fellows B, et al. Opioid epidemic in the United States. *Pain Physician*. 2012;15(suppl 3):ES9–ES38.
32. *Epidemic: responding to America's prescription drug abuse crisis*. Washington, DC: Office of National Drug Control Policy; 2011.
33. Berna C, Kulich RJ, Rathmell JP. Tapering long-term opioid therapy in chronic noncancer pain: evidence and recommendations for everyday practice. *Mayo Clin Proc*. 2015;90(6): 828–842.
34. Walsh KM, Machado AG, Krishnaney AA. Spinal cord stimulation: a review of the safety literature and proposal for perioperative evaluation and management. *Spine J*. 2015;15(8):1864–1869.
35. Lihua P, Su M, Zejun Z, et al. Spinal cord stimulation for cancer-related pain in adults. *Cochrane Database Syst Rev*. 2013;(2):CD009389.
36. Bendersky D, Yampolsky C. Is spinal cord stimulation safe? A review of its complications. *World Neurosurg*. 2014;82(6):1359–1368.
37. Wilkes D. Programmable intrathecal pumps for the management of chronic pain: recommendations for improved efficiency. *J Pain Res*. 2014;7: 571–577.

VI

# 45 CARDIOPULMONARY RESUSCITATION

## Krishna Parekh and David Shimabukuro

Cardiopulmonary resuscitation (CPR) was initially defined nearly 50 years ago, as the administration of mouth-to-mouth ventilation and closed chest cardiac compressions in a pulseless patient. Since that time, significant advances in CPR and cardiovascular life support have been made. Today, the early descriptions of CPR are termed *basic life support* (BLS), whereas adult advanced cardiovascular life support (ACLS) and pediatric advanced cardiovascular life support (PALS) include additional invasive techniques by experienced practitioners.

Out-of-hospital resuscitation is well described, whereas in-hospital resuscitation and life support are less commonly studied. A retrospective analysis of in-hospital CPR found that between 2000 and 2009, 1 in 393 hospitalized patients received CPR, and 23% survived to discharge.[1] Cardiac arrest in the perioperative period is unique in that it can frequently be anticipated, and health care providers and resources are immediately available.

The American Heart Association (AHA), in conjunction with the International Liaison Committee on Resuscitation (ILCOR), published updated guidelines for the administration of CPR and emergency cardiovascular care (ECC) in 2015. These guidelines, revised from the 2010 version, include added emphasis on systems of care in the prehospital, in-hospital, and postresuscitation settings, and on the continued education of CPR techniques to providers. Furthermore, instead of periodic overall updates, new evidence will now be continually evaluated and revised guidelines will be available online.[2,3]

## BASIC LIFE SUPPORT

BLS includes a number of key measures, including recognition of unresponsiveness and cardiac arrest, activation

The editors and publisher would like to thank Dr. Linda Liu for contributing to this chapter in the previous edition of this work. It has served as the foundation for the current chapter.

of an emergency response system, early administration of CPR, and early defibrillation if indicated. In the hospital setting, a health care provider will perform the following sequence of steps, as described by the AHA algorithm: (1) ensure safety; (2) check for response; (3) activate resuscitation team; (4) simultaneously check for adequate breathing and pulse; (5) retrieve automated external defibrillator (AED) and emergency equipment; (6) begin CPR and defibrillate when defibrillator becomes available; and (7) provide two-person CPR as help arrives[4] (Fig. 45.1).

## Recognition

The recognition and management of cardiac arrest in an unresponsive patient differ between laypersons and health care providers. The AHA guidelines recognize this

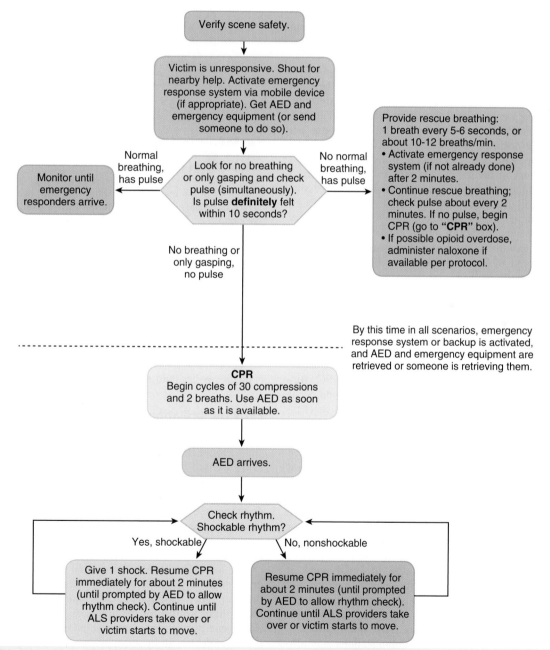

**Fig. 45.1** BLS Healthcare Provider Adult Cardiac Arrest Algorithm—2015 Update. *AED,* Automated external defibrillator; *ALS,* advanced life support; *BLS,* basic life support; *CPR,* cardiopulmonary resuscitation. (©2015 American Heart Association.)

distinction and include increased flexibility in emergency response activation either before or after breathing and pulse assessment for health care providers. The 2015 guidelines also include a larger role for dispatcher-guided CPR for laypersons in treating out-of-hospital cardiac arrest.

Health care providers should check for a pulse while simultaneously evaluating for adequate ventilation. The pulse should be assessed at either the carotid or femoral artery. The elapsed time for the pulse check should not exceed 10 seconds, in order to minimize time to start chest compressions. When monitoring respiration, occasional gasps should not be mistaken for normal breathing.

## Early Cardiopulmonary Resuscitation

When initiating chest compressions, the heel of the hand is placed longitudinally on the lower half of the sternum, between the nipples. The sternum is depressed at least 5 cm (2 inches) at a rate of at least 100 compressions per minute but no faster than 120 compressions per minute. Rates more rapid than 120 compressions per minute lead to a decrease in the depth of compressions.[5] A depth of no more than 6 cm is also recommended, as excessive compression depth has been associated with an increased rate of thoracic injury. Complete chest recoil is necessary to allow for venous return and is important for effective CPR. The pattern is 30 compressions to 2 breaths (30:2 equals 1 cycle of CPR), regardless of whether one or two rescuers are present.

Since 2010, the importance of definitive airway management has taken a secondary role to chest compressions. The old mnemonic ABCD (airway, breathing, circulation, and defibrillation) has given way to CAB (compression, airway, breathing). This is because the early initiation of high-quality chest compressions improves the likelihood of a return of spontaneous circulation (ROSC). Airway maneuvers are still attempted, but they should occur quickly, efficiently, and minimize interruptions in chest compressions. Opening the airway can be achieved by a simple head tilt–chin lift technique (Fig. 45.2). A jaw thrust maneuver can be used in patients with suspected cervical spine injury. Simple airway devices, such as nasal or oral airways, can be inserted to displace the tongue from the posterior oropharynx.

Although several large out-of-hospital studies have demonstrated that chest compression-alone CPR is not inferior to traditional compression-ventilation CPR, health care providers are still expected to provide assisted ventilation.[6,7] Care should be taken to avoid rapid or forceful breaths. Concern exists for reducing preload and cardiac output with excessive positive-pressure ventilation.[8] Establishing an advanced airway during in-hospital cardiac arrest (IHCA) results in fewer interruptions to chest compressions during CPR.[9] Complications may also occur from gastric insufflation and subsequent aspiration of gastric contents. Maximum oxygen concentration

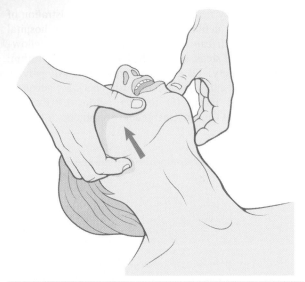

**Fig. 45.2** The head tilt–jaw thrust maneuver provides a patent upper airway by tensing the muscles attached to the tongue, thus pulling the tongue away from the posterior pharynx. Forward displacement of the mandible is accomplished by grasping the angles of the mandible and lifting with both hands, which serves to displace the mandible forward while tilting the head backward.

is administered in order to provide optimally saturated arterial hemoglobin concentrations. Delivered tidal volumes of approximately 400 to 600 mL are given over 1 second and should produce visible chest rise. Once an advanced airway has been established, a respiratory rate of 10 breaths/min is the goal because hyperventilation is detrimental for neurologic recovery. The decreased minute ventilation is also appropriate because cardiac output is much smaller than normal during resuscitation.

## Early Defibrillation

A defibrillator is attached to the patient as soon as possible. Proper electrode pad placement on the chest wall is to the right of the upper sternal border below the clavicle and to the left of the nipple with the center in the midaxillary line (Fig. 45.3). Most electrode pads now come with diagrams showing their correct positioning. Alternative locations include anterior-posterior, anterior–left infrascapular, and anterior–right infrascapular. Right anterior axillary to left anterior axillary is not recommended.

The amount of energy (joules [J]) delivered is dependent on the type of defibrillator used. Two major defibrillator types (monophasic and biphasic) are available. Monophasic waveform defibrillators deliver a unidirectional energy charge, whereas biphasic waveform defibrillators deliver an in-series bidirectional energy charge. Based on evidence from implantable defibrillators, bidirectional energy delivery is probably more successful in in cardiac arrest. However, there may be some benefit in carefully selected patients who suffer from witnessed in-hospital arrest secondary to reversible causes.

## ADULT ADVANCED CARDIAC LIFE SUPPORT

Adult ACLS includes several interventions besides BLS in order to manage cardiac arrest. These interventions can include airway manipulation, medication administration, arrhythmia management, and transition to postresuscitation care. However, the key element of ACLS remains high-quality CPR, which includes correctly performed chest compressions, minimal compression interruption, and early cardiac defibrillation. The additional components of ACLS and specific arrhythmia management will be discussed later. As there were no updates to the bradycardia and tachycardia algorithms from 2010, they will not be reviewed in detail. Figs. 45.4 and 45.5 summarize the management of the patient with bradycardia or tachycardia with a pulse. All algorithms are readily available online.[3]

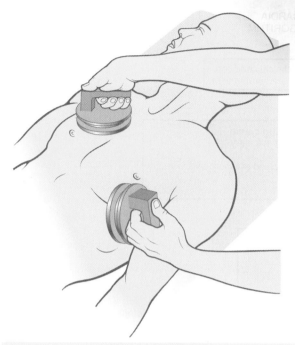

**Fig. 45.3** Schematic depiction of the proper placement of paddle electrodes in an adult.

terminating ventricular tachycardia (VT) and ventricular fibrillation (VF). In addition, biphasic waveform shocks require less energy than traditional monophasic waveform shocks (120 to 200 J vs. 360 J, respectively) and may therefore cause less myocardial damage.

The time until defibrillation is critical to survival, especially because the most frequent initial cardiac rhythm in adult patients is VT/VF. Defibrillation should occur as soon as possible when recognizing a VT/VF arrest. CPR should be initiated while emergency equipment is being retrieved. In one study of IHCAs, 30% of patients received delayed defibrillation. Patients receiving delayed defibrillation have slower rates of ROSC and survival to hospital discharge. Furthermore, each additional minute of delay was associated with worse outcomes.[10] Chest compressions should be resumed immediately following defibrillation.

### Ancillary Devices and Alternative Techniques

The 2015 AHA guidelines reviewed the evidence for ancillary devices used during CPR and found insufficient support to recommend any of the following: impedance threshold device, active compression-decompression CPR with impedance threshold device, mechanical piston device for chest compressions, and load distributing band devices.

There was also insufficient evidence to recommend the routine use of extracorporeal CPR (venoarterial extracorporeal membrane oxygenation [ECMO]) for patients

### Monitoring Cardiopulmonary Resuscitation

A number of physiologic variables can be used to monitor CPR. Continuous monitoring of end-tidal carbon dioxide ($P_{ETCO_2}$) with waveform capnography can be beneficial during resuscitation. In addition to confirmation of advanced airway placement, $P_{ETCO_2}$ can guide the rescuers in adequacy of chest compressions.[11] Alternative physiologic measures during CPR include arterial relaxation diastolic pressure, arterial pressure monitoring, and central venous oxygen saturation. Specific target values during resuscitation are still being evaluated.[12] Furthermore, a prolonged reduction in $P_{ETCO_2}$ should not be used in isolation for prognostication, and it should certainly not be used in patients without an endotracheal tube. Bedside cardiac ultrasound can also be considered when managing cardiac arrest, but its use is not routinely recommended. If it is utilized, an experienced sonographer should perform the ultrasound and interruptions in chest compressions should be minimized.

### Airway Management

The 2015 AHA guidelines, consistent with the ILCOR review, recommend either a bag-mask or advanced airway device (endotracheal tube or supraglottic airway) for providing oxygenation and ventilation during CPR.[13] The choice of technique depends on the skill of the provider. Because chest compressions are often not performed during endotracheal intubation, the rescuer should compare the need for compressions against the need for definitive airway management Chest compressions are not interrupted for longer than 10 seconds during airway management and are resumed immediately following

**VI**

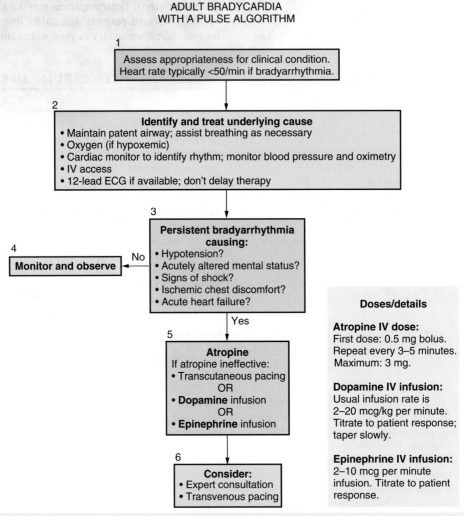

ADULT BRADYCARDIA
WITH A PULSE ALGORITHM

1
Assess appropriateness for clinical condition.
Heart rate typically <50/min if bradyarrhythmia.

2
**Identify and treat underlying cause**
• Maintain patent airway; assist breathing as necessary
• Oxygen (if hypoxemic)
• Cardiac monitor to identify rhythm; monitor blood pressure and oximetry
• IV access
• 12-lead ECG if available; don't delay therapy

3
**Persistent bradyarrhythmia causing:**
• Hypotension?
• Acutely altered mental status?
• Signs of shock?
• Ischemic chest discomfort?
• Acute heart failure?

4
**Monitor and observe** ← No

Yes

5
**Atropine**
If atropine ineffective:
• Transcutaneous pacing
OR
• **Dopamine** infusion
OR
• **Epinephrine** infusion

6
**Consider:**
• Expert consultation
• Transvenous pacing

**Doses/details**

**Atropine IV dose:**
First dose: 0.5 mg bolus.
Repeat every 3–5 minutes.
Maximum: 3 mg.

**Dopamine IV infusion:**
Usual infusion rate is
2–20 mcg/kg per minute.
Titrate to patient response;
taper slowly.

**Epinephrine IV infusion:**
2–10 mcg per minute
infusion. Titrate to patient
response.

**Fig. 45.4** Resuscitation algorithm for bradycardia with a pulse. *ECG*, Electrocardiogram; *IV*, intravenous. (From American Heart Association. Web-based Integrated Guidelines for Cardiopulmonary Resuscitation and Emergency Cardiovascular Care – Part 7: Adult Advanced Cardiovascular Life Support. ECCguidelines.heart.org © Copyright 2015 American Heart Association, Inc.)

endotracheal intubation. If the intubation attempt is unsuccessful, placement of a laryngeal mask airway can be considered (also see Chapter 16). Insertion of an advanced airway can be deferred until after the patient fails to respond to several cycles of CPR and defibrillation. However, the clinical course of the arrest should be considered. For example, a patient with severe pulmonary edema may benefit from endotracheal intubation sooner rather than later. There are no formal recommendations for the timing of advanced airway placement.

Continuous waveform capnography is recommended as the measurement of choice for the assessment of advanced airway placement. Clinical evaluation should also occur, which includes auscultation of bilateral breath sounds and visualization of bilateral chest rise. If capnography is not available, alternative methods include esophageal detector device, nonwaveform capnogram,

and ultrasound. Once the endotracheal tube is confirmed to be in the trachea, it is secured in place. One breath is delivered every 6 seconds (10 breaths/min) without synchronization with compressions.

## Algorithms

### Pulseless Arrest

Cardiac dysrhythmias that produce pulseless cardiac arrest are (1) VF, (2) VT, (3) pulseless electrical activity (PEA), and (4) asystole (Fig. 45.6). During pulseless cardiac arrest, the primary goals are to provide effective chest compressions and early defibrillation if the rhythm is VF or VT. Drug administration is of secondary importance because the efficacy of pharmacologic interventions has been difficult to measure or prove. After initiating CPR and defibrillation, rescuers can then establish intravenous

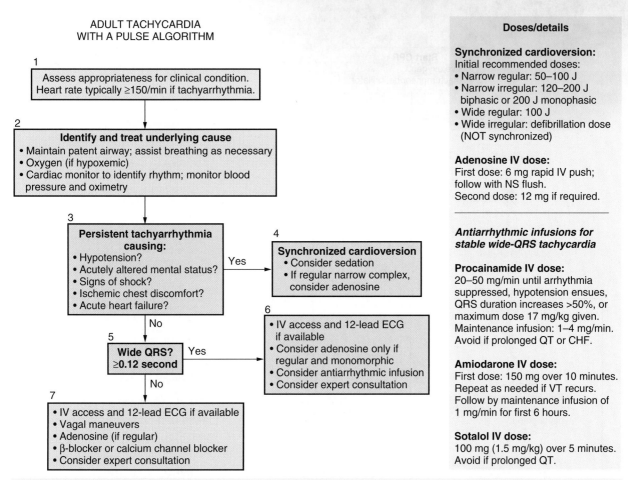

ADULT TACHYCARDIA
WITH A PULSE ALGORITHM

**1**
Assess appropriateness for clinical condition.
Heart rate typically ≥150/min if tachyarrhythmia.

**2**
**Identify and treat underlying cause**
• Maintain patent airway; assist breathing as necessary
• Oxygen (if hypoxemic)
• Cardiac monitor to identify rhythm; monitor blood pressure and oximetry

**3**
**Persistent tachyarrhythmia causing:**
• Hypotension?
• Acutely altered mental status?
• Signs of shock?
• Ischemic chest discomfort?
• Acute heart failure?

Yes →

**4**
**Synchronized cardioversion**
• Consider sedation
• If regular narrow complex, consider adenosine

No ↓

**5**
**Wide QRS?**
**≥0.12 second**

Yes →

**6**
• IV access and 12-lead ECG if available
• Consider adenosine only if regular and monomorphic
• Consider antiarrhythmic infusion
• Consider expert consultation

No ↓

**7**
• IV access and 12-lead ECG if available
• Vagal maneuvers
• Adenosine (if regular)
• β-blocker or calcium channel blocker
• Consider expert consultation

**Doses/details**

**Synchronized cardioversion:**
Initial recommended doses:
• Narrow regular: 50–100 J
• Narrow irregular: 120–200 J biphasic or 200 J monophasic
• Wide regular: 100 J
• Wide irregular: defibrillation dose (NOT synchronized)

**Adenosine IV dose:**
First dose: 6 mg rapid IV push; follow with NS flush.
Second dose: 12 mg if required.

*Antiarrhythmic infusions for stable wide-QRS tachycardia*

**Procainamide IV dose:**
20–50 mg/min until arrhythmia suppressed, hypotension ensues, QRS duration increases >50%, or maximum dose 17 mg/kg given. Maintenance infusion: 1–4 mg/min. Avoid if prolonged QT or CHF.

**Amiodarone IV dose:**
First dose: 150 mg over 10 minutes. Repeat as needed if VT recurs. Follow by maintenance infusion of 1 mg/min for first 6 hours.

**Sotalol IV dose:**
100 mg (1.5 mg/kg) over 5 minutes. Avoid if prolonged QT.

**Fig. 45.5** Resuscitation algorithm for tachycardia with a pulse. *CHF*, Congestive heart failure; *ECG*, electrocardiogram; *IV*, intravenous; J, joule; *NS*, normal saline; *VT*, ventricular tachycardia. (From American Heart Association. Web-based Integrated Guidelines for Cardiopulmonary Resuscitation and Emergency Cardiovascular Care – Part 7: Adult Advanced Cardiovascular Life Support. ECCguidelines.heart.org © Copyright 2015 American Heart Association, Inc.)

access, obtain a more definitive airway, and consider drug therapy, all while providing continued chest compressions and ventilation.

### Ventricular Fibrillation/Ventricular Tachycardia

If the cardiac arrest is witnessed, the health care provider immediately places the defibrillator pads on the patient's chest, determines the rhythm, and delivers a shock if VF or VT is present (see Fig. 45.6). CPR is resumed immediately after delivery of the shock and continued for five cycles or about 2 minutes, followed by reevaluation of the cardiac rhythm. If the patient remains in VF/VT, the defibrillator is charged to the appropriate energy level while CPR is still being performed, as determined by the manufacturer's instructions. A biphasic defibrillator is preferred over monophasic, and a single shock is preferred over sequential (also called *stacked*) shocks.

If VF or VT persists after one to two sets of CPR-defibrillation cycles, a vasopressor is given (Table 45.1). Epinephrine, 1 mg intravenously (IV), may be administered every 3 to 5 minutes. Drug administration is timed to minimize interruptions in chest compressions. If the patient remains in VT/VF, amiodarone, an antiarrhythmic, can improve the likelihood of restoring and maintaining ROSC. The role of antiarrhythmics in improving survival following VF/VT arrest is not clear. A currently ongoing trial, ROC-ALPS seeks to provide information regarding the use of lidocaine, amiodarone, and placebo in managing arrhythmia during cardiac arrest.[14] Magnesium sulfate can be considered if torsades de pointes is suspected.

### Asystole/Pulseless Electrical Activity

Asystole is the absence of any ventricular electrical activity and is usually a moribund rhythm, whereas PEA is

VI

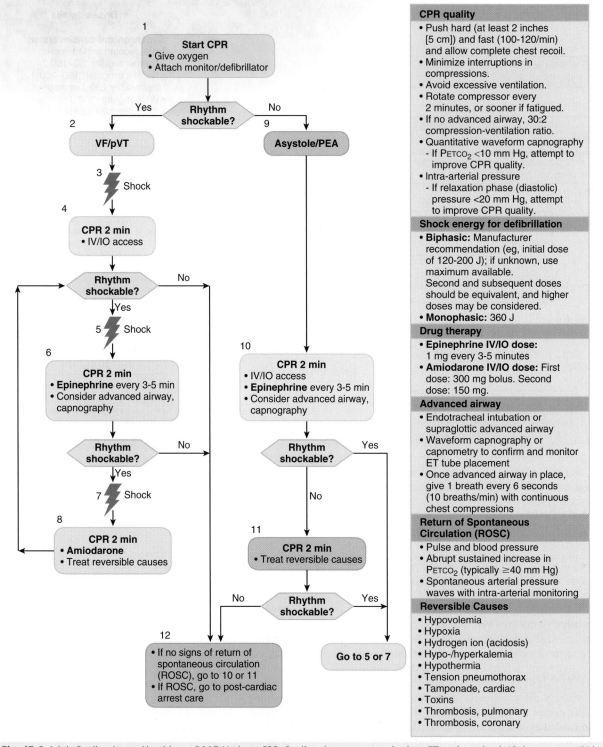

**Fig. 45.6** Adult Cardiac Arrest Algorithm – 2015 Update. *CPR,* Cardiopulmonary resuscitation; *ET,* endotracheal; *IO,* intraosseus; *IV,* intravenous; *PEA,* pulseless electrical activity; *P*ETCO$_2$, partial pressure of end-tidal carbon dioxide; *pVT,* pulseless ventricular tachycardia; *VF,* ventricular fibrillation. (From Link MS, Berkow LC, Kudenchuk PJ, Halperin HR, Hess EP, Moitra VK, Neumar RW, O'Neil BJ, Paxton JH, Silvers SM, White RD, Yannopoulos D, Donnino MW. Part 7: adult advanced cardiovascular life support: 2015 American Heart Association Guidelines Update for Cardiopulmonary Resuscitation and Emergency Cardiovascular Care. *Circulation.* 2015;132(suppl 2):S444–S464. © Copyright 2015 American Heart Association, Inc.)

| Table 45.1 | Drugs Used During Adult Cardiopulmonary Resuscitation | |
|---|---|---|
| **Drug Name** | **Dose** | **Indication** |
| Adenosine | 6 mg IV/IO<br>May repeat 12 mg IV/IO<br>(cut dose in half if using central line) | For stable narrow QRS tachycardia or monomorphic VT (contraindicated with preexcitation syndrome) |
| Amiodarone | 300 mg IV/IO<br>May repeat 150 mg IV/IO<br>150 mg IV/IO over a 10-min period<br>Maintenance infusion of 1 mg/min for 6 h, then 0.5 mg/min<br>Maximum total dose of 2.2 g/24 h | For pulseless VT/VF<br>For stable VT or uncertain wide QRS tachycardia and narrow QRS tachycardias |
| Atropine[a] | 0.5 mg IV/IO<br>May repeat to total dose of 3 mg | For bradycardia |
| Diltiazem | 15 to 20 mg (0.25 mg/kg) IV/IO over a 2-min period<br>May repeat in 15 min at 20-25 mg/kg (0.35 mg/kg)<br>Maintenance infusion of 5-15 mg/h, titrate to heart rate | For stable narrow QRS tachycardia (contraindicated with preexcitation syndrome) |
| Dopamine | 2 to 10 µg/kg/min by infusion | For bradycardia instead of a pacer, while awaiting a pacer, or if a pacer is ineffective or not tolerated |
| Epinephrine[a] | 1 mg IV/IO<br>Repeat every 3 to 5 min<br>2 to 10 µg/min by infusion | For pulseless cardiac arrest<br>For bradycardia instead of a pacer, while awaiting a pacer, or if a pacer is ineffective or not tolerated |
| Esmolol | 0.5 mg/kg IV/IO load, followed by an infusion at 0.05 mg/kg/min<br>May repeat the 0.5-mg/kg bolus and increase the infusion to 0.1 mg/kg/min<br>Maximum infusion of 0.3 mg/kg/min | For stable narrow QRS tachycardias (contraindicated with preexcitation syndrome) |
| Lidocaine[a] | 1 to 1.5 mg/kg IV/IO<br>May repeat 0.5 mg to 0.75 mg/kg<br>Maximum total of three doses or 3 mg/kg | For pulseless VT/VF when amiodarone is NOT available |
| Magnesium | 1 to 2 g IV/IO | For torsades de pointes |
| Metoprolol | 5 mg IV/IO<br>May repeat every 5 min<br>Maximum total dose of 15 mg | For stable narrow QRS tachycardias (contraindicated with preexcitation syndrome) |
| Procainamide | 20 to 50 mg/min IV/IO (max 17 mg/kg) until arrhythmia suppressed<br>Maintenance infusion of 1 to 4 mg/min | For stable wide QRS tachycardia |
| Sotalol | 100 mg (1.5 mg/kg) IV/IO over 5 min | For stable wide QRS tachycardia |
| Verapamil | 2.5 to 5 mg IV/IO over a 2-min period<br>May repeat 5 to 10 mg over a 15- to 30-min period<br>Maximum total dose of 20 mg | For stable narrow QRS tachycardia (contraindicated with preexcitation syndrome) |

[a]Also effectively delivered by tracheal mucosal absorption when administered through an endotracheal tube.

*IO*, Intraosseus; *IV*, intravenous; *VF*, ventricular fibrillation; *VT*, ventricular tachycardia.

often caused by a reversible condition and can be treated if the inciting cause is identified (Table 45.2). These two cardiac rhythms have been combined as the second part of the pulseless arrest algorithm because of similarities in their management (see Fig. 45.6). Neither will benefit from defibrillation; effective CPR with minimal interruptions, identifying and treating reversible causes, and establishing an advanced airway are the primary interventions. A bedside cardiac ultrasound may provide valuable information regarding the cause of arrest. Additionally, the absence of ventricular wall motion on ultrasound predicts an unlikely ROSC.[15] A vasopressor may be administered after initiation of CPR. Epinephrine, 1 mg IV, is given every 3 to 5 minutes. Cardiac rhythm checks

VI

| Table 45.2 | Major Causes of Cardiovascular Collapse in the Perioperative Period |
|---|---|
| **8 Hs** | **8 Ts** |
| **H**ypovolemia | **T**oxins (anaphylaxis/anesthesia) |
| **H**ypoxia | **T**amponade |
| **H**ydrogen ion (acidosis) | **T**ension pneumothorax |
| **H**yperkalemia/hypokalemia | **T**hrombosis in coronary artery |
| **H**ypoglycemia | **T**hrombus in pulmonary artery |
| **H**ypothermia | **T**rauma |
| Malignant **h**yperthermia | Q**T** interval prolongation |
| **H**ypervagal response | Pulmonary hyper**t**ension |

Modified from the 5 Hs and 5 Ts proposed by the American Heart Association (AHA).

are performed after every five cycles or 2 minutes of CPR. The administration of high-quality chest compressions can be monitored by $P_{ETCO_2}$, coronary perfusion pressure, or central venous saturation ($S_{CVO_2}$), if available. If an organized cardiac rhythm is present, the rescuer checks for a pulse. If there is no pulse, CPR should be continued. If a pulse is present, the rescuer identifies the rhythm and treats accordingly.

## Medications

Establishing intravenous access is important, but it should not interfere with CPR and defibrillation. A single, large peripheral intravenous or intraosseus catheter is sufficient for resuscitating most pulseless patients. Drugs are administered rapidly and followed with a 20-mL fluid bolus if given peripherally. If intravenous/intraosseus access cannot be obtained, or is lost, certain drugs (epinephrine, lidocaine, atropine, naloxone) can be given via the endotracheal tube. The endotracheal tube dose is 2 to 10 times the recommended intravenous dose, and the drug is diluted in 5 to 10 mL of sterile water before instillation down the endotracheal tube.

Epinephrine and amiodarone are among the most commonly used drugs in the ACLS algorithms (see Table 45.1) and deserve special attention. Epinephrine is a combined direct α- and β-adrenergic receptor agonist. In multiple animal studies, administration of epinephrine was beneficial in establishing ROSC. Epinephrine can increase diastolic blood pressure and thereby restore coronary perfusion pressure and blood flow back to the myocardium. However, epinephrine also increases myocardial oxygen consumption by increasing heart rate and afterload.

Amiodarone was initially developed as an antianginal drug in the 1950s but was abandoned because of its side effects. Because it has effects on cardiac sodium and potassium channels, as well as α- and β-receptors, amiodarone has been reinvestigated for its antiarrhythmic effects. In this regard, amiodarone prolongs repolarization and refractoriness in the sinoatrial node, the atrial and ventricular myocardium, the atrioventricular (AV) node, and the His-Purkinje cardiac conduction system. Amiodarone can exacerbate or induce arrhythmias especially torsades de pointes. This drug may interact with volatile anesthetics to produce heart block, profound vasodilation, myocardial depression, and severe hypotension. Amidarone has many drug interactions and can prolong the effects of oral anticoagulants, phenytoin, digoxin, and diltiazem. Despite its multiple disadvantages, administration of amiodarone improves survival to hospital admission in adults with out-of-hospital VF/VT arrest when compared with placebo and lidocaine.[8,9] The recommended dose of amiodarone for VF/VT is 300 mg IV. An additional bolus dose of 150 mg IV may be given for persistent VF/VT.

Vasopressin, a nonadrenergic vasopressor, was removed from the 2015 ACLS guidelines because of a lack of demonstrated benefit when compared to epinephrine.[16] Drugs used for ACLS are associated with ROSC but not with improved survival to hospital discharge or neurologic recovery. There are no specific recommendations for timing of ACLS drug delivery, though for a nonshockable rhythm, epinephrine may be given as soon as possible. Administration of steroids along with vasoactive drugs may improve the likelihood of survival and favorable neurologic outcome for IHCAs; however, there is no recommendation for their routine use.[17] Finally, in patients with the potential for cardiac arrest secondary to opioid overdose, administration of naloxone should be considered (see Chapter 9).

## PEDIATRIC ADVANCED CARDIOVASCULAR LIFE SUPPORT

Cardiorespiratory resuscitation of infants and children follows the same basic principles as those for adults (also see Chapter 34). Most pediatric cardiac events are a result of arterial hypoxemia and respiratory compromise, and, thus, airway management and breathing are critical to successful pediatric resuscitation. In contrast, adults tend to experience cardiac arrest as a result of VT or VF secondary to myocardial ischemia. Regardless, pediatric BLS follows the same algorithm as for adults: CAB. Naturally, there are several specific differences between adult and pediatric patients. Infants are younger than 1 year in age, whereas children are between the age of 1 year and adolescence. Adult BLS resuscitation guidelines can be used for adolescent children (Table 45.3). The elements of high-quality CPR in pediatrics remain unchanged from adults and include: (1) adequate chest compression

| | **Recommendations** | | |
|---|---|---|---|
| **Component** | **Adults** | **Children** | **Infants** |
| Recognition | Unresponsive (for all ages) | | |
| | No breathing or no normal breathing (i.e., only gasping) | No breathing or only gasping | |
| CPR sequence | C-A-B | | |
| Compression rate | At least 100-120/min | | |
| Compression depth | At least 2 inches (5 cm) but not more than 2.4 inches (6 cm) | At least one third AP diameter of chest (about 2 inches [5 cm]) | At least one third AP diameter of chest (about 1½ inches [4 cm]) |
| Chest wall recoil | Allow complete recoil between compressions | | |
| Compression interruptions | Minimize interruptions and limit interruptions to <10 s | | |
| Airway | Head tilt–chin lift Jaw thrust, if suspected trauma | | |
| Compression-to-ventilation ratio (until advanced airway is placed) | 30:2 (1 or 2 rescuers) | 30:2 (single rescuer) 15:2 (2 rescuers) | |
| Ventilations: when the rescuer is not proficient | Compressions only | | |
| Ventilations with advanced airway | 1 breath every 6 seconds (10 breaths/min) Asynchronous with chest compressions (about 1 second/breath) Visible chest rise | 1 breath every 6 seconds (10 breaths/min) Asynchronous with chest compressions (about 1 second/breath) Visible chest rise | 1 breath every 6 seconds (8-10 breaths/min) Asynchronous with chest compressions (about 1 second/breath) Visible chest rise |
| Defibrillation | Attach and use AED as soon as available. Minimize interruptions in chest compressions before and after shock. Resume CPR beginning with compressions immediately after each shock. | | |

**Table 45.3** Comparative Resuscitation Techniques Between Adults, Children, and Infants (Summary of Key BLS Components for Adults, Children, and Infants[a])

[a]Excluding the newly born, in whom the cause of an arrest is nearly always asphyxial.
*AED*, Automated external defibrillator; *AP*, anteroposterior; *C-A-B*, compression, airway, breathing; *CPR*, cardiopulmonary resuscitation.
(From 2015 AHA Summary of Key Basic Life Support Components [Adults, Children, Infants].)

rate; (2) adequate chest compression depth; (3) adequate recoil between chest compressions; (4) minimal interruptions to chest compressions; and (5) avoidance of excess ventilation.[18]

## Circulation

In a child, the heel of one or both hands should be placed on the lower half of the sternum, between the nipples, while keeping the fingers off the rib cage and staying above the xiphoid process. In an infant, chest compressions are delivered via the two-finger technique. Two fingers of one hand are placed over the lower half of the sternum approximately one fingerwidth below the intermammary line while keeping above the xiphoid process. For both infants and children, the sternum should be depressed at least one third to one half the anteroposterior diameter of the chest (4 cm infants, 5 cm children) at a rate of 100 to 120 compressions per minute.

Pulse checks and closed chest compressions are performed slightly differently, depending on whether the patient is a child or an infant. In children, the pulse is palpated at the carotid or femoral artery, similar to adults. In infants, the pulse is checked at the brachial or femoral artery. As with adults, $P_{ETCO_2}$ can be used to evaluate the quality of CPR. If invasive monitoring, such as an arterial catheter, is already in place, it may also be used to evaluate and guide CPR.

ECMO can be considered in all pediatric cardiac arrest patients who are refractory to standard conventional therapies.

VI

## Airway

The airway of pediatric patients is slightly different from that of an adult, but head tilt–chin lift is still the technique of choice to open the airway. Children tend to have a larger tongue and epiglottis in relation to the mouth and larynx. In addition, they have a larger head in relation to the body. Overextension or excessive flexion of the head can lead to difficulty visualizing the glottic opening during direct laryngoscopy. Straight laryngoscope blades may be preferred over curved blades to lift the epiglottis anteriorly and away from the glottic opening in young children (also see Chapter 34).

### Breathing

Given the likely causes of pediatric cardiopulmonary arrest, conventional CPR (compressions and ventilation) is recommended over compression-only resuscitation. The pattern should be 30 compressions to 2 breaths (30:2) if there is a single rescuer and 15 compressions to 2 breaths (15:2) if there are two rescuers.

## Defibrillation

In children, defibrillation should be performed when a pulseless shockable rhythm (VT, VF) is present. An initial energy of 2 to 4 J/kg should be attempted, regardless of the waveform type. Subsequent defibrillations should be at least 4 J/kg but should not exceed 10 J/kg. Biphasic AEDs can be used in children older than 1 year old outside the hospital setting. AHA guidelines recommend the use of a pediatric dose attenuator system that will decrease the amount of delivered energy. If one is not available, a standard external defibrillator can be substituted.

## Drugs

Most drug dosages are calculated by using current known weight or ideal body weight based on height. Most pediatric units have resuscitation carts divided by weight to facilitate drug administration in an emergency so that calculations do not need to be performed and valuable time is not wasted. As with adults, epinephrine has been associated with increased rate of ROSC and can be used in cardiac arrest. For refractory VF or pulseless VT in pediatric patients, either lidocaine or amiodarone can be administered.

## POSTRESUSCITATION CARE

After successful resuscitation with ROSC, patients are admitted to the intensive care unit for further definitive and supportive treatment (Fig. 45.7). Post–cardiac arrest care includes improving cardiopulmonary function optimally to ensure adequate organ perfusion. It should be consistent, integrated, and multidisciplinary. If arrest occurs at a center that is not equipped to manage elements of postresuscitation care, transfer to a larger regional center should be considered.[19]

When possible, therapies are administered concurrently. Specifically, percutaneous coronary interventions (PCIs) should not be delayed to institute hypothermia, and the institution of hypothermia should not delay PCI. Often, vasopressors and inotropes need to be administered during the immediate postresuscitation period because of the presence of myocardial stunning and hemodynamic instability. Central venous access for drug administration may be necessary, along with an arterial catheter to facilitate hemodynamic monitoring.

## Acute Coronary Syndrome

An electrocardiogram is obtained as soon as possible after ROSC in order to evaluate for ST-segment elevation myocardial infarction. If acute ST-segment elevation is noted, the patient should be taken for emergent angiography. Some patients with non-ST-segment elevation may also benefit from emergent angiography.[20] These evaluations are made regardless of neurologic status.

## Hemodynamic Goals

Following an ROSC, oxygenation and ventilation should be evaluated and optimized. Advanced airway placement may be considered, and hyperventilation is avoided. The goal for oxygenation is a saturation more than 94% and for ventilation the goal is a $Pa_{CO_2}$ of 35 to 45 mm Hg. A chest radiograph is obtained. Hypotension is treated, avoiding systolic arterial blood pressure less than 90 mm Hg or mean arterial blood pressure less than 65 mm Hg. This can be achieved with a combined administration of intravenous fluids and vasoactive drugs. No specific hemodynamic variables, including arterial blood pressure, cardiac output, venous oxygen saturation, or urine output have been recommended, as these likely vary widely between individual patients. Reversible causes for cardiac arrest are assessed. An electrocardiogram, echocardiogram, and serial cardiac enzymes are obtained. Serum lactate is monitored to assess for adequate tissue perfusion.

## Neurologic Monitoring

In addition to cardiac recovery, neurologic recovery is of vital importance. This is especially true during the immediate postresuscitation phase. An electroencephalogram can be obtained to evaluate for seizure, and anticonvulsants can be administered for status epilepticus.

## Targeted Temperature Management

Temperature should be monitored closely, and hyperthermia is avoided at all times as this can worsen ischemic brain injury (also see Chapter 30). The 2010 ACLS guidelines

ADULT IMMEDIATE POST-CARDIAC ARREST CARE
ALGORITHM - 2015 UPDATE

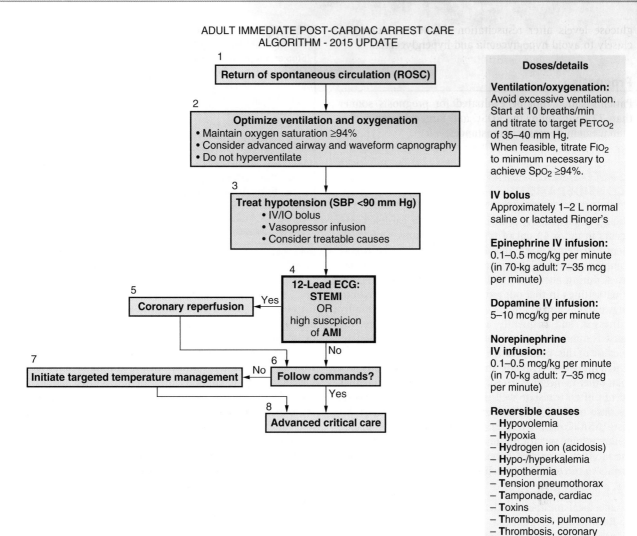

**Fig. 45.7** Algorithm for postcardiac arrest care. *AMI,* Acute myocardial infarction; *ECG,* electrocardiogram; *FiO2,* fraction of inspired oxygen; *IO,* intraosseous; *IV,* intravenous; *PETCO2,* partial pressure of end-tidal carbon dioxide; *SBP,* systolic blood pressure; *SpO2,* pulse oximeter oxygen saturation; *STEMI,* ST-segment elevation myocardial infarction. (From American Heart Association. Web-based Integrated Guidelines for Cardiopulmonary Resuscitation and Emergency Cardiovascular Care – Part 8: Post-Cardiac Arrest Care. ECCguidelines.heart.org. © Copyright 2015 American Heart Association, Inc.)

recommended therapeutic hypothermia of 32° C to 34° C for comatose patients after out-of-hospital VF/VT arrest. Milder therapeutic hypothermia, to 36° C, may confer similar benefit.[21] Temperature management in patients who suffer from IHCA or nonshockable cardiac arrest has not clearly been defined. Given the relative ease and safety of controlling body temperature and the risk of poor neurologic outcome because of hyperthermia, the 2015 guidelines recommend that all comatose patients after cardiac arrest and ROSC be treated with targeted temperature management between 32° C and 36° C. Complications of therapeutic hypothermia include impaired

coagulation and increased risk of infection at lower targeted levels, but are quite minimal at 36° C. Thus, patient factors can be taken into consideration when selecting the targeted temperature. Pre-hospital-induced hypothermia is not recommended.

## Blood Glucose Control

Increased blood glucose concentrations after resuscitation from cardiac arrest are associated with poor neurologic outcome. Yet, tight control of serum glucose has not been verified to improve neurologic outcome. Regardless, glucose levels after resuscitation should be monitored closely to avoid hypoglycemia and hyperglycemia.

## Prognosis

Patients should not be evaluated for prognosis sooner than 72 hours following ROSC and targeted temperature management in most circumstances.

## SPECIAL PERIOPERATIVE CONSIDERATIONS

Though inadequately studied, intraoperative cardiac arrest occurs in up to 43 out of 100,000 procedures. One study identified hemorrhage and anaphylaxis as the two most common causes of intraoperative cardiac arrest.[22] Cardiac arrest during anesthesia is distinct from cardiac arrest in other settings in that our patients have a different pathophysiology. Cardiac arrests during anesthesia are usually witnessed, and frequently anticipated. Furthermore, the cause is often surgical or otherwise more easily reversible. Because of this, perioperative cardiac arrests are associated with a higher survival rate and better neurologic outcomes than other in-hospital arrests.[23] The traditional guidelines do not often translate well into the perioperative setting. Because of that, the American Society of Anesthesiologists (ASA) Committee on Critical Care Medicine published a monograph specific to advanced life support for anesthesia. They expanded common causes of cardiac arrest events to the following categories and factors.[24]

1. Medications: anesthetic overdose, high neuraxial blockade, local anesthetic toxicity, drug administration errors
2. Respiratory: hypoxemia, autopositive end-expiratory pressure (PEEP), acute bronchospasm
3. Cardiovascular: vasovagal, hypovolemic/hemorrhagic shock, distributive shock, obstructive shock, right ventricular failure, left ventricular failure, arrhythmia, acute coronary syndrome

The ASA monograph also suggests the following interventions when performing resuscitation in the operating room: (1) call for help, (2) initiate chest compressions, (3) discontinue anesthetic, (4) discontinue surgery, (5) retrieve emergency equipment, (6) increase fraction of inspired oxygen ($FIO_2$) to 100%, (7) manually ventilate the lungs, (8) open all intravenous lines, and (9) use capnography to assess CPR.

Four unique circumstances to anesthesia providers are detailed in the next paragraphs.

## Anaphylaxis

Minor drug reactions such as a rash are not an uncommon occurrence in the operating room. Major reactions, such as anaphylactic shock, occur much less often. Common

---

**Box 45.1** Treatment of Anaphylaxis

Stop or remove inciting agent or drug
Oxygen at $FIO_2$ 1.0
Intravenous fluids
CPR/ACLS if pulseless
Epinephrine, intravenous
- *Bolus:* 10 to 100 μg—if not pulseless
- *Bolus:* 1-3 mg—if pulseless
- *Infusion:* 4-10 μg/min
Vasopressin, intravenous
- *Bolus:* 0.5 to 2 units—if not pulseless
- *Bolus:* 40 units—if pulseless
$H_1$ blocker, intravenous: diphenhydramine 50 mg
$H_2$ blocker, intravenous: famotidine 20 mg
Steroid, intravenous: hydrocortisone 50 to 150 mg

*ACLS,* Advanced cardiovascular life support; *CPR,* cardiopulmonary resuscitation; $H_1$, $H_2$, histamine receptor types 1 and 2.

---

drugs associated with anaphylaxis are latex, β-lactam antibiotics, succinylcholine, all muscle relaxants, and intravenous contrast material. The treatment of anaphylaxis involves the administration of epinephrine to interrupt the cascade of profound vasodilation and significant vascular leak. If possible, the offending drug should be removed or stopped. Epinephrine and vasopressin can be used to support arterial blood pressure, while steroids and antihistamines are administered to further attenuate the response. Intravenous fluid administration is essential secondary to the vascular leak. CPR and ACLS should be immediately instituted if there is no pulse palpated. In the event of complete cardiovascular collapse, larger doses of epinephrine may be required (Box 45.1).

## Gas Embolism

Although a very rare event, the incidence of gas embolism has the potential to increase in parallel with the worldwide increase in laparoscopic surgical procedures, posterior spine surgery, and endobronchial laser procedures (also see Chapter 30). The initial management includes cessation of the offending cause (i.e., halt insufflation), occlusion of open veins, and flooding the surgical field with saline. Patients should be placed in Trendelenburg position with left side down to keep the gas in the apex of the ventricle and allow for filling. Complete circulatory collapse should be treated with CPR and ACLS.

## Local Anesthetic Systemic Toxicity

Local anesthetics affect sodium channels throughout the body, including the brain and the heart. In general, toxicity occurs in a dose-dependent fashion with cardiovascular collapse occurring at the end of the spectrum (also see Chapter 10). In nonanesthetized patients, central nervous system symptoms are vital to recognize as they tend

---

**Box 45.2** Treatment of Local Anesthetic Toxicity

Stop local anesthetic
CPR/ACLS if pulseless
20% Intralipid IV:
- *Load:* 1.5 mL/kg
- *Infusion:* 0.25 mL/kg/h

Sodium bicarbonate to maintain pH >7.25 in a prolonged resuscitation
Consider transcutaneous or transvenous pacing for brady-cardic rhythms
Continue CPR for at least 60 min

---

*ACLS,* Advanced cardiovascular life support; *CPR,* cardiopulmonary resuscitation; *IV,* intravenous.

to precede cardiac manifestations. Cardiac rhythms can range from premature ventricular contractions to asystole. If possible, the administration of the local anesthetic should be stopped. Intralipid should be given for cardiovascular toxicity.[25] Good neurologic recovery in these patients can occur despite the prolonged resuscitation (Box 45.2). Vasopressin should be avoided, and epinephrine doses should be decreased (<1 μg/kg).[26]

## Cardiovascular Collapse From Neuraxial Anesthesia

Cardiovascular collapse from neuraxial anesthesia has been described but is inadequately understood.[27] It seems to occur in younger, otherwise healthy patients undergoing routine surgical procedures with neuraxial anesthesia (also see Chapter 17). Proposed mechanisms causing the cardiac arrest include a shift in autonomic balance toward the parasympathetic system, a decrease in venous return from pooling in the splanchnic circulation, and activation of baroreceptors that stimulate a paradoxic Bezold-Jarisch response. A high level of spinal anesthesia seems to be the most frequent culprit. Regardless, treatment follows standard CPR and ACLS recommendations.

## SYSTEMS OF CARE

Health care delivery systems differ significantly between out-of-hospital cardiac arrest and IHCAs. The AHA discusses both of these distinct systems; here we will address IHCA and the myriad roles the anesthesia provider may play. A patient at risk of cardiac arrest while in the hospital depends on appropriate surveillance and prevention, prompt recognition and response by a multidisciplinary team, high-quality CPR, early defibrillation, and additional ACLS as needed.[28] Though recovery from IHCA has improved over the last few decades, there remains considerable variability and room for improvement.

The AHA guidelines recommend the establishment of rapid response teams or medical emergency teams in order to reduce the incidence of cardiac arrest in patients who are at increased risk. These patients should be transferred to a higher acuity setting, such as an intensive care unit. Discussions with the patient or family members regarding preference for aggressive resuscitation should ideally be conducted prior to an actual cardiac arrest event. Crisis resource management techniques should be utilized in order to optimize resuscitation team dynamics. These include a designated resuscitation team, with predetermined roles and communication strategies, and a plan for debriefing after an event.

In 2015 the National Academy of Medicine (formerly Institute of Medicine) released a report titled "Strategies to Improve Cardiac Arrest Survival: A Time to Act." This report noted the significant morbidity associated with cardiac arrest, and the need to improve outcomes.[29,30] The report introduced eight recommendations to improve resuscitation practices: (1) robust data collection and dissemination, (2) improved public response, (3) enhanced emergency medical service (EMS) capability, (4) updated national accreditation standards, (5) continuous quality improvement, (6) increased research funding in resuscitative science, (7) increased speed in adopting existing strategies, and (8) establishment of a new nationwide cardiac arrest collaborative. The AHA has responded to this call to action by announcing commitments to improve systems of care, resuscitation research, and creation of a national cardiac arrest collaborative.[31]

## QUESTIONS OF THE DAY

1. What are the components of effective chest compressions in an infant, child, and adult?
2. According to advanced cardiovascular life support (ACLS) guidelines, what is the role of epinephrine, amiodarone, and vasopressin in the management of cardiac arrest?
3. Which patients are most likely to benefit from targeted temperature management after a cardiac arrest?
4. During the perioperative period, what factors are potential contributors to the risk of cardiac arrest?
5. What interventions should be part of cardiac arrest management in the operating room?

VI

## REFERENCES

1. Kazaure HS, Roman SA, Sosa JA. Epidemiology and outcomes of in-hospital cardiopulmonary resuscitation in the United States, 2000-2009. *Resuscitation*. 2013;84(9):1255–1260.

2. Neumar RW, Shuster M, Callaway CW, et al. Part 1: Executive Summary 2015 American Heart Association Guidelines Update for Cardiopulmonary Resuscitation and Emergency Cardiovascular Care. *Circulation*. 2015;132(18 suppl 2):S315–S367.

3. American Heart Association. Emergency Cardiovascular Care (ECC) Guidelines. eccguidelines.heart.org.

4. Kleinman ME, Brennan EE, Goldberger ZD, et al. Part 5: Adult Basic Life Support and Cardiopulmonary Resuscitation Quality 2015 American Heart Association Guidelines Update for Cardiopulmonary Resuscitation and Emergency Cardiovascular Care. *Circulation*. 2015;132(18 suppl 2):S414–S435.

5. Idris AH, Guffey D, Pepe PE, et al. Chest compression rates and survival following out-of-hospital cardiac arrest. *Crit Care Med*. 2015;43(4):840–848.

6. Rea TD, Fahrenbruch C, Culley L, et al. CPR with chest compression alone or with rescue breathing. *N Engl J Med*. 2010;363(5):423–433.

7. Bobrow BJ, Spaite DW, Berg RA, et al. Chest compression-only CPR by lay rescuers and survival from out-of-hospital cardiac arrest. *JAMA*. 2010;304(13):1447–1454.

8. Aufderheide TP, Sigurdsson G, Pirrallo RG, et al. Hyperventilation-induced hypotension during cardiopulmonary resuscitation. *Circulation*. 2004;109(16):1960–1965.

9. Yeung J, Chilwan M, Field R, et al. The impact of airway management on quality of cardiopulmonary resuscitation: an observational study in patients during cardiac arrest. *Resuscitation*. 2014;85(7):898–904.

10. Chan PS, Krumholz HM, Nichol G, Nallamothu BK. American Heart Association National Registry of Cardiopulmonary Resuscitation Investigators. Delayed time to defibrillation after in-hospital cardiac arrest. *N Engl J Med*. 2008;358(1):9–17.

11. Sheak KR, Wiebe DJ, Leary M, et al. Quantitative relationship between end-tidal carbon dioxide and CPR quality during both in-hospital and out-of-hospital cardiac arrest. *Resuscitation*. 2015;89:149–154.

12. Link MS, Berkow LC, Kudenchuk PJ, et al. Part 7: adult advanced cardiovascular life support 2015 American Heart Association Guidelines Update for Cardiopulmonary Resuscitation and Emergency Cardiovascular Care. *Circulation*. 2015;132(18 suppl 2):S444–S464.

13. Callaway CW, Soar J, Aibiki M, et al. Advanced Life Support Chapter Collaborators. Part 4: advanced life support 2015 International Consensus on Cardiopulmonary Resuscitation and Emergency Cardiovascular Care Science With Treatment Recommendations. *Circulation*. 2015;132(16 suppl 1):S84–S145.

14. Kudenchuk PJ, Brown SP, Daya M, et al. Resuscitation Outcomes Consortium-Amiodarone, Lidocaine or Placebo Study (ROC-ALPS): rationale and methodology behind an out-of-hospital cardiac arrest antiarrhythmic drug trial. *Am Heart J*. 2014;167(5):653–659. e4.

15. Blyth L, Atkinson P, Gadd K, Lang E. Bedside focused echocardiography as predictor of survival in cardiac arrest patients: a systematic review. *Acad Emerg Med*. 2012;19(10):1119–1126.

16. Mukoyama T, Kinoshita K, Nagao K, Tanjoh K. Reduced effectiveness of vasopressin in repeated doses for patients undergoing prolonged cardiopulmonary resuscitation. *Resuscitation*. 2009;80(7):755–761.

17. Mentzelopoulos SD, Malachias S, Chamos C, et al. Vasopressin, steroids, and epinephrine and neurologically favorable survival after in-hospital cardiac arrest: a randomized clinical trial. *JAMA*. 2013;310(3):270–279.

18. Atkins DL, Berger S, Duff JP, et al. Part 11: pediatric basic life support and cardiopulmonary resuscitation quality 2015 American Heart Association Guidelines Update for Cardiopulmonary Resuscitation and Emergency Cardiovascular Care. *Circulation*. 2015;132(18 suppl 2):S519–S525.

19. Tagami T, Hirata K, Takeshige T, et al. Implementation of the fifth link of the chain of survival concept for out-of-hospital cardiac arrest. *Circulation*. 2012;126(5):589–597.

20. Callaway CW, Donnino MW, Fink EL, et al. Part 8: post–cardiac arrest care 2015 American Heart Association Guidelines Update for Cardiopulmonary Resuscitation and Emergency Cardiovascular Care. *Circulation*. 2015;132(18 suppl 2):S465–S482.

21. Nielsen N, Wetterslev J, Cronberg T, et al. Targeted temperature management at 33°C versus 36°C after cardiac arrest. *N Engl J Med*. 2013;369(23):2197–2206.

22. Predictors of functional outcome after intraoperative cardiac arrest. http://anesthesiology.pubs.asahq.org/article.aspx?articleid=1921498. Accessed October 24, 2015.

23. Ramachandran SK, Mhyre J, Kheterpal S, et al. Predictors of survival from perioperative cardiopulmonary arrests: a retrospective analysis of 2,524 events from the National Registry of Cardiopulmonary Resuscitation. *Anesthesiology*. 2013;119(6):1322–1339.

24. *Adapting ACLS to the Perioperative Period*. American Society of Anesthesiologists Annual Meeting; 2011. http://www.icaa.ir/Portals/0/Adapting%20ACLS%20to%20the%20Perioperative%20Period.pdf. Accessed August 8, 2016.

25. Rosenblatt MA, Abel M, Fischer GW, et al. Successful use of a 20% lipid emulsion to resuscitate a patient after a presumed bupivacaine-related cardiac arrest. *Anesthesiology*. 2006;105(1):217–218.

26. American Society of Regional Anesthesia and Pain Medicine (ASRA). Checklist for Treatment of Local Anesthetic Systemic Toxicity.pdf. https://www.asra.com/content/documents/checklist-for-local-anesthetic-toxicity-treatment-1-18-12.pdf Accessed October 26, 2015.

27. Kopp SL, Horlocker TT, Warner ME, et al. Cardiac arrest during neuraxial anesthesia: frequency and predisposing factors associated with survival. *Anesth Analg*. 2005;100(3):855–865.

28. Kronick SL, Kurz MC, Lin S, et al. Part 4: systems of care and continuous quality improvement 2015 American Heart Association Guidelines Update for Cardiopulmonary Resuscitation and Emergency Cardiovascular Care. *Circulation*. 2015;132(18 suppl 2):S397–S413.

29. Institute of Medicine. Strategies to improve cardiac arrest survival, a time to act. http://iom.nationalacademies.org/~/media/Files/Report%20Files/2015/Cardiac-Arrest/CardiacArrestReportBrief.pdf; Accessed October 26, 2015.

30. Becker LB, Aufderheide TP, Graham R. Strategies to improve survival from cardiac arrest: a report from the institute of medicine. *JAMA*. 2015;314(3):223–224.

31. Neumar RW, Eigel B, Callaway CW, et al. American Heart Association response to the 2015 Institute of Medicine Report on strategies to improve cardiac arrest survival. *Circulation*. 2015;132(11):1049–1070.

# 46

# OPERATING ROOM MANAGEMENT

## Amr E. Abouleish

*Healing is an art, medicine is a science, and health care is a business.*

Author unknown

Anesthesiologists are in a unique position as physicians. In providing care, anesthesiologists bridge medical and surgical specialties working directly with many specialists, including surgeons, obstetricians and gynecologists, emergency physicians, and other proceduralists including, but not limited to, interventional radiology, gastrointestinal specialists, cardiologists, and hematologists-oncologists. Further, in evaluating patients, anesthesiologists work with primary care physicians and medical specialists to understand underlying comorbid conditions and how to optimize care for these conditions. Because of these many varied relationships with other physicians, anesthesiologists are often identified to help with administrative tasks within a hospital or medical school. Although these positions can be at all levels of administration, the most common administrative role for an anesthesiologist is that of medical director of the operating room (OR), which can include the postanesthesia care unit (PACU) (also see Chapter 39) and day surgery unit (also see Chapter 37). Traditionally, this role has not included administrative roles over OR purchasing and materials management or nursing staff.

On the other hand, the role involves day-to-day case flow management as well as overall governance of block scheduling and staffing. The role also overlaps with anesthesiology group management with decisions of the OR management impacting staffing, billing, income, and, ultimately, the success of the anesthesiology group. The goal of this chapter is to provide a basic discussion of OR management issues that impact the anesthesiology group and that an OR medical director faces daily: (1) staffing, (2) efficiency and utilization, and (3) turnover and OR throughput. At the end of this chapter, additional resources and references are supplied that allow for more in-depth exploration of these issues and other topics.

## PERIOPERATIVE LEADERSHIP

Anesthesiologists can also fill the role of the perioperative physician because of their daily interactions with surgeons and proceduralists, hospitalists and internal medicine physicians, nursing staff, and hospital administrators. Because of the involvement of these different health care clinicians and administrators, the effective anesthesiologist leader needs to be able to work well in teams, to be able to communicate the vision of what the overall goals of the facility are, and to assure that high-quality care remains the first priority.

The physician leader often works directly with a nursing director of perioperative services and an OR governing committee. In this setting, the physician leader uses his or her clinical skills to provide context to policy decisions. In addition, an anesthesiologist may be the only physician who is practiced in all the varied locations (e.g., in the OR, intensive care unit, preoperative evaluation clinic) and, therefore, frequently has the best ability to know how all the different aspects of perioperative care are interconnected. This wide perspective is important when leading work flow improvements, including OR throughput, and developing clinical and hospital policies.

Anesthesiologists who have the interest to be in a leadership and administrative role for their medical group or facility often seek additional education in business and leadership. Although there are physician executive education programs, anesthesiologists in the United States are fortunate to have numerous options targeted specifically to anesthesiologists and perioperative care. These include offerings from the American Society of Anesthesiologists conferences, professional seminars, and certificates in business as well as other conferences and courses offered by business schools.

## ANESTHESIOLOGY STAFFING

In today's health care economy, the cost of anesthesia personnel staffing an OR often exceeds the revenue generated from anesthesia care, creating the need for medical facilities to provide funds for staffing.[1,2] A number of personnel configurations can be used to provide intraoperative anesthesia, including physician anesthesiologists, nurse anesthetists, residents, fellows, and several other types of providers. This variability requires an examination of staffing needs and how such needs are determined and met. The medical center facility, which may be paying for part of the anesthesia staffing, wants to minimize the number of staff members needed, and the anesthesiology group that provides the services wants to ensure that the staff numbers are adequate. Also, legal requirements in various places may vary (i.e., states, countries, regions). This variance leads to a desire from everyone to have an objective manner to determine the actual staff needs.

The various staffing approaches for intraoperative patient care are beginning to be considered by general medical journals. For example, a recent editorial in the *Journal of the American Medical Association*[3] outlines the risks of "concurrent surgeries." Although this editorial was directed to surgeons, the same questions could be addressed to anesthesiologists. One of the important conclusions was that patients should be provided the same type of information regarding their anesthesia. The potential implications for anesthesiologists are clear.

The most logical process is to determine the workload and the average workload per full-time equivalent (FTE). Then simple division will lead to the number of FTEs needed on any given day. (See later discussion about converting FTEs to actual number of providers.)

This logic is often applied to anesthesia-provider staffing. The workload is often used to determine the staffing needs. The problem with this approach becomes evident when simply answering the following question: "For your OR tomorrow, how many people do you need to provide anesthesia at the start of the day?"[4] Unfortunately, the answer rarely includes the number of cases to be performed. Instead, the primary determinants of staffing requirements are the number of clinical sites to be staffed and the staffing ratio (i.e., concurrency). Other determinants include whether or not a second shift is needed in the evening and the number of staff members who are on-call or post-call. In other words, if an anesthesiology group needs to provide care for 20 ORs at 7:30 AM, the number of anesthesia providers required is no different whether all the ORs finish at noon or 3 PM. Therefore, instead of determining staffing needs, workload should be used to determine the appropriate number of ORs needed—assuming this decision is based solely on workload.

A staffing grid, utilizing a spreadsheet, can be used to determine staffing needs[4] (see Additional Resource 1 and online spreadsheet). The spreadsheet has in the first column the types of clinical sites/duties and in the second column the number of anesthesia providers; for care-team model groups, the third and fourth columns are used for the number of anesthesia providers (resident, certified registered nurse anesthetist [CRNA], anesthesiologist assistant [AA]) that are supervised or medically directed by the anesthesiologists (Table 46.1). Several factors will impact the staffing ratio. First, for residents in training, the accrediting rules limit staffing ratio to a maximum of two; that is, one anesthesiologist can cover only two rooms. For Medicare billing of medical direction, the limit is four rooms. Second, the type of surgery may determine the safety of staffing a second room. For example, a neonatal surgery case may not allow the anesthesiologist to cover another room. Third, location of clinical site may not allow for a second room to be covered. Finally, other duties must be considered; for example, the schedule runner (anesthesiologist in charge of the schedule) may be able to cover only one room. All these factors on staffing ratio will need

| Table 46.1 | Example Staffing Grid for an Academic Anesthesiology Department Covering 22 ORs Model: Single Day Shift With Single In-House Call Shift | | | |
|---|---|---|---|---|
| | **ORs Covered** | **Faculty** | **Resident** | **CRNA/AA** |
| **Clinical FTEs Needed** | | | | |
| Medical direction main OR (includes remotes) | 18.0 | 9.0 | 13.0 | 5.0 |
| One-on-one rooms | 1.0 | 1.0 | 1.0 | |
| Faculty rooms in main OR | 2.0 | 2.0 | | |
| Schedule runner main OR | 1.0 | 1.0 | | 1.0 |
| **Total OR sites covered** | **22.0** | | | |
| Preoperative clinic | | 1.0 | 1.0 | |
| Labor and delivery | | 1.0 | 3.0 | |
| Pain management clinic and consults | | 1.0 | 2.0 | |
| Critical care services | | 1.0 | 3.0 | |
| Post call | | 2.0 | 6.0 | |
| **Daily clinical FTEs needed** | | **19.0** | **29.0** | **6.0** |
| **Nonclinical FTEs** | | | | |
| Average clinical FTE % of FTE | | 0.75 | 0.89 | 0.80 |
| **Number of providers that are nonclinical** | | **6.50** | **4.00** | **1.50** |
| **Away FTEs** | | | | |
| Meeting | | 1.15 | 0.21 | 0.19 |
| Vacation | | 2.31 | 1.38 | 0.77 |
| Sick | | 1.00 | 1.00 | 0.50 |
| **Total away FTEs** | | **4.46** | **2.59** | **1.46** |
| **Total FTEs needed in dept.** | | 29.96 | 35.59 | 8.96 |
| **Total on Staff** | | | | |
| Current | | 30 | 36 | 10 |
| Departures | | 5 | 12 | 1 |
| Hires | | 6 | 12 | 0 |
| **Total available FTEs** | | **31** | **36** | **9** |
| **Excess (or deficit) expected** | | **1.04** | **0.41** | **0.04** |

See text for details of the department. Results based on calculations found in the Excel worksheet available as Additional Resource 1 and online. Initial estimates utilized no faculty rooms, but results showed a deficit in residents and nurse anesthetists/AAs. Final estimates include two faculty rooms.
*AA,* Anesthesiologist assistant; *FTE,* full-time equivalent; *OR,* operating room.

to be examined before a final number is determined. For instance, the anesthesiology group might argue that the schedule runner, the anesthesiologist covering radiology, and two other anesthesiologists must be planned for covering only one room with a resident or CRNA, resulting in four clinical sites covered one-on-one. The hospital might argue that only the schedule runner and the radiology anesthesiologist need one-on-one coverage.

The next part of the grid includes the non-OR locations, such as labor and delivery, pain management clinic and procedures, preoperative clinic and consults, and intensive care unit, and for academic departments, resident away rotations. In addition, the number of call providers coming in later in the day and the number who are not available because of post-call status are also listed. The final numbers need to be agreed upon by the anesthesiology group and the hospital.

The staffing grid determines the number of FTEs needed each day. But this number of FTEs cannot be simply converted to determine the number of staff required. For example, 1 FTE anesthesiologist does not work 52 weeks of the year or even all 50 weeks of weekdays remaining after the typical 10 weekday holidays or 2 weeks vacation during a year. Therefore, if 1 FTE is needed, then more than 1 anesthesiologist will be needed on staff. An estimate can be made by determining the number of weeks a full-time anesthesia provider works in the year, or in other words, determining how many weeks off the typical anesthesiologist has in that group. To illustrate with a hypothetical example, suppose each anesthesiologist takes off 2 weeks for hospital holidays, 4 weeks for vacation, 1 week for continuing medical education activity, and 1 week for sick leave, for a total of 8 weeks. Therefore, the typical anesthesia provider in this group works

VI

44 of 52 weeks (or 86%). One way to look at this number is to say that each anesthesiologist represents 0.86 FTE. So, if 6 FTEs are needed, then 7 anesthesiologists will be needed. In addition, for academic departments, the issue of nonclinical rotations also needs to be factored into the calculations. (In Table 46.1, these calculations are at the end of the staffing grid. For more details, see Additional Resource 1 and spreadsheet online). The preceding processes describe only the first steps in determining staffing needs. With daily hour limits, types of shifts people work, the usual inability to hire a fraction of an FTE, and special considerations of the facility, the staffing grid can become complex. But the final message is the same as the initial point: staffing needs are determined by the clinical sites to be covered, not by the workload!

## OPERATING ROOM EFFICIENCY

Because the staffing needs and costs are determined by number of sites to be covered and not by the actual work being done in those sites, then a goal of any OR management is to use the staff efficiently. In other words, if one is going to pay for a person to be there, then the goal is to have that person working rather than simply being available. This is true for the anesthesiology group as well as for the hospital staff (OR nurses and surgical technicians).

The idea that anesthesia staff members should be working (e.g., administering anesthesia) every minute of their shift can actually lead to unintended consequences. The concept of underutilized and overutilized hours is important to understand. An underutilized hour occurs when the staff (and the OR) is not working during the scheduled shift. That is, if the staff is supposed to work until 5 PM, but finishes the last case at 4 PM, then there is 1 underutilized hour. On the other hand, if the last case finishes at 6 PM, there is 1 overutilized hour. In this latter case, one may at first think this is good because the staff worked all of the shift and then some. Unfortunately, that overutilized hour can be costly. For scientific studies, a factor of 1.75 to 2.0 is used to multiply the cost of a regular shift to determine the cost of the overutilized hour. This increased cost may be in direct costs (in compensation) or in indirect costs (for recruitment of new staff to replace former staff members who left because of having to stay late frequently). Therefore, 1 underutilized hour costs less than 1 overutilized hour. A measurement of efficiency would be the sum of underutilized hours and overutilized hours (multiplying by the factor). An efficient OR would be one in which this sum is minimized.[5] Consequently, one of the goals of an efficient staffing system is to match staffing shifts to the actual demand. The work shifts should be aligned among anesthesiologists, the OR staff, and the schedule. For example, if the OR allows for surgeons to schedule cases to finish at 5 PM, then inefficient staffing practice would be to staff the OR until 3 PM and then make

staff stay late. On the other hand, an efficient staffing approach would be to increase staffing by either increasing individual shift hours or planning for a second shift to start later in the day.

Alternatively, efficiency of an OR can be evaluated by how well the OR is running. Macario recommended seven performance measurements in scoring OR efficiencies (Table 46.2).[6] In addition to staffing costs, the measurements also include OR function costs and scheduling costs. Factors such as first-start tardiness, prolonged turnover times, delays, and PACU holds all contribute to an inefficient OR. An infrequent case cancellation and a good prediction of case length are signs of an efficient OR. Finally, measurement of contribution margin (revenue minus costs, including staffing costs) is the best measurement of efficiency for the hospital.

### Operating Room Utilization

Unlike efficiency, utilization is easier to measure and better reported and followed. The simplest definition of utilization is the percentage of time the OR is used for patient care by dividing the time the patient is in the OR by the time that is available for patient care. A more accurate numerator would include setup and cleanup as well as the time the patient is in room time. In addition, determining the denominator correctly—the available time for patient care—is very important. Unfortunately, this definition is not always the same among the OR nursing staff, the hospital administration, the anesthesiology group, and surgeons. From an operational perspective, the utilization of regularly scheduled time is the important number. So inclusion of after-hour shifts can confuse the final calculations. The exercise of determining what the regularly scheduled hours are may in fact point out that staffing shifts do not match the available hours of patient care. For example, surgeons may feel that every OR is staffed and available for surgery till 5 PM each weekday. But in reality, surgical nursing staffs only 40% of the ORs after 3 PM. That is, nursing does not plan or have staff for 60% of ORs from 3 PM to 5 PM. Further, the anesthesia staff may turn over cases to the call team at 4:30 PM with the plan of only staffing a few rooms after this time. Without a consensus of the hours of operation, confusion, dissatisfaction, and frustration will occur. Coming to an agreement of the definition is essential to any OR management team.

But what is a good utilization percentage? Again, this depends on who is answering the question. For example, hospital administrators may feel that 100% utilization should be the goal, whereas nursing and the anesthesiology group would like 75%. Also, the surgeons can benefit from a poor utilization. When a surgeon has an add-on case, the surgeon would like to do it when he or she wants, in the OR he or she wants, and with the staff he or she wants; therefore, poor utilization means the OR is more likely to be open for add-ons). As discussed

**Table 46.2**   A Scoring System for Operating Room (OR) Efficiency[a]

| Metric | Points Scored | | |
|---|---|---|---|
| | 0 | 1 | 2 |
| Excess staffing costs | >10 % | 5-10% | <5% |
| Start-time tardiness—mean tardiness of start times for elective cases per OR per day | >60 min | 45-60 min | <45 min |
| Cancellation rate | >10% | 5-10% | <5% |
| PACU admission delays—% of workdays with at least one delay in PACU admission | >20 % | 10-20% | <10% |
| Contribution margin (mean) per OR per hour | <$1000/h | $1000-$2000/h | >$2000/h |
| Turnover times—mean setup and cleanup turnover time for all cases | >40 min | 25-40 min | <25 min |
| Prediction bias—bias in case duration estimates per 8 hours of OR time | >15 min | 5-15 min | <5 min |
| Prolonged turnovers—% of turnovers that take longer than 60 minutes | >25 % | 10-25% | <10% |

[a]Efficiency scoring system for an OR that takes into account staffing costs, scheduling costs, and functioning costs. For full details of how to use this system, see table source.
PACU, Postanesthesia care unit.
From Macario A. Are your hospital operating rooms "efficient"? A scoring system with eight performance indicators. *Anesthesiology*. 2006;105:237-240.

previously, 100% of regular hours means that no underutilized time exists, but because not all the rooms will finish at the end of regular hours, overutilized hours must exist. This will lead to costly direct staff compensation or indirect costs of having to recruit new staff to replace those who leave in frustration of always working overtime. On the other hand, a utilization of 70% to 80% reflects some underutilized hours that actually might mean a better managed OR. Also, it allows for some leeway for emergency cases.

The most common method of analyzing utilization is by determining block time; that is, the amount of time a surgeon has available to schedule cases. Unfortunately, simply relying on utilization for determination of block time can result in poor OR management decisions. For example, if Surgeon A has utilization of 120% and Surgeon B has utilization of 75%, then the OR management decision based on utilization alone is to give more time to Surgeon A and take time away from Surgeon B. But what if Surgeon A and B are doing the same exact surgical procedures and the same number of patients each day? Surgeon B obviously has shorter surgical durations. If one assumes both surgeons have the same payer mix, then revenue is the same for each, but the costs of Surgeon A would be higher because of more OR time and overtime of OR staff. So the contribution margin (i.e., net profit = revenue minus costs) is better for Surgeon B. An additional benefit of Surgeon B is that there is regular time available for an add-on case. A more detailed tutorial

on the impact of block scheduling, service-specific staffing, and OR productivity will allow further exploration of these issues.[7]

Another use of utilization is to determine if hospital funding is needed to cover costs of anesthesia staffing. This is often seen in negotiated agreements between a hospital and an anesthesiology group when expanding into new clinical sites. The average revenue per hour of care (average revenue per ASA unit and ASA units billed per hour care) can be used to estimate the number of hours of patient care that is needed to cover the staffing costs for one OR. By dividing the number of hours needed by the agreed-upon scheduled staffing hours, a break-even utilization can be estimated. The hospital agreement can state that if utilization is less than this point, the facility will need to help fund the staffing costs. On the other hand, if utilization is above the break-even mark, no facility funding will be necessary.

## Operating Room Throughput and Turnover Time

Once the hospital or facility and the anesthesiology group have agreed to staff a clinical site or an OR, then the goal is to maximize the output for that OR (efficiency) without increasing costs further (e.g., with overtime). Therefore, a common focus of OR management is how to perform more cases per OR, or in other words, how to maximize OR throughput.

VI

A complete examination of OR throughput starts at the beginning of the process, which begins at the time of referral to the surgeon's office. Then, scheduling (including block scheduling), properly predicting surgical duration, and preoperative evaluation and testing (the preoperative clinic) all occur prior to the day of surgery. On the day of surgery, the day surgery unit must prepare the patient and have the patient transported to the OR in a timely fashion. The surgery is completed and then the patient is admitted to the PACU and then either discharged from day surgery or admitted to the hospital. The whole process ends back in the surgeon's office during the postoperative outpatient visit. As one can see, the OR throughput process involves many other departments and personnel than simply the OR staff and anesthesia providers on the day of surgery.[7]

Prolonged turnover time is often stated as the reason more cases cannot be performed. As the previous description of OR throughput demonstrates, this criticism about turnover time is an oversimplification. But why is this criticism so prevalent? The answer is that turnover time is easy to measure and understand. Many of the other parts of OR throughput are complex or involve many different parties, but turnover time is focused on one OR and its small number of staff members, including the anesthesia provider in that one OR. Therefore, OR managers must understand the issues of turnover time, especially as it relates to OR throughput.

### Turnover Time

A commonly stated theme is, "if turnover time were shorter, we could do more cases." Intuitively, it is clear that this is usually not true, and research has established the fact that further reducing reasonable turnover times usually does not increase the number of cases that can be performed in a workday.[8,9] The exception would be if the anesthesia providers and surgeons are unavailable for some reasons. In these instances an excessively long turnaround could result. For example, if the surgical and anesthesia personnel are different than in the first case, they may not be readily available. Turnover time is defined as the time beginning when the preceding patient leaves the OR and the next one enters the OR. For instance, for an OR in a nonambulatory surgical center hospital, a reasonable maximum turnover time between procedures might be 35 minutes. Reducing this number by 20% would only result in a 7-minute time saving between cases. If three cases were done per OR per day, this would mean a 14-minute time saving per day, which is only a fraction of the duration of one case. Therefore, even a good effort of reducing turnover time by 20% will not allow for one more surgical case to be done. Obviously, in an OR where more cases are being performed in a day (e.g., 7 to 10 cataract or pediatric otolaryngology surgeries), reducing turnover time by 7 minutes per case may be significant. But in these specific ORs, the turnover time is already much shorter than in the rest of the ORs (e.g., 15 minutes) and further reduction may not be possible.

Despite the foregoing discussion, evaluation of turnover times has merit. Instead of working on all turnovers, which will result in few benefits, emphasis should be on reducing delays. A delay is a prolonged turnover time that is longer than the reasonable maximum turnover time. Focusing on delays and not all turnovers allows for more potential improvement in the process. For instance, suppose it is decided that the maximum allowed turnover is 35 minutes. Then when a turnover is longer than 35 minutes (a delay), the reasons for the delay must be reported. Avoidable delays are analyzed and often identify system issues that occur not just in this one case but multiple times during the week and even each day. Examples of system issues include (but are not limited to) the preoperative preparation process (anesthesia evaluation), proper surgical paperwork (history and physical examination, informed consent) not completed or available, delayed process of preparing the patient on the day of surgery (from arrival to the hospital to being ready for transport to the holding room), transportation issues, equipment issues (including proper procedure posting), and processes in the OR. By focusing on the delays, more than a handful of minutes per case can be saved that add up over a multitude of cases, in contrast to when all turnovers are examined.

### Throughput on the Day of Surgery
#### Traditional Approach

Traditionally, OR throughput initiatives have focused on how to improve the work processes of the current staff.[10,11] Successful initiatives have involved an interdisciplinary team that includes all personnel involved from physicians (surgeons and anesthesia providers) and nursing staff to transportation staff and environmental service personnel. Surgeons who are technically efficient intraoperatively facilitate throughput of surgical cases. The improvement process looks at work flow assessment and redesign of work. This process works, at least over the short run. Unfortunately, to maintain any gains, the improvement process must include continuous and repeated educational efforts and monitoring. Further, potential gains are limited by the existing staffing levels.

#### Parallel Processing

Additional approaches can improve OR throughput even more, but additional staff and a paradigm shift in the work flow will be needed. Most OR work flow is performed in series. Specifically, one task is completed before the next task is started. For instance, setup for the next case is not performed until the preceding patient is in the PACU and the OR is cleaned. Further, induction of anesthesia in the next patient cannot be performed before the OR surgical equipment is completely set up. In parallel processing, tasks done during the nonoperative time are not

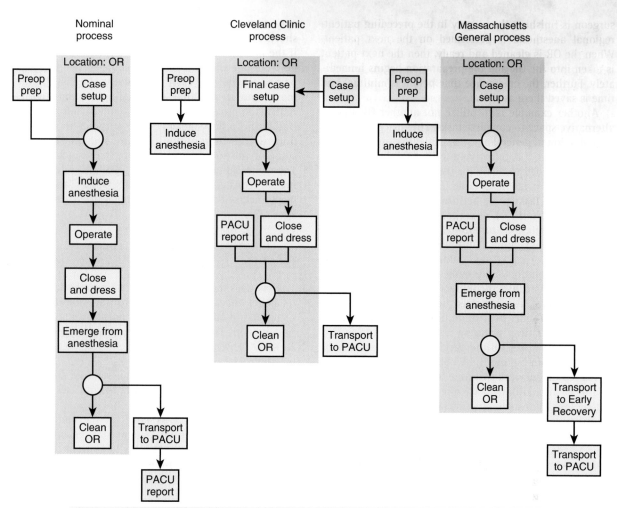

**Fig. 46.1** Flow diagrams of parallel processing for operating room (OR) throughput. Three processes are illustrated. Nominal is the traditional series process in which all activity is done sequentially. The Cleveland Clinic Process (see reference 15) and the Massachusetts General Process (see reference 12) are examples of parallel processes. In both of these processes, nonoperative tasks are not done in series but can be done at the same time (i.e., in parallel) but may require additional staff and space. *PACU,* Postanesthesia care unit. (Redrawn from Sandberg WS. Engineering parallel processing perioperative systems for improved throughput. ASA Monitor. 2010;74(1):26-30. http://monitor.pubs.asahq.org/article.aspx?articleid=2446748&resultClick=3; last accessed February 16, 2017.)

done faster or reduced but are done at the same time. By doing them at the same time, the total nonoperative time is reduced (Fig. 46.1). Parallel processing can be successful in allowing an additional case to be performed.[12-17] In practice, all parallel process solutions will require additional staffing, with the type of staffing dependent on the solution. Parallel processing is used on an increasing frequency in busy tertiary care hospitals.

One example of parallel processing is the practice of providing a surgeon with two ORs. This is such an important concept that this approach was examined in a 2016 issue of JAMA.[3] In these situations, the surgeon's operative time should be the same or less than the nonoperative time (emergence, clean up/setup, and induction) and the surgeon's caseload is sufficient to justify two ORs. In other words, while the surgeon is working in OR A on patient 1, the next patient (patient 2) is induced in OR B. While patient 1 is emerging in OR A and then OR A is cleaned and set up and patient 3 is induced in OR A, the surgeon is completing the procedure on patient 2 in OR B. The surgeon then moves to OR A and begins surgery on patient 3 while patient 2 is emerging in OR B.

Another example of parallel processing is the use of a regional block room. In this situation, the surgeon is working in the OR, but the induction of anesthesia with regional blocks is done in the block room. While the

**VI**

surgeon is finishing the surgery in the preceding patient, regional anesthesia is performed on the next patient. When the OR is cleaned and ready, then the next patient is taken into the OR and the preparation begins immediately. Further, the emergence time period is minimal and time is saved there as well.

Another example is to utilize not another OR but an alternative space to complete tasks. This space may allow for induction of general anesthesia and invasive monitoring to be placed. Alternatively (or in addition), a sterile space is provided to allow for the surgical equipment to be set up on a movable table. Both of these solutions will allow for tasks to be performed while the preceding patient is still in the OR or while the OR is being cleaned.

Several limitations to parallel processing exist. First, all the solutions require additional resources—sometimes physical space, but always additional staff. Economically, these solutions may make sense if the additional revenue is larger than the incremental staffing costs. On the other hand, if overutilized time exists, staffing cost savings may occur even if additional staff members are hired. For instance, hiring an assistant to help the surgical technician set up the surgical equipment may be less costly than having the whole OR staff (including a registered nurse) work overtime. The second limitation is that to do an additional case, the surgical duration must not be long. For example, it makes no sense to implement parallel processing for surgical duration cases of 12 hours, but it may make sense in cases of less than 1 hour. In addition, the surgeon should have the additional patients to fill freed-up OR time. For example, a surgeon

may request two rooms. The operative time needs to be short. Providing a second room seems reasonable. But if the patient volume is too small, then the surgeon will go from one OR with a full schedule to two ORs with a partial schedule in each OR. Finally, the last limitation may occur if the "time-out briefing" is changed. Currently, the process is done immediately before incision. But if the process requires the surgeon to be present prior to induction of anesthesia or regional block, then some of the solutions noted here may not be possible. The technical and clinical skills of all providers, including surgeons, anesthesia providers, nurses, and other OR personnel, are essential components of efficiently managed ORs.

## QUESTIONS OF THE DAY

1. How does the staffing ratio in an anesthesia care team model affect the total number of anesthesia providers needed to administer care in an operating room (OR) suite with 10 ORs?

2. What measurements can be used to assess OR efficiency?

3. Under what circumstances can reduced OR turnover time lead to an increase in number of cases completed in a 10-hour OR day?

4. What is "parallel processing" in the context of OR throughput? Under what circumstances will throughput be improved? What are the limitations to the effectiveness of parallel processing?

## REFERENCES

1. Sandberg WS. Barbarians at the gate. *Anesth Analg.* 2009;109:695–699.
2. Kheterpal S, Tremper KK, Shanks A, et al. Six-year follow-up on work force and finances of the United States anesthesiology training programs: 2000 to 2006. *Anesth Analg.* 2009;109:263–272.
3. Mellow MM, Livingston EH. Managing the risks of concurrent surgeries. *JAMA.* 2016;315:1563–1564.
4. Abouleish AE, Zornow MH. Estimating staffing requirements: how many anesthesia providers does our group need? *ASA Newsletter.* 2001;65:14–16. The 2013 update to this reference can be found at http://monitor.pubs.asahq.org/article.aspx?articleid=2431404&resultClick=3#103544379/; Last Accessed December 15, 2016.
5. Strum DP, Vargas LG, May JH. Surgical subspecialty block utilization and capacity planning. A minimal cost analysis model. *Anesthesiology.* 1999;90:1176–1185.

6. Macario A. Are your hospital operating rooms "efficient"? A scoring system with eight performance indicators. *Anesthesiology.* 2006;105:237–240.
7. McIntosh C, Dexter F, Epstein RH. Impact of service-specific staffing, case scheduling, turnovers, and first-case starts on anesthesia group and operating room productivity: a tutorial using data from an Australian hospital. *Anesth Analg.* 2006;103:1499–1516.
8. Dexter F, Abouleish AE, Epstein RH, et al. Use of operating room information system data to predict the impact of reducing turnover times on staffing. *Anesth Analg.* 2003;97:1119–1126.
9. Dexter F, Macario A. Decrease in case duration required to complete an additional case during regularly scheduled hours in an operating room suite: a computer simulation study. *Anesth Analg.* 1999;88:72–76.

10. Overdyk FJ, Harvey SC, Fishman RL, et al. Successful strategies for improving operating room efficiency at academic institutions. *Anesth Analg.* 1998;86:896–906.
11. Cendan JC, Good M. Interdisciplinary work flow assessment and redesign decreases operating room turnover time and allows for additional caseload. *Arch Surg.* 2006;141:65–69.
12. Sandberg WS, Daily B, Egan M, et al. Deliberate perioperative systems design improves operating room throughput. *Anesthesiology.* 2005;103:406–418.
13. Hanss R, Buttgereit B, Tonner PH, et al. Overlapping induction of anesthesia: an analysis of costs and benefits. *Anesthesiology.* 2003;103:391–400.
14. Torkki PM, Marjamaa RA, Torkki MI, et al. Use of anesthesia induction rooms can increase the number of urgent orthopedic cases completed within 7 hours. *Anesthesiology.* 2005;103:401–405.

15. Smith MP, Sandberg WS, Foss J, et al. High-throughput operating room system for joint arthroplasties durably outperform routine processes. *Anesthesiology*. 2008;109:25–35.

16. Abouleish AE. Increasing operating room throughput: just buzzwords for this decade? *Anesthesiology*. 2008;109:3–4.

17. Sandberg WS. Engineering parallel processing perioperative systems for improved throughput. *ASA Monitor*. 2010;74(1):26–30. http://monitor.pubs.asahq.org/article.aspx?articleid=24467 48&resultClick=3; last accessed February 16, 2017.

## ADDITIONAL RESOURCES

1. Amr Abouleish, Anesthesia Staffing Worksheet. This interactive Excel worksheet allows detailed calculation of staffing requirements of an OR with variable numbers of anesthesiologists, CRNAs, and residents. Worksheets allow entry of faculty nonclinical time and resident away rotations to determine the number of FTEs needed in a department.

2. Sperry RJ. Principles of economic analysis. Basic economic principles written with an anesthesiologist's perspective. *Anesthesiology*. 1997;86:1197–1205.

3. Franklin Dexter. A bibliography of OR management articles can be found at http://www.franklindexter.net/bibliography_TOC.htm; Last Accessed December 15, 2016.

4. ASA Resident Practice Management Tools. Resident Practice Management Education Webpage with podcasts, lectures, and a primer on practice management. Available for ASA members at https://www.asahq.org/about-asa/component-societies/asa-resident-component/resident-resources/resident-practice-management-tools; Last Accessed December 15, 2016.

# 47 AWARENESS UNDER ANESTHESIA

Karen B. Domino and Daniel J. Cole

During interventional/therapeutic procedures, patients may receive drugs that affect the central nervous system (CNS) along a continuum from the awake state to general anesthesia. Dependent upon the nature of the procedure and patient wishes, anesthetic drugs may be given with the intent to produce different levels of sedation or general anesthesia. Patients consenting to receive drugs with the intent to produce only sedation should do so with the understanding that they may have recall of intraoperative events. Conversely, a fundamental component of general anesthesia is unconsciousness and subsequent amnesia. Patients consenting for general anesthesia do so with the expectation that they will not see, hear, feel, or remember intraoperative events.

Amnesia has been a fundamental tenet of training and continuing medical education in anesthesia. Yet, many patients who undergo general anesthesia report preoperative fears of intraoperative awareness, and awareness has been the most important cause of patient dissatisfaction with anesthesia.[1]

## INCIDENCE

Memory consists of explicit, or conscious, memory and implicit, or unconscious, memory. Explicit memory refers to the conscious recollection of previous experiences and is equivalent to remembering. Awareness during anesthesia describes conscious recall (explicit memory) of intraoperative events. However, many more anesthetized patients may respond to commands, yet lack conscious recall of intraoperative events (implicit memory). The anesthetic depth required to block implicit memory is greater than that required to block explicit memory (intraoperative recall).

Intraoperative awareness is best estimated by formally interviewing patients postoperatively, well after discharge from the postanesthesia recovery room.[2] Moreover, memory formation for intraoperative awareness may

| Table 47.1 | Reported Incidence of Intraoperative Awareness | | |
|---|---|---|---|
| Incidence | $N^a$ | Prospective Design | Reference[b] |
| 0.007% | 384,786 | No | 10 |
| 0.1% | 10,811 | No | 2 |
| 0.13% | 18,575 | Yes | 8 |
| 0.15% | 11,785 | Yes | 3 |
| 0.2% | 1000 | Yes | 7 |
| 0.23% | 44,006 | No | 9 |
| 0.41% | 11,101 | Yes | 6 |
| 0.6% | 4001 | Yes | 5 |

[a]Numbers of patients in reported series.
[b]Numbers correspond to references listed at the end of the chapter.

be delayed beyond the immediate recovery period. Sandin and associates[2] reported that only one third of cases of awareness were identified before the patient left the postanesthesia care unit. Often, patients will not voluntarily report awareness if they were not disturbed by it, if embarrassed to do so, or if coping with pain and recovery after major surgery. Therefore, a structured interview (i.e., modified Brice interview) is recommended to evaluate the incidence of awareness[3]:

1. What was the last thing you remember before you went to sleep?
2. What is the first thing you remember after your operation?
3. Can you remember anything in between?
4. Can you remember if you had any dreams during your procedure?
5. What was the worst thing about your procedure?

The methodologies used to assess the incidence of intraoperative awareness are inconsistent, and the results have predictable variation (Table 47.1).[2,4-10] In prospective studies when the Brice interview was used, intraoperative awareness occurred with surprising frequency (1 to 2 per 1000 or greater). The first prospective evaluation of awareness in nearly 12,000 patients undergoing general anesthesia was conducted in Sweden and revealed an incidence of awareness of 0.18% in cases in which neuromuscular blocking drugs were used and 0.10% in the absence of such drugs, for an overall incidence of 0.13% (see Table 47.1).[2] A similar incidence (1 per 1000 patients) was observed in the United States in tertiary care centers. Patients with coexisting morbid conditions tend to have a greater incidence of awareness.[7] Intraoperative awareness and subsequent recall are more likely with a light level of anesthesia, such as occurs during obstetric and cardiac anesthesia.[11] The incidence of awareness is underestimated when assessed using quality improvement and patient self-reporting (see Table 47.1).[8-10,12,13] In 2013, Mashour and associates[14] compared the incidence of awareness in patients who received a standard postanesthesia evaluation to those who received a single modified Brice survey. They found 19 cases of intraoperative awareness out of 19,000 patients were detected by the Brice survey, whereas only 3 were detected by spontaneous report. Significantly, the 3 reported spontaneously were also detected by the Brice survey. It is likely that many patients may have intraoperative awareness that is not detected.

## ETIOLOGY AND RISK FACTORS FOR INTRAOPERATIVE AWARENESS

The three major causes of intraoperative awareness of anesthesia are light anesthesia, increased patient anesthetic requirements, and anesthetic delivery problems.[11,12] Inadequate anesthesia due to reduced anesthetic doses generally occurs because of hemodynamic intolerance of anesthetic drugs or during procedures in which the anesthetic dose is kept deliberately small, such as in cesarean delivery or open heart surgery. Reduced anesthetic doses may be necessary for optimal physiology and safety in patients who are hypovolemic or have limited cardiac reserve. Patients with American Society of Anesthesiologists (ASA) physical status 3 to 5 undergoing major surgery are at increased risk for intraoperative awareness and indeed have a higher incidence of awareness.[7] Patients who experienced intraoperative awareness are more likely to have impaired cardiovascular status, undergo emergency surgery, receive smaller doses of volatile anesthetics, and have experienced an anesthetic with technical difficulties.[15] Children are also more likely to experience awareness.[16]

Anesthetic technique is important in the pathogenesis of awareness during anesthesia. Intraoperative awareness is more likely to occur during induction of anesthesia with nitrous oxide and intravenously administered anesthetics and is less likely to occur when volatile anesthetics are used.[16,17] Use of volatile anesthetics in concentrations at or above 0.7 MAC (minimum alveolar concentration) prevents conscious recall in anesthetized patients similar to that achieved by a brain function monitor of anesthetic depth.[18-20] Unfortunately, neuromuscular blockade prevents an early sign of inadequate anesthesia, namely patient movement. Smaller anesthetic concentrations are needed more to prevent awareness than to render immobility; therefore, an inadequately anesthetized, nonparalyzed patient usually moves first and demonstrates clear evidence of inadequate anesthesia.

Some patients, such as those using alcohol, opioids, amphetamines, and cocaine, may require an increase in anesthetic dose.[11] Moreover, although incompletely

VI

defined, genetic factors may influence anesthetic requirements. Patients with a past history of awareness are more likely to experience awareness compared to patients without a past history of awareness.[21] Finally, equipment problems with the vaporizer or intravenous infusion devices may lead to awareness, although these are less common causes of awareness, especially with use of end-tidal anesthetic gas analysis.[15]

## PSYCHOLOGICAL SEQUELAE

Awareness under general anesthesia can be a traumatic experience, with approximately one third of patients experiencing long-term psychological sequelae.[22-24] However, some patients do not develop long-term psychological sequelae after intraoperative awareness[25] and many patients without awareness have psychological symptoms consistent with posttraumatic stress disorder (PTSD).[23] Some of the most common recalled awareness experiences include auditory sounds, feelings of paralysis, seeing lights, and feelings of helplessness, fear, or anxiety.[26] Pain is less common, although it does occur in some patients, particularly those with complete neuromuscular blockade who are unable to move. Psychological sequelae of recalled memories may include flashbacks, anxiety/nervousness, loneliness, nightmares, and fear/panic attacks that vary from bothersome to distressing.[22,26] Some patients develop severe, persistent symptoms that profoundly interfere with interpersonal relationships and daily activities.[26]

The risk factors for developing PTSD after awareness during general anesthesia are not completely known. An acute emotional reaction to the experience significantly predicted the development of long-term psychological sequelae.[22] Dissociation related to surgery and perceiving that one's life was threatened were associated with PTSD.[23] Paralysis from neuromuscular blockade is particularly traumatic.[27] The role of premorbid depression and other psychological conditions is unclear, but may contribute to risk of PTSD.[23,28] Recurrence of trauma can trigger previous psychological symptoms.

More reporting from patients also increases the understanding of the experiences. In 2007, the ASA established the Anesthesia Awareness Registry to address the concerns of patients with regard to intraoperative awareness.[29] The Registry collected patient self-reports of unintended awareness during general anesthesia to provide a patient perspective on their expectations and experiences of awareness. The Registry was designed to be consistent with "patient-centered" care and focused on patient preferences, needs, and values. Although the Registry relied on patients to volunteer to participate, and therefore had response bias, the results are valid to point out causes and possible solutions to patient dissatisfaction with unexpected recall during surgery.

One finding from the Registry is that patients may have different expectations than anesthesia providers concerning the lack of explicit recall during regional anesthesia or sedation. The Anesthesia Awareness Registry recruited patients who self-identified as having awareness during general anesthesia. However, upon review of the perioperative records, one third of patients had mistakenly believed that they received general anesthesia; instead, they actually received sedation or regional anesthesia.[26] This result shows a disconnect between anesthesia providers' and patients' expectations concerning unconsciousness during surgery. This disconnection may be resolved by improved physician-patient communication concerning the possible recall of events during sedation as well as improved informed consent.

Patients also complain of psychological sequelae after awareness during regional anesthesia or sedation.[8,22,26,27] Some patients may experience psychological consequences because of explicit recall of events during regional anesthesia that were similar to consequences resulting from recall during general anesthesia.[26] Approximately 40% of these patients had persistent psychological sequelae, similar to those with awareness during general anesthesia.[26]

Early psychotherapeutic intervention may reduce the likelihood of acute and long-term psychological sequelae.[23] An explanation or validation of the awareness incident may affect the presence and duration of the psychological consequences. However, if patients do not inform their anesthesia provider of their recall from general anesthesia, they are less likely to know that they should seek psychological therapy.

The Anesthesia Awareness Registry found that most (75%) of the patients with awareness during general anesthesia were dissatisfied with the manner in which their concerns were addressed by their health care providers.[30] Half of the patients reported that neither their anesthesia provider nor the surgeon expressed concern about their awareness experience. Few were offered an apology (10%) or referral for counseling (35%), an explanation (28%), or discussion or follow-up to the awareness episode (26%). Several patients mentioned they were too ill to care about their awareness experience while acutely recovering from surgery or their memory became clearer after days and weeks following surgery. Some patients recommended that anesthesia providers give them a business card to facilitate contact after hospital discharge. Clearly, patients need more systematic responses and follow-up by health care providers.

## PREVENTION OF AWARENESS

Conventional monitoring of anesthetic depth has included rudimentary signs such as patient movement, autonomic changes, tearing, perspiration, and subjective clinical instinct. Autonomic changes, such as an increase in arterial

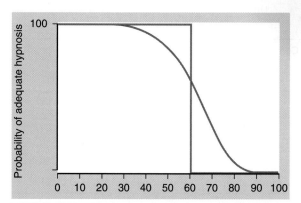

**Fig. 47.1** Probability of adequate hypnosis based upon brain function monitoring index. The straight line is the ideal probability curve with 100% sensitivity and specificity. The curved line is a more realistic expectation of monitoring in which a progressive decrease of the monitored index value correlates with increased probability of adequate hypnosis. (From Cole DJ, Domino KB. Depth of anesthesia: clinical applications, intraoperative awareness and beyond. In Schwartz AJ, ed. *ASA Refresher Courses in Anesthesiology.* Philadelphia: Lippincott, Williams & Wilkins; 2007.)

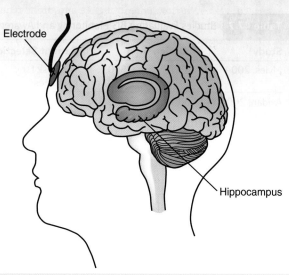

**Fig. 47.2** A brain function monitor typically records cortical electrical activity from a sensor placed on the forehead. Memory is a biochemical function that occurs in the hippocampus, which is some distance from the recording of brain electrical activity.

blood pressure and heart rate, do not reliably predict intraoperative awareness. Indeed, intraoperative awareness can occur in the absence of tachycardia or hypertension.[31] With the advent of anesthetic gas analyzers, anesthetic depth has also been assessed by surrogate data such as determining the dose of volatile anesthetic administered to the patient.[18] In addition, considerable effort has been devoted to establishing a monitor that will reliably determine a patient's depth of anesthesia and hence the risk for intraoperative awareness. Several different devices are commercially available, yet none is 100% effective. These monitors typically collect spontaneous or evoked brain electrical activity, and then process the raw data by a proprietary algorithm and display data to the clinician as a quantitative data point (e.g., number from 0 to 100).

At present there are at least three inherent obstacles to the development of a "foolproof" monitor of anesthetic depth based on electrical activity of the brain and its ability to detect intraoperative awareness. First, at present we have not comprehensively validated a unitary mechanism of general anesthesia, and thus various anesthetics are likely to produce unique electrical activity at a given anesthetic depth. Consequently, a unique algorithm to each specific anesthetic regimen would likely be required for optimal correlation between electrical signals in the brain and anesthetic depth. Second, general anesthesia occurs on a continuum without a quantitative dimension, and there is considerable interpatient pharmacodynamic variability to a specific anesthetic. Attempting to translate a conscious or unconscious state into a quantitative number can at best be limited to the art of probability with an expectation of false positive and false negative data (Fig. 47.1).[32] Finally, there is the likelihood of cortical electrical activity having sensitivity and specificity to a biochemical event that occurs at a distant subcortical structure (hippocampus) that forms memory (Fig. 47.2).

Published suggestions for the prevention of awareness include premedication with an amnestic drug such as a benzodiazepine, giving adequate doses of drugs to induce anesthesia, avoiding muscle paralysis unless necessary, and administering a volatile anesthetic at a dose of 0.7 MAC or more with monitoring of end-tidal levels to ensure delivery of adequate levels of volatile anesthetics.[18,33]

In 2004, the Joint Commission issued a *Sentinel Alert* that contained suggestions for preventing and managing intraoperative awareness.[34] Their recommendations included the development and implementation of an anesthesia awareness policy, including staff education, informed consent for high-risk patients, and timely maintenance of anesthesia equipment. Also advised were postoperative follow-up of all patients who have undergone general anesthesia and postoperative counseling for patients with awareness.

## Brain Function Monitoring

In general, devices that monitor brain electrical activity for the purpose of assessing depth of anesthesia record electroencephalographic (EEG) activity (also see Chapter 20). Some devices process spontaneous EEG and electromyographic activity and others measure evoked responses to auditory stimuli. Most of the research concerning depth of anesthesia has been performed with the bispectral index (BIS) monitor.

The BIS monitor uses a proprietary algorithm to convert a single channel of frontal EEG activities into an index of hypnotic level, ranging from 100 (awake) to 0

**VI**

**Table 47.2** Studies Evaluating BIS Monitoring and Awareness

| Study[a] | Design | n | Patient Selection | Comparison | Findings |
|---|---|---|---|---|---|
| Myles, 2004[35] | RCT | 2500 | High risk for awareness | BIS-guided (40-60) vs. routine care | BIS-guided group reduced awareness (0.17% vs. 0.91%) |
| Avidan, 2008[18] | RCT | 2000 | High risk for awareness | BIS-guided vs. ETAG-guided (0.7-1.3 MAC) | No difference in awareness BIS-guided vs. ETAG-guided (0.2%) |
| Avidan, 2011[19] | RCT | 6041 | High risk for awareness | BIS-guided vs. ETAG-guided (0.7-1.3 MAC) | No difference in awareness BIS-guided vs. ETAG-guided |
| Zhang, 2011[36] | RCT | 5228 | TIVA | BIS-guided (40-60) vs. control group | BIS-guided group reduced awareness (0.14% vs. 0.65%) |
| Mashour, 2012[20] | RCT | 21,601 | Unselected surgical population | BIS-guided vs. anesthetic concentration | No difference in awareness BIS-guided vs. anesthetic concentration (0.08% vs. 0.12%). Post hoc analysis: BIS may decrease awareness compared to routine care. |

[a]Superscript numbers correspond to references listed at the end of the chapter.
*BIS*, Bispectral index; *ETAG*, end-tidal anesthetic gas; *MAC*, minimum alveolar concentration; *RCT*, randomized control trial; *TIVA*, total intravenous anesthesia.

(isoelectric electroencephalogram). Specific ranges of 40 to 60 are recommended to reduce the risk of consciousness during general anesthesia. Five major randomized controlled trials on the incidence of awareness have been performed using the BIS (Table 47.2).[18-20,35,36] Most studies were performed among patients with a high or likely risk for intraoperative awareness (e.g., high-risk cardiac surgery, impaired cardiovascular status, trauma surgery, cesarean section, and patients with chronic benzodiazepine or opioid use, heavy alcohol intake, or prior history of awareness).[18,19,35] Myles and associates[35] compared BIS-guided anesthesia (BIS 40 to 60) to routine care. Intraoperative awareness occurred in 2 patients (0.17%) when BIS monitors were used to guide anesthesia and in 11 patients (0.91%) managed by routine clinical practice ($p < 0.02$).[35] Two subsequent studies, also in high-risk patients,[18,19] compared the incidence of awareness with BIS-guided anesthesia to end-tidal gas–guided anesthesia (0.7% to 1.3% age-adjusted MAC). These studies found no difference in awareness between the two monitoring modalities. During total intravenous anesthesia (TIVA), BIS-guided anesthesia reduced the incidence of awareness compared to routine care.[36] A large effectiveness study in an unselected surgical population found no differences in awareness between BIS-guided and anesthetic concentration-guided anesthesia.[20] However, post hoc analysis suggested that BIS monitoring may decrease awareness compared to routine care. A Cochrane systematic review concluded that BIS-guided anesthesia is superior to care using clinical signs alone, especially in patients receiving TIVA and those at high-risk for awareness.[37] In contrast, BIS-guided anesthesia does not decrease awareness when compared to end-tidal anesthetic gas monitoring.[37]

These findings are not surprising as TIVA is associated with more frequent interindividual variability.[10] Although all of the studies were performed using the BIS monitor, other processed EEG monitors would likely yield the same results for several reasons. Because of the infrequency of intraoperative awareness, the ability of brain monitors to detect or prevent awareness in an individual patient is poor. Accordingly, the cost of monitoring low-risk patients undergoing general anesthesia is high.[38]

## ASA PRACTICE ADVISORY ON INTRAOPERATIVE AWARENESS AND BRAIN FUNCTION MONITORS

The ASA approved a practice advisory on "Intraoperative Awareness and Brain Function Monitoring" in 2005.[33] This advisory has not been updated because the original recommendations are still valid. A practice advisory is a systematically developed report that is intended to assist clinical decision making in areas in which scientific evidence is insufficient to compel a specific decision matrix. Advisories are approved only after a synthesis and analysis of expert opinion, clinical feasibility data are obtained, open-forum commentary is provided, and consensus surveys are acquired. Advisories are not intended as standards or guidelines. The four areas of advice pertain to preoperative evaluation, preinduction phase of anesthesia, intraoperative monitoring, and intraoperative and postoperative management as summarized in Box 47.1.[33]

The preoperative evaluation should involve review of past medical records for potential risk factors for intraoperative awareness. In addition, the patient interview

---

**Box 47.1** Recommendations to Prevent Awareness During General Anesthesia[a]

**Preoperative Evaluation**
- Identify potential risk factors for awareness.
- Interview patient.
- Obtain informed consent for patients at increased risk for awareness.

**Preinduction Phase of Anesthesia**
- Use checklist for machine/equipment check.
- Verify function of intravenous access and infusion equipment.
- Consider preoperative benzodiazepine.

**Intraoperative Monitoring**
- Use multiple modalities to monitor depth of anesthesia.
- Clinical (e.g., purposeful or reflex movement).
- Conventional monitors (e.g., end-tidal anesthetic analyzer, HR, BP).
- Brain function monitoring on a case-by-case basis. Recent studies demonstrate that if a volatile anesthetic is the primary anesthetic, use of end-tidal anesthetic concentration of more than 0.7 age-adjusted MAC in high-risk patients reduces the incidence of awareness. During total intravenous anesthesia, maintaining BIS of 40-60 reduces awareness compared to routine care.

**Intraoperative and Postoperative Management**
- Consider benzodiazepine if patient unexpectedly becomes conscious.
- Speak with patient postoperatively.
- Consider structured interview or Brice questionnaire to determine patient's experience.
- Report occurrence for continuous quality improvement.
- Offer patient psychological counseling.

[a]This practice advisory has not been updated; additional recommendations are based upon multiple randomized controlled trials comparing brain function monitoring using processed electroencephalographic monitoring.
*ASA*, American Society of Anesthesiologists; *BIS*, bispectral index; *BP*, blood pressure; *HR*, heart rate; *MAC*, minimum alveolar concentration. Modified from American Society of Anesthesiologists Task Force on Intraoperative Awareness. Practice advisory for intraoperative awareness and brain function monitoring: a report by the American Society of Anesthesiologists Task Force on Intraoperative Awareness. *Anesthesiology*. 2006;104:847-864.

---

should assess the presence of other potential anesthetic and surgical risk factors. Finally, the advisory recommends that an informed consent discussion include the potential for intraoperative awareness in high-risk patients.[33]

The routine for the preinduction phase of anesthesia should include a checklist protocol for anesthesia machine and equipment and verification of the proper functioning of intravenous access and infusion equipment, including the presence of appropriate backflow check valves. Finally, the anesthesia provider should consider administration of a benzodiazepine on a case-by-case basis for selected patients, especially in patients at increased risk for intraoperative awareness. This recommendation was made even though the data supporting the ability of preoperative benzodiazepines to reduce the incidence of intraoperative awareness are not evident, and preoperative benzodiazepines may convey some risk of postoperative delirium in geriatric patients (also see Chapter 35).

The advisory recommends that multiple modalities be used to monitor depth of anesthesia. These modalities include clinical techniques such as checking for purposeful or reflex movement, conventional monitoring systems (e.g., electrocardiogram, arterial blood pressure monitoring, heart rate), and, finally, analysis of the dose of volatile anesthetic delivered to the patient by an end-tidal anesthetic analyzer. The advisory recommends use of a brain function monitor on a case-by-case basis determined by the individual practitioner for selected patients.[33]

Regarding the intraoperative and postoperative management, the decision to administer a benzodiazepine intraoperatively after a patient unexpectedly becomes conscious should be made on a case-by-case basis.[33] Although a benzodiazepine may be given after such an event, little scientific evidence exists that supports such treatment. The anesthesia provider should speak with patients who report intraoperative awareness to obtain details of the event and to discuss possible reasons for its occurrence. A questionnaire or structured interview may be used to obtain a detailed account of the patient's experience. Once an episode of intraoperative awareness is reported, an occurrence report concerning the event should be completed for the purpose of continuous quality improvement. And finally, the anesthesia provider should offer counseling or psychological support to those patients who report an episode of intraoperative awareness.

## MEDICOLEGAL SEQUELAE OF AWARENESS

As with most complications of anesthesia, the occurrence of an episode of intraoperative awareness does not necessarily mean that a malpractice claim will follow. Only 1 out of 25 patient injuries from negligent care results in a malpractice claim, with even fewer claims arising from injuries owing to standard care.[39] For intraoperative awareness, there is an enormous disparity between the number of patients who might suffer awareness (based upon incidence statistics) and the few awareness claims (approximately 10 per year) that enter the Anesthesia Closed Claims Project database. This database captures claims from liability insurers, which insure approximately one third of anesthesiologists in the United States. This large disparity between the incidence of awareness and malpractice claims is likely due to both the nature and severity of the injuries associated with awareness, as well as the medicolegal and injury compensation systems.

Episodes of awareness that do not result in severe short-term or significant long-term sequelae will not enter the malpractice system. Empathetic explanation of the cause of an awareness episode or an apology may not only be therapeutic, but also helpful in preventing escalation of problems to the point of initiation of a malpractice claim. In addition, malpractice claims are biased by the large prevalence of negligent or substandard care, an essential component of the tort system.

Factors that increase the likelihood that a patient will initiate a claim are poor communication, unmet expectations, and financial pressures on the patient. A study by Huycke and Huycke surveying individuals who had contacted law firms regarding the initiation of malpractice claims found that 50% of these potential plaintiffs felt they had a poor relationship with their physician.[40] Anesthesia providers have a very brief window of opportunity for establishing a good relationship with a patient preoperatively (also see Chapter 13). Compounding the problem of brief preoperative contact are descriptions from closed claims incidences of complaints of patients not having had an opportunity to discuss their intraoperative awareness with their anesthesia provider postoperatively. In addition, their concerns regarding awareness may have been dismissed by health care providers. An insensitive reception to a patient's report of awareness by the anesthesia and other health care providers may exacerbate injury and contribute to a patient's initiation of a malpractice claim. Patients with awareness may avoid situations that trigger painful memories, which the litigation process will certainly emphasize. In addition, most plaintiffs' lawyers work on a contingency-fee basis, taking a percentage of the award as a fee and earning nothing if the plaintiff loses the case. In a system in which plaintiffs' lawyers must bear the initial costs of the litigation, they will weigh the merits of any potential case. It would be poor business practice to take cases with either a small probability of success or with historically limited financial compensation. Therefore, lawyers are the de facto gatekeepers to the legal system.

### Data From the Anesthesia Closed Claims Project

The Anesthesia Closed Claims Project is a structured evaluation of adverse anesthetic outcomes obtained from the files of 20 participating liability insurance companies in the United States. The project contains over 10,000 medical malpractice claims, including 1800 from injuries occurring in the 2000s. The major outcomes in the Anesthesia Closed Claims Project database are death, brain damage, and nerve injury. In contrast, claims for awareness during general anesthesia form a small portion of malpractice claims. Out of 1800 anesthesia claims related to surgical/procedural anesthesia or obstetric anesthesia,

only 2.6% ($n = 46$) were due to awareness during general anesthesia. The majority were female (74%), healthy (57% ASA status 1-2), younger than 60 years old (80%), and underwent elective procedures (83%). These demographics reflect patients at small risk for awareness. One third involved obvious anesthetic delivery problems, including medication errors ($n = 7$), anesthesia delivery problems (vaporizer malfunction [$n = 7$]), and intravenous catheter infiltration ($n = 1$).

Plaintiffs received payment in 63% of the awareness claims, similar to claims for injuries in the Anesthesia Closed Claims Project database. However, payment amounts were smaller for awareness (median payment $78,000 with range of $1000 to $469,000, adjusted for inflation to 2015 dollars) compared to other injuries in the database (median payment $342,000, range $660 to $35.8 million).

## SUMMARY

Amnesia is a fundamental component of general anesthesia. Accordingly, monitoring for depth of anesthesia is an important factor in the anesthetic management of patients. When considering depth of anesthesia as it relates to the risk of intraoperative awareness, the following points are key:

- The incidence as defined by prospective trials is generally accepted to be 1 to 2 per 1000 patients.
- There is the potential for serious psychological and medicolegal sequelae when a patient suffers an episode of awareness under general anesthesia.
- An equipment check is paramount to the prevention of intraoperative awareness.
- Amnestic drugs might be considered for both preventive treatment of intraoperative awareness and as a treatment for patients who have had an episode of inadequate anesthesia (although it should be noted that data supporting such treatment are not available).
- It is advisable to administer additional hypnotics in clinical situations that have a risk for intraoperative awareness (e.g., difficult airway).
- Hemodynamics are unreliable as a predictor of inadequate anesthesia.
- There is no proven awareness monitor that has 100% sensitivity and specificity. Multimodality monitoring is recommended. This should include clinical signs, end-tidal volatile anesthetic gas monitor, and the consideration of a brain function monitor, especially for patients receiving TIVA.
- Consider at least a 0.7 MAC level of a volatile anesthetic.
- Neuromuscular blockers will mask an important indicator of inadequate anesthesia.

## QUESTIONS OF THE DAY

1. What are the major causes of intraoperative awareness during general anesthesia? How does neuromuscular blockade contribute to the risk of awareness?
2. What are the potential psychological sequelae of awareness?
3. How does brain function monitoring or end-tidal anesthetic monitoring compare to routine clinical signs in reducing the risk of intraoperative awareness?
4. What are the major recommendations from the American Society of Anesthesiologists to prevent awareness during general anesthesia?
5. What factors increase the likelihood of a malpractice claim after a patient experiences intraoperative recall?

## REFERENCES

1. Myles PS, Williams DL, Hendrata M, et al. Patient satisfaction after anaesthesia and surgery: results of a prospective survey of 10,811 patients. *Br J Anaesth*. 2000;84:6–10.
2. Sandin RH, Enlund G, Samuelsson P, et al. Awareness during anaesthesia: a prospective case study. *Lancet*. 2000;355:707–711.
3. Brice DD, Hetherington RR, Utting JE. A simple study of awareness and dreaming during anaesthesia. *Br J Anaesth*. 1970;42:535–542.
4. Errando CL, Sigl JC, Robles M, et al. Awareness with recall during general anaesthesia: a prospective observation evaluation of 4001 patients. *Br J Anaesth*. 2008;101:178–185.
5. Xu L, Wu AS, Yue Y. The incidence of intra-operative awareness during general anesthesia in China: a multi-center observational study. *Acta Anaesthesiol Scand*. 2009;53:873–882.
6. Nordstrom O, Engstrom AM, Persson S, Sandin R. Incidence of awareness in total i.v. anaesthesia based on propofol, alfentanil and neuromuscular blockade. *Acta Anaesthesiol Scand*. 1997;41(8):978–984.
7. Sebel PS, Bowdle TA, Ghoneim MM, et al. The incidence of awareness during anesthesia: a multicenter United States study. *Anesth Analg*. 2004;99:833–839.
8. Mashour GA, Wang LY, Turner CR, et al. A retrospective study of intraoperative awareness with methodological implications. *Anesth Analg*. 2009;108:521–526.
9. Pollard RJ, Coyle JP, Gilbert RL, et al. Intraoperative awareness in a regional medical system: a review of 3 years' data. *Anesthesiology*. 2007;106:269–274.
10. Mashour GA, Avidan MS. Intraoperative awareness: controversies and non-controversies. *Br J Anaesth*. 2015;115(suppl 1):i20–i24.
11. Ghoneim MM, Block RI, Haffarnan M, Mathews MJ. Awareness during anesthesia: risk factors, causes and sequelae: a review of reported cases in the literature. *Anesth Analg*. 2009;108(2):527–535.
12. Pandit JJ, Andrade J, Bogod DB, et al. 5th National Audit Project (NAP5) on accidental awareness during general anaesthesia: summary of main findings and risk factors. *Br J Anaesth*. 2014;113:549–559.
13. Pandit JJ, Cook TM, Jonker WR, et al. A national survey of anaesthetists (NAP5 Baseline) to estimate an annual incidence of accidental awareness during general anaesthesia in the UK. *Br J Anaesth*. 2013;68(4):343–353.
14. Mashour GA, Kent C, Picton P, et al. Assessment of intraoperative awareness with explicit recall: a comparison of 2 methods. *Anesth Analg*. 2013;116:889–891.
15. Myles PS. Prevention of awareness during anaesthesia. *Best Pract Res Clin Anaesthesiol*. 2007;21:345–355.
16. Davidson AJ, Smith KR, Blusse von Oud-Ablas HJ, et al. Awareness in children: a secondary analysis of five cohort studies. *Anaesthesia*. 2011;66:446–454.
17. Moerman N, Bonke B, Oosting J. Awareness and recall during general anesthesia. Facts and feelings. *Anesthesiology*. 1993;79:454–464.
18. Avidan MS, Zhang L, Burnside BA, et al. Anesthesia awareness and the bispectral index. *N Engl J Med*. 2008;358:1097–1108.
19. Avidan MS, Jacobson E, Glick D, et al. Prevention of intraoperative awareness in a high-risk surgical population. *N Engl J Med*. 2011;365:591–600.
20. Mashour GA, Shanks A, Tremper KK, et al. Prevention of intraoperative awareness with explicit recall in an unselected surgical population: a randomized comparative effectiveness trial. *Anesthesiology*. 2012;117:717–725.
21. Aranake A, Gradwohl S, Ben-Abdallah A, et al. Increased risk of intraoperative awareness in patients with a history of awareness. *Anesthesiology*. 2013;119:1275–1283.
22. Samuelsson P, Brudin L, Sandin RH. Late psychological symptoms after awareness among consecutively included surgical patients. *Anesthesiology*. 2007;106:26–32.
23. Whitlock E, Rodebaugh T, Hassett A, et al. Pyschological sequelae of surgery in a prospective cohort of patients from three intraoperative awareness prevention trials. *Anesth Analg*. 2015;120:87–95.
24. Leslie K, Chan MT, Forbes A, et al. Post-traumatic stress disorder in aware patients from the B-Aware trial. *Anesth Analg*. 2010;110:823–828.
25. Laukkala T, Ranta S, Wennervita J, et al. Long-term psychosocial outcomes after intraoperative awareness with recall. *Anesth Analg*. 2014;119:86–92.
26. Kent CD, Mashour GA, Metzger NA, et al. Psychological impact of unexpected explicit recall of events occurring during surgery performed under sedation, regional anaesthesia, and general anaesthesia: data from the Anesthesia Awareness Registry. *Br J Anaesth*. 2013;110(3):381–387.
27. Cook TM, Andrade J, Bogod DG, et al. 5th National Audit Project (NAP5) on accidental awareness during general anaesthesia: patient experiences, human factors, sedation, consent, and medicolegal issues. *Br J Anaesth*. 2014;113:560–574.
28. Ranta SO, Laurila R, Saario J, et al. Awareness with recall during general anaesthesia: incidence and risk factors. *Anesth Analg*. 1998;86:1084–1089.
29. Anesthesia Awareness Registry. www.awaredb.org.
30. Kent CD, Posner KL, Mashour GA, et al. Patient perspectives on intraoperative awareness with explicit recall: report from a North American anaesthesia awareness registry. *Br J Anaesth*. 2015;115(suppl 1):i114–i121.
31. Domino KB, Posner KL, Caplan RA, et al. Awareness during anesthesia: a closed claims analysis. *Anesthesiology*. 1999;90:1053–1061.
32. Cole DJ, Domino KB. Depth of anesthesia: clinical applications, intraoperative awareness and beyond. In: Schwartz AJ, ed. *ASA Refresher Courses in Anesthesiology*. vol. 35. Philadelphia: Lippincott, Williams & Wilkins; 2007:51–52.
33. American Society of Anesthesiologists Task Force on Intraoperative Awareness. Practice advisory for intraoperative awareness and brain function monitoring: a report by the American Society of Anesthesiologists Task Force on Intraoperative Awareness. *Anesthesiology*. 2006;104:847–864.
34. The Joint Commission. Preventing, and managing the impact of, anesthesia awareness. *Sentinel Event Alert*; Oct. 6, 2004: 1–3. https://www.jointcommission.org/sentinel_event_alert_issue_32_preventing_and_managing_the_impact_of_anesthesia_awareness. Accessed May 11, 2015.

VI

35. Myles PS, Leslie K, McNeil J, et al. Bispectral index monitoring to prevent awareness during anaesthesia: the B-Aware randomised controlled trial. *Lancet.* 2004;363:1757–1763.

36. Zhang C, Xu L, Ma YQ, et al. Bispectral index monitoring prevent awareness during total intravenous anesthesia: a prospective, randomized, double-blinded, multi-center controlled trial. *Chin Med J.* 2011;124(22):3664–3669.

37. Punjasawadwong Y, Phongchiewboon A, Bunchungmongkol N. Bispectral index for improving anaesthetic delivery and postoperative recovery (review). *Cochrane Database Syst Rev.* 2014;(6): CD003843.

38. O'Connor MF, Daves SM, Tung A, et al. BIS monitoring to prevent awareness during general anesthesia. *Anesthesiology.* 2001;94:520–522.

39. Studdert DM, Mello MM, Gawande AA, et al. Claims, errors, and compensation payments in medical malpractice litigation. *N Engl J Med.* 2006;354:2024–2033.

40. Huycke LI, Huycke MM. Characteristics of potential plaintiffs in malpractice litigation. *Ann Intern Med.* 1994;120:792–798.

# 48 QUALITY AND PATIENT SAFETY IN ANESTHESIA CARE

## Avery Tung

Clinical anesthesia practice is often labeled as a model for quality and safety in medicine. In 1999, the Institute of Medicine (now the Health and Medicine Division of the National Academies) report, "To Err Is Human: Building a Safer Health System," specifically identified anesthesia as "an area in which very impressive improvements in safety have been made." Such attention to a specialty comprising approximately 5% of U.S. physicians highlights the many contributions to overall perioperative quality and safety generated by the specialty of anesthesia. Although actual reductions in anesthesia-specific mortality rates are controversial,[1] ailing patients are anesthetized for more invasive operations than a few decades ago. The principles by which anesthesiologists transformed the inherently dangerous task of reversibly blunting human responses to pain and physical damage and controlling vital life-support functions into a safe and almost routine occurrence should be familiar to all practicing anesthesia providers.

This chapter reviews the history of anesthesia quality and safety, identifies key approaches and strategies that have contributed not only to anesthesia but to other medical specialties, and examines current and future challenges in anesthesia-related quality and safety.

## DEFINITIONS: QUALITY VERSUS SAFETY

Quality and safety are related terms but are not identical. Safety refers to a lack of harm and focuses on avoiding adverse events. If patient injury is avoided, then the process is safe. In contrast, quality refers to the optimal performance of a task, which may refer to outcome,

The editors and publisher would like to thank Drs. Vinod Malhotra and Patricia Fogarty-Mack for contributing to this chapter in the previous edition of this work. It has served as the foundation for the current chapter.

efficiency, cost, satisfaction, or some other metric of performance in addition to avoiding injury.

It is easy to see how quality and safety do not always overlap. As an example, a process can in principle always be made somewhat safer by installing an additional check or adding extra equipment. Taken to its extreme, it can be argued that an anesthesia provider is not fully safe unless a fiberoptic scope is in the operating room for induction of anesthesia. Another example is concluding that safety could be improved by having a second (or third) anesthesia provider in the room as well! Clearly, such an approach could incrementally create more safety but would not necessarily produce more quality. In contrast, quality includes an "optimization" element, so if a process is changed to produce better patient satisfaction, for example, or a shorter length of stay, it represents higher quality but not necessarily better safety.

In the anesthesia realm, the use of ultrasound to place central lines is an example of a strategy that improves both quality and safety. By reducing the incidence of carotid puncture,[2] ultrasound clearly improves safety. By reducing the time to successful insertion (and the number of misses), ultrasound improves quality as well. In contrast, pin indexing backup oxygen tanks adds safety, but does not really change quality.

Historically, advances in anesthesia performance have addressed both quality and safety as described in this chapter.

## SPECIFIC APPROACHES TO ANESTHESIA SAFETY

### Learning From Experience

Because the mechanisms by which most anesthetics exert their effects are not fully understood, and because many intraoperative states (one-lung ventilation, muscle relaxation, cardiopulmonary bypass) are not found in normal human activity, a large component of anesthesia safety is derived from a history of empiric observation and experience. Driven by the goal of minimizing anesthesia-specific fatality and the shockingly high mortality rate during the early years of anesthesia practice,[3] anesthesiologists have over time systematically accumulated an experience base of observations about safety. Emery A. Rovenstine's case series of nine cardiac arrests, published in 1951,[4] is an example of this empiric approach. Although he offered no definitive solution, his practical observations (e.g., cardiac massage through the diaphragm is ineffective, the differential diagnosis of shock versus cardiac standstill can be difficult) allowed anesthesia providers to incrementally and empirically improve anesthesia safety.

Beecher and Todd's exhaustive 1954 study of anesthesia-associated deaths in 10 centers over 4 years stands as a prime example of the empiric approach to anesthesia safety.[3] Involving 21 physicians and 11 secretaries over 5 years, Beecher tracked the outcomes of 599,548 anesthetics, identified 7977 deaths (more than 1 in 100) and cataloged the causes as from patient disease, surgical error, or anesthesia. Their observation that patients who had received neuromuscular blocking drugs had a significantly higher perioperative morbidity rate is still a subject for anesthesia trainees today.

Other examples of empirically derived anesthesia safety observations include the surprising difficulty in detecting esophageal intubation (or arterial desaturation), the tendency of some anesthetics (e.g., desflurane) to trigger hypertensive tachycardic responses,[5] the dangers of circuit disconnection, and the potential for delivery of a hypoxic gas mixture. In all, the anesthesia approach has been to identify and describe such events, determine how they might occur in clinical practice, develop and test countermeasures, and disseminate the results through technical improvements or education. Although most of these anesthesia-related adverse events are by now rare in occurrence, they highlight a key approach: recognize a potentially preventable event, evaluate its likelihood, and systematically develop countermeasures to reduce the incidence. Taken together, observations such as these have led to reductions in anesthesia-related mortality rates, with current estimates ranging from 1:250,000 for healthy patients[6] to 1:1500 for those with complex medical problems.[1]

In addition to empiric observations about patient-related safety, anesthesiologists have addressed safety issues related to provider performance. An everyday example is in the interface between the anesthesia provider and anesthesia delivery system (also see Chapter 15). As in aviation, the human–anesthesia machine interface has been designed specifically to reduce inadvertent errors. In the same way that levers in an airplane for landing gear and flap control have a knob shaped like a wheel and a flap, for example, so is the knob on an anesthesia machine for oxygen gas flow shaped differently from knobs controlling air and nitrous oxide, and it is always located on the right. Similarly, the potentially dangerous delivery of hypoxic gas mixtures is prevented by "linking" the oxygen flow to the nitrous oxide flow so that oxygen is always present in fresh gas flow. Nonuniversal connectors to ensure that oxygen is being delivered through the oxygen flowmeter, and an oxygen analyzer to serve as a final check on the delivered gas mixture are other examples of safety mechanisms designed to avoid the inadvertent delivery of a hypoxic gas mixture.

Even though adverse events due to failure of mechanical ventilation or hypoxic gas delivery have almost been eradicated in anesthesia, this process of empiric observation continues today. Recent awareness of the dangers of anemia during spine surgery (also see Chapter 32),[7] hypotension in the sitting position (also see Chapter 19),[8] or the role of fibrinogen in coagulopathy during maternal hemorrhage (also see Chapter 33)[9] are current examples of issues identified through empiric observation.

## Adoption of Specialty-Wide Standards

Because anesthesia is normally administered in conjunction with therapeutic or diagnostic procedures, identifying adverse outcomes attributable specifically to the anesthesia practice is challenging. In fact, one of Beecher and Todd's explicit goals in their landmark study was to define "the extent of the responsibility which must be borne by anesthesia for failure in the care of the surgical patient."[3] Because adverse events clearly attributed to anesthesia are rare, promulgating appropriate countermeasures across the specialty is difficult. Nevertheless, anesthesia was the first medical specialty to embrace universally applicable standards, developing and promulgating a set of monitoring recommendations with the goal of reducing anesthesia-related adverse events. Driven in part by high malpractice awards, these standards included continuous anesthesiologist presence and vital sign monitoring including blood pressure, heart rate, electrocardiogram, breathing system oxygen concentration, and temperature and were initially published as a research article from a single health care consortium[10] and developed from a database of adverse events.

Although not evidence-based, these standards were incorporated as intraoperative monitoring standards by the American Society of Anesthesiologists (ASA) 2 months later and have remained as one of only three practice standards endorsed by the ASA (the other two being standards for pre- and postoperative care).[11] Since their adoption, conclusive evidence for the efficacy of these standards has remained elusive, but retrospective observations have suggested benefit. In a follow-up study, the authors of the monitoring standards published a case series of 11 major intraoperative accidents attributable to anesthesia from 1976 to 1988, but found that only one occurred after universal adoption of the monitoring standards.[12] Observations from the ASA Closed Claims Project database also suggest a reduction in the number of claims for death or permanent brain damage during that period.[13]

Whether monitoring standards or (possibly) new technologies were responsible for a perceived reduction in adverse events, the willingness of anesthesia providers as a group to adopt practice standards remains an approach almost unique to anesthesiologists and a marker for the priority anesthesiologists put on safety.

## Patient Safety-Focused Programs

A third element characteristic of the anesthesia approach to patient safety is the formation of patient safety-focused specialty entities. Existing only for the promulgation of safety, these societies represent an important aspect of the anesthesia approach to patient safety.

Foremost among these groups is the Anesthesia Patient Safety Foundation (APSF), an independent nonprofit corporation begun in 1985 with the vision "that no patient shall be harmed by anesthesia." Supported by the ASA and corporate sponsors, APSF members include anesthesiologists, nurse anesthetists, manufacturers of equipment and drugs, engineers, and insurers.

The clinical impact of the APSF has been immense. The APSF newsletter, published four times a year,[14] has become one of the most widely circulated anesthesia publications in the world and is dedicated solely to safety. Identifying aspects of anesthesia practice with significant potential for adverse consequences, the APSF newsletter has highlighted diverse issues such as the anesthesia machine checkout, opioid-induced respiratory depression, residual neuromuscular blockade, postoperative visual loss, and emergency manual use. Instructional videos, research grants, and other special conferences are also part of the APSF effort to promote safety.

A second entity with a unique approach to safety is the ASA Closed Claims Project.[13] Operating in cooperation with malpractice lawyers, the Closed Claims Project group reviews data from settled anesthesia lawsuits to identify anesthesia safety concerns that may be amenable to targeted efforts. In a series of academic publications since 1988 and continuing into the present, the Closed Claims Project has investigated a wide range of topics (Table 48.1) focusing on rare events difficult to study systematically. Although such analyses cannot estimate incidences or risk factors, they provide a wealth of descriptive information that has helped anesthesiologists address patient safety issues. Among these are the recognition that listening to the chest may not be a reliable method of detecting esophageal intubation[13] and that a common factor in adverse outcomes due to massive hemorrhage is late recognition.[16]

The Anesthesia Quality Institute (AQI) is the newest and potentially largest patient safety project sponsored by organized anesthesia.[21] Begun in 2008, the goal of the AQI was to "to be the primary source of information for quality improvement in the clinical practice of anesthesiology." Sponsored by the ASA, the AQI administers and supports an Anesthesia Incident Reporting System (AIRS) and the National Anesthesia Clinical Outcomes Registry (NACOR), which currently captures information on approximately 25% of all the anesthetics administered in the United States. The goal is to capture enough anesthetic data that accurate benchmarking of clinical outcomes related to anesthesia can be performed and informed efforts to improve quality can occur.

**Table 48.1** Noteworthy Closed Claims Project Observations

| Year | Title | No. of Claims | Notable Finding(s) |
|---|---|---|---|
| 1988 | Cardiac arrest during spinal anesthesia[17] | 14 | Bradycardia was the most common presenting symptom with hypotension as the second.<br>Epinephrine was not given until 8 minutes (mean) after onset of asystole. |
| 1990 | Adverse respiratory events in anesthesia[15] | 522 | Death/brain damage occurred in 85% of cases.<br>In 48% of esophageal intubations, auscultation of breath sounds was performed and documented. |
| 1999 | Nerve injury associated with anesthesia[18] | 670 | Ulnar nerve injuries were most frequent, were associated with general anesthesia, and occurred predominantly in men. |
| 2006 | Injury associated with monitored anesthesia care[19] | 121 | Monitored anesthesia care claims involved older and sicker patients than general anesthesia claims.<br>Respiratory depression due to sedative/opioid administration was the most common mechanism of damage (21%).<br>The combination of electrocautery and oxygen was a recognized mechanism in 17%. |
| 2014 | Massive hemorrhage[16] | 3211 | 30% of claims involved obstetrics, and thoracic/lumbar spine procedures were also overrepresented.<br>Recognition and initiation of transfusion therapy were commonly delayed. |
| 2015 | Postoperative opioid-induced respiratory depression[20] | 357 | 88% of events occurred within 24 hours of surgery, and somnolence was noted in 62% before the event. |

## FROM SAFETY TO QUALITY: MAKING ANESTHESIA BOTH SAFER AND BETTER

Although most observers believe anesthesia care to be safer today than 50 years ago, whether the quality of anesthesia care has improved is less clear. Incorporating not only safety but efficiency, cost, and patient comfort and satisfaction, anesthesia quality has many more dimensions than the avoidance of adverse outcomes.

Several barriers exist to measuring and improving anesthesia quality. Because the relative contribution of anesthesia to the outcome of surgical procedures is difficult to define, identifying how anesthetic care might have made a difference is likewise challenging. It is easy to see that if a patient goes home a day sooner after a colectomy, for example, determining whether that improvement is due to anesthesia, surgery, or hospital care is extremely difficult. More than likely, this type of improvement is a result of all variables.

### Process Measures

The most significant obstacle to anesthesia quality is knowledge of patient outcomes. Because most of the patient's pre- and postoperative course lies outside the preoperative clinic, operating room, and postanesthesia care unit, understanding how a patient's clinical course is affected by alterations in anesthesia care requires considerable effort to follow patients into the postoperative phase. For this reason, early attempts to improve anesthesia quality focused on perioperative processes rather than outcomes. The Surgical Care Improvement Project, or SCIP, was a national test of this approach. By incentivizing the public reporting of hospital performance on evidence-based process measures such as administering antibiotics in a timely fashion and verifying the continuation of preoperative β-adrenergic blockers into the perioperative period, policymakers hoped to improve quality by improving perioperative processes of care. Puzzlingly, however, over the 8-year history of the SCIP project (2006-2014), performance on nearly all process measures included in the project improved, but outcomes (whether surgical site infections[22,23] or mortality rate[24]) failed to improve. In fact, because of concern regarding adverse outcomes from potentially harmful process measures,[25] several related process measures were also rescinded. Among these were whether β-adrenergic blockers were given to patients within 24 hours of an admission for myocardial infarction[26] and verifying that antibiotics were given within 4 hours of an emergency room visit for pneumonia.[27]

Why implementation of a suite of process measures, all with literature support, have not clearly improved patient outcomes remains a mystery. Clearly, improving quality by mandating specific processes of care is not straightforward and has led quality experts to be much more reluctant to embrace process measures alone as a method of assessing care quality.

## Structural Measures

Measuring structural elements can also provide a glimpse into the presence or absence of quality. Structure refers to the presence or absence of specific organizational features that are considered to be integral to the provision of high-quality care. If present, such features then suggest that the clinical care is of high quality.

Examples of structural elements considered to correlate with quality care include the ready availability of diagnostic radiologic testing, having physicians on call for emergencies, an electronic medical record, and mandating a dedicated intensivist for all critical care units. The presence of an active quality improvement mechanism might also be considered a structural feature of high-quality care. Although structural quality is relatively invisible to trainees unfamiliar with diversity in health care environments, hospital rules governing nurse-patient ratios, timely availability of obstetric anesthesia specialists, and a protocol for hand hygiene are examples.

Although structural measures are generally easy to measure, the link between structure and improved outcomes is often difficult to discern. The availability of in-house critical care attending physicians at night, for example, is intuitively reasonable, and would be a relatively easy structural feature to measure. However, more than one study[28,29] suggests that hospitals that have implemented an in-house night-call system might not see clear improvements in outcomes.

## Outcome Measures

One logical consequence of an inability to identify clinically relevant process measures is to focus instead on outcome. Because there is considerable practice variability in anesthesia,[30,31] variability in outcomes likely exists. In principle, by identifying "bright spot" institutions that have better outcomes, the corresponding best practices can be identified and disseminated. Although NACOR is not yet mature enough to allow outcome analysis, surgical databases are approaching that goal. The Society of Thoracic Surgeons (STS) Adult Cardiac Surgery Database is perhaps the best example, capturing data from more than 90% of all cardiac procedures in the United States.[32] Other databases include the National Surgical Quality Improvement Program (NSQIP) and National Inpatient Sample (NIS). Because sufficiently complete data for outcome reporting has historically not been available, few hospitals have routinely made outcome data available to their clinical care staff. In addition, outcome reporting for anesthesiologists in particular is challenging because events that occur postoperatively may not be related to anesthesia

care per se. Such an approach is changing, however, as hospitals recognize the value of feedback. Monthly central line and catheter-related urinary tract infection rates posted in the intensive care unit or patient satisfaction scores posted in the operating room are examples.

Outcome reporting initially seems straightforward and gives individuals or institutions a benchmark for measuring future performance. But accurately comparing outcomes between individuals or institutions requires some way to adjust for patient conditions unrelated to the anesthesia or surgical (or hospital) care. This "risk adjustment" can be extremely difficult as different adjustment algorithms may produce different results,[33] algorithms may be vulnerable to "gaming" by inducing favorable patient selection,[34] the accuracy of data may be suspect,[35] and the adjustment algorithm itself may not be consistent from year to year.[36]

Current evidence is mixed with regard to whether outcome reporting improves outcomes. Two 2015 studies[37,38] suggest that knowing one's outcomes may not by itself drive improvement. In addition, should a "bright spot" institution with unusually good outcomes be recognized, identifying and disseminating lessons from that institution would likely involve developing a set of process measures, which (as the SCIP program demonstrates) may not have the desired effect.

Nevertheless, the use of both process and outcome measures are key to quality improvement. As the management consultant Peter Drucker once noted, "You can't manage what you can't measure." Yet measurement alone is inadequate. Our current experience with both process and outcome measurement is that neither readily leads to improved quality. Further work is needed to better understand how to use outcome and process measurements to drive quality.

## TOOLS FOR IMPROVING LOCAL OUTCOMES

In addition to empiric observation, improving quality and safety occurs continuously at the local level and is driven by individuals, departments, or hospitals. This section discusses tools in widespread use for quality improvement.

### Structured Quality Improvement Programs: FADE, PDSA, and DMAIC

Because clinical care can be extremely complex and multifaceted, knowing where or how to begin a quality improvement project can be difficult. The acronyms FADE, PDSA, and DMAIC refer to commonly used blueprints for initiating and executing a quality improvement project. Although the letters are different, all three apply the same basic model: evaluate, implement, measure.

FADE stands for Focus/Analyze/Develop/Execute-evaluate. As the words suggest, one should first focus on the process to be improved, analyze data to establish root cases and baseline performance, use the data to develop an action plan, then execute the plan and evaluate the result. PDSA stands for Plan/Do/Study/Act. As one might imagine, the general gist of a PDSA is similar to FADE. DMAIC stands for Define/Measure/Analyze/Improve/Control, which follows essentially the same process.

Because identifying, intervening, and assessing the outcome are core aspects of the anesthesia skill set, anesthesiologists are likely familiar with the general structure of a FADE or PDSA quality improvement program. After all, the simple act of titrating an anesthetic requires that a situational assessment be made, the anesthetic level be adjusted, and the outcome reviewed. However, creating lasting change is more difficult than it appears. A common trap in developing a quality improvement program is to identify an imperfect step and apply a remedy to that specific step without understanding or addressing how that step came to be imperfect. A plan to improve delivery of blood products to the operating room, for example, may be ineffective if the process for ordering blood is not also addressed (also see Chapter 24). Another often missed aspect of quality improvement is the implementation of a change without measuring the result of that change. If an intraoperative handoff tool is implemented, for example, but no improvement in handoff errors results, one possibility is that compliance with the tool is poor. Attention to such details will help optimize the results of any quality improvement project.

## Multidisciplinary Process Improvement: Root Cause Analysis, "Never Events," and Failure Mode Effects Analysis

Root cause analysis (RCA) was developed by manufacturers in the 1950s to better understand industrial events. The goal is, as the title suggests, to identify the primary, or "root," cause of the problem under analysis. One of the first users of this technique was Toyota, who famously used the "5 whys" technique. By asking "why" at least five times during the investigation of a breakdown or undesired event, quality personnel are forced to drill down layer by layer to understand progressively more fundamental causes.

When applied in medicine, the root cause process begins with a multidisciplinary group assembled to evaluate every step of the process that resulted in the event in question. Attention is focused strictly on system processes and not on individual provider behavior. A causal factor chart is often created in skeleton form, with details added as each specialty adds their expertise. Fig. 48.1 depicts a sample factor chart for an intraoperative transfusion reaction[39] (also see Chapter 24).

Although such charts are usually read from left to right, they are often created from right to left, starting with the event and using logic and time information to add relevant causal factors. Note also that the blood bank, hospital engineering, preoperative nursing, anesthesia, and surgery

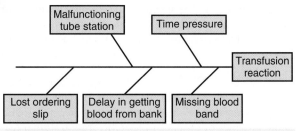

**Fig. 48.1** Sample causal factor chart. (From Tung A. Sentinel events and how to learn from them. *Int Anesthesiol Clin.* 2014;52:53-68.)

---

**Box 48.1** Sentinel Events Related to the Perioperative Period as Defined by The Joint Commission, 2015

- Hemolytic transfusion reaction (also see Chapter 24)
- Invasive procedure on the wrong patient, wrong site, or wrong procedure
- Prolonged fluoroscopy > 1500 rads
- Fire, flame, or unanticipated smoke, heat, or flashes during an episode of patient care
- Any intrapartum maternal death or severe morbidity

*Rads,* Radiation absorbed dose units.

---

are all involved in this particular event, underscoring the multidisciplinary nature of properly performed RCAs.

An RCA is mandated by The Joint Commission, a United States–based nonprofit organization that accredits health care organizations and programs, whenever an accredited hospital experiences one of several prespecified types of adverse events. Such events are called "sentinel" because they expose a dangerous "gap" in care and signal the need for immediate investigation and response. A list of all The Joint Commission–designated events can be accessed at their website.[40] Sentinel events relevant to the perioperative period are listed in Box 48.1.

The Joint Commission also explicitly defines events that do *not* require focused reporting and review. These include any near miss, medication errors that do *not* result in death or functional loss, minor hemolysis, or death or functional loss after leaving against medical advice.

The Joint Commission requires (as a condition of accreditation) that hospitals respond to such events within 45 days by reporting them to The Joint Commission, performing an RCA, and developing an action plan to identify strategies the hospital intends to implement to reduce the risk of similar events in the future. Such a plan must include the action to be taken, who will implement, a time line for implementation, and strategies for measuring the result and sustaining the changes. Although reporting to The Joint Commission is voluntary, identification of such events is a key component of accreditation visits.

Other patient safety organizations have suggested modifications to The Joint Commission list. The National Quality Forum (NQF), for example, endorses a large list of "serious reportable events" that should never occur. Besides The Joint Commission list, the NQF adds "intraoperative death in an ASA class I patient," death/disability from the irretrievable loss of an irreplaceable biologic specimen, and death from electric shock.

Although intuitively reasonable, the real world effectiveness of an RCA can be variable.[41] Adverse events and their investigation are often emotionally charged, and meetings to determine cause can be limited by blame-oriented analysis (which leads to relatively weak "blame and train" remedies). Studies of action plans and implementations suggest that relatively few of these actively target true "root" causes.[42] An inadequate RCA may result from lack of time, inadequate resources, and even disagreement among reviewers with respect to "root" causes.[43] Even when appropriate action plans are created, insufficient resources may prevent effective implementation.

One highly useful outcome of The Joint Commission Sentinel Event program is their series of sentinel event alerts.[44] By maintaining a database of reported events, The Joint Commission can identify trends in safety events and issue bulletins to warn clinicians of potential issues. To date, this program has resulted in more than 50 events including several relevant to anesthesia such as deaths due to concentrated potassium chloride solutions, ventilator-related deaths, medical gas mix-ups, transfusion errors, disruptive behavior, and magnetic resonance imaging accidents. Reports include case descriptions and analysis including the Manufacturer and User Facility Device Experience (MAUDE) database.[45]

One of the major drawbacks to the RCA process is its retrospective nature. Process flaws in care delivery may not be addressed until the event actually occurs and a patient is harmed. To address this problem, the Failure Mode Effects Analysis (FMEA) has been adopted from industry to prospectively identify high-risk aspects of clinical care.

An FMEA is a resource-intensive, comprehensive analysis of a specific process, with the goal of identifying all the potential ways that it can fail. A process to identify and record patient allergies, for example, might fail if the interviewer is unable to accurately identify allergies, if the documentation form is difficult to read or inaccessible, or if medications sound alike. In addition to simulation and imagination, a team should use other sources to identify potential failures including sentinel event alerts, Institute for Safe Medication Practices information, and Food and Drug Administration databases and advisories.

It is easy to see that an FMEA analysis of even a straightforward process is extremely time consuming. Even if most of the relevant failure modes can be identified, implementing effective change can be difficult, in part because no bad event has yet occurred. As a result, FMEA analyses should be reserved for large-volume, high-risk processes for which the risk of catastrophic failure is clear.

## SUMMARY

Anesthesia providers should routinely strive for the highest quality care they can deliver. Because procedures and anesthetic strategies routinely evolve to meet changing needs, quality and safety in anesthesia present by definition a moving target.

Historically, anesthesiologists have led in patient safety by being willing to embrace several practical approaches. Among these are the empiric cataloging of events, a recognition of human-machine interface errors as a significant contributor to adverse events, adoption of strategies from other highly technical fields, and early specialty-wide agreement with respect to practice standards.

Organized patient safety–focused organizations within the specialty have also contributed considerably to anesthesia safety with innovative approaches. These groups include the APSF and the ASA Closed Claims Project.

In part because knowledge regarding care outcomes has been lacking, anesthesiologists have only recently begun to focus in the same way on care quality. The availability not only of specialty registries, such as the STS Adult Cardiac Surgery Database, but of large surgical databases such as NACOR and NSQIP has allowed anesthesiologists to move beyond process and structural measures and toward outcome measurement. Although no "magic bullet" strategy to quality improvement has yet emerged, process, structure, and outcome are all key elements in any comprehensive quality program.

Finally, multiple tools exist at the departmental and institutional level for quality improvement. These tools include blueprints for local quality projects, nationally promulgated sentinel event programs, and root cause and failure mode analyses for adverse events.

Taken together, numerous quality and safety tools and approaches are available to anesthesia teams interested in patient safety. With the growth and maturation of large perioperative databases, and the potential of electronic intraoperative records to shed light into the perioperative period, even more options will become available to make anesthesia practice safer and increased quality in upcoming years.

## QUESTIONS OF THE DAY

1. What is the difference between quality and safety in anesthesia care?
2. What is the rationale for using process measures, structural measures, or outcome measures as a means to improve quality?
3. How can the PDSA (Plan/Do/Study/Act) process be used as a framework for a local quality improvement initiative?
4. What are the key steps in performing an root cause analysis (RCA)? What are the potential benefits and drawbacks to the RCA process?

VI

## REFERENCES

1. Lagasse RS. Anesthesia safety: model or myth? A review of the published literature and analysis of current original data. *Anesthesiology.* 2002;97:1609–1617.
2. Brass P, Hellmich M, Kolodziej L, et al. Ultrasound guidance versus anatomical landmarks for internal jugular vein catheterization. *Cochrane Database Syst Rev.* 2015;1:CD006962.
3. Beecher HK, Todd DP. A study of the deaths associated with anesthesia and surgery: based on a study of 599,548 anesthesias in ten institutions 1948–1952, inclusive. *Ann Surg.* 1954;140:2–35.
4. Ament R, Papper EM, Rovenstine EA. Cardiac arrest during anesthesia; a review of cases. *Ann Surg.* 1951;134:220–227.
5. Ebert TJ, Muzi M. Sympathetic hyperactivity during desflurane anesthesia in healthy volunteers. A comparison with isoflurane. *Anesthesiology.* 1993;79:444–453.
6. Lienhart A, Auroy Y, Péquignot F, et al. Survey of anesthesia-related mortality in France. *Anesthesiology.* 2006;105:1087–1097.
7. Postoperative Visual Loss Study Group. Risk factors associated with ischemic optic neuropathy after spinal fusion surgery. *Anesthesiology.* 2012;116:15–24.
8. Pohl A, Cullen DJ. Cerebral ischemia during shoulder surgery in the upright position: a case series. *J Clin Anesth.* 2005;17:463–469.
9. Butwick AJ. Postpartum hemorrhage and low fibrinogen levels: the past, present and future. *Int J Obstet Anesth.* 2013;22:87–91.
10. Eichhorn JH, Cooper JB, Cullen DJ, et al. Standards for patient monitoring during anesthesia at Harvard Medical School. *JAMA.* 1986;256:1017–1020.
11. American Society of Anesthesiologists. Standards & Guidelines. http://www.asahq.org/quality-and-practice-management/standards-and-guidelines.
12. Eichhorn JH. Prevention of intraoperative anesthesia accidents and related severe injury through safety monitoring. *Anesthesiology.* 1989;70:572–577.
13. Lee LA, Domino KB. The Closed Claims Project. Has it influenced anesthetic practice and outcome? *Anesthesiol Clin North Am.* 2002;20:485–501.
14. APSF Newsletter. http://apsf.org/resources.php.
15. Caplan RA, Posner KL, Ward RJ, et al. Adverse respiratory events in anesthesia: a closed claims analysis. *Anesthesiology.* 1990;72:828–833.
16. Dutton RP, Lee LA, Stephens LS, et al. Massive hemorrhage: a report from the anesthesia closed claims project. *Anesthesiology.* 2014;121:450–458.
17. Caplan RA, Ward RJ, Posner K, et al. Unexpected cardiac arrest during spinal anesthesia: a closed claims analysis of predisposing factors. *Anesthesiology.* 1988;68:5–11.
18. Cheney FW, Domino KB, Caplan RA, et al. Nerve injury associated with anesthesia: a closed claims analysis. *Anesthesiology.* 1999;90:1062–1069.
19. Bhananker SM, Posner KL, Cheney FW, et al. Injury and liability associated with monitored anesthesia care: a closed claims analysis. *Anesthesiology.* 2006;104:228–234.
20. Lee LA, Caplan RA, Stephens LS, et al. Postoperative opioid-induced respiratory depression: a closed claims analysis. *Anesthesiology.* 2015;122:659–665.
21. Anesthesia Quality Institute. www.aqihq.org.
22. Hawn MT, Vick CC, Richman J, et al. Surgical site infection prevention: time to move beyond the surgical care improvement program. *Ann Surg.* 2011;254:494–499.
23. Hawn MT, Richman JS, Vick CC, et al. Timing of surgical antibiotic prophylaxis and the risk of surgical site infection. *JAMA Surg.* 2013;148:649–657.
24. LaPar DJ, Isbell JM, Kern JA, et al. Surgical Care Improvement Project measure for postoperative glucose control should not be used as a measure of quality after cardiac surgery. *J Thorac Cardiovasc Surg.* 2014;147:1041–1048.
25. POISE Study Group, Devereaux PJ, Yang H, Yusuf S, et al. Effects of extended-release metoprolol succinate in patients undergoing non-cardiac surgery (POISE trial): a randomised controlled trial. *Lancet.* 2008;371:1839–1847.
26. Chen ZM, Pan HC, Chen YP. Early intravenous then oral metoprolol in 45,852 patients with acute myocardial infarction: randomised placebo-controlled trial. *Lancet.* 2005;366:1622–1632.
27. Wachter RM, Flanders SA, Fee C, et al. Public reporting of antibiotic timing in patients with pneumonia: lessons from a flawed performance measure. *Ann Intern Med.* 2008;149:29–32.
28. Kerlin MP, Small DS, Cooney E, et al. A randomized trial of nighttime physician staffing in an intensive care unit. *N Engl J Med.* 2013;368:2201–2209.
29. Wallace DJ, Angus DC, Barnato AE, et al. Nighttime intensivist staffing and mortality among critically ill patients. *N Engl J Med.* 2012;366:2093–2101.
30. Lilot M, Ehrenfeld JM, Lee C3, et al. Variability in practice and factors predictive of total crystalloid administration during abdominal surgery: retrospective two-centre analysis. *Br J Anaesth.* 2015;114:767–776.
31. Fleischut PM, Eskreis-Winkler JM, Gaber-Baylis LK, et al. Variability in anesthetic care for total knee arthroplasty: an analysis from the anesthesia quality institute. *Am J Med Qual.* 2015;30:172–179.
32. Jacobs JP, Shahian DM, Prager RL, et al. Introduction to the STS National Database Series: outcomes analysis, quality improvement, and patient safety. *Ann Thorac Surg.* 2015;100(6):1992–2000.
33. Shahian DM, Wolf RE, Iezzoni LI, et al. Variability in the measurement of hospital-wide mortality rates. *N Engl J Med.* 2010;363:2530–2539.
34. Cooper AL, Trivedi AN. Fitness memberships and favorable selection in Medicare Advantage plans. *N Engl J Med.* 2012;366:150–157.
35. Brown ML, Lenoch JR, Schaff HV. Variability in data: the Society of Thoracic Surgeons National Adult Cardiac Surgery Database. *J Thorac Cardiovasc Surg.* 2010;140:267–273.
36. Sigakis MJ, Bittner EA, Wanderer JP. Validation of a risk stratification index and risk quantification index for predicting patient outcomes: in-hospital mortality, 30-day mortality, 1-year mortality, and length-of-stay. *Anesthesiology.* 2013;119:525–540.
37. Etzioni DA, Wasif N, Dueck AC, et al. Association of hospital participation in a surgical outcomes monitoring program with inpatient complications and mortality. *JAMA.* 2015;313:505–511.
38. Osborne NH, Nicholas LH, Ryan AM, et al. Association of hospital participation in a quality reporting program with surgical outcomes and expenditures for Medicare beneficiaries. *JAMA.* 2015;313:496–504.
39. Tung A. Sentinel events and how to learn from them. *Int Anesthesiol Clin.* 2014;52:53–68.
40. The Joint Commission. Patient Safety Systems Chapter, Sentinel Event Policy and RCA2. https://www.jointcommission.org/sentinel_event.aspx.
41. Wu AW, Lipshutz AK, Pronovost PJ. Effectiveness and efficiency of root cause analysis in medicine. *JAMA.* 2008;299:685–687.
42. Wallace LM, Spurgeon P, Adams S, et al. Survey evaluation of the National Patient Safety Agency's Root Cause Analysis training programme in England and Wales: knowledge, beliefs and reported practices. *Qual Saf Health Care.* 2009;18:288–291.
43. Smits M, Janssen J, de Vet R, et al. Analysis of unintended events in hospitals: inter-rater reliability of constructing causal trees and classifying root causes. *Int J Qual Health Care.* 2009;21:292–300.
44. The Joint Commission. Sentinel Event Alert/Topics Library Updates. https://www.jointcommission.org/topics/hai_sentinel_event.aspx.
45. The Joint Commission. Topic Library Resources. https://www.jointcommission.org/topics/default.aspx.

# 49 PALLIATIVE CARE

## Sarah Gebauer

## INTRODUCTION

Patients with serious illnesses often have an intense burden of symptoms that are poorly treated, such as pain, dyspnea, anxiety, and depression.[1] These patients also have frequent but often unsatisfying interactions with the health care team, often due to poor communication.[2] *Palliative care* is "an approach that improves the quality of life of patients and their families facing the problems associated with life-threatening illness, through the prevention and relief of suffering by means of early identification and impeccable assessment and treatment of pain and other problems, physical, psychosocial and spiritual."[3] *Palliative medicine* refers to the medical expertise provided within a palliative care team. Palliative care, with its emphasis on goal setting and symptom management, attempts to improve care for these patients and their families. Many palliative care skills can be used in a variety of settings, and concepts such as shared decision making and a biopsychosocial-spiritual approach should not be reserved only for seriously ill patients.

Modern palliative care started with the hospice movement in the 1960s and has spread to many health systems worldwide. In the United States, at least two thirds of hospitals have palliative care teams,[4] and hospice services are widely available. Despite their common roots, hospice and palliative care are not necessarily interchangeable terms. The meaning of *hospice* and the services offered vary by country, though hospices generally focus on later-stage illnesses. In the United States, hospice refers to an insurance benefit for patients with a life expectancy of less than 6 months. *Palliative care* is a more inclusive term that is appropriate "at any age and any stage in a serious illness, and can be provided together with curative treatment."[5] In the past, there was a perceived binary choice between aggressive curative treatment, then going onto hospice when those treatments failed. Palliative care now provides a more nuanced picture of the time prior to hospice, with patients receiving concurrent palliative and curative treatment with increasing palliative care support if the illness progresses, until hospice services are appropriate (Fig. 49.1).[6] For the purposes of this chapter, palliative care will encompass both palliative and hospice care unless otherwise specified.

Palliative care does not mean giving up, or even providing less aggressive care. It means talking to patients and families, eliciting their values and goals, and making medical recommendations and decisions based on those values and goals. This approach is sometimes referred to as *shared decision making.* It is not uncommon for the palliative care team to advocate for more aggressive treatment, either because it is in line with a patient's wishes and is reasonable medically or because aggressive treatment of specific medical problems can decrease a patient's symptom burden.

Palliative care teams generally approach symptom management by evaluating multiple aspects of a patient's condition, involving both physical and emotional pain. This concept acknowledges that part of the pain a patient feels may be, in part, due to existential or spiritual suffering. This may take the form of a belief that the person's upcoming death is punishment from a higher power, or that the person did not contribute enough to the world. Palliative care specialists attempt to determine what physical or psychosocial factors may be contributing to pain, and use medications or the expertise of other team members such as chaplains, social workers, or art therapists to help alleviate a patient's symptoms, in a broad sense.

Inpatient palliative care teams *reduce costs* while improving patient care. Medical advances and an aging population have led to an increase in the number of patients with serious illnesses. The beneficiaries using the most Medicare dollars include those in the last year of life, even though many people say they do not want to die in a hospital. In 2010, benefits to the most costly 5% of members accounted for 39% of Medicare spending.[7] Not only is the care expensive, but patients and families often describe distressing symptoms, psychosocial needs that go unrecognized, and overall poor care.[8] Hospital costs decrease with palliative care consult services. For example, one study showed an average decrease in cost of $6900 per patient, as well as fewer deaths in the intensive care unit (ICU).[9] Cost reduction is not a primary goal of palliative care. Rather, patients who receive palliative care desire fewer interventions and resources. Importantly, palliative care teams do not increase in-hospital mortality rate.[10] In some situations, palliative care may even *increase survival.* Patients with metastatic lung cancer, for example, lived 2 months longer compared to those receiving standard care.[11]

## What Is Hospice?

In the United States, hospice generally refers to a set of benefits from Medicare or private insurers. More than 40% of all deaths in the United States occur on hospice.[12] Hospice care decreases patient symptom burden, increases patient and family satisfaction, and is associated with cost savings, especially for patients with longer durations of hospice use.[13] Hospice provides patients and families with the most help they can receive when caring for a person at home, including the services listed in Fig. 49.2. Contrary to some patients' beliefs, most hospice services

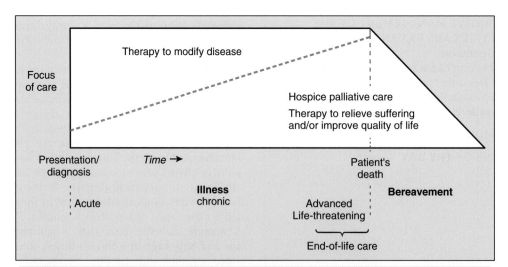

**Fig. 49.1** The role of hospice and palliative care during illness and bereavement. (Redrawn from Ferris FD, Balfour HM, Bowen K, et al. A model to guide patient and family care: based on nationally accepted principles and norms of practice. *J Pain Symptom Manage.* 2002;24:106-123.)

are provided at home and hospice does not pay for care-givers. The hospice nurses and staff teach and support the family in caring for a seriously ill, dying patient, but the families provide the bulk of the care. Some families may opt to have hospice services provided in a nursing home, though the "custodial care," or care of daily needs such as eating and bathing, provided by the nursing home will often not be covered by the patient's insurance. A few patients will qualify for services at an inpatient hospice facility because of specific intractable symptoms such as pain or vomiting, but usually not for the entire time they are receiving hospice (Fig. 49.3).

## Hospice and Palliative Medicine Subspecialty

Hospice and Palliative Medicine is a board-certified sub-specialty that requires a 1-year fellowship for certification. Physicians from 10 medical specialties including anesthesiology are eligible, and more than 100 anesthe-siologists are board certified in Hospice and Palliative

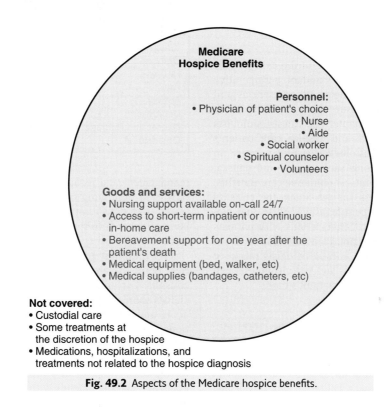

**Fig. 49.2** Aspects of the Medicare hospice benefits.

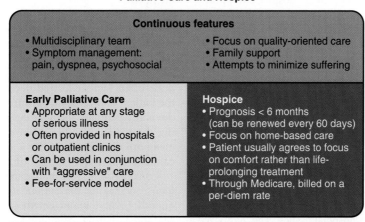

**Fig. 49.3** Features of palliative care and hospice in the United States.

Medicine.[14] Board-certified physicians provide specialist palliative care, which includes refractory symptom management and difficult family meetings.[15] Although most anesthesiologists will not go on to be palliative care physicians, all anesthesiologists should have a familiarity with primary palliative care. This includes goals-of-care conversations and perioperative advance directives, in addition to skills in symptom management for seriously ill patients related to issues commonly seen in anesthesiology practice.[16]

## Anesthesiologists' Contribution to Palliative Care

Anesthesiologists offer specific skills in the care of seriously ill patients in addition to standard perioperative care. Many elderly (also see Chapter 35) and seriously ill people have surgery,[17] pain issues (also see Chapter 44), or critical illness (also see Chapter 41). Anesthesiologists may interact with palliative and hospice care patients in these settings. Anesthesiologists have expertise in the management of symptoms such as pain and nausea, which are frequent complaints of palliative care patients. Crucially, they also possess insight about the risks to the patient for the entire perioperative course and can add valuable information to conversations with patients and families about goals of care. Pain medicine (also see Chapter 44) and critical care anesthesiologists (also see Chapter 41) offer advanced skills and knowledge that can be invaluable in a palliative care patient's care.

## WHAT DO PALLIATIVE CARE TEAMS DO?

Palliative care is an interdisciplinary field involving multiple professionals including physicians, nurses, social workers, chaplains, and others. Palliative care physicians are experts in symptom management and communication for seriously ill patients and their families. Palliative care nurses, including nurses who provide hospice care, practice symptom management, advanced communication skills, and assessment of the psychosocial and spiritual needs of a patient and family.[18] Social workers address the psychosocial needs of patients and families and may assist with complex discharge needs.[19] Chaplains assist patients and families in identifying and addressing spiritual distress related to serious illness and provide or facilitate appropriate spiritual or religious rituals.[20] Anesthesia pain experts may be involved in advanced pain (also see Chapters 40 and 44) management techniques, and anesthesia critical care specialists are often involved in complex goals-of-care discussions.

Palliative care teams assess and treat the patient's symptoms, discuss goals of care, and assess and treat the patient and family's psychosocial issues. The palliative care team takes a biopsychosocial-spiritual approach to

---

**Box 49.1** Common Psychosocial Questions During Palliative Care Consults

"What role, if any, do religion or spirituality play in your life?"
"Where do you live? With whom?"
"What values are important in your life?"
"How do you cope with the changes that are happening?"
"What are your greatest concerns right now?"

---

**Box 49.2** Commonly Assessed Symptoms During a Palliative Care Visit

Insomnia
Dyspnea
Fatigue
Pain
Anxiety
Depression
Nausea and vomiting
Constipation

---

management and recognizes the interplay between these factors in improving overall patient care. Palliative care teams, like consultants, can either focus on a specific issue of concern to the team or perform a comprehensive assessment.

Consultations generally fall into two broad categories: goals-of-care consults and symptom management consults. For goals-of-care consults, palliative care specialists share information, get a sense of what a patient's goals and values are, and make medical recommendations based on those goals and values. For example, one patient's goal might be to stay out of the hospital and spend time with his or her dogs, and another's might be to live until the birth of a grandchild. Others may have goals like making amends with family members, or being able to walk around the house without pain. Palliative care teams also perform an in-depth psychosocial assessment, with questions like those listed in Box 49.1. Talking with patients and families about their understanding of the medical issues, how they want to receive information, and how their home and spiritual lives contribute to their thinking about the medical situation can provide the primary teams with invaluable guidance. These conversations often include shared decision making and helping the patient and family determine a reasonable plan given the many complex factors in every patient's care. Including the patient and family in decision making does not mean offering or agreeing to a plan of care that the medical team believes is harmful or increases suffering.

Consultations for management of symptoms often focus on making the patient more comfortable and frequently involve management of pain or intractable nausea and vomiting. Symptoms that palliative care teams commonly address are listed in Box 49.2. A number of

**Box 49.3** Benefits Associated With Palliative Care in the ICU

- Decreased time in the ICU
- Decreased hospital length of stay
- No increase in mortality rate
- Decreased family member PTSD and anxiety
- Decreased disagreements between families and providers
- Decreased disagreements among providers

*ICU*, Intensive care unit; *PTSD*, posttraumatic stress disorder.
From Aslakson R, Cheng J, Vollenweider D, et al. Evidence-based palliative care in the intensive care unit: a systematic review of interventions. *J Palliat Med.* 2014;17:219-235.

these symptoms require a sophisticated understanding of the patient's underlying pathophysiology. For example, patients with vomiting may have an abdominal tumor, medication effect, or opioid-induced constipation. Patients determined to have intra-abdominal disease affecting the intestinal tract would need to be evaluated for ongoing versus intermittent obstruction and considered for treatment with octreotide or dexamethasone, and possibly a venting gastrotomy tube. Other symptoms close to the end of life like terminal delirium may require treatment with large doses of benzodiazepines or even phenobarbital. For patients whose symptoms do not respond to standard approaches, a palliative care consultation should be obtained.

## Palliative Care in the Intensive Care Unit

Patients in the surgical ICU who stay more than 7 days have a mortality rate of more than 35%[21] and should receive a palliative care consultation.[22] Although some patients routinely stay in the ICU for specific nursing or monitoring needs after surgery, a significant proportion of patients and families will need to make difficult decisions about the treatment plan. Palliative care providers help patients and families determine goals of care, help resolve conflicts, and provide symptom management to patients in critical care units (Box 49.3).[23] Despite palliative care's perceived emphasis on comfort over cure, there is *no increased mortality rate* in patients in the ICU when palliative care teams are introduced (also see Chapter 41).

Communication among patients, families, and providers can be especially difficult in the surgical ICU. The common use of an "open model" ICU in the surgical setting can make it difficult for providers and families to form a cohesive plan.[21] Additionally, what some authors have described as a "surgical covenant" between surgeon and patient, in which the surgeon has "an exaggerated sense of accountability for the patient's outcome," can further complicate the prognosis and make it difficult for all parties to agree on what constitutes a "good" outcome.[21] Though traditional surgical thinking viewed palliative care as being at odds with surgical goals, the

current statement by the American College of Surgeons encourages integration of palliative care of surgical patients who have a range of conditions, not just those at the end of life.[21] Thus, anesthesiologists should work closely with surgeons and palliative care specialists to ensure optimal care during periods of critical illness.

## Withdrawal of Life Support

Many anesthesiologists may be involved in the withdrawal of life support for patients with poor prognoses whose families do not believe continued life-sustaining treatment is compatible with the patients' goals. For these patients, withdrawing life support is the ethical decision. It is important to note and clarify the distinction that family members may perceive when health care personnel discuss withdrawing life support (discontinuing a machine that keeps a patient alive artificially) and withdrawing care (discontinuing all concern about the patient's comfort and well-being). High-quality care and symptom management should be of utmost concern for all patients regardless of the treatment plan, and families should be reassured that the team will continue to care for the patient.

An important example arises in the context of withdrawing ventilator support. Many family members will prefer that the endotracheal tube be removed in addition to the ventilator being discontinued. It is crucial to prepare family members for the process of extubation of the trachea, including the expected coughing and secretions, and to have opioids and sedatives readily available to decrease any perceived discomfort during or after the extubation, such as shortness of breath. Anesthesiologists are experts in the rapid titration of fentanyl and midazolam, which are the most commonly used medications for withdrawal of mechanical ventilator support. A nurse or physician comfortable with administering these medications should be present during ventilator withdrawal in order to decrease signs of distress. Patients should not be paralyzed prior to ventilator withdrawal, as this would make it difficult or impossible to assess for proper titration of opioids and sedatives. Physicians overseeing withdrawal of life support should discontinue any unnecessary tubes and lines, contact the hospital chaplain for help accommodating spiritual care and religious rituals, and ensure family support.

## Spirituality in Serious Illness

Serious illness and possible death often bring up spiritual issues like questioning the meaning of life or beliefs about what happens after death. Many patients say that religion is important in helping them adjust to, and cope with, the diagnosis of a terminal illness. Most physicians do not ask patients about their religious beliefs, though many patients and families describe their religion as being an important

VI

factor in their decisions about medical treatment, and say they want to talk about this topic with their doctor.[24] A simple question like, "What role, if any, do religion or spirituality play in your life?" can help identify patients with unmet needs. There may also be religious rituals, such as the way a patient's body should be handled after death, that are important for the health care team to know.

## PALLIATIVE CARE AND PAIN

Pain management is often an important aspect in the quality of a seriously ill person's life. As experts in pain management, anesthesiologists possess unique skills to contribute to this area. Many seriously ill patients have surgery and may have resulting acute-on-chronic pain (also see Chapter 44).

### Use of Opioids at the End of Life

Some health care professionals may have concerns about the effect of opioids on a patient's time to death and have apprehensions that the medications given are "killing" the patient. The ethical principle of double effect states that a physician can treat symptoms that may hasten death as a secondary effect, as long as the doctor's intention is to have a good outcome, like decreased pain and distress, rather than a bad outcome, like death.[25] Opioids should be administered to these patients in response to signs of pain or discomfort, rather than arbitrarily increased. Opioids do not shorten, and may even increase, the time to death in dying patients.[25] Thus, the appropriate use of opioids at the end of life is indicated from both a medical and ethical standpoint. If, after discussion, a member of the health care team feels significant moral distress in such a situation, another team member should be assigned to the patient.

### Cancer Pain

Cancer pain is the most recognized type of pain for patients with life-threatening illnesses. Most patients with cancer pain can be managed via the World Health Organization's Cancer Pain Stepladder,[26] but some will require the expertise of a pain medicine specialist. A variety of techniques to control cancer pain are available and are covered in Chapter 44, Chronic Pain Management. Important factors to consider in cancer pain are the cause of the pain (such as tumor or chemotherapy-related) and the natural history of cancer pain, which generally gets worse instead of better. The cause of cancer pain is often complex and can be due to the tumor itself, edema around a tumor, or metastases in tissue, nerve, or bone; or it may be related to the cancer treatment itself, such as peripheral neuropathy or radiation-induced brachial plexopathy.[27] Treatment should be targeted to the cause of the pain when possible, and many patients may have pain from multiple sources. Given the complexities of cancer pain, adjunct medications are an important option (Table 49.1).

For some patients, chemotherapy, radiotherapy, or even surgery that aims to decrease the tumor burden may

| Table 49.1 | Adjuvant Analgesic Agents in Management of Cancer Pain, by Conventional Use Category | |
|---|---|---|
| **Category** | **Examples** | **Comment** |
| **Multipurpose Analgesics** | | |
| Glucocorticoids | Dexamethasone, prednisone | Bone pain, neuropathic pain, lymphoedema pain, headache, bowel obstruction |
| **Antidepressants** | | |
| Tricyclics | Desipramine, amitriptyline | Used for opioid-refractory neuropathic pain, first if comorbid depression; secondary amine compounds (e.g., desipramine) have fewer side effects and might be preferred |
| SNRIs | Duloxetine, milnacipran | Good evidence in some conditions, but overall less than for tricyclics; better side-effect profile than tricyclics, however, and often tried first |
| SSRIs | Paroxetine, citalopram | Very scarce evidence, and, if pain is the target, other subclasses are preferred |
| Other | Bupropion | Little evidence for effectiveness, but less sedating than other antidepressants, and often tried early when fatigue or somnolence is a problem |
| $\alpha_2$-Adrenergic agonists | Tizanidine, clonidine | Seldom used systemically because of side effects, but tizanidine is preferred for a trial; clonidine is used in neuraxial analgesia |
| Cannabinoid | THC/cannabidiol, nabilone, THC | Good evidence in cancer pain for THC/cannabidiol; scarce evidence for other commercially available compounds |

**Table 49.1**    Adjuvant Analgesic Agents in Management of Cancer Pain, by Conventional Use Category—cont'd

| Category | Examples | Comment |
|---|---|---|
| **Topical Agents** | | |
| Anesthetic | Lidocaine patch, local anesthetic creams | |
| Capsaicin | 8% patch; 0.25%, 0.75% creams | High concentration patch indicated for postherpetic neuralgia |
| NSAIDs | Diclofenac and others | Evidence in focal musculoskeletal pains |
| Tricyclics | Doxepin cream | Used for itch; can be tried for pain |
| Others | | Compounded creams with varied drugs tried empirically, but no evidence |
| **Used for Neuropathic Pain** | | |
| Multipurpose drugs | As above | As above |
| **Anticonvulsants** | | |
| Gabapentinoids | Gabapentin, pregabalin | Used first for opioid-refractory neuropathic pain unless comorbid depression; may be multipurpose in view of evidence in postsurgical pain; both drugs act at N-type calcium channel in CNS, but individuals vary in response to one or the other |
| Others | Oxcarbazepine, lamotrigine, topiramate, lacosamide, valproate, carbamazepine, phenytoin | Little evidence for all drugs listed; newer drugs preferred because of reduced side-effect liability, but individual variation is great; all drugs considered for opioid-refractory neuropathic pain if antidepressants and gabapentinoids are ineffective |
| **Sodium-Channel Drugs** | | |
| Sodium-channel blockers | Mexiletine, intravenous lidocaine | Good evidence for intravenous lidocaine |
| Sodium-channel modulator | Lacosamide | New anticonvulsant with very scarce evidence of analgesic effects |
| **GABA Agonists** | | |
| GABA$_A$ agonist | Clonazepam | Very scarce evidence, but used for neuropathic pain with anxiety |
| GABA$_B$ agonist | Baclofen | Evidence in trigeminal neuralgia is the basis for trials in other types of neuropathic pain |
| N-methyl-D-aspartate inhibitors | Ketamine, memantine, others | Evidence scarce for ketamine, but positive experience with intravenous use in advanced illness or pain crisis; little evidence for oral drugs |
| **Used for Bone Pain** | | |
| Bisphosphonates | Pamidronate, ibandronate, clodronate | Good evidence; like the NSAIDs or glucocorticoids, usually considered first-line treatment; also reduces other adverse skeletal-related events; concern about osteonecrosis of the jaw and renal insufficiency might restrict use |
| Calcitonin | | Scarce evidence, but usually well tolerated |
| Radiopharmaceuticals | Strontium-89, samarium-153 | Good evidence, but restricted use because of bone-marrow effects and need for expertise |
| **Used for Bowel Obstruction** | | |
| Anticholinergic drugs | Hyoscine compounds, glycopyrronium (aka glycopyrrolate) | Along with a glucocorticoid, considered first-line adjuvant treatment for nonsurgical bowel obstruction |
| Somatostatin analog | Octreotide | Along with a glucocorticoid, considered first-line adjuvant treatment for nonsurgical bowel obstruction |

*CNS,* Central nervous system; *GABA,* γ-aminobutyric acid; *NSAID,* nonsteroidal antiinflammatory drug; *SNRI,* selective noradrenaline reuptake inhibitor; *SSRI,* selective serotonin reuptake inhibitor; *THC,* tetrahydrocannabinol.
From Portenoy RK. Treatment of cancer pain. *Lancet.* 2011;377:2236-2247.

VI

be pursued to decrease pain even when there is no antici-pated increase in life expectancy.[27] Anesthesiologists may be asked to evaluate patients for techniques such as a celiac plexus block, which decreases pain scores but does not change the need for opioids or the quality of life.[28] Bony pain may be due to osteoblastic or osteolytic components, and approaches such as intrathecal catheters, hormonal therapy, bone-modifying agents, or radiotherapy may be helpful. There may also be psychological aspects related to grief, anxiety, or depression that exacerbate a patient's cancer pain. Addressing those issues often enhances the effects of treatments that target physical pain. Similarly, patients with pain that does not respond to traditional pain medications should be screened for spiritual or emo-tional pain, and these patients should be provided with resources and support to address their distress. Treatment of spiritual pain may involve social work, psychiatry, psychology, chaplaincy, integrative medicine, or other fields. With the increasing number of cancer survivors, physicians should be more aware of issues of long-term opioid dependence and addiction.

## Noncancer Pain

Noncancer pain, or pain in patients without cancer, is a major and yet insufficiently studied issue for patients with serious illnesses. Patients with diagnoses other than cancer may have more difficulty achieving pain control owing to lack of physician awareness that pain is associ-ated with the patient's illness. Because anesthesiologists often provide much of the pain management expertise in a hospital, they should be aware of and knowledgeable about pain management in these seriously ill patients. Most patients with dementia have pain at the end of life, though the exact cause of the pain, such as ulcers or musculoskeletal pain, is unknown. Patients with chronic obstructive pulmonary disease (COPD) often have pain, though it is often not treated aggressively, possibly due to anesthesia providers being hesitant to provide opioids to this patient population. However, opioids are consid-ered an accepted part of the treatment of dyspnea for advanced lung disease, as per the American College of Chest Physicians.[29] In this situation, the COPD patient's pain may go untreated because of the physician's con-cern about respiratory depression, despite the evidence in favor of opioids in this patient population. As with all pain, ideally the cause of the pain should be identified, and the treatment should be matched with the cause.

## CHALLENGES IN THE PALLIATIVE CARE PATIENT

### Identifying Palliative Care and Hospice Patients

Knowing which patients are appropriate for pallia-tive care or hospice consultation can be difficult and

may depend on hospital or community norms. Seri-ously ill patients without clear treatment preferences or decision makers should have a palliative care con-sultation, as should patients whose care causes a con-flict among staff members and those with refractory symptoms.[22]

### Inpatient Palliative Care Consults

In general, patients with life-threatening diseases (i.e., metastatic cancer, cirrhosis, or chronic renal failure) or illnesses with a likely probability of death (i.e., multior-gan failure, major trauma, or sepsis) should be considered for a palliative care consultation.[22] Patients who are likely to die in the next year are good candidates for advance care planning. Also, patients with difficult-to-manage symptoms, like pain or nausea, or complex psychosocial or family issues often benefit from palliative care's inter-disciplinary approach.

### Hospice Consults

Hospice consultations should be sought for patients with a life expectancy of 6 months or less who are interested in focusing on symptom-related treatments rather than treatment with curative intent. Hospice services were ini-tially designed primarily for cancer patients, who have relatively predictable courses in the last 6 months of life. However, cancer patients now make up less than half of hospice patients. Deciding which patients should receive hospice is more difficult for dementia, COPD, and chronic heart failure (CHF), which in combination compose the majority of hospice diagnoses, as these diseases lack good prognostic criteria.[12] Hospice referrals are often made very late in the course of illness, and the median time on hospice was only 17 days in 2015.[12] This means that a significant number of patients did not receive hospice services while they were eligible.

Hospice eligibility determinations are often straight-forward but at times can be a challenge even for hospice medical directors. Most patients will fit into disease-specific guidelines created by Centers for Medicare and Medicaid Services (CMS) to help hospice medical directors determine eligibility.[30] For example, a patient with pulmonary disease would be eligible for hospice if he or she had dyspnea at rest, increasing visits to the emergency room or hospitalizations, and an oxygen sat-uration of less than or equal to 88% on room air.[30] How-ever, a patient may be eligible even if he or she does not meet all these criteria if significant comorbid conditions or a rapid functional decline exists.[30] Therefore, there is room for medical interpretation in determining hospice eligibility, and some patients may qualify for enrollment with one hospice service but not with another.

### Outpatient Palliative Care Consults

No clear criteria for outpatient palliative care refer-ral exist. However, patients with complex symptoms, psychosocial issues, or advance care planning needs who are not eligible for hospice are often good candidates.[31] Outpatient palliative care clinics can help patients with advance care planning such as creating advance directives, as well as serve as consultants for patients with difficult to manage symptoms like pain or nausea.

## Prognosis

Inherent in many of the discussions about appropriateness of palliative care and hospice consultations, and the ability of anesthesiologists to discuss goals of care, is the concept of prognosis. Anesthesiologists need to have a general idea of prognosis in order to make appropriate medical recommendations.

### Physician Estimate

Many clinical decisions are influenced by perceived prognosis, such as whether to withdraw the ventilator, give chemotherapy, and proceed with surgery. Despite its importance, prognosis continues to be extremely difficult to determine. Prognostic accuracy tends to be poor, and most physicians tend to overestimate prognosis by a factor of five, with estimates being worse the longer the physician knows the patient.[32] However, ICU physicians

tend to be overly pessimistic about their patients' survival.[33] Nurses and physicians often disagree about the likelihood of a patient's survival and quality of life, with nurses tending to be more pessimistic.[34] One proposed approach is that of the "surprise question." A physician answering "no" to the question, "Would you be surprised if the patient died within the next 12 months?" is a relatively good predictor of patients who are likely to do so.[22] Although this question does not make the future easy to predict or provide clinicians with specifics about how long the patient will live, it can help frame some decisions, such as surgeries or treatments, and can help give families a better sense of what the health care team is thinking.

### Disease Trajectories

It can be helpful for physicians to have and convey a concept of the patient's likely disease trajectory. Patients with most cancers follow a relatively predictable course, whereas those with COPD, for example, tend to have a long course of repeated hospitalizations and associated decline prior to death. These disease trajectories can be useful starting points for discussions with patients and families about what the future is likely to hold (Fig. 49.4).

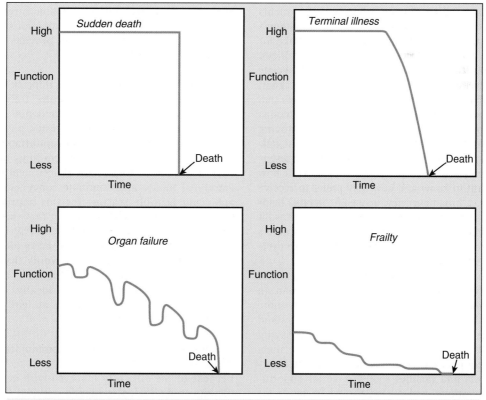

**Fig. 49.4** Trajectories of dying. (Redrawn from Lunney JR, Lynn J, Hogan C. Profiles of older medicare decedents. *J Am Geriatr Soc.* 2002;50:1108-1112.)

VI

## Prognostic Tools

Multiple prognostic tools have been developed, particularly for critically ill patients[35] as well as for patients with other specific conditions. These tools can synthesize broad information about the severity of a patient's disease into a single number or percentile that is easier for caregivers, patients, and families to understand. They can therefore be very useful, but may not take into account all of a patient's comorbid conditions. They cannot predict which individual patients will live or die, which is the information that patients and families really want. Despite these limitations, prognostic calculators can be helpful in framing discussions with families about the patient's likely course.

## Functional Status

Performance status generally correlates quite well with prognosis,[36] with a bedbound patient likely to have a much shorter life span than someone who is ambulatory. For example, a patient who is bedbound and recently stopped eating would likely have days to weeks, whereas a patient with a similar diagnosis who is up in a chair most of the day but needs help with bathing and dressing might have weeks to months.

## Communication

An essential part of discussing medical issues with patients and families is ensuring understanding of a patient's medical issues. Although the medical team may take for granted that a patient starting dialysis has failing kidneys, the patient and family may not automatically associate those two pieces of information. Additionally, different members of the health care team may give patients and families different messages. For example, a cardiologist may inform the family that a patient's heart is improving after a myocardial infarction, while the intensivist tells the family that he is becoming worse because of worsening pneumonia and sepsis. Querying patients about how much they want to know and how they prefer to receive information (i.e., broad overview or specific details) helps to guide these conversation. Some patients may not want to know anything about their illness and can designate a surrogate to receive medical information and make decisions on their behalf.

Asking what the patient and family have been told about the patient's condition can give the clinician an idea about what issues need to be discussed in more detail. "Checking in" with the patient and family about how they are reacting to this information by saying things like, "Is this a surprise for you?" can give them a chance to express their emotions related to new information. Patients and families should have an opportunity to ask questions, and a plan should be made for the patient's care and future meetings, if needed. When possible, family meetings should involve a representative from each specialty taking care of the patient, in addition to the patient or patient's surrogate, as well as other family members requested by the patient or surrogate. Although it can be challenging to find a time for everyone involved in a patient's care to meet, this investment generally leads to a more cohesive, logical care plan for the patient.

Many physicians struggle with how to begin family meetings. Common sense approaches include introducing the family and team members, giving a short explanation for why you are meeting, sitting down with the patient and family, and displaying empathy. A short meeting beforehand with the health care team members can be helpful. Sharing specialty-specific insights and getting a better sense of the decisions that will need to be made during the meeting are also helpful. Nurses, chaplains, social workers, and other professionals should be invited to attend as appropriate.

Occasionally, members of the health care team will disagree about a patient's prognosis, treatment plan, or a variety of other issues. This is expected[34] and should be addressed promptly and professionally. Disagreements that are glossed over can quickly become adversarial and lead to poor patient care and confusion for the family. Many of the same skills in conflict resolution, negotiation, and facilitation that palliative care physicians use in family meetings can be helpful in the setting of provider disagreement. A palliative care consultation should be considered for these situations to help formulate a cohesive care plan and provide the best care possible.

### Physician Tendencies in Addressing Difficult Topics

Most physicians never receive any training in how to discuss difficult topics with patients, yet they are expected to do so routinely. As a result, physicians at all levels of training often feel uncomfortable discussing difficult topics with patients. Recordings of physicians show that they tend to focus on technical detail, avoid emotional topics, and dominate conversations.[37] There are many possible reasons for this approach, including a lack of training and the fact that these behaviors are likely to be coping mechanisms. Physicians should be aware of these tendencies and make efforts to overcome them through the use of words that are understandable, acknowledgment of emotion, and allowing patients and families to speak. Ideally, patients and families should be speaking for at least half of the conversation.

### Patient and Family Wishes About Communicating Prognosis

Because of the difficulty involved with accurately predicting an individual patient's survival, many physicians avoid giving any kind of estimate to avoid being wrong.[38] However, in one study, 87% of surrogate decision makers wanted the physician to give a prognosis, even if it was uncertain.[39] When given a prognosis, though, surrogates tend to be overly optimistic, especially with worse prognoses.[40] Many practitioners choose to state clearly that any estimate is a guess, and use ranges such as hours to days, days to weeks, or weeks to months to convey a general idea of the patient's life expectancy.

### Frameworks for Communicating Difficult Information

Anesthesiologists in the ICU frequently need to communicate sensitive or difficult information about prognosis to patients and families, and it is often necessary in the perioperative or pain settings as well. Ensuring that patients understand their condition is an important part of informed consent for anesthesia. Most of the time, physicians will speak with families because many critically ill patients are unable to participate. Family-clinician communication in the ICU is often inadequate. In one study, only half of families had an adequate understanding of the patient's prognosis, treatments, or diagnoses after a discussion with ICU physicians.[41]

There are several formal frameworks for communicating prognosis to patients and families. The SPIKES protocol[42] (Box 49.4), which includes asking for the patient's or family member's current understanding of the medical issues, responding with empathy, and agreeing on a follow-up plan, was originally described for breaking bad news, but the concepts apply in many instances.

### Discussing Code Status

The palliative-care framework functions in the setting of discussions about resuscitation orders as well. Ideally, discussions about code status should take place in the context of a larger conversation about a patient's overall condition and goals. Between 1 in 1400 and 1 in 1800 patients experiences a cardiac arrest in the operating room.[43] The mortality rate in the immediate perioperative period for these patients is about 60%.[43] This survival rate is markedly better than that among patients who arrest on the floor or out of the hospital, which may be an important part of a patient's decision regarding code status in the perioperative period.

### Time-Limited Trials

A time-limited trial is "an agreement between clinicians and a patient/family to use certain medical therapies over a defined period to see if the patient improves or deteriorates according to agreed-on clinical outcomes."[44] A time-limited trial is a method of dealing with prognostic uncertainty and is a useful tool in family discussions. For example, the family of a patient with a COPD exacerbation and a do not resuscitate (DNR) order may desire a trial of bilevel positive airway pressure (BiPAP) for several days to evaluate whether the patient tolerates

---

| **Box 49.4** A Framework for Breaking Bad News |
| --- |
| **Setting:** Arrange for a quiet, private space large enough for all participants |
| **Perception:** Assess understanding. *"What have the doctors told you about your wife's illness?"* |
| **Invitation:** Ask how much information is desired. *"Some people like all the details, others just like the big picture. What would you like?"* |
| **Knowledge:** Tell what you know. Use language that is easy to understand and avoid using complex medical phrases. |
| **Empathy:** Acknowledge emotions. *"I wish things were different."* |
| **Sequelae:** Agree on next steps. *"Let's meet tomorrow afternoon so I can update you on her condition."* |

From Baile WF, Buckman R, Lenzi R, et al. SPIKES—A six-step protocol for delivering bad news: application to the patient with cancer. *Oncologist.* 2000;5:302-311.

---

the intervention and has improved symptoms.[44] Before starting a time-limited trial of therapy, the medical team should take the following steps: (1) clarify the patient's medical issues and the risks and benefits of any proposed treatments, (2) decide on and discuss with family a reasonable time frame for improvement and reevaluation, (3) implement the trial, and (4) reassess the patient at the end of the agreed-upon time frame. Time-limited trials will not work for every patient, especially those with rapid changes in their clinical conditions, but they can help patients, families, and providers determine a consensus plan when uncertainty or disagreement exists.

### Identifying the Imminently Dying Patient

Anesthesiologists may care for dying patients in the ICU, and patients whose death process has not been identified may occasionally present to the operating room. Thus, anesthesiologists should be able to recognize signs of the dying process in order to provide appropriate care for these patients. Additionally, anesthesiologists should be able to provide information for interested family members about what the dying process looks like. Unfortunately, there are few signs that are both sensitive and specific for impending death. Change of consciousness, dysphagia, and decreased oral intake are sensitive but not specific, for example.[45] Mandibular movement with breathing, peripheral cyanosis, and Cheyne-Stokes breathing are reasonably specific for patient death within 3 days but occur in less than 60% of patients.[45]

## PERIOPERATIVE MANAGEMENT OF THE PALLIATIVE CARE PATIENT

A list of perioperative considerations is provided in Box 49.5.[46]

VI

## Advance Directives

Advance directives encompass a variety of legal documents such as living wills, Five Wishes, or state-specific advance directives, which describe a patient's wishes for medical care. Many of these describe options such as artificial hydration and nutrition or life support, if the patient has no hope of recovery. Although these documents can be useful as a guide, they rarely offer unambiguous guidance for the entirety of the wide range of clinical scenarios.[47] Many clinicians advocate for patients' naming a surrogate and for discussions about values and goals among the patient, surrogate, and health care team.[47] Patients who prepare advance directives are more likely to receive care that aligns with their preferences,[48] and many advance directives include the naming of a surrogate decision maker as part of the form.

## Decision-Making Capacity

Many patients who are in the perioperative period or in the ICU may not have decision-making capacity owing to an inability to communicate, medical issues, or medications.[49] Determining whether a patient has capacity to make medical decisions can be difficult. In fact, identifying patient decision-making capacity[49] can change over time, so physicians must be cognizant that a patient who was previously able to make decisions may have become delirious, for example, and no longer be able to understand the risks of a procedure. The criteria used to decide whether a person has capacity are "the ability to communicate a choice, to understand the relevant information, to appreciate the medical consequences of the situation, and to reason about treatment choices."[49] Asking questions like, "Can you tell me what surgery we are doing and why?" and "Can you tell me the risks of the procedure?" can help clarify whether a patient has decision-making capacity. If the physician is uncertain whether a patient has decision-making capacity, a psychiatric consult may be appropriate. Deciding whether a patient has decisional capacity is a crucial step in the perioperative evaluation. Patients without decisional capacity cannot give informed consent for anesthesia, and a surrogate must be identified for the patient in most cases.

---

**Box 49.5** Perioperative Considerations for Palliative Care Patients

**Preoperative Considerations**

Look in chart for advance directive or documentation of code status

Determine if the patient needs a surrogate, and if so, who that person is

If DNR or other limits on treatment listed, clarify patient's desires based on ASA guidelines[46]:
- Full attempt at resuscitation
- Limited attempt at resuscitation defined with regard to specific procedures
  - Patient or surrogate should be informed about which procedures are essential to providing anesthesia (i.e., an endotracheal tube) and which are not (i.e., chest compressions)
  - *Example:* Patient with extensive rib metastases declines chest compressions but desires other medications and procedures as appropriate
- Limited attempt at resuscitation defined with regard to the patient's goals and values
  - Patient or surrogate allows the medical team to decide which procedures are appropriate
  - *Example:* Patient wants to have issues that seem easily reversible treated (i.e., respiratory depression in the PACU after accidental narcotic overdose) but does not want treatment that may to lead to neurologic compromise (i.e., does not want prolonged CPR)

Document any changes in treatment limitation clearly in the chart
- Include the people present during the discussion

- When the original advance directive will be reinstated
  - Per ASA guidelines, "when the patient leaves the PACU or when the patient has recovered from the acute effects of anesthesia and surgery"

Discuss any changes in treatment limitation with the surgeon, nurse, or other appropriate parties

Ensure that the patient receives any scheduled pain medications preoperatively

Consider involving spiritual care to perform appropriate rituals if there is a high risk of death

Review past medications for agents like Adriamycin and bleomycin

Review records for sites of metastases including lung or brain that may impact physiology

Assess decision-making ability of patients with brain metastases or suspected cognitive impairment

Consider preoperative epidural placement for appropriate patients

Assess baseline functional status and general prognosis

**Intraoperative Considerations**

Take special care in positioning cachectic patients and those with poor skin integrity

Consider PONV prophylaxis for at-risk patients

Communicate any limitations in treatment to oncoming providers

**Postoperative Considerations**

Consider possibly increased postoperative pain requirements in context of baseline opioid use

Ensure availability of rescue antiemetic for at-risk patients

Communicate any limitations in treatment to PACU providers

---

*ASA,* American Society of Anesthesiologists; *CPR,* cardiopulmonary resuscitation; *DNR,* do not resuscitate; *PACU,* postanesthesia care unit; *PONV,* postoperative nausea and vomiting.

## Surrogate Decision Makers

A surrogate decision maker is a person who makes medical decisions on the patient's behalf. Patients may name surrogate decision makers at any point. Patients with decisional capacity may either continue to make their own decisions or defer decisions to their surrogate. Some states have lists that order the priority of surrogates for patients who have not designated one. Surrogates' wishes may not always match those of the patient,[50] so communication about goals and values is crucial. Surrogates should make decisions in the patient's best interest and that are the surrogate's best guess as to what the patient would want, which is not necessarily what the surrogate would choose. Clarifying this distinction with questions like, "What do you think your father would say if he were able to sit with us and understand this information?" can be helpful.

## How to Approach Perioperative DNR Conversations

### Recommendations From the American Society of Anesthesiologists

About 15% of patients who present for surgery have a DNR order,[51] so all anesthesia providers should be well versed in discussing these important issues with patients and families. Additionally, almost 25% of surgical patients with DNR orders die within 30 days of surgery.[52] The American Society of Anesthesiologists (ASA) has published guidelines for care of patients with DNR orders and limitations on treatment.[53] For the purposes of this section, DNR will refer to both DNR orders and other limitations on treatment found in documents such as advance directives. The guidelines emphasize that the automatic and complete suspension of DNR orders (or

other advance directives) may violate the patient's right to self-determination and that a discussion with the patient or surrogate prior to the procedure is essential. The ASA describes three outcomes for discussions for patients with a DNR order who present for surgery (Table 49.2). Importantly, a DNR order may be completely suspended or partially suspended in defined ways to meet patient preferences. An essential part of the ASA guidelines includes discussion and documentation regarding whether, and when, the original DNR order will be reinstated. According to the ASA, "this occurs when the patient leaves the postanesthesia care unit or when the patient has recovered from the side effects of anesthesia/procedure."[53] These discussions should always be clearly documented.

### Recommendations From the American College of Surgeons and the Association of periOperative Registered Nurses

The similarities in recommendations among professional societies of anesthesiologists, surgeons, and nurses are striking (Table 49.3).[54,55] As with the ASA, they recommend a more tailored approach rather than automatic suspension. Despite this, 30% of physicians believe DNR orders should be automatically suspended during surgery, and a large majority of patients want to discuss perioperative changes in DNR orders with their physicians.[56] A study in 2012 demonstrated that only half of surgeons discuss advance directives prior to surgery, and half would not take a patient to the operating room with limitations on treatment.[57]

### Hospice Patients Who Present for Surgery

Hospice patients may decline hospice services at any point. There are cases in which surgery can reduce

---

**Table 49.2** Scenarios for Patients With Perioperative Limitations on Treatment, per the ASA

| Full Attempt at Resuscitation | Limited Attempt at Resuscitation Defined With Regard to Specific Procedures | Limited Attempt at Resuscitation Defined With Regard to the Patient's Goals and Value |
|---|---|---|
| Full suspension of existing DNR. Any procedures may be used. | Specific procedures, for example chest compressions, may not be used. | Anesthesiologist may use clinical judgment to determine which resuscitation procedures are appropriate. |
| | The anesthesiologist should inform the patient which procedures can, or cannot, reasonably be refused during an anesthetic. | Full resuscitation may be desired for events that are likely to be easily reversible, but not those likely to lead to an unwanted outcome. |
| A woman who was recently diagnosed with breast cancer decides to suspend her DNR during the surgery, saying, "I have two kids at home, and I want to live as long as I can for them." | A woman with breast cancer with extensive metastases to her ribs agrees to all interventions except chest compressions, saying, "Even if it worked, I don't want to be on a ventilator with shattered ribs." | A woman with breast cancer whose greatest fear is being unable to recognize her children says, "If you think you can fix the problem and I'll go back to being myself, please do that. If my brain is unlikely to recover, then please don't pursue more aggressive measures." |

*DNR*, Do not resuscitate.
From American Society of Anesthesiologists (ASA). Ethical Guidelines for the Anesthesia Care of Patients with Do-Not-Resuscitate Orders or Other Directives That Limit Treatment. Accessed June 24, 2015. http://www.asahq.org/quality-and-practice-management/standards-and-guidelines.

VI

| Table 49.3 | Comparison of Professional Society Statements Regarding Surgical Patients With DNR Orders | | |
|---|---|---|---|
| Topic | American Society of Anesthesiologists | American College of Surgeons | Association of periOperative Registered Nurses |
| Statement regarding automatic suspension of DNR orders for surgery | "Policies automatically suspending DNR orders or other directives that limit treatment prior to procedures involving anesthetic care may not sufficiently address a patient's rights to self-determination in a responsible and ethical manner" | "Policies that lead to either the automatic enforcement of all DNR orders or to disregarding or automatically cancelling such orders do not sufficiently support a patient's right to self-determination" | "Reconsideration of do-not-resuscitate or allow-natural-death orders is required and is an integral component of the care of patients undergoing surgery or other invasive procedures" |
| Guidelines for the care of surgical patients with DNR orders | "Prior to procedures requiring anesthetic care, any existing directives to limit the use of resuscitation procedures … should, when possible, be reviewed with the patient or designated surrogate"[53] | "The best approach for these patients is a policy of 'required reconsideration' of the existing DNR orders … [with] the patient or designated surrogate and the physicians who will be responsible for the patient's care" | "Health care providers should have a discussion with the patient or patient's surrogate about the risks, benefits, implications, and potential outcomes of anesthesia and surgery in relation to the do-not-resuscitate or allow-natural-death orders before initiating anesthesia, surgery, or other invasive procedures" |

*DNR*, Do not resuscitate.
Data from the American Society of Anesthesiologists,[53] American College of Surgeons,[54] and Association of periOperative Registered Nurses.[55]

suffering, such as the surgical repair of an open fracture after trauma, for example. Surgery for hospice patients should prompt a discussion of the risks and benefits of the procedure, as well as the status of any orders for limitations on perioperative treatment.

## CONCLUSION

Palliative care is a new field that focuses on the relief of suffering in patients with life-limiting conditions. Anesthesiologists have many skills to offer palliative care patients including skills in pain and symptom management and the care of the critically ill. Palliative care should not be reserved only for dying patients. Anesthesiologists should have a working knowledge of what palliative care and hospice offer, how the anesthetic care fits into the patient's overall course, and the legal and ethical issues surrounding perioperative limitations on treatment.

## QUESTIONS OF THE DAY

1. What types of consultations are most often performed by palliative care teams?
2. How can opioids be used in an ethical manner at the end of a patient's life? What is the principle of double effect?
3. What strategies can be used to conduct family meetings for a patient with a life-threatening illness?
4. How can a time-limited trial of therapy be used in the management of a critically ill patient with prognostic uncertainty?
5. How should the anesthesia provider approach perioperative do not resuscitate (DNR) conversations? What are the recommendations of the American Society of Anesthesiologists, American College of Surgeons, and Association of periOperative Registered Nurses?

## REFERENCES

1. Robinson J, Gott M, Ingleton C. Patient and family experiences of palliative care in hospital: what do we know? An integrative review. *Palliat Med.* 2014;28(1):18–33.
2. Nelson JE, Puntillo KA, Pronovost PJ, et al. In their own words: patients and families define high-quality palliative care in the intensive care unit. *Crit Care Med.* 2010;38:808–818.
3. World Health Organization. Definition of Palliative Care. http://www.who.int/cancer/palliative/definition/en/. Accessed July 12, 2016.
4. Morrison RS, Augustin R, Souvanna P, Meier DE. America's care of serious illness: a state-by-state report card on access to palliative care in our nation's hospitals. *J Palliat Med.* 2011;14:1094–1096.
5. Center to Advance Palliative Care. About Palliative Care. http://www.capc.org/about/palliative-care/. Accessed July 12, 2016.
6. Ferris FD, Balfour HM, Bowen K, et al. A model to guide patient and family care: based on nationally accepted principles and norms of practice. *J Pain Symptom Manage.* 2002;24:106–123.

7. Medicare Payment Advisory Commission. *A Data Book: Health Care Spending and the Medicare Program.* www.medpac.gov; 2016.

8. Meier DE. Increased access to palliative care and hospice services: opportunities to improve value in health care. *Milbank Q.* 2011;89(3):343–380.

9. Morrison RS, Dietrich J, Ladwig S, et al. Palliative care consultation teams cut hospital costs for Medicaid beneficiaries. *Health Aff.* 2011;30:454–463.

10. Scheunemann LP, McDevitt M, Carson SS, Hanson LC. Randomized, controlled trials of interventions to improve communication in intensive care: a systematic review. *Chest.* 2011;139:543–554.

11. Temel JS, Greer JA, Muzikansky A, et al. Early palliative care for patients with metastatic non-small-cell lung cancer. *N Engl J Med.* 2010;363:733–742.

12. Rothenberg LR, Doberman D, Simon LE, et al. Patients surviving six months in hospice care: who are they? *J Palliat Med.* 2014;17:899–905. http://www.nhpco.org/sites/default/files/public/Statistics_Research/2015_Facts_Figures.pdf.

13. Kelley AS, Deb P, Du Q, et al. Hospice enrollment saves money for Medicare and improves care quality across a number of different lengths-of-stay. *Health Aff.* 2013;32:552–561.

14. American Board of Internal Medicine. Hospice and Palliative Medicine Policies. http://www.abim.org/certification/policies/imss/hospice.aspx. Accessed June 15, 2015.

15. Quill TE, Abernethy AP. Generalist plus specialist palliative care–creating a more sustainable model. *N Engl J Med.* 2013;368:1173–1175.

16. Gebauer SL, Fine PG. Palliative medicine competencies for anesthesiologists. *J Clin Anesth.* 2014;26:429–431.

17. Kwok AC, Semel ME, Lipsitz SR, et al. The intensity and variation of surgical care at the end of life: a retrospective cohort study. *Lancet.* 2011;378:1408–1413.

18. Hospice and Palliative Nurses Association. http://hpna.advancingexpertcare.org/wp-content/uploads/2014/09/Value-of-Professional-Nurse-in-Palliative-Care-position-statement-080311_062413corrected.pdf. Accessed July 12, 2016.

19. National Association of Social Workers. The Certified Hospice and Palliative Social Worker. http://www.socialworkers.org/credentials/credentials/chpsw.asp. Accessed July 12, 2016.

20. Board of Chaplaincy Certification, Inc. Palliative Care Specialty Certfication Competencies. http://bcci.professionalchaplains.org/content.asp?admin=Y&pl=45&sl=42&contentid=49. Accessed July 12, 2016.

21. Mosenthal AC, Weissman DE, Curtis JR, et al. Integrating palliative care in the surgical and trauma intensive care unit: a report from the Improving Palliative Care in the Intensive Care Unit (IPAL-ICU) Project Advisory Board and the Center to Advance Palliative Care. *Crit Care Med.* 2012;40:1199–1206.

22. Weissman DE, Meier DE. Identifying patients in need of a palliative care assessment in the hospital setting: a consensus report from the Center to Advance Palliative Care. *J Palliat Med.* 2011;14:17–23.

23. Aslakson R, Cheng J, Vollenweider D, et al. Evidence-based palliative care in the intensive care unit: a systematic review of interventions. *J Palliat Med.* 2014;17:219–235.

24. Phelps AC, Maciejewski PK, Nilsson M, et al. Religious coping and use of intensive life-prolonging care near death in patients with advanced cancer. *JAMA.* 2009;301:1140–1147.

25. Mazer MA, Alligood CM, Wu Q. The infusion of opioids during terminal withdrawal of mechanical ventilation in the medical intensive care unit. *J Pain Symptom Manage.* 2011;42:44–51.

26. Zech DF, Grond S, Lynch J, et al. Validation of World Health Organization Guidelines for cancer pain relief: a 10-year prospective study. *Pain.* 1995;63:65–76.

27. Portenoy RK. Treatment of cancer pain. *Lancet.* 2011;377:2236–2247.

28. Wong GY, Schroeder DR, Carns PE, et al. Effect of neurolytic celiac plexus block on pain relief, quality of life, and survival in patients with unresectable pancreatic cancer: a randomized controlled trial. *JAMA.* 2004;291:1092–1099.

29. Romem A, Tom SE, Beauchene M, et al. Pain management at the end of life: a comparative study of cancer, dementia, and chronic obstructive pulmonary disease patients. *Palliat Med.* 2015;29:464–469.

30. Gazelle G. Understanding hospice–an underutilized option for life's final chapter. *N Engl J Med.* 2007;357:321–324.

31. Smith AK, Thai JN, Bakitas MA, et al. The diverse landscape of palliative care clinics. *J Palliat Med.* 2013;16(6):661–668.

32. Christakis NA, Lamont EB. Extent and determinants of error in doctors' prognoses in terminally ill patients: prospective cohort study. *BMJ.* 2000;320:469–472.

33. Rocker G, Cook D, Sjokvist P, et al. Clinician predictions of intensive care unit mortality. *Crit Care Med.* 2004;32:1149–1154.

34. Frick S, Uehlinger DE, Zuercher Zenklusen RM. Medical futility: predicting outcome of intensive care unit patients by nurses and doctors–a prospective comparative study. *Crit Care Med.* 2003;31(2):456–461.

35. Vincent JL, Moreno R. Clinical review: scoring systems in the critically ill. *Crit Care.* 2010;14:207.

36. Olajide O, Hanson L, Usher BM, et al. Validation of the palliative performance scale in the acute tertiary care hospital setting. *J Palliat Med.* 2007;10:111–117.

37. Fine E, Reid MC, Shengelia R, Adelman RD. Directly observed patient-physician discussions in palliative and end-of-life care: a systematic review of the literature. *J Palliat Med.* 2010;13:595–603.

38. Ridley S, Fisher M. Uncertainty in end-of-life care. *Curr Opin Crit Care.* 2013;19:642–647.

39. Evans LR, Boyd EA, Malvar G, et al. Surrogate decision-makers' perspectives on discussing prognosis in the face of uncertainty. *Am J Respir Crit Care Med.* 2009;179:48–53.

40. Zier LS, Sottile PD, Hong SY, et al. Surrogate decision makers' interpretation of prognostic information: a mixed-methods study. *Ann Intern Med.* 2012;156:360–366.

41. Curtis JR, White DB. Practical guidance for evidence-based ICU family conferences. *Chest.* 2008;134:835–843.

42. Baile WF, Buckman R, Lenzi R, et al. SPIKES—A six-step protocol for delivering bad news: application to the patient with cancer. *Oncologist.* 2000;5(4):302–311.

43. Nunnally ME, O'Connor MF, Kordylewski H, et al. The incidence and risk factors for perioperative cardiac arrest observed in the national anesthesia clinical outcomes registry. *Anesth Analg.* 2015;120:364–370.

44. Quill TE, Holloway R. Time-limited trials near the end of life. *JAMA.* 2011;306:1483–1484.

45. Hui D, dos Santos R, Chisholm G, et al. Clinical signs of impending death in cancer patients. *Oncologist.* 2014;19:681–687.

46. Ethical Guidelines for the Anesthesia Care of Patients with Do-Not-Resuscitate Orders or Other Directives That Limit Treatment. http://www.asahq.org/For-Members/Standards-Guidelines-and-Statements.aspx; 2008.

47. Sudore RL, Fried TR. Redefining the "planning" in advance care planning: preparing for end-of-life decision making. *Ann Intern Med.* 2010;153:256–261.

48. Silveira MJ, Kim SY, Langa KM. Advance directives and outcomes of surrogate decision making before death. *N Engl J Med.* 2010;362:1211–1218.

49. Appelbaum PS. Clinical practice. Assessment of patients' competence to consent to treatment. *N Engl J Med.* 2007;357:1834–1840.

50. Shalowitz DI, Garrett-Mayer E, Wendler D. The accuracy of surrogate decision makers: a systematic review. *Arch Intern Med.* 2006;166:493–497.

VI

51. Scott TH, Gavrin JR. Palliative surgery in the do-not-resuscitate patient: ethics and practical suggestions for management. *Anesthesiol Clin.* 2012;30:1–12.

52. Kazaure H, Roman S, Sosa JA. High mortality in surgical patients with do-not-resuscitate orders: analysis of 8256 patients. *Arch Surg.* 2011;146:922–928.

53. American Society of Anesthesiologists. Ethical Guidelines for the Anesthesia Care of Patients with Do-Not-Resuscitate Orders or Other Directives that Limit Treatment. Amended on October 16, 2013. http://www.asahq.org/~/media /sites/asahq/files/public/resourc es/standards-guidelines/ethical-guidelines-for-the-anesthesia-care-of-patients.pdf/.

54. Statement on Advance Directives by Patients. "Do Not Resuscitate" in the Operating Room. American College of Surgeons. https://http://www.facs.org/a bout-acs/statements/19-advance-directives; 2014. Accessed Jul 12, 2016.

55. Association of periOperative Registered Nurses. AORN Position Statement on Perioperative Care of Patients with Do-Not-Resuscitate or Allow-Natural-Death Orders. http://www.aorn.org/g uidelines/clinical-resources/position-statements; 2014. Accessed July 12, 2016.

56. Burkle CM, Swetz KM, Armstrong MH, Keegan MT. Patient and doctor attitudes and beliefs concerning perioperative do not resuscitate orders: anesthesiologists' growing compliance with patient autonomy and self determination guidelines. *BMC Anesthesiol.* 2013;13:2.

57. Redmann AJ, Brasel KJ, Alexander CG, Schwarze ML. Use of advance directives for high-risk operations: a national survey of surgeons. *Ann Surg.* 2012;255:418–423.

# 50 SLEEP MEDICINE AND ANESTHESIA

Mandeep Singh and Frances Chung

## INTRODUCTION

The neurophysiologic mechanisms governing sleep and wakefulness have been identified during recent years. These mechanisms have provided new insights into mechanisms of different arousal states and the impact of different anesthetic drugs on modulation of key components of the sleep-wake neuronal circuits. The similarities and differences between sleep and anesthesia states need to be understood in order to examine a patient's vulnerability to anesthesia and different anesthetic drugs. These differences are also likely to determine the likelihood of complications in one state compared to the other, such as upper airway collapse, hypoventilation, and other respiratory problems.

### Human Sleep

Sleep is defined as a state of decreased arousal that is actively generated by nuclei in the hypothalamus, brainstem, and basal forebrain and is crucial for the maintenance of health.[1,2] Humans spend approximately one third of their lives sleeping. Sleep is described as being under the control of two processes: (1) a circadian clock (the circadian drive) that regulates the appropriate timing of sleep and wakefulness across the 24-hour day and (2) a homeostatic process (the homoeostatic drive) that regulates sleep need and intensity according to the time spent awake or asleep.[3] The daily drive to sleep is modulated by the hypothalamic suprachiasmatic nuclei that coordinate circadian (24-hour) rhythm. The perceived sensation of sleepiness is likely the result of a circadian drive, process C (people tend to get sleepy according to their accustomed sleep times during a 24-hour cycle), along with a homeostatic drive, process S (sleep deprivation leads to increasing sleepiness).[4] These two sleep drives are additive. Also, a temporal organization must be preserved to obtain a subjective experience of being refreshed and

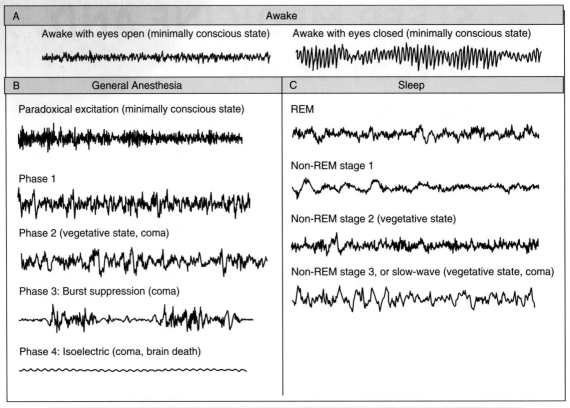

**Fig. 50.1** Electroencephalographic changes seen with different states of consciousness and arousal (awake state, general anesthesia, and sleep stages). *NREM,* Non-rapid eye movement; *REM,* rapid eye movement. (From Brown EN, Lydic R, Schiff ND. General anesthesia, sleep, and coma. *N Engl J Med.* 2010;363(27):2638-2650, used with permission.)

restful.[5,6] For example, patients with chronic insomnia often have difficulties because the two sleep drives are not aligned with each other; in such patients, afternoon naps taken to compensate for sleep deprivation would likely delay sleep onset later in the night).

Normal sleep exhibits a dynamic architecture and is a nonhomogeneous state that can be divided into non–rapid eye movement (NREM) sleep and rapid eye movement (REM) sleep. These two states cycle at an ultradian (less than 24 hour) rhythm of approximately 90- to 120-minute intervals, consolidated in bouts of 6 to 8 hours.[2,5,6]

The American Academy of Sleep Medicine (AASM) has classified wakefulness and sleep into various stages based on characteristic electroencephalogram (EEG) patterns.[7,8] *Wakefulness,* or *stage W,* is characterized by beta activity with eyes open (low amplitude, 12 to 40 Hz) and alpha activity with eyes closed (low amplitude, 8 to 13 Hz). NREM sleep has three distinct EEG stages, based on characteristic patterns on the EEG (Fig. 50.1). *Stage N1 sleep* is characterized by attenuation of alpha activity during wakefulness, to a low amplitude, mixed frequency signal (4 to 7 Hz), and vertex sharp waves (prominent sharp waves lasting <0.5 second and maximal over the central EEG region). *Stage N2 sleep* is characterized by the presence of K-complexes (well-delineated, negative, sharp waves followed by a positive deflection, lasting 0.5 second) and sleep spindles (high-frequency bursts of 11 to 16 Hz, with tapering ends, distinct from the background rhythm and last ≥0.5 second). *Stage N3 sleep* is characterized by the presence of higher-amplitude (75 µV), lower-frequency (0.5 to 2 Hz) rhythms, also known as *delta waves,* accompanied by waxing and waning muscle tone, decreased body temperature, and decreased heart rate.[2] *Stage R,* or *REM sleep,* is characterized by rapid eye movements, dreaming, irregular breathing and heart rate, and skeletal muscle hypotonia.[1] In REM sleep, the EEG shows active high-frequency, low-amplitude rhythms (see Fig. 50.1). This activated EEG pattern has given rise to descriptions of REM sleep as "active" or "paradoxical" sleep and to the NREM phase of sleep as "quiet" sleep.[9,10] Cognitive changes and vivid dreaming are well known to occur during REM sleep.[11]

## General Anesthesia

General anesthesia could be described as a reversible drug-induced coma. Nevertheless, anesthesia providers often refer to the unconsciousness induced by anesthetic drugs as *sleep* because of the negative connotation of the term *coma.* The EEG patterns of general anesthesia-induced consciousness are described in three periods (see Fig. 50.1).

Before *induction of anesthesia,* the patient has a normal, active EEG, with prominent alpha activity (10 Hz) when the eyes are closed. Small doses of hypnotic drugs acting on the γ-aminobutyric acid type A (GABA$_A$) receptors induce a state of sedation in which the patient is calm and easily arousable, with the eyes generally closed. This state is followed by a brief period of paradoxical excitation, characterized by an increase in beta activity on the EEG (13 to 25 Hz).

During the *maintenance* period, four distinct phases have been described.[12] Phase 1, a light state of general anesthesia, is characterized by a decrease in EEG beta activity (13 to 30 Hz) and an increase in EEG alpha activity (8 to 12 Hz) and delta activity (0 to 4 Hz). During phase 2, the intermediate state, beta activity decreases and alpha and delta activity increases, with so-called anteriorization, that is, an increase in alpha and delta activity in the anterior EEG leads relative to the posterior leads. The EEG in phase 2 resembles that seen in stage 3, NREM (or slow-wave) sleep. Phase 3 is a deeper state, in which the EEG is characterized by flat periods interspersed with periods of alpha and beta activity (burst suppression). As this state of general anesthesia becomes more intense, the time between the periods of alpha activity lengthens, and the amplitudes of the alpha and beta activity decrease. Surgery is usually performed during phases 2 and 3. In phase 4, the most profound state of general anesthesia, the EEG is isoelectric (completely flat), indicated in conditions such as induced coma or neuroprotection during neurosurgery (also see Chapter 30).[12]

During *emergence* from general anesthesia, the EEG patterns proceed in approximately reverse order from phase 2 or 3 of the maintenance period to an active EEG that is consistent with a fully awake state. Anesthetic drugs induce unconsciousness by altering neurotransmission at multiple sites in the cerebral cortex, brainstem, and thalamus. Recent advances in spectral EEG analysis have allowed spatiotemporal characterization of the effects of various intravenous and inhaled anesthetics.[13]

## Other Arousal States

Coma is characterized by a state of profound unresponsiveness, which could be drug-induced or a result of brain injury. EEG activity in comatose patients is variable and resembles the high-amplitude, low-frequency activity seen in patients under general anesthesia. The EEG patterns are also dependent on the severity and extent of brain suppression or injury (see Fig. 50.1).[2]

## Sleep and Anesthesia: How Different Are They?

The similarities and differences between sleep and anesthesia states should be understood.[14] Sleep is a natural state of decreased arousal, controlled by circadian and homeostatic

drives. Anesthesia, on the other hand, is a drug-induced state that is independent of these intrinsic rhythms. Sleep states are amenable to disruptive influences such as psychological and environmental factors. Anesthesia, on the other hand, is immune to such influences. Sleep is characteristically a nonhomogeneous state with distinct stages, periodic arousals, and variable body postures, occurring in a cyclic pattern. Anesthesia is a relatively homogeneous state, the depth and duration of which are directly dependent on drug pharmacokinetics and pharmacodynamics. In the presence of significant sensory stimulation, the sleep state gets disrupted and the subject arouses. Yet, a basic tenet of anesthesia is suppression of arousals, rendering the subject insensate to bodily injury during surgery. Sleep state reversal occurs spontaneously after putative restorative functions are completed. However, anesthesia state reversal requires voluntary stoppage of drug administration as well as effective drug elimination.

## FUNCTIONAL NEUROANATOMY OF SLEEP AND AROUSAL PATHWAYS

Common neurophysiologic mechanisms and neural pathways during sleep are also activated by anesthetic drugs.[12,15] Sedative drug requirements decrease with both sleep deprivation and circadian rhythm disruption. Anesthesia on its own, in the absence of surgical stimulation, also has sleep-like restorative properties.[16,17]

Anesthesia-induced loss of consciousness results from interactions of anesthetics with the neural circuits regulating sleep and wakefulness states. Ascending activation of the cerebral cortex by subcortical center activity is important in the maintenance of wakefulness. Deactivation of the thalamus occurs in imaging studies for both the sleep and anesthesia states, indicating that thalamic and extrathalamic pathways are involved in sleep state modulation.[18]

Sleep state modulation is regulated by two groups of neural centers. The wakefulness promoting centers are the locus ceruleus (LC), dorsal raphe (DR), and tuberomammillary nucleus (TMN); and the sleep promoting center is primarily the hypothalamic ventrolateral preoptic nucleus (VLPO).[19,20] One exception is the median preoptic area that contains both wake-active and sleep-active neurons.[19,20] Discrete neurochemical mediators are involved in sleep stage transition during which the cholinergic (in brainstem and forebrain), noradrenergic (in the LC), and serotonergic (in the DR) activity are noted to be less active in NREM sleep; yet, the cholinergic activity increases in REM sleep.[19] The GABAergic/galanin activity from the VLPO is increased in NREM sleep as it inhibits the histaminergic TMN.[19] Orexinergic pathways from the perifornical nucleus are also inactive during NREM sleep and may be the cause of characteristic daytime hypersomnolence and disrupted nocturnal sleep, as noted in narcolepsy.[19]

**VI**

**Waking**  **Non-REM sleep**

Cortical and subcortical areas mediating arousal

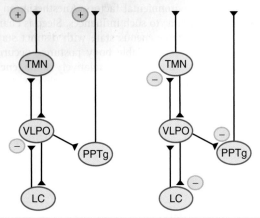

Fig. 50.2 A simplified diagram showing some of the major arousal pathways and their connections with the tuberomammillary nucleus (TMN). *LC,* Locus ceruleus; *PPTg,* pedunculopontine tegmental nuclei; *VLPO,* ventrolateral preoptic nucleus. (From Harrison NL. General anesthesia research: aroused from a deep sleep? *Nat Neurosci.* 2002;5(10):928-929, used with permission.)

During wakefulness, the LC is active and exerts an inhibitory influence on the hypothalamic VLPO. When sleep starts, the LC activity decreases, disinhibiting the VLPO, which now exerts an inhibitory influence on key brainstem and thalamic centers and restrains the ascent of arousal promoting pathways to the cortex through them (Fig. 50.2).[14,20] VLPO projects back onto the LC causing feedback inhibition. Widespread inhibition of ascending arousal promoting pathways occurs, as well as reinforcement of LC output inhibition, resulting in sleep onset. The mutual inhibition between VLPO and LC acts to produce a switch-like, *bistable states* of wakefulness and sleep at a certain threshold.[20] This effect is also caused by anesthetic drugs such as propofol and benzodiazepines, acting on the same target receptors and neural pathways that are integral to sleep and wakefulness.

## SLEEP-DISORDERED BREATHING OR SLEEP-RELATED BREATHING DISORDERS

Sleep-disordered breathing (SDB) is characterized by abnormalities of respiration patterns during sleep. The abnormal patterns of breathing are broadly grouped into obstructive sleep apnea (OSA) disorders, central sleep apnea (CSA) disorders, sleep-related hypoventilation disorders, and sleep-related hypoxemia disorders.[21] OSA disorders are characterized by complete or incomplete upper airway closure during sleep. CSA disorders are characterized by reduction (hypopnea) or cessation (apnea) of airflow due to absent or reduced respiratory effort. Central apnea or

hypopnea may occur in a cyclic, intermittent, or irregular (ataxic) fashion. We will primarily focus on OSA, as this is the most common entity encountered perioperatively.

## OBSTRUCTIVE SLEEP APNEA (OSA)

OSA is characterized by episodes of apnea or hypopnea during sleep, resulting in varying severity of hypoxemia and hypercapnia. The obstructive apnea or hypopnea is caused by repeated episodes of complete or partial closure of the pharynx, accompanied with hypoventilation and desaturation, and terminated by EEG arousal.[22-25]

### Pathophysiology of Upper Airway Collapse in OSA

Upper airway collapsibility and patency are dependent on a continuous balance between collapsing and expanding forces influenced by sleep-wake arousal. Polysomnographic data of important physiologic variables can be used to study characteristic features of an obstructive apnea[26] (Fig. 50.3). During wakefulness, the upper airway stability and patency are achieved by increased genioglossus muscle tone, which pulls the tongue forward.[27] During sleep, upper airway collapse in OSA patients occurs owing to a complex interaction of multiple factors such as loss of upper airway dilating muscle tone, impaired response to mechanoreceptors sensing intrapharyngeal pressures, ventilator overshoot (high loop gain of the respiratory control system), and an increased arousal threshold.[27] Moreover, patients with OSA have an upper airway that is predisposed to collapse, which occurs in the presence of smaller upper airway cross-sectional areas and increased critical closure pressures than those seen in patients without OSA.[28] During NREM sleep and anesthesia, reduction of wakeful cortical influences, reflex gain, and ventilatory drive predispose to upper airway collapse and hypoventilation.[14] These effects are more intense during general anesthesia as the decrease in tonic and phasic muscle activity is profound and abolition of protective arousal response predisposes to prolonged obstruction and more severe oxygen desaturation.

### Clinical Diagnostic Criteria

Classically, the gold standard for the definitive diagnosis of OSA requires an overnight polysomnography (PSG) or sleep study. Based on the AASM recommendations, apneas and hypopneas are defined as a reduction in the rate of airflow from intranasal pressure of at least 90%, or between 50% and 90%, respectively, for at least 10 seconds accompanied by either a 3% to 4% decrease in oxygen saturation or an EEG arousal.[8] Hypopneas are classified as obstructive if thoracoabdominal motion is out of phase or if airflow limitation is observed on the nasal pressure signal, whereas central hypopneas are

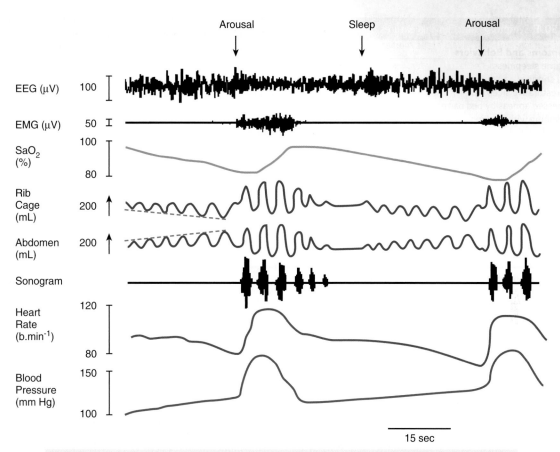

**Fig. 50.3** Polysomnographic recordings of obstructive apnea in a patient with obstructive sleep apnea. Note that during the hypopnea, rib cage and abdominal motion are out of phase (i.e., moving in opposite directions indicating upper airway obstruction). Upper airway obstruction leads to drop in O₂ saturation. The ineffective breathing attempts continue until the patient awakes, as seen by the EEG arousal, and pharyngeal obstruction is relieved. The resuscitative breath now leads to normalization of the oxygen saturation until the next obstructive event ensues. The surge in heart rate and arterial blood pressure occurs along with the arousal, highlighting the activation of sympathetic stimulation in these patients, and placing them at higher risk of long-term cardiovascular complications. The arrows indicate arousals from sleep and sleep onset as determined from the EEG and EMG traces. The sonogram indicates breathing sounds due to snoring. *EEG*, Electroencephalogram; *EMG*, submental electromyogram; *Sao₂*, arterial oxygen saturation. (From Thompson SR, Ackermann U, Horner RL. Sleep as a teaching tool for integrating respiratory physiology and motor control. *Adv Physiol Educ.* 2001;25:101-116, used with permission.)

classified when thoracoabdominal motion is in-phase and there is no evidence of airflow limitation on the nasal pressure signal.[29] Mixed apneas are classified for events that begin as central for at least 10 seconds and end as obstructive, with a minimum of three obstructive efforts. Wherever applicable, ataxic breathing or Cheyne-Stokes type of respiration is also described.[29,30]

The apnea-hypopnea index (AHI) is defined as the average number of abnormal breathing events per hour of sleep. OSA severity is determined by the AHI as follows: mild, 5 to 15 events per hour; moderate, more than 15 to 30 events per hour; and severe, more than 30 events per hour.[8,31] The clinical diagnosis of OSA requires either an AHI of 15 or more, or an AHI more than or equal to 5

events, with symptoms such as excessive daytime sleepiness, unintentional sleep during wakefulness, unrefreshing sleep, loud snoring reported by a partner, or observed obstruction during sleep.[21,32]

## Polysomnography and Portable Devices

A laboratory-based sleep study is set up and analyzed by a registered sleep technologist using standard criteria.[8] All studies are performed using a uniform montage of electrograms including central, occipital, and frontal EEGs; right and left electrooculogram (EOG); chin electromyogram (EMG); electrocardiogram (ECG); and anterior tibialis muscle EMG bilaterally. Thoracoabdominal motion is usually

**Box 50.1** Symptoms and Clinical Features of Obstructive Sleep Apnea (OSA)

| Symptoms and Behaviors | Comorbid Conditions |
|---|---|
| Daytime sleepiness | Obesity |
| Loud snoring | Large neck circumference |
| Nonrestorative sleep | Craniofacial deformities (retrognathia, midfacial hypoplasia) |
| Witnessed apneas by bed partner | Crowded pharynx |
| Awakening with choking | Systemic hypertension |
| Insomnia with frequent brief nocturnal awakenings | Hypercapnia or high serum bicarbonate |
| Lack of concentration | Cardiovascular disease |
| Cognitive deficits | Cerebrovascular disease |
| Changes in mood | Cardiac dysrhythmia |
| Morning headaches | Metabolic syndrome |
| Sleep walking, confusional arousals (arousals from NREM sleep) | Pulmonary hypertension |
| Vivid, strange, or threatening dreams (arousals from REM sleep) | Obesity hypoventilation syndrome |
| Gastroesophageal reflux | Cor pulmonale |
| Nocturia | Polycythemia |
| Drowsy driving, and motor vehicle accidents | Floppy eyelid syndrome |

*NREM*, Non–rapid eye movement; *REM*, rapid eye movement.
Modified from Olson E, Chung F, Seet E. Surgical risk and the preoperative evaluation and management of adults with obstructive sleep apnea. In Post TW, ed. *UpToDate*. Waltham, MA: UpToDate; 2015.

monitored by respiratory inductance plethysmography (RIP), and airflow is monitored using either a nasal pressure transducer or nasal thermistor. Arterial oxygen saturation ($Sao_2$) is monitored by pulse oximetry. Body position and snoring are recorded manually.

Home sleep testing may be a viable alternative to standard PSG for the diagnosis of OSA in certain subsets of patients.[33,34] The Portable Monitoring Task Force of the AASM has classified level 2 (full unattended PSG with seven or more recording channels), level 3 (devices limited to four to seven recording channels), and level 4 (monitors with one to two channels including nocturnal oximetry) devices.[33] In particular, the level 2 portable PSG device has a diagnostic accuracy similar to that of standard PSG,[35] whereas nocturnal oximetry is both sensitive and specific for detecting OSA in high-risk surgical patients.[36] Preoperative overnight oximetry may be a useful screening test (when mean preoperative overnight saturation is less than 93%, oxygen desaturation index more than 29 events per hour, overnight duration of oxygen saturation less than 90% for more than 7% of total sleep time) and predicts postoperative adverse events.[37] Portable devices may be considered when there is high pretest likelihood for moderate to severe OSA without other substantial comorbid conditions[33] and proper standards for conducting the test and interpretation of results are met.[32]

### Prevalence of OSA in the General and Surgical Population

The prevalence of moderate to severe OSA (AHI ≥ 15 events per hour) is 13% among men and 6% among women, respectively, in the general population.[38] The estimates were more frequent with increasing age and body mass index.[39] The difference could be explained

by the underdiagnosis of OSA, as 80% of patients with moderate to severe OSA remain undiagnosed.[38,40] In the general population, OSA diagnosis is an independent risk factor for cardiovascular morbidity and mortality.[41-44]

The prevalence of undiagnosed moderate to severe OSA (AHI > 15 events per hour) among surgical patients is difficult to assess[39] but appears to be higher than that in the general population.[45,46] Sixty percent of patients with moderate to severe OSA (AHI ≥15 events per hour) were not diagnosed by the anesthesia provider preoperatively (also see Chapter 13).[47]

### OSA and Comorbid Conditions

OSA is associated with long-term cardiovascular morbidity including myocardial ischemia, heart failure, hypertension, arrhythmias, cerebrovascular disease, metabolic syndrome, insulin resistance, gastroesophageal reflux, and obesity (Box 50.1).[48] Craniofacial deformities (e.g., macroglossia, retrognathia, midfacial hypoplasia), endocrine disorders (e.g., hypothyroidism, Cushing disease), and demographic (male, age older than 50 years) and lifestyle (e.g., smoking, alcohol consumption) are factors closely associated with OSA.[48] Perioperative physicians (also see Chapter 13) should be aware of the possible coexistence of these medical conditions, which can possibly be improved preoperatively, and risk stratification may be instituted at the time of surgery.

### Surgery and OSA Severity

Factors contributing to the postoperative worsening of OSA have been defined.[49,50] Compared to the preoperative baseline, the AHI significantly increased on the first night, with peak increase occurring on the third night.[49,50]

Preoperative AHI, age, and opioid dosage were significant predictors of postoperative AHI.[50] These findings are clinically significant for surgical patients who may not be monitored as closely during the second and third postoperative nights.

Postoperative complications such as myocardial infarction, congestive heart failure, and pulmonary embolus can be more likely to occur during the second or third postoperative day. According to a 2015 analysis of the American Society of Anesthesiologists (ASA) Closed Claims Project database, 88% of opioid-induced respiratory depression incidents occurred within the first 24 hours of surgery, of which 97% were deemed as preventable.[51] Multiple prescribers (33%), concurrent administration of nonopioid sedating medications (34%), and inadequate nursing assessments or response (31%) were identified as contributory factors.[51] Life-threatening critical respiratory events with opioids occur mostly during the first 24 hours after surgery for all patients[52] and within the first 72 hours for OSA patients.[53] Factors such as OSA, intense levels of sedation, nighttime events, and postoperative acute renal failure are associated with fatality following these events.[54] Increased postoperative complications on the second or third postoperative day may be associated with increased AHI and decreased oxygen saturation.

## OSA and Postoperative Complications

A systematic review of 61 studies[55] and a meta-analysis of 13 studies demonstrated that patients with OSA versus non-OSA were associated with a significantly higher risk of postoperative events, such as acute respiratory failure, desaturation, and intensive care transfer.[56] Large population-based studies have shown that patients with a diagnosis of OSA have an increased risk of perioperative complications, such as the need for emergent endotracheal intubation,[57-59] noninvasive or mechanical ventilation,[57-59] aspiration of gastric contents–induced pneumonia,[58] pulmonary embolism,[58] and atrial fibrillation.[57,59]

Recently, in 2015, a large perioperative database (26,000 patients in 50 U.S. hospitals) was analyzed to determine complications in patients with OSA.[60] Compared with treated OSA, untreated OSA was independently associated with more cardiopulmonary complications, including unplanned reintubation of the trachea and myocardial infarction.[60]

OSA patients who remain undiagnosed at the time of surgery are at increased risk of postoperative complications.[61] Mutter and associates conducted a matched cohort analysis of polysomnography (PSG) data and health administrative data. Patients with undiagnosed OSA were found to have a threefold higher risk of cardiovascular complications, primarily cardiac arrest and shock, compared to diagnosed OSA patients with prescription of continuous positive airway pressure (CPAP)

therapy.[61] Severity of OSA may play an important factor. Patients with severe OSA (AHI >30) had a 2.7-fold increase in postoperative respiratory complications.[61] If available, information on the diagnosis and severity of OSA in the anesthetic assessment may be helpful.

## Clinical Pathways and Principles of Perioperative Management

The perioperative management of OSA patients is challenging, and a sound understanding of the condition is required of anesthesia providers involved in the care of such patients. The 2016 Society of Anesthesia and Sleep Medicine (SASM) guidelines for preoperative screening and assessment of adult patients with OSA recommend that screening for OSA may be useful to provide heightened awareness and potential risk reduction by implementing appropriate interventions[62] (Table 50.1). In addition, the American Society of Anesthesiologists (ASA) updated report on "Practice Guidelines for the Perioperative Management of Patients with Obstructive Sleep Apnea" offers guidance on perioperative management of OSA patients.[63,64] The Society for Ambulatory Anesthesia (SAMBA) consensus statement has provided guidelines addressing the selection of suitable OSA patients for ambulatory surgery.[65] Different clinical pathways and algorithms have been constructed to simplify the approach to OSA patients in the perioperative setting.[63,64,66-68]

### Preoperative Assessment (Also See Chapter 13)
#### Patients With Diagnosed OSA

A thorough history and physical examination are essential. Focused questions regarding nature and severity of OSA symptoms should be asked. Previous consultation with a specialized sleep physician and sleep reports should be reviewed, if possible. (Fig. 50.4).

Patients with long-standing OSA may present with signs and symptoms of significant comorbid conditions including morbid obesity, metabolic syndrome, uncontrolled or resistant hypertension, arrhythmias, cerebrovascular disease, and heart failure.[69] Preoperative assessment should also rule out the presence of significant nocturnal hypoxemia, hypercarbia, polycythemia, and cor pulmonale. Obesity hypoventilation syndrome (OHS) and pulmonary hypertension should be ruled out in OSA patients.[70,71] The likelihood of developing respiratory failure following noncardiac surgery was more than 10-fold in OHS patients with OSA, compared to patients with OSA alone.[72] A serum bicarbonate level of 28 mmol/L or more indicates metabolic compensation for chronic hypercapnia and is a useful screening tool for OHS (Fig. 50.5).[73] A preoperative transthoracic echocardiogram (TTE) may be considered in patients suspected of having severe pulmonary hypertension and if intraoperative acute increases in pulmonary arterial pressures (high-risk or long-duration surgery) are anticipated.[66]

VI

**Table 50.1**   Executive Summary of the Society of Anesthesia and Sleep Medicine (SASM) guidelines

| Recommendations: Executive Summary |
|---|
| • **Patients with obstructive sleep apnea (OSA) undergoing procedures under anesthesia are at increased risk for perioperative complications compared with patients without the disease diagnosis.** Identifying patients at high risk for OSA before surgery for targeted perioperative precautions and interventions may help to reduce perioperative patient complications. |
| • **Screening tools help to risk stratify patients with suspected OSA with reasonable accuracy.** Practice groups should consider making OSA screening part of standard preanesthetic evaluation. |
| • **There is insufficient evidence in the current literature to support canceling or delaying surgery for a formal diagnosis (laboratory or home polysomnography) in patients with suspected OSA,** unless there is evidence of an associated significant or uncontrolled systemic disease or additional problems with ventilation or gas exchange. |
| • The patient and the health care team should be aware that both diagnosed OSA (whether treated, partially treated, or untreated) and suspected OSA may be associated with increased postoperative morbidity. |
| • If available, consideration should be given to obtaining results of the sleep study and, where applicable, the patient's recommended positive airway pressure (PAP) setting before surgery. |
| • If resources allow, facilities should consider having PAP equipment for perioperative use or have patients bring their own PAP equipment with them to the surgical facility. |
| • **Additional evaluation to allow preoperative cardiopulmonary optimization should be considered in patients with diagnosed, partially treated/untreated, and suspected OSA where there is indication of an associated significant or uncontrolled systemic disease or additional problems with ventilation or gas exchange such as: (i) hypoventilation syndromes, (ii) severe pulmonary hypertension, and (iii) resting hypoxemia in the absence of other cardiopulmonary disease.** |
| • **Where management of comorbid conditions has been optimized, patients with diagnosed, partially treated/untreated OSA, or suspected OSA may proceed to surgery provided strategies for mitigation of postoperative complications are implemented.** |
| • The risks and benefits of the decision to proceed with or delay surgery include consultation and discussion with the surgeon and the patient. |
| • **The use of PAP therapy in previously undiagnosed but suspected OSA patients should be considered case by case.** Because of the lack of evidence from randomized controlled trials, we cannot recommend its routine use. |
| • **Continued use of PAP therapy at previously prescribed settings is recommended during periods of sleep while hospitalized, both preoperatively and postoperatively.** Adjustments may need to be made to the settings to account for perioperative changes such as facial swelling, upper airway edema, fluid shifts, pharmacotherapy, and respiratory function. |

From: Chung F, Memtsoudis SG, Ramachandran SK, et al. Society of Anesthesia and Sleep Medicine Guidelines on Preoperative Screening and Assessment of Adult Patients With Obstructive Sleep Apnea. Anesthesia and Analgesia. 2016;123(2):452-473.

OSA patients may be using positive airway pressure (PAP) devices for treatment, such as CPAP, bilevel positive airway pressure (BiPAP), and auto-titrating positive airway pressure (APAP) devices. APAP devices provide upper airway stability during sleep by using airflow measurements, fluctuations in pressure, or airway resistance based on internal algorithms. This approach has the potential to account for night-to-night variability of OSA severity.[74] The SASM guidelines recommend review of sleep study and compliance data from the PAP devices to evaluate information on the current PAP setting, and AHI indicating successful treatment of respiratory events.[62] Per the SASM guidelines, additional evaluation for preoperative cardiopulmonary optimization should be considered in patients who have a known diagnosis of OSA and are nonadherent or poorly adherent to PAP therapy and where there is indication of uncontrolled systemic conditions or additional problems with ventilation or gas exchange. These conditions include, but may not be limited to (1) hypoventilation syndromes, (2) severe pulmonary hypertension, and (3) resting hypoxemia not attributable to other cardiopulmonary disease.[62]

A 2015 meta-analysis of six studies and 904 patients evaluated the use of perioperative CPAP on postoperative outcomes in OSA patients.[75] Perioperative CPAP significantly reduced the postoperative AHI from baseline preoperative AHI, in association with a modest reduction of hospital length of stay.[75]

Patients who are noncompliant to PAP therapy should be counseled to resume therapy preoperatively.[76] Moreover, patients with significant comorbid conditions, a high serum bicarbonate (indicating chronic hypercapnia), and preoperative hypoxemia in the absence of respiratory disease are candidates for preoperative evaluation and initiation of PAP therapy.[76] Current guidelines recommend that surgical patients with moderate or severe OSA who are compliant with PAP therapy should bring the device to the hospital and continue its use.[64] In the general population, mild OSA was not an independent risk factor for higher mortality rate.[42] Patients with mild OSA may not be at a higher risk of undergoing surgery and anesthesia, and preoperative PAP use may not be indicated in these patients.

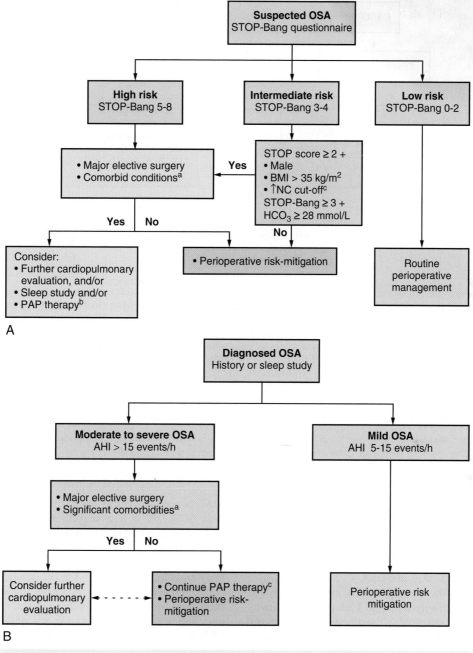

**Fig. 50.4** Preoperative evaluation of a patient with known or suspected obstructive sleep apnea in the pre-admission clinic. (A) Suspected OSA and (B) Diagnosed OSA. A, Per the 2016 SASM guidelines, further cardiopulmonary evaluation may be indicated in patients with uncontrolled systemic disease or additional problems with ventilation or gas exchange, such as hypoventilation syndromes, severe pulmonary hypertension, and resting hypoxemia in the absence of other cardiopulmonary disease.[62] [a]Significant comorbidities: heart failure, arrhythmias, uncontrolled hypertension, cerebrovascular disease, metabolic syndrome, obesity (body mass index >35 kg/m[2]), obesity hypoventilation syndrome, pulmonary hypertension. [b]Positive airway pressure (PAP) therapy: includes continuous PAP, bilevel PAP, and autotitrating PAP. [c]Neck circumference (NC) cut-offs 17 inches/43 cm in male, 16 inches/41 cm in female.[84] *STOP-Bang*, STOP-Bang questionnaire cut-off values.

VI

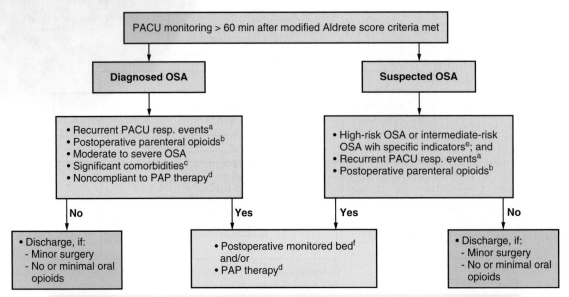

**Fig. 50.5** Postoperative management of the patient with known or suspected obstructive sleep apnea after general anesthesia. [a]Recurrent postanesthesia care unit (PACU) respiratory event: repeated occurrence of oxygen saturation less than 90%, or bradypnea less than 8 breaths/min, or apnea 10 seconds and longer, or pain-sedation mismatch (high pain and sedation scores concurrently).[88] [b]Postoperative parenteral opioid requirement more than the usual standard of care such as multiple routes, long-acting preparations, or high dose infusions. [c]Per the 2016 SASM guidelines, uncontrolled systemic disease or additional problems with ventilation or gas exchange such as: hypoventilation syndromes, severe pulmonary hypertension, and resting hypoxemia in the absence of other cardiopulmonary disease.[62] [d]Positive airway pressure (PAP) therapy: includes continuous PAP, bilevel PAP, or autotitrating PAP. [e]Intermediate-risk and specific indicators include: STOP score $\geq 2$ + male or BMI > 35 kg/m² or ↑NC cutoff (where, NC: neck circumference cut-offs 17 inches/43 cm in male, 16 inches/41 cm in female[82]) and STOP-Bang $\geq 3$ + HCO3 $\geq 28$ mmol/L. [f]Monitored bed: environment with continuous oximetry and the possibility of early medical intervention (e.g., intensive care unit, step-down unit, or remote pulse oximetry with telemetry in surgical ward).

### Methods for Perioperative Screening for OSA

An overnight PSG is the gold standard diagnostic test for OSA. However, routine screening with PSG can be costly and resource intensive. As a result, simple, economical, and sensitive screening tests have been developed to detect patients with suspected OSA.

Preoperatively, the use of sensitive clinical criteria to identify and risk-stratify potential OSA patients is advocated. An updated 2014 ASA Practice Guideline for the perioperative management of patients with obstructive sleep apnea recommends a comprehensive preoperative evaluation including a medical records review, patient/family interview and screening protocol, and physical examination.[63,64] Perioperative risk is predicted by a scoring system based on OSA severity, invasiveness of procedure, and expected postoperative opioid requirement.[64] Other screening tools that have been validated in surgical patients are the STOP-Bang questionnaire,[77] the Berlin Questionnaire,[78] and the Perioperative Sleep Apnea Prediction (P-SAP) score.[79]

The STOP-Bang questionnaire is a concise and easy-to-use screening tool for OSA consisting of eight easily administered questions with the acronym STOP-Bang (Box 50.2).[77,80] It is a self-administered screening tool and includes four "yes/no" questions (*s*noring, *t*iredness, *o*bserved that you stopped breathing, high blood *p*ressure) and questions concerning the demographic data of *b*ody mass index (BMI) (>35 kg/m²), *a*ge (>50 years), *n*eck circumference (>40 cm), and *g*ender (male). Patients are deemed to be at lower risk with scores of 0 to 2, intermediate risk with 3 to 4, and higher risk of OSA with scores of 5 to 8.[77,80-82] The STOP-Bang questionnaire has a high sensitivity and a high negative predictive value for patients with moderate to severe OSA.[77] The sensitivity of a STOP-Bang score of 3 or more to detect moderate to severe OSA (AHI > 15) and severe OSA (AHI > 30) is 93% and 100%, respectively. The corresponding negative predictive values are 90% and 100%. As the STOP-Bang score increases from low risk (0 to 2) to high risk (7 to 8), the probability of moderate to severe OSA increases from 18% to 60%, and the probability of severe OSA increases from 4% to 38%.[81] In patients whose STOP-Bang scores are the mid-range (3 or 4), further criteria are required for classification. For example, a STOP-Bang score of $\geq 2$ +

| Box 50.2   Updated STOP-Bang Questionnaire | |
|---|---|
| **Snoring?** | Do you **Snore Loudly** (loud enough to be heard through closed doors or your bed partner elbows you for snoring at night)? |
| **Tired?** | Do you often feel **Tired, Fatigued, or Sleepy** during the daytime (such as falling asleep during driving)? |
| **Observed?** | Has anyone **Observed** you **Stop Breathing** or **Choking/Gasping** during your sleep? |
| **Pressure?** | Do you have or are you being treated for **High Blood Pressure**? |

**Body Mass Index** more than 35 kg/m²?
**Age** older than 50 years old?
**Neck size** large? (Measured around Adams apple)
For male, is your shirt collar 17 inches/43 cm or larger?
For female, is your shirt collar 16 inches/41 cm or larger?
**Gender:** Male?
Scoring Criteria:
  For general population
  **Low risk of OSA:** Yes to 0-2 questions
  **Intermediate risk of OSA:** Yes to 3-4 questions
  **High risk of OSA:** Yes to 5-8 questions
    or Yes to 2 or more of 4 STOP questions + male gender
    or Yes to 2 or more of 4 STOP questions + BMI > 35 kg/m²
    or Yes to 2 or more of 4 STOP questions + neck circumference large (17 inches/43 cm in male, 16 inches/41 cm in female)

*BMI*, Body mass index; *OSA*, obstructive sleep apnea.
Modified from Chung F, Yegneswaran B, Liao P, et al. STOP questionnaire: a tool to screen patients for obstructive sleep apnea. *Anesthesiology.* 2008;108(5):812-821; Chung F, Subramanyam R, Liao P, et al. High STOP-Bang score indicates a high probability of obstructive sleep apnoea. *Br J Anaesth.* 2012;108:768-775; Chung F, Yang Y, Brown R, et al. Alternative scoring models of STOP-Bang questionnaire improve specificity to detect undiagnosed obstructive sleep apnea. *J Clin Sleep Med.* 2014;10:951-958. Proprietary to University Health Network. www.stopbang.ca.

(BMI > 35 kg/m² or male or neck circumference > 43 cm in males, and > 41 cm in females) or a STOP-Bang score ≥ 3 + serum $HCO_3$ ≥ 28 mmol/L would classify that patient as having a high risk for moderate to severe OSA (Box 50.2 and Fig. 50.4).[81] In addition, patients identified as high risk with a STOP-Bang score of 5-8 have an increased severity of OSA and are at a higher risk of postoperative complications.[83,84]

### Patients With Suspected OSA

In patients suspected of OSA, a focused clinical examination should be performed with emphasis on pertinent symptoms and signs of OSA (Box 50.1). History from the bed partner in the preoperative clinic is useful in the assessment of loud snoring and observed apneic episodes while asleep. In emergency situations, the patient should proceed for surgery, preventing delay of life- or limb-saving surgery. Perioperative risk-mitigation strategies should be implemented based on the clinical suspicion of OSA (Fig. 50.4).[67,85]

For elective non-urgent surgery, the 2016 SASM guidelines state that insufficient evidence exists to support canceling or delaying surgery to formally diagnose OSA in those patients identified as being at intense risk of OSA preoperatively, unless there is evidence of uncontrolled systemic disease or additional problems with ventilation or gas exchange, such as hypoventilation syndromes, severe pulmonary hypertension, and resting hypoxemia, in the absence of other cardiopulmonary disease.[62] (Table 50.1, Fig. 50.4). In these patients, additional cardiopulmonary evaluation is recommended to allow for optimization of the medical conditions and planning of the intraoperative and postoperative management.[63,64] Once the comorbid conditions have been made as optimal as possible, patients with diagnosed, partially treated or untreated OSA, or with suspected OSA may proceed to surgery provided strategies for mitigation of postoperative complications are implemented. The risks and benefits of the decision to proceed with or delay surgery include consultation and discussion with the surgeon and the patient[62] (Table 50.1). If the subsequent intraoperative and postoperative course suggests an increased likelihood of OSA, such as difficult airway,[87] or recurrent postoperative respiratory events, such as desaturation, hypoventilation, or apnea,[88] postoperative referral to a sleep physician may be useful for long term follow-up.

### Perioperative Risk-Mitigation Strategies

Preoperative sedative premedication in an unmonitored setting should be avoided. Intraoperatively, the anesthesia provider should be prepared for difficulties with ventilation via a mask, laryngoscopy, and endotracheal intubation.[89,90] Guidance from the ASA practice guidelines for the management of a difficult airway is useful, and the presence of skilled personnel and advanced airway equipment should be ensured at the time of airway management.[91] Adequate preinduction of anesthesia oxygenation, head-elevated body position, and measures to decrease the risk of aspiration of gastric acid, such as preoperative proton-pump inhibitors, antacids, and rapid sequence induction with cricoid pressure, should be considered.

The use of long-acting anesthetics should be minimized and short-acting drugs such as propofol, remifentanil, and desflurane should be used. Pulmonary hypertension can occur and patients with evidence of right-sided heart failure, and reduced effort tolerance may need additional tests for evaluation. Care should be taken to prevent increased pulmonary artery pressures by avoiding hypercarbia, hypoxemia, hypothermia, and acidosis.

Alveolar hypoventilation in conjunction with central respiratory depression, decreased consciousness, and upper airway obstruction are results of opioid administration and can lead to opioid-induced respiratory depression.[92] Important components of OSA like sleep fragmentation and intermittent hypoxia modulate pain behavior and increase sensitivity to opioid analgesics.[92] Nonopioid analgesics should be used, such as acetaminophen or nonsteroidal antiinflammatory drugs (NSAIDs, celecoxib); partial opioid analgesics (tramadol); anticonvulsants (pregabalin or gabapentin); corticosteroids (dexamethasone); N-methyl-D-aspartate (NMDA); receptor antagonist, ketamine[93]; and the $\alpha_2$-adrenergic agonists, clonidine and dexmedetomidine.[94] Extubation of the trachea should be performed with no residual neuromuscular blockade in an awake, fully conscious patient who is able to obey commands and maintain a patent airway. After extubation of the trachea, patients should be recovered in a nonsupine (semiupright or lateral) position (also see Chapter 13).[64]

Local or regional anesthesia techniques reduce opioid requirements postoperatively and may be of benefit as they avoid manipulation of the airway and reduce the need for postoperative sedating analgesic medications. Patients previously receiving PAP therapy at home may continue using their PAP devices during procedures under mild to moderate sedation.[95] A secured airway is preferred to an unprotected one for procedures requiring deep sedation.[64]

### Postoperative Disposition of OSA Patients (Also See Chapter 39)

The postoperative disposition of the OSA patient depends on the nature of surgery, OSA severity, and the requirement for postoperative parenteral opioids (see Fig. 50.5). A patient with severe OSA who underwent a major surgery and is receiving large-dose intravenous opioids is more likely to require continuous monitoring than another patient with suspected OSA undergoing a superficial cataract surgery via a local anesthetic with minimal opioid analgesic requirements. The attending anesthesia provider is responsible for the final decision, taking into account all patient-related, logistic, and circumstantial factors.

Fig. 50.5 presents a simplified algorithm on the postoperative management of patients with OSA based on recommendations of the 2016 SASM guidelines and expert opinion.[62,67,86] All patients with known or suspected OSA who have received general anesthesia should have extended monitoring in the postanesthesia care unit (PACU) with continuous oximetry. There are currently no evidence-based guidelines addressing the optimal length of monitoring required in the PACU, and some recommendations are difficult to follow, especially in the context of cost and resource management.[95] It is reasonable to observe a suspected or documented OSA patient in the PACU for an additional 60 minutes in a quiet environment after the modified Aldrete criteria for discharge have been met.[67]

The existence of recurrent respiratory events in the PACU is another indication for continuous postoperative monitoring.[88] Recurrent PACU respiratory events are defined as (1) episodes of apnea for 10 seconds or more, (2) bradypnea fewer than 8 breaths per minute, (3) pain-sedation mismatch, and (4) repeated oxygen desaturation to less than 90%. Patients with suspected OSA (i.e., scored as high risk on screening questionnaires) who develop recurrent PACU respiratory events postoperatively are at increased risk of postoperative respiratory complications.[88] Monitoring in surgical wards equipped with continuous oximetry is indicated for these patients. Postoperative PAP therapy may be initiated at an empiric basis to abolish recurrent obstructive events associated with significant hypoxemia.[95] Patients with previously diagnosed OSA already receiving PAP should continue PAP therapy postoperatively.[76]

## CONCLUSION

Understanding the similarities and differences between sleep and anesthesia has enhanced our learning of the neural pathways modulating arousal and the interaction with medications. Common sleep disorders impact this relationship further, and knowledge of timely diagnosis, treatment, and perioperative precautions is necessary for an anesthesiology trainee. Ongoing research and new diagnostic and monitoring technologies will define the change in the diagnosis and management with an impact on health care costs and resource management.

## QUESTIONS OF THE DAY

1. What are the characteristic electroencephalographic (EEG) patterns associated with general anesthesia?
2. What factors contribute to upper airway collapse in a patient with obstructive sleep apnea (OSA)?
3. What is the definition of the Apnea-Hypopnea Index (AHI) during a sleep study? What are the criteria for a clinical diagnosis of OSA based on symptoms and AHI?
4. What are the most common medical conditions associated with OSA?
5. What postoperative events are more likely to occur in a patient with OSA compared to a patient without OSA?
6. What are the components of the STOP-Bang questionnaire for OSA screening? What is the sensitivity of the STOP-Bang score to detect moderate to severe OSA?
7. What strategies can be used to decrease the risk of an adverse outcome during the perioperative period in a patient with OSA?

# REFERENCES

1. McCarley RW. Neurobiology of REM and NREM sleep. *Sleep Med.* 2007;8:302–330.
2. Lydic R, Baghdoyan HA. Sleep, anesthesiology, and the neurobiology of arousal state control. *Anesthesiology.* 2005;103:1268–1295.
3. Borbély AA, Achermann P. Sleep homeostasis and models of sleep regulation. *J Biol Rhythms.* 1999;14:557–568.
4. Borbély AA. A two process model of sleep regulation. *Hum Neurobiol.* 1982;1(3):195–204.
5. Kryger MH, Roth T, Dement WC. *Principles and Practice of Sleep Medicine.* 4th ed. Philadelphia: Elsevier Saunders; 2005:1–1517.
6. Aldrich MS. *Sleep Medicine.* New York: Oxford University Press; 1999:1–382.
7. Berry RB, Budhiraja R, Gottlieb DJ, et al. Rules for scoring respiratory events in sleep: update of the 2007 AASM manual for the scoring of sleep and associated events. *J Clin Sleep Med.* 2012;8:597–619.
8. Iber C, Ancoli-Israel S, Cheeson Jr AL, Quan SF. *For the American Academy of Sleep Medicine. The AASM Manual for the Scoring of Sleep and Associated Events: Rules, Terminology and Technical Specifications.* Westchester, IL: American Academy of Sleep Medicine; 2007.
9. Lydic R, Baghdoyan HA, Hibbard L, et al. Regional brain glucose metabolism is altered during rapid eye movement sleep in the cat: a preliminary study. *J Comp Neurol.* 1991;304:517–529.
10. Nofzinger EA. Functional neuroimaging of sleep disorders. *Curr Pharm Des.* 2008;14(32):3417–3429.
11. Stickgold R, Hobson JA, Fosse R, et al. Sleep, learning, and dreams: offline memory reprocessing. *Science.* 2001;294:1052–1057.
12. Brown EN, Lydic R, Schiff ND. General anesthesia, sleep, and coma. *N Engl J Med.* 2010;363:2638–2650.
13. Purdon PL, Sampson A, Pavone KJ, et al. Clinical electroencephalography for anesthesiologists: part I: background and basic signatures. *Anesthesiology.* 2015;123:937–960.
14. Hillman DR, Eastwood PR. Upper airway, obstructive sleep apnea, and anesthesia. *Sleep Med Clin.* 2015;8:23–28.
15. Allada R. An emerging link between general anesthesia and sleep. *Proc Natl Acad Sci U S A.* 2008;105:2257–2258.
16. Tung A, Lynch JP, Mendelson WB. Prolonged sedation with propofol in the rat does not result in sleep deprivation. *Anesth Analg.* 2001;92:1232–1236.
17. Tung A, Bergmann BM, Herrera S, et al. Recovery from sleep deprivation occurs during propofol anesthesia. *Anesthesiology.* 2004;100:1419–1426.
18. Saper CB, Scammell TE, Lu J. Hypothalamic regulation of sleep and circadian rhythms. *Nature.* 2005;437:1257–1263.
19. Vacas S, Kurien P, Maze M. Sleep and anesthesia. *Sleep Med Clin.* 2015;8:1–9.
20. Harrison NL. General anesthesia research: aroused from a deep sleep? *Nat Neurosci.* 2002;5(10):928–929.
21. American Academy of Sleep Medicine (AASM). *The International Classification of Sleep Disorders*–Third Edition (ICSD-3). Online version. Accessed on July 30, 2014.
22. Remmers JE, DeGroot WJ, Sauerland EK, et al. Pathogenesis of upper airway occlusion during sleep. *J Appl Physiol.* 1978;44:931–938.
23. Mezzanotte WS, Tangel DJ, White DP. Waking genioglossal electromyogram in sleep apnea patients versus normal controls (a neuromuscular compensatory mechanism). *J Clin Invest.* 1992;89:1571–1579.
24. Strollo PJ Jr, Rogers RM. Obstructive sleep apnea. *N Engl J Med.* 1996;334:99–104.
25. Petrof BJ, Hendricks JC, Pack AI. Does upper airway muscle injury trigger a vicious cycle in obstructive sleep apnea? A hypothesis. *Sleep.* 1996;19:465–471.
26. Thompson SR, Ackermann U, Horner RL. Sleep as a teaching tool for integrating respiratory physiology and motor control. *Adv Physiol Educ.* 2001;25:101–116.
27. Eckert DJ, White DP, Jordan AS, et al. Defining phenotypic causes of obstructive sleep apnea. Identification of novel therapeutic targets. *Am J Respir Crit Care Med.* 2013;188:996–1004.
28. Isono S, Remmers JE, Tanaka A, et al. Anatomy of pharynx in patients with obstructive sleep apnea and in normal subjects. *J Appl Physiol.* 1997;82:1319–1326.
29. Yumino D, Bradley TD. Central sleep apnea and Cheyne-Stokes respiration. *Proc Am Thorac Soc.* 2008;5:226–236.
30. Farney RJ, Walker JM, Cloward TV, Rhondeau S. Sleep-disordered breathing associated with long-term opioid therapy. *Chest.* 2003;123(2):632–639.
31. Berry RB, Brooks R, Garnaldo CE, et al. *for the American Academy of Sleep Medicine. The AASM Manual for the Scoring of Sleep and Associated Events: Rules, Terminology and Technical Specification, Version 2.2.* Darien, IL: American Academy of Sleep Medicine; 2015. www.aasmnet.org.
32. Fleetham J, Ayas N, Bradley D, et al. Canadian Thoracic Society 2011 guideline update: diagnosis and treatment of sleep disordered breathing. *Can Respir J.* 2011;18:25–47.
33. Collop NA, Anderson WM, Boehlecke B, et al. Portable Monitoring Task Force of the American Academy of Sleep Medicine. Clinical guidelines for the use of unattended portable monitors in the diagnosis of obstructive sleep apnea in adult patients. *J Clin Sleep Med.* 2007;3:737–747.
34. Collop NA. Home sleep testing: it is not about the test. *Chest.* 2010;138:245–246.
35. Chung F, Liao P, Sun Y, et al. Perioperative practical experiences in using a level 2 portable polysomnography. *Sleep Breath.* 2011;15(3):367–375.
36. Chung F, Liao P, Elsaid H, et al. Oxygen desaturation index from nocturnal oximetry: a sensitive and specific tool to detect sleep-disordered breathing in surgical patients. *Anesth Analg.* 2012;114:993–1000.
37. Chung F, Zhou L, Liao P. Parameters from preoperative overnight oximetry predict postoperative adverse events. *Minerva Anestesiol.* 2014;80(10):1084–1095.
38. Peppard PE, Young T, Barnet JH, et al. Increased prevalence of sleep-disordered breathing in adults. *Am J Epidemiol.* 2013;177:1006–1014.
39. Young T, Evans L, Finn L, et al. Estimation of the clinically diagnosed proportion of sleep apnea syndrome in middle-aged men and women. *Sleep.* 1997;20:705–706.
40. Young T, Palta M, Dempsey J, et al. The occurrence of sleep-disordered breathing among middle-aged adults. *N Engl J Med.* 1993;328:1230–1235.
41. Sánchez-de-la-Torre M, Campos-Rodriguez F, Barbé F. Obstructive sleep apnoea and cardiovascular disease. *Lancet Respir Med.* 2013;1:61–72.
42. Marshall NS, Wong KKH, Liu PY, et al. Sleep apnea as an independent risk factor for all-cause mortality: the Busselton Health Study. *Sleep.* 2008;31:1079–1085.
43. Gami AS, Olson EJ, Shen WK, et al. Obstructive sleep apnea and the risk of sudden cardiac death: a longitudinal study of 10,701 adults. *J Am Coll Cardiol.* 2013;62:610–616.
44. Marin JM, Carrizo SJ, Vicente E, et al. Long-term cardiovascular outcomes in men with obstructive sleep apnoea-hypopnoea with or without treatment with continuous positive airway pressure: an observational study. *Lancet.* 2005;365:1046–1053.
45. Frey WC, Pilcher J. Obstructive sleep-related breathing disorders in patients evaluated for bariatric surgery. *Obes Surg.* 2003;13:676–683.
46. Candiotti K, Sharma S, Shankar R. Obesity, obstructive sleep apnoea, and diabetes mellitus: anaesthetic implications. *Br J Anaesth.* 2009;103(suppl):i23–i30.

**VI**

47. Singh M, Liao P, Kobah S, et al. Proportion of surgical patients with undiagnosed obstructive sleep apnoea. *Br J Anaesth*. 2013;110(4):629–636.

48. Olson E, Chung F, Seet E. Surgical risk and the preoperative evaluation and management of adults with obstructive sleep apnea. In: Post TW, ed. *UpToDate*. Waltham, MA: UpToDate; 2015. (Accessed on October 01, 2015.)

49. Chung F, Liao P, Yegneswaran B, et al. Postoperative changes in sleep-disordered breathing and sleep architecture in patients with obstructive sleep apnea. *Anesthesiology*. 2014;120: 287–298.

50. Chung F, Liao P, Elsaid H, et al. Factors associated with postoperative exacerbation of sleep-disordered breathing. *Anesthesiology*. 2014;120:299–311.

51. Lee LA, Caplan RA, Stephens LS, et al. Postoperative opioid-induced respiratory depression: a closed claims analysis. *Anesthesiology*. 2015;122(3):659–665.

52. Ramachandran SK, Haider N, Saran KA, et al. Life-threatening critical respiratory events: a retrospective study of postoperative patients found unresponsive during analgesic therapy. *J Clin Anesth*. 2011;23:207–213.

53. Gupta RM, Parvizi J, Hanssen AD, et al. Postoperative complications in patients with obstructive sleep apnea syndrome undergoing hip or knee replacement: a case-control study. *Mayo Clin Proc*. 2001;76:897–905.

54. Ramachandran SK, Nafiu OO, Ghaferi A, et al. Independent predictors and outcomes of unanticipated early postoperative tracheal intubation after nonemergent, noncardiac surgery. *Anesthesiology*. 2011;115:44–53.

55. Opperer M, Cozowicz C, Bugada D, et al. Does Obstructive Sleep Apnea Influence Perioperative Outcome? A Qualitative Systematic Review for the Society of Anesthesia and Sleep Medicine Task Force on Preoperative Preparation of Patients with Sleep-Disordered Breathing. *Anesth Analg*. 2016;122(5):1321–1334.

56. Kaw R, Chung F, Pasupuleti V, et al. Meta-analysis of the association between obstructive sleep apnoea and postoperative outcome. *Br J Anaesth*. 2012;109:897–906.

57. Mokhlesi B, Hovda MD, Vekhter B, et al. Sleep-disordered breathing and postoperative outcomes after elective surgery: analysis of the nationwide inpatient sample. *Chest*. 2013;144:903–914.

58. Memtsoudis S, Liu SS, Ma Y, et al. Perioperative pulmonary outcomes in patients with sleep apnea after noncardiac surgery. *Anesth Analg*. 2011;112:113–121.

59. Mokhlesi B, Hovda MD, Vekhter B, et al. Sleep-disordered breathing and postoperative outcomes after bariatric surgery: analysis of the nationwide inpatient sample. *Obes Surg*. 2013;23:1842–1851.

60. Abdelsattar ZM, Hendren S, Wong SL, et al. The impact of untreated obstructive sleep apnea on cardiopulmonary complications in general and vascular surgery: a cohort study. *Sleep*. 2015;38(8):1205–1210.

61. Mutter TC, Chateau D, Moffatt M, et al. A matched cohort study of postoperative outcomes in obstructive sleep apnea: could preoperative diagnosis and treatment prevent complications? *Anesthesiology*. 2014;121: 707–718.

62. Chung F, Memtsoudis SG, Ramachandran SK, et al. Society of Anesthesia and Sleep Medicine Guidelines on Preoperative Screening and Assessment of Adult Patients With Obstructive Sleep Apnea. *Anesthesia and Analgesia*. 2016;123(2):452–473.

63. Gross JB, Bachenberg KL, Benumof JL, et al. Practice guidelines for the perioperative management of patients with obstructive sleep apnea: a report by the American Society of Anesthesiologists Task Force on Perioperative Management of patients with obstructive sleep apnea. *Anesthesiology*. 2006;104:1081–1093. quiz 1117–1118.

64. American Society of Anesthesiologists Task Force. Practice guidelines for the perioperative management of patients with obstructive sleep apnea: an updated report by the American Society of Anesthesiologists Task Force on Perioperative Management of patients with obstructive sleep apnea. *Anesthesiology*. 2014;120:268–286.

65. Joshi GP, Ankichetty SP, Gan TJ, et al. Society for ambulatory anesthesia consensus statement on preoperative selection of adult patients with obstructive sleep apnea scheduled for ambulatory surgery. *Anesth Analg*. 2012;115:1060–1068.

66. Adesanya AO, Lee W, Greilich NB, et al. Perioperative management of obstructive sleep apnea. *Chest*. 2010;138:1489–1498.

67. Seet E, Chung F. Management of sleep apnea in adults—functional algorithms for the perioperative period: continuing professional development. *Can J Anaesth*. 2010;57:849–864.

68. Porhomayon J, El-Solh A, Chhangani S, et al. The management of surgical patients with obstructive sleep apnea. *Lung*. 2011;189:359–367.

69. Bradley TD, Floras JS. Obstructive sleep apnoea and its cardiovascular consequences. *Lancet*. 2009;373:82–93.

70. Chau EH, Lam D, Wong J, et al. Obesity hypoventilation syndrome: a review of epidemiology, pathophysiology, and perioperative considerations. *Anesthesiology*. 2012;117:188–205.

71. Bady E, Achkar A, Pascal S, et al. Pulmonary arterial hypertension in patients with sleep apnoea syndrome. *Thorax*. 2000;55:934–939.

72. Kaw R, Bhateja P, Paz Y, et al. Postoperative complications in patients with unrecognized obesity hypoventilation syndrome undergoing elective non-cardiac surgery. *Chest*. 2016;149(1):84–91.

73. Balachandran JS, Masa JF, Mokhlesi B. Obesity hypoventilation syndrome: epidemiology and diagnosis. *Sleep Med Clin*. 2014;9(3):341–347.

74. Liao P, Luo Q, Elsaid H, et al. Perioperative auto-titrated continuous positive airway pressure treatment in surgical patients with obstructive sleep apnea. *Anesthesiology*. 2013;119:837–847.

75. Nagappa M, Mokhlesi B, Wong J, et al. The effects of continuous positive airway pressure on postoperative outcomes in obstructive sleep apnea patients undergoing surgery. *Anesth Analg*. 2015;120:1013–1023.

76. Chung F, Nagappa M, Singh M, et al. CPAP in the perioperative setting: evidence of support. *Chest*. 2016;149(2):586–597.

77. Chung F, Yegneswaran B, Liao P, et al. STOP questionnaire: a tool to screen patients for obstructive sleep apnea. *Anesthesiology*. 2008;108(5):812–821.

78. Netzer NC, Hoegel JJ, Loube D, et al. Prevalence of symptoms and risk of sleep apnea in primary care. *Chest*. 2003;124:1406–1414.

79. Ramachandran SK, Kheterpal S, Consens F, et al. Derivation and validation of a simple perioperative sleep apnea prediction score. *Anesth Analg*. 2010;110:1007–1015.

80. Chung F, Subramanyam R, Liao P, et al. High STOP-Bang score indicates a high probability of obstructive sleep apnoea. *Br J Anaesth*. 2012;108:768–775.

81. Chung F, Abdullah HR, Liao P. STOP-Bang questionnaire: a practical approach to screen for obstructive sleep apnea. *Chest*. 2016;149(3):631–638.

82. Chung F, Yang Y, Brown R, et al. Alternative scoring models of STOP-BANG questionnaire improve specificity to detect undiagnosed obstructive sleep apnea. *J Clin Sleep Med*. 2014;10:951–958.

83. Chung F, Yegneswaran B, Liao P, et al. Validation of the Berlin questionnaire and American Society of Anesthesiologists checklist as screening tools for obstructive sleep apnea in surgical patients. *Anesthesiology*. 2008;108(5):822–830.

84. Vasu TS, Doghramji K, Cavallazzi R, et al. Obstructive sleep apnea syndrome and postoperative complications: clinical use of the STOP-BANG questionnaire. *Arch Otolaryngol Head Neck Surg.* 2010;136:1020–1024.

85. Olson E, Chung F, Seet E. Intraoperative management of adults with obstructive sleep apnea. In: Post TW, ed. *UpToDate.* Waltham, MA: UpToDate; 2015.

86. Seet E, Han TL, Chung F. Perioperative clinical pathways to manage sleep-disordered breathing. *Sleep Med Clin.* 2013;8:105–120.

87. Chung F, Yegneswaran B, Herrera F, et al. Patients with difficult intubation may need referral to sleep clinics. *Anesth Analg.* 2008;107:915–920.

88. Gali B, Whalen FX, Schroeder DR, et al. Identification of patients at risk for postoperative respiratory complications using a preoperative obstructive sleep apnea screening tool and postanesthesia care assessment. *Anesthesiology.* 2009;110:869–877.

89. Kheterpal S, Martin L, Shanks AM, et al. Prediction and outcomes of impossible mask ventilation: a review of 50,000 anesthetics. *Anesthesiology.* 2009;110: 891–897.

90. Siyam MA, Benhamou D. Difficult endotracheal intubation in patients with sleep apnea syndrome. *Anesth Analg.* 2002;95:1098–1102.

91. Apfelbaum JL, Hagberg CA, Caplan RA, et al. Practice guidelines for management of the difficult airway. *Anesthesiology.* 2013;118:251–270.

92. Lam KK, Kunder S, Wong J, et al. Obstructive sleep apnea, pain, and opioids: is the riddle solved? *Curr Opin Anaesthesiol.* 2016;29(1):134–140.

93. Eikermann M, Grosse-Sundrup M, Zaremba S, et al. Ketamine activates breathing and abolishes the coupling between loss of consciousness and upper airway dilator muscle dysfunction. *Anesthesiology.* 2012;116:35–46.

94. Ankichetty S, Wong J, Chung F. A systematic review of the effects of sedatives and anesthetics in patients with obstructive sleep apnea. *J Anaesthesiol Clin Pharmacol.* 2011;27: 447–458.

95. Sundar E, Chang J, Smetana GW. Perioperative screening for and management of patients with obstructive sleep apnea. *J Clin Outcomes Manage.* 2011;18:399–411.

VI

# NEW MODELS OF ANESTHESIA CARE: PERIOPERATIVE MEDICINE, THE PERIOPERATIVE SURGICAL HOME, AND POPULATION HEALTH

Neal H. Cohen

## GROWTH AND EXPANSION OF ANESTHESIA PRACTICE

Anesthesiology has evolved from a specialty dedicated to the care of patients undergoing surgical procedures in an operating room environment to one devoted to the care of patients receiving a wide variety of clinical services, including anesthesia care in both inpatient and outpatient settings. This expansion in the scope of practice of anesthesiology is largely a result of major advances with anesthetics and other new drugs along with the improved ability of anesthesiologists to assess and better prepare patients for surgery. This aspect includes the capability of more effectively addressing changes in patient physiology during and immediately after surgical procedures and providing improved critical care and pain management.[1] These advances in clinical care and outcomes enable anesthesiologists to care for patients with more complex comorbid conditions who in the past might not have been able to undergo any surgical or other procedure. As a consequence, some anesthesiologists are offering an expanded scope of practice that extends beyond the immediate surgical procedure and that builds on the successes in the operating room environment. These anesthesiologists are working collaboratively with other surgeons and providers to apply some of the lessons learned in the operating room into other aspects of care both within and beyond the hospital environment.

This expansion in scope of anesthesia practice comes at an important time, particularly for the United States. Procedural options have increased the number of patients with underlying comorbid conditions who are able to receive care; simultaneously, the population is aging, creating greater demand for services. The percentage of the U.S. population older than 65 years of age continues to grow, with a projected 21% increase in this population by 2050.[2] To meet the resultant growth in demand for additional health care, the health care workforce will have to increase by 20% to 50%.[3] These demographic changes are occurring in parallel with escalating costs of care and building the pressure on an already strained health care system. Addressing these challenges will necessitate major changes in how health care is delivered—to whom and by whom—and how it is to be financed.

Simultaneously, and in response to the changing patient population and clinical needs, the overall specialty of anesthesiology has expanded its numbers of subspecializations and created other educational and diverse fellowship programs to support the changes in clinical practice. For example, cardiac, pediatric, transplantation, trauma, and neurosurgical anesthesia (also see Chapters 25, 30, 34, 36, and 42) focuses on specific patient populations and the surgical procedures they require; some of the subspecialties have formal fellowship programs that are accredited by the Accreditation Council for Graduate Medical Education (ACGME), whereas others are nonaccredited training programs. The American Board of Anesthesiology (ABA) has implemented certification examinations and provides special qualifications in many of the subspecialties. Besides the expansion of the responsibilities in anesthesia practice, these advances are also redefining and augmenting the scope of the specialty of anesthesiology. Surgeons have been able to apply innovative approaches to surgical management that would otherwise have been impossible. In addition, building on the experiences in the operating room, the practice of anesthesia has extended beyond the traditional setting. More invasive and minimally invasive procedures are being performed outside the operating room environments both within a hospital setting (non–operating room anesthesia, NORA) as well as in ambulatory facilities. Building on the scientific foundation of anesthesia practice in the operating room, anesthesiology has expanded to include acute and chronic pain management (Chapters 40 and 44), critical care medicine (Chapter 41), palliative care (Chapter 49), sleep medicine (Chapter 50), and several other related clinical services. The broadening of the roles and responsibilities is generating tremendous opportunities for anesthesiologists to take advantage of the evolving changes in health care delivery and management and to develop new roles to meet the needs of patients, other providers, hospitals, and health systems.

## CHANGING HEALTH CARE LANDSCAPE

In parallel with the changes in anesthesia practice per se is the increasing emphasis on patient safety, quality, and costs of care, which is fostering a major restructuring of the health care system in the United States as well as in many other countries. These countries are striving to emphasize health, wellness, and preventive measures to reduce burden and its associated costs and improve the overall quality of life for their populations.[4] These goals are challenging to accomplish, particularly with the long history of compartmentalized health care in most countries, and the relatively small investment in public health and prevention over that for treatment. The availability of costly drugs and interventions sounds promising, although in many cases their effect on both quality of life and life span is limited. The recent advances in personalized or precision medicine are also promising but are stressing already overburdened health care systems.

As a consequence of the competing pressures to improve quality and health of the population while reducing costs, the health care system and those who support it are being challenged to redesign the system in major ways. These changes in the organizational approach to the practice of medicine in general and anesthesiology specifically are challenging, rewarding, and sometimes frustrating. They can even be distracting to the quality of anesthesia practice. First, the relationship between hospitals and physicians is changing dramatically *and rapidly*. Hospitals are affiliating or consolidating, creating health care systems that are able to better provide longitudinal care to populations of patients, including out-of-hospital care, high-intensity inpatient services, and coordinated posthospital care (e.g., rehabilitation, skilled nursing care, home health services, telehealth).[5] To successfully expand the scope of care beyond the traditional inpatient focus, hospitals and health care systems are aligning more closely with physicians. In some cases, hospitals hire physicians directly or, when state laws prevent hospitals from doing so, create medical foundations that are "joined at the hip" with the health system. Independent and small group practices are consolidating into single or multispecialty group practices. In the United States, the consolidation into large group practices has been accelerating over the past 5 years,[6] and this growth is impacting the practice of anesthesiology. The consolidation of anesthesia practices allows the group to negotiate from a stronger position than can an individual practitioner or small group practice. In addition, the consolidation of practices, many of which are multispecialty groups, allows anesthesiologists to collaborate with other colleagues more effectively and to negotiate as a group with health care systems and payers.

As the cost of care has continued to increase and the expenditures for health care in the United States in particular have escalated, both government and private payers have been challenged to reduce costs and unnecessary care. Most recently there have been attempts to reduce physician compensation and to increase the percentage of payment based on predefined metrics for quality, patient satisfaction, and cost. One of the most prominent motivators to the changing health care environment in the United States was the implementation of the controversial Affordable Care Act (ACA), which was enacted in 2010.[7] It has a number of provisions that encourage different models of care and collaboration specifically to address quality and value over cost. Another major change that is in part a result of the ACA is the expansion of accountable care organizations (ACOs) to manage and have overall responsibility for providing care to a population of patients.[8,9] To responsibly manage a diverse population of patients, a health system needs to implement different approaches that take into account the continuum of care including inpatient and outpatient care, managing the transitions of care, and putting increased emphasis on prevention and wellness over high-cost, technologically advanced procedural care. Therefore, for an ACO to be successful will require close cooperation, coordination, and communication among physicians, other providers, hospitals, extended care facilities, home health agencies, and other health care organizations to appropriately utilize and rationalize services that fulfill the needs and goals of the patients for whom they assume responsibility.

These major changes in how health care systems have evolved, how services are delivered, and how health care is funded, while challenging, also have significant implications for anesthesia providers. First, and perhaps most difficult for some anesthesia departments to address, is the expansion of clinical services to environments not familiar to most anesthesiologists. The increase in non–operating room locations has been difficult to manage, but also represents an opportunity for anesthesiologists to be more visible members of the health care team beyond the operating room. The expansion of subspecialties, including critical care and pain medicine, has allowed anesthesiologists to address clinical needs not necessarily related to a surgical procedure and to have some experience in dealing with the transitions and continuum of care, though primarily in the inpatient setting. The new models of care allow anesthesia departments to expand their clinical care beyond the operating room suite and procedural areas to other inpatient environments, and in some cases into community settings—with the caveat that in doing so, they do not lose focus on the delivery of high-quality, safe, and value-based perioperative care, which is the mainstay of any anesthesia practice.

## Workforce Changes Affecting the Models of Anesthesia Care

Over the past decade, changes in the workforce have also influenced the role played by physicians in general and

anesthesiologists in particular. As a result of the limitations on duty hours imposed by the ACGME and other changes in care delivery, there are many more transitions of care, most notably during hospitalizations. As clinical demands increase, many surgical services have recruited hospitalists or other providers to help coordinate perioperative care. In many cases anesthesiologists, including critical care anesthesiologists, pain medicine physicians, and others are working with surgeons and hospitalists to optimize overall clinical care beyond the operating room, facilitate the transition to posthospital care and manage outpatient clinical needs to reduce readmissions. These changes have created a variety of clinical and management models, many of which have improved clinical care and outcomes and reduced costs.[10-13] Commensurate with the changing roles for physicians, there has been significant expansion in training of advance practice nurses and physician assistants, including an increase in the number of certified registered nurse anesthetist (CRNA) training programs. In most cases, the advance practice nurses work in close collaboration with physicians and are supervised as part of the clinical care team, particularly for anesthesia practices. There has been some pressure regionally and nationally to allow advance practice nurses to pursue their profession independently. However, for most anesthesia groups, the working relationship between physician anesthesiologists and CRNAs is very good, benefiting patients and ensuring a coordinated approach to clinical management. This collaborative model of care takes advantage of the training and expertise of the CRNAs and the physician anesthesiologists to manage the entire perioperative period, coordinating preoperative management, intraoperative care, and postdischarge clinical needs. The variation in delivery of anesthesia care and how it is organized varies widely internationally.

## New Payment Models

In most countries, financial compensation for anesthesiologists varies widely, ranging from straight salaries to some type of "fee for service" arrangement. In response to the change in focus to value and quality, the payment methods are undergoing dramatic change in the United States. The traditional fee for service payment methods are being challenged; the transition to paying for "value" over volume of care delivered is accelerating for both government and private payers. Most notably, the recent enactment of the Medicare Access and CHIP Reauthorization Act (MACRA) in 2015 has changed the landscape of payment for physician and hospital services. While the details of the implementation are still under discussion,[14] the changes, no matter how they are finally revised, will transition payment from a volume-based fee for service system to one that puts emphasis on value. The details of the MACRA implementation are under review. The primary components of the implementation will require physicians to operate under an incentive-based program (merit-based incentive program, MIPS) or an alternative payment model (APM).[15,16]

The changes in payment methodology from a predominant fee for service model to alternative- and value-based payment models require new approaches to how health care is delivered and how "value" will be defined and influence payment. In addition, physicians and health systems will be expected to share risk and, theoretically, rewards resulting from improved care delivery. Current methods to document quality and value are not sophisticated enough, nor outcome-based, to fulfill these goals. Since Medicare has committed to transitioning about 50% of payment from fee for service to alternative payment models and to linking 90% of payment to value within the next 18 months, each practice will be required to identify specific measures of quality that support payment.

One of the most important changes in payment that will have major impact on the role of each provider is the transition to bundled payments for episodes of care (e.g., 90-day episode of care for a patient undergoing a surgical procedure).[17,18] The goal of bundled approaches to payment is to create financial incentives to encourage coordination of care across the continuum of care and putting the health system rather than Medicare at risk for unnecessary services. Under this model, payment for physician services will be determined based on the "value" each provider or group has contributed to the care of the patient. As a result, anesthesiologists will have to justify why the care they delivered warrants a larger (or smaller) piece of a fixed-bundled payment. To the extent that the anesthesia group is participating broadly in the care of patients throughout the continuum of care (e.g., pre- and postoperative care including critical care and acute pain) and can document quality and cost reduction metrics as a result of the involvement, the group may be able to negotiate from a position of strength for their portion of the payment.

The changes to the health care system, expanding clinical care needs, and the emphasis on value are and will continue to have significant impact on the practice of anesthesiology. They create opportunities to expand the focus of anesthesia care beyond the immediate perioperative period, but also for anesthesiologists to assume a broader role in managing patients throughout the continuum of care, in both inpatient and outpatient settings. Over the past few years, several new models of care have been defined for anesthesiologists, including an expanding role in patient management throughout the perioperative period, administrative roles in perioperative care, and more recently the perioperative surgical home and population health.

## Transitions From Anesthesiology to Perioperative Medicine

The practice of anesthesiology has evolved as a result of the improved clinical capabilities and in response to both the new opportunities and the challenges facing health systems to improve care and control costs. As previously described, the most notable changes in practice have been the expansion of the subspecialties that provide care in the operating room, other procedural areas, and the intensive care unit (ICU), and for both acute and chronic pain. The expansion of anesthesiology to include "perioperative medicine" has been very successful, creating a variety of clinical practice opportunities and management roles for anesthesiologists.[19] In extending the scope of practice to perioperative medicine, particularly with the simultaneous changes in health care delivery, new models of care were required to most effectively meet clinical and administrative needs. For example, the implementation of preoperative clinics (see Chapter 13) was required because fewer patients were admitted prior to the day of surgery. The evolution of preoperative evaluation programs has been successful in many ways. At the same time, fragmentation of care has increased, because the provider completing the preoperative evaluation is generally not the same anesthesia provider who will be delivering care to the patient for a procedure. In some cases, the preoperative evaluation is performed by another physician or an advanced practice nurse rather than an anesthesiologist. The evaluation provides documentation of the patient's history and may include a thorough evaluation of the airway and associated concerns specific to the intraoperative anesthesia care, but may include preoperative optimization of underlying clinical conditions, such as optimizing pulmonary function in a patient with asthma or chronic obstructive pulmonary disease (COPD), controlling blood sugar for a patient with diabetes mellitus, or controlling arterial blood pressure for a patient with hypertension that has been difficult to control. As a result, this approach could necessitate a cancellation on the day of scheduled surgery when the assigned anesthesiologist sees the patient for the first time immediately before surgery and identifies concerns that were not adequately addressed. More important is that this approach does not allow the anesthesia provider to develop a relationship with the patient prior to their meeting either in a preoperative holding area or the operating room.

Similar challenges exist with respect to postoperative care. For most patients, the postoperative care provided by the anesthesiologist includes assessment in the post-anesthesia care unit (PACU) (see Chapter 39) and, if the patient remains hospitalized thereafter, a visit to ensure that the patient has not suffered any immediate complications associated with anesthesia care. For ambulatory patients, a phone call is often made to the patient or family member to ensure that the transition to home

VI

has been without incident. For inpatients, many of whom have either had complex surgical procedures or have underlying medical problems, the care is more often provided by the surgeon with or without the assistance of other physicians and advance practice nurses. In some cases, medical or surgical hospitalists, who have no role in intraoperative management, assume responsibility for postoperative care. In other settings, hospitalists working with surgical services manage underlying or associated medical conditions, while surgical issues are addressed by the surgeon. In other settings, surgical hospitalists have been recruited to help manage the patient during the early postoperative period. While these models may have some advantages, they do not facilitate coordination of care, nor provide seamless transitions through the various stages of perioperative care. In addition, most of these models do not acknowledge the role anesthesiologists can play in extending some of the intraoperative management strategies to the postoperative period. As a result of the intimate knowledge and understanding of a patient's response to anesthetic drugs, changes in intravascular volume, and other intraoperative events, the anesthesiologist often has a great deal of knowledge about the patient's physiology, which can optimize postoperative management. In addition, participation in postoperative care allows a better understanding of the longer-term implications of intraoperative management, such as the effect of intraoperative care on wound healing, the incidence of central line–associated bloodstream infections, the risk of pressure ulcers, pulmonary function, and the integrity of the airway. By redefining anesthesia practice to include perioperative medicine, many anesthesia groups have successfully addressed these issues by creating a cohesive cohort of providers to manage patients through the continuum of their perioperative course. While there are limited data to differentiate outcomes of this model versus the conventional silo approach to care, the importance of anesthesiologists broadening their focus to include perioperative care for the surgical patient has become increasingly important.

Although extending the scope of anesthesia care to include the continuum of the perioperative course for each surgical patient is important, a number of other models of anesthesia care have been implemented or proposed. These models extend the scope of anesthesia practice to incorporate standard, evidence-based practices into perioperative care, development of quality metrics to support clinical management, and new roles for anesthesia providers in both health system management and population health, particularly as it relates to the development of ACOs.

### Enhanced Recovery After Surgery

Enhanced recovery after surgery (ERAS) is one approach that is being utilized to improve clinical care for patients undergoing specific surgical procedures. ERAS utilizes evidence-based practices when they exist to improve outcomes, reduce length of hospital stay, and optimize postoperative care often at reduced overall cost.[20-24] The success of the ERAS programs is based on the principle that a multidisciplinary approach to care that includes anesthesiologists, surgeons, and other appropriate providers will improve both quality and outcome. The specific participants in each ERAS initiative depend on the surgical procedure, anticipated clinical needs, and resources. For example, for patients undergoing laparoscopic surgery, the anesthesia provider coordinates care with physical therapists, dietitians, and others to ensure early ambulation, nutritional support, and return of bowel function. Other approaches to care that have been demonstrated to improve outcome after selected surgical procedures include goal-directed fluid management and multimodal narcotic-sparing approaches to pain management and appropriate selection of antibiotics for perioperative prophylaxis.

### Perioperative Surgical Home

The perioperative surgical home (PSH) is another model of perioperative management that extends some of the concepts of coordinated perioperative care previously described. In many respects, the changing patient population and increasing complexity of perioperative care are creating a demand for better coordination of care and fostering the development of the PSH concept. The development of the PSH is based on the same principles as is the implementation of the patient-centered medical home (PCMH), which is designed to optimize care to patients with complex medical conditions.[25,26] To some extent the PSH is also an extension of some of the basic principles on which ERAS is based. However, although ERAS models have been implemented to optimize the continuum of care related to specific surgical procedures, the concepts behind the PSH extend beyond any single procedure or time period in the perioperative course.[27]

The PSH incorporates clinical management of the patient through the perioperative period to optimize outcomes specifically related to the surgery and addresses other clinical issues to facilitate safe transition from the inpatient hospital setting to home, rehabilitation, or skilled nursing facilities.[28,29] Under this model of care, the anesthesiologist assumes a broader role in clinical management while working collaboratively with the surgeon and other providers to optimize care related to the surgical procedure and underlying or associated clinical problems.

The goals for the PSH include the following:

1. Coordinating the care of a patient scheduled for a surgical procedure and facilitating communication among all providers to ensure that clinical issues are identified and addressed

2. Providing a thorough preoperative assessment and optimizing management of any underlying medical conditions (also see Chapter 13)
3. Defining and implementing appropriate (and evidence-based, when available) approaches to management through the perioperative period
4. Managing clinical care across the continuum
5. Assessing and documenting outcomes and performance on predefined metrics

The PSH concept has been utilized in a variety of different clinical settings with considerable success in terms of efficiency, quality of care, and patient and provider satisfaction.[29] As more experience is gained in the implementation of the PSH and its effect on the management of selected patients, dissemination of best practices should help refine the models to best serve the needs of patients, providers, and health care systems.

### Population Health

Both ERAS and the PSH have had significant impact on the practice opportunities and roles for anesthesiologists and on outcomes of clinical care. At the same time, for the most part, these models focus on acute episodes of care for selected patient populations or procedures. With the changes being imposed by the ACA and other initiatives designed to improve quality and reduce costs, many health systems are developing ACO models designed to manage populations of patients. This transition to population health is having major ramifications for patients, providers, and health systems.[30] The foundation on which "population health" is based assumes that care for a population will be optimized if a health system takes clinical and financial responsibility for managing the wellness of a population as well as coordinating care in every setting.[30-33] In this model, the health system, including the aligned providers, manages all aspects of care including preventive care, wellness, and management of both chronic and acute disease. The concept of population health is creating opportunities for all providers to clarify their value to the health system and its patients, while also to define new roles that not only optimize both acute and chronic care, but also demonstrate value—improved outcomes at reduced cost. To be successful, health systems need to ensure that clinical care is coordinated and collaborative, patient-centric, and that clinical management strategies are based on objective outcome measures of quality and cost.[34]

Although the concept of population health is not evident to many anesthesia practices, population health management provides many opportunities for which anesthesia providers can and do have meaningful roles. The most obvious roles and responsibilities relate to the perioperative course of patients requiring surgical procedures, an extension of the role in perioperative medicine, and the concepts behind both ERAS and the PSH. Beyond these specific roles, however, there are other aspects of anesthesia practice that can be applied to the management of a population of patients. Anesthesiologists can assume a larger role in patient care preoperatively, including managing or coordinating the management of underlying chronic conditions. As an extension of the intraoperative management, anesthesiologists can be more actively involved in coordinating postoperative care, as has been done for some patients in the PSH model of care. Critical care anesthesiologists (also see Chapter 41), pain medicine anesthesiologists (also see Chapters 40 and 44), and palliative care physicians (also see Chapter 49) have important roles in hospital-based care as well as in transitions of care to extended care facilities, skilled nursing homes, and the hospice setting. In some cases, anesthesiologists could serve a meaningful role in working with case managers to identify the appropriate care needs and to facilitate coordination and communication between providers and other facilities.[35]

In addition to the clinically focused roles that anesthesiologists can serve under a population health management strategy, they are often involved in administration and health policy development. Being perioperative medical director with a focus on the efficient management of the operating room suite (also see Chapter 46) is an example. Extending the scope of responsibility for perioperative care to include transitions of care and coordination with providers outside the hospital or health care system will be essential in order to most appropriately coordinate resource use between acute care hospitals and other facilities. Population health management will also require new approaches to pain management for individual patients and to the development of procedures that more effectively utilize multimodal approaches to the care of patients with chronic pain to minimize the use and abuse of opioids (also see Chapters 9 and 44). Critical care anesthesiologists can provide an important perspective in the overall management strategies for patients requiring long-term mechanical ventilatory support and facilitating and coordinating transitions of care to other settings that may be more appropriate for individual patients (also see Chapter 41). Similarly, they can help address how to most effectively manage patients with both acute care needs and extensive rehabilitation, defining the most appropriate management strategies and sites of care. Similarly the anesthesiologist with experience in palliative care can address individual patient goals of care and clinical needs as well as assist the health system in defining how to most appropriately care for this patient population (also see Chapter 49).

Identifying new roles for anesthesiologists in population health has obvious benefits to providers, as well as to patients and to the health system. Because the health system and the providers share the financial risk for the care of the patient population, expanding the scope of practice and documenting the value of these services will be critical to the financial integrity of a department and its

VI

members. Although these expanded roles are important for an anesthesia department as a whole, each member of the department will have a different role in the clinical management of the patients and, for some members, in the administrative functions needed to support the health system. At the same time, the financial underpinnings of population health require that all providers understand the concepts behind population health management and participate in strategies to optimize care and resource use across the continuum based on objective quality metrics and documented outcomes.

## IMPLICATIONS OF NEW MODELS OF CARE ON ANESTHESIA TRAINING PROGRAMS

All of these changes in health care delivery and the new clinical opportunities will have considerable impact on the knowledge and skills required of both anesthesia residents and practicing anesthesiologists. To fulfill the changing needs of patients and health care systems, resident training, ongoing education, and methods to ensure continued competency must incorporate new practices and knowledge to ensure that each anesthesiologist has the full breadth and depth of skills needed to support patient and health system needs.

To address this need, many anesthesia residency programs have incorporated new didactic sessions to address various aspects of perioperative medicine and population health into the curriculum. Many programs have new rotations to provide exposure to the opportunities for anesthesiologists in the evolving health care system. While the specific educational needs will evolve, some core educational needs can be defined. Most residency programs provide some experience in managing a clinical team, supervising other providers, and coordinating care with other specialties. The ACGME core competencies are helpful in ensuring that residents gain knowledge and skills in systems-based practice. Each resident should understand how to develop and implement quality improvement initiatives and how to assess quality of care. This knowledge is essential for every anesthesiologist to understand in order to participate in value-based incentive compensation models. In addition, the need to have objective data to support clinical management decisions will require that each resident has a general understanding of the benefits and limitations of the electronic health record and how to utilize clinical data repositories to assess outcomes, quality, and costs of care. Team and crisis management is particularly important as clinical care has become more complex. More training should be provided in resource utilization, negotiation, conflict management, communication skills, organizational behavior, and other aspects of management, all of which can help optimize clinical care in whatever setting the graduating resident may practice. Because clinical practices will

continue to be evaluated based on evidence-based metrics, the training should include assessment of resource use efficiencies and clinical outcomes, the value of implementing checklists and other ways to ensure standards of care are being met, as well as a general understanding about the value of a root cause analysis and how to assess risk and implement risk reduction strategies. Residency programs should also provide an overview of health care financing, current payment methodologies for anesthesia services (ASA Relative Value Guide), and other physician payment methods (resource-based relative value system, RBRVS), as well as practice in health system management strategies.

The challenge for all programs is to ensure that each resident has broad clinical experiences in all aspects of anesthesia care, subspecialty care, pain medicine, and critical care, while also providing exposure to new clinical and administrative opportunities in anesthesiology. Every residency program will have to find the balance in providing training within the residency and fellowship programs to give each trainee exposure to the breadth and depth of professional opportunities in anesthesiology. A number of anesthesia programs have implemented fellowship training in perioperative medicine, the concepts supporting the PSH, and population health. Additional formal business training may be beneficial for those anesthesiologists interested in pursuing leadership roles in perioperative care or population health within a health system (e.g., certificates or advanced degrees in management science or business administration). As the concepts of the PSH and population health evolve, an assessment of the current educational programs and their scope will be helpful in defining and refining future educational needs for anesthesia providers to successfully fulfill these new roles.

## CONCLUSION

Health care delivery and management are undergoing dramatic changes that will influence the practice of anesthesiology and the future roles for anesthesiologists. In some respects the evolution of perioperative care and its effect on health systems is a result of the advances in anesthesia and its scientific underpinnings. At the same time, the changes taking place are affecting the relationships among providers, patients, and hospitals, all of which are being impacted by the changes in payment methodologies and the transition to a patient-centered and value-based health care system. Despite the challenges facing all providers in the evolving health care delivery system, the development of the PSH and other new models of care create opportunities for anesthesiologists to assume a broader role in clinical care and health system management. In many models, this extended role requires the anesthesiologist to understand the patient population and the anticipated role each provider is expected to play, as well as the capabilities of the department and institution. These new opportunities should be acknowledged as an augmentation and expansion and not a replacement for the core roles most anesthesiologists will have in perioperative care. The advances in anesthesia practice and successes in improving clinical care, quality, and safety have come from the dedicated care provided in the operating room and other procedural locations. Anesthesiologists must continue to have a meaningful and primary role in optimizing perioperative care. At the same time, each practice should identify new roles and opportunities to improve the continuum of care, define how best to take advantage of these opportunities, and as appropriate, acquire the knowledge and skills to manage patients through the continuum of care, with a primary focus on patient-centered, goal-directed, and value-based care.

## QUESTIONS OF THE DAY

1. How have health care workforce changes affected models for anesthesia care?
2. What is a "bundled payment," and how does it differ from fee-for-service billing?
3. What improvements in clinical outcomes have been demonstrated with enhanced recovery after surgery (ERAS) pathways?
4. What are the goals of the perioperative surgical home (PSH) model of care?
5. What is the concept of population health as an approach for a health system to care for its patients?

## REFERENCES

1. Committee on Quality of Care in America, Institute of Medicine. *To Err is Human: Building a Safer Health System.* Washington, DC: National Academy Press; 2000.
2. Administration for Community Living. Administration on Aging. Profile of Older Americans. http://www.aoa.acl.gov/Aging_Statistics/Profile/2015.
3. Kirch DG, Henderson MK, Dill MJ. Physician workforce projections in an era of health care reform. *Annu Rev Med.* 2012;63:435–445.
4. Berwick DM, Nolan TW, Whittington J. The triple aim: care, health and cost. *Health Affairs.* 2008;27:759–769.
5. Cuellar AE, Gertler PJ. Trends in hospital consolidation. The formation of local systems. *Health Affairs.* 2003;23:77–87.
6. Anesthesiology Practice Acquisitions – May 2016. *Special report on mergers and acquisitions of anesthesiology practices.* Haverford Healthcare Advisors; May 2016. www.haverfordhealthcare.com. Accessed July 10, 2016.
7. Read the Law. http://www.hhs.gov/healthcare/about-the-law/read-the-law.
8. Taylor B. Accountable care organizations. *Public Health Rep.* 2011;126:875–878.
9. Fisher ES, Shortell SM. Accountable care organizations: accountable for what, to whom and how. *JAMA.* 2010;304:1715–1716.
10. Cheng HQ. Comanagement hospitalist services for neurosurgery. *Neurosurg Clin North Am.* 2015;26:295–300.
11. Tadros RO, Faries PL, Malik R, et al. The effect of a hospitalist comanagement service on vascular surgery inpatients. *J Vasc Surg.* 2015;61:1550–1555.

12. Kuo YF, Goodwin JS. Effect of hospitalists on length of stay in the Medicare population: variation according to hospital and patient characteristics. *J Am Geriatr Soc.* 2010;58:1649–1657.
13. Auerbach AD, Wachter RM, Cheng HQ, et al. Comanagement of surgical patients between neurosurgeons and hospitalists. *Arch Intern Med.* 2010;170:2004–2010.
14. Medicare Access and CHIP Reauthorization Act of 2015. 42 USC 1305. https://www.congress.gov/114/plaws/publ10/PLAW-114publ10.pdf.
15. Medicare MIPS and APM Proposed Regulations. https://s3.amazonaws.com/public-inspection.federalregister.gov/2016-10032.pdf.
16. Quality Initiatives. https://www.cms.gov/Medicare/Quality-Initiatives-Patient-Assessment-Instruments/Value-Based-Programs/MACRA-MIPS-and-APMs/MACRA-MIPS-and-APMs.html.
17. Creating physician-owned bundled payments. http://catalyst.nejm.org/creating-physician-owned-bundled-payments/. Accessed July 10, 2016.
18. Bozic KJ, Ward L, Vail TP, Maze M. Bundled payments in total joint arthroplasty: targeting opportunities for quality improvement and cost reduction. *Clin Orthop Relat Res.* 2014;472:188–193.
19. Grocott MPW, Pearse RM. Perioperative medicine: the future of anaesthesia? *Br J Anaesth.* 2012;108:723–726.
20. Ljungqvist O. ERAS—enhanced recovery after surgery: moving evidence-based perioperative care to practice. *J Parenter Enteral Nutr.* 2014;38(5):559–566.

21. Oda Y, Kakinohana M. Introduction of ERAS® program into clinical practice: from preoperative management to postoperative evaluation: opening remarks. *J Anesth.* 2014;28:141–142.
22. Fierens J, Wolthuis AM, Penninckx F, D'Hoore A. Enhanced recovery after surgery (ERAS) protocol: prospective study of outcome in colorectal surgery. *Acta Chir Belg.* 2012;112:355–358.
23. Lee L, Li C, Landry T, et al. A systematic review of economic evaluations of enhanced recovery pathways for colorectal surgery. *Ann Surg.* 2015;259:670–676.
24. Varadhan KK, Neal KR, Dejong CH, et al. The enhanced recovery after surgery (ERAS) pathway for patients undergoing major elective open colorectal surgery: a meta-analysis of randomized trials. *Clin Nutr.* 2010;29(4):434–440.
25. Graham J, Bowen TR, Strohecker KA, et al. Reducing mortality in hip fracture patients using a perioperative approach and "Patient-Centered Medical Home" model: a prospective cohort study. *Patient Saf Surg.* 2014;8:7.
26. Schwenk TL. The patient-centered medical home: one size does not fit all. *JAMA.* 2014;311:802–803.
27. Perioperative surgical home. http://www.periopsurghome.info/index.php; asahq.org. Accessed March 28, 2014.
28. Paloski D. Forum Focus—Perioperative surgical home model. American Hospital Association Physician Forum 7/3/13. http://www.ahaphysicianforum.org/news/enews/2013/070313.html. Retrieved March 30, 2014.
29. Vetter TR, Goeddel LA, Boudreaux AM, et al. The perioperative surgical home: how can it make the case so everyone wins? *BMC Anesthesiol.* 2013;13:6.

VI

30. Kindig D, Stoddart G. What is population health? *Am J Public Health.* 2003;93:380–383.
31. Kindig DA. Understanding population health terminology. *Milbank Q.* 2007;85:139–161.
32. Nash DB. Population health: where's the beef? *Popul Health Manag.* 2015;18:1–3.
33. Kindig DA. What are we talking about when we talk about population health?. http://healthaffairs.org/blog/2015/04/06/what-are-we-talking-about-when-we-talk-about-population-health/. Accessed July 10, 2016.
34. Boudreaux AM, Vetter TR. A primer on population health management and its perioperative application. *Anesth Analg.* 2016;123:63–70.
35. Casarett D, Teno J. Why population health and palliative care need each other. *JAMA.* 2016;316(1):27–28.

# INDEX

---

*Note*: Page numbers followed by "b," "f," and "t" indicate boxes, figures, and tables, respectively.

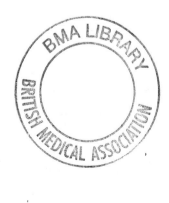